Clinical Laboratory Medicine: Clinical Application of Laboratory Data

Fifth Edition

Clinical Laboratory Medicine: Clinical Application of Laboratory Data

Fifth Edition

Richard Ravel, M.D.
Director of Laboratories
St. Mary Hospital
Quincy, Illinois

Mosby
Year Book

St. Louis Baltimore Boston Chicago London Philadelphia Sydney Toronto

A Year Book Medical Publishers imprint of Mosby-Year Book, Inc.

Mosby-Year Book, Inc.
11830 Westline Industrial Drive
St. Louis, MO 63146

3 4 5 6 7 8 9 0 RM 93 92 91

Library of Congress Cataloging-in-Publication Data

Ravel, Richard, 1932-
Clinical laboratory medicine.

Includes bibliographies and index.
1. Diagnosis, Laboratory. I. Title.
[DNLM: 1. Diagnosis, Laboratory. QY 4 R253c]
RB37.R37 1989 616.07′56 88-26134
ISBN 0-8151-7098-X

Sponsoring Editor: James D. Ryan
Associate Managing Editor, Manuscript Services: Deborah Thorp
Production Manager, Text and Reference/Periodicals: Etta Worthington
Proofroom Manager: Shirley E. Taylor

PREFACE TO THE FIRST EDITION

The clinical laboratory has a major role in modern medicine. A bewildering array of laboratory procedures is available, each of which has its special usefulness and its intrinsic problems, its advantages and its drawbacks. Advances in biochemistry and radioisotopes, to name only two conspicuous examples, are continually adding new tests or modifying older methods toward new usefulness. It seems strange, therefore, that medical education has too often failed to grant laboratory medicine the same prominence and concern that are allotted to other subjects. If ever a comprehensive, systematic and critical teaching system were needed, it is for this complex and heterogeneous topic. It would seem that if one were to consider ordering any laboratory procedure, several things should be known about the test, including:

1. In what situations is the test diagnostic, and in what situations does the test provide information without being diagnostic?

2. What commonly available tests give similar information, and when should one be used in preference to the others?

3. What are the disadvantages of the test and possibilities of error or false results?

The fact that this type of information is not adequately disseminated is quickly brought home to a clinical pathologist, who supervises the clinical laboratory and at the same time acts as liaison to clinicians on laboratory problems. It becomes quickly evident in two ways—the continually rising number of laboratory procedure requests and even a casual inspection of patients' hospital charts. Unnecessary tests represent severe financial and personal inconvenience to the patient; inappropriate tests or tests done under improper conditions mean wasted or misleading information, and often a loss of precious time.

In laboratory medicine, textbooks are available, as in all areas of general medicine considered detailed enough to warrant a specialty status. These fall into two groups: those mainly for the technician and those designed for clinicians. Technician-oriented books necessarily stress the technical aspects of individual tests, with emphasis on cookbook methodology. Textbooks for the clinician vary considerably in approach. Some excellent works concentrate almost exclusively on one subject or subspecialty, such as hematology. Many others combine technician methodology with discussion to varying degrees of the clinical aspects of tests. The latter aspect often suffers due to inevitable limitations imposed by mere length. Some texts which emphasize the clinical approach may be criticized on the grounds that they neglect either adequate attention to possible limitations and sources of error in each particular laboratory procedure, or fail to delineate the background or the technical aspects of the tests enough to provide a clear picture as to just what information the test actually can provide.

This volume attempts to meet these criticisms. Its aim is to provide enough technical and clinical information about each laboratory procedure included so as to allow adequate understanding, selection and interpretation of these procedures. Many of the laboratory tests require varying amounts of individual discussion. Others are noted in the context of the diseases in which they may be useful. In addition, most of the common diseases in which laboratory tests render significant assistance are briefly outlined, and the role of the laboratory in each is explained. Also included are a considerable number of diseases or conditions which are uncommon or even rare, but which may be considered important from various points of view—either as well-known entities, diagnostic problems or cases which may benefit from early diagnosis and therapy.

There is a great temptation for a work of this type to become encyclopedic. Brevity and succinctness are preserved, therefore, at some cost, hopefully with more gain than loss. Probably the most striking examples are the chapters on infectious diseases and parasitology. In most cases, description of clinical syndromes and specific organisms has been eliminated or markedly reduced, because this book is not intended to be a treatise on internal medicine. Emphasis is on material which seems more directly concerned with selection and interpretation of laboratory tests. Nevertheless, a few diseases (such as leptospirosis) are important from the standpoint of laboratory diagnosis because their signs and symptoms mimic other conditions, so the clinical findings are included in some detail. On the other hand, syphilis serology has a chapter to itself due to confusion which surrounds the multiplicity of available tests. Likewise, certain subjects are discussed at unusual length. These are topics which, in my experience, seem to be common problem areas. The aim is to provide a reasonably thorough, yet compact survey of laboratory medicine. This book is meant to provide some area of assistance to anyone who is engaged in clinical medicine, and to provide, in a sense, a reasonably comprehensive course in clinical pathology.

It is anticipated that the style and format of this book may be criticized; either because the uninitiated reader might gain an impression that laboratory medicine can be reduced to a relatively few rules or protocols, or that one approach to diagnosis is presented as though all others were invalid. Such inferences are not intended.

It should be obvious that no person could write a book covering clinical pathology entirely from his own experience. On the other hand, adequate citation of references would be a tremendous undertaking in itself. A compromise is therefore offered. At the ends of the chapters there are lists of suggested readings, composed of selected references which include textbooks with general or specific coverage, papers on certain specific subjects and occasionally an article selected because of an unusually inclusive bibliography. Due to space considerations, those references with more than two authors have been listed in the first author's name only. This book is only a beginning; the reader is urged to consult these papers and others on individual subjects in order to broaden the information presented here, and to evaluate contrasting points of view.

An Appendix is provided, in order to include certain information which is useful but which seemed better presented separately from the regular text. Much of this is in tabular form.

I wish to express my deep appreciation to the following members of the University of Miami Medical School faculty, and to several others, who critically reviewed portions of the manuscript and made many valuable suggestions:

J. Walter Beck, Ph.D., Associate Professor of Pathology, Department of Parasitology.

George W. Douglas, Jr., M.D., Chief, Microbiology Section, Communicable Disease Center, U.S. Public Health Service.

N. Joel Ehrenkranz, M.D., Professor of Medicine, Division of Infectious Diseases.

Mary J. Harbour, M.D., Instructor, Department of Radiology.

Martin H. Kalser, M.D., Ph.D., Professor of Medicine, Division of Gastroenterology.

Robert B. Katims, M.D., Assistant Professor of Medicine, Division of Endocrinology.

Howard E. Lessner, M.D., Associate Professor of Medicine, Division of Hematology.

Joel B. Mann, M.D., Assistant Professor of Medicine, Division of Renal Disease and Endocrinology.

Leslie C. Norins, M.D., Chief, Venereal Disease Research Laboratory, Communicable Disease Center, U.S. Public Health Service.

William L. Nyhan, M.D., Ph.D., Professor of Pediatrics.

John A. Stewart, M.D., Assistant Chief, Virology Section, Communicable Disease Center, U.S. Public Health Service.

Thomas B. Turner, M.D., Director, John Elliot Blood Bank, Miami, Fla.

Richard Ravel, M.D.

PREFACE TO THE FIFTH EDITION

This book was written to provide as much information as possible that can help in understanding, selecting, and interpreting laboratory tests for patient care. In this edition I have used a slightly different format in order to help find each test more quickly and locate certain information about the different tests more easily. Once again, whenever possible I have included approximate expected percentages from the literature when discussing the frequency of an abnormal test result in a particular disease. Most textbooks state that a test value is either "increased" or "decreased" in a certain disease or that it is increased or decreased "sometimes," "frequently," or "usually." One then reviews the literature and finds that "usually" may represent 60% of cases: that is, 40% of patients have normal test results. This means that an abnormal test result will not be present in a large number of patients and that a normal result is meaningless. Without this knowledge, one might assume that "is increased in" or "usually increased" means "almost always." I think that this information can be extremely useful, and hope that the frequent appearance of these numbers is not annoying or overwhelming. In most cases, I have included the range of test result percentages I found in the literature in order to provide a better evaluation of the approximate expected percentage or the percentage found in some individual report in the literature. One frequently finds that the data from one article may not be representative of what can be expected from the majority of laboratories.

All areas of this book have been completely updated and many sections have been rewritten. More than 50 tests have been added since the previous edition. Some examples (not a complete listing) include: HIV and HTLV virus infection; AIDS and tests for HIV antigen and antibody; delta hepatitis; nucleic acid ("DNA") probes; *Campylobacter pyloridis*; Lyme disease; *Cryptosporidium*; coagulation proteins C and S; "lupus anticoagulant" and antiphospholipid antibodies; D-dimer assay; RBC distribution width measurements; CPK-MM isoforms; fructosamine assay; microalbuminuria in diabetics; bentiromide (PABA) test of pancreatic function; hydrogen breath test in lactase deficiency; clonidine stimulation in pheochromocytoma and in growth hormone testing; ultrasensitive TSH assays; tests for circulating immune complexes; revised FAB criteria for myelodysplastic syndromes; chromosome abnormalities in leukemia (including the bcr gene rearrangement assay); lymphocyte immunotyping; flow cytometry; prostate-specific antigen; cancer antigens 19-9, 15-3, 125, and 549; detection of cocaine, marijuana, and nicotine; digoxin antibody fragment therapy; cyclosporine and tricyclic antidepressent assay; and the NIH Consensus and NCEP criteria for hypercholesterolemia.

Richard Ravel, M.D.

CONTENTS

Preface to the First Edition v

Preface to the Fifth Edition vii

1 / Interpretation of Laboratory Test Data 1
2 / Basic Hematologic Tests and Classification of Anemia 9
3 / Factor Deficiency Anemia 23
4 / Production-Defect Anemia 36
5 / Depletion Anemia 42
6 / White Blood Cells 61
7 / Leukemia, Lymphomas, and Myeloproliferative Syndromes 69
8 / Blood Coagulation 90
9 / Immunohematology: Antibody Detection, Blood Group Antigens, and Pretransfusion Tests 118
10 / Blood Transfusions 129
11 / Undesirable Effects of Blood or Blood Product Transfusion 139
12 / Urinalysis and Renal Disease 153
13 / Renal Function Tests 175
14 / Bacterial Infectious Diseases (Including *Chlamydia* and *Mycoplasma* Infections) 188
15 / Mycotic Infections 237
16 / Viral and Rickettsial Infectious Diseases 244
17 / Medical Parasitology 276
18 / Cerebrospinal Fluid Examination 285
19 / Liver and Biliary Tract Tests 299
20 / Cardiac, Pulmonary, and Miscellaneous Diagnostic Procedures 320
21 / Serum Proteins 342
22 / Bone and Joint Disorders 369
23 / Acid-Base and pH Measurements 392
24 / Serum Electrolytes and Protein-Calorie Malnutrition 404
25 / Gastrointestinal Function 437
26 / Pancreatic Function 453
27 / Tests for Diabetes and Hypoglycemia 461
28 / Thyroid Function Tests 482
29 / Adrenal Function Tests 509
30 / Pituitary and Gonadal Function Tests; Tests in Obstetrics 530
31 / Tests for Syphilis 561

32 / Laboratory Aspects of Cancer 569

33 / Genetic Disorders 593

34 / Laboratory Analysis of Therapeutic and Toxic Substances 612

35 / Special Category Tests 640

36 / Appendix: A Compendium of Useful Data and Information 674

Index 709

1 Interpretation of Laboratory Test Data

Interpretation of laboratory test results is much more complicated than simply comparing the test result against a so-called normal range, labeling the test values normal or abnormal according to the normal range limits, and then fitting the result into patterns that indicate certain diseases. Certain basic considerations underlie interpretation of any test result and often are crucial when one decides whether a diagnosis can be made with reasonable certainty or whether a laboratory value should alter therapy.

SENSITIVITY AND SPECIFICITY

All laboratory tests have certain attributes. Sensitivity refers to the ability of the test to detect patients with the disease in question (i.e., how often false negative results are encountered). A test sensitivity of 90% for disease Z indicates that in 10% of patients with disease Z, the disease will not be detected. Specificity describes how well test abnormality is restricted to those persons who have the disease in question (i.e., how often false positive results are produced). A specificity of 90% for disease Z indicates that 10% of results suggestive of disease Z will, in fact, not be due to disease Z.

PREDICTIVE VALUE

In recent years, Galen and Gambino have popularized the concept of predictive value, formulas based on Bayes' theorem that help demonstrate the impact of disease prevalence on interpretation of laboratory test results (Table 1–1). *Prevalence* is the incidence of the disease (or the number of persons with the disease) in the population being tested. Briefly, predictive value helps dramatize the fact that the smaller the number of persons with a certain disease in the population being tested, the lower will be the proportion of persons with an abnormal test result who will be abnormal because they have the disease in question (i.e., the higher will be the proportion of false positive results). For example, if test Y has a sensitivity of 95% and a specificity of 95% for disease Z (both of which would usually be considered quite good), and if the prevalence of disease Z in the general population is 0.1% (1 in 1,000 persons), the predictive value of a positive (abnormal) result will be 1.9%. This means that of 100 persons with abnormal test results, only 2 will have disease Z, and 49 of 50 abnormal test results will be false positive. On the other hand, if the prevalence of disease Z were 10% (as might happen in a group of persons referred to a physician's office with symptoms suggesting disease Z), the predictive value would rise to 68%, meaning that 2 out of 3 persons with abnormal test results would have disease Z.

Predictive value may be applied to any laboratory test to evaluate the reliability either of a positive (abnormal) or a negative (normal) result. Predictive value is most often employed to evaluate a positive result; in that case the major determinants are the incidence of the disease in question for the population being tested and the specificity of the test. However, predictive value is not the only criterion of laboratory test usefulness and may at times be mis-

TABLE 1–1.
Influence of Disease Prevalence on Predictive Value of a Positive Test Result*

Prevalence of Disease in Population Tested (%)	Predictive Value (%) for Test With 95% Sensitivity and 95% Specificity
1	16
5	50
10	68
20	83
50	95

*Percentage of patients with a positive test result who actually have the disease being tested for.

leading if used too rigidly. For example, a test may have excellent characteristics as a screening procedure in terms of sensitivity, low cost, and ease of technical performance and may also have a low positive predictive value. Whether or not the test is useful would depend on other factors, such as the type and cost of follow-up tests necessary in case of an abnormal result and the implications of missing a certain number of persons with the disease if some less sensitive test were employed.

There may be circumstances in which predictive value is misleading or difficult to establish. If one is calculating the predictive value of a test, one must first know the sensitivity and specificity of that test. This information requires that some accurate reference method for diagnosis must be available other than the test being evaluated, that is, a standard against which the test in question can be compared (a gold standard). This may not be possible. There may not be a more sensitive or specific test or test combination available; or the test being evaluated may itself be the major criterion by which the diagnosis is made. In other words, if it is not possible to detect all or nearly all patients with a certain disease, it will not be possible to provide a truly accurate calculation of sensitivity, specificity, or predictive value for tests used in the diagnosis of that disease. The best one could obtain are estimates, which vary in their reliability.

REPRODUCIBILITY AND ACCURACY

Reliability of laboratory tests is quite obviously affected by technical performance within the laboratory. The effect of these technical factors is reflected by test reproducibility and accuracy. Reproducibility (precision or inherent error) is a measure of how closely the laboratory can approach the same answer when the test is performed repeatedly on the same specimen. Theoretically, exactly the same answer should be obtained each time, but in actual practice this does not happen due to equipment and human imperfection. These deviations from the same answer are usually random and thereby form a random or gaussian distribution (Fig 1–1). Variation from the average (mean) value is expressed in terms of standard deviation (SD). The laboratory frequently converts the standard deviation figure to a percentage of the mean value and calls this the coefficient of variation (CV). The majority of tests in a good laboratory can be shown to have reproducibility—expressed as coefficient of variation—in the neighborhood of 4% (some may be a little better and some a little worse). This means that two thirds of the values obtained are actually somewhere between 4% above and 4% below the true value. Since ±2 SD (which includes 95% of the values) is customarily used to define acceptable limits (just as in determination of normal ranges), plus or minus twice the CV similarly forms the boundaries of permissible technical error. Returning to the 4% CV example, a deviation up to ±8% would therefore be considered technically acceptable. In some assays, especially if they are very complicated and automated equipment cannot be used, variations greater than ±8% must be permitted. The experience and integrity of the technical personnel, the reagents involved, and the equipment used all affect the final result and influence reproducibility expressed as CV. In general, one can say that the worse the reproducibility (as reflected in higher CVs), the less chance for accuracy (the correct result), although good reproducibility by itself does not guarantee accuracy.

These considerations imply that a small change in a test value may be difficult to evaluate since it could be due to laboratory artifact rather than to disease or therapy. Larger alterations or a continued sequence of change are much more helpful.

Accuracy is defined as the correct answer (the result or value the assay should produce). Besides inherent error, there is the possibility of unexpected error of various kinds, such as human mistake when obtaining the specimen, performing the test, or transcribing the result.

Investigators have reported erroneous results in 0.2%–3.5% of reports from one or more areas of the laboratory. The laboratory analyzes so-called control specimens (which have known assay values of the material to be tested) with each group of patient specimens. The assumption is that any technical factor that would produce erroneous patient results would also produce control specimen results different from the expected values. Unfortunately, random inaccuracies may not affect all of the specimens and thus may not alter the control specimens. Examples of such problems are a specimen from the wrong patient, the effect of specimen hemolysis or lipemia, inaccurate pipetting, and insufficient mixing when the assay method uses a whole blood specimen. In addition, clerical errors occasionally occur. In my experience, the majority of clerical difficulties are associated with patients who have the same last name, patients who have moved from one room to another, decimal point mistakes, transcription of results onto the wrong person's report sheet, and placement of one person's report sheet into the chart of someone else. These considerations imply that unexpected laboratory abnormalities (or sometimes even the degree of abnormality) should be interpreted in the context of the clinical picture. This does not imply that unexpected test values should be ignored, but if there is doubt, or if the result would call for extensive workup or therapeutic action, it may be advisable to have the test repeated. If possible, the repeat should be performed on the original specimen or, if that is no longer available, on a new specimen obtained without delay. The more time lapse between the original and the new specimen, the more problem in differentiating an error in the original specimen from true change that occurred before the next specimen. One of the more frustrating duties of a laboratory director is to receive a question or complaint about a laboratory test result several days or even weeks after the test was performed, when it is usually too late for a proper investigation.

NORMAL RANGES

The most important single influence on laboratory test interpretation is the concept of

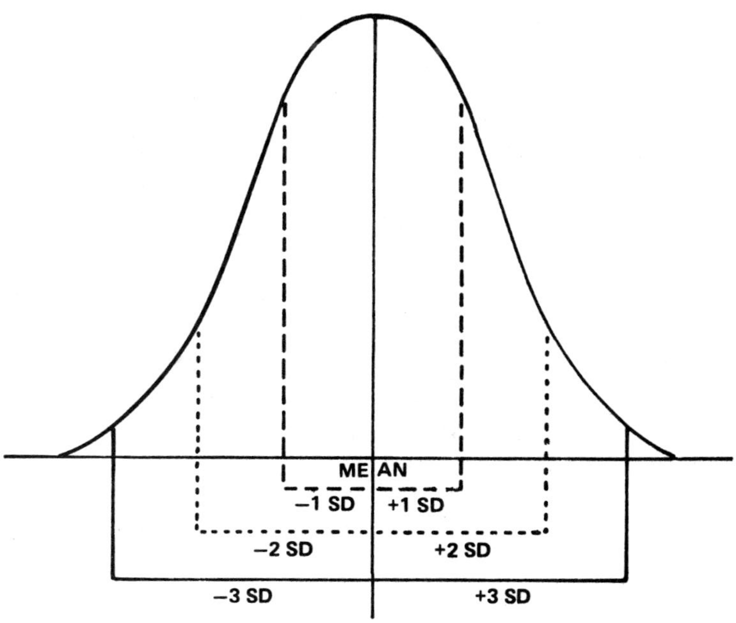

FIG 1–1.
Gaussian (random) value distribution with a visual display of the area included within increments of standard deviation *(SD)* above and below the mean: ± 1 SD = 68% of total values; ± 2 SD = 95% of total values; ± 3 SD = 99.7 % of total values.

a normal range, within which test values are considered normal and outside of which they are considered abnormal. The criteria and assumptions used in differentiating normal from abnormal in a report, therefore, assume great importance. The first step usually employed to establish normal ranges is to assume that all persons who do not demonstrate clinical symptoms or signs of any disease are normal. For some tests, normal is defined as no clinical evidence of one particular disease or group of diseases. A second assumption commonly made is that test results from those persons considered normal will have a random distribution; in other words, no factors that would bias a significant group of these values toward either the low or the high side are present. If the second assumption is correct, a gaussian (random) distribution would result, and a mean value located in the center (median) of the value distribution would be obtained. Next, the average deviation of the different values from the mean (SD) can be calculated. In a truly random or gaussian value distribution, 68% of the values will fall within 1 SD above and below the mean, 95% within ±2 SD, and 99.7% within ±3 SD (see Fig 1–1). The standard procedure is to select ±2 SD from the mean value as the limits of the normal range.

Accepting ±2 SD from the mean value as normal will place 95% of clinically normal persons within the normal range limits. Conversely, it also means that 2.5% will have values above and 2.5% will have values below this range. Normal ranges created in this way represent a deliberate compromise. A wider normal range (e.g., ±3 SD) would ensure that almost all normal persons would be included within normal range limits and thus would increase the specificity of abnormal results. However, this would place additional diseased persons with relatively small test abnormality into the expanded normal range and thereby decrease test sensitivity for detection of disease.

Problems Derived From Use of Normal Ranges

1. A small but definite group of clinically normal persons may have subclinical or undetected disease and may be inadvertently included in the supposedly normal group used to establish normal values. This has two consequences. There will be abnormal persons whose laboratory value will now be falsely considered normal, and the normal limits may be influenced by the values from persons with unsuspected disease, thereby extending the normal limits and accentuating overlap between normal and abnormal persons. For example, we tested serum specimens from 40 clinically normal blood donors to obtain the normal range for a new serum iron kit. The range was found to be 35–171 μg/dl, very close to the values listed in the kit package insert. We then performed a serum ferritin assay (the current gold standard for iron deficiency, see chapter 3) on the 10 serum samples with the lowest serum iron values. Five had low ferritin levels suggestive of iron deficiency. After excluding these values, the recalculated serum iron normal range was 60–160, very significantly different from the original range. The kit manufacturer conceded that their results had not been verified by serum ferritin or bone marrow.

2. Normal ranges are sometimes calculated from a number of values too small to be statistically reliable.

3. Various factors may affect results in nondiseased persons. The population from which specimens are secured for normal range determination may not be representative of the population to be tested. There may be differences due to age (see Table 36–1), sex, locality, race, diet, posture (Table 1–2), specimen storage time, and so forth. An example is the erythrocyte sedimentation rate (ESR) in which the normal values by the Westergren method for persons under age 60 years, corrected for ane-

TABLE 1–2.

Decrease in Test Values After Change From Upright to Supine Position*

Test	% Decrease
Hemoglobin	4 (0–17)
Hematocrit	6 (4–9)
Potassium	1 (0–3)
Calcium	4 (2–6.8)
Total protein	9 (7–10)
Albumin	9 (6.2–14)
Cholesterol	9 (5–15)
Triglyceride	10 (3–20)
Alkaline phosphatase	9 (5–11)
Alanine aminotransferase (SGPT)	7 (4–14)

*Average percent change with range of values found in the literature.

mia, are 0–15 mm/hour for men and 0–20 mm/hour for women, whereas in persons over age 60, normal values are 0–25 mm/hour for men and 0–30 mm/hour for women. There may even be significant within-day or between-day variation in some substances in the same person.

4. Normal values obtained by one analytical method may be inappropriately used with another method. For example, there are several well-accepted techniques for assay of serum albumin. The assay values differ somewhat because the techniques do not measure the same thing. Dye-binding methods measure dye-binding capacity of the albumin molecule, biuret procedures react with nitrogen atoms, immunologic methods depend on antibodies against antigenic components, and electrophoresis is influenced primarily by the electric charge of certain chemical groups in the molecule. In fact, different versions of the same method may not yield identical results, and even the same version of the same method, when performed on different equipment, may display variance.

5. As pointed out previously, normal values supplied by the manufacturers of test kits rather frequently do not correspond to the results obtained on a local population by a local laboratory, sometimes without any demonstrable reason. The same problem is encountered with normal values obtained from the medical literature. In some assays, such as fasting serum glucose using so-called true glucose methods, there is relatively little difference in normal ranges established by laboratories using the same method. In other assays there may be a significant difference. For example, one reference book suggests a normal range for serum sodium by flame photometry of 136–142 mEq/L, whereas another suggests 135–155 mEq/L. A related problem is the fact that normal ranges given in the literature may be derived from a laboratory or group of laboratories using one equipment and reagent system, whereas results may be considerably different when other equipment and reagents are used. The only way to compensate for this would be for each laboratory to establish its own normal ranges. Since this is time-consuming, expensive, and a considerable amount of trouble, it is most often not done; and even laboratories that do establish their own normal ranges are not able to do so for every test.

6. Population values may not be randomly distributed and may be skewed toward one end or the other of the range. This would affect the calculation of standard deviation and distort the normal range width. In such instances, some other way of establishing normal limits, such as a nonparametric method, would be better, but this is rarely done in most laboratories.

One can draw certain conclusions about problems derived from the use of the traditional concept and construction of normal ranges:

1. Some normal persons may have abnormal laboratory test values. This may be due to ordinary technical variables. An example is a person with a true value just below the upper limit of normal that is lifted just outside of the range by laboratory method imprecision. Another difficulty is the 2.5% of normal persons arbitrarily placed both above and below normal limits by using ±2 SD as the limit criterion. It can be mathematically demonstrated that the greater the number of tests employed, the greater the chance that at least one will yield a falsely abnormal result. In fact, if a physician uses one of the popular 12-test biochemical profiles, there is a 46% chance that at least one test result will be falsely abnormal. Once the result falls outside normal limits, without other information there is nothing to differentiate a truly abnormal from a falsely abnormal value, no matter how small the distance from the upper normal limit. Of course, the farther the values are from the normal limits, the greater the likelihood of a true abnormality. Also, if two or more tests that are diagnosis-related in some way are simultaneously abnormal, it reinforces the probability that true abnormality exists. Examples could be elevation of aspartate aminotransferase (SGOT) and alkaline phosphatase levels in an adult nonpregnant woman, a combination that suggests liver disease, or elevation of both blood urea nitrogen (BUN) and creatinine levels, which occurring together strongly suggest a considerable degree of renal function impairment.

2. Persons with disease may have normal test values. Depending on the width of the normal range, considerable pathologic change in the assay value of any individual person may occur without exceeding normal limits of the population. For example, if the person's test value is normally in the lower half of the population limits, his or her test value might double or undergo even more change without

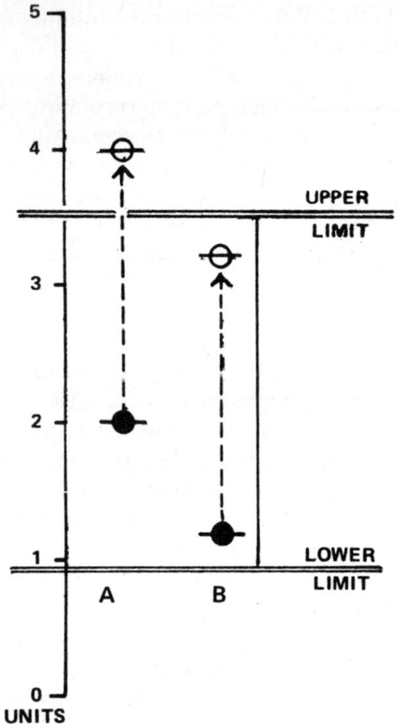

FIG 1–2.
How patient abnormality may be hidden within population reference ("normal") range. Patients A and B had the same degree of test increase, but the new value for patient B remains within the reference range because the baseline value was sufficiently low.

exceeding population limits (Fig 1–2). Comparison with previous baseline value would be the only way to demonstrate that substantial change had occurred.

Due to the various considerations outlined previously, there is a definite trend toward avoiding the term "normal range." The most frequently used replacement term is *reference range* (or *reference limits*). Therefore, the term "reference range" will be used throughout this book instead of "normal range."

PROBLEMS WITH LABORATORY SPECIMENS

Specimen collection and preservation may create laboratory problems (see Table 36–40). Probably the most frequent offender is contamination of urine from female patients by vaginal or labial secretions. Using more than 10 squamous epithelial cells per low-power field in a centrifuged urine sediment as the index of probable contamination, my surveys have found this present in 20%–30% of female random voided or midstream ("clean catch") specimens. These secretions may add red blood cells, white blood cells, protein, and bacteria to the urine. Nonfasting blood specimens may occasionally be troublesome, particularly for blood glucose and the effect of lipemia. This is most frequent in patients who are admitted in the afternoon and in outpatients. We have had some success in alleviating this problem by requesting that physicians ask elective presurgical patients either to have admission laboratory tests drawn fasting prior to admission or to come to the hospital for admission after fasting at least 3 hours. Certain tests, such as blood gas analysis, biochemical acid phosphatase assay, and plasma renin assay, necessitate special preservation techniques to be reliable.

One of the most well-known specimen collection problems is that of ensuring completeness of 24-hour urine specimens. Some patients are not informed that the 24-hour collection begins only after a urine specimen has been voided and discarded. It is frequently helpful to give the patient written instructions as to how a clean-voided specimen may be obtained and how the 24-hour specimen is collected. The two standard criteria used to evaluate adequacy of collection are the specimen volume and the urine creatinine content. Specimen volume is helpful only when the volume is abnormally low (e.g., <400 ml/24 hours in adults). A small volume that does not have maximal concentration (as evidenced by a high specific gravity or osmolality) suggests incomplete collection. However, renal disease, medications such as diuretics, and other conditions may prevent concentration, so this criterion is difficult to apply unless the patient is known to have good renal function. The second criterion is a normal quantity of urine creatinine. Creatinine is derived from muscle metabolism and has a reasonably constant daily excretion. However, creatinine production and excretion are dependent on body muscle mass. It has also been shown by several investigators that even in the same individual, daily creatinine excretion may vary 5%–25%, with an average variation of about 10%. Meat, especially when cooked for a long time, may increase creatinine excretion up to 40% for short periods of time and possibly 10%–20% over a 24-hour period.

Since creatinine excretion correlates with muscle mass, it might be helpful to compare measured creatinine excretion with calculated ideal excretion based on body height and ideal body weight (see Table 36–19). This would be only a rough benchmark, but it might be more helpful than the population reference range, which is rather wide.

EFFECTS OF PHYSIOLOGIC VARIABLES

Physiologic differences between groups of persons may affect test results. These deviations may be attributable to normal metabolic alterations in certain circumstances. Some examples are age (e.g., an increase in alkaline phosphatase levels in children compared with adult values) (see Table 36–1), sex (e.g., higher values for serum uric acid in males than in females), race (e.g., higher values for creatine phosphokinase in black men than in white men); time of day (e.g., higher values for serum cortisol in the morning than in the evening), meals (e.g., effect on blood glucose), and body position (e.g., change in values shown in Table 1–2 due to change in posture, resulting in possible decrease in many serum test values when an ambulatory outpatient becomes a hospital inpatient).

EFFECTS OF MEDICATIONS

The effect of medications is a major problem since a patient may be taking several drugs or may be taking over-the-counter pharmaceuticals without reporting them to the physician. Medication effects (see Table 36–2) may be manifest in several ways: drug-induced injury to tissues or organs (e.g., isoniazid-induced hepatitis), drug-induced alterations in organ function (e.g., increase in γ-glutamyltransferase produced by phenytoin microsomal induction in liver cells), drug competition effect (e.g., displacement of thyroxine from thyroxine-binding proteins by phenytoin), and interference by one drug with the analysis method of another (e.g., decrease in serum glucose using glucose oxidase when large doses of vitamin C are ingested).

EFFECTS OF HOSPITAL WORKING PROCEDURES

Several common hospital conditions may affect laboratory results without such alteration being recognized by the physician. These include intravenous fluids running at the time the test specimen is drawn, the effect of dehydration, the effect of heparin flushes on some tests, the effects of various medications, and in certain cases the administration of medication at a time different from that expected or recorded. The last item refers to the common situation in which several patients are scheduled to receive medication at the same time (e.g., 8 A.M.). Although administration to each may be charted as being the same time,the actual time that any individual receives the medication may vary significantly.

Another frequent problem is defective communication between the physician and the laboratory. In some cases this takes the form of incorrectly worded, ambiguous, or illegible orders. Nursing or secretarial personnel can easily misinterpret such orders and relay them incorrectly to the laboratory. Nonstandard test abbreviations or acronyms created from the names of new tests not familiar to nursing personnel also cause difficulties. In some cases the physician should supply at least a minimal amount of pertinent clinical information to obtain better service. This information is most vitally needed in the microbiology department. The microbiology technologist must know from what area the specimen was obtained, exactly what type of culture is desired, and especially, whether any particular organism is suspected so that special growth media or special handling may be employed if necessary. Basic clinical information is even more essential to the surgical pathologist and the radiologist. The surgical pathologist must at least know where the tissue specimen originated, and both the pathologist and radiologist can do a much better job providing an answer to the clinician if they could only know what the clinician's question is (i.e., for what reason is he or she requesting the study).

A word must be said about stat orders. *Stat* means emergency to the laboratory. Someone must stop whatever he or she is doing and perform the stat analysis immediately, possibly having to obtain the specimen first. After analysis the report must be delivered immediately.

During this time that laboratory person may not do any other work. Stat tests result in great decrease of laboratory efficiency and cost effectiveness. The most efficient and least expensive way to perform tests is to analyze several patient specimens at the same time, so that the initial setup and quality control portions of the test need be performed only once and all specimens can be incubated simultaneously. Extra speed is obtained when a test is ordered stat, but results for everyone else are delayed. Unfortunately, many stat requests, sometimes even the majority, are ordered for reasons other than a true emergency need for the result. In some cases the order orginates from nursing service because someone neglected to send a requisition for a routine test to the laboratory. In other cases the order is made stat because of convenience to the physician or the patient. Stat orders for these purposes at best are inconsiderate, wasteful, and disruptive. The physician should consider whether some other action-producing order category could be substituted, such as "as soon as possible." If the actual problem is that of unacceptable turnaround time for routine tests, this is a matter to be discussed with the laboratory director rather than evaded by stat orders.

LABORATORY TESTS AND THE MEDICAL LITERATURE

One of the more interesting phenomena in medicine is the scenario under which new tests or new uses for old tests are introduced. In most cases the initial reports are highly enthusiastic. Also in most cases there is eventual follow-up by other investigators who either cannot reproduce the initial good results or who uncover substantial drawbacks to the test. In some cases the problem lies in the fact that there may not be any way to provide an unequivocal standard against which test accuracy can be measured. An example is acute myocardial infarction, because there is no conclusive method to definitively separate severe myocardial ischemia from early infarction (i.e., severe reversible change from irreversible change). Another example is acute pancreatitis. In other cases the initial investigators may use analytical methods (e.g., "homemade" reagents) that are not identical to those of subsequent users. Other possible variances include different populations tested, different conditions under which testing is carried out, and effects of medication. Historical perspective thus suggests that initial highly enthusiastic claims about laboratory tests should be received with some caution.

Additional information relevent to this chapter is found in Chapter 35.

BIBLIOGRAPHY

Frazer CG: The application of theoretical goals based on biological variation data in proficiency testing. *Arch Pathol Lab Med* 1988; 112:404.

Lacher DA: Predictive value derived from likelihood ratios. *Am J Clin Pathol* 1987; 87:673.

Villa B: Statistical measures in methods evaluation: A brief review. *Lab Mgmt* 1987; 25(7):49.

Rasmussen P: Use of the laboratory in patient management. *Am Fam Physician* 1987; 35:214.

Sox HC: Probability theory in the use of diagnostic tests. *Ann Intern Med* 1986; 104:60.

Lum G, Beeler MF: Reference groups: Comparing oranges with oranges and apples with apples. *JAMA* 1983; 249:1890.

Zweig MH, Robertson EA: Why we need better test evaluations. *Clin Chem* 1982; 28:1272.

Young DS: What to make of the borderline test result. *Diagnosis* 1982; 4:21.

Beck JR: Quantitative logic and new diagnostic tests. *Arch Intern Med* 1982; 142:681.

Harris JM: The hazards of bedside Bayes. *JAMA* 1981; 246:2602.

Riegelman RK: The limits of the laboratory: Nuances of normality. *Postgrad Med* 1981; 70:203.

Barr JT: A priori considerations when using laboratory determinations in cost-effectiveness and clinical decision analysis. *Am J Med Technol* 1981; 47:619.

Dix D: On the interpretation of diagnostic tests: A common logical fallacy. *Clin Chem* 1981; 27:776.

Ash KO: Reference intervals (normal ranges): A challenge to laboratorians. *Am J Med Technol* 1980; 46:504.

Galen RS: New math in the lab: Notions of normality. *Diagn Med* 1980; 3(4):59.

Galen RS: New math in the lab: Predictive value theory. *Diagn Med* 1979; 2(1):23.

Rossing RG, Hatcher WE: Percentiles as reference values for laboratory data. *Am J Clin Pathol* 1979; 72:94.

2 Basic Hematologic Tests and Classification of Anemia

The major emphasis in hematology is placed on the three cellular elements of the blood—red blood cells (RBCs), white blood cells (WBCs), and platelets. Each of these elements will be discussed subsequently in separate chapters, beginning with disorders of the RBCs. The noncellular elements of the blood (fluid, electrolytes, plasma proteins, and other constituents) will be included in later chapters.

Several tests form the backbone of laboratory diagnosis in hematology.

HEMOGLOBIN

Hemoglobin is the oxygen-carrying compound contained in RBCs. The amount of hemoglobin per 100 ml of blood can be used as an index of the oxygen-carrying capacity of the blood. Total blood hemoglobin depends primarily on the number of RBCs (the hemoglobin carriers) but also, to a much lesser extent, on the amount of hemoglobin in each RBC. Depending on the method used and the care with which the laboratory checks its instruments, manual hemoglobin methods using a spectrophotometer are accurate to 4%–5%, and automated cell counters are accurate to about 2%–3%.

Reference values are most frequently quoted as 14–18 gm/100 ml (140–180 g/L) for men and 12–16 gm/100 ml (120–160 g/L) for women (100 ml = 1 dl; 1 gm/100 ml = 1 gm/dl = 1 gm%). Some reports indicate lower values, especially in women, so it might be better not to consider a patient anemic until the hemoglobin level is less than 13 gm/100 ml in men and 11 gm/100 ml in women. Infants have different reference limits (see Table 36–3). Both boys and girls have about the same hemoglobin levels until approximately age 11, after which male values slowly become higher. In one study, adult levels were attained at age 15 in women and at age 18 in men. Reference values for blacks average 0.5–1.0 gm (5–10 g/L) less than values for whites at most ages. The reason for this difference, and how much of it (if any) can be explained by a higher incidence of chronic iron deficiency, is still undecided. In addition, several investigators have found a significant decrease in hemoglobin levels (as much as 1.0 gm) between a sample obtained after some time in the upright position and another obtained later after overnight bed rest (see Table 1–2). There is some evidence that heavy smokers have increased hemoglobin concentration compared with nonsmokers; reported increases range from 0.5–2.2 gm/100 ml (5–20.2 g/L). In pregnancy, the hemoglobin concentration slowly decreases because of dilution from increasing plasma volume, with values as low as 10.0 gm/100 ml (100 g/L) being considered normal in the third trimester. There is controversy whether hemoglobin and hematocrit reference values should be lower in the elderly. At present the majority of investigators would not use a different reference range.

In newborns, capillary (heelstick) hemoglobin and hematocrit values are higher than venous blood values. The average neonatal difference between capillary and venous hemoglobin levels is 3.5 gm/dl (30.5 g/L) but varies from 1–10 gm/dl, with a corresponding difference in the hematocrit values. The increase in capillary hemoglobin concentration tends to be greater in smaller and sicker infants. The difference between heelstick and venous hemoglobin levels becomes less each day and virtually disappears by the fifth day of life. Neonatal hemoglobin concentration depends to some extent on the amount of blood received from the umbilical cord before the cord is clamped.

RED BLOOD CELL COUNT

The number of RBCs per cubic millimeter gives an indirect estimate of the hemoglobin content of the blood. Manual blood cell counting chamber (hemocytometer) methods give errors of 7%–14% or even more, depending on the experience of the technician. Automatic counting machines reduce this error to about 4%. However, many smaller laboratories do not have these machines. Reference values are 4.5–6.0 million/cu mm (4.5–6.0 × 10^6/L) for men and 4.0–5.5 million/cu mm (4.0–5.5 × 10^6/L) for women.

HEMATOCRIT

After centrifugation, the height of the RBC column is measured and compared with the height of the column of original whole blood. The percentage of RBC mass to original blood volume is the hematocrit. Anticoagulated whole blood is centrifuged in a special tube. Since whole blood is made up essentially of RBC and plasma, the percentage of packed RBCs after centrifugation gives an indirect estimate of the number of RBCs/100 ml of whole blood (and thus, in turn, is an indirect estimate of the amount of hemoglobin). Hematocrit thus depends mostly on the number of RBCs, but there is some effect (to a much lesser extent) from the average size of the RBC. In most automated cell counting systems the hematocrit is not measured directly but is calculated from the RBC count value and the mean corpuscular volume (MCV) value obtained from electric pulse height sizing of the RBCs. Reference values are 40%–54% for men and 37%–47% for women. The average error in hematocrit procedures is about 1%–2%. Microhematocrits are generally as accurate as the older standard Wintrobe (macrohematocrit) technique. The hematocrit may be decreased when going from upright to recumbent position and increased (1.5%–5.8% units) by heavy smoking in the same manner as the hemoglobin.

Useful relationships between Hb, Hct, and RBC count include:

Traditional Units	SI Units
Hb × 3 = Hct	Hb × .003 = Hct
RBC (millions) × 3 = Hb	RBC (10^6/L) × 30 = Hb
RBC (millions) × 9 = Hct	RBC (10^6/L) × .09 = Hct

INDICES (WINTROBE INDICES)

Wintrobe introduced a very useful method to demonstrate certain characteristics of RBCs.

Mean Corpuscular Volume

Measurement of the MCV utilizes the effect of the average RBC size on the hematocrit. If the average RBC size is increased, the same number of RBCs will have a slightly larger cell mass and thus a slightly increased hematocrit reading; the opposite happens if the average RBC size is smaller than normal. The MCV is calculated by dividing the hematocrit value by the RBC count.

There is some disagreement in the literature on MCV reference ranges. Older sources and Coulter Company printed values are approximately 80–94 femtoliters (fL) for men and 81–99 fL for women. More recent reports are in substantial agreement on 80–100 fL for both sexes. Heavy smoking may increase the MCV as much as 3 fL.

Conditions that increase the MCV are listed in Table 2–1. In my experience, the most common etiology of macrocytosis is alcoholism with or without cirrhosis. The major causes for folic acid deficiency are dietary deficiency or malabsorption; for vitamin B12 deficiency, pernicious anemia; and for substantial degrees of reticulocytosis, acute bleeding or hemolytic anemia. Occasionally there are mixed disorders; for example, some patients with alcoholism, malignancy, myxedema, and drug-induced macrocytosis have folic acid deficiency, and some patients with sideroblastic or sideroachrestic anemia have pyridoxine deficiency.

It must be emphasized that a substantial number of patients with disorders associated with macrocytosis will not display an elevated MCV when first seen by a physician. For ex-

TABLE 2–1.

Some Causes of Increased Mean Corpuscular Volume (Macrocytosis)

Causes	% of All Macrocytosis Patients*	% of Macrocytosis in Each Disease†
Common		
Folate or B12 deficiency	20–30 (5–50)‡	80–90 (4–100)
Chronic liver disease	15–20 (6–28)	30–40 (8–65)
Chronic alcoholism	10–12 (3–15)	60 (26–90)
Cytotoxic chemotherapy	10–15 (2–20)	30–40 (13–82)
Cardiorespiratory abnormality	8 (7–9.5)	?
Reticulocytosis	6–7 (0–15)	Depends on severity
Myelodysplastic syndromes	Frequent over age 40	>60 in RAEB and RARS§
Unexplained	25 (22.5–27)	—
Less common	<4%	
Noncytotoxic drugs		
Phenytoin		12–15 (11–55)
Hypothyroidism		10–15 (8–29)
Chronic leukemia/myelofibrosis		
Radiotherapy for malignancy		
Chronic renal disease		
Distance-runner macrocytosis		
Down's syndrome		
Artifactual		

*Percentage of all patients with macrocytosis.
†Percentage of patients with each condition listed who have macrocytosis.
‡Numbers in parentheses are literature range.
§RAEB, refractory anemia with excessive blasts; RARS, refractory anemia with ring sideroblasts (formerly called IASA, or idiopathic acquired sideroblastic anemia).

ample, the incidence of macrocytosis in megaloblastic anemia (folate or B12 deficiency) is about 80%–90% (literature range, 4%–100%); in alcoholism, about 60% (range, 6%–90%); in liver disease, about 25%–30% (range, 8%–65%); in hypothyroidism, about 20%–30% (range, 8%–55%); in phenytoin (Dilantin) anticonvulsant therapy, about 30% (range, 14%–50%), and in patients with malignancy undergoing cytotoxic therapy, about 30%–40% (range, 12.5%–82%).

TABLE 2–2.

Some Causes of Decreased Mean Corpuscular Volume (Microcytosis)

Common	Less Common
Chronic iron deficiency	Some cases of polycythemia
Alpha or beta thalassemia (minor)	Some cases of lead poisoning
Anemia of chronic disease	Some cases of congenital spherocytosis
	Some cases of sideroblastic anemia
	Certain abnormal Hbs (Hb E, Hb Lepore)

Conditions that decrease MCV are listed in Table 2–2; the most frequent (in the U.S. population) is chronic iron deficiency. The incidence of decreased MCV in chronic iron deficiency ranges from 27%–76% (averaging about 65%), depending considerably on the degree of deficiency. Thalassemia minor (alpha or beta) comprises about 15% of patients with microcytosis but may be less frequent in some populations. The anemia associated with various chronic diseases (uremia, rheumatoid-collagen diseases, severe chronic infection, etc.) is usually normocytic; but according to the literature, it can be microcytic in about 15% of patients (range, 0%–36%). In my experience, however, incidence has been 7% (100 patients). Differential diagnosis of these conditions is discussed in the section on chronic iron deficiency.

Some reports in the literature indicate discrepancies when MCV data from microhematocrits are compared with results from automated cell counters such as the Coulter Counter. For example, one report noted that more than 30% of specimens in which the MCV fell below the lower reference range limit of 80

TABLE 2–3.
Some Conditions That Affect the Mean Corpuscular Hemoglobin Concentration (MCHC)*

MCHC Increased	MCHC Decreased
Spherocytosis	Chronic iron deficiency
Free plasma hemoglobin (intravascular hemolysis)	Sideroachrestic (sideroblastic) anemia
High-titer cold agglutinins	Anemia of chronic disease
Severe plasma lipemia	
Heavy smoking (mild effect)	

*Depends to some extent on the particular methodology used.

fL by Coulter Counter measurement were still within reference range when microhematocrits were used for the calculation. Another investigator found that macrocytes were reported on peripheral blood smear in only 65% of patients with elevated MCV by Coulter Counter measurement. These studies suggest that MCV values obtained using an automated cell counter are more sensitive to abnormality than other common hematologic parameters. On the other hand, in approximately 10%–20% of patients with an elevated MCV there was no adequate explanation for the abnormality (these patients usually had relatively small elevations, but small elevations do not imply nonsignificance). Also, a patient may have macrocytes in the peripheral blood smear with a normal MCV, since the MCV represents only the average RBC size.

Mean Corpuscular Hemoglobin

The mean corpuscular hemoglobin (MCH) is based on estimates of the quantity (weight) of hemoglobin in the average RBC. Calculation is done by dividing the blood hemoglobin level by the RBC count. Reference values are 27–31 pg by manual methods and 26–34 pg by Coulter Counter.

The MCH is influenced by the size of the RBC; a large RBC with normal hemoglobin content will contain a greater weight of hemoglobin than a smaller cell with a normal hemoglobin content. The MCH also depends on the amount of hemoglobin in relation to the size of the cell; a hypochromic cell has a smaller weight of hemoglobin than a normochromic cell of equal size. In general, the MCH level is increased in macrocytosis and decreased in microcytosis and in hypochromia, but there is some variation because of the interplay between the two factors of cell size and concentration of hemoglobin.

Recent articles have pointed out that MCH values from automated counting instruments closely parallel MCV, significantly more so than by calculation from manual measurements. Therefore, MCH levels from automated cell counters are said to add little if any useful information to that available from the MCV.

Mean Corpuscular Hemoglobin Concentration

The MCH concentration (MCHC) estimates the average concentration of hemoglobin in the average RBC. The MCHC depends on the relationship of the amount of hemoglobin to the volume of the RBC. Thus, the MCHC does not depend on cell size alone; a macrocyte with a normal amount of hemoglobin has a normal MCHC. The MCHC is calculated by dividing the hemoglobin value by the hematocrit value. Reference values are 32%–36% (320–360 g/L) (manual methods) or 31%–37% (Coulter Counter). Conditions that affect the MCHC are listed in Table 2–3.

Red Blood Cell Distribution Width

Some of the newer electronic cell counting machines are able to sort out RBCs of different sizes and group them according to size (size histogram) as well as calculate the mean corpuscular volume (MCV). Normally, most RBCs are approximately equal in size, so that only one gaussian-type histogram peak is generated. Disease may change the size of some RBCs, for example, by fragmentation of RBCs (e.g., in hemolysis) or by a gradual process of size change in newly produced RBCs (e.g., in folic acid or iron deficiency). In most cases the abnormal cell population coexists with normal (or at least, less affected) RBCs. The difference in size between the abnormal and less abnormal RBCs produces either more than one histogram peak or a broadening of the normal peak. The cell counting machines can calculate an index of the RBC size differences (anisocytosis) using data from the histogram and the MCV, called the RBC distribution width (RDW). Although the degree of abnormality determines whether or not the index value exceeds index population reference range, in general the RDW is elevated in factor deficiency (iron, folate, or B12), RBC fragmentation, and homozygous hemoglobinopathies (hemoglobin [Hb] S, C, and H) and is normal in thalassemia minor, anemia of chronic disease, and heterozygous trait combinations of abnormal hemoglobins with normal Hb A. The RDW index is never decreased. The RDW (like the MCV) is sometimes abnormal before anemia appears and may be abnormal even before the MCV. Different automated cell counters differ in the way they measure cell size and compute the index, and there may be differences in sensitivity of the index between instruments of different manufacturers and even between different instrument models of the same manufacturer (providing one source of confusion when data are evaluated in the literature and in patient reports). Also, reports differ in percentage of patients with different diseases who have abnormal RDW (e.g., reports of elevated RDW in untreated pernicious anemia range from 69% to 100%). Differentiation between various disorders affecting RBC using MCV and RDW are outlined in Table 2–4 (the diseases listed in each category do not include all patients with that disease).

FACTORS THAT AFFECT INTERPRETATION OF RED BLOOD CELL INDICES

1. As an index of RBC hemoglobin, the MCHC was often more reliable than the MCV when manual counting methods were used, because manual RBC counts are relatively inaccurate. Since this is not a problem with automated cell counters, MCHC is not frequently helpful except to raise the question of spherocytosis if the MCHC is elevated. Increase in MCHC is usually limited to relatively severe RBC abnormalities. Elevated MCHC may be a clue to a false increase in MCV and decrease in hematocrit due to cold agglutinins or to a false increase in hemoglobin level due to hyperlipemia. However, different counting instruments react differently to cold agglutinins.

2. The MCV, MCH, and MCHC are affected only by average cell measurements either of size or of quantity of hemoglobin. This is especially noticeable in the indices dependent on average RBC size (MCV and, to some extent, MCHC). There may be considerable variation in size between individual RBCs (anisocytosis), but average measurement indices do not reflect this, since they take into account only the average size.

3. Although careful examination of a well-made peripheral blood smear yields a considerable amount of the same information as RBC indices, abnormality may be indicated by one and not by the other, so that the two techniques are complementary.

4. Reference values for hemoglobin, hematocrit, and indices for infants and children differ from adult values (see Table 36–3). There is some discrepancy in the literature regarding pediatric reference range values, more so than

TABLE 2–4.
Red Blood Cell Distribution Width and Mean Cell Volume

NL* RDW, low MCV	NL RDW, NL MCV	NL RDW, high MCV
Thalassemia minor	Chronic disease (90%)	Aplastic anemia
Chronic disease (10%)	Hb AS, AC	Myelodysplastic syndrome
	Hereditary spherocytosis	Alcoholism
	Acute bleeding	
	Cirrhosis	
	Uremia	
High RDW, low MCV	**High RDW, NL MCV**	**High RDW, high MCV**
Iron deficiency	Early factor deficiency	B12 or folate deficiency
S-thalassemia	SS disease†	Autoimmune hemolytic anemia
Hb H	SC disease‡	Cold agglutinins
RBC fragmentation	Myelofibrosis	Newborn
	Sideroblastic anemia	

*NL, normal.
†SS disease means that sickle hemoglobin (Hb S) is present on both genes (SS).
‡SC disease means that one gene for Hb S is combined with one gene for Hb C.

for adult reference ranges. Some of the reasons may be a more limited number of patients and the discrepancy between data derived from manual methods and data derived from automated cell counters.

5. It usually is not necessary to repeat RBC indices for screening or diagnostic purposes after one set of values has been obtained.

CELL COUNTING INSTRUMENT ARTIFACTS

Many laboratories perform hemoglobin, RBC, and WBC determinations on electronic particle counting instruments. In certain cases, artifacts may falsely alter results.

1. When WBC counts are substantially greater than 50,000/cu mm, the hemoglobin, hematocrit, RBC, MCV, and MCH values may be falsely increased unless corrective measures are taken (the word "increase" as used here means increase from true values, which may or may not place the values outside of reference limits).

2. Peripheral blood nucleated RBCs in substantial numbers will produce false increases of the WBC count unless manually corrected.

3. Marked hyperlipidemia (> 2,000 mg/dl of triglyceride) may increase hemoglobin, MCH, and MCHC values.

4. High titers of cold agglutinins may decrease the hematocrit and RBC count and increase MCV, MCH, and MCHC values. However, not all counting instruments react the same to cold agglutinins.

5. Cryoglobulins may falsely increase the WBC count.

6. Marked erythrocytosis may falsely decrease the RBC count and the hematocrit from true levels and falsely elevate MCH and MCHC values.

EXAMINATION OF WRIGHT-STAINED PERIPHERAL BLOOD SMEAR

This procedure gives a vast amount of information. It allows visual estimation of the amount of hemoglobin in the RBCs and the overall size of the RBCs. In addition, alterations in size, shape, and structure of individual RBCs or WBCs are visible, which may have diagnostic significance in certain diseases. Pathologic early forms of the blood cells are also visible. Finally, a good estimate of the platelet count can be made in most cases from the peripheral smear alone (normal is 7–25 platelets per oil immersion field, using 10 × oculars).

TABLE 2–5.
Causes of Spherocytosis

ABO hemolytic disease of newborn
Acute transfusion reactions (especially ABO type)
Hereditary spherocytosis
Transfused stored bank blood
Autoimmune hemolytic anemia
Thermal injury, especially in first 24 hr
Physical RBC injury (as a component of microangiopathic hemolytic anemia)
Toxins (*Clostridium welchii* sepsis and certain snake venoms)
Hereditary elliptocytosis (10%–20% of cases)
Occasionally in severe Heinz body hemolytic anemias

Peripheral Smear Abnormalities

Hypochromia (an increase in the RBC central clear area) raises the question of chronic iron deficiency (chapter 3).

Macrocytes in considerable numbers suggest a differential diagnosis of megaloblastic anemia vs. the other etiologies of increased MCV (see Table 2–1). Macrocytes in small numbers suggest reticulocytosis as the most likely etiology. Some hematologists differentiate between types of macrocytes: oval macrocytes (folic acid or vitamin B12 deficiency; myeloid metaplasia) and round macrocytes (alcoholism; cirrhosis; reticulocytosis; aplastic anemia).

Microcytes are small RBCs caused by any of the conditions listed under decreased MCV (see Table 2–2). Hypochromic microcytes suggest a differential diagnosis of chronic iron deficiency vs. thalassemia minor or anemia of chronic disease.

Spherocytes are a type of microcyte in which the cell is round and lacks the central clear area. Spherocytes are a feature of congenital spherocytosis (chapter 5) and are also found to varying degrees in certain other conditions (Table 2–5).

Polychromatophilic RBCs (discussed later) are reticulocytes, a sign of markedly increased RBC production, and therefore may be present in patients with acute bleeding, hemolytic processes, hematopoietic and nonhematopoietic malignancies, and factor deficiency anemia responding to therapy (see Table 2–7). Sometimes a few polychromatophilic RBC may be present without a definite etiology.

Schistocyte ("broken cell"; also called schizocyte) is a term given to a deformed or broken RBC. In general, the cells are smaller than normal, are misshapen, and have one or more sharp points protruding from the periphery. Names have been applied to various subgroups of misshapen RBCs, such as "burr cell," "acanthocyte," and "helmet cell." Unfortunately, some of these names, especially burr cell, have been applied to different cells by different investigators, so that in most instances it might be preferable to use the noncommittal term, schistocyte. Some conditions associated with schistocytes are listed in Table 2–6.

Acanthocytes are a subgroup of schistocytes consisting of small spherical cells with several finger-like projections from the RBC surface distributed in an irregular manner. The ends of the projections tend to be slightly thickened. Acanthocytes are typically found in large numbers in hereditary abetalipoproteinemia (Bassen-Kornsweig disease, chapter 21), in moderate numbers in severe liver disease or in anorexia nervosa, and in small numbers in association with schistocytes of other types in other conditions.

Red blood cell crenation (echinocytes) are RBCs that appear normal except for uniform small triangular projections arranged in a uniform manner around the circumference of the cell, like the outer edge of a gearwheel. When most of the RBCs have this appearance, they are most commonly artifactual; but in lesser numbers they may be found in liver disease, renal disease, hyperlipidemia, and in some RBC enzymopathies.

Bite cells (degmacytes) are RBCs with a semicircular defect in one area of the outer edge. When present in significant number, bite cells are suggestive of hemolytic anemia due to an oxidizing agent (Heinz body anemia).

Sickle cells are crescent-shaped RBCs pointed at one or both ends found in some patients with homozygous sickle cell anemia (chapter 5). Hemoglobin SC disease may sometimes display stubby sickled cells with a short thick bar protruding from the center that represents an Hb C crystal.

Elliptocytes (ovalocytes) are oval RBCs found in varying numbers in persons with congenital elliptocytosis and occasionally in small numbers in normal persons. When seen on edge, the cells may look somewhat like short rods and, rarely, may superficially resemble an atypical sickle cell.

Target cells consist of a peripheral ring and central disk of Hb. Target cells are found in large numbers in Hb C disease (chapter 5) and in lesser numbers with certain other abnormal hemoglobins, in thalassemia, and in chronic liver disease.

Teardrop cells look like RBCs in which one side has been gently pulled out to a sharp point while the opposite side is still rounded. These cells are most characteristically associated with myeloid metaplasia (myelofibrosis, chapter 7) but can also be present in lesser numbers in other myeloproliferative syndromes, such as chronic myelocytic leukemia.

Stomatocytes are RBCs that have a rectangular or slit-like central pallor configuration. This may be due to hereditary stomatocytosis or may be drug induced. A few stomatocytes

TABLE 2–6.

Some Conditions Associated With Schistocytes

Many	Few to Moderate Number
RBC fragmentation syndromes	Any condition with RBC injury
Disseminated intravascular coagulation	Many hemolytic anemias
Hemolytic-uremic syndromes	Septicemia
Thrombotic thrombocytopenic purpura	Some patients with malignancy
Mechanical RBC injuries (e.g., prosthetic heart valves)	Renal failure
	Alcoholism
Severe extensive burns	Cirrhosis
Zieve's syndrome	Hypothyroidism
Abetalipoproteinemia (acanthocytes)	Unknown cause

may be found in normal persons and in a variety of diseases.

Rouleaux are RBCs partially adhering to each other with the overall appearance of a partially spread out stack of coins. The RBC central clear area is usually absent. This appearance is similar to that normally seen in the very thick areas of a peripheral blood smear. However, with rouleaux there are a moderate number of free single RBCs intermingled with the RBC stacks, whereas there are no free RBCs in thick areas of the smear. Considerable rouleaux formation suggests the possibility of abnormal serum proteins (such as the monoclonal proteins of multiple myeloma).

Red Blood Cell Inclusions

Basophilic stippling describes a moderate number of small dark blue dotlike structures scattered fairly uniformly throughout the hemoglobinated area of the RBC. Stippling is derived from nuclear remnants, so that the cell represents a reticulocyte and thus may be seen in many of the same conditions as polychromatophilic RBCs. However, stippling is especially associated with lead poisoning (chapter 34).

Howell-Jolly bodies are small, round, blue-black inclusions that are considerably larger than basophilic stippling and ordinarily occur only one to an RBC. Howell-Jolly bodies may be present in any severe anemia but are more likely to be seen in severe hemolytic anemias and after splenectomy.

Pappenheimer bodies are small dark-staining granular inclusions that tend to occur in small numbers, are irregularly distributed, and often occur in small groups. They actually are hemosiderin granules that can be confirmed with ferricyanide iron stains. They are found after splenectomy, in some patients with sideroblastic anemias, and occasionally in patients with severe hemolytic anemia.

Three types of RBC inclusions cannot be seen with Wright's or Giemsa stain. All three require supravital staining techniques or other special procedures. Reticulocytes (discussed in detail later) are the stage in RBC maturation just before full maturity. Their number serves as an index of bone marrow RBC production. Hemoglobin H inclusions can sometimes be seen on a reticulocyte preparation as uniformly distributed small round dots somewhat resembling basophilic stippling but of slightly differing sizes. If a reticulocyte is affected, the Hb H inclusions coexist with the more irregular and more linear reticulum structures. Heinz bodies also require a special staining procedure and may need RBC pretreatment with a strong oxidizing agent such as phenylhydrazine. Heinz body formation is most often found in anemias due to RBC enzyme defects, "unstable" hemoglobins (chapter 5), and certain uncommon hemoglobins such as hemoglobin Koln and Zurich. The Heinz bodies are small, scattered, dotlike structures of varying size in the RBC derived from denatured hemoglobin.

Limitations of the Peripheral Blood Smear Examination

The peripheral smear is one of the most useful laboratory procedures in hematology. There obviously are many limitations; for example, a peripheral smear cannot demonstrate the presence of anemia per se, which must be detected by means of either the hemoglobin level, hematocrit value, or RBC count. Also, many etiologies of anemia are associated with nonspecific peripheral blood changes. In some cases in which the peripheral smear is highly suggestive, it may not be so in early stages of the disease. Even if characteristic cell changes are present, there may be different underlying causes for the same morphologic type of anemia, different causes that call for different treatment. Finally, some conditions produce anemia without any demonstrable morphologic changes in the RBC on the peripheral smear. The same comments about RBCs are also generally applicable to the WBCs of the peripheral smear. However, it is often possible to predict leukocytosis by comparing the overall visual ratio of WBCs to RBCs. A differential count of the various WBC forms is done from the peripheral smear.

RETICULOCYTE COUNT

Reticulocytes occupy an intermediate position between nucleated RBCs in the bone marrow and mature (nonnucleated, fully hemoglobinated) RBCs. After the normoblast (metarubricyte) nucleus is extruded from the cell, some cytoplasmic microsomes and ribosomes remain for 1–2 days that are not ordinarily visible on peripheral blood smears using Wright's or Giemsa stain but that can be seen by using vital staining techniques and dyes such as methylene blue or cresyl blue. The material then is seen microscopically in the form of dark blue dots or thin short irregular linear structures arranged in loose aggregates or reticulum. The reticulocyte count is an index of the production of mature RBCs by the bone marrow. Increased reticulocyte counts mean an increased number of RBCs being put into the peripheral blood in response to some stimulus. In exceptionally great reticulocyte responses, there may even be nucleated RBCs pushed out into the peripheral blood due to massive RBC production activity of the bone marrow. Except in a very few diseases, such as erythroblastosis, peripheral blood nucleated RBCs are usually few in number and of a later maturity stage when they do appear. Reticulocytes are not completely mature RBCs; therefore, when reticulocytes appear in the peripheral blood, they may be slightly larger than normal RBCs and may be sufficiently large to be recognizable as macrocytes. When present in sufficient numbers, these macrocytes may increase the MCV index. Early reticulocytes sometimes appear blue-gray or gray with Wright's stain in contrast to the red-orange appearance of the normal RBC; this phenomenon is called *polychromatophilia* and is produced by immature bluish cytoplasmic material to which reddish staining hemoglobin is added. In some conditions a reticulocyte may display small, evenly distributed dotlike aggregates of cytoplasmic ribosomes visible with Wright's stain, a phenomenon known as *basophilic stippling*.

Reference limits for the reticulocyte count are usually considered to be 0.5%–1.5%. Some investigators have reported somewhat higher values, especially in women. There is a substantial problem concerning reproducibility of reticulocyte counts, with statistical variation on the order of ±1 reticulocyte percent unit at normal reticulocyte levels of 0.5%–1.5% and somewhat greater variation at levels of 5% or more.

Reticulocytes are reported as a percentage of total RBCs (total RBC includes both mature RBCs and reticulocytes). In some clinical situations the number of mature RBCs may decrease while the absolute (total) number of reticulocytes remains the same; this increases the reticulocyte percentage and gives a false impression of increased reticulocyte production. Therefore, some authorities recommend that reticulocyte counts be corrected for effects of anemia. This may be done by multiplying the reticulocyte count (percent) by the patient hematocrit and dividing the result by an average normal hematocrit (47 for men and 42 for women). An alternate method is to obtain the absolute number of circulating reticulocytes by multiplying the patient RBC count by the reticulocyte count (after converting reticulocyte % to a decimal fraction). If polychromatophilic RBCs are present, some experts recommend that the (already) corrected reticulocyte count be divided by 2 to correct for the longer stay of younger reticulocytes in the peripheral blood.

TABLE 2–7.
Most Common Causes of Reticulocytosis

Hemolytic anemia, chronic or acute (antibody-induced, drug-induced, associated with abnormalities in hemoglobin or RBC structure, etc.)
Acute bleeding
After treatment of vitamin B12/folate/iron deficiency

As noted previously, reticulocyte counts are used as an index of bone marrow activity. Any substantial change in bone marrow RBC production theoretically should be reflected in reticulocyte count change. Important causes of elevated reticulocyte counts are listed in Table 2–7. A normal reticulocyte count has traditionally been considered evidence against a substantial degree of hemolytic anemia and can be used as an index of success in therapy for factor-deficiency anemia (therapeutic trial, chapter 35). One difficulty is that it usually takes 48–96 hours, sometimes even longer, to establish a reticulocyte count elevation following acute episodes of blood loss, onset of hemolysis, or beginning of factor therapy. Also, reticulocyte counts are not above reference range in some patients with hemolytic anemia (as many as 20%–25% in some studies, depending on the etiology of the disorder), with the degree of reticulocyte response having some correlation with the severity of the hemolytic process. In some cases, failure to obtain expected degrees of reticulocyte response may be due to superimposed factor deficiency (e.g., iron or folate). Another problem may be failure to suspect a hemolytic process or blood loss because the hemoglobin level may remain within population reference range if increased RBC production balances RBC loss or destruction.

In certain hemolytic anemias such as sickle cell anemia and congenital spherocytosis, temporary aplastic "crises" may develop in which the anemia worsens due to a halt in RBC production rather than an increase in rate of hemolysis. These crises are sometimes due to parvovirus B-19 infection. The reticulocyte count will become normal or decrease after time is allowed for reticulocytes already in the peripheral blood to disappear.

In certain anemias caused by ineffective erythropoiesis, the reticulocyte count is normal or decreased unless therapy is given. Some examples include deficiencies of iron, folic acid, vitamin B12, or pyridoxine, or in many patients with anemia associated with chronic disease. In the case of factor deficiency, blood transfusion or hospital diet may contain a sufficient quantity of the deficient factor to increase RBC production.

WHITE BLOOD CELL COUNT

White blood cell counts may be done either manually using a hemocytometer or with automated cell counters. The error produced by hemocytometer counts is about 4%–8% but may be higher with inexperienced personnel. Automated counters have approximately 2%–4% error. The machine has the disadvantage that WBC counts more than 100,000/cu mm become increasingly inaccurate unless a dilution is used. In addition, some of the abnormal lymphocytes of lymphocytic leukemia are exceptionally fragile and may be destroyed when the specimen is prepared for a machine count, thus giving a reading falsely lower than the true value. With either hemocytometer or machine counting, nucleated RBCs are counted as WBCs, and a correction must be made on the basis of the percentage of nucleated RBCs (to 100 WBCs) found on the peripheral smear.

Reference values are most often quoted as 5,000–10,000/cu mm (5–10 × 10^9/L). Several studies suggest that 4,500–11,000/cu mm would be more correct. However, there is a significant overlap of normal and abnormal between 4,500–5,000/cu mm and 10,000–11,000/cu mm, especially in the latter area. There is some evidence that the normal range for blacks may be at least 500/cu mm (.5 × 10^9/L) lower than the normal range for whites. Alterations in WBC levels are discussed in chapter 6.

PLATELET COUNT

The manual procedure that employs a hemocytometer counting chamber and a standard microscope has approximately a 10%–20% error. A somewhat similar method that makes use of a phase contrast microscope has a reported error of about 8%. Platelet counting machines can reduce the error even further. Reference values are 150,000–400,000/cu mm (150–400 × 10^9/L) for direct counts.

BONE MARROW ASPIRATION

Bone marrow aspiration is of help in several situations: (1) to confirm the diagnosis of megaloblastic anemia; (2) to establish the diagnosis of leukemia or multiple myeloma; (3) to determine whether deficiency of one or more of the peripheral blood cellular elements is due to a deficiency in the bone marrow precursors (bone marrow hypoplasia); (4) to document a deficiency in body iron stores in certain cases of suspected iron deficiency anemia; and (5) in certain cases, to demonstrate metastatic neoplasm or some types of infectious disease (culture or histologic sections may be preferred to routine Wright-stained smears).

COMMENTS ON HEMATOLOGIC TESTS

The nine procedures previously described are the basic tests of hematology. Careful selection and interpretation of these procedures can go far toward solving the vast majority of hematologic problems. Other tests may be ordered to confirm or exclude a diagnosis suggested by the results of preliminary studies. These other tests will be discussed in association with the diseases in which they are useful.

However, once again certain points should be made. Laboratory tests in hematology are no different from any other laboratory tests. Two or more tests that yield essentially the same information in any particular situation should not be ordered. For example, it is rarely necessary to order hemoglobin and hematocrit determinations and RBC count all together unless indices are needed. In fact, either the hemoglobin or the hematocrit alone is usually sufficient, although initially the two are often ordered together as a check on each other (because it is the least accurate, the RBC count is rarely helpful). Both the WBC count and differential are usually done initially. If both are normal, there usually is no need to repeat the differential count if the total WBC count remains normal and there are no morphologic abnormalities of the RBCs and WBCs.

Another point to be stressed is the proper collection of specimens. The timing of collection may be extremely important. Transfusion therapy may cause a megaloblastic bone marrow to lose its diagnostic megaloblastic features, sometimes in as little as 12 hours. On the other hand, transfusion will not affect a bone marrow that has no iron. Capillary blood (finger puncture) is best for making peripheral blood smears because oxalate anticoagulant causes marked artifacts in WBC morphology and even will slightly alter the RBC. Ethylenediamine tetraacetic acid (EDTA) anticoagulant will cause a false decrease in hematocrit (hemoglobin is not affected) if the amount of blood collected is less than one half the proper volume (for the amount of EDTA in the tube). When capillary (finger puncture) blood is used to obtain the hematocrit or hemoglobin values or the cell counts, too much squeezing of the finger or other poor technique may result in falsely low values caused by dilution of the blood by tissue juice. On the other hand, dehydration may result in hemoconcentration and produce falsely high values. This may mask an anemia actually present; or another determination after the patient is properly hydrated may give the false impression of a sudden drop in values, as might otherwise come from an acute bleeding episode. Very severe hemoconcentration may simulate polycythemia.

ANEMIA

Although anemia may be defined as a decrease in hemoglobin concentration, it may result from a pathologic decrease in the RBC count. Since mature RBCs are fully saturated with hemoglobin, such a decrease means that total blood hemoglobin value will also be affected.

Before commencing transfusion therapy or an extensive workup for the etiology of anemia, one should consider the possibility of *pseudoanemia* (Table 2–8). Pseudoanemia may be associated with either a hemoglobin value below reference range limits or a drop in hemoglobin level of 2 gm/100 ml (20 g/L) or more from a previous value. Accuracy of the values, especially those below the reference range, should be verified by redrawing the specimen. It is also possible that a patient could have true anemia simultaneously with one of the conditions in Table 2–8.

One frequently overlooked cause of hemoglobin decrease is iatrogenic blood loss due to laboratory test specimens. Several studies document that a surprising amount of blood can be withdrawn, especially in critically ill patients or those with diagnostic problems. Whereas the majority of patients contributed an average of 10–20 ml of blood per day, those in critical care units may average 40–50 ml/day and sometimes even as much as 150–500 ml per patient per day for several days' time. In some cases this may total more than 1,000 ml during the hospital stay. (The data sometimes include blood withdrawn to clear arterial lines and sometimes not; this blood also may represent a considerable total quantity.)

Classification of Anemia

Classification of anemia is helpful because it provides a handy reference for differential diagnosis. There are several possible classifications; each is helpful in some respects.

Anemia may be classified by pathogenesis. According to pathogenesis, three mechanisms may be responsible.

1. Deficiency of vital hematopoietic raw material *(factor deficiency anemia)*. The most common causes of factor deficiency anemia are iron deficiency and deficiency of vitamin B12, folic acid, or both.

TABLE 2–8.

Some Conditions That Produce or Contribute to False Anemia

Some Conditions That Produce or Contribute to False Anemia
Overhydration or rehydration of a dehydrated patient
Specimen obtained with intravenous (IV) fluid running
Fluid retention
Pregnancy
Hypoalbuminemia
Posture changes (from upright to recumbent)
Laboratory variation in hemoglobin assay (approximately ± 0.5 gm/dl) or laboratory error

2. Failure of the blood-forming organs to produce or to deliver mature RBCs to the peripheral blood *(production-defect anemia)*. This may be due to (1) replacement of marrow by fibrosis or by neoplasm (primary or metastatic); (2) hypoplasia of the bone marrow, most commonly produced by certain chemicals; or (3) toxic suppression of marrow production or delivery without actual marrow hypoplasia, found to a variable extent in some patients with certain systemic diseases. The most common of these diseases are severe infection, chronic renal disease, widespread malignancy (without extensive marrow replacement), rheumatoid-collagen diseases, and hypothyroidism. (These conditions may sometimes be associated with an element of hemolytic anemia.)

3. Red blood cell loss from the peripheral blood *(depletion anemia)*. This is commonly due to (1) hemorrhage, acute or chronic (causing escape of RBCs from the vascular system); (2) hemolytic anemia (RBCs destroyed or RBC survival time shortened within the vascular system); or (3) hypersplenism (splenic sequestration).

A second classification is based on RBC morphology. Depending on the appearance of the RBC on a peripheral blood smear, Wintrobe indices, or both, anemias may be characterized as microcytic, normocytic, or macrocytic. They may be further subdivided according to the average amount of RBC hemoglobin, resulting in hypochromia or normochromia. (Macrocytic RBCs may appear hyperchromic on peripheral smear, but this is an artifact due to enlarged and thicker cells that, being thicker, do not transmit light through the central portion as they would normally.) Table 2–9 lists the more common etiologies.

TABLE 2–9.
Some Common Causes of Anemia According to Red Blood Cell Morphology*

Microcytic
- Hypochromic
  - Chronic iron deficiency (most frequent cause)
  - Thalassemia
  - Occasionally in chronic systemic diseases
- Normochromic
  - Some cases of chronic systemic diseases
  - (May be simulated by spherocytosis or polycythemia in some patients)

Normocytic
- Hypochromic
  - Some cases of anemia due to systemic diseases
  - Many cases of lead poisoning
- Normochromic
  - Many cases of anemia due to systemic disease (most common cause)
  - Many cases of anemia associated with pituitary, thyroid, or adrenal disease
  - Acute blood loss
  - Hemolytic anemia
  - Bone marrow replacement or hypoplasia
  - Hypersplenism
  - Distance-runner anemia

Macrocytic
- Hypochromic
  - Some cases of macrocytic anemia with superimposed iron deficiency
- Normochromic
  - Vitamin B12 or folic acid deficiency
  - Malabsorption (vitamin B12 or folic acid)
  - Chronic alcoholism
  - Reticulocytosis
  - Some cases of chronic liver disease and some cases of hypothyroidism
  - Myelodysplasia syndromes/aplastic anemia

*All patients with any disease do not fit into any one category.

Investigation of a Patient With Anemia

Anemia is a symptom of some underlying disease and is not a diagnosis. There always is a cause, and most of the causes can be discovered by a relatively few simple procedures. Knowing the common causes of anemia, getting a good history, doing a thorough physical examination, and ordering a logical sequence of laboratory tests based on what the clinical picture and other findings suggest provide the greatest assistance in identifying which underlying disease is responsible. When anemia is discovered (usually by the appearance of a low hemoglobin or hematocrit value), the first step is to determine whether anemia really exists. The abnormal result should be confirmed by drawing a second specimen. Then, if the patient is not receiving excess IV fluid that might produce hemodilution, the next step is to obtain a WBC count, differential, RBC indices, reticulocyte count, and a description of RBC morphology from the peripheral smear. It is wise for the physician to personally examine the peripheral smear, because many technicians do not routinely pay much attention to the RBCs. A careful history and physical examination must be performed. To some extent, the findings on peripheral smear and RBC indices (including the RDW, if available) help suggest areas to emphasize:

1. If the RBCs are microcytic, the possibility of chronic blood loss must always be carefully excluded.

2. If the RBCs are macrocytic, the possibility of megaloblastic anemia or reticulocytosis due to acute bleeding must always be investigated.

3. If the RBCs are not microcytic, if megaloblastic anemia is ruled out in patients with macrocytosis, and if the reticulocyte count is significantly elevated, two main possibilities should be considered: acute blood loss and hemolytic anemia. The reticulocyte count is usually 5% or higher in these cases. However, the possibility of a deficiency anemia responding to therapy should not be forgotten.

4. In a basically normocytic-normochromic anemia without significant reticulocytosis and in which either leukopenia or thrombocytopenia (or both) is present, hypersplenism, bone marrow depression, or a few systemic diseases (e.g., systemic lupus erythematosis) are the main possibilities. In patients over age 40 with normocytic-normochromic anemia and without WBC or platelet decrease, myeloma should be considered, especially if rouleaux or other abnormalities are present that are commonly associated with myeloma. The possibility of chronic iron deficiency should not be forgotten, even though the typical RBC morphology of iron deficiency is microcytic-hypochromic. Occasionally, patients with B12 or folate deficiency have an MCV in the upper normal range.

5. Appearance of certain RBC abnormalities in the peripheral blood suggests certain diseases. A considerable number of target cells suggests one of the hemoglobinopathies or chronic liver disease. Marked basophilic stippling points toward lead poisoning or reticulocytosis. Sickle cells mean sickle cell anemia. Nucleated RBCs indicate either bone marrow replacement or unusually marked bone marrow erythropoiesis, most commonly seen in hemolytic anemias. Significant rouleaux formation suggests monoclonal gammopathy or hyperglobulinemia. Spherocytes usually indicate an antigen-antibody type of hemolytic anemia but may mean congenital spherocytosis or a few other types of hemolytic anemia. Schistocytes (burr cells) are usually associated with microangiopathic hemolytic anemias or with uremia, alcoholism, and hypothyroidism. Macrocytes are frequently produced by reticulocytosis but are also associated with megaloblastic anemias, cirrhosis, chronic alcoholism, hypothyroidism, and aplastic anemia.

Once the basic underlying process is identified, the etiology can usually be identified by using selected laboratory tests with the help of history, physical findings, and other diagnostic procedures. In general it is best to perform diagnostic laboratory studies before giving blood transfusion, although in many cases the diagnosis can be made despite transfusion. Blood specimens for the appropriate tests can usually be obtained before transfusion is actually begun, since blood for type and crossmatching must be drawn first. Serum can be saved or frozen for additional studies, if needed.

BIBLIOGRAPHY

Saxena S, et al: Red blood cell distribution width in pernicious anemia. *Am J Clin Pathol* 1988; 89:660.

Zauber NP, Zauber AG: Hematologic data of healthy very old people. *JAMA* 1987; 257:2181.

Brittenham GM, Koepke JA: Red blood cell volume distributions and the diagnosis of anemia. *Arch Pathol Lab Med* 1987; 111:1146.

Flynn MA, et al: Limitations in red blood cell distribution width (RDW) in evaluation of microcytosis. *Am J Clin Pathol* 1986; 85:445.

Bell A, Lofness KG: A photo essay on red cell morphology. *J Med Technol* 1986; 3:85.

Henry ML, et al: Iatrogenic anemia. *Am J Surg* 1986; 151:362.

Krause JR: Red-cell abnormalities in the blood smear: Disease correlations. *Lab Mgmt* 1985; 23(10):29.

Scamurra D, Davey FR: Anemias associated with spherocytic erythrocytes. *Lab Med* 1985; 16:83.

Dallman PR, et al: Prevalence and causes of anemia in the United States 1976 to 1980. *Am J Clin Nutr* 1984; 39:437.

Fishleder AJ, Hoffman GC: Automated hematology: Counts and indices. *Lab Mgmt* 1984; 22(12)21.

Walsh JR: Borderline anemia in old age. *Geriatr Med Today* 1983; 2(3):25.

Bessman JD, et al: Improved classification of anemia by MCV and RDW. *Am J Clin Pathol* 1983; 80:322.

Steinberg MH, Dreiling BJ: Microcytosis: Its significance and evaluation. *JAMA* 1983; 249:85.

Fisher SL, Fisher SP: Mean corpuscular volume. *Arch Intern Med* 1983; 143:282.

Thomas WJ, Collins TM: Comparison of venipuncture blood counts with microcapillary measurements in screening for anemia in one-year-old infants. *J Pediatr* 1982; 101:32.

Shanahan MB: Reticulocyte counts. *Arch Intern Med* 1982; 142:1585.

Nathan DG, Oski FA (eds): *Hematology of Infancy and Childhood,* ed 2. Philadelphia, WB Saunders Co, 1981.

Soloway HB: The diagnosis is microcytosis: Now what? *Diagn Med* 1981; 4:39.

Graitcer PL, et al.: Hemoglobins and hematocrits: Are they equally sensitive in detecting anemias? *Am J Clin Nutr* 1981; 34:61.

Markman M: Falling hematocrit value on cessation of smoking. *JAMA* 1981; 245:1314.

Crosby WHP: Red cell mass: Its precursors and its perturbations. *Hosp Pract* 1980; 15:71.

Kough RH: Pattern recognition—the key to office Dx of anemia. *Modern Med* 1980; 48:69.

Marchand A: Restoring energy to a tired anemia diagnosis. *Diagn Med* 1980; 3:23.

Freedman ML, Marcus DL: Anemia and the elderly: Is it physiology or pathology? *Am J Med Sci* 1980; 280:81.

Fairbanks VF: Nonequivalence of automated and manual hematocrit and erythrocyte indices. *Am J Clin Pathol* 1980; 73:55.

Galen RS: Abnormal MCHC. *Med Lab Observer* 1980; 12:13.

Carmel R, et al: Anemia: Textbook vs. practice. *JAMA* 1979; 242:2295.

Chanarin I: Alcohol and the blood. *Br J Haematol* 1979; 42:333.

Peck TM, Arias F: Hematologic changes associated with pregnancy. *Clin Obstet Gynecol* 1979; 22:785.

3 Factor Deficiency Anemia

IRON METABOLISM

Hemoglobin contains about 70% of the body iron, and storage iron accounts for most of the remainder. One gram of hemoglobin contains 3.4 mg of iron, and 1 ml of packed red blood cells (RBCs) contains about 1 mg of iron. Iron intake averages about 10 mg/day, of which about 10% is absorbed. Iron loss averages about 1 mg/day in men and nonmenstruating women and about 2 mg/day in menstruating women. There is an additional iron requirement for pregnant and lactating women.

Most body iron originates from dietary iron in the ferric state, which is converted to the ferrous state after ingestion and absorbed predominantly in the duodenum and jejunum. Iron circulates in the blood coupled to a beta globulin, transferrin. Bone marrow RBC precursors utilize a portion of the available iron; about 60% of the remainder is stored within reticulum cells in bone marrow, liver, and spleen as ferritin and about 40% as hemosiderin. Iron from ongoing RBC death and hemoglobin breakdown is the primary source of iron storage material.

Approximately 50% more oral iron is absorbed if taken 45–60 minutes before food ingestion than if taken with food. Meat inhibits absorption less than dairy products or foods with high fiber content. Coffee and tea also inhibit absorption, whereas vitamin C (given with iron) enhances absorption. Iron in human milk is absorbed much more readily than that in cow's milk.

IRON DEFICIENCY

Iron deficiency may be produced in three ways: (1) iron intake not sufficient to replace normal iron losses, (2) iron not available for erythropoiesis despite adequate body iron, and (3) increased loss of body iron (blood loss) not adequately replaced by normal intake.

Acute blood loss can usually be handled without difficulty if the bleeding episode is not too prolonged and if tissue iron stores are adequate. The anemia that develops from acute bleeding is normocytic and normochromic and is not the type characteristic of chronic iron deficiency (acute changes in hematocrit are discussed elsewhere [blood volume, chapter 11]). Chronic bleeding, however, is often sufficient to exhaust body iron stores from continued attempts by the bone marrow to restore the blood hemoglobin level. If this occurs, a hypochromic-microcytic anemia eventually develops. Chronic bleeding may be in the form of slow, tiny, daily losses, intermittent losses of small to moderate size not evident clinically, or repeated, more widely spaced, larger bleeding episodes. Chronic iron deficiency may develop with normal diet but is hastened if the diet is itself borderline or deficient in iron.

Chronic iron deficiency is common among infants, usually from deficient dietary intake. The infant grows rapidly and must make hemoglobin to keep up with expanding blood volume. Most of the infant's iron comes from fetal hemoglobin present at birth. Since premature infants have a smaller birth weight on the average, they also tend to have a smaller hemoglobin mass than term infants. The premature infant is thus more likely than the term infant to develop clinical iron deficiency at age 6 months to 2 years, when the demands of rapid growth are most likely to produce iron depletion. Breast milk contains a marginally adequate iron content, but cow's milk is definitely low in available iron. Whether iron deficiency results will therefore depend on infant birth weight, the type of milk received, and the length of milk feeding before supplementation or replacement by other foods. It has been estimated that 15%–20% of infants between 9 and 12 months of age have some degree of iron deficiency and possibly up to 50% in low socioeconomic groups.

In adults, iron deficiency from inadequate diet alone more frequently is subclinical rather than severe enough to produce anemia. However, poor iron intake may potentiate the effects of iron deficiency from other etiologies, such as menstruation. In one study, about 5% of clinically healthy white female adolescents were found to have chronic iron deficiency anemia, with about 9% of others having nonanemic iron deficiency. Iron deficiency is frequent in malabsorption diseases such as sprue, which, strictly speaking, represents inability to use available dietary iron rather than a true dietary deficiency. A common etiology is pregnancy, in which iron deficiency is caused by maternal iron utilization by the fetus superimposed on previous iron deficiency due to excessive menstrual bleeding or multiple pregnancies. About 50% of chronic alcoholics and 20%–40% of patients with megaloblastic anemia are said to have some degree of iron deficiency. An interesting related condition is long-distance runner or jogger anemia, said to occur in about 40% of women active in these sports, and to be caused by a combination of iron deficiency from poor diet, gastrointestinal bleeding, hematuria, and hemolysis.

By far the most common cause of chronic iron deficiency in adolescents or adults severe enough to cause anemia is excessive blood loss. In men, this is usually from the gastrointestinal (GI) tract. In women it may be either GI or vaginal bleeding. It has been estimated that 20%–50% of women in the menstrual age group have some degree of iron deficiency; menstrual loss is frequently aggravated by poor diet. Therefore, careful inquiry about the frequency, duration, and quantity of menstrual bleeding is essential in treating women. An estimate of quantity may be made from the number of menstrual pads used. Gastrointestinal bleeding is most frequently due to peptic ulcer in men and women below age 40. After age 40 GI carcinoma is more common and should always be ruled out. Hemorrhoids are sometimes the cause of chronic iron deficiency anemia, but since hemorrhoids are common it should never be assumed that the anemia is due only to hemorrhoids.

If excessive vaginal bleeding is suspected, a careful vaginal/uterine examination with a Papanicolaou smear should be done. If necessary, a gynecologist should be consulted. For possible GI bleeding an occult blood test on a stool sample should be ordered on at least three separate days. However, one or more negative stool guaiac results do not rule out GI cancer or peptic ulcer, since these lesions may bleed intermittently (see chapter 25). If a patient is over age 40 and stool guaiac results are negative, many gastroenterologists recommend a barium enema and possibly sigmoidoscopy or colonoscopy. If the barium enema or endoscopy result is negative, and no other cause for the iron deficiency anemia can be demonstrated, they recommend repeating the barium enema in 3–4 months in case a lesion was missed. Lower GI tract studies are particularly important for detection of carcinoma because colon carcinoma has an excellent cure rate if discovered in its early stages. Gastric carcinoma, on the other hand, has a very poor cure rate by the time it becomes demonstrable. The detection of peptic ulcer and the differential diagnosis of GI tract lesions by selection of appropriate laboratory tests are discussed in more detail in chapter 26. In addition to peptic ulcer, gastric hiatal hernia is sometimes associated with iron deficiency anemia.

LABORATORY TESTS FOR CHRONIC IRON DEFICIENCY

Several laboratory tests are commonly used to screen for or establish a diagnosis of chronic iron deficiency. The sequence in which abnormal test results appear is given in Table 3–1. In a normal adult on a normal diet made iron deficient by repeated phlebotomy (for experimental reasons), it takes about 3 months before

TABLE 3–1.
Sequence of Test Abnormalities in the Evolution of Chronic Iron Deficiency

Early preclinical changes
Negative iron balance
Decreased bone marrow hemosiderin
Decreased serum ferritin
Later preclinical changes
Increased RBC protoporphyrin levels
Increased total iron-binding capacity
Decreased serum iron
Relatively late changes
RBC microcytosis
RBC hypochromia
Anemia

significant anemia (Hb more than 2 gm/dl below normal) appears. The first laboratory indication of iron deficiency is lack of marrow iron on bone marrow aspiration. The next test to become abnormal is the serum iron level. When anemia becomes manifest, it is moderately hypochromic but only slightly microcytic; marked hypochromia and microcytosis are relatively late manifestations of iron deficiency. When the anemia is treated, results of these tests return to normal in reverse order. Even with adequate therapy it takes several months before bone marrow iron appears again.

Peripheral Blood Smear.—The peripheral blood smear in chronic iron deficiency anemia typically shows RBC hypochromia. There is also microcytosis, but lesser degrees of microcytosis are more difficult to recognize than hypochromia. Some of the peripheral blood changes may appear before actual anemia. However, examination of the peripheral blood smear cannot be depended on to detect iron deficiency, since changes suggestive of chronic iron deficiency either may not be present or may be missed. In one study the peripheral blood smear did not show typical RBC changes in as many as 50% of patients with chronic iron deficiency anemia. This happens more often in patients with mild anemia. Even if hypochromia is present, iron deficiency must be differentiated from other conditions (see Table 3–1) that also may produce hypochromic RBC. In severe anemia there is anisocytosis and poikilocytosis in addition to microcytosis and rather marked hypochromia. The anisocytosis means that the RBCs may not all be microcytes. The microcytes of iron deficiency must be differentiated from spherocytes; such distinction is usually not difficult, since in chronic iron deficiency even the microcytes are hypochromic. Bone marrow aspiration reveals mild erythroid hyperplasia and no marrow iron (using iron stains).

Red Blood Cell Indices.—The mean corpuscular volume (MCV) typically is decreased below reference range lower limits, and the RBC distribution width (RDW) is increased by the time iron deficiency anemia has appeared. However, the few studies available indicate that the MCV is normal in about 30%–35% (range 24%–55%) of patients. The mean corpuscular hemoglobin (MCH) is normal in about 20%. There is considerable disagreement on MCH concentration (MCHC) values, with a decrease reported in 21%–81% of patients. Although various factors could have biased these studies, it is probable that chronic iron deficiency will not be detected by RBC indices in a significant number of patients with chronic iron deficiency anemia. Some of these patients, but not all, may have other superimposed conditions that mask the morphologic effects of iron deficiency. Even if the MCV is decreased, iron deficiency must be differentiated from various other conditions (see Table 2–2) that also produce microcytosis.

Reticulocytes.—The reticulocyte count is normal in uncomplicated chronic iron deficiency anemia. Superimposed acute blood loss or other factors, such as adequate iron in the hospital diet, may cause reticulocytosis. For a short time following recent (acute) hemorrhage, the Wintrobe MCV may be normal or even increased due to the reticulocytosis. The reticulocyte response to iron therapy (3%–7%) is somewhat less than that seen with treatment of megaloblastic anemia.

Serum Iron.—Serum iron levels fall sometime between depletion of tissue iron stores and development of anemia. Therefore, the serum iron value should be a sensitive indicator of possible iron deficiency by the time a patient has anemia. Unfortunately, about 10%–15% (literature range 0%–32%) of serum iron measurements in patients with iron deficiency anemia remain in the lower half of the reference range.

Conditions That Affect Serum Iron Levels.—The first is transferrin levels. Serum iron measurement predominantly reflects iron bound to serum proteins. Under usual conditions, most iron is bound to transferrin. Normally, transferrin is about one third saturated. Therefore, serum iron values depend not only on the quantity of iron available but also on the amount of transferrin present. (If transferrin is increased, the serum iron measurement reflects not only the quantity of iron bound to the normal amount of protein but also the iron bound to the additional protein. The opposite happens when transferrin is decreased.) Second is the time of day. There is a 20%–30% diurnal variation in serum iron levels (literature range 2%–69%); the time of day at which the peak value appears is most often in the morning, but it may occur in the early or late afternoon. In one study the peak was found at 8 A.M. in 72% of 25 patients and at 4 P.M. in 28%. Therefore, in some patients the time of day that the specimen is obtained can materially influence whether a result is interpreted as mildly decreased or still within the lower reference range. Third, it has also been found that serum iron displays considerable day-to-day variation among individuals, with changes averaging 20%–30% but in some cases varying over 100%. Finally, in some cases there may be some degree of iron contamination of laboratory materials.

Serum Iron Decrease in Various Conditions.—Serum iron levels may be decreased in other conditions besides iron deficiency; the most frequent is probably the anemia associated with severe chronic disease such as the rheumatoid-collagen diseases, extensive malignancy, uremia, cirrhosis, and severe chronic infection (Table 3–2). There is usually a slight increase in serum iron levels in the first trimester of pregnancy, since increased estrogens tend to increase transferrin. However, by the third trimester the effect of estrogens is reversed, partially by hemodilution but also from utilization of maternal iron by the fetus. This leads to a decrease in serum iron in the third trimester. Severe stress (surgery, infection, myocardial or cerebral infarction) frequently produces a considerable decrease in serum iron (in one study by an average of 65% with a range of 38%–93%), which begins within 24 hours of the onset of the stress (sometimes as early as 4–6 hours). Its nadir occurs between 24 and 48 hours and recovery begins toward baseline about 6–7 days after the original decrease.

Serum Iron Increase.—Serum iron levels may be increased in hemolytic anemia, iron overload conditions, estrogen therapy (due to an increase in transferrin), acute hepatitis, and parenteral iron therapy. The effects of intramuscular iron-dextran (Imferon) administration persist for several weeks. The serum iron level is normal or increased in thalassemia minor without coexisting iron deficiency.

Serum Iron in Megaloblastic Anemia.—When megaloblastic anemia is treated, the serum iron level temporarily falls due to marked utilization of previously unused available iron. On the other hand, a significant minority of patients with megaloblastic anemia (20%–40%) have coexisting iron deficiency that eventually will be unmasked by correction of the folate or B12 deficiency. Since megaloblastic anemia can interfere with interpretation of tests for iron deficiency, it has been recommended that follow-up studies be done 1–3 months after the beginning of folate or B12 therapy to rule out iron deficiency.

Serum Total Iron-Binding Capacity.—Serum total iron-binding capacity (TIBC) is an approximate estimate of serum transferrin. Assay is usually performed by adding an excess of iron to serum to saturate serum transferrin, removing all iron not bound to protein, and then measuring the serum iron (which is as-

TABLE 3–2.
Hypochromic Anemias

Common	Less Common
Chronic iron deficiency	*Lead poisoning*
Chronic diseases	*Sideroachrestic anemias*
Chronic infection	
Chronic alcoholism	
Chronic noninfective inflammatory conditions	
Uremia	
Malignancy	
Rheumatoid-collagen diseases	
Chronic liver disease	
Protein malnutrition	
Thalassemias	

sumed to be mostly bound to transferrin under these conditions). Since transferrin is not the only protein that can bind iron, the TIBC is not an exact measurement of transferrin and tends to be even less representative in cases of iron overload and certain other conditions.

Serum TIBC is increased in uncomplicated chronic iron deficiency, most studies indicating abnormality at the same time as a decrease in serum iron levels or even before. Unfortunately, the TIBC is not elevated above reference limits in 30%–40% (29%–68%) of patients with chronic iron deficiency anemia. In the best-known study published, 69% of iron deficiency anemia patients with low serum iron levels had an elevated TIBC, 11% had a TIBC within reference limits, and an additional 21% had decreased TIBC values. Transferrin is a "negative" acute-phase reaction protein and decreases both with various acute diseases and with severe chronic diseases (the same chronic diseases that decrease serum iron levels). Decrease in transferrin depresses TIBC to low or low-normal levels. Hypoproteinemia and iron overload conditions are also associated with a decreased TIBC. Unfortunately, conditions that decrease TIBC can mask the TIBC elevation of coexisting chronic iron deficiency. Some conditions increase transferrin levels and therefore increase TIBC; these include pregnancy, estrogen therapy, alcoholism, and acute hepatitis.

Transferrin Saturation.—The textbook pattern of iron tests in chronic iron deficiency shows a decrease in serum iron levels and an increase in TIBC. This will increase the unsaturated binding capacity of transferrin and decrease the percent of transferrin that is bound to iron (percent transferrin saturation, or %TS). A %TS of 15% or less is the classic finding in chronic iron deficiency anemia. The %TS is said to be a more sensitive screening test for chronic iron deficiency than either serum iron levels or the TIBC, since a decreased serum iron level that still remains in the lower end of the reference range plus a TIBC still in the upper end of the TIBC reference range may produce a %TS below 15%. A decrease in %TS is also found in many patients with anemia of chronic disease, so that decreased %TS is not specific for iron deficiency. Also, about 15% (10%–34%) of patients with iron deficiency have a %TS greater than 15%, especially in the early stages or when iron deficiency is superimposed on other conditions. The %TS is increased in hemolytic or megaloblastic anemia, sideroblastic anemia, and iron overload states and is normal or increased in thalassemia minor (Table 3–3; a more complete list of conditions that affect TIBC and %TS is included in Table 36–4).

TABLE 3–3.

Serum Iron and Total Iron-Binding Capacity Patterns

SI* ↓	TIBC ↓	Chronic diseases (see Table 3–2) Uremia
SI ↓	TIBC ↑	Chronic iron deficiency anemia Pregnancy in third trimester
SI ↑	TIBC ↓	Hemachromatosis Iron therapy overload (TIBC may be normal) Hemolytic anemia; thalassemia; lead poisoning; megaloblastic anemia; aplastic, pyridoxine deficiency, or other sideroachrestic anemias
SI ↑	TIBC ↑	Oral contraceptives Acute hepatitis (some report TIBC is low normal)

*SI, serum iron.

Serum Ferritin.—Ferritin is the major body iron-storage compound. Routine tissue or bone marrow iron stains, however, detect hemosiderin but not ferritin. Ferritin in serum can be measured by radioassay or enzyme immunoassay. A serum ferritin level decrease accompanies a decrease in tissue ferritin level, which, in turn, closely mirrors decrease of body iron stores in iron deficiency. The decrease in tissue ferritin occurs before changes in serum iron tests, changes in RBC morphology, or anemia. Except for bone marrow iron stains, serum ferritin is currently the most sensitive test available for detection of iron deficiency. The major factors that modify its efficacy as an indicator involve the technical aspects of present-day ferritin immunoassay kits, some of which have less than desirable reproducibility and accuracy at the low end of the reference range. A major reason for this is the fact that the lower edge of the reference range (20–150 ng/ml or μg/L) is not far from zero. Another problem is the extreme difficulty most laboratories have in establishing their own ferritin reference range, since there is no good way to exclude subclinical iron deficiency from the clinically "normal" population without performing bone marrow aspiration. A third problem, partially arising from inadequately validated reference ranges, is disagreement in the literature as to what cutoff level should be used to confirm or exclude iron deficiency. The majority of investigators use 12 ng/ml as the cutoff level (literature range 10–20 ng/ml). A fourth problem (discussed later) is increase in ferritin levels by various conditions that may coexist with iron deficiency.

Ferritin levels at birth are very high and are the same for boys and girls. Ferritin values decrease rapidly by age 3 months and reach their lowest point at about age 9 months. At some time during the teenage years the reference ranges for boys and girls begin to diverge somewhat, with the lower limit of the reference range for girls being approximately 10 ng/100 ml lower than that for boys. The upper limit in men tends to increase slowly until old age, whereas the upper limit in women tends to remain relatively stationary until menopause and then slowly increases. The lower limits of reference ranges for both sexes are affected only to a small degree by age. There is approximately a 10%–15% average daily variation in ferritin values in the same individual; about one half the variation is due to fluctuation in serum iron values.

Interpretation of Serum Ferritin Results.—A serum ferritin level less than 12 ng/ml is considered almost diagnostic of iron deficiency. Presumably false positive results in the literature based on bone marrow iron stains (displaying decreased serum ferritin levels with bone marrow iron present) range from 0%–4% of cases. False negative results have been reported in 2.6% of bone marrow–proven uncomplicated iron-deficient cases. However, if iron deficiency coexists with a condition that raises the serum ferritin, the ferritin value in a substantial number of patients may be higher than the cutoff value for iron deficiency. Serum ferritin level is decreased to a variable degree during pregnancy; the amount of decrease may be reduced as much as 50% if iron supplements are given.

Many conditions can elevate ferritin levels. Serum ferritin is one of a group of proteins that become elevated in response to acute inflammation, infection, or trauma; elevation begins between 24 and 48 hours, peaks in about 3 days, and lasts 5 days–5 weeks. In addition, a more sustained increase in ferritin levels may be produced by various chronic diseases (see Table 3–2), including those that decrease serum iron and serum TIBC values. Fortunately, some patients with coexisting chronic disease and iron deficiency still have decreased serum ferritin levels. Ferritin values may also be increased in some patients who have had blood transfusions, in megaloblastic anemia, and in hemolytic anemias. Ferritin is greatly increased in iron overload states such as hemochromatosis and acute iron poisoning.

The serum ferritin level has been used in chronic renal failure to monitor iron status. Because chronic disease raises serum ferritin levels, the ferritin lower limit used for this purpose (approximately 100 ng/ml) is much higher than the lower limit of reference range used for the general population.

Free Erythrocyte Protoporphyrin (Zinc Protoporphyrin).—This test is discussed in detail in chapter 20. The last step in heme synthesis occurs when the heme precursor protoporphyrin IX forms a complex with an iron atom with the help of the enzyme ferrochelatase (see Fig. 20–3). If iron is not available, or if ferrochelatase is inhibited (as occurs in lead poisoning), a zinc ion becomes complexed with protoporphyrin IX (zinc protoporphyrin; ZPP) instead of iron. When ZPP is assayed using manual biochemical techniques, the zinc ion is removed during acid extraction of RBC hemoglobin, and the metal-free substance measured is then called free erythrocyte protoporphyrin. Zinc protoporphyrin can be measured directly and quickly using one or two drops of whole blood by means of a small commercially available instrument called a hematofluorometer.

Zinc Protoporphyrin in Iron Deficiency.—Zinc protoporphyrin levels are elevated in iron deficiency and in lead poisoning. In iron deficiency, ZPP levels become elevated after several weeks of deficient iron stores and return to normal only after 2–3 months of iron therapy. In two studies, elevated ZPP levels detected 83%–94% of patients who were iron-deficient on the basis of low serum ferritin levels.

Problems With Zinc Protoporphyrin Assays.—Some hematofluorometers report ZPP per unit of whole blood; this reporting system may be affected by changes in hematocrit values. This problem is avoided with instruments that report results as a ZPP/heme ratio. Another potential difficulty is falsely decreased results due to a shift in the protoporphyrin fluorescent maximal absorption peak if the hemoglobin is not fully oxygenated. This can be avoided in several ways. More troublesome is ZPP elevation by acute or chronic infections, noninfectious inflammation, various malignancies, chronic liver disease, and moderate or severe hemolytic anemias. Therefore, ZPP levels are elevated in many of the same conditions that falsely elevate serum ferritin levels. Although ZPP is a good screening method for iron deficiency and lead poisoning, most laboratories do not own a hematofluorometer.

Bone Marrow Iron Stain.—The gold standard for chronic iron deficiency has been bone marrow aspiration or biopsy with Prussian blue chemical reaction for iron (hemosiderin). Although there is some disagreement, a clot section is generally considered more reliable for iron staining than an aspiration smear. Bone biopsy specimens must be decalcified, and some decalcifying reagents (but not others) may destroy some iron. The major problem with bone marrow aspiration has been reluctance of patients to undergo the procedure. Bone marrow aspiration may be necessary to diagnose occasional patients with hypochromic anemia without clear-cut evidence from other tests for or against iron deficiency. However, a therapeutic trial of iron might provide the same information.

DIAGNOSIS OF CHRONIC IRON DEFICIENCY

The usual signals of iron deficiency are a decreased MCV (or anemia with a low-normal MCV) or elevated RDW. Hypochromia with or without microcytosis on peripheral blood smear is also suspicious. Conditions frequently associated with chronic iron deficiency (e.g., malabsorption, megaloblastic anemia, pregnancy, infants on prolonged milk feeding) should also prompt further investigation. The major conditions to be considered are chronic iron deficiency, thalassemia minor, and anemia of chronic disease. The most frequently used differential tests are the serum iron plus TIBC (considered as one test) and the serum ferritin. Although the serum ferritin test alone may be diagnostic, the test combination is frequently ordered together to save time (since the results of the serum ferritin test may not be conclusive), to help interpret the values obtained, and to provide additional information. Low serum iron levels plus low TIBC suggests chronic disease effect (Tables 3–2 and 3–3). Low serum iron levels with high-normal or elevated TIBC suggest possible iron deficiency. If the serum iron level and %TS are both low, it is strong evidence against thalassemia minor. Laboratory tests for thalassemia minor are discussed elsewhere in more detail (chapter 5). If the serum ferritin level is low, this is diagnostic of chronic iron deficiency and excludes both thalassemia and anemia of chronic disease, unless they are coexisting with iron deficiency. If iron deficiency is superimposed on another condition, the iron deficiency can be treated first and the other condition diagnosed later. In some cases there may be a question whether chronic iron deficiency is being obscured by chronic disease elevation of the serum ferritin value. In some of these instances there may be indication for a bone marrow aspiration or a therapeutic trial of oral iron.

Since RBC indices and peripheral blood smear may appear to be normal in some patients with chronic iron deficiency, it may be rational and justifiable to perform a biochemical screening test for iron deficiency (serum iron or serum ferritin) in patients with normocytic-normochromic anemia. In fact, no single biochemical test, not even serum ferritin determination, will rule out iron deficiency simply because the test result is normal. In 42 of our patients with chronic iron deficiency anemia, 9% had an MCV of 90–100 fl and 45% overall had a normal MCV. Fifteen percent had normal serum iron levels and 65% had normal TIBC. Ten percent had a serum iron level and TIBC pattern suggestive of anemia of chronic disease (presumably coexistent with the iron deficiency). Thirty percent had a serum ferritin level greater than 15 ng/100 ml (although all but one were less than 25 ng).

VITAMIN B12 DEFICIENCY

Vitamin B12 (cyanocobalamin) is necessary for adequate DNA synthesis through its role in folic acid metabolism. Vitamin B12 transforms metabolically inactive 5-methyl-tetrahydrofolate to tetrahydrofolate, which can then be converted to an active coenzyme. Vitamin B12 also acts as a single-carbon transfer agent in certain other metabolic pathways, such as metabolism of propionic acid. Vitamin B12 is absorbed through the ileum with the aid of "intrinsic factor" produced by parietal cells in the fundus of the stomach.

Vitamin B12 deficiency may be produced in three ways. The most common cause is deficiency of intrinsic factor, leading to pernicious anemia. The second most common are malabsorption syndromes involving the ileum mucosa or B12 absorption by the ileum. Besides direct damage to ileal mucosa, various causes of vitamin B12 malabsorption include bacterial overgrowth in the intestine (blind loop syndrome), infestation by the fish tapeworm, severe pancreatic disease, and interference by certain medications (chapter 36). Finally, there is dietary B12 deficiency, which is rare and found mainly in strict vegetarians.

Vitamin B12 Assay.—Vitamin B12 deficiency can usually be proved by serum B12 assay. Therefore, a therapeutic trial of oral B12 (chapter 35) is seldom needed. In patients with severe anemia of unknown etiology it is often useful to freeze a serum specimen before blood transfusion or other therapy begins, since vitamin B12 and folic acid measurements (or other tests) may be desired later. Chloral hydrate is reported to increase B12 levels in some patients using certain assay kits but not others. Pregnancy, large doses of vitamin C, and folic acid deficiency may be associated with reduced B12 assay levels. Achlorhydria is reported to produce decreased release or utilization of vitamin B12 from food, although intestinal absorption of vitamin B12 is not affected. Vitamin B12 deficit may be accompanied by folic acid deficiency in some conditions and by chronic iron deficiency.

Vitamin B12 is transported in serum bound to several serum proteins, among which the most important are transcobalamin and "R-protein." Severe liver disease or myeloproliferative disorders with high white blood cell (WBC) counts produce elevated vitamin B12–binding protein levels and falsely raise total serum B12 values. In 1978, reports were published demonstrating that certain metabolically inactive analogues of B12 were present in serum bound to R-protein. It was found that commercial vitamin B12 assay kits contained varying amounts of R-protein in the material used to segregate patient B12 for measurement and that the B12 analogues could bind to the reagent R-protein and be included with active B12 in the measurement, thereby falsely increasing the apparent B12 value. A low vitamin B12 value could be elevated into the reference range. Most manufacturers have redesigned their B12 assay kits to eliminate the effects of R-protein. Nevertheless, case reports of patients with symptoms of B12 deficiency but normal-range serum B12 assay results continue to appear. In these cases some additional test, such as intrinsic factor antibodies or methylmalonic acid excretion (chapter 35) or a therapeutic trial with B12, may be desirable.

A decreased B12 level does not guarantee that actual B12 deficiency exists. Several investigators have reported that less than 50% of their patients with decreased serum B12 levels had proven B12 deficiency.

Megaloblastic Changes.—Deficiency of either vitamin B12 or folic acid eventually leads to development of megaloblastic anemia. Vitamin B12 deficiency may take 1–2 years for the MVC to become elevated and megaloblastic changes to appear. The RBC precursors in the marrow become slightly enlarged, and the nuclear chromatin develops a peculiar sievelike appearance, referred to as *megaloblastic change*. This affects all stages of the precursors. The bone marrow typically shows considerable erythroid hyperplasia as well as megaloblastic change. Not only RBCs are affected by folate or B12 deficiency but also WBCs and platelets. Actual anemia develops 6–18 months later (2–3 years after the original disease onset). In far-advanced megaloblastic anemia there are peripheral blood leukopenia and thrombocytopenia in addition to anemia; in early cases there may be anemia only. The bone marrow shows abnormally large metamyelocytes and band neutrophils. Macrocytes are usually present in the peripheral blood, along with considerable anisocytosis and poikilocytosis. Hypersegmented polymorphonuclear neutrophils are characteristically found in the peripheral smear, though their number may be few or the degree of hypersegmentation (five lobes or more) may be difficult to distinguish from normal variation. The reticulocyte count is normal.

Bone Marrow Examination.—The diagnosis of megaloblastic anemia is made from bone marrow aspiration. Now that B12 and folate assays are available, some physicians no longer obtain bone marrow aspiration. The major difficulty occurs if megaloblastic anemia is strongly suspected and the B12 and folate assay results are within normal limits. To be useful, a bone marrow aspiration should be performed as early as possible and definitely before blood transfusion. Blood transfusion, hospital diet, or vitamin B12 administered as part of a Schilling test may considerably reduce or eliminate diagnosable megaloblastic change from the bone marrow in as little as 24 hours' time, even though the underlying body deficiency state is not cured by the small amount of B12 and folate in blood transfusion.

Megaloblastic changes in the bone marrow are not diagnostic of folic acid or vitamin B12 deficiency. Some cytologic features of megaloblastic change ("megaloblastoid" or "incomplete megaloblastic" change) may appear whenever intense marrow erythroid hyperplasia takes place, such as occurs in severe hemolytic anemia. Similar changes may also be found in chronic myelofibrosis, in sideroblastic anemias, in myelodysplasia syndromes and Di Guglielmo's syndrome, in some patients with neoplasia, cirrhosis, and uremia, and in association with certain drugs, such as phenytoin (Dilantin), methotrexate, and alcohol (most of which affect folate metabolism).

Red Blood Cell Indices.—The MCV in megaloblastic anemia is usually elevated. However, 15%–25% of patients (0%–96%) with folic acid or B12 deficiency, more often folic acid deficiency, had an MCV in the upper half of the reference range. In some patients normal MCV was probably due to early or mild disease. In others, these findings were explained on the basis of a coexisting condition that produced microcytosis (most commonly chronic iron deficiency, thalassemia minor, and anemia of infection, and less commonly malnutrition. In one study, 21% of patients with pernicious anemia had a significant degree of iron deficiency. If chronic iron deficiency coexists, therapy for megaloblastic anemia alone may only partially (or not at all) correct the anemia but will unmask the chronic iron deficiency picture. If the iron deficiency alone is treated, the megaloblastic defect is unmasked (unless it is a deficiency that is inadvertently treated by hospital diet or vitamins).

The MCV is less likely to be elevated in B12 deficiency without anemia. In one study, only 4% of nonanemic patients with decreased serum B12 during one time period had elevated MCV. On the other hand, the MCV may become elevated before there is hemoglobin decrease to the level of anemia; therefore, an elevated MCV, with or without anemia, should not be ignored.

Serum Lactic Dehydrogenase.—Serum lactic dehydrogenase (LDH) levels are elevated in most patients with hemolytic anemia and in 85% or more of patients with megaloblastic anemia. The electrophoretically fast-migrating LDH fraction 1 is found in RBCs, myocardial muscle cells, and renal cortex cells. Megaloblastic change induces increased destruction of RBCs within bone marrow, which is reflected by the increase in serum LDH levels. If the LDH is included in patient admission chemistry screening panels, an LDH elevation might provide a clue to the type of anemia present. In hemolytic and megaloblastic anemia, LDH isoenzyme fractionation typically displays elevated LDH fraction 1 with fraction 1 greater than fraction 2 (reversal of the LDH-1/LDH-2 ratio). However, the usefulness of serum LDH or LDH isoenzymes is limited by their nonspecificity (since LDH fraction 1 is not specific for RBCs, and other LDH isoenzymes are present in other tissues such as liver) and by the fact that the degree of LDH change is roughly proportional to the severity of anemia, so that patients with mild cases may have total LDH or fraction 1 values still within reference range.

Schilling Test.—Pernicious anemia is caused by lack of intrinsic factor produced by parietal cells of the stomach. Intrinsic factor is necessary for vitamin B12 absorption, which takes place in the terminal ileum. Patients with pernicious anemia have atrophic gastritis, which, in turn, is manifest by achlorhydria, a complete lack of free hydrochloric acid production, even when stimulated by potent agents such as betazole (Histalog) or pentagastrin. The defect in vitamin B12 absorption leads to megaloblastic anemia, which in its classic form includes pancytopenia, macrocytosis with an elevated MCV, a normal reticulocyte count, and megaloblastic bone marrow.

The definitive diagnosis of pernicious anemia is made by the Schilling test with and without intrinsic factor, as described in chapter 25. The classic Schilling test response in pernicious anemia is low absorption (positive test result) without intrinsic factor and normal absorption when intrinsic factor is added; whereas primary small bowel disease or most other malabsorption etiologies produce impaired vitamin B12 absorption both with and without intrinsic factor. Some patients with pernicious anemia are reported to have a Schilling test response typical of primary small bowel malabsorption; after treatment for 1–2 months with parenteral B12, the Schilling test results become typical of pernicious anemia.

Reticulocyte Response.—Treatment with oral vitamin B12 plus intrinsic factor evokes a reticulocyte response of 5%–15%. The same response occurs after a Schilling test due to the nonisotopic B12 given parenterally. One B12 therapeutic or Schilling test dose is sufficient to produce a reticulocyte response in patients with folic acid deficiency, and therapeutic doses of folate can produce a reticulocyte response in B12 deficiency. In addition, folate therapy can increase serum levels of B12.

Diagnosis of Vitamin B12 Deficiency.—Laboratory tests available for the diagnosis of pernicious anemia include complete blood cell count, platelet count, reticulocyte count, serum LDH level, serum B12 assay, gastric aspiration for gastric acid with stimulation, bone marrow aspiration, and the Schilling test. Of these, the hemoglobin level, WBC count, platelet count or estimate of platelets from the peripheral smear, MCV, and the reticulocyte count are extremely useful in suggesting the possibility of megaloblastic anemia. Presence of anemia is the usual stimulus for investigation, although occasionally an elevated MCV may occur when the hemoglobin level is still within reference range. A reticulocyte count is helpful in differentiating macrocytosis due to increased RBC production, as seen in hemolytic anemia (elevated reticulocyte count), from that due to megaloblastic anemia (normal reticulocyte count). Pancytopenia or a decrease in WBC count or in platelets is other evidence in favor of megaloblastosis. However, pancytopenia and a normal reticulocyte count are not diagnostic of megaloblastosis, since they may occur in other conditions such as cirrhosis with hypersplenism. An elevated serum LDH level is found in 85% or more of patients with megaloblastic anemia and, if present, adds some additional support to the diagnosis (since LDH is elevated in hemolytic anemia, a reticulocyte count is necessary to interpret the data). Once pernicious anemia is suspected, a Schilling test is the method of choice for diagnosis.

The place of gastric aspiration, bone marrow aspiration, and serum B12 assay in the diagnosis of pernicious anemia is somewhat controversial. If facilities exist to perform the Schilling test, there seems little need for gastric aspiration, which is not a popular technique with patients. If the Schilling test result is equivocal or if the test cannot be carried out satisfactorily for any reason, gastric aspiration becomes more important. Bone marrow aspiration is another unpleasant procedure for patients. Bone marrow aspiration documents the presence of megaloblastic changes and is helpful in establishing the diagnosis when other evidence fails to do so with sufficient certainty. Bone marrow aspiration can also demonstrate chronic iron deficiency, which may coexist with megaloblastic anemia. Bone marrow findings cannot differentiate vitamin B12 deficiency from folate deficiency. Serum B12 assay is another procedure that is not necessary if a Schilling test is performed. The major difficulty in deciding what to do first is that once blood transfusions are administered (especially multiple units) or a Schilling test is performed, bone marrow studies and B12 assay are no longer helpful. This could be a problem if the Schilling test is inadequate, and timing of the bone marrow aspiration and B12 assay must take this into consideration. In the case of B12 assay, one could obtain and freeze a serum specimen as soon as possible after admission in case B12 (or folate) assay is required later. Some physicians routinely obtain a serum (or RBC) folate specimen for assay before the Schilling test is started, since most megaloblastic anemias are due to folate rather than B12 deficiency.

FOLIC ACID DEFICIENCY

Folic acid (folate) is necessary for adequate synthesis of certain purines and pyrimidines, which, in turn, are precursors of cell DNA. Folate is also necessary for methionine synthesis, histadine catabolism, and metabolism of serine and glycine. Vitamin B12 converts inactive 5-methyl-tetrahydrofolate to tetrahydrofolate, which is able to transfer one-carbon groups.

Folic acid deficiency causes a megaloblastic anemia that may be indistinguishable from pernicious anemia in every laboratory test except the Schilling test without intrinsic factor. It may also be indistinguishable clinically, except that neurologic symptoms do not occur from folic acid deficiency. Folic acid therapy improves most hematologic abnormalities of pernicious anemia, even though the pernicious anemia defect is a deficiency of vitamin B12, not folic acid, but folic acid therapy alone can worsen pernicious anemia neurologic damage. Therefore, it is necessary to differentiate B12 from folic acid problems.

Causes of Folic Acid Deficiency.—The most frequent cause of folic acid deficiency is dietary deficiency. This is especially common in chronic alcoholics. However, some investigators report that alcohol can inhibit folate absorption and interfere with folate metabolism. Another important etiology is malabsorption, especially that category due to primary small bowel disease (chapter 25). Ten percent to 25% of pregnant women are reported to have some degree of folic acid deficiency, although by far the most common cause of deficiency anemia in pregnancy is iron deficiency. Folic acid deficiency in pregnancy may be due to dietary defect plus fetal demands; sometimes no good explanation is available. Uncommonly ($< 5\%$) a more severe folate deficiency state can occur in the last half of the third trimester. Some reports suggest that oral contraceptive pills can be associated with folic acid and vitamin B6 deficiency, but this is disputed by others. Drug-induced folate deficiency includes several drug categories. Certain cytotoxic medications such as methotrexate exert antitumor effect by interfering with folate metabolism. Anticonvulsant drugs, especially phenytoin (about 30% of cases, range 14%–50%) and primidone (Mysoline), frequently show macrocytosis without anemia, but in a few patients induce a macrocytic megaloblastic anemia that responds best to folic acid. Phenytoin is associated with some degree of folate deficiency in about 40% of patients (27%–76%). It should be noted that megaloblastic anemia due to diet, pregnancy, or anticonvulsant drugs shows normal Schilling test results. Sulfasalazine (Azulfidine), used in therapy of ulcerative colitis, is also sometimes associated with macrocytosis due to folic acid deficiency. Colchicine, para-aminosalicylic acid (PAS), and neomycin interfere with folate absorption in some patients.

Serum Folate Assay.—Folic acid deficiency can be proved by serum folic acid measurement. If the test is done by the original microbiologic assay system, any antibiotic therapy must cease for a full week before the serum is drawn. Radioimmunoassay (RIA) is less complicated than bacterial methods and is not affected by antibiotics; therefore, RIA has made folate measurement more practical. Unfortunately, because serum folate measurement is not ordered frequently, smaller laboratories will probably not do the test for economic reasons. Serum folate levels fall below normal limits 3–4 weeks after dietary or absorption-induced deficiency begins. Tissue folate levels (measured by RBC folate assay) become abnormal about 3 months later than serum folate and also return to normal after therapy somewhat later than serum folate. Anemia may not develop until 5 months after onset of deficiency in folate. In some patients with folate deficiency from deficient diet, a few meals with adequate folic acid may elevate serum folate values into the folate reference range, but RBC folate levels may still be low. My personal experience, as well as that of some others, indicates that RBC folate levels are more frequently low than serum folate levels in patients with suspected folate deficiency. Another problem with serum folate is a decreased level sometimes found in patients with severe liver or kidney disease. However, the RBC folate method also has its difficulties. Some manufacturers have kits that permit B12 and folate assay to be performed simultaneously on the same serum specimen (thus saving time and money), whereas RBC folate assay requires a different specimen and different processing than does serum B12 assay. Another problem is that B12 deficiency interferes with incorporation of folate into RBC. Therefore, B12 deficiency without folate deficiency can produce low RBC folate levels even though the serum folate level is normal; the combination of low serum B12 and low RBC folate levels might be misinterpreted as the combined B12 and folate deficiency seen in malabsorption.

The therapeutic trial and certain other tests are discussed in chapter 35.

PYRIDOXINE

Pyridoxine (vitamin B6) is necessary for synthesis of δ-aminolevulinic acid, a precursor of heme. Pyridoxine-deficient patients develop anemia with microcytic-hypochromic RBCs that can simulate chronic iron deficiency. Both hereditary and acquired (secondary) forms exist. The hereditary form is rare and the acquired form is uncommon, with the most frequently mentioned secondary type being due to tuberculin therapy with isoniazid (INH).

Sideroblastic Anemias.—Pyridoxine deficiency anemia is included in the sideroblastic anemias. These conditions by definition have conversion of at least 20% of all bone marrow nucleated RBC to ringed sideroblasts. Ring sideroblasts are normoblasts with abnormal numbers of iron-stainable cytoplasmic granules that appear to form a ring around the nucleus when stained with iron stains. The sideroblastic anemia group includes the rare hereditary form that frequently responds to pyridoxine and a secondary or acquired category that includes various conditions that may be associated with sideroblastic marrows (Table 3–4). Of these, the most likely to have sideroblastic marrows are alcoholism, thalassemia, and some of the myelodysplastic syndromes. Hematologically, the sideroblastic anemias are characterized by hypochromic RBCs, sometimes predominate and sometimes coexisting with a minority or majority population of nonhypochromic RBC ("dimorphic" RBC population). If the hypochromic microcytic RBC are predominate, the MCV may be decreased. There typically is an elevated serum iron level with increased saturation of iron-binding capacity.

Additional tests relevant to factor deficiency anemia are described in chapter 35.

TABLE 3–4.
Sideroblastic Anemias*

Hereditary (sideroachrestic)
Acquired
Idiopathic
Alcoholism (most common etiology)
Lead poisoning
Drug induced (isoniazid, cycloserine, chloramphenicol)
Some patients with various diseases
Thalassemia
Other hemolytic anemias
Megaloblastic anemia
Rheumatoid-collagen
Myeloproliferative and myelodysplastic disorders
Lymphomas/carcinomas/myeloma
Infection
Uremia
Hypothyroidism or hyperthyroidism

*Marrow sideroblasts more than 20% of nucleated RBC.

BIBLIOGRAPHY

Lindenbaum J, et al: New assays for cobalamin deficiency. *Lab Mgmt* 1988; 26:44.

Piomelli S: The diagnostic utility of measurements of erythrocyte porphyrins. *Hematol Oncol Clin North Am* 1987; 1:419.

Thompson WG, Babitz L, Cassino C, et al: Evaluation of current criteria used to measure vitamin B_{12} levels. *Am J Med* 1987; 82:291.

Liu PI, Lim JY: Sideroblastic anemia. *JAMA* 1987; 257:2814.

Carmel R, et al: Iron deficiency occurs frequently in patients with pernicious anemia. *JAMA* 1987; 257:1081.

Karnaze DS, Carmel R: Low serum cobalamin levels in primary degenerative dementia. *Arch Intern Med* [illegible].

Magnus EM: Cobalamin and unsaturated transcobalamin values in pernicious anemia: relation to treatment. *Scand J Haematol* 1986; 36:457.

Cooper BA, et al: Recognition of deficiency of vitamin B12 using measurement of serum concentration. *J Lab Clin Med* 1986; 107:447.

Hitzhusen JC, Taplin ME, Stephenson WP, et al: Vitamin B_{12} levels and age. *Am J Clin Pathol* 1986; 85:32.

Witte DA, et al: Prediction of bone marrow iron findings from tests performed on peripheral blood. *Am J Clin Pathol* 1986; 85:202.

Witte DA: Laboratory tests to confirm or exclude iron deficiency. *Lab Med* 1985; 16:671.

Cooper BA: Megaloblastic anemia. *Drug Therapy* 1984; 14(4):65.

Jacob RA: Vitamin B12. *Clin Chem News* 1984; 10(4):8.

Slingerland DW, Cardarelli JA, Burrows BA, et al: The utility of serum gastrin levels in assessing the significance of low serum B_{12} levels. *Arch Intern Med* 1984; 144:1167.

King CE, Toskes PP: Evolution of protein-bound cobalamin malabsorption. *Arch Intern Med* 1983; 143:2219.

Fairbanks VF, Elveback LR: Tests for pernicious anemia: Serum vitamin B_{12} assay. *Mayo Clin Proc* 1983; 58:135.

Schilling RF: Vitamin B12: Assay and absorption testing. *Lab Mgmt* 1982; 20:31.

Finch CA, Huebers H.: Perspectives in iron metabolism. *N Engl J Med* 1982; 306:1520.

Halliday JW, Powell LW: Iron overload. *Semin Hematol* 1982; 19:42.

Cook JD: Clinical evaluation of iron deficiency. *Semin Hematol* 1982; 19:6.

Spivak JL: Masked megaloblastic anemia. *Arch Intern Med* 1982; 142:2111.

Berlin NI, et al: Recommended methods for the measurement of vitamin B12 absorption. *J Nucl Med* 1981; 22:1091.

Garry PJ: Ferritin test for iron disorders. *Clin Chem News* 1981; 7:18.

Pilon VA, et al: Day-to-day variation in serum ferritin concentration in healthy adults. *Clin Chem* 1981; 27:78.

Witherspoon LR: Vitamin B12: Are serum radioassay measurements reliable? *J Nucl Med* 1981; 22:474.

Fitzsimons EJ, Kaplan K: Rapid drop in serum iron concentration in myocardial infarction. *Am J Clin Pathol* 1980; 73:552.

Reeves WB, Haurani FI: Clinical applicability and usefulness of ferritin measurements. *Ann Clin Lab Sci* 1980; 10:529.

Scott JM, Weir DG: Drug-induced megaloblastic change. *Clin Haematol* 1980; 9:587.

Herbert V: The nutritional anemias. *Hosp Pract* 1980; 15:65.

Dawson DW, Chang J: Megaloblastic anaemia with normal mean cell volume. *Lancet* 1979; 1:675.

Peck TM, Arias F: Hematologic changes associated with pregnancy. *Clin Obstet Gynecol* 1979; 22:785.

4 Production-Defect Anemia

Anemia due to inadequate erythropoiesis without factor deficiency may be classified in several ways. One system is based on the mechanism involved, including (1) marrow failure to incorporate adequate supplies of hematopoietic raw materials (e.g., iron) into red blood cell (RBC) precursors, (2) failure to release mature RBCs from the marrow, or (3) destruction of RBC precursors in the marrow. From a clinical point of view, it is easier to divide production-defect anemias into two categories: those due to a hypoplastic bone marrow and those with normally cellular marrow that are associated with certain systemic diseases.

HYPOPLASTIC MARROW

Conditions that produce a hypoplastic marrow affect the bone marrow directly either by actual replacement or by toxic depression of RBC precursors. Bone marrow examination is the main diagnostic or confirmatory test.

Replacement of Marrow by Fibrosis.—This condition, commonly termed *myelofibrosis*, is usually idiopathic and leads to a clinical syndrome called *myeloid metaplasia*. The peripheral blood picture is similar in many ways to that of chronic myelogenous leukemia. Many include this condition with the myeloproliferative syndromes (see chapter 6).

Replacement of Marrow by Neoplasm.—The types of tumors most commonly metastatic to bone marrow, the laboratory abnormalities produced, and the main hematologic findings are described in chapter 32. The anemia of neoplasia is usually normocytic and normochromic. Iron deficiency anemia secondary to hemorrhage may be present if the tumor has invaded or originated from the gastrointestinal (GI) tract. Besides extensive marrow replacement *(myelophthisic anemia)*, neoplasia may produce anemia with minimal bone involvement or even without any marrow metastases; in these patients, there seems to be some sort of toxic influence on the marrow production and release mechanism. In occasional cases of widespread neoplasm, a hemolytic component (shortened RBC life span) has been demonstrated.

Multiple myeloma is a neoplasm of plasma cells that is difficult to distinguish for classification purposes from leukemia on one hand and malignant lymphoma on the other. Myeloma initially or eventually involves the bone marrow and produces a moderate normocytic-normochromic anemia. The diagnosis of multiple myeloma is covered in chapter 21. Despite proliferation of plasma cells in the bone marrow, appearance of more than an occasional plasma cell in the peripheral blood is very uncommon. Peripheral blood RBCs often display the phenomenon of rouleau formation, a piling up of RBCs like a stack of coins. This is not specific for myeloma and is most often associated with hyperglobinemia.

Aplastic Anemia.—Aplastic anemia is defined as peripheral blood pancytopenia (decrease in RBCs, white blood cells [WBCs], and platelets below population reference range) due to below-normal numbers and function of bone marrow cell precursors without cytologic marrow abnormality or marrow replacement by fibrosis or malignancy. Among the various etiologies are agents that predictably damage the bone marrow (e.g., radiation, certain chemicals such as benzene, and certain cytotoxic antitumor drugs). Another category, sometime called idiosyncratic or acquired aplastic anemia, includes medications or chemicals that ordinarily do not produce cytopenia. Effects of some medications in this group are dose-related (e.g., chloramphenicol) and in others occur completely unpredictably. A third category of aplasia appears to have some autoimmune component. This includes aplasia (usually temporary) that uncommonly occurs in association with certain viral infections (e.g., parvovirus B-19, Epstein-Barr, rubella, herpes zoster–varicella) and a permanent type rarely seen in non-A, non-B (type C) hepatitis virus infection. A fourth category, probably related to category 3, might include aplasia associated with pregnancy or thymoma (the latter most often affecting RBCs only). The aplastic "crisis" of sickle cell anemia might also fit here. Some of these temporary aplastic crises may be due to parvovirus B-19 infection. A fifth category includes congenital diseases in which aplasia appears with varying frequency, of which the best known are Fanconi's syndrome and the Diamond-Blackfan syndrome. Finally, some investigators create a more controversial category into which they place certain conditions involving bone marrow that frequently, but not always, develop into typical hematopoietic malignancies (the myelodysplastic syndromes, discussed in chapter 7). Even more controversial is the status of other hematopoietic or nonhematopoietic malignancies that affect bone marrow function without actual marrow involvement.

About 50% (in some reports, up to 70%) of aplastic anemia cases are unexplained or the cause is unproven. To make matters even more difficult, in some cases marrow aplasia may develop days or weeks after beginning treatment or exposure to the causative agent; and in some cases it may appear some time after exposure has ceased (in the case of radiation, even years later). Also, certain other conditions, such as hypersplenism, megaloblastic anemia, or marrow replacement by tumor, can simulate aplastic anemia.

A great variety of drugs and chemicals have been reported to cause idiosyncratic reactions. The effects range from pancytopenia to any combination of single or multiple blood element defects. Bone marrow aspiration usually shows a deficiency in the particular cell precursor involved, although, especially with megakaryocytes, this is not always true. Patients most often recover if they can be supported long enough, although a considerable number die of superimposed infection.

The drugs most often implicated in idiosyncratic reaction aplastic change are listed here according to blood element defect:

Pancytopenia.—Chloramphenicol (Chloromycetin), phenylbutazone (Butazolidin), indomethacin, mephenytoin (Mesantoin), gold preparations, nitrogen mustard compounds (e.g., busulfan [Myleran]) and other antileukemic drugs. In addition, chloramphenicol may produce the "gray syndrome" in premature infants and newborns.

Leukopenia.—Chlorpromazine (Thorazine), promazine (Sparine), phenylbutazone, thiouracil, antileukemic drugs, sulfonamides.

Thrombocytopenia.—Quinidine, nitrofurantoin (Furadantin), sulfonylureas, chlorothiazide.

Aplastic anemia is most often normocytic-normochromic. Reticulocyte counts are usually low (although they sometimes are slightly elevated if the patient is in a recovery phase). About one third of aplastic anemia patients have a macrocytic peripheral blood smear.

As noted, bone marrow aspiration is usually essential for diagnosis and can be used to follow any response to therapy. However, certain problems are associated with this method of diagnosis and must be taken into account. A false impression of marrow hypocellularity may be produced by hemodilution of the marrow specimen, by aspiration at a place that has unusually large amounts of fatty tissue, and by poor slide preparation technique. An occasional completely dry puncture may occur in normal persons due to considerable variability in the bone marrow distribution. Therefore, the diagnosis should never be made on the basis of a single failure to obtain marrow. Also, a bone marrow biopsy specimen, or at least a clot section (clotted marrow aspirate, processed as an ordinary histologic specimen), is more reliable than a smear for estimating cellularity. This is especially true for megakaryocytes. On the other hand, a smear is definitely more valuable for demonstrating abnormal morphology.

Both can usually be done at the same time.

Certain conditions may be associated with episodes of transient bone marrow RBC hypoplasia. These include congenital spherocytosis, sickle cell anemia, and RBC hypoplasia associated with thymoma. Aplastic pancytopenia may occur in paroxysmal nocturnal hemoglobinuria, either preceding onset of the disease or after onset as a transient episode.

Pancytopenia in children may be caused by Fanconi's anemia or Diamond-Blackfan congenital hypoplastic anemia. Fanconi's anemia is an autosomal recessive disorder characterized by pancytopenia and congenital abnormalities such as short stature, web neck, cleft lip, mental retardation, and renal anomalies. More than 10% of peripheral blood lymphocytes display chromosome abnormalities. Anemia may appear in children up to age 10 years with the disease. Diamond-Blackfan syndrome also has an autosomal recessive inheritance pattern and displays congenital anomalies, but it consists of pure RBC aplasia, and onset of anemia occurs either at birth or by age 6 months.

In children, apparent aplastic anemia or pancytopenia must be differentiated from acute leukemia.

ANEMIA ASSOCIATED WITH SYSTEMIC DISEASE

As noted in chapter 3, anemia associated with various chronic diseases is usually normocytic and either normochromic or hypochromic. The serum iron and total iron-binding capacity (TIBC) are typically both decreased. In 100 consecutive patients in our hospital who had chronic disease and red cell or iron-related biochemical abnormalities, 68 had anemia with normal MCV, decreased iron, and decreased TIBC; 7 had no anemia; 9 had normal iron levels; 6 had normal TIBC; and 7 had decreased MCV (with normal serum ferritin levels).

Chronic Renal Disease

Anemia of moderate degree is frequently found in association with uremia. Some investigators claim it is almost always present when the blood urea nitrogen (BUN) level is persistently more than twice normal, and it often appears before this level is reached. Patients with prolonged but potentially reversible azotemia (e.g., acute renal failure) often develop anemia until the kidneys recover. Transient types of azotemia usually do not produce anemia unless azotemia is prolonged or due to the underlying cause itself. The anemia of actual renal insufficiency develops regardless of the cause of the uremia.

The peripheral blood RBCs are usually normocytic-normochromic; there is often mild to moderate anisocytosis. Varying numbers of burr cells (triangular shrunken RBCs with irregular pointed projections from the surface (chapter 2) are found in some patients. In some cases there is mild hypochromia and, occasionally, some degree of microcytosis. On the other hand, mild macrocytosis may be present in a few patients.

Bone marrow usually shows normal cellularity, although in some cases there is mild RBC hypoplasia. Marrow iron is adequate. The serum iron level is usually normal, but about 20%–30% of patients have low serum iron levels even though they do not have iron deficiency. Most of these patients also have a low or low-normal TIBC typical of chronic disease anemia (chapter 3). Reticulocyte counts are usually normal; occasionally, they may be slightly elevated.

The pathophysiology involved is not well understood. The primary known abnormality is a lack of incorporation of iron into RBCs within the bone marrow. There is depression both of hemoglobin synthesis and of formation and release of mature RBCs into the peripheral blood. In 10%–15% of patients there is also decreased RBC survival in the peripheral blood, although the hemolytic aspect is usually not severe. There is, however, a rare condition known as the *hemolytic-uremic syndrome* that features a severe microangiopathic (RBC fragmentation) hemolytic anemia. Patients in the late stages of uremia may have a bleeding tendency due to coagulation defects, most commonly thrombocytopenia. Platelet function may be abnormal even with normal numbers of platelets. The effect of hemorrhage, if it occurs, is separate and additional to the anemia of chronic renal disease.

Anemia of Neoplasia

Anemia develops in 60%–90% of patients with moderate or far-advanced cancer. The anemia of neoplasia is usually normocytic with normal reticulocyte counts, unless there is hemorrhage or chronic blood loss. Cytotoxic chemotherapy is accompanied by a macrocytic mean corpuscular volume (MCV) in 30%–40% (12%–82%) of patients. A hemolytic component is present in a considerable minority of patients, but hemolysis is generally mild and is not detectable except with radioisotope RBC survival procedures. Occasionally, hemolysis may be severe, especially in patients with chronic lymphocytic leukemia and malignant lymphomas. In one series, anemia was ascribed to a combination of decreased RBC survival and decreased marrow production in 56% of patients, to blood loss in 29%, and to marrow metastases by the tumor in 13%. Thrombocytopenia may be found in certain types of leukemia and in myelophthisic anemias. Fibrinolysins appear in occasional cases of widespread malignancy, most often prostate carcinoma.

Anemia of Infection

Mild to moderate anemia is frequently associated with subacute or chronic infection. The mechanism of this anemia is not well understood, but there seems to be a decreased rate of erythropoiesis, coupled in some patients with slightly shortened RBC survival time and failure to utilize iron normally. The anemia of infection usually does not develop unless the infection lasts 1 month or more, although it may develop rapidly in patients with severe acute infection such as septicemia. Chronic infection producing anemia generally is of at least moderate severity. Infections in which anemia is likely to develop include bronchiectasis, salpingitis, abscess of visceral organs or body cavities, and severe pyelonephritis. Anemia is a common finding in subacute bacterial endocarditis and in the granulomatous diseases such as tuberculosis and sarcoidosis. The anemia is usually normocytic and normochromic, but sometimes it is hypochromic. Reticulocyte counts are usually normal, although occasionally they may be slightly increased. Bone marrow aspiration shows either normal marrow or hyperplasia of the granulocytes. The serum iron level is usually low or low-normal, and plasma TIBC is reduced (in iron deficiency anemia the TIBC is elevated).

Aplastic anemia is a rare complication of type C (non-A, non-B) hepatitis virus infection.

Rheumatoid-Collagen Disease Group

Rheumatoid-collagen diseases are frequently associated with mild to moderate normocytic anemia. In one study 40% of males and 63% of females with rheumatoid arthritis were anemic. Active disease is more likely to produce anemia. Incidence of coexistent iron deficiency ranges from 10%–30%. Reticulocytes are usually normal, and the bone marrow is unremarkable. In many patients there apparently is decreased erythropoiesis with a slightly shortened RBC survival time, but there is some disagreement regarding frequency of decreased RBC survival. About 5%–10% of patients with rheumatoid arthritis have splenomegaly, which may be associated with cytopenias.

Chronic Liver Disease

The type and frequency of anemia in liver disease vary with the type and severity of hepatic dysfunction, but anemia has been reported in up to 75% of patients. It is most frequently seen in far-advanced cirrhosis. Extensive metastatic carcinoma of the liver may produce the same effect, although it is difficult to say whether the liver involvement or the neoplasm itself is the real cause. About 30%–50% (8%–65%) of patients with anemia have macrocytosis; about one third are normocytic. Some have hypochromia due to GI blood loss. Target cells in varying numbers are a frequent finding on peripheral blood smear.

Macrocytic anemia in liver disease is most often found in severe chronic liver damage; this type of anemia is not frequent in acute liver disease, even when severe, or in chronic disease of only slight or mild extent. A small but significant percentage of hepatic macrocytic anemias are megaloblastic, usually secondary to folic acid dietary deficiency, although most are not megaloblastic and are not corrected by folic acid treatment. A peripheral blood smear may be macrocytic even when there is a normal hemoglobin or hematocrit, and sometimes even with a normal MCV.

Gastrointestinal bleeding occurs in a considerable number of cirrhotic patients; often it is very slight and intermittent. Esophageal varices are present in some. Other lesions may be demonstrated in other patients. In a considerable proportion of cases the source of bleeding cannot be located.

Hypersplenism occurs in some patients with portal vein hypertension and its resulting splenic congestion. Thrombocytopenia, usually mild, is reported to occur in up to 50% of patients with cirrhosis, and other cytopenias may sometimes develop. In severe chronic (or massive acute) liver disease, coagulation problems may result from insufficient hepatic synthesis of several blood coagulation factors.

Some liver-diseased patients have shortened RBC survival demonstrated only by using radioactive isotope studies and show no evidence of GI bleeding. There is no clinical or laboratory evidence of hemolysis otherwise. About 3%–5% develop *Zieve's syndrome*, a combination of hyperlipemia, cirrhosis, and microangiopathic hemolytic anemia. This hemolytic anemia is associated with reticulocytosis and the other classic features of hemolysis.

Unless blood loss is a factor, and excluding megaloblastic anemia, the bone marrow is unremarkable in liver disease and the reticulocyte count is usually close to normal. Not all cases of anemia associated with liver disease can be explained.

Hypothyroidism

Anemia is found in 30%–50% (21%–60%) of hypothyroid patients. About 15% (8%–20%) of the anemic patients have macrocytosis, most of the remainder having either normocytic-normochromic or normocytic-hypochromic indices. A small percentage have hypochromic-microcytic RBCs.

The hypochromic anemia of hypothyroidism responds to a combination of iron and thyroid hormone preparation. The iron deficiency component is frequently produced by excessive menstrual bleeding. In patients without demonstrable blood loss it is speculated that decreased intestinal iron absorption may occur, since thyroid hormone is known to affect intestinal carbohydrate absorption. Most of the macrocytic cases respond only to thyroid hormone. In these patients the bone marrow is not megaloblastic and is sometimes slightly hypocellular. The reticulocyte count is usually normal. Isotope studies reportedly show normal RBC survival time in most cases. Lack of thyroid hormone seems to have a direct effect on erythropoiesis, since thyroid hormone therapy cures both the myxedema and the anemia (unless there is superimposed iron deficiency). A minority of patients with macrocytic anemia have folic acid or vitamin B12 deficiency, presumably secondary to decreased intestinal absorption. Thyroid hormone is required in addition to folic acid or vitamin B12. About 5% have actual pernicious anemia, with megaloblastic bone marrow.

Comments on Chronic Disease Anemia

To conclude this discussion, it should be noted that the normocytic-normochromic anemia of systemic disease has often been called "simple chronic anemia," although the pathophysiology is far from simple. The disease categories listed in this chapter are only the most common. In many cases, the diagnosis is one of exclusion; the patient has anemia for which no definite etiology can be found, so whatever systemic disease he or she has is blamed for the anemia. Some investigators restrict the diagnosis of chronic disease anemia to those who have decreased serum iron and TIBC. Regardless, it is important to rule out treatable serious diseases. This is especially true for hypochromic anemias (in which blood loss might be occurring) and macrocytic anemias (which may be due to vitamin B12 or folic acid deficiency). A normocytic-normochromic anemia may be due to an occult underlying disease, such as malignant lymphoma or multiple myeloma.

BIBLIOGRAPHY

Glader BE: Diagnosis and management of red cell aplasia in children. *Hematol Oncol Clin North Am* 1987; 1:431.

International Agranulocytosis and Aplastic Anemia Study: Risks of agranulocytosis and aplastic anemia: A first report of their relation to drug use with special reference to analgesics. *JAMA* 1986; 256:1749.

Gordon-Smith EC: Treatment of aplastic anemias. *Hosp Pract* 1985; 20:69.

Zeldis JB, et al: Aplastic anemia and non-A, non-B hepatitis. *Am J Med* 1983; 74:64.

Casale TB: Aplastic anemia. *Postgrad Med* 1982; 71:59.

Miale JB: *Laboratory Medicine—Hematology*, ed 6. St Louis, CV Mosby Co, 1982.

Sexauer CL, Matson JR: Anemia of renal failure. *Ann Clin Lab Sci* 1981; 11:484.

Wintrobe MM, et al: *Clinical Hematology*, ed 8. Philadelphia, Lea & Febiger, 1981.

Barton JC: Clinical approach to pancytopenia. *Ala J Med Sci* 1981; 18:248.

Lipton JM, Nathan DG: Aplastic and hypoplastic anemia. *Pediatr Clin North Am* 1980; 27:217.

Buehler BA: Hematologic aberrations in metabolic diseases. *Ann Clin Lab Sci* 1980; 10:500.

Heimpel H, Heit W: Drug-induced aplastic anaemia: Clinical aspects. *Clin Haematol* 1980; 9:641.

Yunis AA, Salem Z: Drug-induced mitochondrial damage and sideroblastic change. *Clin Haematol* 1980; 9:607.

Bateman CJ: Sideroblastic anemia. *Arch Intern Med* 1980; 140:1278.

Goldstein M: The aplastic anemias. *Hosp Pract* 1980; 15:85.

Leland J, MacPherson B: Hematologic findings in cases of mammary cancer metastatic to bone marrow. *Am J Clin Pathol* 1979; 71:31.

5 Depletion Anemia

Two types of depletion anemia are possible: (1) abnormal loss of red blood cells (RBCs) from the circulation and (2) abnormal destruction of RBCs within the circulation. Red blood cell loss due to hemorrhage has been covered elsewhere (blood volume, chapter 11; iron deficiency anemia, chapter 4). Intravascular or intrasplenic RBC destruction is called *hemolytic anemia.* There are two clinical varieties of hemolytic anemia. In one type, RBC destruction is relatively slow. Although RBC survival is shortened, the only laboratory test that demonstrates this fact is radioisotope study using tagged RBCs. In the other variety, hemolysis or shortened RBC life span is sufficient to cause abnormality on one or more standard laboratory test results.

Two etiologic groups comprise most of the hemolytic anemias: those due primarily to intracorpuscular RBC defects and those due primarily to extracorpuscular agents acting on the RBCs. This provides a rational basis for classification of the hemolytic anemias, as follows.

Due Primarily to Intracorpuscular Defects

1. Hemoglobin structure abnormalities (e.g., sickle cell and Hb C disease)
2. Hemoglobin synthesis abnormalities (e.g., thalassemia)
3. RBC enzyme deficiencies (e.g., glucose-6-phosphate dehydrogenase deficiency)
4. RBC membrane abnormalities (e.g., congenital spherocytosis)

Due Primarily to Extracorpuscular Defects

1. Isoimmune antibodies (e.g., ABO transfusion reactions)
2. Autoimmune antibodies (e.g., cold agglutinins)
3. Drug-induced (e.g., α-methyldopa–induced hemolytic anemia)
4. Traumatic ("microangiopathic") (e.g., disseminated intravascular coagulation)
5. Abnormal interaction with activated complement (e.g., paroxysmal nocturnal hemoglobinuria)
6. Toxins (e.g., lead, bacterial toxins)
7. Parasites (e.g., malaria)
8. Hypersplenism

LABORATORY TESTS IN HEMOLYTIC ANEMIAS

Certain laboratory tests are extremely helpful in suggesting or demonstrating the presence of hemolytic anemia. Which tests give abnormal results, and to what degree, depends on the severity of the hemolytic process and possibly on its duration.

Reticulocyte Count.—Reticulocyte counts are nearly always elevated in moderate or severe active hemolytic anemia, with the degree of reticulocytosis having some correlation with the degree of anemia. The highest counts appear after acute hemolytic episodes. Hemolytic anemia may be subclinical, detected only by RBC survival studies, or it may be more overt but of minimal or mild intensity. In overt hemolytic anemia of mild intensity the reticulocyte count may or may not be elevated. Studies have found reticulocyte counts within reference range in 20%–25% of patients with hemolytic anemia, most often of the idiopathic autoimmune type. In one study of 35 patients with congenital spherocytosis, reticulocyte counts were normal in 8.5% of patients; and in one study of patients with thalassemia minor, reticulocyte counts were less than 3% in one half of the patients. Nevertheless, the reticulocyte count is a valuable screening test for active hemolytic anemia, and reticulocyte counts of more than 5% should suggest this diagnosis. Other conditions that give similar reticulocyte response are acute bleeding and deficiency anemias after initial treatment (sometimes the treatment may be dietary only). It usually takes 2–3 days after acute hemolysis or bleeding for the characteristic reticulocyte response to appear, and occasionally 4 or 5 days if the episode is relatively mild.

Lactic Dehydrogenase.—Total serum lactic dehydrogenase (LDH) consists of a group of enzymes (isoenzymes) that appear in varying amounts in different tissues. The electrophoretically fast-migrating fraction LDH-1 is found in RBCs, myocardial muscle fibers, and renal cortex cells. RBC hemolysis releases LDH-1, which elevates LDH-1 values and usually increases total LDH values. The LDH measurement is a fairly sensitive screening test in hemolytic disease, probably as sensitive as the reticulocyte count, although some investigators believe that LDH results are too inconsistent and unreliable in mild disease. Other conditions that increase LDH-1 levels include artifactual hemolysis from improper venipuncture technique or specimen handling, megaloblastic anemia, and acute myocardial infarction. In addition, the total LDH value may be elevated due to an increase in one of the other LDH isoenzymes, especially the liver fraction. Therefore, nonspecificity has limited the usefulness of total LDH values in the diagnosis of hemolytic anemia. The LDH-1 assay is more helpful. A normal total LDH value, however, would assist in ruling out hemolytic anemia if the degree of anemia were substantial.

Serum Haptoglobin.—Haptoglobin is an alpha-2 globulin that binds any free hemoglobin released into the blood from intravascular or extravascular RBC destruction. Haptoglobin can be estimated in terms of haptoglobin-binding capacity or measured by using antihaptoglobin antibody techniques (chapter 10). Under ordinary conditions a decreased serum haptoglobin level suggests that hemolysis has lowered available haptoglobin through binding of free hemoglobin. Total haptoglobin levels decrease within 8 hours after onset of hemolysis.

The usefulness of serum haptoglobin levels in the diagnosis of hemolytic conditions is somewhat controversial, although the haptoglobin level is generally considered to have a sensitivity equal to or better than that of the reticulocyte count. The actual sensitivity for minimal or mild hemolytic disease is not well established. There are reports that haptoglobin values may be normal in 10%–20% of cases. Serum haptoglobin levels have been used to differentiate reticulocytosis due to hemolytic anemia from reticulocytosis due to acute bleeding or iron deficiency anemia under therapy. However, some reports indicate that haptoglobin levels may be mildly decreased in occasional patients with iron deficiency anemia not known to have hemolytic anemia. Most patients with megaloblastic anemia have decreased haptoglobin levels. Haptoglobin levels also may be decreased in severe liver disease, from extravascular hematomas (due to absorption of hemoglobin into the vascular system), and with estrogen therapy. Congenital absence of haptoglobin occurs in approximately 3% of blacks and rarely in whites. Haptoglobin is one of the "acute-phase reaction" serum proteins that are increased in conditions such as severe infection, tissue destruction, acute myocardial infarction, burns, and some patients with cancer; these conditions may increase the haptoglobin level sufficiently to mask the effect of hemolytic anemia or a hemolytic episode.

Plasma Methemalbumin.—After the binding capacity of haptoglobin is exhausted, free hemoglobin combines with albumin to form a compound known as methemalbumin. This can be demonstrated with a spectroscope. The presence of methemalbumin means that intravascular hemolysis has occurred to a considerable extent. It also suggests that the episode was either continuing or relatively recent, because otherwise the haptoglobins would be replenished and would once again take over the hemoglobin removal duty from albumin.

Free Hemoglobin in Plasma or Urine.—Circulating free hemoglobin occurs when all of the plasma protein-binding capacity for free hemoglobin is exhausted, including albumin. Normally there is a small amount of free hemoglobin in the plasma, probably because some artifactual hemolysis is unavoidable in drawing blood and processing the specimen. This is less when plasma is used instead of serum. If increased amounts of free hemoglobin are found in plasma, and if artifactual hemolysis due to poor blood-drawing technique (very frequent, unfortunately) can be ruled out, a relatively severe degree of intravascular hemolysis is probable. Marked hemolysis is often accompanied by free hemoglobin in the urine (hemoglobinuria). In chronic hemolysis, the urine may contain hemosiderin, located in urothelial cells or casts.

Direct Coombs' Test.—This test is helpful when a hemolytic process is suspected or demonstrated. It detects a wide variety of both isoantibodies and autoantibodies that have attached to the patient's RBCs (see chapter 10). The indirect Coombs test is often wrongly ordered in such situations. The indirect Coombs test belongs to a set of special techniques for antibody identification and by itself is usually not helpful in most clinical situations. If antibody is demonstrated by the direct Coombs test, an antibody identification test should be requested. The laboratory will decide what techniques to use, depending on the situation.

Serum Unconjugated (Indirect-Acting) Bilirubin.—The serum unconjugated bilirubin level is often elevated in hemolysis of at least moderate degree. Slight or mild degrees of hemolysis often show no elevation. The direct-acting (conjugated) fraction is usually elevated to less than 1.2 mg/100 ml (2.05 μmol/L) and less than 30% of total bilirubin unless the patient has coexisting liver disease. Except in blood bank problems, serum bilirubin is not as helpful in diagnosis of hemolytic anemias as most of the other tests and often shows equivocal results.

Red Blood Cell Survival Studies.—Red blood cell survival can be estimated in vivo by tagging some of the patient's RBCs with a radioactive isotope, such as chromium 51, drawing blood samples daily for isotope counting, and determining how long it takes for the tagged cells to disappear from the circulation. Survival studies are most useful to demonstrate low-grade hemolytic anemias, situations in which bone marrow production is able to keep pace with RBC destruction but is not able to keep the RBC count at normal levels. Low-grade hemolysis often presents as anemia whose etiology cannot be demonstrated by the usual methods. There are, however, certain drawbacks to this procedure. If anemia is actually due to chronic occult extravascular blood loss, radioisotope-labeled RBCs will disappear from the circulation by this route and simulate decreased intravascular survival. A minor difficulty is the fact that survival data are only approximate, because certain technical aspects of isotope RBC tagging limit the accuracy of measurement.

HEMOGLOBIN STRUCTURE ABNORMALITIES

Hemoglobin consists of one heme unit (a complex of one iron atom within four protoporphyrin structures) plus one globin unit (consisting of two pairs of polypeptide chains, one pair known as *alpha* and the other pair called *beta*). The heme units are identical in each hemoglobin molecule; changes in amino acid sequence in the globin chains result in different hemoglobins.

The major hemoglobin structural abnormalities can be divided into two groups: the hemoglobinopathies, consisting of amino acid substitutions in the globin beta chain; and the unstable hemoglobins, which have focal structural abnormality in the globin chains of a different type than the hemoglobinopathies, predisposing the hemoglobin molecule to denaturation.

The Hemoglobinopathies

At birth, approximately 80% of the infant's hemoglobin is fetal-type hemoglobin (Hb F), which has a greater affinity for oxygen than the adult type. By age 6 months, all except 1%–2% is replaced by adult hemoglobin (Hb A). Persistence of large amounts of Hb F is abnormal. There are a considerable number of abnormal hemoglobins that differ structurally and biochemically, to varying degrees, from normal Hb A. The clinical syndromes produced in persons having certain of these abnormal hemoglobins are called the hemoglobinopathies. The most common abnormal hemoglobins in the Western Hemisphere are sickle hemoglobin (Hb S) and hemoglobin C (Hb C). Hemoglobin E is comparably important in Southeast Asia. All the abnormal hemoglobins are genetically transmitted, just as normal Hb A is. Therefore, since each person has two genes for each trait (e.g., hemoglobin type), one gene on one chromosome received from the mother and one gene on one chromosome received from the father, a person can be either homozygous (two genes with the trait) or heterozygous (only one of the two genes with the trait). The syndrome produced by the abnormal hemoglobin is usually much more severe in homozygous persons than in heterozygous persons. Less commonly, a gene for two different abnormal hemoglobins can be present in the same person (double heterozygosity).

Sickle Hemoglobin

Several disease states may be due to the abnormal hemoglobin gene called sickle hemoglobin (Hb S). When Hb S is present in both genes (SS), the disease produced is called *sickle cell anemia*. When Hb S is present in one gene and the other gene has normal Hb A, the disease is called *sickle trait*. Hemoglobin S is found mostly in blacks, although it may occur in populations along the northeastern Mediterranean and in India. In blacks in the United States, the incidence of sickle trait is about 8% (literature range 5%–14%) and of sickle cell anemia less than 1%. The S gene may also be found in combination with a gene for another abnormal hemoglobin, such as Hb C.

Tests to Detect Sickle Hemoglobin.—Diagnosis rests on first demonstrating the characteristic sickling phenomenon and then doing hemoglobin electrophoresis to find out if the abnormality is SS disease or some combination of another hemoglobin with the S gene. Bone marrow shows marked erythroid hyperplasia, but bone marrow aspiration is not helpful and is not indicated for diagnosis of suspected sickle cell disease.

Peripheral Blood Smear.—Sickled cells can be found on a peripheral blood smear in many patients with SS disease but rarely in sickle trait. The peripheral blood smear is much less sensitive than a sickle preparation. Other abnormal RBC shapes may be confused with sickle cells on the peripheral smear. The most common of these are ovalocytes and schistocytes (burr cells). Ovalocytes are rod-shaped RBCs that, on occasion, may be found normally in small numbers but that may also appear due to another genetically inherited abnormality, hereditary ovalocytosis. Compared with sickle cells, the ovalocytes are not usually curved and are fairly well rounded at each end, lacking the sharply pointed ends of the classic sickle cell. Schistocytes (schizocytes, chapter 2) may be found in certain severe hemolytic anemias, usually of toxic or antigen-antibody etiology. Schistocytes are RBCs in the process of destruction. They are smaller than normal RBCs and misshapen and have one or more sharp spinous processes on the surface. One variant has the form of a stubby short crescent; however, close inspection should differentiate these without difficulty from the more slender, smooth, and regular sickle cell.

Screening Tests.—When oxygen tension is lowered, Hb S becomes less soluble than normal Hb A and forms crystalline aggregates that distort the RBC into a sickle shape. A sickle preparation ("sickle cell prep") may be done in two ways. A drop of blood from a finger puncture is placed on a slide, coverslipped, and the edges are sealed with petrolatum. The characteristic sickle forms may be seen at 6 hours (or earlier) but may not appear for nearly 24 hours. A more widely used procedure is to add a reducing substance, 2% sodium metabisulfite, to the blood before coverslipping. This speeds the reaction markedly, with the preparation becoming readable in 15–60 minutes. Many laboratories have experienced difficulty with sodium metabisulfite, since it may deteriorate during storage, and occasionally the reaction is not clear-cut, especially in patients with sickle trait.

Differential Hemoglobin Solubility Tests.—A second sickle prep method involves deoxygenation of Hb S by certain chemicals such as dithionate; Hb S then becomes insoluble and precipitates in certain media. These chemical tests, sold under a variety of trade names (usually beginning with the word "sickle"), are easier to perform than the coverslip methods and have replaced the earlier coverslip methods in most laboratories. These tests are generally reliable, but there are certain drawbacks. False negative results may be obtained in patients whose hemoglobin level is less than 10 gm/100 ml (or hematocrit 30%) unless the hematocrit is adjusted by removing plasma. Reagents may deteriorate and inactivate. Dysglobulinemia (myeloma, Waldenstrom's macroglobulinemia, or cryoglobulinemia) may interfere.

Both the coverslip and chemical sickle preps may yield false negative results in infants less than 4–6 months old because Hb F is not yet completely replaced by Hb A. Neither the coverslip nor the chemical tests can differentiate between homozygous SS disease and heterozygous combinations of S with normal A Hb (sickle trait) or with another hemoglobin. These methods are positive at Hb S levels greater than 8%, but they cannot quantitate Hb S. Neither the coverslip nor the chemical tests are completely specific for Hb S, because several rare non-S hemoglobins (e.g., C-Harlem) will produce a sickle reaction with metabisulfite or dithionate. None of the tests will detect other abnormal hemoglobins that may be combined with Hb S in heterozygous patients. Thus, these tests are screening procedures, and abnormal results should be confirmed with more definitive techniques.

Immunoassay.—A third sickle screening method, recently made commercially available, is an enzyme immunoassay (JOSHUA) that is specific for Hb S and therefore is not affected by Hb F or the hematocrit level.

Definitive Diagnosis.—Hemoglobin electrophoresis produces good separation of Hb S from Hb A and C. In cord blood, sickle cell anemia (SS) infants demonstrate an Hb F plus S (FS) pattern, with Hb F comprising 60%–80% of the total. A cord blood FSA Hb mixture suggests either sickle trait or sickle thalassemia (S-thalassemia). After age 3–6 months the SS infant's electrophoretic pattern discloses 80%–90% Hb S with the remainder being Hb F. Sickle trait patients have more than 50% Hb A with the remainder Hb S (therefore more A than S), whereas S-(beta) thalassemia has 50% or more Hb S with about 25% Hb A and less than 20% Hb F (therefore more S than A and more A than F). Hemoglobin electrophoresis is most often done using cellulose acetate or agarose media at alkaline pH. Some hemoglobins migrate together on cellulose acetate or agarose under these conditions, most important, Hb C, E, and A_2 together and Hb S and D together (see Fig 36–2). In some systems, Hb A and F cannot be reliably separated. Citrate agar at a more acid pH has separation patterns in some respects similar to cellulose acetate, but Hb D, E, and G migrate with A on citrate, whereas they travel with S on cellulose acetate. Likewise, Hb C and A_2 migrate separately on citrate, whereas they migrate together on cellulose acetate. Thus, citrate agar electrophoresis can be used after cellulose acetate for additional information or as a confirmatory method. In addition, citrate agar gives a little better separation of Hb F from A in newborn cord blood, and some investigators prefer it for population screening. Isoelectric focusing electrophoresis is available in some specialized laboratories. This procedure gives very good separation of the major abnormal hemoglobins plus some of the uncommon variants. No single currently available method will identify all of the numerous hemoglobin variants that have been reported. Hemoglobin F can be identified and quantitated by the alkali denaturation procedure or by a suitable electrophoretic method.

Sickle Cell Anemia.—Homozygous sickle cell (SS) disease symptoms are not usually noted until age 6 months or later. On the other hand, a considerable number of these patients die before age 40. Anemia is moderate or severe in degree, and the patient often has slight jaundice (manifest by scleral icterus). The patients seem to adapt surprisingly well to their anemic state and, apart from easy fatigability or perhaps weakness, have few symptoms until a sickle cell "crisis" develops. The painful crisis of sickle cell disease is often due to small-vessel occlusion producing small infarcts in various organs, but in some cases the reason is unknown. Abdominal pain or bone pain are the two most common symptoms, and the pain may be extremely severe. There usually is an accompanying leukocytosis, which, if associated with abdominal pain, may suggest acute intra-abdominal surgical disease. The crisis ordinarily lasts 5–7 days. In most cases, there is no change in hemoglobin levels during the crisis. Patients may have nonpainful transient crises involving change in level of anemia. Children less than 5 years of age may have episodes of RBC splenic sequestration, frequently associated with a virus infection. There may be bone marrow aplastic crises in which marrow RBC production is sharply curtailed, also frequently associated with infection (e.g., parvovirus B-19). Uncommonly there may be crisis due to acceleration of hemolysis.

Infection, most often pneumococcal, is the greatest problem in childhood, especially in the early age group from 2 months to 2 years. Because of this, an NIH Consensus Conference (1987) recommended neonatal screening for SS disease in high-risk groups, so that affected infants can be treated with prophylactic antibiotics. After infancy, there is still some predisposition toward infection, with the best-known types being pneumococcal pneumonia and staphylococcal or *Salmonella* osteomyelitis.

Other commonly found abnormalities in sickle cell disease are chronic leg ulcers (usually over the ankles), hematuria, and a loss of urine-concentrating ability. Characteristic bone abnormalities are frequently seen on x-ray films, especially of the skull, and avascular necrosis of the femoral head is relatively common. Gallstone frequency is increased. There may be various neurologic signs and symptoms. The spleen may be palpable in a few patients early in their clinical course, but eventually it becomes smaller than normal due to repeated infarcts. The liver is palpable in occasional cases. Obstetric problems are common for both the mother and the fetus.

Hematologic Findings.—As previously mentioned, anemia in SS disease is moderate to severe. There is moderate anisocytosis. Target cells are characteristically present but constitute less than 30% of the RBCs. Sickle cells are found on peripheral blood smear in many, although not all, patients. Sometimes they are very few and take a careful search. There are usually nucleated RBCs of the orthochromic or polychromatophilic normoblast stages, most often ranging from 1–10/100 white blood cells (WBCs). Polychromatophilic RBCs are usually present. Howell-Jolly bodies appear in a moderate number of patients. The WBC count may be normal or there may be a mild leukocytosis, which sometimes may become moderate in degree. There is often a shift to the left in the WBC maturation sequence (in crisis, this becomes more pronounced), and sometimes even a few myelocytes are found. Platelets may be normal or even moderately increased.

The laboratory features of active hemolytic anemia are present, including moderate or even marked reticulocytosis.

Sickle Cell Trait.—As mentioned earlier, sickle cell trait is the heterozygous combination of one gene for Hb S with one gene for normal Hb A. There is no anemia and no clinical evidence of any disease, except in two situations: some persons with S trait develop splenic infarcts under hypoxic conditions, such as flying at high altitudes in nonpressurized airplanes; and some persons develop hematuria. On paper electrophoresis, 20%–45% of the hemoglobin is Hb S and the remainder is normal Hb A. The metabisulfite sickle preparation is usually positive. Although a few patients have been reported to have negative results, some believe that every person with Hb S will have a positive sickle preparation if it is properly done. The chemical sickle tests are perhaps slightly more reliable in the average laboratory. The peripheral blood smear rarely contains any sickle cells.

Sickle Hemoglobin–Hemoglobin C Disease.—As previously mentioned, in this disease one gene for Hb S is combined with one gene for Hb C. About 20% of patients do not have anemia and are asymptomatic. In the others a disease is produced that may be much like SS disease but is usually milder. Compared with SS disease, the anemia is usually only of mild or moderate degree, although sometimes it may be severe. Crises are less frequent; abdominal pain has been reported in 30%. Bone pain is almost as common as in SS disease but is usually much milder. Idiopathic hematuria is found in a substantial minority of cases. Chronic leg ulcers occur but are not frequent. Skull x-ray abnormalities are not frequent but may be present.

Hemoglobin SC disease differs in some other respects from SS disease. In SC disease, aseptic necrosis in the head of the femur is common; this can occur in SS disease but not as frequently. Splenomegaly is common in SC disease, with a palpable spleen in 65%–80% of the patients. Finally, target cells are more frequent on the average than in SS disease (due to the Hb C gene), although the number present varies considerably from patient to patient and cannot be used as a distinguishing feature unless more than 30% of the RBCs are involved.

Nucleated RBCs are not common in the peripheral blood. Sickle cells may or may not be present on the peripheral smear; if present, they are usually few in number. White blood cell counts are usually normal except in crises or with superimposed infection.

Sickle preparations are usually positive. Hemoglobin electrophoresis establishes a definitive diagnosis.

Hemoglobin C

The C gene may be homozygous (CC), combined with normal Hb A (AC), or combined with any of the other abnormal hemoglobins (e.g., SC disease).

Hemoglobin C Disease.—Persons with Hb C disease are homozygous (CC) for the Hb C gene. The C gene is said to be present in only about 3% of blacks in the United States, so homozygous Hb C (CC) disease is not common. Episodes of abdominal and bone pain may occur but usually are not severe. Splenomegaly is generally present. The most striking feature on the peripheral blood smear is the large number of target cells, always more than 30% and often close to 90%. Diagnosis is by means of hemoglobin electrophoresis.

Hemoglobin C Trait.—Persons with Hb C trait have one Hb C gene and the normal Hb A gene. There is no anemia or any other symptom. The only abnormality is a variable number of target cells on the peripheral blood smear.

Definitive Diagnosis.—Diagnosis of Hb C is made using hemoglobin electrophoresis. As noted previously, on cellulose acetate or agar electrophoresis, Hb C migrates with Hb A_2. Hemoglobin A_2 is rarely present in quantities greater than 10% of total hemoglobin, so that hemoglobin migrating in the A_2 area in quantity greater than 10% is suspicious for Hb C.

Comments on Detection of the Hemoglobinopathies

To conclude this discussion of the hemoglobinopathies, I must make certain observations. First, a sickle screening procedure should be done on all black patients who have anemia, hematuria, abdominal pain, or arthralgias. This should be followed up with hemoglobin electrophoresis if the sickle screening procedure is positive or if peripheral blood smears show significant numbers of target cells. However, if the patient has had these studies done previously, there is no need to repeat them. Second, these patients may have other diseases superimposed on their hemoglobinopathy. For example, unexplained hematuria in a person with Hb S may be due to carcinoma and should not be blamed on the hemoglobinopathy without investigation. Likewise, when there is hypochromia and microcytosis, one should rule out chronic iron deficiency (e.g., chronic bleeding). This is especially true when the patient has sickle trait only, since this does not usually produce anemia. The leukocytosis found as part of SS disease (and to a lesser degree in SC and S-thalassemia) may mask the leukocytosis of infection. As mentioned, finding significant numbers of target cells suggests one of the hemoglobinopathies. However, target cells are often found in chronic liver disease, may be seen in any severe anemia in relatively small numbers, and are sometimes produced artifactually at the thin edge of a blood smear.

The Unstable Hemoglobins

The unstable hemoglobins are characterized by a focal amino acid mutation that permits hemoglobin denaturation under certain conditions (e.g., heat or oxidation), with the formation of Heinz bodies. There are several different abnormalities, and either the alpha or beta hemoglobin chain may be affected. Unstable hemoglobin variants are rare; the best known are Hb-Köln, Hb-Zurich, and Hb-Gun Hill. They are usually inherited as autosomal dominant traits. Depending on the hemoglobin variant, clinical and laboratory evidence of hemolytic anemia varies from normality to severe hemolytic disease. In some types that normally are subclinical, such as Hb-Köln and Hb-Zurich, hemolysis may be precipitated by infection or oxidizing medications. Laboratory diagnosis is accomplished with a Heinz body test; if the results are positive for hemolytic disease, a heat stability test or isopropanol precipitation test is called for. In those patients with acute hemolytic episodes, glucose-6-phosphate dehydrogenase (G-6-PD) deficiency may have to be differentiated. Heinz body formation is not specific for the unstable hemoglobins but may appear in patients with G-6-

PD or certain other RBC enzyme defects when hemolysis is precipitated by chemicals and in alpha or beta thalassemia trait.

HEMOGLOBIN SYNTHESIS ABNORMALITIES

Thalassemia

Strictly speaking, there is no thalassemia hemoglobin. Thalassemia comprises a complex group of genetic abnormalities in globin chain synthesis. There are three major clinical categories: thalassemia major, associated with severe and often life-threatening clinical manifestations; thalassemia minor, with mild or minimal clinical manifestations; and a combination of the thalassemia gene with a gene for another abnormal hemoglobin.

The genetic situation is much more complicated than arbitrary subdivision into the major clinical syndromes would imply.

The globin portion of normal hemoglobin (Hb A_1) is composed of two pairs of polypeptide (amino acid) chains, one pair called alpha (α) and the other beta (β). All normal hemoglobins have two alpha chains, but certain hemoglobins have polypeptide chains with amino acid sequences different from those of beta chains that replace one or both of the beta chains. Thus, Hb A_2 has two delta (δ) chains, and Hb F has two gamma (γ) chains in addition to the two alphas. All three of these hemoglobins (A_1, A_2, and F) are normally present in adult RBCs, but A_2 and F normally are present only in trace amounts. One polypeptide chain from each pair of alpha and beta chains is inherited from each parent, so that one alpha chain and one beta chain are derived from the mother and the other alpha and beta chain from the father. The thalassemia gene may involve either the alpha or the beta chain. In the great majority of cases, the beta chain is affected; genetically speaking, it would be more correct to call such a condition a beta thalassemia. If the condition is heterozygous, only one of the two beta chains is affected; this usually leaves only one beta chain (instead of two) available for Hb A_1 synthesis and yields a relative increase in Hb A_2. This produces the clinical picture of thalassemia minor. In a homozygous beta thalassemia, both of the beta chains are affected; this apparently results in marked suppression of normal Hb A_1 synthesis and leads to a compensatory increase in gamma chains; the combination of increased gamma chains with the nonaffected alpha chains produces marked elevation of Hb F. This gives the clinical syndrome of thalassemia major. It is also possible for the thalassemia genetic abnormality to affect the alpha chains. The genetics of alpha thalassemia are more complicated than those of beta thalassemia, because there are two alpha-globin gene loci on each of the two globin-controlling body chromosomes, whereas for beta-globin control there is one locus on each of the two chromosomes. In alpha thalassemia trait ("silent carrier"), one gene locus on one chromosome only is deleted or abnormal (one of the four loci). In alpha thalassemia minor, two of the four loci are affected. This may be produced either by deletion or abnormality in both loci on one of the two chromosomes (a genotype called *alpha-thalassemia-1*, more common in Asians), or by deletion of one of the two loci on each of the two chromosomes (a genotype called *alpha-thalassemia-2*, more common in Africans and those of Mediterranean descent). Hemoglobin A_1 production is mildly curtailed, but no Hb A_2 or F increase occurs because they also need alpha chains. Hemoglobin H disease results from deletion or inactivation of three of the four loci. All four globin chains of Hb H are beta chains. Hemoglobin H disease occurs mostly in Asians but occasionally is found in persons from the Mediterranean area. The most serious condition is that resulting from deletion or inactivation of all four alpha-globin gene loci; if this occurs, the hemoglobin produced is called Bart's hemoglobin, and all four globin chains are the gamma type. In most cases functional hemoglobin production is curtailed enough to be lethal in utero or neonatal life. Another abnormal hemoglobin that should be mentioned is Hb-Lepore, which is called a *fusion hemoglobin*, and which consists of two normal alpha chains and two nonalpha fusion chains, each containing the amino terminal portion of a delta chain joined to the carboxy terminal portion of a beta chain.

Thalassemia Major (Cooley's Anemia).— This globin variant is the homozygous form of beta thalassemia and consists of two alpha chains and two gamma chains. The condition generally does not become evident until substantial changeover to adult hemoglobin at about

2–3 months of age and clinically is manifest by severe hemolytic anemia and a considerable number of normoblasts in the peripheral blood. The nucleated RBCs are most often about one-third or one-half the number of WBCs but may even exceed them. There are frequent Howell-Jolly bodies and considerable numbers of polychromatophilic RBCs. The mature RBCs are usually very hypochromic, with considerable anisocytosis and poikilocytosis, and there are moderate numbers of target cells. The mean corpuscular volume (MCV) is microcytic. White blood cell counts are often mildly increased, and there may be mild granulocytic immaturity, sometimes even with myelocytes present. Platelets are normal. Skull x-ray films show abnormal patterns similar to those in sickle cell anemia but even more pronounced. Death most often occurs in childhood or adolescence.

Diagnosis.—Diagnosis is suggested by a severe anemia with very hypochromic RBCs, moderate numbers of target cells, many nucleated RBCs, and a family history of Mediterranean origin. The sickle preparation is negative. Definitive diagnosis depends on the fact that in thalassemia major, Hb F is elevated (10%–90% of the total hemoglobin, usually > 50%). Hemoglobin F has approximately the same migration rate as Hb A_1 on paper electrophoresis but may be separated by other electrophoretic techniques. In addition, Hb F is much more resistant to denaturation by alkali than is Hb A_1. This fact is utilized in the alkali denaturation test. The hemoglobin solution is added to a certain concentration of sodium hydroxide (NaOH), and after filtration the amount of hemoglobin in the filtrate (the undenatured hemoglobin) is measured and compared with the original total quantity of hemoglobin. One report cautions that if the RBCs are not washed sufficiently before the hemoglobin solution is prepared, reagents of some manufacturers may produce a false apparent increase in Hb F.

The gene producing the Mediterranean type of homozygous beta thalassemia does not synthesize any beta chains and is sometimes referred to as β°. Homozygous beta thalassemia may occur in blacks, in whom the gene is apparently slightly different because small amounts of beta chains may be produced as well as the predominant gamma chains. This gene is referred to as β^+, and the degree of anemia tends to be less severe than in the Mediterranean β° type.

Thalassemia Minor.—This clinical subgroup of the thalassemias is most frequently the heterozygous form of beta thalassemia (beta thalassemia trait). Besides a relatively high incidence (1%–10%) in Americans of Mediterranean extraction, there is an estimated frequency of 1% (0.5%–2%) in American blacks. About 75% of patients have anemia, which is usually mild; fewer than 10% of patients with anemia have hemoglobin levels less than 10 gm/100 ml. Patients with beta thalassemia trait have microcytic MCV values in a great majority of cases (87%–100%) whether or not anemia is present. The mean corpuscular hemoglobin (MCH) value is also decreased below reference range in almost all cases. Peripheral blood smears typically contain hypochromic and somewhat microcytic RBCs, usually with some target cells and frequently with some RBCs containing basophilic stippling. Nucleated RBCs are not present. The reticulocyte count is frequently elevated (50% of patients in one study had reticulocytosis > 3%).

The main laboratory abnormality in beta thalassemia trait is an increased amount of Hb A_2 (A_2 is not elevated in alpha thalassemia trait). As noted previously, A_2 is a variant of adult Hb A and is normally present in quantities up to 2.5% or 4%, depending on the method used. In beta thalassemia trait, A_2 is elevated to some degree with a maximum of approximately 10%. (If > 10% is reported using cellulose acetate electrophoresis, this suggests another Hb migrating in the A_2 area, such as Hb C.) Hemoglobin F is usually normal but can be present in quantities up to 5%. Hemoglobin A_2 cannot be identified on paper electrophoresis, and demonstration or quantitation necessitates cellulose acetate or polyacrylamide gel electrophoresis or resin column methods.

Thalassemia minor due to alpha thalassemia trait is probably more common in the United States than previously recognized. There is a relatively high incidence in persons of Southeast Asian origin and in blacks. (Limited studies have detected 6%–30% affected persons from U.S. blacks.) There is also a significant incidence in persons of Mediterranean extraction. The majority of affected persons do not exhibit any clinical symptoms or any anemia, and of the minority that do, symptoms or anemia are most often relatively mild. In one limited study of blacks in Los Angeles, the majority of affected persons had decreased MCV but only about 10% were anemic. The average MCH value was about 2 pg less than the average value for normal persons, and the average MCH concentration (MCHC) was about the same as that of normal persons. There is no current easy laboratory method to diagnose genetic alpha-globin abnormality. However, in the newborn's cord blood, Bart's hemoglobin is generally elevated (by electrophoresis) in rough proportion to the severity of the alpha thalassemia syndrome. Bart's hemoglobin thus constitutes about 25% (range 20%–40%) in Hb H disease, about 5% (range 2%–10%) in alpha thalassemia trait, and about 1%–2% in the silent carrier state. After about 4 months (range 4–6 months) of age, Bart's hemoglobin has mostly disappeared. Thereafter, globin chain synthesis studies or restriction endonuclease studies are the current methods used, but these techniques are available only in research laboratories. Hemoglobin H inclusions in RBCs can be seen using standard reticulocyte count methods, but their sensitivity is disputed (especially in alpha thalassemia trait), possibly due in part to differences in methodology. Hemoglobin H disease can be detected by appropriate hemoglobin electrophoretic techniques. Hemoglobin H disease is mostly restricted to Asians and is manifest by a chronic hemolytic anemia of moderate degree (which may, however, be mild rather than moderate). There is also an acquired form of Hb H disease, reported in some patients with myelodysplastic or myeloproliferative syndromes.

Thalassemia Minor vs. Chronic Iron Deficiency.—Thalassemia minor must sometimes be differentiated from iron deficiency anemia because of the hypochromic-microcytic status of the RBCs. Certain guidelines have been suggested to increase suspicion for thalassemia minor or to presumptively rule it out in patients with microcytic anemia. The RBC distribution width (RDW; chapter 2) is usually normal in uncomplicated thalassemia minor and elevated in chronic iron deficiency anemia. Uncomplicated thalassemia minor typically has an RBC count greater than 5 million/cu mm in spite of decreased MCV. Uncomplicated thalassemia minor very uncommonly has a hemoglobin level less than 9.0 gm/100 ml (90 g/L) and usually has a MCHC of 30% or greater (adult reference range, 33%–37% or 330–370 g/L), whereas 50% of patients with chronic iron deficiency anemia have a hemoglobin level less than 9.0 gm (90 g/L), and 50% or more have an MCHC less than 30% (300 g/L). There are also several formulas to segregate thalassemia trait from chronic iron deficiency, of which the best known is the discriminant function of England and Frazer. Unfortunately, there is enough overlap to severely limit the usefulness of these formulas for any individual patient. Serum iron is usually decreased in uncomplicated chronic iron deficiency anemia or anemia of chronic disease and is usually normal in uncomplicated beta thalassemia trait. An elevated TIBC suggests iron deficiency, and a decreased TIBC suggests chronic disease. Serum ferritin is decreased in uncomplicated chronic iron deficiency and is normal in uncomplicated beta thalassemia trait. Bone marrow iron is absent in iron deficiency and normal or increased in thalassemia trait. The word "uncomplicated" is stressed because patients with beta thalassemia trait may have concurrent chronic iron deficiency and because anemia of chronic disease may be concurrent with either condition. The anemia of chronic disease may itself be microcytic and hypochromic in about 10% of cases.

Definitive diagnosis of beta thalassemia trait involves measurement of Hb A_2, which is increased in uncomplicated beta thalassemia trait but not in chronic iron deficiency or chronic disease. However, chronic iron deficiency decreases Hb A_2 levels so that iron deficiency coexistent with beta thalassemia trait could lead to falsely normal Hb A_2 results. In one study, 15% of children with beta thalassemia minor initially displayed normal A_2 levels that became elevated after 2 months of therapy with oral iron. Conditions other than beta thalassemia that raise Hb A_2 levels include folate or B12 deficiency, increase in Hb F level, and the presence of certain abnormal hemoglobins that migrate with A_2, the particular variety of interfering hemoglobin being dependent on the A_2 assay method used.

Sickle Thalassemia.—This combination produces a condition analogous to SC disease, clinically similar in many respects to SS anemia but considerably milder. Sickle cell test results are positive. There frequently are considerable numbers of target cells. Approximately 60%–80% of the hemoglobin is Hb S. In the S-thalassemia β° (S-Thal-β°) type, most of the remaining hemoglobin is Hb F, so that the pattern resembles SS anemia. However, S-Thal-β° is clinically milder, and the peripheral smear may display RBCs that are more hypochromic than one would expect with SS disease. Also, Hb A_2 is increased. The S-thalassemia β^+ (S-Thal-β^+) pattern might be confused with the SA pattern of sickle trait. However, in sickle trait Hb A predominates rather than Hb S, so that an electrophoretic SA pattern in which more than 50% of the total Hb is Hb S suggests S-thalassemia.

Screening for Thalassemia.—Several reports indicate that a decreased MCV detected by automated hematology cell counters is a useful screening method for thalassemia as well as for chronic iron deficiency anemia. One report suggests an 85% chance of thalassemia when there is a combination of MCV of less than 75 femtoliters (fL) with a RBC count of more than 5 million/cu mm (5×10^6/L). A hemoglobin level less than 9.0 gm/100 ml (90 g/L) plus an MCHC less than 30% suggests chronic iron deficiency rather than thalassemia. As noted previously, cord blood has been used for detection of the alpha thalassemias. It is now becoming possible to screen for homozygous hemoglobinopathies and severe forms of thalassemia in utero employing DNA analysis of a chorionic villus biopsy at 8–10 weeks or amniotic fluid cells from amniocentesis at 16–18 weeks.

RED BLOOD CELL ENZYME DEFICIENCIES

These conditions are sometimes called *congenital nonspherocytic anemias*. The RBC contains many enzymes involved in various metabolic activities. Theoretically any of these may be affected by congenital or possibly by acquired dysfunction. The most frequent congenital abnormalities are associated with enzymes that participate in metabolism of glucose. After glucose is phosphorylated to glucose-6-phosphate by hexokinase, about 10% of the original molecules follow the oxidative hexose monophosphate (pentose) pathway and about 90% traverse the anaerobic Embden-Meyerhof route. The only common defect associated with clinical disease is produced by G-6-PD deficiency, which is a part of the hexose monophosphate shunt. The primary importance of this sequence is its involvement with metabolism of reduced glutathione (GSH), which is important in protecting the RBC from damage by oxidizing agents. The next most frequent abnormality, pyruvate kinase defect, a part of the Embden-Meyerhof pathway, is very uncommon, and other enzyme defects are rare. The various RBC enzyme defects (plus the unstable hemoglobins) are sometimes collectively referred to as the congenital nonspherocytic anemias.

Red blood cell enzyme defects of the hexose monophosphate shunt and others involved in glutathione metabolism are sometimes called *Heinz body anemias*. The term also includes many of the unstable hemoglobins and a few idiopathic cases. Heinz bodies are small, round, dark-staining, intraerythrocytic inclusions of varying size that are visualized only when stained by supravital stains (not ordinary Wright's or Giemsa). In most cases, the Heinz bodies must be induced by oxidizing agents before staining.

Glucose-6-Phosphate Dehydrogenase Defect

Glucose-6-phosphate dehydrogenase defect is a sex-linked genetic abnormality carried on the female (X) chromosome. To obtain full expression of its bad effects, the gene must not be opposed by a normal X chromosome. Therefore, the defect is most severe in males (XY) and in the much smaller number of females in whom both X chromosomes have the abnormal gene. Those females with only one abnormal gene (carrier females) have varying expressions of bad effect ranging from completely asymptomatic to only moderate abnormality even under a degree of stimulation which is greater than that needed to bring out the defect clinically in affected males or homozygous females.

The G-6-PD defect is found mainly in blacks and to a lesser extent in persons whose ancestors came from Mediterranean countries such as Italy or Greece. The defect centers in the key role of G-6-PD in the pentose phosphate glucose metabolic cycle of RBCs. As RBCs age, they normally are less able to utilize the pentose phosphate (oxidative) cycle, which is an important pathway for utilization of glucose, although secondary to the Embden-Meyerhof (nonoxidative) glycolysis cycle. When defective G-6-PD status is superimposed on the older erythrocyte, utilization of the pentose phosphate shunt is lost. This cycle is apparently necessary to protect the integrity of the RBCs against certain chemicals. Currently it is thought that these chemicals act as oxidants and that reduced nicotinamide-adenine dinucleotide phosphate (NADPH) from the pentose cycle is the reducing agent needed to counteract their effects. At any rate, exposure to certain chemicals in sufficient dosage results in destruction of erythrocytes with a sufficiently severe G-6-PD defect. About 11% of American black males are affected. Their defect is relatively mild, since the younger RBCs contain about 10% of normal enzyme activity, enough to resist drug-induced hemolysis. As the RBCs age they lose nearly all G-6-PD activity and are destroyed. In affected persons of Mediterranean ancestry, all RBCs regardless of age contain less than 1% G-6-PD activity.

As previously noted, susceptible persons do not have anemia before drug exposure. After a hemolytic drug is given, acute hemolysis is usually seen on the second day, but sometimes not until the third or fourth day. All the classic laboratory signs of nonspecific acute hemolysis are present. The degree of anemia produced in blacks is only moderate, because only the older cell population is destroyed. If the drug is discontinued, hemolysis stops in 48–72 hours. If the drug is continued, anemia continues at a plateau level, with only a small degree of active hemolysis taking place as the RBCs advance to the susceptible cell age. Whites have a more severe defect and therefore more intense hemolysis, which continues unabated as long as the drug is administered.

Many drugs have been reported to cause this reaction in G-6-PD-defective persons. The most common are the antimalarials, sulfa drugs, nitrofurantoin (Furadantin) family, aspirin, and certain other analgesics such as phenacetin. Hemolysis induced by various infections has been frequently reported and may also occur in uremia and diabetic acidosis.

Screening Tests for G-6-PD Deficiency.— Several different tests are available, among which are methemoglobin reduction (Brewer's test), glutathione stability, dye reduction, ascorbate test, and fluorescent spot tests. Glucose-6-phosphate dehydrogenase assay procedures can also be done. During hemolytic episodes in blacks, dye reduction and glutathione stability tend to give false normal results. Blood transfusions may temporarily invalidate all tests for G-6-PD deficiency in blacks and whites.

The same caution applies to G-6-PD that was applicable to the hemoglobinopathies. Hemolytic anemia in populations known to have a high incidence of G-6-PD defect should always raise the suspicion of its presence. However, even if a patient has the defect, this does not exclude the possibility that the actual cause of hemolysis was something else.

Other Red Blood Cell Enzyme Deficiencies

There are numerous enzymes in both the anaerobic Embden-Meyerhof glycolytic pathway and the aerobic pentose phosphate shunt. Deficiency in any of these enzymes could result in clinical abnormality. After G-6-PD deficiency, by far the most common is pyruvate kinase deficiency, accounting for 90% of those hemolytic anemias from congenital RBC enzyme defects that are not produced by G-6-PD. Actually, pyruvate kinase deficiency is uncommon, and clinical abnormality from pyruvate kinase or other glycolytic enzymes is rare. Clinical abnormality from pyruvate kinase or other Embden-Meyerhof glycolytic enzyme deficiencies is usually manifest as a Coombs-negative hemolytic anemia without the relationship to drugs or infections that is associated with G-6-PD.

RED BLOOD CELL MEMBRANE ABNORMALITIES

The major conditions in this category are congenital spherocytosis and hereditary elliptocytosis. Also included in this group are the uncommon conditions abetalipoproteinemia and the extremely rare hereditary stomatocytosis.

Congenital Spherocytosis

Congenital spherocytosis is one of the more common hereditary hemolytic anemias after the hemoglobinopathies and G-6-PD deficiency. Most patients are English or northern European. About 75% of cases manifest an autosomal dominant inheritance pattern, with about 25% apparently being sporadic.

Symptoms may develop at any time. Splenomegaly is found in approximately 50% of young children with the disease and in about 80% of older children and adults (literature range 72%–95%). About 50% develop jaundice, which is usually intermittent. Jaundice occurs in a substantial minority of patients in the first 48 hours of life but occasionally may appear after the first week. Gallstones develop in 55%–75% of patients by the time of old age and even during childhood in a few cases.

Hematologic Findings.—Some degree of ongoing hemolysis is present in more than 90% of cases. However, about 50%–60% of patients are able to compensate by continued bone marrow hyperactivity and do not manifest anemia except during crises. When anemia is present, it is usually mild or moderate, and hemoglobin values are normally more than 8 gm/100 ml. Patients who are symptomatic and thus are diagnosed during childhood tend to have more pronounced anemia than those diagnosed in adulthood. Reticulocyte counts are elevated in approximately 90% of patients, with a mean count of approximately 9%. The MCV and MCH values are within reference range in about 80% of cases; in the remaining 20% these values may be increased or decreased. The MCHC is also more often within reference range, but 20%–50% of affected persons may have an increased value, and an increased MCHC is a finding that suggests the possibility of congenital spherocytosis. Peripheral blood spherocytes are the trademark of congenital spherocytosis. The number of spherocytes varies and in 20%–25% of cases are few in number and frequently not recognized. Spherocytes are not specific for congenital spherocytosis and may be found in ABO transfusion reactions as well as in some patients with widespread malignancy, *Clostridium welchii* septicemia, severe burns, some autoimmune hemolytic anemias, and after transfusion with relatively old stored blood.

Patients with congenital spherocytosis may experience two different types of crises, which are self-limited episodes in which the anemia becomes significantly worse. The most common type is an increased degree of hemolysis (hemolytic crisis), which is frequently associated with viral infections and in which the decrease in hemoglobin level is usually not severe. The other type is the aplastic crisis, sometimes accompanied by fever and abdominal pain, lasting 6–14 days, in which bone marrow production of WBCs, RBCs, and platelets comes to a halt and during which the hemoglobin level drops to nearly one half previous values. Folic acid deficiency leading to megaloblastic anemia has also been described in congenital spherocytosis.

The spherocytes are not destroyed in the bloodstream but are sequestered, removed, and destroyed in the spleen. Splenomegaly usually is present. Splenectomy satisfactorily cures the patient's symptoms because increased marrow RBC production can then compensate for the presence of spherocytes, which have a shorter life span than normal RBCs.

Diagnosis of Congenital Spherocytosis.—The most useful diagnostic test in congenital spherocytosis is the osmotic fragility test. Red blood cells are placed in bottles containing decreasing concentrations of sodium chloride (NaCl). When the concentration becomes too dilute, normal RBCs begin to hemolyze. Spherocytes are more susceptible to hemolysis in hypotonic saline than normal RBCs, so that spherocytes begin hemolyzing at concentrations above normal range. This occurs when there are significant degrees of spherocytosis from any cause, not just congenital spherocytosis. Incidentally, target cells are resistant to hemolysis in hypotonic saline and begin to hemolyze at concentrations below those of normal RBCs. Osmotic fragility is not reliable in the newborn unless the blood is incubated at 37°C for 24 hours prior to testing. Incubation is also necessary in 20%–25% of adults, so that a normal nonincubated osmotic fragility result does not rule out congenital spherocytosis.

In the great majority of patients with congenital spherocytosis, the nonincubated or the incubated osmotic fragility tests yield clear-cut positive results. In a few cases the results are equivocal, and in rare cases they are negative. In these few cases the autohemolysis test may be helpful. Congenital spherocytosis produces a considerable increase in hemolysis under the conditions of the test, which can be corrected to a considerable degree by addition of glucose to the test media. The autohemolysis test was originally proposed as a general screening procedure for genetic hemolytic disorders, but problems with sensitivity and specificity have led some investigators to seriously question its usefulness except when osmotic fragility tests fail to diagnose a case of possible congenital spherocytosis.

Spherocytes are often confused with nonspherocytic small RBCs (microcytic RBCs). A classic spherocyte is smaller than normal RBCs, is round, and does not demonstrate the usual central clear area. (The relatively thin center associated with normal biconcave disk shape is lost as the RBC becomes a sphere.)

Hereditary Elliptocytosis (Ovalocytosis)

Hereditary elliptocytosis is found in Europeans and blacks. It is inherited as a dominant trait. Eighty percent to 90% of affected persons have mild compensated hemolysis either without anemia or with a mild anemia. Reticulocyte counts are usually slightly elevated but are not greatly increased. More than 40% of the RBCs are elliptocytes. These are oval RBCs that look like thick rods when viewed from the side. Normal persons reportedly may have up to 15% elliptocytes. There are several uncommon variants of hereditary elliptocytosis in which hemolysis is more pronounced, and moderate or severe anemia may be present; these include a variant of severe neonatal hemolytic anemia with jaundice in which anisocytosis and poikilocytosis are prominent but elliptocytosis is not. Infants with this variant slowly revert to the more usual mild elliptocytic clinical and hematologic picture by age 6–12 months. There is also a form called *hemolytic hereditary elliptocytosis with spherocytosis* in which there is mild anemia and another very similar form called *homozygous hereditary elliptocytosis* in which anemia is severe. Both variants demonstrate spherocytes as well as elliptocytes.

Abetalipoproteinemia (Bassen-Kornsweig Syndrome)

Patients with abetalipoproteinemia totally lack chylomicrons, very low-density lipoproteins, and low-density lipoproteins (chapter 21) and have only high-density lipoproteins in fasting plasma. There is associated fat malabsorption, various neuromuscular abnormalities (especially ataxia), retinitis pigmentosa, and presence of acanthocytes (chapter 2) constituting 40%–80% of the peripheral blood RBCs. There is mild to moderate anemia with mild to moderate reticulocytosis. A peripheral smear picture simulating abetalipoproteinemia may be present in Zieve's syndrome (hemolytic anemia with hypertriglyceridemia in alcoholic liver disease).

Congenital Stomatocytosis (Stomatocytic Elliptocytosis)

Congenital stomatocytosis is found in certain Pacific Ocean populations, is inherited as an autosomal recessive trait, consists clinically of mild anemia, and demonstrates slightly elliptocytic stomatocytes on peripheral smear. Stomatocytes are RBCs with the central clear area compressed to a linear rodlike shape. Stomatocytes may also be found in association with alcoholism and liver disease.

HEMOLYTIC ANEMIAS DUE TO EXTRACORPUSCULAR AGENTS

Anemias Due to Isoagglutinins (Isoantibodies)

These anemias are hemolytic reactions caused by antibodies within the various blood group systems. The classification, symptomatology, and diagnostic procedures necessary for detection of such reactions and identification of the etiology are discussed in chapter 11.

Anemias Due to Autoagglutinins (Autoantibodies)

Autoagglutinins are antibodies produced by an individual against certain of his or her own body cells. This discussion concerns autoantibodies produced against his or her own RBCs. The anemia associated with this condition has been called *autoimmune hemolytic anemia* or *acquired hemolytic anemia*.

Autoantibodies of the autoimmune hemolytic anemias form two general categories: those that react best in vitro above room temperature (37°C, warm autoantibodies) and those that react best in vitro at cold temperatures (cold autoantibodies or cold agglutinins). For each type there are two general etiologies, idiopathic and secondary to some known disease.

Warm autoantibodies are IgG antibodies usually directed against Rh antigens on the RBC membrane. Clinical disease from warm autoantibodies is more frequent than clinical abnormality from cold autoantibodies, and the idiopathic variety is twice as frequent as that secondary to known disease. Clinically, anemia due to warm-reacting autoantibodies appears at any age and may be either chronic or acute. When chronic, it is often low grade. When acute, it is often severe and fatal. The laboratory signs are those of any hemolytic anemia and depend on the degree of anemia. Thus, there are varying degrees of reticulocyte elevation. The direct Coombs test result is usually, although not always, positive. Most patients have spherocytes in peripheral blood, especially if the anemia is acute, and splenomegaly is frequent.

Cold agglutinins are IgM antibodies usually directed against the I antigen on RBC membranes. Clinical disease from cold-reacting agglutinins is seen much less frequently than hemolytic disease from warm-reacting autoantibodies. Cold agglutinin disease is seen predominantly in adults, particularly in the elderly. The most common cause of symptomatic hemolytic anemia induced by cold agglutinins is mycoplasma infection. After mycoplasma-induced disease, the idiopathic and the secondary forms occur in nearly equal incidences. Clinically, the disease is often worse in cold weather. Raynaud's phenomenon is common. Splenomegaly is not common. Laboratory abnormalities are not as marked as in the warm autoantibody type, except for a usually positive direct Coombs' test result, and the anemia tends to be less severe. The reticulocyte count is usually increased but often only slightly. Spherocytes are more often absent than present. White blood cells and platelets are usually normal unless altered by underlying disease. However, exceptions to these statements may occur, with severe hemolytic anemia present in all its manifestations. As noted in the discussion of mycoplasma pneumonia (chapter 14), cold agglutinins may occur in many normal persons but only in titers up to 1:32. In symptomatic anemia due to cold agglutinins the cold agglutinin titer is almost always more than 1:1,000.

Paroxysmal Cold Hemoglobinuria

Paroxysmal cold hemoglobinuria is a rare syndrome in which an antibody (Donath-Landsteiner antibody) of the IgG class binds to and sensitizes RBCs at cold temperatures and then produces complement-activated RBC lysis at warmer temperatures. Paroxysmal cold hemoglobinuria was originally associated with syphilis, but more cases occur idiopathically or following viral infection than from syphilis. Hemoglobinuria is produced after patient exposure to cold temperatures and may be accompanied by back or leg pain, chills, and cramps, similar to symptoms of hemolytic transfusion reaction. The IgG-specific Coombs' reagent produces positive direct Coombs' test results at cold temperatures and Coombs' reagents containing non-gamma non-IgG-specific antibody (sometimes called *broad-spectrum Coombs' reagent*) produces positive direct Coombs' test results at the usual Coombs' test temperature of 37°C. The major diagnostic procedure for paroxysmal cold hemoglobinuria is the Donath-Landsteiner test, in which the development of hemolysis in patient and normal blood is compared at cold temperature.

Secondary Acquired Autoimmune Hemolytic Anemia

The causes of acquired hemolytic anemia of the secondary type, either warm or cold variety, can be divided into three main groups. The first group in order of frequency is leukemia and lymphoma; most often chronic lymphocytic leukemia, to a lesser extent lymphocytic lymphoma, and occasionally Hodgkin's disease. The second group in order of frequency is collagen disease, notably lupus erythematosus. The third group is a miscellaneous collection of systemic diseases in which overtly hemolytic anemia rarely develops but may do so from time to time. These diseases include viral infections, severe liver disease, ovarian tumors, and carcinomatosis. It should be emphasized that in all three disease groups, anemia is a common or even frequent finding, but the anemia is usually not hemolytic, at least not of the overt or symptomatic type.

Drug-Induced Hemolytic Anemia

Drug-induced hemolytic anemia is sometimes included with the autoimmune hemolytic anemias. However, in most cases antibodies are formed primarily against the drug, and action against the RBC is secondary to presence of the drug on the RBC surface.

There are four basic mechanisms proposed, as follows:

1. Combining of the drug with antidrug antibody to form an immune complex that is adsorbed onto RBCs, often activating complement. Quinidine is the best-known drug of this type. The antiquinidine antibody is of the IgM class.

2. Binding of the drug to the RBC membrane and acting as a hapten. Penicillin (in very large doses, ≥ 10 million units/day for 7 days or more) is the major drug of this type, although abnormality develops in fewer than 3% of these cases.

3. Nonspecific coating of RBC by drug with adsorption of various proteins. The antibiotic cephalothin has been shown to act by this mechanism. A positive direct Coombs' test result is produced by antibodies against proteins adsorbed onto the cell or onto cephalothin. There is no hemolysis, however. Cephalothin may occasionally act as a hapten and in these cases may be associated with hemolytic anemia.

4. Unknown mechanism. α-Methyldopa is the predominant drug of this type and may be the most common agent associated with drug-induced hemolytic anemia. The antimethyldopa antibody is of the IgG class and usually has Rh group specificity. Besides coating of RBCs, α-methyldopa-treated patients may have circulating autoantibodies demonstrated by an indirect Coombs test, which is unusual for other drugs. Patients taking α-methyldopa may also develop a syndrome resembling systemic lupus erythematosus, with antinuclear antibodies and lupus erythematosus cells (chapter 22). Up to 25% of patients (literature range 10%–36%) develop a positive direct Coombs' test, and about 1% (literature range 0%–5%) develop hemolytic anemia. The direct Coombs' test result remains positive 1–24 months after the end of therapy.

Laboratory investigation of possible drug-induced hemolytic anemia is usually difficult for the ordinary laboratory. The procedure usually involves washing off (eluting) the antibody from the RBC, if possible, and trying to determine whether the antibody has specificity against drug-coated RBCs rather than normal RBCs.

Traumatic (Microangiopathic) Hemolytic Anemia

This category includes several diseases that produce hemolytic anemia with many schistocytes, the schistocytes being formed through some kind of trauma. Representative conditions are disseminated intravascular coagulation and thrombotic thrombocytopenic purpura (in which RBCs strike fibrin clots in small vessels), the hemolytic-uremic syndrome (thrombi in renal glomerular capillaries and small vessels), the cardiac prosthesis syndrome (in which RBCs are damaged while passing through the artificial heart valve), and hemolytic anemia associated with vascular grafts and some long-term indwelling catheters. The same type of hemolytic anemia may be found in a few patients with malignancy (most commonly gastric carcinoma), in Zieve's syndrome associated with cirrhosis, in the first few hours after extensive severe burns, and in *C. welchii* septicemia. As noted in chapter 2, schistocytes can be found in smaller numbers in other conditions. Microangiopathic hemolytic anemia is discussed in greater length in chapter 8.

Paroxysmal Nocturnal Hemoglobinuria

Patients with paroxysmal nocturnal hemoglobinuria (PNH) develop an acquired blood cell membrane defect in which RBCs, WBCs, and platelets demonstrate abnormal sensitivity to the effect of activated serum complement. This is manifest by hemolytic anemia, granulocytopenia, and thrombocytopenia. Not all patient RBCs have the same degree of abnormality, and resistance to lysis varies from relatively normal to markedly abnormal. It is often associated with aplastic anemia and is said to develop in 5%–10% of these patients without regard to the etiology of the marrow depression (with the exception that PNH is not associated with radiation marrow damage). It may appear either at the beginning of aplasia, during the aplastic period, or during recovery. About 50% of cases develop without prior evidence of aplastic marrow. It may also develop in some patients with erythroleukemia, myelofibrosis, or refractory anemia.

Red blood cells that are abnormally sensitive to complement have markedly decreased acetylcholinesterase levels, but this is not thought to be the cause of the defect in PNH.

Paroxysmal nocturnal hemoglobinuria most often affects young or middle-aged adults, with the usual age range being 10–60 years. The disease presents as hypoplastic anemia in about 25% of cases, as an episode of abdominal pain in about 10%, and with hemoglobinuria in about 50%. Clinically, there is a chronic hemolytic anemia, with crisis episodes of hemoglobinuria occurring most often at night. However, hemoglobinuria is present at disease onset only in about 50% of cases. Another 20% develop it within 1 year, and eventually it occurs in more than 90% of patients. Anemia is usually of moderate degree except during crisis, when it may be severe. A crisis is reflected by all the usual laboratory parameters of severe hemolysis, including elevated plasma hemoglobin levels. No spherocytosis or demonstrable antibodies are present. The disease gets its name because hemoglobinuric episodes turn urine collected during or just after sleep to red or brown due to large amounts of hemoglobin. Urine formed during the day is clear. Stimuli known to precipitate attacks in some patients include infections, surgery, and blood transfusion.

Laboratory Findings.—In addition to anemia, leukopenia (granulocytopenia) is present in about 50% of patients, and some degree of thrombocytopenia is present in about 70%. This is in contrast to most other hemolytic anemias, in which hemolysis usually provokes leukocytosis. The MCV is elevated in about 83%, normal in about 13%, and decreased in about 5%. The reticulocyte count is elevated in about 90%. Loss of iron in the urine (in the form of hemoglobin and hemosiderin) leads to chronic iron deficiency in some patients. For some reason the kidney in PNH is not damaged by the hemoglobin or by renal tubular cell deposition of hemosiderin.

Venous thrombosis is frequent in PNH, and patients have a considerably increased tendency toward infection (predominantly lung and urinary tract). There may be episodes of abdominal pain related to venous thrombosis.

Tests for Paroxysmal Nocturnal Hemoglobinuria.—A good screening test is a urine hemosiderin examination. However, a positive urine hemosiderin value may be obtained in many patients with chronic hemolytic anemia of various types and also may be produced by frequent blood transfusions, especially if these are given over periods of weeks or months. A much more specific test is the acid hemolysis (Ham) test. The RBCs of PNH are more susceptible to hemolysis in acid pH. Therefore, serum is acidified to a certain point that does not affect normal RBCs but will hemolyze the RBCs of PNH. Another widely used procedure is the sugar-water (sucrose hemolysis) test, which is easier to perform than the Ham test and may be more sensitive. It is based on evidence that RBCs in PNH are more susceptible to hemolysis in low ionic strength media than normal RBCs. Many laboratories screen with the sugar-water test and confirm a positive result with the Ham test. The sugar-water test is apt to produce more weak positive reactions in patients who do not have verifiable PND than does the Ham test. In my experience (also reported by others) there occasionally is discrepancy between results of the sugar-water test and the Ham test in the same patient, resulting in diagnostic problems.

Hemolytic Anemia Due to Toxins

Chemical.—Lead poisoning is the most frequent cause in this group. Ingestion of paint containing lead used to be frequent in children and still happens occasionally. Auto battery lead, gasoline fumes, and homemade whiskey distilled in lead-containing apparatus are the most common causes in adults. It takes several weeks of chronic exposure to develop symptoms unless a large dose is ingested. The anemia produced is most often mild to moderate, and the usual reason for seeking medical treatment is development of other systemic symptoms, such as convulsions from lead encephalopathy, abdominal pain, or paresthesias of hands and feet. The anemia is more often hypochromic but may be normochromic; it is usually normocytic. Basophilic stippling of RBCs is often very pronounced and is a classic diagnostic clue to this condition. Basophilic stippling may occur in any severe anemia, especially the hemolytic anemias, but when present to an unusual degree should suggest lead poisoning unless the cause is already obvious. The stippled cells are reticulocytes, which, for some unknown reason, appear in this form in these patients. However, in some patients, basophilic stippling is minimal or absent. Tests useful in lead poisoning for screening purposes or for diagnosis are discussed in chapter 34.

Other chemicals were mentioned in the discussion of G-6-PD deficiency anemia. Benzene toxicity was discussed in the section on hypoplastic bone marrow anemias. Other chemicals that often produce a hemolytic anemia if taken in sufficient dose include naphthalene, toluene, phenacetin, and distilled water given intravenously. Severe extensive burns often produce acute hemolysis to varying degrees.

Bacterial.—*Clostridium welchii* septicemia often produces a severe hemolytic anemia with spherocytes. Hemolytic anemia is rarely seen with tuberculosis. The anemia of infection is usually not overtly hemolytic, although there may be a minor hemolytic component (not demonstrable by the usual laboratory tests).

Hemolytic Anemia Due to Parasites

Among hemolytic anemias due to parasites, malaria is by far the most frequent. It must be considered in persons who have visited endemic areas and who have suggestive symptoms or no other etiology for their anemia. The diagnosis is made from peripheral blood, best obtained morning and afternoon for 3 days. Organisms within parasitized RBCs may be few and often are missed unless the laboratory is notified that malaria is suspected. A thick-drop special preparation is the method of choice for diagnosis. With heavy infection, the parasites may be identified on an ordinary (thin) peripheral blood smear. A hemolytic anemia is produced with the usual reticulocytosis and other laboratory abnormalities of hemolysis. Most patients have splenomegaly. *Bartonella* infection occurs in South America, most often in Peru. This is actually a bacterium rather than a parasite, but in many textbooks it is discussed in the parasite category. The organisms infect RBCs and cause hemolytic anemia clinically similar to malaria. *Babesiosis* is an uncommon protozoan infection of RBC similar in some respects to malaria. This condition is discussed in chapter 17.

Hypersplenism

Hypersplenism is a poorly understood entity whose main feature is an enlarged spleen associated with a deficiency in one or more blood cell elements. The most common abnormality is thrombocytopenia, but there may be a pancytopenia or any combination of anemia, leukopenia, and thrombocytopenia. Hypersplenism may be primary or, more commonly, secondary to any disease that causes splenic enlargement. However, splenic enlargement in many cases does not produce hypersplenism effects. Portal hypertension with secondary splenic congestion is the most common etiology; the usual cause is cirrhosis. If anemia is produced in hypersplenism, it is normocytic and normochromic without reticulocytosis. Bone marrow examination in hypersplenism shows either mild hyperplasia of the deficient peripheral blood element precursors or normal marrow.

Several mechanisms have been proposed to explain the various effects of hypersplenism. To date, the weight of evidence favors sequestration in the spleen. In some cases, the spleen may destroy blood cells already damaged by immunologic or congenital agents. In some cases, the action of the spleen cannot be completely explained.

BIBLIOGRAPHY

Abbondanzo SL, et al: Myelodysplastic syndrome with acquired hemoglobin H disease. *Am J Clin Pathol* 1988; 89:401.

NIH Consensus Conference: Newborn Screening for sickle cell disease and other hemoglobinopathies. *JAMA* 1987; 258:1205.

Fishleder AJ, Hoffman GC: A practical approach to the detection of hemoglobinopathies: I. *Lab Med* 1987; 18:368.

Hall FW, Lundgrin DB: Screening for alpha-thalassemia in neonates. *Am J Clin Pathol* 1987; 87:389.

Jacobs S, et al: Newborn screening for hemoglobin abnormalities. *Am J Clin Pathol* 1986; 85:713.

LeCrone CN, Detter JC: Screening for hemoglobinopathies and thalassemia. *J Med Technol* 1985; 2:389.

Hazelwood L: Isoelectric focusing of hemoglobin variants. *Clin Lab Prod* 1985; 14(3):29.

Hansen RM, et al: Failure to suspect and diagnose thalassemic syndromes. *Arch Intern Med* 1985; 145:93.

Florane RK: Hemolytic manifestations of an RBC defect. *Diagn Med* 1983; 6(3):99.

Marchand A: Immune hemolytic anemia: Test procedures and strategy. *Diagn Med* 1983; 6(2):25.

Marchand A: Immune hemolytic anemia: Classification, manifestations, and mechanisms of destruction. *Diagn Med* 1982; 5(8):51.

Choi ESK, Necheles TS: Thalassemia among Chinese-Bostonians: Usefulness of the hemoglobin H preparation. *Arch Intern Med* 1983; 143:1713.

Johnson CS, et al: Alpha-thalassemia: Prevalence and hematologic findings in American blacks. *Arch Intern Med* 1982; 142:1280.

Travis SF, Delivoria-Papadopoulos M: Red cell enzymopathies in the newborn: I. Evaluation of red cell metabolism. *Ann Clin Lab Sci* 1982; 12:89.

Fehr J: Haptoglobin and hemolytic disease. *JAMA* 1981; 245:2028.

Rossi EC, et al: Platelets and the hemolytic-uremic syndrome. *Ann Clin Lab Sci* 1981; 11:269.

Ohene-Frempong K, Schwartz E: Clinical features of thalassemia. *Pediatr Clin North Am* 1980; 27:403.

Vichinsky EP, Lubin BH: Sickle cell anemia and related hemoglobinopathies. *Pediatr Clin North Am* 1980; 27:429.

Vichinski EP, Lubin BH: Unstable hemoglobins, hemoglobins with altered oxygen affinity, and M-hemoglobins. *Pediatr Clin North Am* 1980; 27:421.

Schrieber AD: Autoimmune hemolytic anemias. *Pediatr Clin North Am* 1980; 27:253.

Sullivan DW, Glades BE: Erythrocyte enzyme disorders in children. *Pediatr Clin North Am* 1980; 27:449.

Lux SE, Wolfe LC: Inherited disorders of the red cell membrane skeleton. *Pediatr Clin North Am* 1980; 27:463.

Marchand A, et al: The predictive value of serum haptoglobin in hemolytic disease. *JAMA* 1980; 243:1909.

Forget BG: Hemolytic anemias, congenital and acquired. *Hosp Pract* 1980; 15:67.

Horwitz C: Autoimmune hemolytic anemia: 1. Warm antibody type. *Postgrad Med* 1979; 66:167.

Horwitz C: Autoimmune hemolytic anemia: 3. Cold antibody type. *Postgrad Med* 1979; 66:189.

Antman KH, et al: Microangiopathic hemolytic anemia and cancer: A review. *Medicine* (Baltimore) 1979; 58:377.

Beutler E: Red cell enzyme defects as nondiseases and as diseases. *Blood* 1979; 54:1.

Morrison JC: Hemoglobinopathies and pregnancy. *Clin Obstet Gynecol* 1979; 22:819.

6 White Blood Cells

White blood cells (WBCs, leukocytes) form the first line of defense of the body against invading microorganisms. Neutrophils and monocytes respond by phagocytosis; lymphocytes and plasma cells apparently produce antibodies. In addition to a nonspecific response to bacterial or viral infection, there are alterations in the normal leukocyte blood picture that may provide diagnostic clues to specific diseases, both benign and malignant. Nonneoplastic leukocyte alterations may be quantitative, qualitative, or both; qualitatively, leukocytes may demonstrate an increased degree of immaturity, morphologic alteration in cellular structure, or the increased production of less common types of WBCs.

WBC MATURATION SEQUENCE

Normal WBC maturation sequence begins with the blast form, derived from hematopoietic stem cells that, in turn, are thought to be derived from tissue reticulum cells (Table 6–1). In the myelocytic (granulocytic or neutrophilic) series, the blast is characterized by a large nucleus with delicate very uniform-appearing light-staining chromatin and with one or more nucleoli. Typically, a blast has relatively scanty basophilic cytoplasm without granules, but the French-American-British (FAB) group (chapter 7) describes a category of blasts with cytoplasm that may contain a few "azurophilic" granules. Next in sequence is the progranulocyte (promyelocyte), which is similar to the blast but has a variable number of cytoplasmic granules. The promyelocyte gives rise to the myelocyte. Myelocyte nuclear chromatin is more condensed, there is no nucleolus, and the nucleus itself is round or oval, sometimes with a slight flattening along one side. The cytoplasm is mildly basophilic and is granular to varying degrees, although sometimes granules are absent. Often there is a small, localized, pale or clear area next to the flattened portion (if present) of the nucleus, called the *myeloid spot*. Next, the nucleus begins to indent; when it does, the cell is called a *metamyelocyte* (juvenile). As the metamyelocyte continues to mature, the nucleus becomes more and more indented. The nuclear chromatin becomes more and more condensed, clumped, and darkly stained, and the cytoplasm becomes progressively less basophilic. The entire cell size becomes somewhat smaller, with the nucleus taking up increasingly less space. Finally, the band (stab) neutrophil stage is reached. There is some disagreement as to what constitutes a band as opposed to a metamyelocyte or band as opposed to an early mature polymorphonuclear leukocyte. Basically, a band is distinguished from a late metamyelocyte when the nucleus has indented more than one half its diameter and has formed a curved rod structure that is roughly the same thickness throughout. As the band matures, nuclear indentation continues and may also occur in other areas of the nucleus. When at least one area of nuclear constriction becomes a thin wire, the cell has reached the final stage of maturity, called the *polymorphonuclear* (poly) or *segmented neutrophil*. The nucleus has segmented into two or more lobes, at least one of which is connected only by a threadlike filament to the next. The nuclear chromatin is dense and clumped. The cytoplasm is a very slightly eosinophilic color, or at least there is no basophilia. There usually are small irregular granules, which often are indistinct.

In some cases there may be a problem dif-

TABLE 6–1.
Terminology of Blood Cells

Series	Classic Terminology	Synonyms
Granulocytic	Myeloblast	
	Promyelocyte	Progranulocyte
	Myelocyte	
	Metamyelocyte	Juvenile cells
	Band granulocyte	Stab cells
	Segmented granulocyte	Polymorphonuclear cells
	Hypersegmented granulocyte	
Erythroid	Pronormoblast	Rubriblast
	Basophilic normoblast	Prorubricyte
	Polychromatophilic normoblast	Rubricyte
	Orthochromic normoblast	Metarubricyte
	Reticulocyte	
	Erythrocyte	
Lymphocytic	Lymphoblast	
	Prolymphocyte	
	Lymphocyte	
Plasmocytic	Plasmablast	
	Proplasmocyte	
	Plasmocyte	Plasma cell
Monocytic	Monoblast	
	Promonocyte	
	Monocyte	

ferentiating bands from segmented neutrophils when a bandlike nucleus is folded over itself in such a way as to hide the possibility of a thin wirelike constricted area. The majority of investigators classify this cell as a segmented form. However, many laboratorians consider these cells bands; unless the reference range takes into account the way these cells will be interpreted, the number of bands reported can differ considerably between persons or between laboratories and could lead to incorrect diagnosis. When there is multiple nuclear segmentation and the lobes connected only by a thin wire number more than five, the cell is termed *hypersegmented.* Some investigators believe that hypersegmentation is present if more than 5% of the neutrophils have five lobes. Naturally, there are transition forms between any of the maturation stages just described (Fig 6–1).

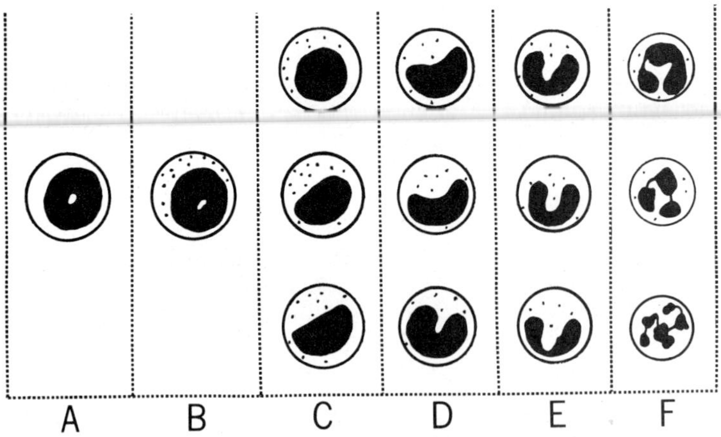

FIG 6–1.
Maturation sequence of granulocytic (myelocytic) series. *A,* blast; *B,* promyelocyte; *C,* myelocyte (*top,* early stage; *bottom,* late stage); *D,* metamyelocyte (*top,* early stage; *bottom,* late stage); *E,* band granulocyte (*top,* early stage; *bottom,* late stage); *F,* segmented granulocyte (*top,* early stage; *bottom,* hypersegmented late stage).

Monocytes are often confused with metamyelocytes or bands. The monocyte tends to be a larger cell. Its nuclear chromatin is a little less dense than chromatin of the myeloid cell and tends to have a strandlike configuration of varying thickness rather than forming discontinuous masses or clumps. The nucleus typically has several pseudopods, which sometimes are obscured by being superimposed on the remainder of the nucleus and must be looked for carefully. Sometimes, however, a monocyte nuclear shape that resembles a metamyelocyte is found. The monocyte cytoplasm is light blue or light gray, is rather abundant, and frequently has a cytoplasm border that appears frayed or has small irregular tags or protrusions. The granules of a monocyte, when present, usually are tiny or pinpoint in size, a little smaller than those of a neutrophil. In some cases, the best differentiation is to find undisputed bands or monocytes and compare their nucleus and cytoplasm with that of the cell in question.

The reference range for peripheral blood WBCs is 4,500–10,500/cu mm (4.5–10.5 × 10^9/L). Most persons have WBC counts of 5,000–10,000/cu mm, but there is significant overlap between normal and abnormal in the wider range, especially between 10,000 and 11,000/cu mm. There is some evidence that mean WBC counts in blacks are at least 500/cu mm (0.5 × 10^9/L) less than those in whites, with some investigators reporting differences as much as 3,500/cu mm. This difference would be important, since it would produce a greater than expected incidence of apparent leukopenia and less than expected leukocyte response to infection and inflammation. However, not all reports agree that there is a consistent difference between blacks and whites. Normal WBC differential values are listed here:

Total neutrophils	50%–70%
Segmented neutrophils (polys)	50%–70%
Bands (stabs)	0%–5%*
Metamyelocytes (juveniles)	0%–1%
Lymphocytes	20%–40%
Monocytes	0%–7%
Eosinophils	0%–5%
Basophils	0%–1%

*Range, 0%–9% (conservative criteria).

The value for each cell type traditionally is known as the cell "count" (i.e., band count), although the findings are expressed as a percentage of 100 WBCs rather than the actual cell number counted.

Some investigators report a diurnal variation for neutrophils and eosinophils. Neutrophil peak levels were reported about 4 P.M. and lowest values reported about 7 A.M., with an average change of about 30%. Eosinophil levels roughly paralleled serum cortisol levels, with highest values about 7 A.M. and lowest values about 4 P.M. The average change was about 40%. The remainder of this chapter describes anomalies of WBC morphology or count and associated disease states.

PELGER-HUËT ANOMALY

Of various hereditary abnormalities of WBC morphology, the most important is the Pelger-Huët nuclear anomaly. This is manifested by WBC nuclear hyposegmentation. In the neutrophil series, many of the segmented cells appear to have bilobed nuclei shaped like a dumbbell or a pair of eyeglasses. There is also an increase in bandlike forms and forms with round or oval nuclei resembling myelocytes. Eosinophils normally may have a bilobed nuclear form. Although occasional normal neutrophils may have this nuclear shape, it is not a common finding, and more than two or three neutrophils with a bilobed nucleus per 100 WBCs would be unusual. The Pelger-Huët anomaly may be congenital, inherited as a mendelian dominant trait; the congenital form is not common and is asymptomatic. An increased number of neutrophils with similar appearance may represent an acquired change (known as pseudo-Pelger-Huët), most often seen in myeloproliferative disorders, myeloid leukemia, and agranulocytosis, in some patients with metastatic tumor to bone marrow, or under conditions of drug toxicity. Neutrophils of the Pelger-Huët anomaly must be differentiated from true neutrophil immaturity such as that seen with infection or chronic myelogenous leukemia.

NEONATAL LEUKOCYTOSIS

At birth, there is a leukocytosis of 18,000–22,000/cu mm (18–22 × 10^9/L) for the first 1–3 days. This drops sharply at 3–4 days to levels between 8,000 and 16,000/cu mm. At roughly 6 months, approximately adult levels are reached, although the upper limit of normal is more flexible. Although the postnatal period is associated with neutrophilia, lymphocytes slightly predominate thereafter until about age 4–5 years, when adult values for total WBC count and differential become established (see Table 36–3). Capillary (heelstick) blood WBC reference values are about 20% higher than venous WBC values on the first day of life and about 10% higher on the second day.

NEUTROPHILIC LEUKOCYTOSIS DUE TO INFECTION AND INFLAMMATION

Inflammation is the most frequent condition associated with neutrophilic leukocytosis. Besides an increase in total neutrophil count, there often is some degree of immaturity ("shift to the left"*). Usually a shift to the left involves an increase in the early segmented and the band neutrophil stages. Occasionally even some earlier cells (metamyelocytes or even myelocytes) may appear; this is known as *leukemoid* reaction. Leukocytosis is most often seen with bacterial infection; viral infections tend to be associated with normal counts or even leukopenia. The granulomatous infections (tuberculosis, sarcoidosis) most often have normal WBC counts, but tuberculosis occasionally demonstrates a leukocytosis. Typhoid fever is a bacterial infection that usually does not have a WBC increase; on the other hand, a neutrophilic leukocytosis may be present in 30% or more of persons with severe enteric cytopathic human orphan (ECHO) virus infection. Overwhelming infection, particularly in debilitated persons or the elderly, may fail to show leukocytosis.

Deviation From Usual WBC Pattern in Infection

The classic WBC picture of acute bacterial infection is leukocytosis with an increased percentage of neutrophils and band forms. Unfortunately, leukocytosis may be absent in approximately 15%–30% of cases (literature range, 10%–45%), and band forms may remain within reference limits in approximately 30%–40% (range, 21%–61%) of cases. The band count variation can be attributed at least partially to differences in individual technologist interpretation of folded bands vs. segmented neutrophils (referred to previously), failure of individual laboratories to establish their own band reference range (rather than using values found in some publication), technical variance such as irregular distribution of cell types on the peripheral smear due to technique in making the smear and the areas chosen for cell counting, and very poor reproducibility (50%–200% variation reported) due to the small numbers involved and the other factors just cited. In general, absolute values (total number of neutrophils or bands per cubic millimeter) are more reliable than values expressed as a percent of the total WBC count, since the percentage of one cell type may reflect a change in the number of another cell type rather than a strict increase or decrease of the cell type in question. Total neutrophil count (percentage) is also more reliable because there is a minimum of subjective interpretation needed. To illustrate this, I studied hematologic findings that were obtained on the same day as the urine culture in 64 consecutive cases of well-documented urinary tract infection. In 9% of these cases, WBC count, total neutrophil count, and band count were all normal. White blood cell count was normal in 34% of cases, total neutrophil count in 19%, and band count in 50%. In only 5% of cases was the band count elevated when both the WBC count and total neutrophil count were normal. In summary, the total neutrophil percentage appears to be the most sensitive and useful parameter of infection, while the band count is the least reliable.

Automated Cell Counter Differential Counts

Certain newer automated cell counters can produce a limited differential in percent and absolute numbers. These instruments have better reproducibility than manual differential cell counts. However, to date each of these instruments has some omissions compared to manual differentials, such as lack of a band count, fail-

*The maturation sequence of Schilling used to be diagrammed with the immature and less mature forms on the left progressing to the more mature forms on the right.

ure to note WBC and red blood cell (RBC) inclusions, and failure to detect certain abnormally shaped RBCs.

Special Problems in Neonates and Younger Children

First, age-related reference values are essential. However, reference values for neonates from different sources vary even more than those for adults. Second, as noted previously, total WBC and neutrophil values rise sharply after birth and then fall. Most, although not all, investigators do not consider total WBC or absolute neutrophil values reliable in the first 3 days of life. After that time, absolute neutrophil values are said to be more reliable than total WBC counts. However, although elevated results are consistent with bacterial infection, there may be substantial overlap with WBC values seen in nonbacterial infection, and values within the reference range definitely do not exclude bacterial infection. In fact, it has been reported that neonates with sepsis are more likely to have normal range or low WBC counts than elevated ones. It has been reported that violent crying can temporarily increase WBC and band counts over twice baseline values for as long as 1 hour.

Neutrophil Cytoplasmic Inclusions.—Certain neutrophil cytoplasmic inclusions are associated with infection (although they are also seen in tissue destruction, burns, and similar toxic states); these include toxic granulation and Döhle bodies. Toxic granulation is accentuation of normal neutrophilic cytoplasm granules, which become enlarged or appear as short, rod-shaped structures of irregular width, either dark blue-black or the same color as the nucleus. Döhle bodies are moderate-sized, light blue structures most frequently located next to the cytoplasmic border. The presence of vacuoles in the cytoplasm of peripheral blood neutrophils has repeatedly been cited as a clue to septicemia. However, although there is a strong association with bacteremia or septicemia, neutrophil cytoplasmic vacuoles may occur in patients without definite evidence of bacterial infection.

Neutrophilic Leukocytosis Due to Tissue Destruction.—Tissue destruction may be due to burns, abscess, trauma, hemorrhage, infarction, carcinomatosis, active alcoholic cirrhosis, or surgery and is often accompanied by varying degrees of leukocytosis. The leukocytosis varies in severity and frequency according to the etiology and amount of tissue destruction.

Neutrophilic Leukocytosis Due to Metabolic Toxic States.—The most frequent metabolic toxic states are uremia, diabetic acidosis, acute gout attacks, and convulsions. A similar effect under nontoxic circumstances is seen after severe exercise and during the last trimester of pregnancy. During labor there is often a neutrophil leukocytosis that increases with duration of labor; in one report the majority of patients had total WBC counts less than 18,000/cu mm (18×10^9/L), but some rose as high as 24,000/cu mm. In 100 consecutive obstetrical patients admitted to our hospital for childbirth, 38% had a count between 10,500 and 18,000/cu mm. The highest WBC count was 23,000/cu mm. Twenty percent had elevated band counts and 26% had elevated total neutrophil counts.

Neutrophilic Leukocytosis Due to Certain Drugs and Chemicals.—Adrenal cortical steroids even in relatively low doses often produce a considerable increase in mature segmented neutrophils, with total WBC counts rising within 48 hours to levels that are often double baseline values. Peak counts remain for 2–3 weeks and then slowly decline somewhat, although not to baseline. Therapy with lithium carbonate for psychiatric depression produces an average WBC elevation of about 30%. Epinephrine therapy for asthma frequently produces a significant leukocytosis. Poisoning by various chemicals, especially lead, is another cause of leukocytosis. On the other hand, certain drugs may cause leukopenia from idiosyncratic bone marrow depression.

Neutrophilic Leukocytosis Due to Other Etiologies.—Cigarette smokers, especially heavy smokers, are reported to have total WBC counts that average 1,000/cu mm (1.0×10^9/L) or even more above those for nonsmokers. Other causes of neutrophilic leukocytosis are acute hemorrhage or severe hemolytic anemia (acute or chronic), myelogenous leukemia, and the myeloproliferative syndromes, including some cases of polycythemia vera.

MONOCYTOSIS

Monocytosis may occur in the absence of leukocytosis. Monocytosis is most frequently found in subacute bacterial endocarditis (about 15%–20% of patients), disseminated TB (15%–20% of patients), during the recovery phase of various acute infections, in many types of hematologic disorders (including nonmonocytic leukemias, myeloma, and hemolytic anemias), in malignant lymphomas and carcinomas, in rheumatoid-collagen diseases, and in typhoid fever. Malaria and leishmaniasis (kala-azar) are frequent causes of monocytosis outside the United States. Monocytic leukemia and myelodysplastic syndromes (chapter 7) also enter the differential diagnosis.

EOSINOPHILIA

Parasites.—Eosinophilia is most often associated with roundworms and infestation by various flukes. In the United States, roundworms predominate, such as *Ascaris, Strongyloides,* and *Trichinella (Trichina).* The condition known as *visceral larva migrans,* caused by the nematode *Toxocara canis* (common in dogs) is sometimes seen in humans. In *Trichinella* infection an almost diagnostic triad is bilateral upper eyelid edema, severe muscle pain, and eosinophilia. (Eosinophilia, however, may be absent in overwhelming infection.)

Acute Allergic Attacks.—Asthma, hay fever, and other allergic reactions may be associated with eosinophilia.

Certain Extensive Chronic Skin Diseases.—Eosinophilia is often found in pemphigus; it also may appear in psoriasis and several other cutaneous disorders.

Certain Bacterial Infections.—Eosinophilia may occur in scarlet fever and brucellosis.

Miscellaneous Conditions.—Eosinophilia is reported in 20% of polyarteritis nodosa cases and 25% of sarcoidosis patients. It also has been reported in up to 20% of patients with Hodgkin's disease, but the degree of eosinophilia is usually not impressive. Eosinophilia is associated with certain types of pneumonitis such as Löffler's syndrome and the syndrome of "pulmonary infiltration with eosinophilia." Eosinophilia may occur with various types of cancer, but the overall incidence is less than 1%. A substantial number of patients undergoing peritoneal dialysis for chronic renal failure are reported to have intermittent eosinophilia (about 60% of cases in one report), most often following insertion of the dialysis catheter. A number of other diseases have been reported to produce eosinophilia, but either the diseases are rare or there is a low incidence of eosinophilia.

BASOPHILIA

Basophilia is most frequently found in chronic myelogenous leukemia. Basophils may be increased in the other "myeloproliferative" diseases and occasionally in certain nonmalignant conditions.

LEUKEMOID REACTION

Leukemoid reaction is usually defined as a nonleukemic WBC count more than 50,000/cu mm (50×10^9/L) or a differential count with more than 5% metamyelocytes or earlier cells. It is basically a more severe or pronounced form of ordinary nonneoplastic granulocyte reaction. Some conditions associated with leukemoid reaction are severe bacterial infections, severe toxic states (burns, tissue necrosis, etc.), extensive bone marrow replacement by tumor, severe hemolytic anemia, severe acute blood loss, and juvenile rheumatoid arthritis.

LYMPHOCYTOSIS

Lymphocytosis is most commonly associated with a normal or a decreased total WBC count. The most common etiology is viral infection. The lymphocytosis seen in the majority of viral infections is actually a relative type due to a decrease in granulocytes while total (absolute) lymphocyte numbers remain constant. The same phenomenon is found in Addison's disease and in drug-induced agranulocytosis. A real (absolute) lymphocytosis with leukocytosis occurs in pertussis, infectious lymphocytosis, lymphocytic leukemia, and in some infants with adenovirus infection. Infectious mononucleosis, adult cytomegalovirus infection, and sometimes hepatitis virus infection are associated with absolute lymphocytosis and atypical lymphocytes; there may be leukopenia in the early stages, which is followed by leukocytosis. Toxoplasmosis sometimes produces absolute lymphocytosis. One report indicates that severe trauma may be associated with absolute lymphocytosis that changes to lymphopenia accompanied by increased granulocytes within 24 hours.

NEUTROPENIA (GRANULOCYTOPENIA)

Neutropenia is usually defined as a WBC count less than 4,000/cu mm. Some conditions associated with neutropenia include (1) Conditions associated with pancytopenia, such as megaloblastic anemia, aplastic anemia, acute or aleukemic leukemia, hypersplenism of varying etiology (e.g., cirrhosis, systemic lupus, Gaucher's disease), and paroxysmal nocturnal hemoglobinuria; (2) drug-induced neutropenia (agranulocytosis); (3) certain infections, such as typhoid, some viral infections (e.g., Epstein-Barr, in the first week of illness, and the hepatitis viruses), overwhelming bacterial infection (septicemia, miliary tuberculosis); and (4) cyclic and chronic idiopathic neutropenia.

LEUKOERYTHROBLASTOSIS

Leukoerythroblastosis can be defined as the presence of both immature WBCs (metamyelocytes or earlier cells) and nucleated RBCs in the peripheral blood smear. Although the relative frequency of etiologies is different in different reports, approximately 25%–30% of patients with leukoerythroblastosis have metastatic tumor in the bone marrow, about 20% have leukemia, about 10% have myeloid metaplasia or polycythemia vera, and about 8% have hemolytic anemia. Severe infection, megaloblastic anemia, and severe acute hemorrhage account for about 5% each. There is a miscellaneous nonneoplastic group with relatively few cases of any single etiology comprising 5%–15% of the total.

BIBLIOGRAPHY

Shapiro MF, Greenfield S: The complete blood count and leukocyte differential count. *Ann Intern Med* 1987; 106:65.

Strausbaugh L: Hematologic manifestations of bacterial and fungal infections. *Hematol Oncol Clin North Am* 1987; 1:185.

Baranski B, Young N: Hematologic consequences of viral infections. *Hematol Oncol Clin North Am* 1987; 1:167.

Pierre RV, et al: Comparison of four leukocyte differential methods with the national committee for clinical laboratory standards (NCCLS) reference method. *Am J Clin Pathol* 1987; 87:201.

Arkin CF, et al: The white blood cell differential. Evaluation of rapid impression scanning versus the routine manual count. *Am J Clin Pathol* 1987; 87:628.

Drewinko B, et al: Analytical errors of manual and automated white blood cell differential counts. *Am J Clin Pathol* 1987; 87:418.

Kalish RJ, Becker K: Evaluation of the Coulter S-Plus V three-part differential in a community hospital. *Am J Clin Pathol* 1986; 86:751.

Frymark WB, Jonasson O: Acute appendicitis in the elderly. *Illinois Med J* 1986; 169:159.

Thommasen HV, et al: Absolute lymphocytosis associated with nonsurgical trauma. *Am J Clin Pathol* 1986; 86:480.

Van Assendelft OW: Reference values for the total and differential leukocyte count. *Blood Cells* 1985; 11:77.

Acker DB, et al: The leukocyte count in labor. *Am J Obstet Gynecol* 1985; 153:737.

Rainey P: Utility of the leukocyte differential in the diagnosis of bacterial infection. *Pathologist* 1985; 39(7):38.

Deitch E: Peritoneal lavage and abdominal trauma. *JAMA* 1983; 249:640.

May ME, Waddell CC: Basophils in peripheral blood and bone marrow. *Am J Med* 1984; 76:509.

Rock WA, Grogan JE: Demand v. need v. physician prerogatives in the use of the WBC differential. *JAMA* 1983; 249:613.

Sadowitz PD, Oski FA: Differences in polymorphonuclear cell counts between healthy White and Black infants: Response to meningitis. *Pediatrics* 1983; 72:405.

Rich EC, et al: Effectiveness of differential leukocyte count in case finding in the ambulatory care setting. *JAMA* 1983; 249:633.

Statland BE: Preanalytic sources of variation in healthy subjects: II. *Diagn Dialog* 1982; 4(1):8.

Fauci AS, et al: The idiopathic hypereosinophilic syndrome. *Ann Intern Med* 1982; 97:78.

Parmley RT, Crist WM: Childhood neutropenia. *Ala J Med Sci* 1982; 19:249.

Peevy KJ, et al: Capillary-venous differences in neonatal neutrophil values. *Am J Dis Child* 1982; 136:357.

Bower RJ, et al: Diagnostic value of the white blood count and neutrophil percentage in the evaluation of abdominal pain in children. *Surg Gynecol Obstet* 1981; 152:424.

Floranc RK: A most uncommon eosinophilia. *Diagn Med* 1981; 4(1):68.

Weetman RM, Boxer LA: Childhood neutropenia. *Pediatr Clin North Am* 1980; 17:361.

Young GAR, Vincent PC: Drug-induced agranulocytosis. *Clin Haematol* 1980; 9:483.

Spry CJF: Eosinophilia and allergic reactions to drugs. *Clin Haematol* 1980; 9:521.

Friedenberg WR, Marx JJ: The effect of lithium carbonate on lymphocyte, granulocyte, and platelet function. *Cancer* 1980; 45:91.

Ward PCJ: The myeloid leukocytoses. *Postgrad Med* 1980; 67:219.

Ward PCJ: The lymphoid leukocytoses. *Postgrad Med* 1980; 67:217.

Christensen RD, Rothstein G: Pitfalls in the interpretation of leukocyte counts of newborn infants. *Am J Clin Pathol* 1979; 72:608.

Morens DM: WBC count and differential: Value in predicting bacterial diseases in children. *Am J Dis Child* 1979; 133:25.

Dale DC, et al: Chronic neutropenia. *Medicine* (Baltimore) 1979; 58:128.

Malcolm ID, et al: Vacuolization of the neutrophil in bacteremia. *Arch Intern Med* 1979; 139:675.

Delsol G, et al: Leukoerythroblastosis and cancer frequency, prognosis, and physiopathologic significance. *Cancer* 1979; 44:1009.

7 Leukemia, Lymphomas, and Myeloproliferative Syndromes

A consideration of tho origin and maturation sequence of white blood cells (WBCs) is helpful in understanding the classification and behavior of the leukemias and their close relatives, the malignant lymphomas. Most authorities agree that the basic cell of origin is the fixed tissue reticulum cell. Figure 7–1 shows the normal WBC development sequence. The corresponding malignancy is given in parentheses at each stage.

Malignancy may occur at each major stage in the development sequence of the blood cells. In general, the earlier the stage at which the cell is involved by malignancy, the worse the prognosis. Thus, a leukemia whose predominant cell is the myeloblast has a much worse prognosis (if untreated) than one whose predominant cell is the myelocyte.

Leukemia is a term that denotes malignancy of WBCs, although its definition is often extended to include malignancy of any type of blood cell. In many patients with leukemia (including the majority of those with the chronic leukemias), the total number of WBCs in the peripheral blood is increased above the reference range. *Acute leukemia* was originally defined as a leukemia that, if untreated, would be expected to permit an average life span of less than 6 months. The predominant cell is usually the blast (or closely related cells such as the promyelocyte). In most cases there are more than 25% blasts in the peripheral blood, and for many years this criterion was the usual basis for suggesting the diagnosis of acute leukemia. The major exception was *monocytic leukemia*, which behaves like acute leukemia even though the number of monoblasts may be very low. Definitive diagnosis was usually made by bone marrow aspiration; this is a necessity when using the French-American-British (FAB) classification system (discussed later). *Chronic leukemia* is a leukemia that, if untreated, would be expected to permit an average life span of more than 1 year. The predominant cell forms are more mature; generally, the prognosis is best for chronic leukemias involving the most mature forms. Thus, chronic lymphocytic leukemia (CLL) has a better prognosis than chronic granulocytic (myelocytic) leukemia (CGL).

Subleukemic leukemia is sometimes used to refer to a leukemia in which the total peripheral blood WBC count is within the reference range but a significant number of immature cells (usually blasts) are present.

Aleukemic leukemia is the term used when the peripheral blood WBC count is normal (or, more often, decreased) and no abnormal cells are found in the peripheral blood. The diagnosis of subleukemic or aleukemic leukemia is made by bone marrow examination. More than 30% blasts in the bone marrow usually means leukemia; 10–30% suggests the dysmyelopoietic syndrome (discussed later).

Stem cell leukemia or *acute blastic leukemia* are terms often applied when nearly all the WBCs are blasts and no definite differentiating features are present. Myeloblasts and lymphoblasts are morphologically very similar on peripheral blood smears, and reliable differentiation by morphologic appearance alone is sometimes not possible even by experts. In some cases differentiation is made on the basis of other information, such as the age of the patient and the types of cells accompanying the blasts. Cytochemical stains (discussed later) are very helpful. *Auer rods* are small rod-shaped

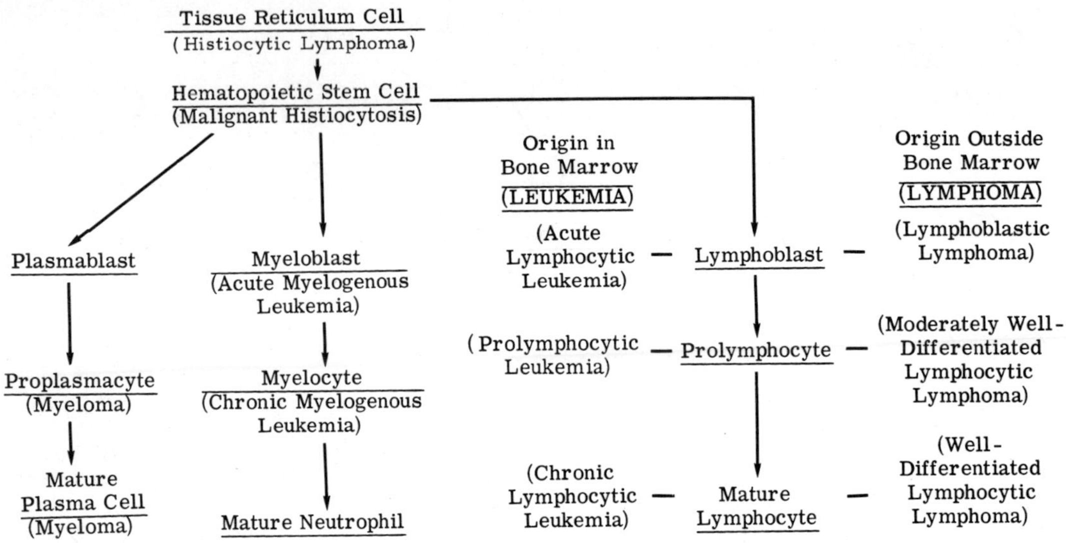

FIG 7–1.
Relationship of leukemia and malignant lymphoma to normal WBC maturation sequence.

structures that sometimes are present in the cytoplasm of blasts. Auer rods are diagnostic of myeloid cells, either myeloblasts or the myelomonocytic form of monocytic leukemia.

Both the lymphocytic leukemias and the malignant lymphomas are derived from lymphocytes or lymphocyte precursors; but the leukemias originate in bone marrow, whereas the lymphomas originate outside the marrow, usually in lymph nodes. The lymphomas and their close relative, Hodgkin's disease, will be discussed later.

ACUTE LEUKEMIA

About 80%–90% of acute leukemia in childhood is acute lymphocytic leukemia (ALL), and about 85%–90% in adults is acute nonlymphocytic leukemia (most commonly acute myelogenous leukemia and myelomonocytic leukemia). Peak incidence in childhood is 3–10 years, whereas it is most common in adults after age 50. Acute leukemia usually has more than 25% blasts in the peripheral blood and by FAB criteria must have more than 30% blasts in the bone marrow. Sometimes the peripheral blood has fewer than 25%, especially if there is a leukopenia or if the patient has monocytic leukemia. The peripheral blood WBC count typically is mildly to moderately elevated (15,000–50,000/cu mm; 15–50 × 10^9/L), but nearly one half of the patients either have WBC mal range or have leukopenia. About 10% have counts in the normal range or have leukopenia. About 10% have WBC counts more than 100,000/cu mm (100 × 10^9/L). Anemia is present in about 90% of patients and is generally of moderate to severe degree. If not present initially, it develops later. Thrombocytopenia is reported in 80%–85% of patients (range, 72%–90%); about 40% have a platelet count of 50,000/cu mm or less. Childhood acute leukemia may be associated with meningeal involvement in as many as 50% of patients.

Lymphadenopathy, usually of mild degree, is present in about 50% of patients, and splenomegaly, also usually minimal or mild, is reported in about 65% (range, 50%–76%). Generally speaking, enlargement of visceral organs is related to the duration of leukemia, so that the chronic leukemias are usually much more likely than the acute leukemias to be associated with marked organomegaly or with adenopathy. A significant number of patients with acute leukemia develop ulcerative lesions in the oral mucous membranes or gums and occasionally elsewhere, as in the gastrointestinal tract. Hemorrhagic phenomena (petechiae or localized small hemorrhages) are frequent, due to thrombocytopenia. Superimposed infection is common and is probably the most frequent cause of death.

French-American-British Classification of Acute Leukemias

In 1976 a group of French, American, and

TABLE 7–1.
French-American-British Classification of Acute Leukemia

FAB Designation*	Description	Appearance†
M1	Acute myelocytic without maturation	Predominantly myeloblasts; other immature granulocytes absent
M2	Acute myelocytic with maturation	Myeloblasts with other immature granulocytes
M3	Acute promyelocytic	Predominantly promyelocytes with heavy granulation‡
M4	Acute myelomonocytic	Predominantly cells with monocytic-type nucleus and myelocytic-type cytoplasm
M5	Acute monocytic with maturation	Predominantly nonblastic monocytic cells without granulocytic-type cytoplasm ("pure monocytic")
M5A	Acute monoblastic without maturation	Predominantly monoblasts (without granulocytic-type cytoplasm)
M6	Erythroleukemia	Megaloblastoid pronormoblasts and myeloblasts present with other cells
L1	Homogeneous small blast type	Predominantly small blasts, fairly uniform appearance
L2	Heterogeneous blast type	Mixed blast size and appearance; typically with nuclear clefting or irregularity
L3	Homogeneous large blast type ("Burkitt's cell")§	Uniform large blasts with intensely basophilic cytoplasm that usually contains vacuoles

*M, myeloid; L, lymphoid.
†Bone marrow lower limit for acute leukemia diagnosis is at least 30% blasts and/or promyelocytes. Up to 10% of cells may deviate from standard morphologic criteria.
‡A small subgroup of promyelocytic leukemia without heavy granulation exists. It is assigned to category M2 by some investigators and to M3 by others.
§A subgroup of cases is similar in morphology but displays heterogeneity of cell size ("non-Burkitt's cells").

British hematologists proposed a system for classification of acute leukemia based primarily on morphologic and cytochemical criteria. The FAB classification has been widely adopted as the basis for standardization of diagnosis and comparing results of therapy (Table 7–1). During this time there have been several minor modifications. The classification can be applied only before initial therapy is begun. There are two categories, acute lymphocytic leukemia (ALL, FAB prefix L) and acute non-lymphocytic leukemia (ANLL, FAB prefix M). The latter includes myelocytic, myelomonocytic, monocytic, and erythroid leukemic subcategories. The panel stated that great caution was required before diagnosing leukemia in hypocellular bone marrow aspirates. It is worth noting that using morphologic study alone, even experts reached complete agreement only in about 80% of cases submitted for diagnosis.

Cytochemical Stains

The FAB group found that cytochemical stains were extremely helpful in categorizing some cases of acute leukemia, especially those that are relatively undifferentiated. Results of the Sudan black B stain are usually positive in myelocytic and myelomonocytic leukemia but negative in lymphocytic or other types of monocytic leukemia. The myeloperoxidase stain gives results similar to Sudan black B but is more technique dependent and thus less reliable in many laboratories. Nonspecific esterase stains are used to diagnose the monocytic leukemias. Results of alpha-naphthylbutyrate esterase are positive only in monocytic cells, whereas NASD-acetate esterase is positive in both myeloid and monocytic cells but is inhibited by fluoride in monocytic but not in myeloid cells. In a few cases none of the special stains produce diagnostic results. In categories not supposed to display special stain reaction, up to 3% reactive cells is permitted.

Terminal deoxynucleotidyl transferase (TdT) enzyme reaction is normally present (positive reaction) in nuclei of thymus cells and a few lymphocytic bone marrow cells but is not present in normal lymph node lymphocytes, peripheral blood lymphocytes, or B-cell lymphocytic malignancies (e.g., chronic lymphocytic leukemia, well-differentiated and poorly differentiated lymphocytic lymphoma, or myeloma). Terminal deoxynucleotidyl transferase enzyme activity is present in 90% or more (88%–

95%) of ALL patients, comprised mostly of T-cell and non-B, non-T phenotypes. The equivalent malignant lymphoma category (T-cell/lymphoblastic lymphoma) is also TdT positive. Therefore, TdT positivity has been used to differentiate ALL from ANLL. However, there are exceptions; FAB L3 (B-cell ALL) and the equivalent malignant lymphoma (Burkitt's lymphoma) are usually TdT negative. About 5%–10% of AML are reported to be TdT positive. About one third of patients in the blast crisis of chronic myelogenous leukemia (CML) may have a positive TdT reaction, even some who have the Philadelphia chromosome.

Acute Nonlymphocytic Leukemia

In adults, approximately 80% of acute leukemia cases are the ANLL type. Of the adult ANLL cases, about 30% each are FAB-M1, M2, or M4. About 5% are FAB-M3, known as *acute progranulocytic leukemia*. This category, especially the so-called hypergranular variant, is associated with an unusually high incidence of coagulation disorders, particularly disseminated intravascular coagulation (DIC). In childhood, about 20% of acute leukemia is ANLL; roughly 60% of these are M4 and about 25% are M1 or M2.

Acute Lymphocytic Leukemia

About 20% of adult acute leukemia is ALL; of these patients, about 65% are FAB-L2. About 80% of children with acute leukemia have ALL, and about 15% have the nonlymphocytic form. About 50% of childhood ALL cases occur between ages 3 and 7, whereas the age incidence of ANLL is more evenly distributed. Childhood ALL and ANLL occur predominantly (> 80%) in whites. About 5% have CNS involvement at the time of diagnosis, and the CNS is eventually involved in about 50% unless prophylactic therapy is given. About 80% of childhood ALL cases are the FAB-L1 type. About 2% of childhood cases and less than that of adult cases are FAB-L3. Morphologically, FAB-L3 leukemia resembles the malignant lymphoma known as *Burkitt's lymphoma* and currently has the worst prognosis of the ALL categories.

Lymphocyte Immunophenotyping

Lymphocytes can be divided into two types: B (bone marrow) lymphocytes and T (thymus) lymphocytes. B lymphocytes progress through a sequence of changes to a cell capable of antibody (immunoglobulin) production. Plasma cells are derived from B lymphocytes. T lymphocytes also undergo a series of changes, resulting in cells that are directly involved in cell-mediated immunologic reactions (graft-vs.-host; delayed hypersensitivity) and host defense against certain bacteria and fungi (frequently producing granulomatous reactions). There are two major subsets of T lymphocytes: helper (inducer) cells, which stimulate B lymphocytes to produce antibodies and differentiate into plasma cells; and suppressor (cytotoxic) cells, which inhibit B-cell production of immunoglobulin and also can attack target cells that contain antigen that previously had sensitized the body immune system. There is also a third class of lymphocytes, so-called non-T, non-B cells, some of which are natural killer (NK) cells that can attack target cells without prior sensitization and some of which are killer (K) cells that attack antibody-coated target cells. In normal adult peripheral blood there are about 60%–80% T lymphocytes, about 5%–15% B lymphocytes, and about 10%–20% nontypeable (non-T, non-B) lymphocytes.

Identification of B and T Lymphocytes.—B lymphocytes are usually identified by immunofluorescent methods that demonstrate presence of immunoglobulin on the surface of the cytoplasm membrane. T cells are usually identified by the erythrocyte (E) rosette technique in which sheep red blood cells (RBCs) spontaneously aggregate around the T cell to form a "rosette." The classic procedure for measuring T-cell function is the migration inhibition factor (MIF) assay.

Monoclonal Antibody Identification of Lymphocyte Subgroups.—Besides surface immunoglobulin and E-rosette tests, various monoclonal antibodies are now available (with more being developed) that can help identify the major lymphocyte classes, their functional subclasses, and their stage of maturation. A monoclonal antibody is an antibody specially produced to detect a single limited antigen. Some of these antibodies detect surface (cytoplasmic membrane) immunoglobulins, some detect surface epitopes (antigen sites), some detect antigens present in the various stages of cell maturation, and some detect enzymes. Certain manufacturers have produced entire families of such monoclonal antibodies (e.g., the OKT/B, the Leu, and the CD series); many of the antibodies in each family react with identical antigens, and some react with either related or different antigens. Detection methods include manual methods, generally with a fluorescent or peroxidase enzyme antibody label, and electronic (or laser) cell-sorting equipment (flow cytometry), which can isolate certain cells by size, staining, or antibody reaction and quantitate each group isolated. Cell nuclei can be stained for DNA and then analyzed to see if the cells have normal (diploid) or abnormal (aneuploid) DNA patterns. In general, manual methods are more often used with the lymphocytic leukemias and flow cytometry with malignant (Non-Hodgkin's) lymphomas or nonlymphoid tumors.

Immunologic Classification of Acute Lymphocytic Leukemia

Both ALL and the non-Hodgkin's malignant lymphomas have been classified according to the immunologic type of lymphocyte involved. Acute lymphocytic leukemia has been subdivided by immunologic techniques into three categories: B cell, T cell, and non-B, non-T. *B-cell ALL* displays surface immunoglobulin production and comprises about 2% (range 1%–5%) of ALL cases. Morphology is usually FAB-L3 and resembles Burkitt's lymphoma. *T-cell ALL* demonstrates a positive spontaneous E rosette test. Two categories of T-cell ALL have been reported; the "idiopathic" type and the "endemic" type. The idiopathic type comprises about 20% (10%–28%) of ALL in the United States. It tends to occur in later childhood or in adolescents and has male predominance. Approximately 75% have a mediastinal mass due to lymphadenopathy; this group resembles the type of malignant lymphoma called lymphoblastic in the Rappaport classification. The endemic type is most frequent in Japan and the Caribbean islands and is apparently caused by human T-cell leukemia virus-I (HTLV-I) retrovirus infection. This type is more frequent in adults, has about equal male-female incidence, does not have a high incidence of prominent mediastinal lymphadenopathy, has leukemic cells with convoluted nuclei, and has a relatively high incidence of skin involvement and also of hypercalcemia (about 25% of cases, but ranging up to 70% in some series). Non-T, non-B ALL comprises about 70%–80% of ALL patients; these patients have blasts that do not possess surface immunoglobulins and have a negative E rosette test result. Non-B, non-T can be further subdivided into four groups. About 75%–80% (range, 65%–90%) of non-B, non-T patients, constituting about 65% (range, 50%–76%) of all ALL cases, have blasts with a surface antigen that reacts with antibody prepared against non-B, non-T lymphocytes (*common ALL antigen* or CALLA). This group is often designated "common" ALL. Another subset of about 10%–20% (constituting about 10%–15% of all ALL cases) demonstrate intracytoplasmic immunoglobulin production but not surface (membrane) immunoglobulin and are said to have *pre-B-cell ALL*. A few patients have blasts that react with antisera to T-lymphocyte surface antigens but that have negative E rosette test results. These patients are said to have *pre-T-cell ALL*. Finally, there are about 10%–15% of patients with blasts that do not react with any of the tests mentioned. These patients are said to have *null cell ALL*. Originally, all four subcategories of patients whose blasts did not react with surface immunoglobulin or have positive E rosette test results (therefore, non-B non-T ALL) were included in the null cell group. Thus, when the designation "null cell ALL" is used, it may be difficult to tell whether the entire non-B, non-T group is meant or just the relatively small category of patients whose cells are nonreactive with all the various techniques.

Monocytic Leukemia

Monocytic leukemia has the clinical and laboratory aspects of acute leukemia and is included in the FAB classification of acute leukemia as categories M4 and M5. In monocytic leukemia, however, the number of actual blasts may be low in both the peripheral blood and bone marrow. Instead of blasts there are cells resembling monocytes. In FAB category M4 the cells have a monocytic nucleus and cytoplasm containing granules resembling those found in granulocytes rather than those of monocytes (myelomonocytic leukemia, originally known as monocytic leukemia of Naegeli). In FAB category M5 the cells have both nucleus and cytoplasm resembling a monocyte ("pure" monocytic leukemia, originally known as monocytic leukemia of Schilling). Diagnosis of M5 requires 80% or more of the nonerythroid nucleated cells in the bone marrow to be monocytes, promonocytes, or monoblasts. There are two FAB subdivisions: 5A, in which more than 80% of the marrow monocytic cells are monoblasts, and 5B, in which less than 80% of the marrow monocytic cells are monoblasts.

Myelomonocytic leukemia is by far the most frequent type of monocytic leukemia. It actually is a form of myelogenous leukemia in which the leukemic cells have cytoplasmic features of the more differentiated myeloid line and nuclear characteristics of the more primitive histiocytic precursors of the myeloid cells. There may be accompanying myeloid cells that are nonmonocytic, less immature forms; if so, this helps suggest the diagnosis. Sometimes the monocytic cells are indistinguishable from those of pure monocytic leukemia (Schilling type), but eventually some of them develop myeloid cytoplasmic features. If Auer rods are found, this establishes the myeloid derivation of the cells. According to the revised FAB criteria, if there is peripheral blood absolute monocytosis, M4 can be diagnosed if more than 20% of the bone marrow nucleated cells are monocytic. Cytochemical tests for monocytes may be needed. If peripheral blood monocytes are not increased, more than 20% of the bone marrow nucleated cells must be monocytic either confirmed by cytochemical stains or by elevated serum lysozyme (an enzyme associated with histiocytes or monocytes).

Diseases accompanied by peripheral blood monocytosis sometimes raise the question of monocytic leukemia. Bone marrow aspiration provides the differentiation. The most common of these diseases are subacute bacterial endocarditis, typhoid fever, and tuberculosis.

Erythroleukemia

Erythroleukemia (FAB M6) was formerly known as *Di Guglielmo's syndrome*. Some considered Di Guglielmo's a single entity (erythroleukemia) and others included at least two categories: erythroleukemia and a syndrome comprising one or more disorders now included in myelodysplasia (discussed later). Erythroleukemia constitutes about 8% (range, 3.3%–13%) of acute leukemia cases. Sixty-five percent to 71% of patients are male. The mean age at diagnosis is in the forties and fifties, but patients from age 2–85 have been reported. Splenomegaly is reported in 10%–20% of patients, hepatomegaly in 0%–18%, and lymphadenopathy in 2%–43%. Various cytogenetic abnormalities have been found in about 60% of cases. At the time of diagnosis, all patients have anemia, most often moderate or severe, either normocytic or macrocytic. Leukopenia is reported in 25%–86% of cases, and thrombocytopenia is found in about 75%. A monocytosis may be present in occasional patients.

The disease is reported to progress in three bone marrow stages: (1) an erythroproliferative phase with abnormalities largely confined to the erythroid line; (2) a mixed erythroid-myeloid dysplastic phase; and (3) a transition to ANLL. Therefore, in erythroleukemia there is abnormality in both the RBC and the myeloid precursors. The peripheral blood typically contains varying numbers of nucleated RBCs and immature granulocytes. In classic cases there are some peripheral blood myeloblasts and rubriblasts (pronormoblasts), but in some patients there are only a few nucleated RBCs, and rubriblasts are not seen. There may be increased numbers of monocytes. There is most often leukocytosis, but the WBC count may be normal or decreased. A normocytic (or slightly macrocytic) and normochromic anemia is present with considerable RBC anisocytosis and often with some oval macrocytes. The platelet count may be normal or decreased. The bone marrow shows overall increase in cellularity with hyperplasia of both the granulocytic and the erythroid series. The erythroid hyperplasia usually predominates, typically producing a reversal of the myeloid to erythroid (M/E) ratio (the normal M/E ratio is 3:1 or 2:1). The erythroid precursors are usually megaloblastic or, at least, megaloblastoid, are often bizarre in appearance, and may exhibit erythrophagocytosis (40%–50% of patients); frequently there are increased (> 2%) numbers of multinucleated RBC precursors. Ringed sideroblasts are usually present. The FAB criteria for M6 diagnosis are nucleated RBCs comprising more than 50% of all marrow nucleated cells, and at least 30% of the nonerythrocytic nucleated cells must be blasts. In most patients the marrow picture eventually progresses to ANLL of the M1, M2, or M4 type.

Differential Diagnosis of Acute Leukemia

Several diseases can simulate part of the clinical or laboratory picture of acute leukemia.

Infectious mononucleosis is frequently a

problem because of the leukocytosis (or initial leukopenia) plus atypical lymphocytes. However, infectious mononucleosis is almost never associated with anemia and only rarely with thrombocytopenia. The bone marrow of infectious mononucleosis is normal and is not infiltrated by significant numbers of atypical lymphocytes. Results of the Paul-Bunnell test for heterophil antibodies (chapter 16) are positive with infectious mononucleosis but negative in leukemia.

Pancytopenia or other peripheral blood cytopenias (Chapter 6) may raise the question of possible acute leukemia, since acute leukemia may present in this way. Aplastic anemia is one of the more frequent causes for concern. The bone marrow, however, is usually hypoplastic, and the number of blasts is not significantly increased. Patients with agranulocytosis have leukopenia and often have mouth lesions, thereby clinically simulating monocytic leukemia, but do not have anemia or thrombocytopenia or increased number of blasts in their bone marrow.

Certain viral diseases, such as mumps, measles, and pertussis, are occasionally associated with considerably elevated WBC counts. There may be occasional atypical lymphocytes. There is no anemia or thrombocytopenia. A disease called *infectious lymphocytosis* occurs in children but is uncommon. White blood cell counts may be 40,000–90,000, with most WBCs being mature lymphocytes. This condition lasts only a few days. There are no abnormal cells and no anemia or thrombocytopenia, and the bone marrow is normal.

Overwhelming infection may cause immature cells and even a few blasts to appear in the peripheral blood of infants and young children, and sometimes other toxic bone marrow stimulation has the same effect. Anemia is frequent, and sometimes there is thrombocytopenia. Bone marrow aspirates may be hypercellular and show marked myeloid hyperplasia but do not usually contain the number of blasts found in leukemia. There are usually less than 5% blasts in the peripheral blood. They decrease in number and disappear when the underlying disease is treated.

MYELODYSPLASTIC SYNDROMES

The myelodysplastic syndromes are a group of disorders with a varying number of features that may raise the question of early, borderline, or atypical acute leukemia but that do not satisfy FAB criteria for leukemia (especially, the FAB cutoff level of 30% blasts in the bone marrow). The disorders included in this category by the FAB group have certain common features: insufficient blasts in bone marrow to be diagnosed as acute leukemia; some degree of abnormality in at least two cell lines (RBC, WBC, or platelets), a high incidence of pancytopenia or cytopenia of less than three cell lines, frequent normocellular or hypercellular bone marrow in spite of peripheral blood pancytopenia, and a relatively high rate of progression to acute nonlymphocytic leukemia (roughly 15%–45%, depending on the particular subgroup of the FAB classification). Some or all of these disorders were previously considered a subgroup of Di Guglielmo's syndrome by some investigators and were called "preleukemia" by others. Some believe that these disorders represent a leukemic cell clone or clones that for some reason have a relatively slow or variable progression. These syndromes can be idiopathic or preceded (and presumably induced) by bone marrow injury from toxins or radiation. The myelodysplastic syndrome occurs predominantly in persons over age 50 (reported mean ages varying between 60 and 80). Men are affected more frequently than women in some studies but not in others. Chromosome abnormalities have been reported in 35%–50% of cases, with the most common being the 5q – abnormality (deletion of a large part of the long arm of chromosome 5).

The peripheral blood frequently contains some abnormal cells such as oval macrocytes; moderate anisocytosis and poikilocytosis; a few nucleated RBCs; myeloid cells with Pelger-Huët nuclear changes, abnormal granulation, or abnormal granules; and abnormal platelets. There may be a few blasts, but less than 5%. Bone marrow shows various combinations of myeloid immaturity (but < 30% blasts), increased monocytes, megaloblastic or megaloblastoid

RBC precursor change, ring sideroblasts, and abnormal megakaryocytes in addition to changes similar to those of the peripheral blood. Table 7–2 lists the major differences between subgroups of the myelodysplastic syndrome.

HAIRY CELL LEUKEMIA

This disease has now been classified as a B-lymphocyte disorder. A few variant patients, such as rare patients with T-cell characteristics, have been reported. A few cases have been reported in association with retrovirus HTLV-II infection. Hairy cell leukemia was originally called *leukemic reticuloendotheliosis*. It affects primarily men (male/female ratio 4:1) between ages 40 and 60 (range, 24–80) years. The clinical course if untreated is usually described as chronic but progressive (mean 4 years, range < 1 to > 20 years). The most common cause of death is infection (55%–65% of patients). There is splenomegaly in 80%–90% of cases; about 20% have spleens with enlargement to palpation of less than 5 cm, whereas about 15% are more than 15 cm. In the typical patient there is splenomegaly without lymphadenopathy; lymphadenopathy actually does occur in approximately 30% of cases but is usually not prominent. Mild hepatomegaly is found in approximately 20%.

Laboratory Picture.—About 70% of patients with hairy cell leukemia (literature range, 59%–90%) present with pancytopenia; about 10%–15% have WBC counts greater than 10,000/cu mm (10×10^9/L). A relative lymphocytosis is frequently present. The anemia is normocytic-normochromic. Serum alkaline phosphatase levels are elevated in about 20% of cases. Hairy cells are present in the peripheral blood in approximately 90% of patients, although the number of such cells varies considerably. In most cases there are relatively few hairy cells; in 10% of cases more than one half of all leukocytes are hairy cells. Hairy cells are present in the bone marrow and spleen as well as the peripheral blood. The hairy cell is similar to a lymphocyte in appearance but the cytoplasm appears frayed or has irregular, narrow, hair-like projections. The hairy cytoplasm appearance is not specific; it may occasionally be seen in a few persons with other conditions or as an artifact (usually only a few cells are affected).

Bone marrow aspiration is diagnostic in 70%–80% of cases in which marrow is ob-

TABLE 7–2.
French-American-British Classification of Myelodysplastic Syndromes

	Peripheral Blood	Bone Marrow
Refractory anemia (RA)*	Not > 1% blasts Reticulocytopenia Presence of abnormal RBCs Variable WBC and platelets, usually normal	Not > 5% blasts Normocellular or hypercellular WBCs and megakaryocytes normal
Refractory anemia with ringed sideroblasts (RARS)	Same as RA	Not > 5% blasts Ringed sideroblasts comprise > 15% of all nucleated cells
Refractory anemia with excess blasts (RAEB)	Cytopenia in at least two cell lines < 5% blasts Morphologic abnormalities in all three cell lines	Between 5% and 20% blasts Granulocyte maturation to promyelocytes and myelocytes (or further)
Chronic myelomonocytic leukemia (CMML)	Persistent absolute monocytosis Not > 5% blasts	Resembles RAEB < 20% blasts No increase in monocytes but may have some increase in promonocytes
RAEB in transformation	1. > 5% blasts 2. < 5% blasts 3. Auer rods present	1. < 30% blasts 2. 20%–30% blasts 3. < 30% blasts

*About 5% of patients categorized as RA are not anemic but have only neutropenia, thrombocytopenia, or both. This condition is sometimes called "refractory cytopenia."

tained; no marrow can be aspirated in 30%–50% of patients, and a bone biopsy is then necessary. Some investigators believe that bone marrow is nearly always diagnostic if the correct specimen in sufficient quantity is obtained and adequate testing is done. Clot sections as well as smears should be prepared if marrow is aspirated, and slide imprints should be made if a bone biopsy is performed. The bone marrow is usually hypercellular but occasionally may be normocellular or even hypocellular. Some patients develop varying degrees of marrow fibrosis, which could lead to a misdiagnosis of myeloid metaplasia. Marrow infiltration by hairy cells begins in small patches that eventually become confluent and finally become generalized. Spleen sections typically show involvement of the red pulp rather than the malpighian corpuscles, and spleen sections may contain diagnostic pseudosinuses lined by hairy cells.

Acid Phosphatase Stain.—Hairy cells typically demonstrate a positive cytoplasmic acid phosphatase cytochemical reaction, which is resistant to tartrate. This reaction was originally thought to be specific for hairy cells but has since been found (more often with weak reactivity) in some patients with B-cell or T-cell CLL, prolymphocytic leukemia, adult T-cell leukemia, Sézary syndrome, and occasionally in acute myeloblastic leukemia and acute monoblastic leukemia. On the other hand, the number of hairy cells that exhibit a positive tartrate-resistant acid phosphatase reaction is variable (5%–95% of the hairy cells), and in about 5% (range, 5%–10%) of patients all peripheral blood and bone marrow cells may be normal. A few patients become diagnostic problems, and electron microscopy (ribosomal-lamellar complex in 60%) or testing for certain antigens (e.g., HLA-DR) may be helpful.

CHRONIC LYMPHOCYTIC LEUKEMIA

The lymphocytes of CLL are B lymphocytes, although there are about 2%–3% (range, 2%–5%) of cases that consist of T lymphocytes. The disease is usually found after the age of 50. It is twice as common in men than in women. Average survival is 3–7 years after diagnosis, with an appreciable number of patients alive at 8–10 years. Various chromosome abnormalities are reported in about 50% of patients. Total WBC counts are usually elevated; in one study about 10% were normal; about 45% were between 10,000 and 50,000/cu mm ($10–50 \times 10^9$/L), about 15% were between 50,000 and 100,000/cu mm, and about 35% were more than 100,000/cu mm. The majority (frequently, the great majority) of the WBCs are lymphocytes; of these, most (often nearly all) are mature types. In some patients there may be a considerable number of prolymphocytes and even some blasts, but this is not common. There is mild to moderate normocytic-normochromic anemia, usually without reticulocytosis. Platelets are decreased in approximately 40% of cases, but this may not occur until late in the disease. The bone marrow contains at least 20% lymphocytes and usually more than 50%. There is splenomegaly in 65%–75% of cases, usually to at least moderate degree, and moderate adenopathy in 65%–85% of cases. Hepatomegaly is found in approximately 50% of patients. Occasionally the splenomegaly and adenopathy are marked. There is a considerable tendency to infection, and this is often the cause of death. A Coombs-positive autoimmune hemolytic anemia is reported in about 10% (5%–20%) of cases; a Coombs-negative hemolytic anemia, often without a reticulocytosis, eventually develops in 15%–25% of cases. About 50% (40%–77%) of patients eventually develop some degree of hypogammaglobulinemia, with any or all of the major immunoglobulins (IgG, IgA, and IgM) being involved. There is some disagreement as to which of the three is most frequently decreased. Up to 5% of CLL patients develop a serum monoclonal protein like those produced in myeloma.

In the majority of patients with CLL the disease is relatively benign and only slowly progressive over a period of several years. In approximately 20% the disease is more aggressive. Whether this represents a distinct subset of CLL or simply diagnosis relatively late in the course of their disease is still being debated. Patients with CLL have an increased chance of developing a second malignancy, most often a carcinoma. This tendency is disputed by some but has been reported to be as high as 34%. One well-recognized condition is called Richter's syndrome, in which approximately 5% (literature range, 3%–15%) of CLL cases evolve into or develop non-Hodgkin's lymphoma, most commonly the large cell type (histiocytic lymphoma in the Rappaport classification). About 1.5% (0%–6.9%) of CLL cases terminate in a "blast crisis." The majority are ALL, but acute myeloblastic leukemia (AML) and others have been reported. Finally, a few patients with CLL develop transformation to prolymphocytic leukemia, which is more aggressive. Prolymphocytic leukemia can also exist without known previous CLL but is very uncommon.

CHRONIC MYELOGENOUS (GRANULOCYTIC) LEUKEMIA

Chronic myelogenous leukemia is most common between the ages of 20 and 50 and is rare in childhood. There is an increased (total) peripheral WBC count in more than 95% of patients, with about 70% more than 50,000/cu mm (50×10^9/L) and about 45% more than 100,000/cu mm. There is usually a predominance of myeloid cells having intermediate degrees of maturity, such as the myelocyte and early metamyelocyte. In fact, the peripheral blood smear often looks like a bone marrow aspirate. Anemia is usually present, although initially it is often slight. Later, anemia becomes moderate. There may be mild reticulocytosis with polychromatophilia, and occasionally there are a few nucleated RBCs in the peripheral blood. Platelets are normal in about 75% of patients and increased in the remainder, with about 8% having thrombocytosis more than 1,000,000/cu mm. Average patient survival is 2–4 years after onset. Terminally, 70%–80% of patients develop a picture of acute leukemia (the blast crisis); about 70% of these are AML and about 30% are ALL or rarely some other type.

Bone marrow aspiration in CML shows a markedly hypercellular marrow due to the granulocytes, with intermediate degrees of immaturity. In this respect, it resembles the peripheral blood picture. Some patients develop varying degrees of marrow fibrosis and can therefore simulate myelofibrosis (myeloid metaplasia, discussed later).

On physical examination there are varying degrees of adenopathy and organomegaly. The spleen is often greatly enlarged, and the liver may be moderately enlarged. Lymph nodes are often easily palpable but generally are only slightly to moderately increased in size.

Many patients with CML have an increased number of basophils in the peripheral blood. The reason for the basophilia is not known.

An interesting aspect of CML is the presence of a specific chromosome abnormality called the *Philadelphia chromosome* in the leukemic cells of most patients. No other neoplasm thus far has such a consistent cytogenetic abnormality. The abnormality involves the breaking off of a portion of the long arm of chromosome number 22 (formerly thought to be number 21) of the 21-22 group in the Denver classification (G group by letter classification); the broken-off chromosome segment is usually translocated to chromosome number 9. The abnormal chromosome 22 (Philadelphia chromosome) is found in approximately 85%–90% of patients with CML (reported range, 60%–95%). Those not having it seem as a group to have a worse prognosis. Interestingly, the Philadelphia chromosome has also been reported in about 25% of patients with adult-onset ALL and in some patients with the ALL variant of CML blast crisis.

Philadelphia chromosome detection usually involves cytogenetic chromosome analysis, that is, separating the chromosomes from several body cells and visually inspecting each chromosome for abnormality. It is now possible to use the nucleic acid probe (see "DNA Probe," chapter 14) technique for the same purpose. There is a gene area called bcr (breakpoint cluster region) in chromosome 22 that develops a crack or fissure to which a genetic area called c-abl (located at one end of the long arm of chromosome 9) becomes attached and fused. The restructured chromosome 22 with the grafted DNA material from chromosome 9 now has a hybrid gene bcr-abl at the fusion area. There is some evidence that this abnormal hybrid gene may have a role in the events that lead to the development of CML (therefore acting as an oncogene). A DNA probe can be constructed to detect the new hybrid gene; this has been called by some "bcr gene rearrangement assay." The DNA probe method has certain advantages over the cytogenetic method. The DNA probe can be used on peripheral blood specimens, does not require bone marrow, does not need dividing cells, and analyzes thousands of cells—vs. less than 20 by cytogenetic analysis. In addition, the DNA probe is claimed to be a little more sensitive than cytogenetic analysis.

At present, the bcr rearrangement assay is only available in a very few laboratories.

AGNOGENIC MYELOID METAPLASIA

A disease that is often very difficult to separate from CML is agnogenic (idiopathic) myeloid metaplasia (AMM). It is most common in persons aged 50–60 years. The syndrome results from bone marrow failure and subsequent extramedullary hematopoiesis on a large scale in the spleen and sometimes in the liver and lymph nodes. Actually, the extramedullary hematopoiesis is compensatory and therefore is not idiopathic (agnogenic), but the bone marrow failure is agnogenic. The bone marrow typically shows extensive replacement by fibrous tissue (myelofibrosis), but in an early stage AMM may present with a normally cellular or even hypercellular marrow and such minimal fibrosis that reticulum stains are required to demonstrate abnormality. The average life span after diagnosis is 5–7 years. One percent to 5% of patients eventually develop acute leukemia.

Although marrow fibrosis is typically associated with AMM, varying degrees of fibrosis have been reported in 15%–30% of patients with polycythemia vera and in some patients with CML, hairy cell leukemia, acute leukemia, metastatic carcinoma to bone marrow, and multiple myeloma.

In AMM there is a normochromic anemia of mild to moderate degree and usually a moderate degree of reticulocytosis. The peripheral blood smear typically contains a moderate number of polychromatophilic RBCs and varying numbers of later-stage nucleated RBCs as well as moderate RBC anisocytosis and poikilocytosis. Teardrop RBCs are characteristic of AMM and are usually (although not always) present in varying numbers. The WBC counts in AMM are most often in the 12,000–50,000/cu mm (12–50 × 10^9/L) range (approximately 40% of cases), but a substantial proportion of patients have counts within reference limits (20%–35% of cases), and a significant number have leukopenia (10%–30% of cases). About 7% have WBC counts over 50,000/cu mm (literature range 0%–18%). Peripheral blood differential counts usually show mild or moderate myeloid immaturity centering on metamyelocytes and band forms with some myelocytes present, similar to the picture of CML. The number of basophils is increased in approximately 35% of cases. The number of platelets is normal in 40%–50% of cases, increased in approximately 40% (literature range, 8%–48%), and decreased in 20%–25% (literature range, 10%–40%). Giant platelets are often found. Splenomegaly is present in more than 95% of cases (literature range, 92%–100%), and hepatomegaly is also common (approximately 75% of cases; literature range, 55%–86%). Splenomegaly is present even when the WBC count is relatively low. Lymphadenopathy is not common (approximately 10% of cases; literature range, 0%–29%).

One uncommon variant of AMM has been reported under the name of "acute myelofibrosis." The typical picture is pancytopenia, normal peripheral blood RBC morphology, lack of splenomegaly, and typical myelofibrosis on bone marrow examination. Most of the patients were over age 50, and most died in less than 1 year. All of the patients had blast cells in the peripheral blood, in most cases less than 15% but occasionally in greater numbers. Cases of acute myelofibrosis are difficult to separate from atypical cases of AMM (which occasionally terminates in a blast crisis, like CML), atypical cases of AML (in which a fibrotic bone marrow occasionally develops), and some patients with CML who develop some degree of marrow fibrosis and then progress to a blast crisis.

LEUKEMOID REACTION

Leukemoid reaction is an abnormally marked granulocytic response to some bone marrow stimulus, most commonly infection. Leukemoid reaction is basically the same process as an ordinary leukocytosis except in the degree of response. The expected peripheral blood WBC count response is even more marked than usual and may reach the 50,000–100,000/cu mm (50–100 × 10^9/L) range in some cases. Instead of the mild degree of immaturity expected, which would center in the band neutrophil stage, the immature tendency ("shift to the left"; see chapter 6) may be extended to earlier cells, such as the myelocyte. The bone marrow may show considerable myeloid hyperplasia with unusual immaturity. However, the number of early forms in either the peripheral blood or bone marrow is not usually as great as in classic CML. There is no basophilia, although the increased granulation often seen in neutrophils during severe infection ("toxic granulation") is sometimes mistaken for basophilia. The bone marrow in leukemoid reaction is moderately hyperplastic and may show mild immaturity but, again, is not quite as immature as in CML. Splenomegaly and lymphadenopathy may be present in a leukemoid reaction due to the underlying infection, but the spleen is usually not as large as in classic CML.

One other phenomenon that could be confused with CML is the so-called leukoerythroblastic marrow response (chapter 6) seen with moderate frequency in widespread involvement of the bone marrow by metastatic cancer and occasionally in diseases such as severe hemolytic anemia, severe hemorrhage, and septicemia. Anemia is present, and both immature WBCs and nucleated RBCs appear in the peripheral blood.

DIFFERENTIAL DIAGNOSIS OF CHRONIC MYELOGENOUS LEUKEMIA, AGNOGENIC MYELOID METAPLASIA, AND LEUKEMOID REACTION

When CML has the typical picture of a WBC count more than 100,000/cu mm (100×10^9/L) with myelocytic predominance, increased platelets, and basophilia, the diagnosis is reasonably safe. Otherwise, the two conditions that most frequently enter the differential diagnosis are agnogenic myeloid metaplasia and leukemoid reaction. Chronic myelogenous leukemia tends to have a greater degree of leukocytosis than AMM or leukemoid reactions, so that WBC counts more than 100,000/cu mm are more likely to be CML. An increased basophil count is more likely to occur in CML than in AMM and is not expected in leukemoid reactions. More than an occasional teardrop cell is more often seen in AMM than in CML, whereas teardrop cells are not expected in leukemoid reactions.

Bone marrow examination is a valuable differentiating procedure for CML, AMM, and leukemoid or leukoerythroblastic reactions. Chronic myelogenous leukemia has a hypercellular marrow with a moderate degree of immaturity; AMM most often has a marrow with varying degrees of fibrosis (although a hypercellular marrow may occur); and bone marrow in leukoerythroblastic reactions due to metastatic tumor frequently contains tumor cells. Clot sections as well as smears are desirable to increase diagnostic accuracy. In some patients with AMM and occasionally in patients with bone marrow tumor metastasis, no marrow can be obtained by aspiration, and a bone biopsy is necessary to be certain that the problem was not due to technical factors but to actual absence of marrow.

Although these distinguishing features suggest that differentiation between CML and AMM should be easy, the differences may be slight and the differentiating elements may at times appear in either disease. In fact, CML and AMM have been classified together under the term "myeloproliferative syndrome." Some workers include the whole spectrum of leukemic-type proliferations of granulocytes, RBCs, and platelets within this term.

Leukocyte alkaline phosphatase (LAP) stain is the second useful test for differentiating leukemoid reaction, CML, and AMM. A fresh peripheral blood smear is stained with a reagent that colors the alkaline phosphatase granules normally found in the cytoplasm of mature and moderately immature neutrophils. One hundred neutrophils are counted, each neutrophil is graded 0 to 4+, depending on the amount of alkaline phosphatase it possesses, and the total count (score) for the 100 cells is added up. In most patients with leukemoid reaction or simple leukocytosis due to infection, or leukocytosis of pregnancy or estrogen therapy (birth control pills), and in 80%–90% of patients with polycythemia vera, the score is higher than reference range. About two thirds of patients with AMM have elevated values, about 25% have values within normal limits, and about 10% have low values. In CML, about 90% of patients have below-normal values, but 5%–10% reportedly have normal values. Values may be normal in CML during remission, blast crisis, or superimposed infection. In acute leukemia, each cell type differs in percentage of LAP values that are low, normal, or high, but results are not sufficiently clear cut to provide adequate cell type diagnosis. Overlap and borderline cases limit the usefulness of LAP in establishing a definitive diagnosis; however, values that are elevated are substantial evidence against CML, whereas values that are definitely low suggest CML rather than AMM. An experienced technician is needed to make the test reliable because the test reagents often give trouble, and the reading of the results is subjective and sometimes is not easy. Therefore, diagnosis should not be based on this test alone. In obvious cases, there is no need to do this test.

The LAP value is elevated in many patients with "active" Hodgkin's disease. Infectious mononucleosis in early stages is associated with low or normal values in 95% of cases. In sickle cell anemia, LAP values are decreased even though WBCs are increased; however, if infection is superimposed, there may be an LAP increase (although a normal LAP value does not rule out infection). Low values are found in paroxysmal nocturnal hemoglobinuria.

A cytogenetic or DNA probe study for the Philadelphia chromosome is a third test that may be helpful in occasional diagnostic problems. Presence of the Philadelphia chromosome in a clinical and laboratory setting suspicious for chronic leukemia would be strong evidence in favor of CML.

POLYCYTHEMIA

Polycythemia is an increase in the total blood RBCs over the upper limit of the reference range. This usually entails a concurrent increase in hemoglobin and hematocrit values. Since various studies disagree somewhat on the values that should be considered the upper limits of normal, partially arbitrary criteria are used to define polycythemia. A hemoglobin level more than 18 gm/100 ml (180 g/L) for men and 16 gm/100 ml (160 g/L) for women with a hematocrit of more than 55% for men and 50% for women are generally considered consistent with polycythemia.

Polycythemia may be divided into three groups: primary (polycythemia vera), secondary, and relative.

Polycythemia vera has sometimes been included with CML and AMM as a myeloproliferative disease. Polycythemia vera is most frequent in persons between ages 40 and 70 years. Splenomegaly occurs in 60%–90% of patients and is more common in those with leukocytosis. Hepatomegaly is less frequent but still common (40%–50%). Polycythemia vera is reported to progress to myelofibrosis with myeloid metaplasia in about 20%–25% (range, 15%–30%) of cases, usually in 5–15 years. Five percent to 6% of polycythemia vera cases terminate in acute leukemia; this is more frequent after therapy with radioactive phosphorus (average, 10%–20% of cases) or after chlorambucil chemotherapy. The incidence of acute leukemia after phlebotomy therapy is not known with certainty but is believed to be considerably less than that associated with radioactive phosphorus. Clinically, there is an increased incidence of peptic ulcer and gout and a definite tendency toward the development of venous thrombosis.

Laboratory Picture.—In classic cases, peripheral blood WBC counts and platelets are also increased with the RBC counts; however, this is not always found. The peripheral blood WBC count is more than 10,000/cu mm (10×10^9/L) in 50%–70% of the cases. About 20%–30% of patients have leukocytosis of more than 15,000/cu mm with relatively mature forms; about 10% have leukocytosis of more than 15,000/cu mm with a moderate degree of neutrophil immaturity (myelocytes and metamyelocytes present). Platelets are elevated in about 25% of cases. There may be small numbers of polychromatophilic RBCs in the peripheral blood, but these are not usually prominent. Bone marrow aspirates usually show marrow hyperplasia with an increase in all three blood element precursors—WBCs, RBCs, and megakaryocytes and with absent marrow iron. A marrow section is much more valuable than marrow smears to demonstrate this. The serum uric acid level is elevated in up to 40% of cases due to the increased RBC turnover.

The classic triad of greatly increased RBC mass (hemoglobin and hematocrit), leukocytosis with thrombocytosis, and splenomegaly makes the diagnosis obvious. However, the hemoglobin and hematocrit values are often only moderately elevated, and one or both of the other features may be lacking. The problem then is to differentiate between polycythemia vera and the other causes of polycythemia.

True polycythemia refers to an increase in the total RBC mass (quantity). *Relative polycythemia* is a term used to describe a normal total RBC mass that falsely appears increased due to a decrease in plasma volume. Dehydration is the most common cause of relative polycythemia; in most cases, the hematocrit value is high-normal or only mildly increased, but occasionally it may be substantially elevated. In simple dehydration, the values of other blood constituents, such as the WBCs, electrolytes, and blood urea nitrogen, also tend to be (falsely) elevated. The most definitive test is a blood volume study (chapter 11), which will demonstrate that the RBC mass is normal. Stress polycythemia (Gaisböck's syndrome) also is a relative polycythemia due to diminished plasma volume. Most persons affected are middle-aged men; there is a strong tendency toward mild degrees of hypertension, arteriosclerosis, and obesity.

Secondary polycythemia is a true polycythemia, but, as the name implies, there is a specific underlying cause for the increase in RBC mass. The most common cause is either hypoxia (due to chronic lung disease but sometimes to congenital heart disease or life at high altitudes) or heavy cigarette smoking ("smoker's polycythemia," due to carboxyhemoglobin formation). In some cases associated with heavy smoking the RBC mass is within reference limits but the plasma volume is reduced, placing this group into the category of relative polycythemia. Cushing's syndrome is frequently associated with mild, sometimes moderate, polycythemia. A much less common etiology is tumor, most frequently renal carcinoma (hypernephroma) and hepatic carcinoma (hepatoma). The incidence of polycythemia is 1%–5% in renal carcinoma and 3%–12% in hepatoma. The rare tumor cerebellar hemangioblastoma is associated with polycythemia in 15%–20% of cases. There are several other causes, such as marked obesity (pickwickian syndrome), but these are rare.

Laboratory Tests Useful to Differentiate Secondary and Relative Polycythemia From Polycythemia Vera

1. *Blood volume measurements* (RBC mass plus total blood volume) can rule out relative polycythemia. In relative polycythemia there is a decreased total blood volume (or plasma volume) and a normal RBC mass.

2. Arterial blood oxygen saturation studies frequently help to rule out hypoxic (secondary) polycythemia. Arterial oxygen saturation should be normal in polycythemia vera and decreased in hypoxic (secondary) polycythemia. Caution is indicated, however, since patients with polycythemia vera may have some degree of lowered PO_2 or oxygen saturation from a variety of conditions superimposed on the hematologic disease. In smoker's polycythemia, arterial blood oxygen saturation measured directly by a special instrument is reduced, but oxygen saturation estimated in the usual way from blood gas data obtained by ordinary blood gas analysis equipment is normal. In heavy smokers with polycythemia, a blood carboxyhemoglobin assay may be useful if arterial oxygen saturation values are within reference limits. A carboxyhemoglobin level more than 4% is compatible with smoker's polycythemia (although not absolute proof of the diagnosis).

3. *Leukocyte alkaline phosphatase* is elevated in approximately 90% of patients with polycythemia vera; the elevation occurs regardless of the WBC count. Elevated LAP is unlikely in other causes of polycythemia unless infection or inflammation is also present.

4. *Bone marrow aspiration or biopsy* is often useful, as stated earlier. If aspiration is performed, a marrow section (from clotted marrow left in the syringe and fixed in formalin or Bouin-type fixatives, then processed like tissue biopsy material) is much better than marrow smears for this purpose. However, even bone marrow sections are not always diagnostic. In one study, about 5% of patients had normal or slightly increased overall marrow cellularity in conjunction with normal or only slightly increased numbers of megakaryocytes.

5. *Erythropoietin hormone assay* may be needed in a few equivocal cases (in most instances this would not be necessary). In polycythemia vera, erythropoietin levels are decreased, whereas in relative or secondary polycythemia, erythropoietin levels are normal or increased.

6. An elevated *serum uric acid level* without other cause favors the diagnosis of polycythemia vera, since secondary polycythemia is associated with normal uric acid values. However, since uric acid is normal in many cases of polycythemia vera, a normal value is not helpful.

MALIGNANT LYMPHOMAS

The malignant lymphomas include Hodgkin's disease and non-Hodgkin's lymphomas; both are derived from lymphoid tissue, predominantly from lymph nodes. Lymph nodes are composed of two parts, germinal centers and lymphoreticular tissue. The germinal centers contain lymphoblasts and reticulum cells;

these produce the mature lymphocytes and reticulum cells that form the remainder of the lymphoid tissue. Therefore, three main cell types exist in lymph nodes (and other lymphoid tissue): reticulum cells, lymphoblasts, and lymphocytes. Malignancy may arise from any of these three cell types.

Histologic Classification of the non-Hodgkin's Lymphomas

Rappaport's Classification

In Rappaport's classification, the non-Hodgkin's lymphomas are divided into three types based on whatever cell of origin is suggested by the microscopic appearance: lymphocytic lymphoma, histiocytic lymphoma (originally called *reticulum cell sarcoma*), and undifferentiated. Lymphocytic lymphoma (originally called *lymphosarcoma*) may, in turn, be subdivided into well-differentiated and poorly differentiated (lymphoblastic) types, depending on the predominant degree of differentiation of the lymphoid cells (Table 7–3). Besides the degree of differentiation, malignant lymphomas may exist in two architectural patterns, nodular and diffuse. In the nodular type, the lymphomatous tissue is distributed in focal aggregates or nodules. In the diffuse type, the lymphomatous cells diffusely and completely replace the entire lymph node or the nonlymphoid area invaded. Hodgkin's disease, which will be discussed later, also exists in a nodular or diffuse form, although the nodular variety is rare. In the malignant lymphomas as a group, the diffuse pattern is more frequent than the nodular one.

In general, the nodular pattern carries a better prognosis than the corresponding diffuse pattern. The better the cell differentiation, the better the prognosis, just as in the leukemias. The most frequent histologic types of non-Hodgkin's lymphoma are poorly differentiated lymphocytic and mixed types.

Histiocytic lymphoma may be found with different nuclear types, but the various possible subclassifications all have roughly the same prognosis. Untreated histiocytic lymphoma has a prognosis comparable with that of acute leukemia. The same is true for the poorly differentiated lymphocytic lymphomas.

The nodular form of lymphoma has been called *Brill-Symmer's disease*, or *giant follicular lymphoma*. This was originally thought to have a relatively good prognosis. However, many believe that this terminology should be abandoned, since evidence exists that prognosis depends as much on the cell type as on the architectural pattern. This would suggest that the poorly differentiated or more primitive cell types do not have a good prognosis even when they appear in a nodular ("follicular") form.

It is interesting that 20%–30% of non-Hodgkin's lymphomas of the nodular or the better differentiated type are reported to eventually undergo change to a diffuse pattern or a less favorable nuclear type.

Rappaport's classification has been criticized by various investigators. Some wish to include more subclassifications, whereas others believe that the terminology does not reflect cell origin correctly. The majority of cases that would be classified as histiocytic by Rappaport's criteria have been shown to display reactions to special stains or certain antibodies that are more typical of lymphoid cells than histiocytes. Nevertheless, Rappaport's classification is the one most frequently used in the United States and seems to provide a fairly reliable index of prognosis.

TABLE 7–3.
Histologic Classification of Non-Hodgkin's Malignant Lymphomas (Rappaport Modified)

Cell Type	Histologic Tissue Pattern
Lymphocytic lymphoma	
Well differentiated	All types: nodular or diffuse (nodular type rare in well-differentiated lymphocytic lymphoma and Burkitt's)
Moderately well differentiated*	
Poorly differentiated	
Lymphoblastic*	
Histiocytic lymphoma	
Mixed cell (lymphocytic-histiocytic)	
Undifferentiated	
Burkitt's*	
Non-Burkitt's*	

*Subcategories added since the original publication.

Immunologic Characterization of Malignant Lymphomas

Most classifications of hematopoietic malignancies are based on cell morphology and tissue pattern (often including interpretation of cell origin or even cell function as estimated from morphology). Work that characterizes malignancies involving lymphocytes according to phylogenetic origin of the cells (referred to previously in the section on acute leukemia) has been presented. Lymphocytes have two origins: thymus-derived (T) cells, which functionally are responsible for delayed hypersensitivity cell-mediated immune reactions; and bone marrow–derived (B) cells, which are involved with immune reactions characterized by immunoglobulin (antibody) production. T cells in lymph nodes are located in the deep layers of the cortex and in a thin zone surrounding the germinal centers. B cells are located in germinal centers and in the outer cortex of lymph nodes; they are precursors of plasma cells. In general, most work to date indicates that multiple myeloma, 98% of CLL, Burkitt's lymphoma, and approximately 75% of lymphocytic lymphomas (especially the better-differentiated varieties) are of B-cell origin. In childhood ALL about 20% of cases are T cell, about 2% are B cell, and 75% are non-T, non-B and do not react in E rosette or surface immunoglobulin tests. The T-cell subgroup of childhood ALL has many clinical features in common with a subgroup of the non-Hodgkin's lymphomas (the lymphoblastic lymphoma of Rappaport's classification or the convoluted lymphocytic lymphoma of the Lukes-Collins classification; the same neoplasm was referred to in the older literature as Sternberg's sarcoma). These features include presence of a mediastinal tumor mass, onset in later childhood or adolescence, predominance in males, and poor prognosis. Other T-cell malignancies include mycosis fungoides and the Sézary syndrome, both sometimes referred to as "cutaneous lymphomas."

TABLE 7–4.
Lukes-Collins Classification of Non-Hodgkin's Lymphomas

I. U-cell (undefined cell) type
II. T-cell types
  1. Mycosis fungoides and Sézary's syndrome
  2. Convoluted lymphocyte
  3. Immunoblastic sarcoma of T cells
III. B-cell types
  1. Small lymphocyte (CLL)
  2. Plasmacytoid lymphocyte
  3. Follicular center cell (FCC) types (follicular, diffuse, follicular and diffuse, and sclerotic patterns)
    a. Small cleaved
    b. Large cleaved
    c. Small noncleaved
    d. Large noncleaved
  4. Immunoblastic sarcoma of B cells
IV. Histiocytic type
V. Unclassifiable

Lukes-Collins Classification

Lukes and Collins have published a classification of non-Hodgkin's lymphomas based on results of immunologic testing of lymphomas, the morphologic appearance of the cell nucleus plus cell size, and their concept of lymphoid cell maturation (Table 7–4). This classification has proved attractive to many institutions because it places those lymphomas of Rappaport's "histiocytic" category that are actually lymphocytic rather than histiocytic into the lymphocytic lymphoma category and emphasizes cell appearance rather than prediction of cell type. The major problem with the Lukes-Collins classification is that it is frequently difficult to decide whether to assign cells with large noncleaved nuclei to the category of large noncleaved follicular center cells or to the category of immunoblastic sarcoma.

National Cancer Institute Lymphoma Panel Working Formulation

In 1980, a panel of well-known authorities on histopathology of malignant lymphomas, collectively known as the National Cancer Institute (NCI) Non-Hodgkin's Lymphoma Pathologic Classification Project, met in Palo Alto, California, and by 1982 developed a new classification of non-Hodgkin's lymphoma (Table 7–5), which they called the "Working Formulation." This classification combines some features of Rappaport's classification (nodular and diffuse patterns, mixed cell pattern) with the basic nuclear morphologic descriptive terms of Lukes and Collins, plus subdivision by degrees of malignancy as found in the British and Kiel (German) classifications. Although the NCI Working Formulation has somewhat improved pathologist agreement in lymphoma classification, even experts in lymphoma pathology do not unanimously agree in about 15% of cases.

Burkitt's Lymphoma

Burkitt's lymphoma is a B-cell variant of malignant lymphoma that was originally reported in African children. It is now known to occur in children elsewhere in the world. In African Burkitt's lymphoma, about 50%–70% of affected persons have involvement of the jaw, a site rarely affected by other lymphomas. In non-African Burkitt's lymphoma, the jaw area is involved in only 12%–18% of patients, a tumor mass is frequently located in the abdomen, single peripheral lymph node groups are involved in about 30% of patients, and widespread peripheral lymphadenopathy is rare. Histologically, the cell nuclei are rather uniform in appearance, and sheets of these cells characteristically include scattered single cells exhibiting phagocytosis ("starry sky appearance"). Appearance of individual Burkitt's cells resembles that of the FAB acute leukemia B-cell category, and occasional Burkitt's lymphoma patients in the United States have developed ALL. In addition, occasional patients in the United States have been young adults rather than children. There is a strong association with Epstein-Barr virus infection in African Burkitt's but much less evidence of Epstein-Barr in American Burkitt's lymphoma.

TABLE 7–5.

Classification of Non-Hodgkin's Lymphomas: Non-Hodgkin's Lymphoma Pathologic Classification Project

Low grade
Small (noncleaved) lymphocytic
Follicular* lymphoma, predominantly small cleaved cell
Follicular lymphoma, mixed small cleaved and large cell
Intermediate grade
Follicular lymphoma, predominantly large cell
Diffuse small cleaved cell
Diffuse mixed small and large cell
Diffuse large cell (cleaved/noncleaved)
High grade
Diffuse large cell of immunoblastic type
Lymphoblastic (convoluted/nonconvoluted)
Small noncleaved cell (Burkitt's/non-Burkitt's)

*Follicular = nodular.

Hodgkin's Disease

Hodgkin's disease is usually considered a subgroup of the malignant lymphomas. The basic neoplastic cell is the malignant reticulum cell. Some of these malignant reticulum cells take on a binucleated or multinucleated form with distinctive large nucleoli and are called *Reed-Sternberg* (R-S) cells. These are the diagnostic cells of Hodgkin's disease.

Other types of cells may accompany the R-S cells. Therefore, Hodgkin's disease is usually subdivided according to the cell types present (Fig 7–2). Besides R-S cells there may be various combinations of lymphocytes, histiocytes, eosinophils, neutrophils, plasma cells, and reticulum cells. The main histologic forms of Hodgkin's disease are the following (using a classification developed by the U.S. Armed Forces Institute of Pathology):

1. Paragranuloma: Lymphocytes only (plus R-S cells)
2. Lymphohistiocytic: Lymphocytes and histiocytes (plus R-S cells)
3. Granuloma: At least three different cell types (plus R-S cells)
4. Nodular sclerosing: A peculiar variation of granuloma that occurs predominantly in the mediastinum and cervical lymph nodes, characterized by a nodular pattern, the nodules separated by bands of fibrous tissue
5. Sclerosing: Rare; granuloma that is mostly replaced by spontaneous fibrosis
6. Sarcoma: Predominantly malignant reticulum cells (including R-S cells)

The most widely accepted pathologic classification today is the one developed by Lukes and co-workers at the Rye Conference in 1965 (see Fig 7–2). This classification combines certain histologic tissue patterns having similar prognosis, resulting in four groups instead of six. Of the groups, lymphocytic predominance comprises about 12% (range, 5%–17%) of patients with Hodgkin's disease, nodular sclerosing about 45% (27%–73%), mixed cellularity about 30% (16%–37%), and lymphocytic depletion about 10% (3%–23%). Prognosis is relatively good for untreated lymphocytic predominance (9–15 years' average survival after onset). Lymphocytic depletion behaves like histiocytic lymphoma or acute leukemia, with an average survival of 1 year or less. Mixed cellularity has an intermediate prognosis (average, 2–4 years' survival). The nodular sclerosing category as a group has a prognosis

LEUKEMIA, LYMPHOMAS, AND MYELOPROLIFERATIVE SYNDROMES

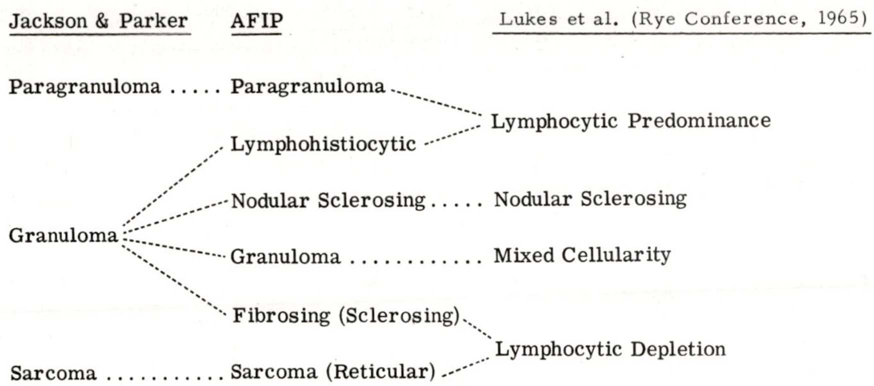

FIG 7–2.
Various histologic classifications of Hodgkin's disease.

between that of lymphocytic predominance and mixed cellularity with much individual variation; a considerable number of patients achieve the survival time of patients with lymphocytic predominance Hodgkin's disease. Life expectancy in Hodgkin's disease is quite variable, even without treatment, and some patients live for many years with the lymphocytic predominance, nodular sclerosing, and even the mixed cellularity forms.

Also of great importance, especially for therapy, is the degree of spread when the patient is first seen (Table 7–6). Localized Hodgkin's disease has an encouraging possibility of cure by adequate radiotherapy. There is considerable correlation between the tissue histologic patterns and the clinical stage (degree of localization) of disease when first seen.

TABLE 7–6.
Clinical Staging of the Malignant Lymphomas*†

Stage I	Localized in one group of lymph nodes
IE	Localized involvement (one area) of one extralymphatic organ or site
Stage II	Localized in two separate groups of lymph nodes on the same side of the diaphragm
IIE	Localized in one group of lymph nodes plus localized involvement of one extralymphatic organ or site (including spleen) on the same side of the diaphragm
Stage III	Involving components of the lymphoid system (including spleen) on both sides of the diaphragm
IIIE	Involving components of the lymphoid system on both sides of the diaphragm plus localized involvement of one extralymphatic organ or site
Stage IV	Diffuse or disseminated involvement of one or more extralymphatic organs or sites with or without lymph node involvement.

*Ann Arbor revision of Peter's classification.
†In Hodgkin's disease, patients are additionally subclassified as A or B, according to whether systemic symptoms are absent (A) or present (B).

Clinical Findings in Malignant Lymphoma

Clinically, malignant lymphoma is more common in males. The peak incidence for Hodgkin's disease is age 20–40, and age 40–60 for other malignant lymphomas. Lymph node enlargement is found in the great majority of cases but may not become manifest until later. Fever is present at some time in at least one half of patients. Staging laparotomy has shown that splenic Hodgkin's disease occurs in 35%–40% of cases; if this occurs, para-aortic nodes are usually involved. Liver metastasis is found in 5%–10% of cases; if the liver is involved, the spleen is always invaded. In non-Hodgkin's lymphoma, laparotomy discloses splenic involvement in 30%–40% and hepatic metastasis in 10%–20% of cases, with rather wide variation according to histologic classification. Splenomegaly is not reliable as a criterion for presence of splenic tumor. Bone marrow metastasis is present at the time of diagnosis in 10%–60% of cases of non-Hodgkin's lymphoma and 5%–30% of cases of Hodgkin's disease. Lymphocytic lymphoma has a greater tendency to reach bone marrow, liver, or spleen than histiocytic lymphoma, and the nodular form is more likely to metastasize to these organs than the diffuse type.

Laboratory Findings in Malignant Lymphoma

Anemia is found in 33%–50% of cases and is most common in Hodgkin's disease and least common in histiocytic lymphoma. Occasionally, this anemia becomes overtly hemolytic. The platelet count is usually normal unless the bone marrow is extensively infiltrated. The WBC count is usually normal in non-Hodgkin's lymphoma until late in the disease; in Hodgkin's disease, it is more often mildly increased but may be normal or decreased. White blood cell differential counts are usually normal in malignant lymphoma unless malignant cells disseminate into the peripheral blood or, more commonly, if some other condition is superimposed, such as infection. In Hodgkin's disease, eosinophilia may occur; in late stages, leukopenia and lymphopenia may be present. Bone marrow needle biopsy in both Hodgkin's and non-Hodgkin's lymphoma demonstrates bone marrow involvement more frequently than clot sections or smears. A second biopsy increases the yield by 10%–20%.

Diagnosis of Malignant Lymphoma

Diagnosis of the malignant lymphomas is established by tissue biopsy, usually lymph node biopsy. The particular node selected is important. The inguinal nodes should be avoided, if possible, because they often contain changes due to chronic inflammation that tend to obscure the tissue pattern of a lymphoma. If several nodes are enlarged, the largest one should be selected; when it is excised, the entire node should be taken out intact. This helps to preserve the architectural pattern and permits better evaluation of possible invasion outside the node capsule, one of the histologic criteria for malignancy.

Differential Diagnosis of Malignant Lymphoma

Several diseases enter into the differential diagnosis of malignant lymphoma. Tuberculosis, sarcoidosis, and infectious mononucleosis all produce fever, lymphadenopathy, and, frequently, splenomegaly. The atypical lymphocytes of infectious mononucleosis (chapter 16) may simulate lymphocytic lymphoma cells, since both are abnormal lymphocytic forms. Usually lymphoma cells in the peripheral blood are either more immature or more distorted than the average infectious mononucleosis (virocyte) cell. Nevertheless, since infectious mononucleosis patients are usually younger persons, the finding of lymphadenopathy and a peripheral blood picture similar to infectious mononucleosis in a patient over age 40 would suggest lymphosarcoma (if some other viral illness is not present). Suspicion is intensified if results of the Paul-Bunnell (heterophil) test (chapter 16) are less than 1:28 or are 1:28–1:112 with a normal differential absorption pattern (two different determinations normal, done 2 weeks apart to detect any rising titer). Occasionally, rheumatoid-collagen diseases create a clinical picture suggestive of either an occult malignant lymphoma or its early stages. Phenytoin (Dilantin), smallpox vaccination, and certain skin diseases may produce a lymphadenopathy, which creates difficulty for both the clinician and the pathologist. Malignant lymphoma often enters into the differential diagnosis of splenomegaly, especially if no other disease is found to account for the splenomegaly.

LANGERHANS' CELL HISTIOCYTOSIS (HISTIOCYTOSIS X)

This term was coined to describe three closely related disorders characterized by proliferation of the Langerhans cell, a type of histiocyte. Histiocytosis X was the original term used for this group of diseases. The group comprises three well-known disorders and several rarer ones. *Letterer-Siwe disease* is a rapidly progressive, fatal condition that is seen mostly in early childhood and infancy. There is widespread involvement of bone, skin, visceral, and reticuloendothelial organs by atypical histiocytes, with accompanying anemia and thrombocytopenia. Bone marrow aspiration or, occasionally, lymph node biopsy is the usual diagnostic procedure. *Eosinophilic granuloma* is the benign member of the triad. It is seen most often in later childhood and most commonly presents as isolated bone lesions. These usually are single but may be multiple. The lungs are occasionally involved. The lesion is composed of histiocytes with many eosinophils and is diagnosed by direct biopsy. *Hand-Schüller-Christian disease* is somewhat intermediate between the other two in terms of chronicity and histology. Bone lesions, often multiple, are the major abnormalities. Soft tissue and reticuloendothelial organs may be affected. There may be very few systemic symptoms, or there may be anemia, leukopenia, and thrombocytopenia. The lesions are composed of histiocytes containing large amounts of cholesterol in the cytoplasm and accompanied by fibrous tissue and varying numbers of eosinophils. Diagnosis usually is by direct biopsy of a lesion.

Additional tests relevant to this chapter are described in chapter 35.

BIBLIOGRAPHY

Kantarjian HM, et al: Characteristics of accelerated disease in chronic myelogenous leukemia. *Cancer* 1988; 61:1441.

Najean Y, et al: Acute leukemia and myelodysplasia in polycythemia vera. *Cancer* 1988; 61:89.

Koeffler HP: Syndromes of acute nonlymphocytic leukemia. *Ann Intern Med* 1987; 107:748.

Kantarjian HM: Chronic myelogenous leukemia in blast crisis. *Am J Med* 1987; 83:445.

Dekmezian R, et al: The relevance of reticulin stain-measured fibrosis at diagnosis in chronic myelogenous leukemia. *Cancer* 1987; 59:1739.

Nanba K, et al: Agreement rates and American-Japanese pathologists' comparability of a modified Working Formulation for non-Hodgkin's lymphomas. *Cancer* 1987; 59:1463.

Kiyokawa T, et al: Hypercalcemia and osteoclast proliferation in adult T-cell leukemia. *Cancer* 1987; 59:1187.

bcr-abl in chronic myelogenous leukemia (editorial). *Lancet* 1986; 2:258.

Heim S, Mitelman F: Chromosome abnormalities in the myelodysplastic syndromes. *Clin Haematol* 1986; 15:1003.

York JC, et al: TdT in leukemia and lymphoma: I. Historic and pathophysiologic aspects. *Lab Mgmt* 1986; 24(1):39.

York JC, Nasrallah AG: TdT in leukemia and lymphoma: II. Applications. *Lab Mgmt* 1986; 24(3):53.

Bennett JM: Classification of the myelodysplastic syndromes. *Clin Haematol* 1986; 15:909.

Jacobs A, Clark RE: Pathogenesis and clinical variations in the myelodysplastic syndromes. *Clin Haematol* 1986; 15:925.

Kantarjian HM: Clinical and prognostic features of Philadelphia chromosome-negative chronic myelogenous leukemia. *Cancer* 1986; 58:2023.

Silver RT, Gale RP: Chronic myeloid leukemia. *Am J Med* 1986; 80:1137.

Burkart PT: Advances in the management of acute leukemia in adults. *Curr Concepts Oncol* 1986; 8(3):10.

Hait WN, et al: Non-Hodgkin's lymphoma for the nononcologist. *JAMA* 1985; 253:1431.

Bennett JM, et al: Proposed revised criteria for the classification of acute myeloid leukemia. *Ann Intern Med* 1985; 103:620.

Gale P, et al: Chronic lymphocytic leukemia. *Ann Intern Med* 1985; 103:101.

Waller KW, Bruzzese DB: Flow cytometry in the clinical laboratory. *Lab Med* 1985; 16:480.

Sariban E, et al: Jaw involvement in American Burkitt's lymphoma. *Cancer* 1984; 53:1777.

Wolde-Mariam W, Peter JB: Recent diagnostic advances in cellular immunology. *Diagn Med* 1984; 7(3):25.

Westbrook CA, Golumb HM: Hairy cell leukemia. *Curr Concepts Oncol* 1984; 6(4):4.

Pedraza MA, et al: Acute leukemias: Ultrastructural, cytochemical, and immunologic diagnostic approaches. *Lab Med* 1983; 14:45.

Varki A, et al: The syndrome of idiopathic myelofibrosis. *Medicine* (Baltimore) 1983; 62:353.

Rowe JM: Clinical and laboratory features of the myeloid and lymphocytic leukemias. *Am J Med Technol* 1983; 49:103.

Ruddles RA: Surface markers in non-Hodgkin's lymphomas. *Hosp Pract* 1983; 18:161.

Bartl R, et al: Bone marrow histology in Hairy Cell leukemia. *Am J Clin Pathol* 1983; 79:531.

Non-Hodgkin's Lymphoma Pathologic Classification Project: National Cancer Institute sponsored study of classifications of non-Hodgkin's lymphomas: Summary and description of a working formulation for clinical use. *Cancer* 1982; 49:2112.

Rupani M: Acute myelofibrosis. *Am J Clin Pathol* 1982; 77:475.

Roggli VL, Saleem A: Erythroleukemia. *Cancer* 1982; 49:101.

Foucar K, Goeken JA: Clinical application of immunologic techniques to the diagnosis of lymphoproliferative and immunodeficiency disorders. *Lab Med* 1982; 13:403.

Colby TV, et al: Hodgkin's disease: A clinicopathologic study of 659 cases. *Cancer* 1981; 49:1848.

Ziegler JL: Burkitt's lymphoma. *N Engl J Med* 1981; 305:735.

Nathwani BN: Lymphoblastic lymphoma. *Cancer* 1981; 48:2347.

Foucar K: Acute leukemias: Part 1. Acute lymphoblastic leukemias. *Lab Med* 1981; 12:404.

Foucar K: Acute leukemias: Part 2. Acute nonlymphocytic leukemias. *Lab Med* 1981; 12:473.

Golde DW, et al: Polycythemia: Mechanisms and management. *Ann Intern Med* 1981; 95:71.

Clark MA, et al: Pseudoleukemia. *Arch Pathol Lab Med* 1981; 105:122.

Kobrinsky NL, et al: Acute non-lymphocytic leukemia. *Pediatr Clin North Am* 1980; 27:345.

Glick AD: Acute leukemia of adults. *Am J Clin Pathol* 1980; 73:459.

Miller DR: Acute lymphoblastic leukemia. *Pediatr Clin North Am* 1980; 27:269.

Foucar K, Rydell RE: Richter's syndrome in chronic lymphocytic leukemia. *Cancer* 1980; 46:118.

McBride PA, et al: Polycythemia vera with myelofibrosis and myeloid metaplasia. *Am J Clin Pathol* 1980; 74:693.

Lukes RJ: The immunologic approach to the pathology of malignant lymphomas. *Am J Clin Pathol* 1979; 72:657.

8 Blood Coagulation

Normally, blood remains fluid within a closed vascular system. Abnormalities of blood coagulation take two main forms: failure to clot normally (and thus to prevent abnormal degrees of leakage from the vascular system) and failure to prevent excessive clotting (and thus to maintain the patency of the blood vessels). Most emphasis in clinical medicine has been on the diagnosis and treatment of clotting deficiency. To understand the various laboratory tests designed to pinpoint defects in the coagulation mechanism, we must outline the most currently accepted theory of blood coagulation (Fig 8–1).

BLOOD COAGULATION THEORY

According to current theories of blood coagulation, the clotting mechanism is activated in two ways. The first activation pathway begins either when the endothelial lining of a blood vessel is damaged or when blood comes into contact with certain types of foreign surfaces. This activating sequence is begun by substances normally present within blood and is therefore called the *intrinsic system pathway*. The second trigger is a substance, tissue thromboplastin, which is not present in blood but which can be released from endothelial cells or other body tissues, usually when the tissue cells are injured. Tissue thromboplastin, sometimes called *factor III*, initiates the *extrinisic system pathway*. Activation of the clotting sequence by extrinsic system thromboplastin bypasses the first half of the intrinsic system pathway, although both systems share several final pathway coagulation factor reaction sequences.

Extrinsic System

The extrinsic system tissue thromboplastin forms a complex with calcium ions and a proenzyme known as *factor VII*. Factor VII is normally inactive but now becomes activated by tissue thromboplastin. The thromboplastin complex with activated factor VII converts another inactive enzyme (proenzyme), *factor X*, to an active form. Activated factor X with two cofactors (phospholipid from tissue thromboplastin and activated factor V) in the presence of calcium ions converts prothrombin to thrombin. Thrombin, in turn, converts fibrinogen to fibrin monomer. Fibrin monomer polymerizes; the polymer then becomes "stabilized" (resistant to dissociation) by adding cross-linkages between molecules with the assistance of activated factor XIII. The stabilized fibrin also becomes insoluble in certain substances such as urea.

Intrinsic System

The intrinsic system is triggered by contact between blood and a suitable foreign surface. Within vessels, this usually occurs at a break in the vascular endothelial lining where collagen is exposed. Platelets adhere to the exposed collagen and release a phospholipid called *platelet factor 3*, or PF-3. In addition, a proenzyme in serum called *factor XII* becomes activated by exposure to the collagen. Activated factor XII initiates a side reaction involving high molecular weight kininogen (HMWK) as a cofactor, which converts a proenzyme called *prekallikrein*, to kallikrein which, in turn, helps convert more factor XII to its active form. The major consequence of activated factor XII is conversion of inactive factor

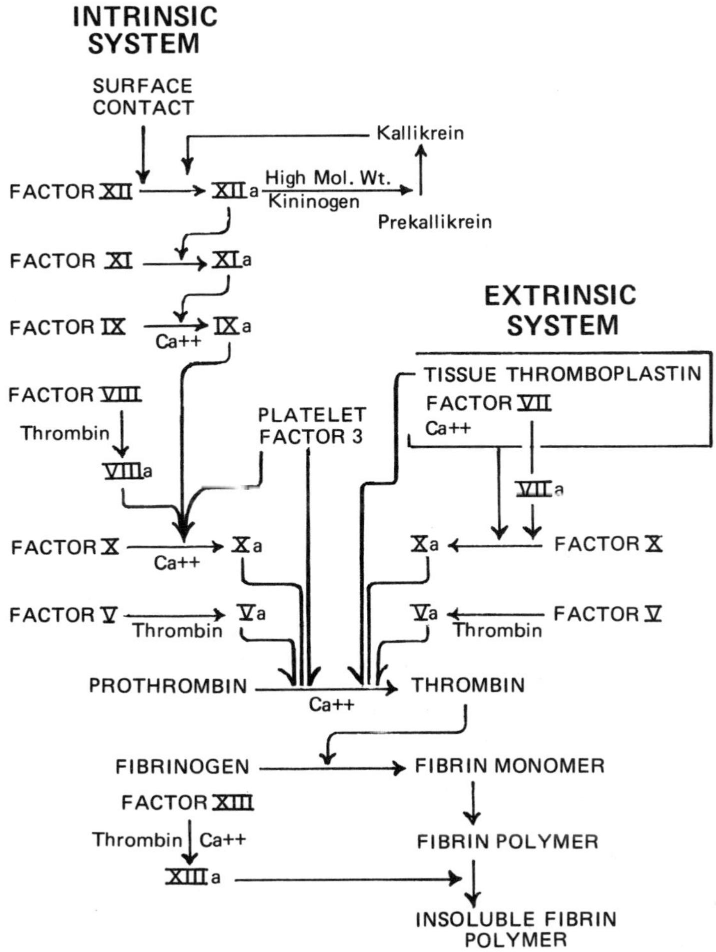

FIG 8–1.
Blood coagulation pathways.

XI to its active form, which, in turn, converts factor IX to its active form. Activated factor IX converts factor X to activated factor X with the assistance of activated factor VIII and PF-3 in the presence of calcium ions. (Thus, activated factors VIII and IX plus PF-3 produce the same effect as the tissue thromboplastin complex and activated factor VII. Tissue thromboplastin supplies phospholipid to the extrinsic system and PF-3 does so for the intrinsic system.) Activated factor X plus activated factor V and PF-3 convert factor II (prothrombin) to thrombin, leading to conversion of fibrin to fibrinogen. The steps subsequent to formation of active factor X are the same in both the extrinsic and the intrinsic pathway ("final common pathway"), except that in the intrinsic system PF-3 supplies phospholipid cofactor for conversion of prothrombin to thrombin, whereas the phospholipid component of tissue thromboplastin performs this function for the extrinsic system.

Nine of the 13 coagulation factors are proenzymes that must be activated. Exceptions are factor I (fibrinogen), which is not an enzyme; factor III (tissue thromboplastin), which is a complex rather than a single protein; factor IV (calcium); and factor VI, which currently is a number that is not in use.

BASIC TESTS IN HEMORRHAGIC DISORDERS

History.—A history of easy bleeding or easy bruising should lead to further investigation.

Platelet Count.—Platelet disorders will be discussed later. Using the direct count (reference values 150,000–400,000/cu mm; 150–400 × 10^9/L), a platelet count less than 100,000/cu mm indicates moderate thrombocytopenia, and one less than 50,000/cu mm indicates severe thrombocytopenia. Platelet number can be estimated with a reasonable degree of reliability from a well-made peripheral blood smear.

Clot Retraction.—Platelets have a major role in clot retraction. The clot shrinks and pushes out serum that was trapped within as the blood clotted. The shrunken clot is much firmer than it was originally. Normally, clot retraction begins at approximately 1 hour and usually is complete (a firm clot with about 50% serum and 50% clot) by 24 hours. There is deficient clot retraction in all types of thrombocytopenia and in Glanzmann's thrombasthenia, but clot retraction is usually normal in other varieties of platelet function abnormality. Clot retraction is rarely used today because of wider availability of accurate platelet counts and also platelet function tests.

Tourniquet Test.—This test demonstrates capillary abnormality due either to an intrinsic defect in the capillary walls (capillary fragility) or to some types of thrombocytopenia. The tourniquet test is usually abnormal in immunologic thrombocytopenias such as idiopathic thrombocytopenic purpura (ITP) and drug-induced thrombocytopenia. It produces variable results, more often normal, in thrombocytopenia of other etiologies. It is usually normal in disorders that do not entail increased capillary fragility or thrombocytopenia, but occasionally it may be abnormal in patients with hemophilia or vitamin K disorders. The test is abnormal in hereditary telangiectasia. The tourniquet test is another procedure that is rarely used today since platelet counts are readily available, but it could be helpful in some instances of nonthrombocytopenic purpura if capillary fragility is suspected.

Bleeding Time.—The template (Mielke) modification of the Ivy technique is now the standard procedure for the bleeding time test. The template procedure, however, requires that a 9-mm long, 1-mm deep incision be made, which may leave a scar. Many laboratories (including my own) use commercial modifications of this technique such as Surgicutt or Simplate, a disposable spring-driven small lancet in a plastic case, which makes a uniform and reproducible incision 5 mm long and 1 mm deep with minimal pain or sequelae. There are some technical factors that influence results; for example, an incision parallel to the antecubital fossa produces a longer bleeding time than one oriented perpendicular to that line. The bleeding time is most helpful as an indicator of platelet abnormality, either in number or function. The bleeding time is usually normal when the platelet count is decreased but still more than 100,000/cu mm (100 × 10^9/L). With platelet counts less than 100,000/cu mm, there is a rough correlation between severity of thrombocytopenia and degree of bleeding time prolongation. The bleeding time is usually abnormal in congenital defects of platelet function such as Glanzmann's thrombasthenia. The bleeding time is frequently abnormal in acquired platelet function abnormality such as that seen in uremia and the myeloproliferative syndromes. In uremia, there frequently are demonstrable abnormalities in platelet function tests but not sufficient to entirely explain bleeding problems. In addition, up to 50% of uremic patients develop some degree of thrombocytopenia. In one study, about 45% of uremic patients had elevated bleeding times; the occurrence and degree of bleeding time elevation did not correlate well with the blood urea nitrogen (BUN) level since elevated bleeding times occurred at BUN levels as low as 50 mg/100 ml (18 mmol/L) (although more often > 100 mg/100 ml), whereas patients with normal bleeding times had BUN values as high as 180 mg/100 ml (64 mmol/L). The majority of studies report that actual bleeding in uremia is infrequent unless the bleeding time is elevated, but some studies do not agree. Reports indicate that the uremic bleeding tendency can be corrected by fresh frozen plasma, cryoprecipitate, or a synthetic analog of vasopressin (antidiuretic hormone, ADH) named 1-deamino-8-D-arginine vasopressin, or desmopressin (DDAVP).

Certain drugs interfere with platelet function and can produce a prolonged bleeding time (Table 36–2, V-D), the most common and important being aspirin. After a single small dose of aspirin, prolongation of the bleeding time over baseline is present by 2 hours or less, with maximum effect at about 24 hours. Whether the bleeding time exceeds population normal limits depends on whether the preaspirin value was in the lower or the upper half of the reference range and on individual susceptibility to aspirin. In one study, bleeding times that exceeded the reference range upper limit occurred in about 50% of clinically normal persons even with a relatively small aspirin dose such as 10 grains (two adult tablets); sometimes even with one 5-grain tablet. About 5% of the population appear to be hyperresponders, producing relatively large and prolonged bleeding time elevations. Aspirin permanently affects all platelets in circulation; platelet life span is 7–10 days, and about 10% of the circulating platelets are replaced each day. After aspirin is stopped, it takes 2–3 days (range, 1–8 days) for sufficient production of new (nonaffected) platelets to reduce an elevated bleeding time to normal. Ethyl alcohol ingested with aspirin is reported to increase the magnitude and duration of the bleeding time prolongation. Pretreatment with aspirin (aspirin tolerance test) increases the sensitivity of the bleeding time to platelet function defects such as occur in von Willebrand's disease. Even without aspirin the bleeding time is usually, although not always, abnormal in von Willebrand's disease (discussed later). The bleeding time may be abnormal in a variable number of patients with capillary fragility problems. The bleeding time typically is normal in the hemophilias and the vitamin K or fibrinogen deficiencies but may be abnormal in severe (or sometimes even in moderately severe) cases. The bleeding time is elevated in about 20% (range, 0%–65%) of hemophilia A patients. In one study, the Ivy bleeding time was consistently normal even though the Simplate method was abnormal in a significant number of patients.

There is disagreement in the literature as to the clinical significance of a prolonged bleeding time as a predictor of hemorrhage during surgery. There definitely is not a good linear correlation between degree of elevated values and probability of hemorrhage. In general, however, when the bleeding time is 1.5 times the upper limit of the reference range, the possibility of excessive bleeding during surgery is somewhat increased. When the bleeding time is more than twice the upper reference limit, there is definitely an increased risk of excess bleeding. There is also disagreement as to the surgical risk after ingestion of aspirin or aspirin-containing compounds. In the majority of patients there does not seem to be a greatly increased risk. However, some patients develop a greater degree of platelet dysfunction than the average, so that the bleeding time is useful in uncovering these cases.

Prothrombin Time.—A "complete" tissue thromboplastin plus calcium is added to the patient's plasma (complete thromboplastin contains tissue-derived material that activates the extrinsic coagulation system plus phospholipid that acts as a platelet substitute). Formation of a fibrin clot is the end point. The prothrombin time (PT) mainly indicates defects in the extrinsic coagulation system (prothrombin and factors V, VII, and X). If defect in fibrinogen is severe, it also will produce abnormal PT test results, since the test depends on an intact fibrin mechanism to generate the clot end point. However, the fibrinogen level usually must be less than 100 mg/100 ml (reference range, 200–400 mg/100 ml; 2–4 g/L) before hypofibrinogenemia affects the PT. Platelet or intrinsic system factor defects prior to the prothrombin to thrombin stage do not affect the PT because a complete thromboplastin reagent activates the extrinsic coagulation system and bypasses the intrinsic system.

Because the coagulation theory designates conversion of prothrombin to thrombin as the major reaction directly affected by thromboplastin activity, prothrombin is commonly considered the principal agent measured by the PT. Actually, the test is much more sensitive to factor VII than to prothrombin. Clinically this makes little difference, since both factor VII and prothrombin are altered by the same two major conditions affecting the extrinsic system—liver parenchymal disease (most often cirrhosis) and vitamin K deficiency. Vitamin K abnormality is most often drug-induced (coumarin anticoagulation or, less frequently, use of certain cephalosporin antibiotics) or secondary to malabsorption. In some cases low vitamin K intake due to anorexia or use of prolonged intravenous (IV) feeding because of serious illness may accentuate previous subclinical degrees of vitamin K deficiency or the action of medications that affect vitamin K metabolism.

The PT can be affected by heparin if the blood level is high enough. Levels ordinarily associated with continuous IV heparin usually do not prolong the PT significantly. With intermittent bolus or subcutaneous full-dose heparin, heparin blood levels are relatively high (often sufficiently high to prolong the PT) shortly after administration; they decline thereafter. Coagulation monitoring may not adequately demonstrate this heparin effect since the tests are customarily not done until approximately 1 hour or less before the next heparin dose, thereby not reflecting peak heparin sodium activity. When heparin and warfarin sodium (Coumadin) are given together, heparin (even continuous IV heparin) affects the PT due to the additive effect of coumadin on the PT. To obtain a valid PT, one must wait until the heparin effect has disappeared (5 hours after IV bolus injection and 12–24 hours after subcutaneous injection). Heparin blood levels are increased in patients with a high hematocrit (the same dose in a smaller plasma volume). This is especially important in neonates, who normally have a relatively high hematocrit.

The effect of sodium warfarin on the PT can be influenced by the amount of vitamin K in the diet. Some other factors include the effect of previous low tissue vitamin K stores (potentiated by low dietary intake), impaired vitamin K absorption, or action of broad-spectrum antibiotics on gastrointestinal (GI) tract bacteria. In one report, antibiotic therapy superimposed on IV feeding was said to precipitate vitamin K deficiency in as little as 48 hours after admission. Certain antibiotics (cefamandole, cefoperazone, and moxalactam) frequently produce a prolongation of the PT time that is reversible with parenteral vitamin K. The effect of heparin can be neutralized in vivo and in laboratory specimens with protamine (1 mg of protamine sulfate given intravenously for every 100 mg of heparin in the last dose). Excess protamine should be avoided since protamine itself may elevate the PT. Other ways to eliminate heparin from laboratory specimens are neutralization with hexadimethrine bromide (Polybrene) or absorption onto a special cellulose material (Heparsorb). Warfarin effect can be treated by parenteral administration of vitamin K, after which the PT should return to normal within 6–24 hours. In bleeding emergencies, fresh frozen plasma can be used.

Activated Partial Thromboplastin Time.— The precursor of the activated partial thromboplastin time (APTT) was the partial thromboplastin time (PTT). An "incomplete" thromboplastin reagent plus calcium is added to patient plasma, and the time necessary to form a fibrin clot is measured. The partial thromboplastin reagent is only a phospholipid platelet substitute without any of the other components of thromboplastin. The PTT was useful in detecting intrinsic factor abnormalities but was relatively insensitive to effects of heparin. Adding certain "contact activators" (usually chemicals or particulate matter, such as kaolin) to the PTT reagent was found to activate factor XII (contact factor) swiftly and uniformly and thus eliminate another variable in the clotting process. In addition, the APTT was found to be sensitive to heparin. The APTT is very sensitive to coagulation factor deficiencies within the intrinsic system prior to the prothrombin to thrombin stage. It may also be abnormal in prothrombin or fibrinogen deficiencies but only if the defect is relatively severe (prothrombin or fibrinogen/fibrin abnormalities may affect the test because the test depends on fibrin clot formation as the reaction end point). The APTT is not as sensitive to prothrombin abnormalities as the PT because the extrinsic thromboplastin used in the PT test is more powerful than the intrinsic system prothrombin activator complex generated by the APTT, thus enabling the PT to demonstrate relatively smaller defects in prothrombin. Platelet abnormalities do not influence the APTT.

Advantages of the APTT are adequate reproducibility (< 10% variation), speed (reaction time of about 30–50 seconds), ease of performance, and suitability for automation. Disadvantages are:

1. Blood levels of heparin that are very much above anticoagulant range cause the APTT to become nonlinear, excessively prolonged, and unreliable.
2. Various techniques and equipment are used for the APTT readout (clot detection); the different machines as well as different companies' reagents may produce results that deviate significantly on the same specimen. This may cause problems in comparing values from different laboratories.
3. The APTT is not affected by platelets, whereas platelets do influence heparin activity in vivo (platelets contain platelet factor 4 [PF-4], which inhibits the anticoagulant activity of heparin).
4. The APTT is affected by warfarin. When the PT is in the warfarin thera-

peutic range, the APTT is also prolonged and may even be above the APTT therapeutic range for heparin.

Certain technical problems affect interpretation of PT and APTT test results. The labile factors are preserved better in citrate than in oxalate anticoagulant. Once exposed to air, citrated plasma is stable for only 3 hours at room temperature and 6 hours in the refrigerator at 4°C. If collected in a vacuum tube and if the top has not been opened, the plasma is stable for a longer time. Excess anticoagulant relative to the amount of plasma may affect results. Insufficient blood drawn in the tube means that less plasma is available for the amount of anticoagulant present, and the test results may be falsely prolonged. The same thing may occur in blood that has a high hematocrit, since in that case the excess red blood cells (RBCs) are replacing some of the plasma. When 3.8% sodium citrate (the most commonly used anticoagulant) is used to prepare plasma, both the PT and APTT may be affected (prolonged) when the hematocrit reaches 50%, and prolongation may become marked with a hematocrit more than 60%. The APTT is affected more than the PT. The hematocrit effect is especially troublesome in neonates, since a newborn normally has a relatively high hematocrit. A hematocrit of 20% or less may produce a false decrease in the PT and APTT. If 3.2% sodium citrate is used, the effect of hematocrit is reported to be considerably less. One of the most frequent etiologies for falsely elevated APTT (and sometimes PT) arises from attempts to keep IV lines open by heparin flushes. Usually this is not known to the phlebotomist. One report indicates that heparin tends to adhere to the wall of catheters (depending to some extent on the chemical composition of the catheter), which can affect results from specimens drawn from the catheter. In patients on constant-infusion heparin therapy, faulty or improperly calibrated delivery systems may be the reason for otherwise inexplicable APTT fluctuations. Technical considerations are important even in patients not known to be receiving anticoagulants; according to one report, 40% of abnormal APTT results in these patients were eventually interpreted as being false elevations due to technical factors. Another report found a 2% incidence of false elevations in clinically normal persons and 11% in patients being evaluated for bleeding. Recollection by an experienced technologist has solved many problems. Other possible causes for unexpected APTT elevation are circulation factor inhibitors or the lupus anticoagulant (discussed later).

Activated Whole Blood Clotting Time.— Whole blood is drawn into a vacuum tube containing a contact factor activator. The tube is incubated in a heat block at 37°C and tilted every 5 seconds. The normal upper limit is about 2 minutes. The test is claimed to be very reproducible. It can be used for coagulation defect screening and to monitor heparin therapy. It is said to have approximately the same sensitivity as the APTT in coagulation defects, and in heparin assay it is more linear than APTT at greater heparin effects. Many coagulation experts prefer this test to the APTT when monitoring heparin therapy. Disadvantages are the need for a portable heating unit and inability to automate the procedure (that the test is done at the bedside is considered by its proponents to be an advantage). The test is not sensitive to platelet variations.

Venous Clotting Time.—The Lee-White method is preferred for venous clotting time (VCT). Technique is extremely important. When the usual three test tubes are used, number 3 is filled first, since the last blood to enter the syringe is probably least contaminated with tissue juice. If glass syringes are used, the test timing should be started as soon as blood enters the syringe. If plastic syringes are used, one can wait until blood enters tube number 3 (the first tube filled) to start the test timing, because clotting time in plastic material is prolonged. The tubes should be incubated at 37°C. The VCT is affected mainly by defects in the intrinsic pathway factors prior to prothrombin and by defects in fibrinogen/fibrin. It is not sensitive to platelet abnormalities and is relatively insensitive to abnormalities of prothrombin or factor VII (in which severe deficiency is required to produce significant VCT abnormality). In deficiencies of the intrinsic pathway factors or fibrinogen, the test is only moderately sensitive, requiring considerable deficiency to cause abnormal test results. The VCT is reasonably sensitive to heparin effect and was the original test used to monitor heparin therapy.

Disadvantages of the VCT are relative lack

of reproducibility (> 15% variation in most laboratories when the test is repeated on the same patient), necessity for 37°C incubation and careful technique (hardly ever observed by the average technologist), relatively long reaction time (5–15 minutes), the fact that each test must be done separately at the patient's bedside, and the fact that platelets do not affect the test. The VCT has been replaced in most laboratories by the APTT or some other method that is more reproducible and more easily controlled.

Thrombin Time.—If commercially supplied thrombin is added to patient plasma, the time required to form a clot can be used to estimate the rate of fibrin formation. Variables include the amount of patient fibrinogen available and whether any inhibitors are present. The inhibitors could either be fibrin split products (which interfere with fibrin monomer polymerization) or antithrombins (e.g., heparin). Some manufacturers market reagents based on certain snake venoms that directly convert fibrinogen to fibrin without being affected by heparin. Fibrinolysins can also produce abnormality both by destroying fibrin or fibrinogen and by producing fibrin split products. The thrombin time is therefore used as a test for abnormalities in the fibrinogen/fibrin stage of coagulation. The test is not as widely used as some of the other coagulation procedures.

Plasma Fibrinogen.—There are several methods for measuring plasma fibrinogen levels. The oldest methods ("clottable protein") involved precipitating a fibrin clot from plasma either by adding thrombin or by recalcifying the plasma (adding enough calcium to neutralize the chelating effect of the laboratory anticoagulant used to obtain the plasma). The fibrin clot was then assayed chemically by one of several indirect methods, or the change in optical density of the clot was measured. Newer techniques consist of immunologic methods using antibodies against fibrinogen and methods based on a modified thrombin time principle. At present, the most widely used is the thrombin time technique. Most of the techniques are not reliable when high titers of fibrinolysins are present or when heparin is present. Fibrinogen can be measured using certain snake venom reagents (Reptilase or Ancrod) instead of thrombin, which convert fibrinogen to fibrin and are not affected by heparin. True low plasma fibrinogen levels may be due to high titers of fibrinolysin (when fibrinolysins are present in high titer, fibrinogen may be attacked as well as fibrin) or to the disseminated intravascular coagulation (DIC) syndrome. Disseminated intravascular coagulation is by far the more common cause. A thromboplastin tissue substance or substance with equivalent action is liberated in the bloodstream and causes fibrin deposition (clots) in small blood vessels.

It might be useful to compare the results of some laboratory tests just discussed in the various phases of blood coagulation:

Test Result* Affected by Abnormality in:

	Platelets	Intrinsic Pathway†	Prothrombin	Fibrinogen or Fibrin
PT	No	No	VS	Ins
APTT	No	VS	Ins	Ins
VCT	No	Mod S	Ins	Mod S

*VS = very sensitive; Ins = insensitive; Mod S = moderately sensitive; No = not affected.

†Factors XIII, IX, X, XI, and XII (not including platelets or common pathway.

In hemophilia (factor VIII defect), the various tests have approximately the following sensitivity:

PT—normal at all levels of factor VIII C deficiency.

VCT—normal until factor VIIIC activity levels are less than 2% of normal.

APTT—normal until factor VIII activity levels are less than 30%–35% of normal.

Note that normal persons may have 50%–150% of "normal" levels on factor VIII activity assay.

COAGULATION PATHWAY FACTORS

In this section the various coagulation pathway factors will be discussed individually, with emphasis on abnormalities for which laboratory tests are useful.

Factor I (Fibrinogen)

Fibrinogen is a glycoprotein that is synthesized in the liver, the liver being a major source of many coagulation factors. Conversion of fibrinogen to fibrin under the influence of thrombin is the final major step in coagulation. Besides its role in coagulation, fibrinogen is an important part of the body's "acute-phase" reaction to trauma or to a variety of severe illnesses; this initial response to illness results in fibrinogen production increase and therefore serum level increase. Decreased plasma fibrinogen levels may occur from decreased liver production, from the action of fibrinolysins (enzymes that destroy fibrin and may attack fibrinogen), and from conversion of fibrinogen to fibrin that is too extensive to permit adequate replacement of the fibrinogen. Decreased fibrinogen production is usually due to liver cell damage, as occurs in acute hepatitis or cirrhosis. However, production mechanisms are efficient, and a severe degree of liver damage is required before significant hypofibrinogenemia develops. Fibrinolysins may be primary or secondary. Primary fibrinolysins are rare and usually attack only fibrinogen. Secondary fibrinolysins are more common and attack primarily fibrin but can attack fibrinogen. Fibrinolysins are discussed in more detail in the section on anticoagulants. The major etiology of hypofibrinogenemia other than severe liver disease is fibrinogen depletion caused by disseminated intravascular coagulation (DIC).

Current therapeutic sources of fibrinogen are fresh frozen plasma or cryoprecipitate (chapter 11).

Factor II (Prothrombin)

Prothrombin is a proenzyme synthesized by liver cells. That portion of the prothrombin molecule that permits the molecule to function in the coagulation pathway is formed with the help of vitamin K. Without vitamin K a variety of prothrombin molecules are produced that are inactive. Vitamin K exists in two forms, one of which is preformed in green vegetables and certain other foods and one of which is synthesized by GI tract bacteria. Both forms are fat soluble and depend on bile salts for absorption. A deficiency of vitamin K may thus result from malabsorption of fat (as seen with lack of bile salts in obstructive jaundice, or primary malabsorption from sprue; see chapter 20) or from failure of GI tract bacteria to synthesize this substance (due to prolonged oral antibiotic therapy). It usually takes more than 3 weeks before the body vitamin K stores are exhausted and the deficiency of available vitamin K becomes manifest. Dietary lack may be important but ordinarily does not cause a severe enough deficiency to produce clinical abnormality unless other factors (e.g., the anticoagulant vitamin K inhibitors) are present.

Neonatal hemorrhage due to vitamin K deficiency may occur during the first 24 hours of life, from 1–7 days after birth, and uncommonly, 1–3 months later. Neonatal deficiency may be idiopathic or associated with certain maternal medications (anticonvulsants, warfarin, antibiotic therapy). It has been reported that up to 3% of infants at birth are vitamin K deficient. Thereafter, diet is important. Breast milk and certain infant milk formulas are relatively low in vitamin K and predispose to clinical deficiency. One dose of vitamin K at birth is frequently used as a prophylactic measure.

Assuming that normal supplies of vitamin K are available, the other main limiting factor in prothrombin formation is the ability of the liver to synthesize it. In severe liver disease (most often far-advanced cirrhosis), enough parenchyma is destroyed to decrease prothrombin formation in a measurable way, eventually leading to a clinical coagulation defect. Whereas a deficiency of available vitamin K responds promptly to administration of parenteral vitamin K, hypoprothrombinemia due to liver parenchymal disease responds poorly, if at all, to parenteral vitamin K therapy.

Vitamin K is also necessary for synthesis of factors VII, IX, and X. The greatest effect seems to be on prothrombin and factor VII.

Factor III (Tissue Thromboplastin)

Tissue thromboplastin is composed of phospholipids and lipoproteins and can be extracted from most tissues. Tissue thromboplastin forms a complex with factor VII and calcium ions that initiates the extrinsic coagulation pathway. This complex is used as the reagent for the PT test.

Factor IV (Calcium Ions)

Calcium is necessary as a cofactor in several steps of the coagulation pathway. The common hematology and blood bank anticoagulants oxalate, ethylenediamine tetraacetic acid (EDTA), and citrate exert their anticoagulant effect by blocking calcium function through chelation of the calcium ions.

Factor V (Labile Factor)

Factor V is synthesized by the liver and is decreased in severe liver disease. Factor V is found in plasma but not in serum. Factor V is unstable and becomes markedly reduced in 2–3 days when refrigerated anticoagulated blood is stored in the blood bank. Refrigeration helps preserve factor V in laboratory specimen plasma, but even at 4°C factor V is considerably reduced within 24 hours, and freezing soon after the specimen is obtained is necessary to maintain activity. In factor V deficiency the PT is abnormal; the APTT test is abnormal in severe deficiency but may be normal in mild deficiency.

Factor VII (Stable Factor)

Factor VII is synthesized in the liver and is dependent on vitamin K for its activity. The biologic half-life of factor VII is only 4–6 hours, making it the shortest lived of the vitamin K–dependent coagulation factors. The coumarin vitamin K antagonists produce a more rapid and profound depressive effect on factor VII than on any of the other vitamin K–dependent factors. Factor VII is present in plasma and in serum and is stable in both. In factor VII deficiency the PT is abnormal; the APTT and bleeding time are normal.

Factor VIII/von Willebrand Factor Complex

Nomenclature of Factor VIII/von Willebrand factor (factor VIII/vWF) complex has been confusing. Until recently, the entire complex was known as "Factor VIII." In 1985 the International Committee on Thrombosis and Haemostasis proposed a new nomenclature system that is adopted here. Research on Factor VIII over many years demonstrated that the factor was not a single molecule but a complex with at least two components. One is the substance whose deficiency produces classic hemophilia. This component previously was called antihemophilic globulin (AHG) and is now called factor VIII (or antihemophilic factor). For coagulation test purposes, factor VIII (antihemophilic factor) is separated into (1) the factor protein molecule, and (2) its coagulant activity. Antibodies have been produced against the factor VIII protein, and this antigen is now called factor VIII antigen, or VIII:Ag (formerly this was designated VIIIC:Ag). The coagulant activity of factor VIII is now designated VIII:C. The second component of the complex is associated with von Willebrand's disease and is called von Willebrand factor, or vWf (formerly, this was called factor VIII–related antigen, or VIIIR). Antibodies have been produced against von Willebrand factor protein, and this antigen is now called von Willebrand factor antigen, or vWf:Ag (formerly, this was called VIIIR:Ag). In addition, the von Willebrand factor has at least two coagulant actions or activities: an effect on platelet adhesion demonstrated by the glass bead column retention test and an effect on platelet aggregation demonstrated by the ristocetin test. The von Willebrand–ristocetin effect on platelets was formerly called the von Willebrand ristocetin cofactor and designated VIIIR:RC; but in the new nomenclature system no formal name or abbreviation is assigned to any vWf function such as the ristocetin cofactor or the vWf effect on platelet adhesion. The site where factor VIII is synthesized in humans is not known, but the von Willebrand factor is apparently synthesized in endothelial cells and megakaryocytes.

The hemorrhagic disease known as hemophilia is usually associated with factor VIIIC deficiency. A similar disease may result from factor IX deficiency (and a similar, but milder, disease from factor XI deficiency), so factor VIIIC deficiency is sometimes referred to as hemophilia A and factor IX deficiency as hemophilia B. About 90% of clinical hemophilia cases are due to hemophilia A and about 9% to hemophilia B.

The gene for factor VIII is located on the female sex chromosome and is transmitted as a sex-linked recessive trait. Females with the hemophilia A gene are usually carriers (heterozygous, xX), and males with the gene have clinical disease (xY, the hemophilic x gene not being suppressed by a normal X gene as it is in a carrier female). However, sporadic cases occur without known inheritance. The gene for vWf is usually transmitted as an autosomal incomplete dominant trait and uncommonly as an autosomal recessive trait. Rare cases of x-linked recessive inheritance have also been reported.

The VIII/vWf complex is found in plasma but not in serum. Both VIII:C and vWf activity (or vWf:RC) are unstable. Refrigeration helps preserve factor VIII activity (VIII:C), but even at 4°C the coagulant activity decreases considerably within 24 hours in laboratory plasma specimens. Freezing maintains factor VIII:C activity if it is done within a short time after the specimen is obtained.

Differentiation of Hemophilia A and von Willebrand's Disease.—Male patients with hemophilia A have decreased factor VIII coagulant activity, whereas vWf coagulant activity, as measured by platelet function tests, is normal. Factor VIII:Ag is decreased by antibody techniques, whereas vWf:Ag levels are normal. The majority of female hemophilia A carriers have also been shown to have reduced VIII:Ag levels, although usually not depressed to a marked degree (since one chromosome has a normal X gene and apparently can ensure some production of factor VIII). In contrast to hemophilia, patients with classic von Willebrand's disease have both reduced VIII:C activity and vWf activity of about equal degree and demonstrate corresponding decreases in both antigens using antibody techniques. Further discussion of von Willebrand's disease will be deferred to the section on platelet disorders.

Clinical Aspects of Hemophilia A.—Hemophilia A exists in varying degrees of factor VIII:C activity deficiency that roughly correlate with clinical severity. Severe (classic) hemophiliacs have less than 2% of normal factor VIII:C activity levels on assay, moderate hemophiliacs have 2%–5%, and mild hemophiliacs have 5%–25% of normal levels. Hemophilia with levels between 25% and 50% of normal is sometimes called *subhemophilia* or *borderline hemophilia*. About two thirds of factor VIII:C–deficient patients have classic (severe) hemophilia. About one third of carrier females have factor VIII:C activity levels similar to those in the mildly decreased group, although usually the carriers are asymptomatic. Occasional female carriers have been reported to have clinical disease when their factor VIII:C activity is unusually low, and rare homozygous (xx) females with classic disease have been described.

The major symptom of hemophilia is excessive bleeding. Most bleeding episodes follow trauma. In classic cases the trauma may be very slight. In mild cases the trauma must usually be more significant, such as a surgical operation or dental extraction. Bleeding into joints (hemarthrosis) is a characteristic finding in classic and moderate factor VIII:C activity deficiency, with the more repeated and severe hemorrhagic episodes being found in the more severely factor-deficient patients. Bleeding from the mouth, urinary tract, and GI tract and intracranial hemorrhage are also relatively common in severe cases. In mild cases there may be only an equivocal history of excessive bleeding or no history at all before severe trauma or a surgical procedure brings the condition to light. Another complication of severe hemophilia is hepatitis virus infection from factor replacement therapy. Before laboratory screening of donor blood was possible, transmission of human immunodeficiency virus-I (HIV-I, formerly called HTLV-III) infection through blood product transfusion affected many hemophiliacs.

The biologic half-life of factor VIII:C activity is approximately 8–12 hours. Factor VIII:C activity is unstable, and in freshly drawn and anticoagulated blood stored in the refrigerator the activity decreases to 40% by 24 hours. The current therapeutic sources of factor VIII:C include fresh frozen plasma, factor VIII:C concentrate, and cryoprecipitate (chapter 11). Factor VIII:C in therapeutic material is measured in terms of units that equal the amount of factor VIII:C activity in 1 ml of normal plasma. As a rule of thumb, one factor VIII unit in therapeutic material per kilogram of body weight should increase factor VIII activity levels by 2% of normal with a half-life of 12 hours. About 10% of patients with hemophilia A develop antibodies against transfused factor VIII. Factor IX (prothrombin complex) concentrate has been used with some success in these patients on an empirical basis.

Mild hemophilia A (factor VIII levels > 5%) can also be treated with desmopressin (DDAVP), which was found to act as a stimulant to factor VIII and to vWf production. Intravenous injection of desmopressin produces peak action in about 30 minutes, resulting in average twofold increases in factor VIII that last about as long as the effect of cryoprecipitate. Since desmopressin is synthetic, the possible infectious complications of blood products are avoided. However, patients with severe hemophilia A cannot respond sufficiently.

Laboratory Tests in Hemophilia A.—The major screening test for hemophilia A is the APTT. The APTT becomes abnormal when factor VIII:C activity is less than 30%–35% of normal, so that the APTT should detect 99%–100% of patients with severe and moderate factor VIII:C activity deficiency. In mild cases, reported detection rate varies from 48%–100% (depending on the particular reagents used and the population selected). Therefore, some of the milder ("subhemophilia") cases produce borderline or normal results. Definitive diagnosis of hemophilia A usually requires assay of factor VIII:C activity. This used to require the thromboplastin generation test (TGT, chapter 35) but now is ordinarily carried out with the APTT test and commercially obtained factor VIII–deficient plasma reagent. There is a substantial variation in results in average laboratories, and the reference range is usually considered to be 50%–150% of a normal pooled plasma. Studies using a combination of factor VIII:C activity assay and vWf protein assay (obtaining a ratio of the two results) are more sensitive than standard factor VIII activity assays alone in detection of hemophilia A, with results of the combined studies (ratio) positive in approximately 50%–75% of female carriers (literature range, 48%–94%), whereas factor VIII:C activity assays alone detect only about one third of female carriers. Increased estrogen levels (pregnancy or estrogen-containing contraceptive medication) increase factor VIII:C activity and could mask a mild deficiency. Factor VIII protein is one of the so-called "acute reaction" proteins (Chapter 21) whose synthesis is increased in response to acute illness or stress. Surgery, acute bleeding, pregnancy, severe exercise, inflammation (infectious or noninfectious), and severe stress of other types may raise factor VIII:C activity levels somewhat (within 1–2 days after stress onset) and may temporarily mask a mild factor deficiency state if testing is delayed that long. Another problem is therapy given before test specimens are obtained. There are some technical details that affect tests for factor VIII:C activity. The specimen must be fresh or preserved by short-term refrigeration or by freezing. Most methods quantitate results by comparing the patient results against those of a reference plasma. Commercially available lyophilized reference plasma gives more reliable results than fresh "normal" plasma. Photooptical instruments in general give better results than mechanical clot timers. Prothrombin time test results are normal in all factor VIII:C activity–deficient groups. The bleeding time is usually normal, but it will be elevated in about 20% of patients, more often those with severe deficiency.

Factor IX (Plasma Thromboplastin Component)

Factor IX deficiency is inherited as an X-linked recessive trait. Deficiency occurs in variable degree, and clinical severity varies accordingly, similar to hemophilia due to factor VIII deficiency. Factor IX deficiency produces a hemophilia syndrome comparable to that of factor VIIIC deficiency, but hemorrhage into joints is not as frequent as in factor VIIIC deficiency, even in the severe form of factor IX disease. The factor IX deficiency syndrome is also called hemophilia B, or Christmas disease (named after the first patient studied in detail). Factor IX is found in plasma or serum and is stable in either.

Diagnosis is similar to that of factor VIII deficiency. The APTT test is the standard screening method and also is used for diagnosis and quantitative activity assay with factor IX–deficient plasma reagent. As in factor VIII deficiency, the PT is normal. Quick differentiation of factor IX deficiency from factor VIII deficiency can be provided by addition of normal serum or normal fresh plasma to patient serum; the APTT abnormality is corrected by serum in factor IX deficiency, whereas fresh plasma but not serum is required to correct a factor VIII deficiency. Increased estrogens may falsely increase factor IX.

Current therapeutic sources of factor IX include ordinary blood bank plasma, fresh frozen plasma, and factor IX (prothrombin complex) concentrate. Cryoprecipitate is not useful because it does not contain any factor IX. As a rule of thumb, one unit of factor IX in therapeutic material per kilogram of body weight should increase factor IX levels by 1% of normal with a half-life of 24 hours. Occasional patients develop antibodies against transfused factor IX.

Factor X (Stuart Factor)

This factor is a part of both the extrinsic and the intrinsic coagulation pathways. Deficiency is rare and is inherited as an autosomal recessive trait. The clinical syndrome produced is usually mild compared with classic hemophilia A. Factor X is present in plasma and in serum and is stable in both. Both the APTT and the PT are abnormal; the bleeding time is normal.

Factor XI (Plasma Thromboplastin Antecedent)

This factor deficiency is uncommon and is inherited as an autosomal incompletely recessive trait. Deficiency varies in degree according to whether the patient is homozygous or heterozygous. Clinical symptoms from either degree of deficiency are milder than those of comparable cases of hemophilia A or B. Factor XI is present in plasma and serum and is stable in both. The APTT is abnormal; the PT and bleeding time are normal.

Factor XII (Hageman Factor)

Factor XII deficiency is very uncommon and is inherited as an autosomal recessive trait. Clinical manifestations (bleeding) are rare, and most of the interest in this disorder derives from the role of factor XII as a surface contact activator of the intrinsic coagulation pathway. The extrinsic pathway is not affected. Factor XII deficiency produces clotting deficiency on laboratory tests that is particularly marked when activation enhancement materials are included in coagulation test reagents (such as the APTT) or glass tubes are used (glass ordinarily would strongly activate factor XII). The APTT and whole blood clotting time are abnormal; the PT and the bleeding time are normal. Diagnosis can be confirmed by means of the APTT with commercial factor XII–deficient plasma reagent. It has been reported that patients with factor XII deficiency have an increased incidence of myocardial infarction and thrombosis.

High Molecular Weight Kininogen (HMWK; Fitzgerald Factor)

This factor is a part of the kallikrein system, which affects factor XII in the coagulation intrinsic pathway and also plays a role in the body inflammatory response. Deficiency of HMWK is rare, and no clinical bleeding is induced. The APTT and whole blood clotting time are abnormal; the PT and bleeding time are normal.

Prekallikrein (Fletcher Factor)

This proenzyme is the central part of the kallikrein system. Prekallikrein deficiency does not predispose to abnormal bleeding. The whole blood clotting time is abnormal; the PT and bleeding time are normal. The APTT is abnormal if particulate activators such as silica or kaolin are used but is normal if soluble activators such as ellagic acid are used. The APTT abnormality with particle activators may be corrected by prolonged incubation (10–15 minutes vs. the usual 1–3 minutes).

Factor XIII (Fibrin Stabilizing Factor)

Factor XIII deficiency is transmitted as an autosomal recessive trait. Bleeding frequently is first noted in newborns. In later life bleeding episodes are usually mild except when related to severe trauma or surgery. Secondary deficiency may occur in a variety of conditions, especially malignancy or severe liver disease, but abnormality is usually subclinical. All of the usual coagulation tests (PT, APTT, and bleeding time) are normal, even in congenital deficiency. Diagnosis can be made because fibrin clots from factor XIII–deficient persons are soluble in certain concentrations of urea, whereas clots from normal persons are not. Several other assay methods have been reported.

ANTICOAGULANT SYSTEMS

Coumarin Anticoagulants

Liver cells produce certain coagulation factors that require vitamin K for synthesis into a form that can be activated. Drugs of the coumarin family inhibit vitamin K utilization by liver cells. The vitamin K–dependent factors, listed in order of decreasing sensitivity to coumarin, are factor VII, factor IX, factor X, and prothrombin. Factor VII has the shortest half-life (4–6 hours) and is decreased first and most severely, with activity levels less than 20% of baseline by 24 hours after coumarin intake. The other factor activities decrease somewhat more slowly and less profoundly. As noted earlier in this chapter, vitamin K metabolism may be affected by intake (low intake potentiates the effect of coumarins and unusually high intake antagonizes that effect), absorption (availability of bile salts and necessity for an intact duodenal mucosal cell absorption mechanism), and utilization by hepatic cells (number and health of liver cells).

There are several members of the coumarin family derived from the original drug dicumarol, of which the most commonly used in the United States is warfarin sodium. Warfarin is water soluble, and oral doses are nearly completely absorbed by the small intestine. Maximal plasma concentration is reached 1–9 hours after ingestion. It is 95%–97% bound to albumin after absorption and is metabolized by the hepatic cell microsome system. The half-life of warfarin varies greatly among individuals (mean value 35–45 hours, range 15–60 hours). With an initial dosage of 10 mg once each day, it takes 5–10 days (five half-lives) to reach equilibrium. Coumarin drugs usually take 36–48 hours to develop measurable effect on the PT time, and between 3 and 5 days to develop maximal anticoagulant effect. Duration of action is 4–5 days. Warfarin effect can be terminated by parenteral vitamin K. The dose needed has some relationship to the degree of PT elevation. Normalization of the PT ordinarily occurs in 6–24 hours.

Monitoring Coumarin Anticoagulants.— Anticoagulation by coumarin-type drugs is best monitored by the PT, although the PT is not affected by factor IX, one of the four vitamin K–dependent coagulation factors. Until recently, the most commonly accepted PT therapeutic range was 2.0–2.5 times a control value derived from normal pooled plasma. A recent National Conference on Antithrombotic Therapy recommended that PT therapeutic ranges of 1.3–1.5 times control value be used rather than 2.0–2.5 times control if the PT reagent is derived from rabbit brain or is a rabbit brain-lung combination (these are the most common PT reagents in the United States). With the usual reference range of 11–13 seconds, this would be roughly equivalent to an anticoagulant range of 15–20 seconds. An anticoagulant range of 1.5–2.0 times control was recommended for prosthetic valve prophylaxis against thrombosis. When one considers the large number of patients anticoagulated with coumarin drugs, it is surprising what little information is available from human studies regarding clinical evaluation of different therapeutic levels. Reporting PT results in terms of seconds compared with control is preferred to results in terms of percentage of normal, because percentage must be based on dilution curves, which are frequently inaccurate. An international committee has recommended that PT results be reported as the international normalized ratio (INR). This is the patient PT divided by a control plasma PT; the result is then adjusted by being multiplied by an exponent derived by comparison of the thromboplastin reagent being used with an international standard. A calculator is needed for this mathematical task. This standardizes PT results and permits a patient to have a PT performed with a comparable result in any laboratory using this system. Coumarin drugs present increased risk in pregnancy due to increased congenital malformations and undesirable effects on early fetal bone development and due to increased possibility of fetal or maternal hemorrhage at or near birth. Various medications affecting warfarin are listed in Table 36–2, V.

Heparin/Antithrombin III System

Antithrombin III

Heparin acts predominantly as an antithrombin, but it also inhibits most of the other coagulation factors, with greatest effect on activated factors IX and X. Heparin requires a cofactor, antithrombin III (AT-III), to produce anticoagulation; and it is now believed that AT-III provides most of the anticoagulant effect, whereas heparin serves primarily as the catalyst for AT-III activation. It is thought that AT-III is synthesized by the liver. Antithrombin III concentrations are decreased in the first 6 months of life and in hereditary AT-III deficiency. Concentrations may be secondarily decreased in severe liver disease, extensive malignancy, the nephrotic syndrome, deep venous thrombosis, malnutrition, septicemia, after major surgical operations, and in DIC. Antithrombin III is also decreased 5%–30% by pregnancy or use of estrogen-containing oral contraceptives. Although there is not a good linear correlation between AT-III levels and demonstrated risk of venous thrombosis, in general a considerably decreased AT-III level tends to predispose toward venous thrombosis. This is most evident in hereditary AT-III deficiency, which is uncommon, is transmitted as an autosomal dominant, and is associated with a very high risk of venous thrombosis. A decreased AT-III level also decreases the apparent effect of standard doses of heparin as measured by coagulation tests and thus produces the appearance of "heparin resistance." In general, patients respond to heparin when AT-III activity levels are more than 60% of normal and frequently do not respond adequately when AT-III activity levels are less than 40% of normal. Warfarin increases AT-III levels somewhat.

Antithrombin III Assay.—AT-III can be assayed by several techniques. In general, these can be divided into two groups: those that estimate AT-III activity ("functional" assay) using coagulation factor or synthetic AT-III substrates; and those that measure the quantity of AT-III molecules present ("immunologic" assay) by means of antibody against AT-III. The results of the two assays do not always correlate in clinical situations, since AT-III normally has little inhibitory effect until it is activated (as with heparin) and since the conditions of AT-III activation and AT-III binding to affected coagulation factors may vary.

Heparin

Heparin is not consumed during its coagulation activity. It is degraded primarily in reticuloendothelial and vessel endothelial cells. Protamine and polybrene are specific neutralizing agents for heparin (1 mg of protamine for each 100 units of heparin). Platelets contain a heparin-neutralizing factor, PF-4. Severe thrombocytopenia may increase sensitivity to heparin. Heparin therapy induces thrombocytopenia in about 10%–15% of patients (range 1%–31%), generally occurring 5–7 days (range 2–15 days) after onset of therapy. Heparin therapy in pregnancy is reported to be associated with a considerably increased incidence of congenital malformations.

Monitoring of Heparin Therapy.—Anticoagulation by heparin is monitored by the APTT (or the activated clotting time or by one of the other procedures described in chapter 35). The Lee-White whole blood clotting time was originally used but proved too cumbersome, insensitive, and nonreproducible. The therapeutic range is usually stated as 1.5–2.5 times the APTT upper reference limit, but it is better to perform a pretherapy APTT test and use that value as the reference point for determining the therapeutic range. Heparin is usually administered either by continuous IV infusion or by intermittent injection. With constant IV infusion, heparin anticoagulant response is theoretically uniform, and the APTT test theoretically could be performed at any time. However, several studies have reported a heparin circadian rhythm, even with constant IV infusion; the peak effect occurring between 7 P.M. and 7 A.M., with maximum about 4 A.M., and the trough effect occurring between 7 A.M. and 7 P.M., with the maximum effect about 8 A.M. When intermittent injection is used, peak heparin response is obtained 30 minutes to 1 hour after IV injection or 3–4 hours after subcutaneous injection. In the average person, using a single small or moderate-sized heparin dose, anticoagulant effect decreases below the threshold of measurement by 3–4 hours after IV injection and by 6 hours after subcutaneous injection. Most believe that the optimum time to monitor therapy is 1 hour before the next dose. At this time the APTT should be at least 1.5 times the upper normal limit or pretherapy value. There is controversy as to whether the peak of the response should also be measured. If low-dose therapy is used, many clinicians do not monitor blood levels at all. However, in such cases it may be desirable to perform an AT-III assay since there would be no way to know if an unsuspected low AT-III level were present that would prevent any heparin effect.

Different commercial APTT reagents differ in their sensitivity and linearity of response to heparin effect. Some APTT reagents have shown rather poor sensitivity, and most are not very linear in response once the upper limit of anticoagulant range is exceeded. Variation in reagent sensitivity is a problem because APTT therapeutic limits obtained with one manufacturer's reagent might not be applicable to another manufacturer's reagent and could lead to overdosage or underdosage of heparin. Results of various comparative studies have not unanimously shown any single manufacturer's product to have clear superiority. Results of comparative studies have also been difficult to interpret because of changes in different manufacturers' reagents over the years. Various other tests that are claimed to provide better results in monitoring heparin therapy (chapter 35) have been introduced. Of these, the activated whole blood clotting time is probably the most widely used.

Protein C/Protein S Anticoagulant System

Protein C

Protein C is a proteolytic enzyme of the serine protease type that produces anticoagulant action by inactivating previously activated factor V and factor VIII. The plasma half-life of protein C is 6–8 hours. Protein C is produced in the liver, is vitamin K–dependent, and circulates as an inactive preenzyme (zymogen). Activation is dependent on a protein called thrombomodulin, which is located on the cell membrane of blood vessel endothelial cells. Thrombomodulin binds thrombin and induces thrombin to attack inactive protein C (rather than the usual thrombin target fibrinogen), converting inactive protein C to active protein C. Activated protein C then attacks both activated factor VIII from the intrinsic factor pathway and activated factor V from the extrinsic factor pathway. Both actions inhibit conversion of prothrombin to thrombin (this end result is similar to the end result of warfarin action, although the mechanism is different). To reach maximum effect, protein C needs a cofactor, called protein S. Protein S is also synthesized in the liver and is also vitamin K dependent. Since protein C is a naturally occurring anticoagulant and protein S is necessary for protein C action, sufficient decrease in either protein C or S may result in a tendency for increased or recurrent vascular thrombosis. Protein C deficiency can be congenital or acquired. The congenital form is transmitted as an autosomal dominant trait. Individuals genetically heterozygous for protein C deficiency have protein C levels about 50% of normal (range, 25%–70%). Some, but not all, of these patients develop recurrent thrombophlebitis or pulmonary embolism. This usually does not occur before adolescence and is often associated with a high-risk condition such as surgery, trauma, or pregnancy. Homozygous protein C deficiency has been reported mostly in newborns, in which case protein C levels are close to zero and symptoms occur soon after birth and are much more severe.

Acquired protein C deficiency can be associated with parenchymal liver disease, vitamin K deficiency, DIC (especially when DIC occurs with neoplasia), and with certain medications, particularly coumarin anticoagulants. Warfarin reduces protein C activity levels about 40% (and also protein S) in addition to its action on the other vitamin K–dependent coagulation factors. Since protein C has a short plasma half-life, if protein C is already decreased before warfarin is administered, protein C decrease sufficient to induce thrombosis may occur before maximal decrease of factor VII, resulting in thrombosis before the anticoagulant effect of warfarin is manifest.

Protein C has an additional anticoagulation effect by increasing production of an enzyme called tissue plasminogen activator (t-PA) that initiates activity of the plasmin fibrinolytic system (discussed later).

Assay for Protein C.—Protein C can be assayed by quantitative immunologic or immunoelectrophoretic methods or by somewhat complex functional methods. Immunologic methods quantitate total amount of protein C. However, in some cases protein C is normal in quantity but does not function normally. Therefore, some investigators recommend functional assay rather than immunologic assay for screening purposes. If it is desirable to assay protein C (and protein S) quantity or function, they should be assayed before coumarin therapy is started because coumarin drugs decrease both antigen quantity and activity values.

Protein S

As noted previously, protein S is a vitamin K–dependent cofactor for protein C. Protein S exists about 40% in active form and about 60% bound to a protein belonging to the complement group. Total protein S is measured using quantitative immunologic or immunoelectrophoretic methods similar to those used for protein C.

Plasmin/Fibrinolysin Anticoagulants

Fibrinolysins are naturally occurring or acquired enzymes that attack and destroy either fibrinogen or fibrin or both. Fibrinolysins may be either primary or secondary. *Primary fibrinolysins* are acquired (not normally present), are rare, attack fibrinogen as their primary target, and are most often seen in association with malignancy or after extensive and lengthy surgery (most often lung operations). *Secondary fibrinolysins* are a part of normal body response to intravascular clotting, which consists of an attempt to dissolve the clot. The fibrinolysin produced is called plasmin, which is generated from an inactive precursor called plasminogen. Certain enzymes, such as streptokinase or urokinase, catalyze the reaction. Plasminogen also can be activated by t-PA, which is regulated by another enzyme called plasminogen activator inhibitor. Protein C exerts its action on this system by inhibiting plasminogen activator inhibitor, which, in turn, releases t-PA to activate more plasminogen to become plasmin. Plasmin attacks the fibrin clot and splits the fibrin into various fragments ("split products," or "fibrin degradation products"; FDPs). The FDP can interfere with polymerization of fibrin monomer (which ordinarily becomes fibrin polymer) and thus complement the fibrin-dissolving action of plasmin by helping to retard further clotting. Secondary fibrinolysin usually does not attack fibrinogen, although it may do so if the concentration of fibrinolysin (plasmin) is high enough. Primary fibrinolysin seems to be very similar, if not identical, to plasmin. Primary fibrinolysins circulate without clotting being present, so that primary fibrinolysins ordinarily attack fibrinogen rather than fibrin.

In addition to plasminogen activator inhibitor, there is an enzyme that directly inhibits plasmin called alpha-2 antiplasmin. This substance prevents plasmin from prematurely dissolving vessel thrombi that are preventing injured vessels from bleeding. Alpha-2 antiplasmin forms a covalent complex with plasmin that inactivates plasmin and thereby prevents fibrin clot dissolution and formation of FDP.

Tests for Fibrinolysins.—Various tests available to screen for fibrinolysins include the clot lysis test, fibrinogen assay, thrombin time, PT, APTT, and tests for FDPs. The clot lysis test is the oldest. Patient plasma is added to the blood clot of a normal person, and the clot is observed for 6–24 hours for signs of clot breakdown. This procedure is slow and fails to detect weak fibrinolysins. Thrombin time, PT, and PTT depend on formation of fibrin from fibrinogen as the test end point and thus will display abnormal results if there is sufficient decrease in fibrinogen or sufficient interference with the transformation of fibrinogen to fibrin. Fibrinogen assay was discussed previously; fibrinogen can be measured either directly, by immunologic methods, or indirectly, by measuring fibrin after inducing transformation of fibrinogen to fibrin. These methods are all moderately sensitive to fibrinolysins but still fail to detect some low-grade circulating anticoagulants. The most sensitive tests currently available are those that detect FDP; these will be discussed in detail next.

Fibrinogen/Fibrin Split Products.—Normally, thrombin catalyzes conversion of fibrinogen to fibrin by splitting two fibrinopeptide molecules, known as fibrinopeptide A and B, from the central portion of fibrinogen. This action exposes polymerization sites on the remaining portion of the fibrinogen molecule, which is now called fibrin monomer. Fibrin monomers spontaneously aggregate together in side-to-side and end-to-end configurations to form a fibrin gel. Thrombin also activates factor XIII, which helps introduce cross-linking isopeptide bonds between the fibrin monomers to form stabilized insoluble fibrin polymer. Fibrin polymer forms the scaffolding for blood clots. Fibrinolysins may attack either fibrinogen or fibrin, splitting off FDPs, which, in turn, are broken into smaller pieces. These split products may form a complex with fibrin monomers and interfere with polymerization. Fibrinogen degradation products can be produced by action of primary fibrinolysin on fibrinogen and also by action of plasmin on fibrinogen and fibrin monomers or fibrin clots formed in a variety of conditions, normal and abnormal. Plasmin attacks intravascular blood clots formed as part of normal hemostasis (e.g., trauma or surgery) as well as blood clots that produce disease (e.g., thrombosis or embolization). In addition, FDPs can be associated with intravascular clots composed of fibrin (e.g., DIC) and some partially extravascular conditions such as extensive malignancy, tissue necrosis and infarcts, infection, and inflammation.

Protamine Sulfate Test.—Protamine sulfate in low concentration is thought to release fibrin monomers from the split-product complex and allow the monomers to polymerize. The test result is positive in conditions producing secondary fibrinolysin and is negative with primary fibrinolysin. Primary fibrinolysin will not induce a protamine sulfate reaction because the end point of this test depends on the presence of fibrin monomers produced by the action of thrombin. Primary fibrinolysin is not ordinarily associated with activation of the thrombin clotting mechanism.

Since DIC is the major condition associated with substantial production of secondary fibrinolysin, various studies endorse protamine sulfate as a good screening test for DIC. Negative results are strong evidence against DIC. Various modifications of the protamine sulfate method have been introduced. These vary in sensitivity, so that it is difficult to compare results in diseases other than DIC. Any condition leading to intravascular clotting may conceivably produce secondary fibrinolysin; these conditions include pulmonary embolization, venous thrombosis, infarcts, and either normal or abnormal postoperative blood vessel clots in the operative area. Occasional positive results have been reported without good explanation.

Immunologic Fibrin Degradation Product Assay.—When fibrinogen or fibrin monomers are attacked by plasmin, a large fragment called X is broken off. In turn, X is split into a larger fragment Y, a smaller fragment D, and the smallest fragment of all, E. Therefore, intermediate products are fragments X and Y, and final products are two fragment Ds and one fragment E. The split products retain some antigenic determinants of the parent fibrinogen molecule. Antibody to certain of these fragments can be produced and, as part of an immunologic test, can detect and quantitate these fragments. Since the antibodies will react with fibrinogen, fibrinogen must be removed prior to the test, usually by clotting the blood with thrombin. Heparin may interfere with the action of thrombin, which, in turn, leads to residual fibrinogen, producing false apparent FDP elevation. The earliest immunologic FDP test in general use was the "Fi test," a slide latex agglutination procedure detecting mainly intermediate fragments X and Y, which was shown to be insufficiently sensitive. Another test, the tanned RBC hemagglutination–inhibition test (TRCHII), detected fragments X, Y, and D and was sensitive enough but too complicated for most laboratories. A newer 2-minute latex agglutination slide procedure (Thrombo-Wellcotest) has immunologic reactivity against fragments D and E and seems to have adequate sensitivity and reliability. The Thrombo-Wellcotest is replacing protamine sulfate in many laboratories. All of the FDP tests are usually abnormal in the various conditions that affect the protamine sulfate test. Titers of 1:10 or less on the Thrombo-Wellcotest are considered normal. Occasional clinically normal persons have titers between 1:10 and 1:40. Patients with venous thrombosis develop a secondary fibrinolysin body response that can produce an abnormal Thrombo-Wellcotest result. In most of these cases the titer is greater than 1:10 but less than 1:40, but a minority of patients may have a titer of 1:40 or greater. Classic DIC induces a strong secondary fibrinolysin response producing large quantities of split products with a Thrombo-Wellcotest titer over 1:40. However, mild cases of DIC may have a titer in the equivocal zone between 1:10 and 1:40. Thus, there is overlap between normal and abnormal between 1:10 and 1:40. In addition, it is necessary to add a plasmin inhibitor (e.g., aprotinin [Trasylol]) to the patient sample soon after collection to prevent continued breakdown of fibrinogen or fibrin, which could result in falsely elevated FDP levels.

D-Dimer Test.—Another type of FDP test detects breakdown products of plasmin action on fibrin clots. Since cross-linkage has already occurred, the degradation fragments also have some degree of residual cross-linkage and are called cross-linked FDP, or D-dimer (since fragment D is the major constituent). D-dimer assay is abnormal in nearly all of the same conditions as protamine sulfate or Thrombo-Wellcotest. However, D-dimer assay (like protamine sulfate) is normal with primary fibrinolysins, since D-dimers can be produced only after fibrin formation and cross-linking.

Disseminated Intravascular Coagulation

The most common serious condition associated with fibrinolysin is DIC. Tissue thromboplastin or unknown substances with similar effect are liberated into the bloodstream and result in deposition of fibrin and fibrin clots in many small blood vessels, thus depleting plasma of the fibrin precursor substance fibrinogen (defibrination syndrome). Originally considered an obstetric disease associated with premature separation of the placenta and amniotic fluid embolism, DIC is now attributed to a growing list of etiologies, among which are septicemia, surgery complicated by intraoperative or postoperative shock, severe burns or trauma, extensive cancer, and newborn respiratory distress syndrome; and it is occasionally seen in many other conditions such as virus infection. Shock is the best common denominator but is not always present, nor has it been definitely proved to be either a cause or an effect.

Clinically, DIC is manifested by coagulation problems, which may be severe. Blood oozing from tissues during surgery is a frequent warning sign. Shock, acute renal failure, and acute respiratory failure are common in severe cases. Vascular thrombi and focal tissue infarction are also relatively frequent. Purpura fulminans refers to the rare cases in which bleeding into the skin dominates the clinical picture. Hemoglobin levels may be within reference range initially or may be decreased. Peripheral smear in classic cases displays many schistocytes, producing the picture of microangiopathic hemolytic anemia. Platelets are usually, although not always, decreased. Differential diagnosis is discussed later in the section on thrombotic thrombocytopenic purpura.

Laboratory Diagnosis.—Various laboratory tests have been advocated for the diagnosis of DIC, many of which have been discarded as newer tests are announced or older ones reevaluated. At present, hypofibrinogenemia and thrombocytopenia are the two best-established findings, which, occurring together, are considered strongly suggestive of DIC. The PT and APTT are usually both abnormal. Milder forms of DIC have been reported, however, in which one or all of these tests may be normal. The most sensitive and widely used tests for DIC screening are the protamine sulfate test and the immunologic FDP tests (e.g., the Thrombo-Wellcotest). The Thrombo-Wellcotest has been more reliable than protamine sulfate in my experience, but there are not sufficient comparison studies in the literature to permit definitive judgment between the two procedures. Since the two procedures give similar information, there is no need to use both for the diagnosis of DIC. D-dimer assay should give results similar to the Thrombo-Wellcotest.

Primary vs. Secondary Fibrinolysin.—Occasionally it is necessary to distinguish between primary and secondary etiologies for a fibrinolysin. The protamine sulfate test and D-dimer assay are normal with primary fibrinolysins and abnormal with secondary fibrinolysins. This occurs because the protamine sulfate test needs fibrin monomers (and the D-dimer assay needs cross-linked fibrin) to produce a positive reaction, whereas with primary fibrinolysins, since the clotting (thrombin) mechanism is not ordinarily activated, no fibrin monomers or cross-linked fibrin molecules are present and FDPs are generated from fibrinogen rather than fibrin. Primary fibrinolysins can be treated with ϵ-aminocaproic acid, or EACA (Amicar), but EACA is contraindicated in DIC, since inhibition of secondary fibrinolysin generation would aggravate the clotting disorder.

Immunologic-Type Coagulation Factor Inhibitors

There are several antibody-type inhibitors of coagulation factors. The most common are the "lupus inhibitors" (or "lupus anticoagulant") and the antibodies that may develop against factor VIIIC. Lupus inhibitors were originally found in systemic lupus erythematosus (about 10%–15% of cases; range, 0.4%–65%) but have subsequently been reported in occasional cases of severe chronic inflammatory disease, various malignancies, rheumatoid-collagen diseases, pregnancy, acquired immunodeficiency syndrome (AIDS) (usually during opportunistic infections), and in association with certain drugs such as chlorpromazine, procainamide, or penicillin derivatives. In some cases no cause is found. Clinical bleeding is uncommon unless some other coagulation abnormality is present (e.g., thrombocytopenia, present in about 20% of cases, range 14%–63%). In fact, vascular thrombosis is often associated with the lupus inhibitor (about 30%–40% of cases, range 14%–60%) rather than hemorrhage. The lupus inhibitor is antibody of either IgM or IgG immunoglobulin directed against certain phospholipids. These antiphospholipid antibodies interfere with coagulation factor assays that use phospholipid reagents or phospholipid-dependent procedures such as the APTT as part of the test method, even though the antiphospholipid antibody does not directly affect the actual coagulation factor activity the test is supposed to be measuring.

Laboratory Diagnosis.—The APTT is elevated in about 90% of patients with the lupus inhibitor. In fact, unexpected APTT elevation is the usual way the inhibitor is detected. Factor assays that use the APTT as part of the assay method are also abnormal. Different APTT reagents have varying phospholipid composition and quantity and therefore do not all have the same sensitivity for the lupus inhibitor. The PT is typically normal, although the PT can be elevated in about 20% (range 10%–27%) of the patients. The thrombin time is normal. The cardiolipin tests for syphilis (rapid plasma reagin, VDRL) are positive in about 20%–40% (range 0%–87%) of cases. The easiest diagnostic test for the lupus inhibitor consists of diluting the patient's plasma with an equal portion of fresh normal plasma. This will correct the APTT when the problem is a factor deficiency or antifactor antibody, but the APTT should not decrease substantially in the presence of a lupus inhibitor. Unfortunately, there are varying criteria in the literature as to what constitutes substantial correction. Also, there may be interpretive difficulty when the APTT elevation is less than 10 seconds. To further complicate matters, about 15% of lupus inhibitor cases are reported to demonstrate substantial or complete correction. In some of these cases there may be time-dependent inhibition, that is, the APTT corrects but slowly becomes abnormal again 1–2 hours later (this behavior is more typical of a factor VIII inhibitor). Tests reported to be more sensitive and reliable for definitive diagnosis, although not widely available, include the platelet neutralization procedure or anticardiolipin antibody radioimmunoassay.

Factor VIII Antibody.—Antibodies against factor VIII develop in approximately 10% of patients with hemophilia A (literature range 5%–25%). Similar antibodies occasionally have been reported in rheumatoid-collagen diseases, in ulcerative colitis, and after administration of certain drugs. Clinically, bleeding may occur similar to the coagulation defect of hemophilia. The results of standard laboratory tests resemble the pattern of hemophilia A, with the APTT being abnormal and the PT and bleeding time being normal. Factor VIII activity assay shows decreased factor VIII activity levels. If fresh normal plasma is added to patient plasma and the factor VIII activity assay is repeated, the defect is partially corrected (the degree of correction depending on the factor VIII level before normal plasma was added). This is the expected finding in hereditary factor VIII deficiency (hemophilia A). However, if the mixture of patient plasma and normal plasma is incubated for 1 hour and factor VIII activity is again assayed, in hemophilia A no significant further decrease in activity occurs, but with antibodies against factor VIII there should be a considerable further decrease in activity. Another way to suggest the diagnosis is a screening test like that described with the lupus inhibitor. If equal parts of patient plasma and fresh normal plasma are mixed, the APTT abnormality seen with patient plasma will be corrected both in hemophilia A and with a Factor VIII inhibitor. However, if the mixture is allowed to incubate for 1 or 2 hours (at 37°C), the presence of a factor VIII inhibitor will cause the APTT to increase again to abnormal levels, whereas little change should occur in hemophilia A. Although this time-dependent inhibition is suggestive of a factor VIII inhibitor, it is not completely specific, since about 10%–15% of patients with the lupus inhibitor are reported to display some degree of time-dependent inhibition.

Miscellaneous Anticoagulants

Medications.—Various drugs may affect coagulation. Aspirin and certain others have direct effects on clotting. Aspirin inhibits platelet adhesion and thus may potentiate a tendency to hemorrhage when a patient is receiving anticoagulant therapy. Other medications may act indirectly by enhancing or inhibiting the effects of anticoagulants (see Table 36–2).

Dysproteinemia.—Some persons with abnormal serum proteins, most frequently persons with myeloma or one of the macroglobulinemias, have interference with conversion of fibrinogen to fibrin despite normal fibrinogen levels. This is manifested by poor clot stability and failure of clot retraction and may cause a hemorrhagic tendency or purpura.

Thrombolytic Therapy.—Various conditions predispose to thrombosis (Table 8–1). Antithrombin III, protein C and S, and t-PA were discussed earlier. Many of the other conditions are discussed elsewhere. Stasis, vessel narrowing, and hyperviscosity are the most common etiologic problems. Cancer is a surprisingly important cause of thrombosis and embolization, especially in persons without evidence of the usual predisposing conditions. According to several studies about 5%–15% (range, 1%–34%) of cases of pulmonary embolization or deep vein thrombosis are associated with cancer, the cancer usually becoming manifest in less than 2 years. Gastrointestinal tract adenocarcinoma (especially pancreas), lung, and ovary are the most common primary tumors.

TABLE 8–1.
Some Conditions That Predispose to Thrombosis

Vessel lumen narrowing (e.g., atherosclerosis)
Vessel wall damage (e.g., vasculitis)
Stasis (e.g., congestive heart failure, immobile extremity)
Increased platelets (thrombocythemia)
Heparin-induced thrombocytopenia
Polycythemia
Serum hyperviscosity (e.g., Waldenström's macroglobulinemia)
Deficiency of AT-III, protein C, or protein S
Pregnancy
Oral (estrogen-containing) contraceptives
Lupus anticoagulant
Fibrin thrombi (e.g., DIC)
Platelet thrombi (thrombotic thrombocytopenic purpura [TTP])
Paroxysmal nocturnal hemoglobinuria
Malignancy (e.g., pancreatic carcinoma)

Various forms of therapy have been used to dissolve thrombi. Heparin has been used the longest, but heparin therapy has several problems (discussed earlier) and is better in preventing clot propagation than in dissolving the clot. Fibrinolysin (plasmin) can be used therapeutically to lyse intravascular thrombi and has produced better results than heparin. The most common indications are coronary artery thrombi, deep vein thrombosis (femoral, iliac, or popliteal veins), and large pulmonary emboli. A plasminogen activator can be administered to generate endogenous plasmin. To date, these activators include streptokinase (SK), urokinase (UK), t-PA, anisoylated plasminogen–streptokinase activator complex (AP-SAC), and pro-urokinase (P-UK). Streptokinase is a protein that is produced by beta-hemolytic streptococci. It forms a complex with plasminogen; this complex then activates noncomplexed plasminogen (either circulating or fibrin bound) to form plasmin. However, this process has the potential of overactivating the system, depleting plasminogen, and producing hemorrhage. Also, there is a tendency to form anti-SK antibodies. Urokinase produces therapeutic results at least as good as those of SK and is less antigenic. It directly activates plasminogen. However, it is very expensive. Tissue plasminogen activator acts on plasminogen by forming a complex with plasminogen that is bound to fibrin. Therefore, t-PA preferentially acts on plasminogen at the site of clotting rather than circulating plasminogen, which is a major advantage. Disadvantages of t-PA include a very short half-life (2–5 minutes), which necessitates substantial doses for best results; an extremely high cost per dose at present; and reports of some systemic fibrinolytic effect when administered in large doses. Better therapeutic results are being reported for t-PA (at least for coronary artery thrombus dissolution) than results for SK and UK. Anisoylated plasminogen–streptokinase activator complex is a modified SK-tPA complex that can circulate without activating plasminogen. However, when the complex meets fibrin, such as a blood clot, the complex binds to the fibrin and then activates plasminogen that is also bound to the fibrin. Pro-urokinase is the inactive precursor of urokinase and circulates in the blood. When clotting occurs, it attaches to fibrin and forms (activated) urokinase there. Action is specific for fibrin, and the half-life of P-UK is considerably longer than t-PA, so that a smaller dose is needed. Once the decision is made to use a thrombolytic agent, current practice is to obtain a baseline blood specimen for either the APTT or the thrombin time. A second specimen is obtained 3–4 hours following administration of the thrombolytic agent. The desired result is a value sufficiently elevated above baseline so that there is no question of a true increase. The reason for testing is to prove that a thrombolytic effect has been obtained; other than this, the degree of test abnormality is not helpful since it does not correlate well with the actual amount of fibrinolysis taking place.

PLATELET DEFECTS

Platelet-associated abnormality is most commonly produced by decreased number (thrombocytopenia) or defective function (thrombocytopathia). A bleeding tendency may also appear with a greatly increased platelet count (thrombocytosis), usually not until the count exceeds 1 million/cu mm. Clinically, purpura is the hallmark of platelet abnormality. Most other types of coagulation disorders do not cause purpura.

Thrombocytopenia

Decrease in number is the most common platelet abnormality. In general, such conditions may be classified according to etiology:

1. Immunologic thrombocytopenia
   Drug-induced thrombocytopenia
   Idiopathic thrombocytopenia
   Posttransfusion thrombocytopenia
   Other thrombocytopenias with an immunologic component
2. Hypersplenism
3. Bone marrow deficiency
4. Other causes

Immunologic Thrombocytopenia

Drug-Induced Thrombocytopenia.—This syndrome occurs due to idiosyncratic hypersensitivity to certain drugs. It may develop during initial, continued, or intermittent use of the drug. Once hypersensitivity begins, platelet depression follows swiftly. The bone marrow most often shows a normal or increased number of megakaryocytes, which often display degenerative changes. The most frequently associated drugs are heparin, quinidine, quinine, cimetidine, and various sulfonamide derivatives; but other drugs (potassium chloride and furosemide, among others) have been incriminated in rare instances. Of course, this effect is uncommon even with the relatively frequent offenders. Platelet antibodies have been demonstrated in many cases. Heparin-induced thrombocytopenia is reported in about 10%–15% of patients (range, 1%–30%). In fact, it has been estimated that 33%–66% of patients who receive heparin intravenously develop some degree of platelet decrease from baseline levels. Thrombocytopenia may occur with either IV or subcutaneous therapy and has even been reported with heparin flushes. Decrease in platelets occurs about 5–7 days (range, 2–15 days) after start of therapy. The degree of thrombocytopenia is most often mild or moderate but in some cases may be less than 50,000/cu mm. Diagnosis of immune thrombocytopenia can be assisted by platelet-associated IgG measurement in the presence of the offending drug. However, at present none of the methods is easy; none detects all cases; false positive results are sometimes reported in nonimmune thrombocytopenias, and small degrees of hemolysis may interfere.

Idiopathic Thrombocytopenic Purpura.—Idiopathic thrombocytopenic purpura may exist in either an acute or chronic form. The acute form is usually seen in children, has a sudden onset, lasts a few days to a few weeks, and does not recur. The majority of cases follow infection, most often viral, but some do not have a known precipitating cause. The chronic form is more common in adults; however, onset is not frequent after age 40. There are usually remissions and exacerbations over variable lengths of time. No precipitating disease or drug is usually found. Platelet antibodies have been demonstrated in 80%–90% of patients with chronic ITP. The methods used are generally based on measurement of platelet-associated IgG. Some patients eventually are found to have systemic lupus erythematosus or other diseases.

Clinically, there is purpura or other hemorrhagic manifestations. The spleen is usually not palpable, and an enlarged spleen is evidence against the diagnosis of ITP. Bone marrow aspiration shows a normal or increased number of megakaryocytes, although not always.

Posttransfusion Purpura.—Platelets contain certain blood group and tissue antigens on their surface; the most important of these are ABO, HLA, and platelet-specific antigen (PLA). Posttransfusion purpura usually (not always) occurs in patients whose platelets are PLA1 negative, who have been sensitized to the PLA1 antigen by previous transfusions or by pregnancy, and who are then administered blood products containing PLA1-positive platelets. An alloantibody is formed in response to sensitization. Once the antibody is formed, it exhibits rather unusual behavior for an alloantibody since it attacks both PLA1-positive or negative platelets, whether belonging to the patient or a donor. The syndrome is uncommon in spite of the fact that about 2% of Europeans are PLA1 negative. The great majority of reported patients have been female. Onset of thrombocytopenia most often occurs about 7 days after transfusion (range 2–14 days). Thrombocytopenia is often severe. The episodes last about 3 weeks, with a range of 4–120 days. They may or may not recur with future transfusion. If massive transfusions with stored bank blood are given during a short time period, thrombocytopenia frequently develops, usually ascribed to dilutional factors and to the low functional platelet content of stored bank blood. This takes at least five units of blood and usually more than 10, given within 1–2 days' time, and may or may not be accompanied by a bleeding tendency. However, stored blood deficiency of factors V and VIII (the unstable clotting factors) may contribute to any bleeding problem.

Other Thrombocytopenias With an Immunologic Component

Neonatal thrombocytopenia may be due to antiplatelet antibodies in maternal blood that cross the placenta to the fetus. These antibodies are most commonly PLA1 alloantibodies or antibodies associated with ITP. The mother's platelet count does not reliably predict the infant's count. In one study, about 25% of women with autoimmune thrombocytopenia and platelet counts more than 100,000/cu mm (100 $\times 10^9$/L) delivered infants with platelet counts less than 50,000/cu mm. Neonatal thrombocytopenia may also be due to other causes, such as intrauterine viral infection or neonatal sepsis. *Narcotic addicts* and *clinically healthy homosexual males* have a high incidence of thrombocytopenia. Most, but not all, display reactive screening tests for HIV-I (HTLV-III) infection. Some have demonstrable antiplatelet antibodies and some do not.

Hypersplenism

Hypersplenism was discussed in chapter 5. The syndrome may be primary or secondary; if secondary, it is most commonly due to portal hypertension caused by cirrhosis. There may be any combination of anemia, leukopenia, or thrombocytopenia, but isolated thrombocytopenia is a fairly frequent manifestation. The spleen is usually palpable, but not always. Bone marrow megakaryocytes are normal or increased. The thrombocytopenia seen in lupus erythematosus is usually associated with antiplatelet antibodies, but there may be an element of splenic involvement even though the spleen is often not palpable.

Bone Marrow Deficiency

This condition and its various etiologies were discussed in chapter 4, the principal causes being metastatic tumor to bone, aplastic anemia, and myelofibrosis. This group forms a large and important subgroup of the thrombocytopenias and is the reason why bone marrow examination is frequently indicated in a patient with thrombocytopenia.

Thrombocytopenia is a very frequent feature of acute leukemia and monocytic leukemia, even when the peripheral blood WBC pattern is aleukemic. It may also occur in the terminal stages of chronic leukemia.

Other Causes of Thrombocytopenia

A miscellaneous group remains that includes various unrelated disorders, some of which will be discussed.

Thrombotic Thrombocytopenic Purpura (Moschcowitz's Disease).— This is a very uncommon disorder that occurs most frequently in young adults, although it may occur at any age. There is a characteristic triad of severe microangiopathic hemolytic anemia (96%–98% of cases), thrombocytopenia (83%–96%), and neurologic symptoms (84%–92%) which typically are multiple and shifting. About 75% of patients have the complete triad. Some also include renal disease (76%–88%) and fever (59%–98%). Hemoglobin is less than 10 gm/100 ml in about 90% of cases. The peripheral blood usually contains many schistocytes. Nucleated RBCs are present in about 20%. The direct Coombs test is positive in 6% (0%–7%). The white blood cell count is increased in about 55%. Serum bilirubin levels are elevated to some degree in about 80% with the unconjugated fraction predominating. Serum LDH levels are increased, and haptoglobin levels are decreased. In textbook cases, PT, APTT, fibrinogen, and FDP are all normal. However, in several series about 18% had elevated PT; 7% had elevated APTT; 7% decreased fibrinogen; and about 25% elevated FDP.

Thrombi composed of platelets with some fibrin occur in capillaries and small arterioles. Diagnosis is most definitively made through biopsy. Renal biopsy was the original recommended procedure; however, gingival or skin biopsy (if possible, of a petechia) is more common now. However, diagnostic yield from these sources is less than 40%. Differential diagnosis includes the other microangiopathic hemolytic anemias (DIC, Zieve's syndrome, the hemolytic-uremic syndrome, the prosthetic valve hemolytic syndrome, and sepsis). Systemic lupus, autoimmune hemolytic anemia, and Evan's syndrome also enter consideration of hemolytic anemia, but these anemias usually are not microangiopathic, and the results of the Coombs test are usually positive.

Megaloblastic Anemia.—Thrombocytopenia occurs as a frequent manifestation of untreated well-established B12 and folic acid deficiency anemias, sometimes even when the anemia is mild. In chronic iron deficiency anemia, platelet counts are normal and may at times actually be somewhat increased.

Infections.—Thrombocytopenia has been reported in 18%–77% of patients with bacteremia. Neonatal thrombocytopenia always raises the question of sepsis. However, thrombocytopenia is not limited to actual septicemia. In one study of patients who had surgery because of intestinal perforation with peritonitis, all patients showed platelet count decrease that reached its lowest point 3–5 days postoperatively at mean platelet levels about 55,000/cu mm. This was followed by slow platelet count increase that reached the 100,000/cu mm level about postoperative day 10. This thrombocytopenia did not seem to produce an increased tendency to bleed and was not related to DIC, although DIC can develop in septic patients. Thrombocytopenia can occur in nonbacterial infections. It is especially associated with the congenital rubella syndrome and with later (AIDS) stages of HIV-I (HTLV-III) virus infection. However, thrombocytopenia may occasionally and transiently be found in the early stages of other virus infections such as Epstein-Barr infectious mononucleosis.

Rheumatoid-Collagen Diseases.—Thrombocytopenia is reported in about 15% (range 5%–26%) of patients with systemic lupus.

Hypertension of Pregnancy.—Thrombocytopenia has been associated with preeclampsia (pregnancy-induced hypertension). Some patients have microangiopathic peripheral smear changes with relatively normal coagulation studies, a laboratory picture similar to TTP

Thyrotoxicosis.—Some degree of thrombocytopenia has been reported in 14%–43% of patients with Graves' disease. Severe thrombocytopenia with bleeding is uncommon.

Uremia.—As noted in the discussion of the bleeding time test, up to 50% of patients in uremia are reported to have some degree of thrombocytopenia in addition to various platelet function defects.

Artifactual Thrombocytopenia.—Apparent thrombocytopenia is occasionally encountered when platelet counts are performed by particle-counting machines. Some of the causes are platelet satellitosis around neutrophils in EDTA-anticoagulated blood, many giant platelets, improperly prepared specimens (platelet aggregates), and platelet cold agglutinins. Peripheral blood smears may also falsely suggest some degree of thrombocytopenia due to platelet clumping or uneven distribution if the slide is not properly made.

Platelet Function Defects

Platelet function usually refers to the role of platelets in blood coagulation. To carry out this role, platelets go through a series of changes, partially morphologic and partially biochemical. Abnormality may develop at various stages in this process, and platelet function tests have been devised to detect abnormality in certain of these stages. These are special procedures not available in most laboratories and include techniques designed to evaluate platelet factor release (PF-3 or serotonin), platelet aggregation (adenosine diphosphate, thrombin, collagen, epinephrine) and platelet adhesion (glass bead retention). These tests are useful primarily to categorize platelet action abnormality rather than to predict the likelihood of bleeding. The bleeding time test is probably the best procedure to evaluate degree of clinical abnormality.

Hereditary disorders of defective platelet action with normal platelet count is uncommon, the most famous of this group being Glanzmann's disease (hereditary thrombasthenia). Platelets in Glanzmann's disease have abnormal aggregation and glass bead retention. The clot retraction test result is abnormal, whereas the results are normal in other thrombopathic (platelet function abnormality) disorders. Tourniquet test results are variable.

Defective platelet function has been observed in many patients with uremia and some patients with chronic liver disease, even without the thrombocytopenia that occasionally may develop. Cryoprecipitate or desmopressin can correct the bleeding time elevation in uremia. Many other conditions can sometimes be associated with platelet function test abnormalities, including leukemias and myeloproliferative disorders, dysproteinemias such as myeloma, and systemic lupus. Giant platelets may be found in certain conditions, especially in myeloid metaplasia (less often in chronic myelocytic leukemia), but this does not seem to produce a clinical bleeding tendency.

Certain drugs may interfere with platelet function, as noted earlier. Aspirin affects platelet factor release and also platelet aggregation. Other drugs may interfere with one or more platelet function stages.

von Willebrand's Disease

von Willebrand's disease combines platelet function abnormalities with deficiency in factor VIII activity. The clinical disease produced has been called "pseudohemophilia." Although there used to be considerable argument as to just what this disease should include, it is now generally restricted to a hereditary disorder of the von Willebrand factor portion of the factor VIII/vWf complex. As described in the section on factor VIII deficiency, the factor VIII/vWf complex consists of two components, the hemophilia A factor VIII portion and the von Willebrand factor portion. Factor VIII controls factor VIII activity within the coagulation intrinsic pathway system. In hemophilia A, VIII antigenic material is present but is nonfunctional, so that VIII:C activity is decreased. The vWf portion of the complex is normal both in quantity and function. That part of the complex comprising vWf controls at least two aspects of platelet function. In von Willebrand's disease the vWf antigen is decreased, and platelets display decreased adhesiveness (manifested by decreased retention in glass bead columns) and also decreased platelet agglutination under the stimulus of the antibiotic ristocetin. In addition, the vWf is thought to stabilize factor VIII levels, so that a decrease in vWf leads to a decrease in factor VIII levels, both in the quantity of factor VIII as well as its activity. Thus, the entire factor VIII complex is decreased.

Classic von Willebrand's disease (and all but one variant forms) is transmitted as an autosomal dominant trait (in contrast to hemophilia A, which is transmitted as a sex-linked recessive trait). Most patients with von Willebrand's disease are heterozygous and have a clinically mild hemorrhagic disorder. Most of the serious bleeding episodes are induced by trauma or surgery. Uncommonly, the patient is homozygous for von Willebrand factor deficiency, and these patients have a severe hemorrhagic disorder. In a third variant, also uncommon, vWf is present in normal quantity but is nonfunctional or only partially functional; these patients have normal factor VIII activity and normal vWf antigen by immunoassay but low ristocetin cofactor and platelet glass bead retention activity and an abnormal bleeding time.

Acquired von Willebrand's Disease.—A few patients have been reported who had clinical and laboratory findings consistent with von Willebrand's disease but had no evidence of hereditary transmission. These patients had a variety of diseases but most often seemed to have lymphoma, carcinoma, autoimmune disorders, and conditions associated with monoclonal gammopathies.

Laboratory Diagnosis.—The various forms of von Willebrand's disease as well as the expected results of the various diagnostic tests are summarized in Table 8–2. As noted previously, there is a wide spectrum of clinical severity and also degree of laboratory test abnormality in patients with von Willebrand's disease. In the usual ("classic") type, factor VIII activity is variably decreased, the bleeding time is prolonged, and platelet function by glass bead column retention and ristocetin aggregation is abnormal. However, even in the classic form,

TABLE 8–2.
von Willebrand's Disease Variant Forms*

	Type I†	Type IIA	Type IIB	Type IIC‡	Type III
vWf:Ag	D	N/D	N/D	N	D
vWf:C	D	D	N/D	D	D
vWf:R	D/N	D	I	D	D
VIII:C	D	D/N	D/N	N	D
Inheritance	Dom	Dom	Dom	Rec	Rec

*D, decreased; N, normal; underline, most common; Dom, dominant; Rec, recessive.
†Type I (IA) is the classic and most common form. There is also a type IB, which differs from IA predominantly by multimeric pattern.
‡There is also a type IID, which differs from IIC by inheritance pattern (dominant) and by multimeric pattern.

some patients display bleeding times that may intermittently be normal. In some patients factor VIII:C activity is normal but the bleeding time is prolonged. In others the disease is so mild that even the bleeding time is normal, but pretreatment with aspirin can uncover the bleeding time defect. As noted in the section on factor VIII, the factor VIII/vWf complex is one of the so-called acute reaction protein group, so that vWf can be increased to some degree in surgery, infection or noninfectious inflammation, severe exercise, and severe stress of other types and in mild cases may temporarily correct the bleeding time and factor VIII/vWf assay results. Increased estrogens (pregnancy or use of estrogen-containing contraceptives) can increase factor VIII activity and vWf antigen levels in some patients with von Willebrand's disease even though the bleeding time may continue to be abnormal. In a few cases, especially when laboratory results are conflicting or equivocal, it may be necessary to obtain multimeric analysis (analysis of the factor VIII/vWf complex structure fraction sizes by special gel electrophoresis).

Therapy.—Fresh frozen plasma or cryoprecipitate contain the factor VIII complex and can temporarily correct vWf deficiency. Administration of desmopressin can temporarily stimulate factor VIII/vWf production (to levels about twice baseline) and correct the bleeding time, as was discussed in the section on hemophilia A therapy. However, desmopressin effect on vWf lasts only about 3–6 hours, which is somewhat less prolonged than the effect on factor VIII.

Thrombocytosis

Certain diseases are associated with increased numbers of platelets. About 25%–35% of cases have malignancy. Less frequent but still important causes are acute bleeding, acute infection, postsplenectomy, collagen diseases, and the myeloproliferative syndromes (including polycythemia vera). In most cases there is no clinical problem until the platelet count exceeds 1 million/cu mm. When that happens there is an increased tendency to bleed and also to develop thrombosis. The most common diseases associated with very high platelet counts are idiopathic thrombocythemia and the myeloproliferative syndromes.

Vascular Defects

Senile purpura is a frequent nonhereditary type of vascular fragility problem, manifested by localized purpuric lesions or small bruises developing on the extremities of older persons. The only laboratory abnormality is a positive tourniquet test result in some cases. A somewhat similar clinical condition is the easy bruising found in some young adult persons, especially women. All results of standard laboratory tests are usually normal, except for an occasionally positive tourniquet test result. Some of these persons have abnormal platelet function test results; in the majority, however, the reason for abnormality is not known. It should be mentioned that continued or intermittent bleeding from a small localized area is most often due to physical agents (e.g., repeated trauma) or to a local condition (e.g., scar tissue) that prevents normal small-vessel retraction and subsequent closure by thrombosis.

Allergic (anaphylactoid) purpura is characterized by small blotchy hemorrhages over the extremities, frequently accompanied by ankle edema, produced by an allergic capillary or small-vessel vasculitis. Many patients also have glomerulonephritis. *Henoch's purpura* is a subdivision in which the bleeding occurs mainly in the GI tract. Schönlein's purpura features the skin manifestations without GI involvement. The tourniquet test result is usually positive. Platelet counts and other laboratory test results are normal. Diagnosis is made through biopsy of a fresh small purpuric area.

Embolic purpura can simulate capillary fragility defects, although the skin lesions may resemble petechiae more than the larger lesions of purpura. There may, however, be some component of capillary fragility. These disorders include subacute bacterial endocarditis, fat embolism, and some cases of septicemia (although other cases of septicemia also have thrombocytopenia). The tourniquet test result is often positive and the bleeding time is variable. Other coagulation defect test results are normal (except in septicemia complicated by DIC). When the patient is seriously ill with disease of acute onset, purpura raises the question of meningococcemia.

Laboratory Investigation of Purpura

The etiologic diagnosis of purpura should begin with a platelet count and a complete blood count, with special emphasis on the peripheral blood smear. If the platelet count discloses thrombocytopenia, depending on the clinical circumstances a bone marrow aspiration may be justified, utilizing preferably both a clot section and a smear technique. The clot section affords a better estimate of cellularity. The smear permits better study of morphology. This is true for megakaryocytes as well as for other types of cells. Investigation of purpura without thrombocytopenia should include a bleeding time (for overall platelet function). In a few cases a tourniquet test might be considered to test for abnormal capillary fragility. If necessary, platelet function tests may be done. These tests are not indicated in already known thrombocytopenia, because their results would not add any useful information. The other tests for hemorrhagic disease must have previously ruled out abnormality in other areas. Occasional cases of nonthrombocytopenic purpura are caused by abnormal serum proteins, which may be demonstrated by serum protein electrophoresis (then confirmed by other tests, described in chapter 22).

Usually a bleeding tendency does not develop in thrombocytopenia until the platelet count is less than 100,000/cu mm (100×10^9/L) (direct method) and most often does not occur until the platelet count is less than 50,000/cu mm. The 20,000/cu mm value is usually considered the critical level. However, some patients do not bleed even with platelet counts near zero, whereas occasionally there may be trouble with patients with counts more than 50,000/cu mm. Most likely there is some element of capillary fragility involved, but the actual reason is not known at this time.

BLEEDING PROBLEMS IN SURGERY

Bleeding constitutes a major concern to surgeons. Problems may arise during operation or postoperatively, and bleeding may be concealed or grossly obvious. The major causes are:

1. Physical defect in hemostasis—improper vessel ligation, overlooking a small transected vessel or other failure to achieve adequate hemostasis, or postoperative tissue devitalization and release of a vessel ligature.
2. Unrecognized preoperative bleeding problem—a coagulation defect is present but was not recognized prior to surgery. This may be congenital (e.g., hemophilias), secondary to a disease that the patient has (e.g., cirrhosis), or due to medications (e.g., aspirin or anticoagulant therapy).
3. Transfusion reactions or complications from massive transfusion.
4. Intraoperative DIC.
5. Unexplained bleeding difficulty.

Unusual bleeding has some correlation with the type (magnitude) of the operative procedure, the length of the operation, and the particular disease involved. The more that any of these parameters is increased, the more likely that excessive bleeding may occur. In most cases, the defect can be traced by means of laboratory tests or, retrospectively, by reestablishing physical hemostasis. In some cases laboratory workup is hindered by transfusions administered before a coagulation problem was considered. Sometimes the source of bleeding is never uncovered, even after thorough investigation. This fact cannot be used as an excuse for inadequate workup, because proper therapy depends on finding the etiology. This is why some knowledge of blood coagulation mechanisms is necessary.

INVESTIGATION OF BLEEDING DISORDERS

There is no standardized protocol for workup of bleeding problems. Also, one should differentiate between workup of a patient who is actively bleeding and the use of screening tests in persons who are not bleeding. Any algorithm presented could be criticized by someone who prefers a different approach or different test procedures. Nevertheless, I will present one possible workup for persons who are actively bleeding. This includes bleeding time (to test for platelet and capillary fragility abnormalities), inspection of a peripheral blood smear for platelets and RBC morphology, APTT (to test for intrinsic pathway abnormalities), PT (to test for extrinsic pathway abnormalities), and FDP test (for DIC). If bleeding time is abnormal, a platelet count should be done. If the PT and PTT results are both abnormal, the fibrinogen level should be determined. If the APTT is the only abnormal finding, a simple correction experiment is done using the APTT and patient plasma diluted 1:1 with fresh normal plasma. If the APTT is corrected, the defect is presumed to be a factor deficiency within the intrinsic pathway. If the abnormal APTT is not corrected, or if there is time-dependent noncorrection, a circulating anticoagulant or an inhibitor should be suspected. If the PT is the only abnormal finding, liver disease or unsuspected coumarin intake should be suspected. If both the APTT and PT results are abnormal, unsuspected heparin effect (e.g., heparin flushes) are possible, as well as DIC, coumarin therapy, severe liver disease, and circulating antithrombins or fibrinolysins. The results from the FDP test should help support or rule out DIC.

If at all possible, the results of abnormal screening tests should be verified by a redrawn blood specimen, since a frequent cause of incorrect results is a nonoptimal specimen.

A frequent obstacle to correct diagnosis is transfusion of blood or blood products before a bleeding disorder is suspected, or empirical attempts at therapy before diagnostic tests are ordered or a consultation is obtained. If there is any question of abnormal bleeding, a citrate anticoagulant coagulation test tube, an EDTA-anticoagulated hematology test tube, and a nonanticoagulated serum tube should be obtained in case coagulation tests are needed later. The citrate tube should be kept in the refrigerator.

Additional tests relevant to this chapter are described in chapter 35.

BIBLIOGRAPHY

Clyne LP, et al: Time dependency of lupus-like anticoagulants. *Arch Intern Med* 1988; 148:1060.

High KA: Antithrombin III, protein C, and protein S. *Arch Pathol Lab Med* 1988; 112:28.

Rao AK, et al: Thrombolysis in myocardial infarction (TIMI) trial—Phase I: Hemorrhagic manifestations and changes in plasma fibrinogen and the fibrinolytic system in patients treated with recombinant tissue plasminogen activator and streptokinase. *J Am Coll Cardiol* 1988; 11:1.

Brandt JT, et al: Factor VIII assays. *Arch Pathol Lab Med* 1988; 112:7.

Rao KPP, et al: Acquired von Willebrand's syndrome associated with an extranodal pulmonary lymphoma. *Arch Pathol Lab Med* 1988; 112:47.

Blatt PM, Martin SE: The lupus anticoagulant. *Arch Pathol Lab Med* 1987; 111:113.

Lottenberg R, et al: Acquired hemophilia. *Arch Intern Med* 1987; 147:1077.

Brandt JT, et al: The sensitivity of different coagulation reagents to the presence of lupus anticoagulants. *Arch Pathol Lab Med* 1987; 111:120.

Hathaway, WE: New insights on vitamin-K. *Hem/Oncol Clin North Am* 1987; 1:367.

Gottschall JL: Effect of hemolysis on apparent values of platelet-associated IgG. *Am J Clin Pathol* 1987; 87:218.

Greenberg CS, et al: Measurement of plasma fibrin D-dimer levels with the use of a monoclonal antibody coupled to latex beads. *Am J Clin Pathol* 1987; 87:94.

Marder VJ, et al: Rapid lysis of coronary artery thrombi with anisoylated plasminogen:streptokinase activator complex. *Ann Intern Med* 1986; 104:304.

Conroy JD, Kahn SB: Agents for antithrombotic therapy. *Am Fam Physician* 1986; 34:192.

Kasper CK, Ewing NP: Acquired inhibitors of plasma coagulation factors. *J Med Technol* 1986; 3:431.

Straight DL: The physiologic inhibitors of blood coagulation and fibrinolysis. *J Med Technol* 1986; 3:443.

Hundley JM: Idiopathic (autoimmune) thrombocytopenic purpura. *J Med Technol* 1986; 3:285.

Iberti TJ, et al: Thrombocytopenia following

peritonitis in surgical patients. *Ann Surg* 1986; 204:341.

Vogelsang G, et al: Post-transfusion purpura. *Am J Hematol* 1986; 21:259.

Suchman AL, Griner PF: Diagnostic uses of the activated partial thromboplastin time and prothrombin time. *Ann Intern Med* 1986; 104: 810.

Bjornsson TD, et al: Variability in heparin sensitivity of APTT reagents. *Am J Clin Pathol* 1986; 86:199.

Marder VJ, et al: Standard nomenclature for factor VIII and von Willebrand factor: A recommendation by the International Committee on Thrombosis and Haemostasis. *Thromb Haemost* 1985; 54:871.

International Committee for Standardization in Haematology: International normalized ratio. *Am J Clin Pathol* 1985; 83:779.

Kulkarni GA, et al: Thrombotic thrombocytopenic purpura. *Am Fam Physician* 1985; 31:141.

Schafer AI: The hypercoagulable states. *Ann Intern Med* 1985; 102:814.

Smith PS, et al: The prolonged bleeding time in hemophilia A: Comparison of two measuring technics and clinical associations. *Am J Clin Pathol* 1985; 83:211.

Elmer O, et al: Impairment of primary hemostasis and platelet function after alcohol ingestion in man. *Haemostasis* 1984; 14:223.

Lind SE: Prolonged bleeding time. *Am J Med* 1984; 77:305.

Marlar RA, et al: Comparison of the sensitivity of commercial APTT reagents in the detection of mild coagulopathies. *Am J Clin Pathol* 1984; 82:436.

Finley PR, Fletcher C: Laboratory tests in immune thrombocytopenia. *J Med Technol* 1984; 1:709.

Warrier AI, Lusher JM: DDAVP: A useful alternative to blood components in moderate hemophilia A and von Willebrand disease. *J Pediatr* 1983; 102:228.

McGann MA, Triplett DA: Laboratory evaluation of the fibrinolytic system. *Lab Med* 1983; 14:18.

Adrouny A, et al: Variable presentation of thrombocytopenia in Graves' disease. *Arch Intern Med* 1982; 142:1460.

Wilson JJ, et al: Infection-induced thrombocytopenia. *Semin Thromb Hemost* 1982; 8:217.

Triplett DA: Anticoagulant therapy: Monitoring techniques. *Lab Mgmt* 1982; 20(8):31.

Dale NL, Schumacher HR: Platelet satellitism: New spurious results with automated instruments. *Lab Med* 1982; 13:300.

Hoyer LW: Pseudo-von Willebrand's disease. *N Engl J Med* 1982; 306:360.

Caprini JA, Seners SF: Altered coagulability in cancer patients. *CA* 1982; 32:162.

Deykin D, et al: Ethanol potentiation of aspirin-induced prolongation of the bleeding time. *N Engl J Med* 1982; 306:852.

Adrouny A, et al: Variable presentation of thrombocytopenia in Graves' disease. *Arch Intern Med* 1982; 142:1460.

Hoyer LW: The factor VIII complex: Structure and function. *Blood* 1981; 58:1.

Rodriguez-Erdmann F, et al: Interaction of antibiotics with vitamin K. *JAMA* 1981; 246:937.

Entes K: Fletcher factor deficiency, source of variations of the activated partial thromboplastin time test. *Am J Clin Pathol* 1981; 75:626.

Kitchens CS, Smith LS: Evaluation of the prolonged partial thromboplastin time. *Cont Ed Fam Physician* 1981; 15:51.

Ridolfi RL, Bell WR: Thrombotic thrombocytopenic purpura. *Medicine (Baltimore)* 1981; 60:413.

Miescher PA, Graf J: Drug-induced thrombocytopenia. *Clin Haematol* 1980; 9:505.

Colman RW: Patho-physiology of kallikrein system. *Ann Clin Lab Sci* 1980; 10:220.

Hattersley PG, et al: Sources of error in heparin therapy of thromboembolic disease. *Arch Intern Med* 1980; 140:1173.

Steiner RW, et al: Bleeding time in uremia: A useful test to assess clinical bleeding. *Am J Hematol* 1979; 7:107.

Mant MJ, King EG: Severe, acute disseminated intravascular coagulation. *Am J Med* 1979; 67:557.

Marder V: The use of thrombolytic agents: Choice of patient, drug administration, laboratory monitoring. *Ann Intern Med* 1979; 90:802.

9 Immunohematology: Antibody Detection, Blood Group Antigens, and Pretransfusion Tests

Before this subject is discussed, it is useful to give some definitions:

Antigen: Any substance that causes formation of antibodies to it. The most common antigens are protein, but certain carbohydrate polysaccharides may act in a similar manner. Lipid may be combined with either. Each antigen has a certain chemical configuration that gives it antibody-provoking ability. This specific chemical group may become detached from its carrier molecule and temporarily lose antigenic power; it is then called a *hapten.* Attachment of a hapten to another suitable molecule leads to restoration of antigenic properties.

Antibody: Proteins of the globulin class, most often gamma globulins, produced by lymphocytes and plasma cells in response to antigenic stimulation. They may be specific, combining only with specific antigen molecules, or nonspecific, combining with a variety of antigens. Presumably, nonspecific antibodies attack a variety of molecules because similar hapten groups may be present even though the carrier molecule is different (cross reactivity).

Agglutinogen: Antigen on the surface of a red blood cell (RBC).

Agglutinin: Antibody that attacks RBC antigens and manifests this activity by clumping the RBCs.

Hemolysin: Same as an agglutinin, except that lysis of affected erythrocytes takes place.

Isoantibodies (alloantibodies): Antibodies produced against antigens coming from genetically different individuals of the same species. These "foreign" antigens are usually introduced into the body by transfusion or by pregnancy (if fetal RBCs containing antigens that the mother lacks reach the maternal circulation). When isoantibodies are produced, they do not cause disease unless RBCs containing antigens that the antibodies recognize subsequently come in contact with these antibodies.

Autoantibodies: Antibodies produced by the body against one or more of its own tissues. These antibodies are associated with autoimmune disorders and may cause clinical disease.

There are several types of antibodies, depending on their occurrence and laboratory characteristics:

Complete (bivalent) antibodies: These usually will directly agglutinate appropriate RBCs. In vitro tests for these antibodies tend to demonstrate better reaction in saline medium at room temperature (20°C) or lower. They often require complement.

Incomplete (univalent) antibodies: These

usually cannot directly agglutinate appropriate RBCs but only coat their surface. In vitro tests for these antibodies tend to show better reaction at higher temperatures, such as 37°C, and in high-protein medium.

Warm antibody: Reacts best in vitro at 37°C.

Cold antibody: Reacts best at 4°C–10°C.

ANTIBODY DETECTION METHODS

There are two methods of detecting and characterizing antibodies: (1) the direct Coombs test and (2) a group of procedures that try to determine if an antibody is present, and if present, attempt to identify the antibody by showing what the antibody will do in various controlled conditions.

Direct Coombs Test

To prepare reagents for the Coombs test, human globulin, either gamma (IgG), nongamma (IgM), or a mixture of the two, is injected into rabbits. The rabbit produces antibodies against the injected human globulin. Rabbit serum containing these antihuman globulin antibodies is known as Coombs serum. Since human antibodies are globulin, usually gamma globulin, addition of Coombs serum (rabbit antibody against human gamma globulin) to anything containing human antibodies will result in the combination of the Coombs rabbit antibody with human antibody. There also has to be some indicator system that reveals that the reaction of the two antibodies has taken place. This can be seen visually if the Coombs rabbit antibody has been tagged with a fluorescent dye; or if the reaction takes place on the surface of RBCs, lysis or agglutination of the RBC can be produced.

The direct Coombs test demonstrates that in vivo coating of RBCs by antibody has occurred. It does not identify the antibody responsible. It is a one-stage procedure. The Coombs serum reagent is simply added to a preparation of RBCs after the RBCs are washed to remove nonspecific serum proteins. If the RBCs are coated with antibody, the Coombs reagent will attack this antibody on the RBC and will cause the RBCs to agglutinate to one another, forming clumps. The antibody on the RBC is most often univalent but sometimes is polyvalent. Although antibodies on RBCs that are detected by the direct Coombs test are most often antibodies to RBC blood group antigens, certain medications (e.g., methyldopa and levodopa) in some patients may cause autoantibodies to be produced against certain RBC antigens. Also, in some cases antibodies not directed against RBC antigens can attach to RBCs, such as antibodies developed in some patients against certain medications such as penicillin or autoantibodies formed in the rheumatoid-collagen diseases or in some patients with extensive cancer. In addition, some reports indicate an increased incidence of apparently nonspecific positive direct Coombs reactions in patients with elevated serum gamma globulin levels.

The reagent for the direct Coombs test can be either polyspecific or monospecific. The polyspecific type detects not only gamma globulin but also the C3d subgroup of complement. Complement may be adsorbed onto RBCs in association with immune complexes generated in some patients with certain conditions, such as the rheumatoid-collagen diseases and certain medications, such as quinidine and phenacetin. Monospecific Coombs reagents are specific either for IgG immunoglobulin (and therefore, for antibody) or for complement C3d. If the polyspecific reagent produces a positive result, use of the monospecific reagents (plus elution techniques discussed later) can narrow down the possible etiologies.

The direct Coombs test may be done by either a test tube or a slide method. The direct Coombs test must be done on clotted blood and the indirect Coombs test on serum, since laboratory anticoagulants may interfere. A false positive direct Coombs test result may be given by increased peripheral blood reticulocytes using the test tube method, although the slide technique will remain negative. Therefore, one should know which method the laboratory uses for the direct Coombs test.

In summary, positive direct Coombs test results can be due to blood group incompatibility, may be drug induced, may be seen after cardiac valve operations, and may appear in rheumatoid-collagen diseases, malignancy, idiopathic autoimmune hemolytic anemia, and other conditions. The overall incidence of a positive direct Coombs test result in hospitalized patients is reported to be about 7%–8% (range 1%–15%).

The main indications for the direct Coombs test include the following (most are discussed later in detail):

1. The diagnosis of hemolytic disease of the newborn.
2. The diagnosis of hemolytic anemia in adults. These diseases include many of the acquired autoimmune hemolytic anemias of both idiopathic and secondary varieties. Results of the direct Coombs test at normal temperatures are usually negative with cold agglutinins.
3. Investigation of hemolytic transfusion reactions.

In these clinical situations the indirect Coombs test should not be done if the direct test result is negative, since one is interested only in those antibodies that are coating the RBCs (and thus precipitating clinical disease).

Antibody Detection and Identification

Indirect Coombs Test

The indirect Coombs test is a two-stage procedure. The first stage takes place in vitro and may be done in either of two ways:

1. Red blood cells of known antigenic makeup are exposed to serum containing unknown antibodies. If the antibody combines with the RBCs, as detected by the second stage, this proves that circulating antibody to one or more antigens on the RBC is present. Since the RBC antigens are known, this may help to identify that antibody more specifically.
2. Serum containing known specific antibody is exposed to RBCs of unknown antigenic makeup. If the antibody combines with the RBCs, as detected by the second stage, this identifies the antigen on the RBCs.

The second stage consists in adding Coombs serum to the RBCs after the RBCs have been washed to remove nonspecific unattached antibody or proteins. If specific antibody has coated the RBCs, Coombs serum will attack this antibody and cause the cells to agglutinate. The second stage is thus essentially a direct Coombs test done on the products of the first stage.

Therefore, the indirect Coombs test can be used either to detect free antibody in a patient's serum or to identify certain RBC antigens, depending on how the test is done.

The major indications for the indirect Coombs test are:

1. Detection of certain weak antigens in RBCs, such as D^u or certain RBC antigens whose antibodies are of the incomplete type, such as Duffy or Kidd (see chapter 10).
2. Detection of incomplete antibodies in serum, either for pretransfusion screening or for purposes of titration.
3. Demonstration of cold agglutinin autoantibodies.

The indirect Coombs test is almost never needed routinely. In most situations, such as cold agglutinins or antibody identification, simply ordering a test for these substances will automatically cause an indirect Coombs test to be done. The indirect Coombs test should be thought of as a laboratory technique rather than as an actual laboratory test.

False positives and false negatives may occur with either the direct or indirect Coombs technique due to mixup of patient specimens, clerical error when recording results, technical error (too much or not enough RBC washing; also failure to add reagents or adding the wrong reagent), contamination by 5% or 10% glucose in water (but not glucose in saline) from intravenous tubing, and, rarely, use of faulty commercial Coombs reagent.

Antibody Elution

When a direct Coombs test yields positive results, especially when the cause is thought to be a blood group–specific antibody, it is desirable to attempt elution (removal or detachment) of the antibody from the RBC to determine the antigen against which it is reacting. This is usually done by changing the physical conditions surrounding the antibody to neutralize the attachment forces. The most common current methods are heat, freeze-thaw, and chemical. Once the antibody is isolated from the RBCs, it can be tested with a panel of RBCs containing known antigens to establish its identity.

AUTOANTIBODIES

Autoantibodies present an interesting problem, both in their clinical manifestations and in the difficulty of laboratory detection and identification. They may be either the warm or cold type and may be complete or incomplete.

Warm autoantibodies react at body temperature and are most often of the incomplete type. They comprise about 70% of autoantibodies. They may be idiopathic or secondary to certain diseases. The main disease categories responsible are leukemias and lymphomas (particularly chronic lymphocytic leukemia and Hodgkin's disease); collagen diseases (especially disseminated lupus); and, uncommonly, a variety of other diseases, including cirrhosis and extensive carcinoma. Results of the direct Coombs test are usually but not always positive, both in the "idiopathic acquired" and the secondary autoimmune hemolytic anemias. In one report, 2%–4% of patients with autoimmune hemolytic anemia had a negative direct Coombs test result. If the Coombs test result is negative, demonstration of warm autoantibodies is very difficult, often impossible.

Cold autoantibodies react at 4°C–20°C and are found so frequently in normal persons that titers up to 1:32 are considered normal. They are hemagglutinating and are believed to be due to infection by organisms having antigenic groups similar to some of those on the RBCs. These antibodies behave mostly as bivalent types and require complement for reaction. In normally low titer they need refrigerator temperatures to attack RBCs. In response to a considerable number of diseases, these cold agglutinins are found in high titer, sometimes very high, and may then attack RBCs at temperatures approaching body levels, causing hemolytic anemia. High-titer cold agglutinins may be found in nonbacterial infections, especially mycoplasma pneumonia (primary atypical pneumonia), influenza, and infectious mononucleosis; in collagen diseases, including rheumatoid arthritis; in malignant lymphomas; and occasionally in cirrhosis. Fortunately, even when cold autoantibodies are present in high titer there usually is no trouble, and generally only very high titers are associated with in vivo erythrocyte agglutination or hemolytic anemia. This is not always true, however. The direct Coombs test result is usually negative. When cold agglutinin studies are ordered, an indirect Coombs test is generally done, with the first stage being incubation of RBCs and the patient's serum at 4°C–10°C.

ABO BLOOD GROUP SYSTEM

The ABO blood group system is a classic example of agglutinogens and their corresponding isoantibodies. There are three of these antigens—A, B, and O—whose genes are placed in one locus on each of two paired chromosomes. These genes are alleles, meaning that they are interchangeable at their chromosome location. Therefore, each of the paired chromosomes carries any one of the three antigen genes. This makes four major phenotype groups possible—A, B, AB, and O—since A and B are dominant over O. A and B are strong antigens, whereas O is so weak an antigen that for practical purposes it is considered nonantigenic. Furthermore, it is a rule that when either A or B antigen is present on an individual's RBCs, the corresponding isoantibodies anti-A or anti-B will be absent from his or her serum; conversely, if an individual lacks either A or B antigen, his or her serum will contain the isoantibody to the missing isoantigen. Therefore, a person who is AA or AO will have anti-B isoantibodies in his or her serum, a person who is OO will have both anti-A and anti-B isoantibodies, and so on. Why the body is stimulated to produce antibodies to the missing AB antigens is not completely understood, but apparently antigens similar to ABO substances exist elsewhere in nature and somehow cause a natural sensitization.

Anti-A and anti-B are bivalent antibodies that react in saline at room temperature. Ordinarily, little difficulty is encountered in ABO typing. There is, however, one potentially serious situation that arises from the fact that subgroups of agglutinogen A exist. These are called A_1, A_2, and A_3. The most common and strongest of these is A_1. A_2 is troublesome because it is sometimes so weak that some commercial anti-A serums fail to detect it. This may cause A_2B to be falsely typed as B or A_2O to be falsely typed as O. Fortunately, this situation is not frequent with present-day potent typing serums. Group A subgroups weaker than A_2 exist but are rare. They are easily missed, even with potent anti-A typing serums. The main importance of the A_2 subgroup is that persons with A_2 sometimes have antibodies to A_1 (the most common subgroup of A).

SIMPLIFIED REPRESENTATION OF WIENER AND FISHER-RACE THEORIES
(schematic)

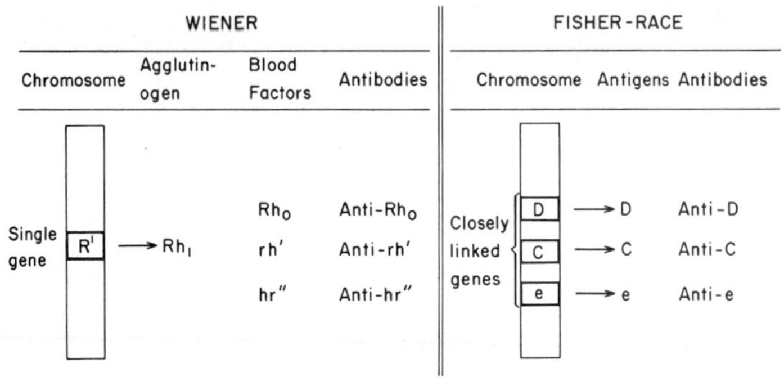

COMPARISON OF THE WIENER MULTIPLE ALLELE THEORY
AND THE FISHER-RACE LINKED GENE THEORY

WIENER			FISHER-RACE	
Gene	Corresponding agglutinogen	Blood factors	Genes	Corresponding antigens
r	rh	hr′ and hr″	*cde*	c,d,e
r'	rh′	rh′ and hr″	*Cde*	C,d,e
r''	rh″	rh″ and hr′	*cdE*	c,d,E
r^y	rh_y	rh′ and rh″	*CdE*	C,d,E
R^o	Rh_o	Rh_o, hr′ and hr″	*cDe*	c,D,e
R^1	Rh_1	Rh_o, rh′ and hr″	*CDe*	C,D,e
R^2	Rh_2	Rh_o, rh″ and hr′	*cDE*	c,D,E
R^z	Rh_z	Rh_o, rh′ and rh″	*CDE*	C,D,E

FIG 9–1.
Comparison of the Fisher-Race and Wiener nomenclatures. (From *Hyland Reference Manual of Immunohematology,* ed. 2. Los Angeles, Hyland Division of Travenol Laboratories, 1964, pp 38–39. Reproduced by permission.)

Rh BLOOD GROUP SYSTEM

The next major blood group is the Rh system. There is considerable controversy over nomenclature of the Rh genetic apparatus between advocates of the English Fisher-Race CDE-cde nomenclature and the American Wiener's Rh-hr labeling (Fig 9–1).

According to Wiener, the Rh group is determined by single genes, each chromosome of a pair containing one of these genes. In most situations each gene is expected to determine one antigen, to which there may develop one specific antibody. In Wiener's Rh system theory, each gene does, indeed, control one antigen. However, each of these antigens (agglutinogens) gives rise to several different blood factors, and it is antibodies to these factors that are the serologic components of the Rh system. There are eight such agglutinogens, each associated with certain specific blood factors. In most situations, specific antibodies are produced when a person is stimulated by a specific antigen that he or she lacks. In the Rh system, most people respond to stimulation by specific Rh system agglutinogens by producing certain specific blood factors. In a few persons, a blood factor different from the expected ones may be produced, along with some or all of the expected blood factor antibodies to one of the specific agglutinogens. Since this rare factor is inherited as one of a specific group of factors dependent on a specific agglutinogen, new antibodies can be added to Wiener's Rh system and assigned to one of the agglutinins by statistical computation of inheritance patterns.

According to the Fisher-Race theory, there are three sets of two allelic genes, Cc, Dd, and Ee, and one gene from each of the three pairs is linked together in one single locus on each of two paired chromosomes. The result is CDE, each letter of which can be either big or little, on each of the two chromosomes.

In the Fisher-Race system a single gene controls one single antigen, which controls one single antibody. This means that three genes would be present on each chromosome of a chromosome pair and that the three-gene group is inherited as a unit. New antibodies are assumed to be due to mutation or defective separation of the genes that make up the gene group during meiosis ("crossover" rearrangement).

At present, most experts believe that Wiener's theory fits the actual situation better than the Fisher-Race theory. The main drawback to Wiener's theory is its cumbersome terminology. Actually, in the great majority of situations, the much simpler Fisher-Race terminology is adequate, because the antibodies that it names by its special letters are the same as the basic blood factors of Wiener's system. It is only in unusual or rare situations that the Wiener system becomes indispensable. The Fisher-Race terminology has persisted because, for most practical work, one can use it while ignoring the underlying theory of gene inheritance. In the literature one often finds both the Fisher-Race and the Wiener nomenclatures, one of them being given in parentheses.

Of the Rh antigens, D (Rh_o) is by far the most antigenic, and when it is present on at least one chromosome, the patient types as Rh positive. Only 20% of the population lack D (Rh_o) completely and is therefore considered Rh negative. Of the other antigens, c (hr′) is the next strongest, although much less important than D.

Rh antigens lack corresponding naturally occurring antibodies in the serum. Therefore, when antibodies appear, they are of the immune type and are the result of sensitization caused by Rh antigen stimulation on receipt of RBCs of another person. This may happen from transfusion or in pregnancy. It is now well documented that RBCs from the fetus escape the placenta into the bloodstream of the mother. In this way the mother can develop Rh antibodies against the Rh antigen of the fetus. One exception to this occurs when the mother's serum contains antibodies against the ABO group of the fetus, for example, if the mother is group O and the fetus group B. In these cases the fetal RBCs are apparently destroyed in the maternal circulation before Rh sensitization can proceed to a significant extent, although this does not always happen. The syndrome of Rh-induced erythroblastosis will be discussed later. Rh incompatibility was a major cause of blood transfusion reactions, although these reactions occur much less often than ABO transfusion reactions. Rh antibody transfusion reactions may occur by transfusion of donor blood containing Rh antibodies or by previous sensitization of a recipient, who now will have the antibodies in his or her own serum.

Rh antigen may be typed using commercial antiserum. Preliminary screening is only for antigen D, which establishes a person as Rh positive or negative. If a person is Rh negative, further studies with antiserum to other components of the Rh group may be done, depending on the situation and the individual blood bank. In particular, there is a weak subgroup of D (Rh_o) called D^u (Rh_o variant), which is analogous to the weak A_2 subgroup of A in the ABO system. D^u blood often fails to give a positive reaction with some commercial Rh anti-D typing serums and so may falsely type as Rh negative. Therefore, many large blood banks screen Rh-negative RBCs for D^u as well as for c (hr′) and E (rh″), the most antigenic of the minor Rh antigens.

Rh antibodies are usually univalent and react best in vitro at 37°C in high-protein medium. Large blood banks screen donor serum for these antibodies using a variety of techniques. When Rh antibodies attack RBCs in vivo, whether in transfusion or in hemolytic disease of the newborn, they coat the surface of the RBCs in the usual manner of univalent antibodies and then get a positive result with the direct Coombs test (until the affected RBCs are destroyed).

OTHER BLOOD GROUP ANTIGEN SYSTEMS

Besides the ABO and the Rh system there are a number of other unrelated blood group antigen systems that have some importance, either for medicolegal parenthood studies or because sensitization to these antigens causes transfusion reactions or hemolytic disease of the newborn. The most important of these systems is Kell (K), a well-recognized blood bank problem. The Kell antibodies are similar in characteristics and behavior to the Rh system D (Rh_o) antibody. Fortunately, only about 10%

of whites and 2% of blacks have the Kell antigen and are thus Kell positive, so that opportunities for sensitization of a Kell-negative person are not great. Kell antibody is univalent and, like Rh, acts best in vitro in a high-protein medium at 37°C. If reactions to Kell antibodies occur, results of the direct Coombs test are positive (until the affected RBCs are destroyed). A similar situation exists for the rare Duffy (Fy) and Kidd (jK) systems. There are other systems that resemble the ABO system in their antibody characteristics, and these include the MN, P, Lewis (Le), and Lutheran (Lu) systems. They are primarily bivalent antibodies and react best in vitro in a saline medium at room temperature or below. They are rare causes of transfusion reactions, and when difficulties arise, they are clinically milder than the problems associated with the univalent antibody systems.

There are a large number of so-called minor blood group antigens. The most important is the I-i, or IH, system. This system is very weak in newborn RBCs and becomes established at approximately age 2 years. Anti-I (or anti-IH) antibodies are IgM cold agglutinins. Anti-I antibody is a frequent cause of viral or mycoplasma-associated cold agglutinins or idiopathic cold autoimmune hemolytic anemia. Some of the other systems include "public," or "universal," antigens, such as the Vel system. Nearly all persons have the antigen on their RBCs, so the chance is extremely small that any individual would not have the antigen and thereby would be capable of producing antibody to the antigen. Another group includes the "private," or "low-incidence," antigens, the most common of which is the Wright (Wr^a) antigen-antibody system. Very few persons have the low-incidence antibody on their RBCs, so risk of encountering the antigen is extremely small. Yet another antigen group is the "high titer–low avidity" type of antibody, which is occasionally responsible for weakly positive Coombs test results in recipient or donor antibody screens. In the vast majority of cases other than high-titer anti-I antibodies, the minor group antigens or antibodies are not clinically significant. However, they are a great source of frustration to the blood bank when they occur, because any unexpected antibody must be identified and because they interfere with the crossmatch and cause donor bloods to appear incompatible with the recipient.

ANTIBODY SCREEN

Even if major blood group typing has been done, transfusion reactions can occur due to unexpected antibodies in the serum of the recipient or due to incorrect RBC typing. To prevent reactions, the concept of a crossmatch evolved. The basic procedure is the "major" crossmatch, in which RBCs of the donor are placed into the serum of the recipient under standard conditions. Previously, the "minor" crossmatch (RBCs of the recipient matched with the serum of the donor) was also a standard procedure, but most blood banks no longer perform this test, and in addition, the American Association of Blood Banks (AABB) recommends that the test not be done. Even if the donor serum contains antibodies to one or more of the RBC antigens of the recipient, the relatively large blood volume of the recipient in most cases should dilute the relatively small volume of donor serum to a point at which it is harmless. The minor crossmatch has been replaced by an antibody screen on recipient serum. The antibody screen consists of the recipient serum and a commercially supplied panel of different blood group O RBCs that contain various other blood group antigens. If there is free antibody in the patient serum (other than ABO antibody), it either will coat or will agglutinate the test RBC so that the presence of the antibody will be detected. Detection is carried out by incubation at 37°C (usually with some enhancing agent, e.g., albumin or low ionic strength medium), followed by a direct Coombs test. The antibody screen does not detect errors in ABO typing, since the reagent RBCs are all group O and thus nonreactive with anti-A or anti-B antibody. Once an unexpected antibody is discovered, the type of antibody has to be identified. This can usually be deduced by the pattern of reaction with the various RBCs of the test panel. In a few cases the specimen must be sent to a reference laboratory for special tests.

MAJOR CROSSMATCH

The purpose of the major crossmatch is to detect unexpected antibodies in the serum of the recipient, so that it acts as a check on a previous antibody screen. It also serves as a check on ABO typing, since a mistake in ABO typing may result in RBCs from the donor being incompatible with naturally occurring ABO antibodies in the serum of the recipient. Unfortunately, it will not detect the most common ABO incompatibility errors, which are patient identification mistakes, either crossmatch specimens obtained from the wrong patient or properly crossmatched blood transfused into the wrong patient. Also, the procedure will not detect errors in Rh typing if no Rh antibodies are present in donor or recipient blood. Since Rh antibodies do not occur naturally, either donor or recipient would have to be previously sensitized before Rh or similar antibodies would appear. Without antibodies present the crossmatch does not demonstrate antigens and thus will not prevent immunization (sensitization) of the recipient by Rh or other non-ABO blood groups. This can be done only by proper typing of the donor and recipient cells beforehand.

The crossmatch is usually carried out in several steps using several techniques to detect groups of antibodies that have different temperature and reaction medium requirements. Occasionally the laboratory is asked to do an emergency crossmatch. One or more steps in the crossmatch procedure can be eliminated to gain speed, but each omission produces a small but definite risk of missing an unexpected antibody that is present.

In summary, RBC typing is ordinarily designed to show what ABO and Rh antigens are on the RBC and thus what blood group RBCs can be given to a recipient, either without being destroyed by antibodies the recipient is known to possess or without danger of sensitizing the recipient by introducing antigens that he or she might lack and against which he or she might produce antibodies. Antibody screening is designed to demonstrate unexpected antibodies in the serum of the recipient that may destroy donor RBCs thought to be compatible as a result of RBC blood group typing. The major crossmatch is performed to verify the antibody screening result as well as the correctness of the ABO and Rh typing.

The most widely used crossmatch technique from approximately 1960 to 1980 consisted of three sequential parts. The first was incubation at room temperature in saline diluent to detect bivalent antibodies. Next was incubation at 37°C with 22% albumin added (or other albumin concentration), with the albumin acting to enhance agglutination of univalent antibodies such as the Rh group. Finally, a Coombs test that detected weaker univalent antibodies was performed. The AABB no longer recommends the room temperature incubation phase of the procedure since non-ABO bivalent antibodies rarely produce clinical difficulty (other than high-titer cold agglutinins), and most transfusion reactions produced by ABO incompatibility are caused by drawing the recipient crossmatch specimen from the wrong patient or transfusion of already crossmatched blood into the wrong recipient, neither of which can be detected in the crossmatch. Many laboratories are substituting low ionic strength saline (LISS) reagent for albumin, which decreases incubation time from 30 minutes to 15 minutes. It has the same or slightly better sensitivity as the albumin reagent, with a minor disadvantage that LISS detects more antibodies that turn out to be clinically unimportant than does albumin.

The AABB, in their 1984 Blood Bank Standards, have gone even further and permit omission of the Coombs (antiglobulin) stage of the crossmatch as well as the high-protein (or LISS) stage, relying instead on ABO and Rh typing and the antibody screen of the recipient serum plus an "immediate spin" saline crossmatch procedure for possible ABO incompatibility. The immediate spin method entails centrifugation and examination without incubation, which takes only about 5 minutes. A traditional crossmatch procedure would be performed only when the antibody screen detected abnormality. This protocol saves a significant amount of time and money, since ABO typing and recipient serum antibody screen are usually performed well in advance of the actual order to transfuse. Studies indicate that about 0.06% (range 0.01%–0.4%) of recipient units will contain antibody that will be missed (although the majority of these would not be likely to produce life-threatening hemolysis). Other studies found that crossmatch alone detected about 4% (range 1%–11%) of total antibodies detected by combined antibody screen and crossmatch. However, there is still considerable debate about how far to go in altering the traditional crossmatch procedure and whether or not to perform it in all cases. Although there is no doubt that abbreviating the crossmatch saves time, there is some controversy whether the risk is sufficiently compensated for by the speed of blood availability and the amount of cost reduction. This would depend to some extent on how much of the traditional crossmatch procedure is being performed.

PRETRANSFUSION TEST CONSIDERATIONS

A word must also be said regarding a few patients whose blood presents unexplained difficulty in crossmatching. The laboratory should be allowed to solve the problem and possibly to obtain aid from a reference laboratory. During this time 5% serum albumin or saline may temporarily assist the patient. In the absence of complete crossmatching, blood is given as a calculated risk.

If blood is needed for emergency transfusion without crossmatch, a frequent decision is to use group O Rh-negative blood. The rationale is that no recipient (whether group O or any other ABO group) would have antibodies against group O cells, and any unexpected antibodies in donor serum against recipient RBCs would be diluted by the blood volume of the recipient. Even so, there is risk involved, since the recipient may possess antibody to some RBC non-ABO blood group antigen of the donor (e.g., anti-Rh or anti-Kell). A crossmatch would detect this. Moreover, the anti-A or anti-B antibodies in group O blood may be in high titer, and transfusion reactions may occur when this blood is used in recipients who are group A, B, or AB. Many blood banks maintain a certain amount of low-titer O-negative blood for use in emergencies. Titers over 1:50 are considered too high for this purpose. In addition, A and B group–specific substance (Witebsky substance) may be added to the donor blood to partially neutralize anti-A and anti-B antibodies. These substances are A and B antigens manufactured from animal sources and, being foreign antigens, may sensitize the patient.

Rather than use group O Rh-negative blood in a blind fashion for emergencies, a better method is to use blood of the same ABO and Rh type as the patient's blood. ABO and Rh typing can be done in 5 minutes using anticoagulated specimens of the patient's blood. This avoids interpretation problems produced by putting group O cells into a group A or B patient and subsequently attempting crossmatches for more blood.

When repeated transfusions are needed, a new specimen should be drawn from the patient (recipient) for crossmatching purposes if blood was last given more than 48 hours earlier. Some patients demonstrate marked anamnestic responses to RBC antigens that they lack and may produce clinically significant quantities of antibody in a few hours. This antibody is not present in the original specimen from the patient.

TYPE AND SCREEN

Current recommended procedure for pretransfusion testing, as previously described, is to obtain the ABO and Rh type of the recipient RBCs and perform an antibody screen on the serum of the recipient. This has become known as type and screen. This is followed by a crossmatch on blood units actually transfused; only the immediate spin procedure is mandated by AABB rules, but testing can be more extensive. Except in certain emergencies, physicians who anticipate need for blood order an estimated amount (number of units) to be processed in case they are needed. For many years, all of these units were typed and crossmatched immediately. Some institutions now maintain a "maximum surgical blood order schedule" in which the average blood need for various surgical procedures is calculated and crossmatch is performed routinely only on these units, with others subjected only to type and screen unless actually needed. In other institutions, only type and screen is done routinely, but when the order to actually transfuse is given, a crossmatch is performed. In either case, since many blood units are ordered that are never transfused, type and screen decreases the number of crossmatches required. Some blood bankers maintain that even the immediate spin can be eliminated with acceptable safety, thereby transfusing without any crossmatch.

WHITE BLOOD CELL ANTIGENS

The RBC ABO surface antigens are found in most tissues except the CNS. Some of the other RBC antigens, such as the P system, may occur in some locations outside the RBCs. White blood cells also possess a complex antigen group that is found in other tissues, more specifically, in nucleated cells. This is called the human leukocyte-A (HLA) system and is found in one site (locus) on chromosome number 6. Each locus is composed of four subloci. Each of the four subloci contains one gene. Each sublocus (gene) has multiple alleles (i.e., a pool of several genes), any one of which can be selected as the single gene for a sublocus. The four major subloci are currently designated A, B, C, and D. There is possibly a fifth sublocus, designated DR (D-related), either close to the D locus or part of it.

HLA-A, B, and C are known as class I antigens. They have similar structure, including one polypeptide heavy chain, and can be identified using standard antiserum (antibody) methods. HLA-D is identified by the mixed lymphocyte culture test in which reagent lymphocytes with HLA-D antigen fail to stimulate proliferation of patient lymphocytes when patient lymphocytes have the same HLA-D antigen but will stimulate proliferation if the patient HLA-D antigens are not compatible. HLA-DR is classified as a class II antigen with a structure that includes two polypeptide heavy chains. It includes a group of antigens found on the surface of B lymphocytes (B antigen) and also in certain other cells such as monocytes but not in most T lymphocytes. HLA-DR is currently tested for by antibody methods using patient lymphocytes and antibody against DR antigen (microcytotoxicity test). Two other antigen groups, MB and MT, which are closely associated with HLA-DR, have been described.

The four subloci that form one locus are all inherited as a group (linked) in a manner analogous to the Fisher-Race theory of Rh inheritance. Again analogous to Rh, some HLA gene combinations are found more frequently than others.

The HLA system has been closely identified with tissue transplant compatibility to such a degree that some refer to HLA as histocompatibility leukocyte-A. It has been shown that HLA antigens introduced into a recipient by skin grafting stimulate production of antibodies against the antigens that the recipient lacks, and that prior sensitization by donor leukocytes produces accelerated graft rejection. In kidney transplants from members of the same family, transplant survival was found to correlate with closeness of HLA matching between donor and recipient. On the other hand, there is evidence that HLA is not the only factor involved, since cadaver transplants frequently do not behave in the manner predicted by closeness of HLA typing using HLA-A and B antigens. There is some evidence that HLA-D, DR, and MB antigens may also be important in renal transplant compatibility.

Platelets contain HLA antigens, and patients who receive repeated transfusions of platelets may become refractory to such transfusions due to immunization against HLA antigens. Transfusion of HLA-A and B compatible platelets improves the success rate of the platelet units. However, about one third of platelet transfusion units containing well-matched HLA-A and B platelets will not be successful once the patient is sufficiently immunized.

HLA antigens on each chromosome are inherited as a unit in a mendelian dominant fashion. Therefore, HLA typing has proved very useful in paternity case investigations.

Besides their association with immunologic body defenses, certain HLA antigens have been found to occur with increased frequency in various diseases. The B27 antigen is associated with so-called rheumatoid arthritis (RA) variants (chapter 22). In ankylosing spondylitis, Reiter's syndrome, and Yersinia enterocolitica arthritis, HLA-B27 occurs in a very high percentage of cases. The incidence of HLA-B27 in ankylosing spondylitis is 90%–95% (literature range 83%–96%) in whites and approximately 50% in American blacks. In Reiter's syndrome the incidence is 80%–90% (literature range 63%–100%) in whites and approximately 35% in blacks. In juvenile rheumatoid, psoriatic, and enteropathic (ulcerative colitis and Crohn's disease) arthritis, the incidence of HLA-B27 depends on the presence of spondylitis or sacroiliitis. In all RA-variant patients, those with spondylitis or sacroiliitis have B27 in more than 50% of cases (some report as high as 70%–95%); without clinical disease in these locations, B27 is found in less than 25%. Increased frequency of the B27 antigen was also reported in close relatives of patients with ankylosing spondylitis.

An increased incidence of certain other HLA antigens has been reported in celiac disease (HLA-B8), chronic active hepatitis, and multiple sclerosis (as well as in various other diseases) but with lesser degrees of correlation than in the RA variants. The significance of this is still uncertain, and verification is needed in some instances.

BIBLIOGRAPHY

Kuriyan M, Kim DU: The maximum surgical blood order schedule: Choice of methods used in its development. *Lab Med* 1988; 19:156.

Heddle NM, et al: Hypergammaglobulinemia can be associated with a positive direct antiglobulin test, a nonreactive eluate, and no evidence of hemolysis. *Transfusion* 1988; 28:29.

Kickler TS: Platelet-compatibility testing: An update. *Lab Mgmt* 1987; 25(9):33.

Ludvigsen CW, et al: The failure of neonates to form red blood cell alloantibodies in response to multiple transfusions. *Am J Clin Pathol* 1987; 87:250.

Mitten EA: Double failure of the type and screen. *Am J Clin Pathol* 1987; 87:252.

Shulman IA, Nelson JM: The pros and cons of abbreviating the major crossmatch. *J Med Technol* 1986; 3:417.

Mougey R: Are HTLA antibodies clinically significant? *Lab Med* 1986; 17:132.

Rolih SD: Enhancement techniques for antigen-antibody interactions. *Lab Med* 1986; 17:203.

Schmidt PJ, et al: Rational reduction in pretransfusion testing. *Transfusion* 1986; 26:217.

Lincoln PJ, Jenkins GC: Blood transfusion. *Clin Anaesth* 1986; 4:481.

Arnett FC: HLA genes and predisposition to rheumatic diseases. *Hosp Pract* 1986; 21:89.

Winchester RJ: The HLA system and susceptibility to diseases: An interpretation. *Clin Aspect Autoimmun* 1986; 1:9.

Kaplan HS, Garratty G: Predictive value of direct antiglobulin test results. *Diagn Med* 1985; 8(1):29.

Snyder EL, Falast GA: Significance of the direct antiglobulin test. *Lab Med* 1985; 16:89.

Shulman IA: Experience with a cost-effective crossmatch protocol. *JAMA* 1985; 254:93.

Branch DR: Blood transfusion in autoimmune hemolytic anemias. *Lab Med* 1984; 15:402.

Calin A: HLA-B27 in 1982: Reappraisal of a clinical test. *Ann Intern Med* 1982; 96:114.

Noto TA: How to interpret a positive DAT. *Diagn Med* 1982; 5(6):59.

Grindon AJ, Wilson MJ: False-positive DAT caused by variables in sample procurement. *Transfusion* 1981; 21:313.

Lipman AG: Which drugs can induce a positive direct Coombs test? *Mod Med* 1980; 48:157.

10 Blood Transfusions

Blood transfusions may consist of whole blood, blood substitutes, or various blood fractions. Whereas chapter 11 discusses problems resulting from transfusion, this chapter will discuss substances used for transfusion.

WHOLE BLOOD

Useful Life.—Whole blood is collected in a citrate anticoagulant-preservative solution. The original acid-citrate-dextrose (ACD) formulation was replaced by citrate-phosphate-dextrose (CPD), which has a storage limit of 21 days when refrigerated between 1°C and 6°C. Addition of adenine (CPDA-1) increased the shelf-life to 35 days. More recently, other nutrient-additive solutions (e.g., AS-1, Adsol) have extended storage capability to 42-49 days, at which time there is at least 70% red blood cell (RBC) viability 24 hours after transfusion. AS-1 is currently approved only for packed RBCs, not for whole blood.

Platelets in Whole Blood.—Platelets devitalize rapidly on storage in refrigerated whole blood (discussed in greater detail in chapter 11). Platelets in fresh whole blood are about 60% effective at 24 hours and almost completely ineffective after 48 hours. Ordinary stored whole blood or packed RBCs, therefore, essentially have no functioning platelets even though the platelet count may be normal. This may produce difficulty in massive transfusions using stored whole blood or packed RBCs, although there is usually no problem when administration takes place over longer periods of time.

Transfusion Indications.—The traditional cutoff point for transfusion, especially when a patient is undergoing surgical procedures, is a hemoglobin level of 10.0 gm/100 ml (100 g/L) or a hematocrit of 33%. Based in part on experience from open-heart surgery, use of this level has recently been challenged, and a hemoglobin level of 9.0 gm/100 ml (or hematocrit of 25%–30%) is being advocated to replace the old standard.

Whole blood is used for restoration of blood volume due to acute simultaneous loss of both plasma and RBCs. This is most frequently seen in acute hemorrhage, both external and internal. Stored blood is adequate for this purpose in most cases. Actually, packed RBCs are being used in many of these patients.

Transfusion Speed.—Under usual circumstances, the American Association of Blood Banks (AABB) recommends that one unit of whole blood or packed cells be administered in 1.5 hours. The infusion rate should be slower during the first 15 minutes (100 ml/hour), during which time the patient is observed for signs and symptoms of transfusion reaction. One unit of whole blood or packed cells raises the hemoglobin level approximately 1 gm/100 ml and hematocrit approximately 3 percentage units. (Various factors can modify these average values.) Red blood cells will hemolyze when directly mixed with 5% dextrose in either water or 0.25% saline or with Ringer's solution.

Fresh whole blood is used within 2 days and preferably 1 day after collection. Platelets are still viable, and the labile coagulation factor VIII (antihemophilic globulin) and factor V still retain nearly normal activity. Most other disadvantages of prolonged storage are obviated. Obviously, donor and administrative problems greatly limit use and availability of fresh blood. Also, there is usually not sufficient time to perform screening tests for hepatitis B virus or human immunodeficiency virus-I (HIV-I; previously called HTLV-III). Current official policy of the AABB states that there are no valid indications for specifically ordering fresh whole blood. Specific blood components would be more effective. In a few circumstances when whole blood is useful but long-term storage is undesirable (e.g., infant exchange transfusion), blood less than 4–5 days old is acceptable.

BLOOD DONATION

The standard time interval between blood donations is 8 weeks. However, most healthy persons can donate one unit every 5–7 days for limited periods of time (1–2 months), assisted by oral iron supplements.

Since the use of blood transfusion has increased dramatically over the years, maintenance of adequate donor sources has been a constant problem. In Russia, cadaver blood apparently has been used to a limited extent. If collected less than 6 hours postmortem, it does not differ significantly from stored (bank) blood, except that anticoagulation is not required. A few experimental studies have been done in the United States, with favorable results.

Autotransfusion (autologous transfusion) is the collection and subsequent transfusion of the patient's own blood. This avoids all problems of transfusion reaction or transfusion-related infection, and in addition is useful in patients whose religious beliefs preclude receiving blood from others. Depending on the circumstances, one or more units may be withdrawn at appropriate intervals (every 5–7 days) before elective surgery and either preserved as whole blood, as packed RBCs, or in long-term storage as frozen RBCs, depending on the time interval between processing and transfusion. Another type of autotransfusion consists of equipment that enables operating room personnel to reclaim suctioned blood from operative sites and recyle it back into the patient as a transfusion.

PACKED RED BLOOD CELLS

Packed RBCs consist of refrigerated stored blood with about three fourths of the plasma removed. Packed cells help avoid the problem of overloading the patient's blood volume and instigating pulmonary edema. This is especially useful in patients with anemias due to destruction or poor production of RBCs, when the plasma volume does not need replacement. In fact, when anemia is due to pure RBC deficiency, plasma volume becomes greater than usual, because extracellular fluid tends to replace the missing RBC volume to maintain total blood volume. Packed cells are sometimes used when the donor RBCs type satisfactorily but antibodies are present in donor plasma. Packed cell administration also helps diminish some of the other problems of stored blood, such as elevated plasma potassium or ammonium levels. Packed RBCs retain about 20%–25% of the plasma and most of the white blood cells (WBCs) and platelets.

Leukocyte-Poor Packed Cells.—Techniques are available to remove 70%–90% of the WBCs, depending on the method used. The RBCs have normal preservation, but nearly 20% are lost in processing. This type of preparation is indicated when a patient has reactions due to leukoagglutinins.

Washed Red Blood Cells.—Washed RBCs are packed cells that have received several washes with saline. This removes more than 90% of the WBCs with most of the platelets and plasma proteins. About 10%–20% of the RBCs are lost. Indications for washed cells are relatively few. Cell washing removes donor antibodies and is useful in IgA immune reactions. Washed RBCs are traditionally used in patients with paroxysmal nocturnal hemoglobinuria. Washed cells are reported to cause fewer leukoagglutinin reactions than ordinary leukocyte-poor RBCs and could be tried in patients who continue to have leukoagglutinin reactions even when leukocyte-poor blood is used. The saline wash process reduces but does not completely eliminate the risk of viral hepatitis.

Washed RBCs must be discarded if not transfused within 24 hours after preparation (washing). No more units should be ordered than definitely will be used.

Frozen Red Blood Cells.—Fresh citrate-anticoagulated RBCs may have their storage life greatly prolonged by freezing. Glycerol is added to packed RBCs to protect them during freezing; this substance prevents intracellular fluid from becoming ice. The blood is slowly frozen and is maintained at below-zero temperatures until ready for use. Thereafter it must be thawed, after which the glycerol is removed (to avoid osmotic hemolysis), and the cells are suspended in saline. This technique will maintain packed RBCs for up to 5 years. Advantages to the blood bank include the ability to maintain a much larger inventory of blood types without fear of outdating and better control over temporary fluctuations in donor supply or recipient demand. It also permits stockpiling of rare RBC antigen types. Advantages to the patient include approximately 95% elimination of leukocytes, platelets, and plasma proteins, thus removing sources of immunization and febrile reactions; removal of most potassium, ammonium, and citrate, three substances that might be undesirable in large quantities; and considerable reduction of risk for viral hepatitis. Unfortunately, risk of viral hepatitis or HIV-I (HTLV-III) infection is not completely eliminated.

Disadvantages include considerably greater cost; significant time lost in thawing and preparing the RBCs (1 hour or more); equipment limitation on the number of units that can be prepared simultaneously, which might cause difficulty in emergencies; the fact that once thawed, cells must be used within 24 hours (by current AABB rules; some data suggest this period could be extended); and the presence of variable amounts of free hemoglobin, which might be of sufficient quantity to be troublesome if tests are needed for possible hemolytic transfusion reaction.

Frozen RBCs are becoming more widely available as larger blood banks acquire the necessary equipment. In addition to use in persons with rare blood types, current practice favors their use in some circumstances with greater attendant risk of immunohematologic sensitization. These circumstances include repeated transfusions or exposure to blood, as is frequently necessary in leukemia, chronic hemolytic anemias, bone marrow suppression, in patients undergoing renal dialysis, during elective multiple unit transfusion (e.g., cardiac surgery), and in patients with leukoagglutinins.

Irradiated Red Blood Cells.—Donor lymphocytes can induce the graft-vs.-host reaction (chapter 10) in recipients who are severely immunocompromised. Gamma radiation (at doses of 1500–2500 rad) affects lymphocytes but not RBCs, granulocytes, or platelets. Such radiation substantially reduces the risk of graft-vs.-host reaction. Radiation of this magnitude will not inactivate viral hepatitis or HIV-I. If blood product irradiation is necessary, all blood products that contain any lymphocytes must be irradiated; these include whole blood, the various RBC preparations (including frozen RBCs), platelet concentrates, and granulocyte concentrates.

PLATELETS

Platelets are supplied in units that are equivalent to the number of platelets in one unit of whole blood (about 5.5×10^{10}). These are obtained as single platelet units from random-donor whole blood units or as multiple platelet units from a single donor by means of platelet apheresis. Platelets are stored at room temperature up to 5 (sometimes 7) days. One single-donor unit ordinarily is expected to raise the platelet count 7,000–11,000/cu mm/sq of body surface (equivalent to 5,000–10,000/cu mm in an average-size adult). It has been suggested that platelets should be transfused as soon as possible after collection to retain maximum function and that infusions should be rapid (10 ml/min). Some also suggest a microaggregate filter (usually 40-μ size) if platelet storage has been more than 24 hours from time of collection. Platelet concentrates prepared by ordinary methods usually contain some plasma (about 50 ml/platelet unit) and some WBCs.

Platelet Antigens.—Platelets themselves contain various antigens, including ABO and HLA. Single-donor platelets can be transfused without typing (similar to random-donor platelets) or can be typed (usually ABO and HLA) for recipient compatibility before administration. Platelet ABO incompatibility usually has only a minor effect on donor platelet survival. HLA incompatibility may become a more serious problem. After repeated transfusions with random-donor nonmatched platelets about 50%–70% of patients (range 10%–100%) become sensitized to platelet HLA antigens (or sometimes, to platelet-specific antigens), and these patients usually become refractory to additional platelet transfusions. Most can still be transfused with HLA-matched platelets. Siblings have the best chance of providing HLA-compatible blood, although nonsiblings often match adequately. Some institutions administer only HLA-matched platelets when long-term need for platelets is anticipated. However, the AABB currently recommends that patients receive non-HLA-matched platelets initially, with HLA-matched platelets reserved for those who become refractory. Some investigators perform a 1-hour and a 24-hour platelet count after transfusion. Low 1-hour recovery is said to suggest platelet antigen sensitization. When conditions that decrease platelet survival (e.g., fever, infection, or disseminated intravascular coagulation [DIC]) are present, the 1-hour count shows normal recovery but the 24-hour count is low. One report suggests that a platelet count 10 minutes after transfusion provides the same platelet values as the 1-hour count.

Indications for Platelet Transfusion.— Platelet transfusion can be therapeutic or prophylactic. Therapeutic transfusions are indicated when severe acute bleeding occurs and the patient is severely thrombocytopenic (< 50,000 platelets/cu mm). When the patient has thrombocytopenia but has very minor bleeding or is not bleeding, the question of prophylactic platelet transfusion may arise. The decision is usually based on the degree of risk and the type of disorder being treated. According to most authorities, high-risk patients are those with platelet counts less than 20,000/cu mm (some use a cutoff value of 10,000/cu mm); moderate-risk patients (transfusion only if clinically indicated) are those with counts of 20,000–50,000/cu mm; and low-risk patients include those with counts over 50,000/cu mm. The bleeding time has also been used as a guide to therapy; a bleeding time value of less than twice the upper limit of the reference range would not ordinarily need platelet transfusion. In patients with conditions that require multiple platelet transfusions over relatively long time periods, an additional consideration is the probability of developing antiplatelet antibodies that would interfere with therapy if actual bleeding developed later. In idiopathic thrombocytopenic purpura, antiplatelet antibodies that destroy donor platelets are already present, so that transfusion is useless unless the patient is actively bleeding. In drug-induced thrombocytopenia, transfusion is useless if the drug is still being given; after medication has been discontinued, transfusion can be helpful since a normal platelet count will usually return in about 1 week and transfused platelets survive about 1 week.

GRANULOCYTES (NEUTROPHILS)

White blood cell transfusions are being used for treatment of infections not responding to antibiotics in patients with severe leukopenia due to acute leukemia or bone marrow depression. The AABB recommends 500 granulocytes/cu mm (or per microliter) as the cutoff point defining severe leukopenia. Clinical improvement has been reported in some of these patients but not all. Most large blood banks have the equipment to offer granulocyte transfusion as a routine procedure. The granulocytes are usually collected by apheresis methods and stored at room temperature. The AABB recommends that granulocytes be transfused within 24 hours after collection.

PLASMA

Plasma itself may be either stored or fresh frozen. Stored plasma until the early 1970s was the treatment of choice for blood volume depletion in burns and proved very useful as an initial temporary measure in hemorrhagic shock while whole blood was being typed and crossmatched. It was also useful in some cases of shock not due to hemorrhage. Stored plasma may be either from single donors, in which case it must be crossmatched prior to transfusion, or more commonly from a pool of many donors. Pooled plasma dilutes any dangerous antibodies present in any one of the component plasma units, so that pooled plasma may be given without crossmatch. For many years it was thought that viral hepatitis in plasma would be inactivated after storage for 6 months at room temperature. For this reason, pooled stored plasma was widely used. In 1968 a study reported a

10% incidence of subclinical hepatitis even after storage for prescribed time periods. The National Research Council Committee On Plasma And Plasma Substitutes then recommended that 5% albumin solution be used instead of plasma whenever possible.

Fresh Frozen Plasma.—Fresh frozen plasma is prepared from fresh whole blood within 6 hours after collection. Fresh frozen plasma used to be the treatment of choice for coagulation factor deficiencies such as factor VIII (hemophilia A), von Willebrand's disease, or fibrinogen. Since large volumes were often required for hemophilia A, methods were devised to concentrate factor VIII. Concentrated factor VIII solutions and cryoprecipitate are both available commercially and have largely superseded the use of fresh frozen plasma in hemophilia A. All of these products, unfortunately, may transmit infection by viruses, including the hepatitis viruses and HIV-I (HTLV-III). Heat treatment in conjunction with donor testing has nearly eliminated HIV-I infectivity of factor VIII concentrate and greatly reduced hepatitis B virus infections.

CRYOPRECIPITATE

Cryoprecipitate is prepared from fresh frozen plasma; it is the material that does not become totally liquid when fresh frozen plasma is slowly thawed and the major part has liquefied. Cryoprecipitate contains about 50% of the original factor VIII and von Willebrand factor activity, about 20%–40% of the fibrinogen and some factor XIII. The major advantage over fresh frozen plasma is reduction in the total volume of fluid that is transfused. Transfusion of one unit of cryoprecipitate carries about the same risk of hepatitis or HIV-I infection as transfusion of one unit of fresh frozen plasma or one unit of whole blood. Cryoprecipitate can also transmit infection by cytomegalovirus and Epstein-Barr virus. The amount of factor VIII activity in each unit of cryoprecipitate is reported to be highly variable (from approximately 25–150 units), although each bag is supposed to contain at least 80 units. Each unit contains about 150 mg of fibrinogen. Cryoprecipitate is useful in treating von Willebrand's disease as well as hemophilia A. Some reports suggest that cryoprecipitate, for unknown reasons, has some corrective activity in uremic patients with a bleeding tendency. If many units of cryoprecipitate are administered, some believe that ABO-compatible units should be used, since cryoprecipitate is a plasma preparation and could contain anti-A and anti-B antibodies. These antibodies could produce a positive direct Coombs test result on recipient RBC, which would be confusing. However, the need for ABO compatibility has been disputed. Large amounts of cryoprecipitate might elevate plasma fibrinogen levels and through this mechanism could produce a temporary elevation of the RBC sedimentation rate.

SPECIAL COAGULATION FACTOR MATERIALS

Factor VIII concentrate differs from cryoprecipitate in several ways. It is prepared from a pool of donors and is lyophilized. The two major advantages are that factor VIII activity has been assayed by the manufacturer for each concentrate bag and that heat treatment (when coupled with donor testing) can virtually eliminate infectivity by hepatitis B virus and HIV-I. However, there is still a greater risk of non-A, non-B (type C) hepatitis than with cryoprecipitate, and other viral infections can still be transmitted. Factor VIII concentrate is not reliable for therapy of von Willebrand's disease.

Hemophilia A patients who develop factor VIII inhibitors and become refractory to ordinary factor VIII therapy have been treated with some success using a commercial product known as *prothrombin complex concentrate.* This was originally developed for use in factor IX deficiency. A newer product known as *activated prothrombin complex concentrate* (or anti-inhibitor coagulant complex) is said to be more effective.

Factor IX concentrate (prothrombin complex concentrate) is available for therapy of factor IX deficiency (hemophilia B; Christmas disease). There is a high risk of hepatitis virus infection. Fresh frozen plasma can be used in mild cases.

Factor XI deficiency is usually treated with fresh frozen plasma, although some factor XI is present in all blood or blood products.

Antithrombin III (AT-III) deficiency or protein C deficiency (chapter 8) are usually treated with fresh frozen plasma, although AT-III activity is fairly stable in plasma that is present in any blood product. Cryoprecipitate also contains AT-III, but the amount per unit is not large. *Fibronectin* is a plasma glycoprotein thought to play a role in phagocytosis by acting as a nonspecific opsonin. Fibronectin is said to be fairly stable in plasma contained in any blood product, but the usually recommended therapeutic source is cryoprecipitate.

FIBRINOGEN

Fibrinogen is a blood fraction that is essential for clotting. It is decreased in two ways, both relatively uncommon: (1) by intravascular deposition of fibrin in the form of small clots (DIC) and (2) by inactivation in the presence of primary fibrinolysin. Fibrinogen concentrates used to be prepared commercially but are no longer available due to the considerable risk of hepatitis. Cryoprecipitate contains 150 mg or more of fibrinogen per bag and is the most commonly used source of therapeutic fibrinogen.

ALBUMIN AND PURIFIED PLASMA PROTEIN FRACTION

As mentioned in the earlier discussion about plasma, 5% albumin can be used instead of plasma to restore colloid oncotic pressure, mainly in hypovolemic shock due to massive acute blood loss or extensive burns. About 40% of body albumin is intravascular, with the remainder being in extracellular fluid. In a normal-sized person, 500 ml of blood contains about 11 gm of albumin, which is about 3.5% of total body albumin and about 70% of the albumin synthesized daily by the liver. Therefore, the albumin lost in three or four units of whole blood would be replaced in about 3 days of normal production. The AABB and other investigators believe that albumin has been overutilized in bleeding persons. They discourage use of albumin infusions in persons with hypoalbuminemia due to chronic liver disease or albumin loss through the kidneys or gastrointestinal tract on the grounds that such therapy does not alter the underlying disease and has only a very short-term effect. They are also critical of therapeutic albumin in hypoalbuminemia due to nutritional deficiency, which should be treated with parenteral hyperalimentation or other nutritional therapy. Purified plasma protein fraction (PPPF) can be used in most cases instead of albumin but has few advantages. It is not recommended when rapid infusion or large volumes are needed since it may have a hypotensive effect under these conditions. Albumin and PPPF do not transmit viral hepatitis because they are pasteurized.

RED BLOOD CELL SUBSTITUTES

Attempts have been made to find an RBC substitute that will not require crossmatching, can be stored conveniently for long periods of time, can be excreted or metabolized in a reasonable period of time, is relatively nontoxic, and can provide an adequate delivery of oxygen to body tissues and return carbon dioxide to the lungs. Thus far, no perfect answer has emerged. The current two leading candidates have been hemoglobin solutions (free of RBC stroma) and synthetic substances, of which the most promising to date are fluorocarbon compounds. However, major problems still remain. Free hemoglobin can precipitate in the tubules of the kidney or alter renal function. Another difficulty involves a generalized and a coronary artery vasoconstrictor effect. Fluorocarbons usually must be oxygenated for maximum effectiveness, most commonly by having the patient breathe 100% oxygen. Elimination of fluorocarbons from the body is fairly rapid (the half-life is about 24 hours), which sometimes would necessitate continued administration. Thus far, none of these blood substitute preparations has proved entirely successful.

OTHER PROCEDURES RELEVANT TO TRANSFUSION THERAPY

Apheresis

Apheresis is a technique in which blood is withdrawn from a donor, one or more substances are removed from the blood, and the blood is then returned to the donor. Most present-day apheresis equipment is based on separation of blood components by differential centrifugation. Apheresis has two major applications. One is the removal of certain blood components (e.g., platelets) to be used for transfusion into another patient. Apheresis has permitted collection of blood components in greater quantity and more frequently than ordinary phlebotomy. In addition, when all components come from the same donor, the risk of hepatitis is less than if blood from multiple donors is used. This technique is the major source of many rare blood group antibodies and certain blood components. The second major use of apheresis is the direct therapeutic removal of harmful substances or blood components from a patient. The most common application is removal of abnormal proteins from serum by plasmapheresis in patients with the hyperviscosity syndrome (associated with Waldenström's macroglobulinemia or myeloma). Apheresis has also been used to remove immune complexes from patients with various disorders associated with autoimmune disease. However, use of apheresis in many of these conditions is considered experimental.

Blood Transfusion Filters

For many years it has been the custom during blood transfusion to place a filter with a 170-μ pore size between the blood donor bag and the patient. This trapped any blood clots large enough to be visible that might have formed in the donor bag. In the 1960s it was recognized that nonvisible clots or microaggregates of platelets, fibrin, degenerating leukocytes, and other debris frequently were present in stored bank blood and could produce microembolization with pulmonary and cerebral symptoms. The most severe condition was pulmonary insufficiency associated with open-heart surgery or massive blood transfusion for severe trauma. It was found that microfilters with pore sizes of 20–40 μ could trap most of these microaggregates. Some publications advocated using such a filter for every transfusion (the filter can accept 5–10 units of whole blood or packed cells before it must be replaced). Others believe that transfusions limited to one or two units do not subject the lungs to sufficient embolized material to necessitate use of a microfilter. Originally there was a flow rate problem with the 20-μ filters, but newer models have better flow characteristics. A substantial number of platelets are trapped by filter sizes less than 40 μ. However, blood more than 2 days old does not contain viable platelets.

Blood Volume Measurement

Blood volume measurement is useful in certain circumstances: (1) to differentiate anemia due to hemodilution from anemia due to RBC deficiency, (2) to differentiate polycythemia from dehydration, and (3) to quantitate blood volume for replacement or for therapeutic phlebotomy purposes. Blood volume measurement is discussed in this chapter since the most frequent indication for transfusion therapy is to replace depleted blood volume. This most commonly arises in association with surgery or from nonsurgical blood loss, acute or chronic. Immediately after an acute bleeding episode, the hemoglobin and hematocrit values are unchanged (because whole blood has been lost), even though the total blood volume may be greatly reduced, even to the point of circulatory collapse (shock). With the passage of time, extracellular fluid begins to diffuse into the vascular system to partially restore total blood volume. Since the hematocrit is simply the percentage of RBCs compared with total blood volume (total blood volume being the RBC mass plus the plasma volume), this dilution of the blood by extracellular fluid means that the hematocrit eventually decreases, even while total blood volume is being increased (by extracellular fluid increasing plasma volume). Hemodilution (and thus the drop in hematocrit) may be hastened if the patient has been receiving intravenous (IV) fluids. Serial hematocrit determinations (once every 2–4 hours) may thus be used as a rough indication of blood volume changes. It usually takes at least 2 hours after an acute bleeding episode for a significant drop in hematocrit to be demonstrated. Sometimes it takes longer, even as long as 6–12 hours. The larger the extracellular blood loss, the sooner a significant hematocrit change (> 2%) is likely to appear.

Previous dehydration, a low plasma protein level, or both will tend to delay a hematocrit drop. Besides the uncertainty introduced by time lag, other conditions may affect the hematocrit and thus influence its interpretation as a parameter of blood volume. Anemias due to RBC hemolysis or hematopoietic factor deficiencies such as iron may decrease RBC mass without decreasing plasma or total blood volume. Similarly, plasma volume may be al-

TABLE 10–1.
Factors That Can Adversely Affect the Conditions Necessary for Accurate Blood Volume Results

1. All isotope must be delivered into the fluid volume being measured:
   - Extravasation outside vein (falsely increased result)
2. Need uniform mixing of isotope throughout fluid volume being measured:
   - Capillary sequestration in shock
   - Slow mixing in congestive heart failure
   - Focal sequestration in splenomegaly
3. Need correct normal reference values for individual patient:
   - Male vs. female
   - Obesity or malnourishment

tered in many situations involving fluid and electrolyte imbalance without changing the RBC mass. Obviously, a need exists for accurate methods of measuring blood volume.

Blood Volume Methods.—The first widely used direct blood volume measurement technique was Evan's Blue dye (T-1824). After IV injection of the dye, the amount of dilution produced by the patient's plasma was measured, and from this the plasma volume was calculated. At present, radioisotopes are the procedure of choice. These methods also are based on the dilution principle. Chromium 51 can be used to tag RBCs; a measured amount of the tagged RBCs is then injected into the patient. After equilibration for 15 minutes, a blood sample is obtained and radioactivity is measured. Since the tagged RBCs have mixed with the patient's RBCs, comparison of the radioactivity in the patient's RBCs with the original isotope specimen that was injected reveals the amount that the original isotope specimen has been diluted by the patient's RBCs; thus, the patient's total RBC mass (RBC volume) may be calculated. If the RBC mass is known, the plasma volume and total blood volume may be derived using the hematocrit value of the patient's blood. Another widely used method uses serum albumin labeled with radioactive iodine (RISA). This substance circulates in the plasma along with the other plasma proteins. Again, a measured amount is injected, a blood sample is withdrawn after a short period of equilibration, and the dilution of the original injected specimen is determined by counting the radioactivity of the patient's plasma. Plasma volume is provided by RISA measurement; RBC volume must be calculated using the patient's hematocrit. There is no doubt that isotope techniques are much more accurate than the hematocrit for estimating blood volume. Nevertheless, there are certain limitations to isotope techniques in general and specific limitations to both ^{51}Cr and RISA (Table 10–1).

Assay Problems.—The main drawback of blood volume techniques is the lack of satisfactory reference values. Attempts have been made to establish reference values for males and females in terms of height, weight, surface area, or lean body mass. Unfortunately, when one tries to apply these formulas to an individual patient, there is never any guarantee that the patient fits whatever category of normal persons that the formula was calculated from. The only way to be certain is to have a blood volume measurement from a time when the patient was healthy or prior to the bleeding episode. Unfortunately, this information is usually not available. Another drawback is the fact that no dilution method can detect bleeding that is going on during the test itself. This is so because whole blood lost during the test contains isotope in the same proportion as the blood remaining in the vascular system (a diminished isotope dose in a diminished blood volume) in contrast to the situation that would prevail if bleeding were not going on, when the entire isotope dose would remain in a diminished blood volume. Fortunately, such active bleeding would have to be severe for test results to be materially affected. Another problem is dependence on hematocrit when results for RISA are used to calculate RBC mass or data from ^{51}Cr are used to obtain plasma volume. It is well established that hematocrit values from different body areas or different-sized vessels can vary considerably, and disease may accentuate this variation. The venous hematocrit may therefore not be representative of the average vascular hematocrit.

Single-Tag vs. Double-Tag Methods.—All authorities in the field agree that blood volume determination combining independent measurement of RBC mass by ^{51}Cr and plasma volume by RISA is more accurate than the use of either isotope alone. Nevertheless, because both isotopes must be counted separately with special equipment, most laboratories use only a single isotope technique. Most authorities concede that ^{51}Cr has a slightly better overall accuracy than RISA, although some dispute this strongly. However, most ^{51}Cr techniques call for an extra venipuncture to obtain RBCs from the patient for tagging, plus an extra 30-minute wait while the actual tagging of the cells takes place. In addition, tagged RBCs (and their radioactivity) remain in the circulation during the life span of the cells. The main advantages of RISA are the need for one less venipuncture than ^{51}Cr and the fact that RISA procedures can be done in less than half the time of ^{51}Cr studies. The error with RISA blood volume has reached 300 ml in some studies, although most determinations come much closer to double-isotope results. In patients with markedly increased vascular permeability, significant quantities of RISA may be lost from blood vessels during the test, which may produce additional error. Severe edema is an example of such a situation. Nevertheless, even under adverse conditions, RISA (and ^{51}Cr) represents a decided advance over hematocrit values for estimating blood volume.

Central Venous Pressure Measurement.— Central venous pressure (CVP) is frequently used as an estimate of blood volume status. However, CVP is affected by cardiac function and by vascular resistance as well as by blood volume. Circumstances in which the CVP does not accurately reflect the relationship between blood quantity and vascular capacity include pulmonary hypertension (emphysema, embolization, mitral stenosis), left ventricular failure, and technical artifacts due to defects in catheter placement and maintenance.

BIBLIOGRAPHY

McGrath K, et al: Detection of HLA antibodies by platelet crossmatching techniques. *Transfusion* 1988; 28:214.

O'Connell B, et al: The value of 10-minute posttransfusion platelet counts. *Transfusion* 1988; 28:66.

McMican A: Neonatal transfusion therapy. *Lab Med* 1988; 19:353.

Walker RH: Special report: Transfusion risks. *Am J Clin Pathol* 1987; 88:374.

Alsop KS, Condie RM: Current status of hemoglobin-based resuscitative fluid. *Lab Med* 1987; 18:444.

McMican A, et al: Practical aspects of blood irradiation. *Lab Med* 1987; 18:299.

Aster RH, et al: Consensus Conference: Platelet transfusion therapy. *JAMA* 1987; 257:1777.

Kieckbusch ME, et al: Platelet crossmatch evaluation in refractory hematologic patients. *Mayo Clin Proc* 1987; 62:595.

Coffin CM: Current issues in transfusion therapy: 2. Indications for use of blood components. *Postgrad Med* 1987; 81:343.

AMA Council on Scientific Affairs: Autologous blood transfusions. *JAMA* 1986; 256:2378.

Prince AM: Effect of heat treatment of lyophilised blood derivatives on infectivity of human immunodeficiency virus. *Lancet* 1986; 1:1280.

NIH Consensus Conference: The utility of therapeutic plasmapheresis for neurological disorders. *JAMA* 1986; 256:1333.

Gould SA, et al: Fluosol-DA as a red-cell substitute in acute anemia. *N Engl J Med* 1986; 314:1653.

AMA Council on Scientific Affairs: Current status of therapeutic plasmapheresis and related techniques. *JAMA* 1985; 253:819.

Tullis JL, et al: Consensus Conference: Fresh-frozen plasma. *JAMA* 1985; 253:551.

Popovsky MA, et al: Intraoperative autologous transfusion. *Mayo Clin Proc* 1985; 60:125.

Boral LI: Platelet transfusion therapy. *Lab Med* 1985; 16:221.

Graze PR: How fast should platelets be transfused? *Diagn Med* 1984; 7(9):15.

Braunstein AH, Oberman HA: Transfusion of plasma components. *Transfusion* 1984; 24:281.

Wooten MJ: Leukocyte-poor, washed red blood cells in transfusion therapy. *Lab Med* 1984; 15:42.

Domen RE: Transfusion therapy of the oncology patient. *Lab Med* 1984; 15:251.

Theil KL, Kennedy MS: Corrected count increment: A measure to detect platelet alloimmunization. *Diagn Med* 1984; 7(10):8.

Insalaco SJ: Massive transfusion. *Lab Med* 1984; 15:325.

Sehgal LR, et al: Appraisal of red cell substitutes: Hemoglobin solution and perfluorochemical emulsions. *Lab Med* 1983; 14:545.

Lerner KG: Autotransfusion. *Lab Med* 1983; 14:273.

Simpson S: A survey of blood-ordering practices for elective surgical procedures. *Lab Med* 1982; 13:357.

Feng CS: Therapeutic plasmapheresis. *Postgrad Med* 1982; 72:251.

Maierhoter W, et al: Treatment of the bleeding tendency in uremia with cryoprecipitate. *N Engl J Med* 1981; 305:645.

Noto TA, Steib MD: Use of exchange transfusions in neonatology. *Lab Med* 1981; 12:609.

International Committee for Standardization in Haematology: Recommended methods for measurement of red-cell and plasma volume. *J Nucl Med* 1980; 21:793.

Alexander MR, et al: Therapeutic use of albumin. *JAMA* 1979; 241:2527.

11 Undesirable Effects of Blood or Blood Product Transfusion

Transfusion reactions occur in a certain percentage of blood transfusions. The three main types are hemolytic, febrile, and allergic. Although there is some overlap with topics discussed in chapter 8 (blood coagulation), chapter 9 (immunohematology), and chapter 10 (blood transfusion), this chapter will provide a more in-depth discussion of transfusion-related problems.

HEMOLYTIC REACTIONS

Hemolytic reactions may be caused by either complete or incomplete antibodies. In reactions caused by complete antibodies, such as occur in the ABO blood group system, there is usually intravascular hemolysis. The amount of hemolysis depends on several factors, such as quantity of incompatible blood, antibody titer, and the nature of the antibody involved. However, there is an element of individual susceptibility; some patients die after transfusion of less than 100 ml of incompatible blood, whereas others survive transfusion of several times this amount. The direct Coombs test result is often positive, but this depends on whether all the RBCs attacked by the complete antibody have been lysed, whether more antibody is produced, and, to some extent, on how soon the test is obtained. If the sample is drawn more than 1 hour after the ABO transfusion reaction is completed, the chance of a positive direct Coombs test result is much less. A Coombs reagent acting against both gamma globulin and complement (broad spectrum) is needed; most laboratories now use this type routinely. Free hemoglobin is released into the plasma from lysed RBCs and is carried to the kidneys, where it is excreted in the urine. Some of the intravascular hemoglobin is converted to bilirubin in the reticuloendothelial system so that the serum nonconjugated (indirect) bilirubin level usually begins to increase. In reactions caused by incomplete antibodies, such as the Rh system, there is sequestration of antibody-coated cells in organs such as the spleen, with subsequent breakdown by the reticuloendothelial system. With incomplete antibody reactions, RBC breakdown is extravascular rather than intravascular; in small degrees of reaction, plasma free hemoglobin levels may not rise, although indirect bilirubin levels may eventually increase. In more extensive reactions, the plasma hemoglobin level is often elevated, although the elevation is sometimes delayed in onset. The direct Coombs test should be positive in hemolytic reactions due to incomplete antibodies (unless all affected RBCs have been destroyed).

Hemolytic transfusion reactions are usually caused by incompatible blood but are occasionally caused by partial hemolysis of the RBCs before administration, either before leaving the blood bank or just prior to transfusion if the blood is warmed improperly. Analysis of fatal cases of hemolytic transfusion reaction reported to the Food and Drug Administration in 1976–1983 shows that almost 65% were due to problems of mistaken identity and about 9% were due to clerical error. Only about 18% were due to error while performing blood bank tests.

Frequent mistakes included transfusion into one patient of blood meant for another patient, obtaining a recipient crossmatch specimen from the wrong patient, mixup of patient crossmatch specimens in the blood bank, and transcription of data belonging to one patient onto the report of another.

The great majority of hemolytic transfusion reactions occur during transfusion. Symptoms and laboratory evidence of hemolysis usually are present by the time transfusion of the incompatible unit is completed, although clinical symptoms or laboratory abnormalities may sometimes be delayed for a few minutes or even a few hours. Occasionally, hemolytic reactions take place after completion of transfusion. In one kind of delayed reaction, the reaction occurs 1–5 days following transfusion and is due to anamnestic stimulation of antibodies that were already present but in very low titer. The Kidd (Jk) system is frequently associated with this group. The intensity of the reaction may be mild or may be clinically evident, but most are not severe. In a second kind of delayed reaction, the reaction occurs several weeks after transfusion and is due to new immunization by the transfused RBC antigens with new antibody production. This type of reaction is usually mild and subclinical. In both types of reaction, and occasionally even in an immediate acute reaction, a hemolytic reaction may not be suspected and the problem is discovered accidentally by a drop in hemoglobin level or by crossmatching for another transfusion.

Symptoms of hemolytic transfusion reaction include chills, fever, and pain in the low back or legs. Jaundice may appear later. Severe reactions lead to shock. Renal failure (acute tubular necrosis) is common due either to shock or to precipitation of free hemoglobin in the renal tubules. Therefore, oliguria develops, frequently accompanied by hemoglobinuria, which is typically manifest by red urine or nearly black "coffee ground" acid hematin urine color.

Tests for Hemolytic Transfusion Reaction

These tests include immediate rechecking and comparison of patient identification and the unit or units of transfused donor blood. Tubes of anticoagulated and nonanticoagulated blood should be drawn. The anticoagulated tube should be centrifuged immediately and the plasma examined visually for the pink or red color produced by hemolysis. A direct Coombs test and crossmatch recheck studies should be performed as soon as possible. A culture and Gram stain should be done on the remaining blood in the donor bag.

Plasma Free Hemoglobin

The presence of free hemoglobin in plasma is one of the most valuable tests for diagnosis of acute hemolytic transfusion reaction. Most cases of severe intravascular hemolysis due to bivalent antibodies such as the ABO group produce enough hemolysis to be grossly visible. (Artifactual hemolysis from improperly drawn specimens must be ruled out.) If chemical tests are to be done, plasma hemoglobin is preferred to serum hemoglobin because less artifactual hemolysis takes place before the specimen reaches the laboratory. Although hemolytic reactions due to incomplete antibodies, such as Rh, have clinical symptoms similar to those of ABO, direct signs of hemolysis (e.g., free plasma hemoglobin) are more variable or may be delayed for a few hours, although they become abnormal if the reaction is severe. Another drawback in the interpretation of plasma hemoglobin values is the effect of the transfusion itself. The older erythrocytes stored in banked blood die during storage, adding free hemoglobin to the plasma. Therefore, although reference values are usually considered to be in the range of 1–5 mg/100 ml, values between 5 and 50 mg/100 ml are equivocal if stored blood is given. Hemolysis is barely visible when plasma hemoglobin reaches the 25–50 mg/100 ml range. Frozen blood has a greater content of free hemoglobin than stored whole blood or packed cells and may reach 300 mg/100 ml.

Additional Tests

If visual inspection of patient plasma does not suggest hemolysis and the direct Coombs test result is negative, additional laboratory tests may be desirable to detect or confirm a hemolytic transfusion reaction. Procedures that may be useful include serum haptoglobin measurement, both immediately and 6 hours later; serum indirect bilirubin measurement at 6 and 12 hours; and urinalysis.

A pretransfusion blood specimen, if available, should be included in a transfusion reaction investigation to provide baseline data when the various tests for hemolysis are performed.

Urinalysis.—Urine can be examined for hemoglobin casts, red blood cells (RBCs), and protein and tested for free hemoglobin. Red blood cells and RBC casts may be found in hemolytic reactions since the kidney is frequently injured. If no hematuria or free hemoglobin is found, this is some evidence against a major acute hemolytic transfusion reaction. Abnormal findings are more difficult to interpret unless a pretransfusion urinalysis result is available for comparison, since the abnormality might have been present before transfusion. In addition, abnormal urine findings could result from hypoxic renal damage due to an episode of hypotension during surgery rather than a transfusion reaction.

Hemoglobin passes through the glomerular filter into the urine when the plasma hemoglobin level is above 125 mg/100 ml. Therefore, since hemolysis should already be visible, the major need for urine examination is to verify that intravascular hemolysis occurred rather than artifactual hemolysis from venipuncture or faulty specimen processing. Conversely, unless the plasma free hemoglobin level is elevated, urine hemoglobin may represent lysed RBCs from hematuria unrelated to a hemolytic reaction. However, if sufficient time passes, the serum may be cleared of free hemoglobin while hemoglobin casts are still present in urine. Hemosiderin may be deposited in renal tubule cells and continue to appear in the urine for several days.

Serum Haptoglobin.—Haptoglobin is an alpha globulin that binds free hemoglobin. Two types of measurements are available: haptoglobin-binding capacity and total haptoglobin. Binding capacity can be measured by electrophoresis or chemical methods. Total haptoglobin is usually estimated by immunologic (antibody) techniques; a 2-minute slide test is now commercially available. The haptoglobin-binding capacity decreases almost immediately when a sufficient quantity of free hemoglobin is liberated and remains low for 2–4 days. Stored banked blood, fortunately, does not contain enough free hemoglobin to produce significant changes in haptoglobin-binding capacity. The total haptoglobin level decreases more slowly than the binding capacity after onset of a hemolytic reaction and might not reach its lowest value until 6–8 hours later. Haptoglobin assay is much less helpful when frozen RBCs are transfused due to the normally increased free hemoglobin in most frozen RBC preparations. Bilirubin determinations are not needed if haptoglobin assay is done the same day.

In common with other laboratory tests, serum haptoglobin levels may be influenced by various factors other than the one for which the test is ordered. Haptoglobin levels may be decreased by absorption of hemoglobin from an extravascular hematoma and also may be decreased in severe liver disease, hemolytic or megaloblastic anemia, estrogen therapy, and pump-assisted open heart cardiac surgery. Haptoglobin is one of the body's "acute-phase reactant" proteins that are increased by infection, tissue injury or destruction, widespread malignancy, and adrenocorticosteroid therapy. Therefore, a mild decrease in haptoglobin level could be masked by one of these conditions.

Sensitivity of Tests in Hemolytic Reaction

Data regarding frequency of test abnormality in transfusion reaction are difficult to obtain. In one series, comprising predominantly hemolytic reactions not due to ABO antibodies, free hemoglobin was detected in plasma or urine in 88% of cases involving immediate reactions and in 52% of cases involving incomplete antibodies or delayed reactions. Serum haptoglobin levels were decreased in 92% of the patients in whom it was assayed. Various factors influence this type of data, such as the amount of incompatible blood, the antibody involved, the time relationship of specimen to onset of reaction, and the test method used.

Nursing Station Action in Possible Hemolytic Reaction

Transfusion should be stopped at the first sign of possible reaction and complete studies done to recheck compatibility of the donor and recipient blood. If these are still satisfactory, and if results of the direct Coombs test and the studies for intravascular hemolysis are negative, a different unit can be started on the assumption that the symptoms were pyrogenic rather than hemolytic. Whatever unused blood remains in the donor bottle, the donor bottle pilot tube, and a new specimen drawn from the patient must all be sent to the blood bank for recheck studies. Especially dangerous situations exist in transfusion during surgery, where anesthesia may mask the early signs and symptoms of a reaction. Development during surgery of a marked bleeding or oozing tendency at the operative site is an important danger signal. A hemolytic transfusion reaction requires immediate mannitol or equivalent therapy to protect the kidneys.

Hemolytic Disease of the Newborn

The other major area where blood banks meet blood group hemolytic problems is in hemolytic disease of the newborn (HDN). It may be due to ABO, Rh, or (rarely) minor group incompatibility between fetal and maternal RBCs. ABO and the Rh antigen D (Rho) are by far the most common causes. The Rh antigen c and the blood group Kell antigen are next most important. Hemolytic disease of the newborn results from fetal RBC antigens that the maternal RBCs lack. These fetal RBC antigens provoke maternal antibody formation when fetal RBCs are introduced into the maternal circulation after escaping from the placenta. The maternal antibodies eventually cross the placenta to the fetal circulation and attack the fetal RBCs.

Hemolytic Disease of the Newborn Due to Rh

Hemolytic disease of the newborn due to Rh incompatibility varies in severity from subclinical status, through mild jaundice with anemia, to the dangerous and often fatal condition of erythroblastosis fetalis. The main clinical findings are anemia and rapidly developing jaundice. Reticulocytosis over 6% accompanies the anemia, and the jaundice is mainly due to unconjugated (indirect) bilirubin released from the reticuloendothelial sequestration and destruction of RBCs. The direct Coombs test result is positive. In severe cases there are usually many nucleated RBCs in the peripheral blood. Jaundice is not present at birth (since the mother excretes bilirubin produced by the fetus) but develops several hours later or even after 24 hours in mild cases. Diseases that cause jaundice in the newborn, often accompanied by anemia and sometimes a few peripheral blood nucleated RBCs, include septicemia, cytomegalic inclusion disease, toxoplasmosis, and syphilis. Physiologic jaundice of the newborn is a frequent benign condition that may be confused with hemolytic disease or vice versa. There is, however, no significant anemia. A normal newborn has a (average) hemoglobin value of 18 gm/100 ml (see Table 36–3), and a value less than 15 gm/100 ml (150 g/L) indicates anemia. Anemia may be masked if heelstick (capillary) blood is used, since neonatal capillary hemoglobin values are higher than venous blood values.

Hemolytic disease due to Rh incompatibility occurs in an Rh-negative mother whose fetus is Rh positive. The mother develops antibodies against the RBC Rh antigen after being exposed to Rh-positive RBCs. This may occur due to pregnancy, abortion, ectopic pregnancy, amniocentesis (or other placental trauma), blood transfusion with Rh-positive RBCs, or transfusion of certain RBC-contaminated blood products such as platelets. The most common maternal contact with Rh-positive RBCs occurs during pregnancy when fetal RBCs escape through the placenta into the maternal circulation. This may happen at any time after the 16th week of pregnancy, and both the quantity of cells and the frequency of exposure increase until delivery. The largest single dose of fetal RBCs occurs during delivery. Not all mothers have detectable fetal RBCs in their circulation, and of those who do, not all become sensitized during any one pregnancy. There is approximately a 10%–13% risk of sensitization in previously nonsensitized Rh-incompatible pregnancies. When fetal-maternal ABO incompatibility (with the mother being group O) is present, the usual risk for Rh sensitization is decreased, presumably because sufficient fetal cells are destroyed that the stimulus for sensitization is reduced below the necessary level.

The first child is usually not affected by Rh hemolytic disease if the mother has not been exposed to Rh-positive RBCs before pregnancy, and full sensitization usually does not develop until after delivery in those mothers who become sensitized. However, occasional firstborn infants are affected (5%–10% of HDN infants) either because of previous maternal exposure (e.g., a previous aborted pregnancy) or because of unusually great maternal susceptibility to Rh stimulus during normal pregnancy. Once maternal sensitization takes place, future exposure to Rh antigen, as during another pregnancy with an Rh-positive fetus, results in maternal antibody production against the Rh antigen, which can affect the fetus.

Current recommendations of the American College of Obstetricians and Gynecologists (ACOG) are that every pregnant woman should have ABO and Rh typing and a serum antibody screen as early as possible during each pregnancy. If results of the antibody screen are negative and the mother is Rh positive, the antibody screen should be repeated early in the third trimester. Theoretically, if the mother is Rh positive, or if the mother is Rh negative and the father is also Rh negative, there should be no risk of Rh-induced fetal disease. However, the antibody screen is still necessary to detect appearance of non-Rh antibodies. If results of the antibody screen are negative and the mother is Rh negative, the father should be typed for Rh and the antibody screen should be repeated at 28 weeks' gestation. If the antibody screen results are still negative, a prophylactic dose of Rh immune globulin is recommended (discussed later). If the antibody screen detects an antibody, subsequent testing or action depends on whether the antibody is Rh or some other blood group and whether or not this is the first pregnancy that the antibody was detected. The father should be tested to see if he has the antigen corresponding to the antibody. If the antibody is one of the Rh group, antibody titers should be performed every 2 weeks. Titers less than 1:16 suggest less risk of fetal hazard. Titer equal to or greater than 1:16 is usually followed by amniocentesis for amniotic fluid spectrophotometric examination (as early as 24 weeks' gestation). Antibodies that are not Rh are managed by amniotic fluid examination without antibody titers, since there is inadequate correlation of titers to fetal outcome.

Rh Immune Globulin

Studies have now proved that nearly all nonsensitized mothers with potential or actual Rh incompatibility problems can be protected against sensitization from the fetus by means of a "vaccine" composed of gamma globulin with a high titer of anti-Rh antibody (RhIg). This exogenous antibody seems to prevent sensitization by destroying fetal RBCs within the mother's circulation and also by suppressing maternal antibody production. Abortion (spontaneous or induced), ectopic pregnancy, amniocentesis, and platelet or granulocyte transfusions (which may be contaminated with Rh-positive RBCs) may also induce sensitization and should be treated with RhIg. Current ACOG recommendations are to administer one unit (300 μg) of RhIg to all Rh-negative women at 28 weeks of gestation and a second unit within 72 hours after delivery. A minidose of 50 μg is often used rather than the standard dose when abortion occurs before 12 weeks' gestation. Although 72 hours after delivery is the recommended time limit for RhIg administration, there is some evidence that some effect may be obtained up to 7 days after delivery. Untreated Rh-negative women have about a 10%–13% incidence of Rh antibody production (sensitization). When RhIg is administered postpartum it reduces incidence to about 1%–2%, and antepartum use combined with postpartum use reduces the incidence to about 0.1%–0.2%. It will produce a positive Rh antibody screening test result if present in sufficient titer, so that antibody screening should be performed before administration rather than after. The half-life of exogenous gamma globulin (which applies to RhIg) is about 25 days (range 23–28 days). Injected RhIg may be detected in maternal blood after intramuscular injection within 24–48 hours with a peak at about 5 days and may still be detectable for as long as 3 months. Detection after 6 months postpartum suggests patient sensitization (failure of the RhIg). There have been a few reports that some Rh-positive infants whose mother received antepartum RhIg had a weakly positive direct Coombs test result at birth due to the RhIg. The blood bank should always be informed if RhIg has been given antepartum to properly interpret laboratory test results. The standard dose of 300 μg of RhIg neutralizes approximately 15 ml of Rh-positive RBCs (equivalent to 30 ml of fetal whole blood). In some patients the RBCs received from the fetus may total more than 15 ml. There are several methods used to quantitate fetal RBCs in the maternal circulation, none of which are considered ideal. The Kleihauer acid elution test is a peripheral smear technique that stains the hemoglobin F (Hb F) of fetal RBCs. Other tests that have been used are the D^u test read microscopically (to detect the mixed field agglutination of the relatively small number of fetal RBCs involved) and the RhIg crossmatch technique. None of these three procedures has proved adequately sensitive. For example, a proficiency survey in 1980 found that about 10% of the laboratories using acid elution or microscopic D^u techniques failed to detect the equivalent of 30 ml of fetal RBCs (twice the significant level). When a normal blood sample was tested, about 10% of those using microscopic D^u obtained false positive results, and those using acid elution had 40% or more false positive results (especially with one commercial adaptation of the acid elution technique called Fetaldex). Also, false positive acid elution test results can be produced if increased maternal Hb F is present, as seen in beta thalassemia minor and in hereditary persistence of fetal hemoglobin. Newer procedures, such as the erythrocyte rosette test, have proved much more sensitive and somewhat more reproducible. However, the rosette test is not quantitative, so that screening is done with the rosette test (or equivalent) and a positive result is followed by quantitation with the acid elution procedure. If the quantitative test for fetal RBCs indicates that more than 15 ml is present, additional RhIg should be administered. If this is not done, failure rates for RhIg of 10%–15% have been reported; if it is done, the failure rate is approximately 2%. The current American Association of Blood Banks (AABB) recommendation is to administer twice the dose of RhIg indicated by formulas, depending on the percent of fetal RBCs detected by acid elution methods. This is done because of variation above and below the correct result found on proficiency surveys.

Laboratory Tests in Hemolytic Disease of Newborns (HDN)

When an infant is affected by Rh-induced HDN, the result of the direct Coombs test on cord blood is nearly always positive. In ABO-induced HDN the direct Coombs test result on cord blood is frequently positive. The direct Coombs test result on infant peripheral blood is usually positive in Rh-induced disease but is frequently negative in ABO-induced disease, especially when done more than 24 hours after delivery. The direct Coombs test should be performed in all cases of possible HDN, because incomplete antibodies occasionally coat the surface of fetal RBCs to such an extent as to interfere with proper Rh typing. Cord blood bilirubin is usually increased and cord blood hemoglobin is decreased in hemolytic disease of the newborn. It has been reported that the cord blood hemoglobin level has a better correlation with disease severity than the cord blood bilirubin or infant venous or capillary hemoglobin. Infant hemoglobin tends to be higher than cord hemoglobin if blood from the cord and placenta is allowed to reach the infant after delivery.

ABO-Induced Hemolytic Disease of the Newborn

Fifty percent or more of HDN is due to ABO incompatibility between mother and fetus. Most cases are found in mothers of blood group O with infants of other blood groups. Infant anti-A and anti-B production begins between 3 and 6 months after birth. Until then, ABO antibodies in the infant's serum originate from the mother. If the mother possesses antibodies to the A or B RBC antigens of the fetus, hemolytic disease of the fetus or newborn may result, just as if the fetus or newborn had received a transfusion of serum with antibodies against his or her RBCs. Nevertheless, although 20%–25% of all pregnancies display maternal-fetal ABO incompatibility, only a small number of these infants develop clinically evident hemolytic disease. In those who do, the condition is usually clinically milder than its counterpart caused by Rh incompatibility. The incidence of clinically evident disease is about the same as that of Rh, although even severe cases are relatively milder than the comparable Rh cases. Some infants, however, will die or suffer cerebral damage if treatment is not given. Therefore, the diagnosis of ABO disease and its differential diagnosis from the other causes of jaundice and anemia in the newborn are of great practical importance.

There are two types of ABO antibodies: the naturally occurring complete saline reacting type discussed earlier and an immune univalent (incomplete) type produced in some unknown way to fetal A or B antigen stimulation. In most cases of clinical ABO disease the mother is group O and the infant is group A or B. The immune anti-A or anti-B antibody, if produced by the mother, may cause ABO disease, because it can pass the placenta. Maternal titers of 1:16 or more are considered dangerous. The saline antibodies do not cross the placenta and are not significant in HDN.

Results of the direct Coombs test done on the infant with ABO hemolytic disease are probably more often negative than positive, and even when positive the test tends to be only weakly reactive. Spherocytes are often present but the number is variable. Good evidence for ABO disease is detection of immune anti-A or anti-B antibodies in the cord blood of a newborn whose RBCs belong to the same blood group as the antibody. Detection of these antibodies only in the serum of the mother does not conclusively prove that ABO disease exists in the newborn.

Laboratory Criteria for Hemolytic Disease of the Newborn

Infants with HDN can frequently be saved by exchange transfusion. Commonly accepted indications for this procedure are:

1. Infant serum indirect bilirubin level more than 20 mg/100 ml (342 μmol/L) or, in premature infants, 15 mg/100 ml (257 μmol/L).
2. Cord blood indirect bilirubin level more than 3 mg/100 ml (51 μmol/L) (some require 4 mg/100 ml).
3. Cord blood hemoglobin level less than 13 gm/dl (130 g/L) (literature range 8–14 gm/100 ml).
4. Maternal Rh antibody titer of 1:64 or greater, although this is not an absolute indication if the bilirubin does not rise very high.

Bilirubin Levels in Hemolytic Disease of the Newborn.—Most infants with HDN can be treated effectively enough that exchange transfusion is not needed. The level of infant bilirubin is generally used as the major guideline for decision and to monitor results of other treatment such as phototherapy. An infant total bilirubin level greater than 12 mg/100 ml (205 μmol/L) is the most commonly accepted value at which therapy is begun. However, there is surprising variation in the levels quoted in various medical centers. Also, kernicterus has been reported at bilirubin levels of 9.5 mg/100 ml (and even as low as 6 mg/100 ml), although this is uncommon. Most infants who develop kernicterus with bilirubin levels less than 20 mg/100 ml have been premature, and those with kernicterus at levels less than 10 mg/100 ml were very ill. The rapidity with which the bilirubin level rises is also a factor. One report suggests that exchange transfusion be initiated if the serum indirect bilirubin level is 15 mg/100 ml rather than 20 mg/100 ml if this level is reached within 48 hours after delivery and even at 10 mg/100 ml if this level is reached within 24 hours after delivery. To further complicate matters, autopsy studies have shown yellow staining of brain tissue typical of kernicterus in some infants who did not have clinical symptoms of kernicterus. Therefore, it may be necessary to retrospectively correlate predictive levels of bilirubin with clinical symptoms rather than with gross autopsy findings. Another problem concerns interpretation of total bilirubin levels during phototherapy. Light breaks down bilirubin into nontoxic bilirubin isomers, which, however, are measured and included with unconjugated bilirubin in standard bilirubin assays. Finally, it must be mentioned that bilirubin is one of the least accurate of frequently or routinely performed chemistry assays, with proficiency surveys consistently showing between-laboratory coefficients of variation of 10% or more. To this is added variances due to specimens obtained under different conditions (venous vs. capillary or heelstick), state of infant hydration, and differences between laboratories because of different methodologies. At present, the bilirubin measurement within the capability of most laboratories that is considered to best correlate with clinical kernicterus is unconjugated (indirect) bilirubin. In HDN, most of the bilirubin will be unconjugated. Therefore, it usually is sufficient to obtain total bilirubin levels in order to follow the patient's progress. If there is a question about the diagnosis, one request for conjugated/unconjugated fractionation is sufficient. A definite consideration is the additional blood needed to assay both the conjugated and unconjugated fractions since large specimens may be difficult to obtain from an infant heel puncture.

Albumin-Bound Bilirubin.—Unconjugated bilirubin is presumed to be the cause of kernicterus. However, unconjugated or total bilirubin levels do not always correlate well with development of kernicterus. Most of the unconjugated bilirubin in serum is tightly bound to serum albumin, with a small portion being loosely bound ("free"). Since the free portion rather than the tightly bound portion theoretically should be the most important element in kernicterus, various methods have been devised to assay free unconjugated bilirubin rather than total bilirubin. Until approximately 1980, direct measurement was difficult, and most attention was given to indirect methods, chiefly estimation of the bilirubin-binding capacity of albumin. In general, when more bilirubin binds to albumin, the residual binding capacity becomes smaller and less binding of serum free bilirubin takes place. Therefore, free bilirubin levels are more likely to increase. Several methods have been proposed to measure albumin-binding capacity; the most popular involved a Sephadex resin column. Sephadex resin competes with albumin for loosely bound bilirubin. When unconjugated bilirubin levels exceed the bilirubin-binding capacity of albumin, the excess binds to the sephadex column. There are conflicting reports in the literature on the value of the albumin-binding capacity assay. Some reports indicated that it was very helpful; others found that results from individual patients were either too often borderline or did not correlate sufficiently well with the clinical picture. More recently, an instrument called the hematofluorometer that measures total bilirubin-binding capacity (TBBC) has become available. Total bilirubin-binding capacity as measured by the hematofluorometer is reported to correlate well with unbound bilirubin. In summary, although a total bilirubin level of 20 mg/100 ml is a reasonably good cutoff point for substantial risk of kernicterus in full-term infants, no adequate cutoff point has been found for sick premature infants; nor has consideration of risk factors such as septicemia, acidosis, hypothermia, hypoxia, hypoalbuminemia, or bilirubin-binding capacity led to safe criteria for therapy vs. nontherapy.

Role of Amniocentesis in Hemolytic Disease of the Newborn.—Amniocentesis has been advocated in selected patients as a means of estimating risk of severe HDN while the fetus is still in utero. A long needle is introduced into the amniotic fluid cavity by a suprapubic puncture approach in the mother. The amniotic fluid is subjected to spectrophotometric estimation of bilirubin pigments. Markedly increased bilirubin pigment levels strongly indicate significant degrees of hemolytic disease in the fetus. If necessary, delivery can be induced prematurely once the 32nd week of gestation has arrived. Before this, or if the fetus is severely diseased, intrauterine exchange transfusion has been attempted using a transabdominal approach. The indications for amniocentesis are development of significant titer of Rh antibody in the mother or a history of previous erythroblastosis. Significant maternal antibody Rh titers do not always mean serious fetal Rh disease, but absence of significant titer nearly always indicates a benign prognosis. Also, if initial amniocentesis at 32 weeks does not suggest an immediately dangerous situation, even though mild or moderate abnormalities are present, a fetus can be allowed to mature as long as possible (being monitored by repeated studies) to avoid the danger of premature birth.

GRAFT-vs.-HOST DISEASE

This syndrome results from introduction of sufficient HLA-incompatible immunologically competent donor lymphocytes into a recipient who is sufficiently immunodeficient that the incompatible donor cells cannot be destroyed. Current reports indicate that 60%–70% of patients with bone marrow grafts from HLA-compatible siblings develop some degree of graft-vs.-host symptoms, and 10%–20% of marrow transplant patients die from it. In other patients, transfusion is the usual cause. Patients at risk are those receiving intrauterine or neonatal exchange transfusions, and in congenital immunodeficiency syndromes, malignancy undergoing intensive chemotherapy (especially when combined with radiotherapy), and aplastic anemia. Incidence of post-transfusion graft-vs.-host syndrome in these conditions is not known with certainty but varies from 0%–8%, depending on the disease, therapy, and institution. The highest incidence appears to be in malignant lymphoma. In classic cases the syndrome develops 1–2 weeks (range 3 days–6 weeks) after transfusion and consists of fever, severe diarrhea, pancytopenia, hepatitis, and skin rash. Up to 90% of patients with a transfusion-related full-blown syndrome die, usually from infection. This syndrome can be prevented by gamma radiation treatment of the blood product being transfused, in dosage sufficient to affect lymphocytes but not other blood cells (usually 1,500–2,500 rad). Red blood cell transfusion itself has immunologic effects on the recipient. It has been shown that random-donor blood transfusions prior to renal transplant decrease the incidence of graft rejection. Some institutions use RBC transfusion for this purpose. It is reported that transfusion therapy depresses natural killer cell function in these patients but the T4/T8 cell ratio remains normal. In addition, some studies report a somewhat greater incidence of recurrences or decreased overall survival in colon cancer patients who had multiple transfusions compared with those without transfusion, although this is disputed by other investigators.

PLATELET REACTIONS

Blood platelets contain at least three antigen systems capable of producing a transfusion reaction. The first is the ABO (ABH) system, also found on RBCs; for that reason the AABB recommends that single-donor platelet units be typed for the ABO group before being transfused. Platelets do not contain the Rh antigen; however, since platelet units may be contaminated by RBCs, it is safer to type for D (Rh_o) antigen in addition to ABO typing. The majority of investigators believe that ABO-Rh typing is useful only to avoid possible sensitization of the recipient to RBCs and that recipient anti-A or anti-B antibody will not destroy ABO-incompatible platelets. There are platelet-specific antigens (PLA1 group, also called Zw^a, and several others) that are found in high incidence and thus rarely cause difficulty. However, PLA1 antibodies have been implicated in a syndrome known as posttransfusion purpura (chapter 8). Finally, there is the histocompatibility leukocyte antigen (HLA-A) group. This tissue compatibility system has been incriminated in patients who become refractory to repeated platelet transfusions (i.e., in whom the platelet count fails to rise) and in those who develop a febrile reaction after platelet administration. Persons who are HLA-A compatible (usually siblings) as a rule are able to donate satisfactorily. The HLA-A antigens are also present on white blood cells (WBCs). Finally, other types of antiplatelet antibodies may appear, such as those of chronic idiopathic thrombocytopenia. In this situation, transfused platelets are quickly destroyed, making the transfusion of little value unless the patient is actively bleeding (chapter 10).

FEBRILE REACTIONS

A febrile transfusion reaction is usually defined as a nonhemolytic reaction that includes fever as one symptom.

Leukoagglutinin Reaction.—Probably the most common variety of transfusion reaction is a febrile episode during or just after transfusion due to patient antibodies (leukoagglutinins) against donor leukocytes. Before leukoagglutinins were recognized, these episodes were included among the pyrogenic reactions (discussed later). Fever may be the only symptom but there may be others, such as chills, headache, malaise, confusion, and tachycardia. In a small number of cases a syndrome known as transfusion-related acute lung injury is produced. It includes febrile reaction symptoms plus dyspnea and tachycardia; the chest x-ray film has a characteristic pattern described as numerous hilar and lower lobe nodular infiltrates without cardiac enlargement or pulmonary vessel congestion. In some cases the clinical picture includes marked hypoxemia and also hypotension and thus strongly resembles the adult respiratory distress syndrome. However, symptoms usually substantially improve or disappear in 24–48 hours (81% of patients in one report), but the radiologic abnormalities may persist for several days. Some patients have eosinophilia, but others do not. The syndrome has been called "noncardiac pulmonary edema," a somewhat unfortunate term since pulmonary edema is not present, although many clinical findings simulate pulmonary edema. Most cases with leukoagglutinin lung involvement follow transfusion of whole blood. At least some of these reactions have been traced to HLA antigen system incompatibility.

Most patients produce leukoagglutinins due to previous transfusion or from fetal antigen sensitization in pregnancy. The more transfusions, the greater the likelihood of sensitization.

Reactions due to leukoagglutinins are usually not life threatening but are unpleasant to the patient, physician, and laboratory. Since clinical symptoms are similar to those of a hemolytic reaction, each febrile reaction must be investigated to rule out RBC incompatibility, even if the patient is known to have leukoagglutinins. Leukoagglutinin reactions may be reduced or eliminated by the use of leukocyte-poor packed cells, washed cells, or frozen RBCs (chapter 10). There are specialized tests available to demonstrate leukoagglutinin activity, but most laboratories are not equipped to perform them. The diagnosis, therefore, is usually a presumptive one based on history and ruling out hemolytic reaction.

Washed or frozen RBCs contain fewer WBCs than the average leukocyte-poor packed cell preparation. However, since washed or frozen RBCs must either be transfused within 24 hours after preparation or be discarded, one must be certain that a need for transfusion exists sufficient to guarantee that the blood will actually be administered before these blood products are ordered.

Immunoglobulin A Antigen Reactions.—Immunoglobulin A (chapter 21) is the principal immunoglobulin in such human secretions as saliva, bile, and gastric juice. *Class-specific* anti-IgA occurs in patients who lack IgA; these persons may be clinically normal or may have such disorders as malabsorption syndrome, autoimmune disease, or recurrent sinus or pulmonary infection. *Limited specificity* anti-IgA occurs in persons who have normal IgA levels but who become sensitized from exposure to human plasma proteins from blood transfusion or pregnancy. Anti-IgA antibodies produce reaction only in transfusions that include human plasma proteins. Symptoms consist of tachycardia, flush, headache, chest pain, dyspnea, and fever. Severe episodes may include hypotension. Again, these are nonspecific symptoms that could be produced by leukoagglutinins or hemolytic reactions. Tests to prove IgA incompatibility are available only in a few medical centers; therefore, the diagnosis is rarely made. Reactions of this type can be avoided by eliminating plasma proteins through the use of washed cells or frozen cells.

Pyrogenic Reactions.—These result from contamination by bacteria, dirt, or foreign proteins. One frequently cited study estimates that nearly 2% of donor blood units have some degree of bacterial contamination, regardless of the care taken when the blood was drawn. Symptoms begin during or shortly after transfusion and consist of chills and fever; the more severe cases often have abdominal cramps, nausea, and diarrhea. Very heavy bacterial contamination may lead to shock. Therefore, in a patient with transfusion-associated reaction that includes hypotension, a Gram-stained smear should be made from blood remaining in the donor bag without waiting for culture results.

Allergic Reactions.—Allergic reactions are presumably due to substances in the donor blood to which the recipient is allergic. Symptoms are localized or generalized hives, although occasionally severe asthma or even laryngeal edema may occur. There is usually excellent response to antihistamines or epinephrine.

INFECTIONS TRANSMITTED BY TRANSFUSION

Bacterial infection from contaminated blood or blood products is rare as long as continuous adequate refrigeration is provided. Platelets are especially apt to develop bacterial growth when stored at room temperature. The spirochetes of syphilis usually die after refrigerated storage for 4–5 days. Virus infections are a much greater problem. These infections are discussed in detail in chapter 16 and will be mentioned only briefly here.

Hepatitis Virus Infection.—Transfusion-related hepatitis virus infection occurs in about 10% of transfused patients (range 0.02%–25%) and as high as 50% in those who receive many transfusions. However, only about 10% of these infections are symptomatic. Currently, about 85%–90% of hepatitis virus infections are due to non-A, non-B (type C) hepatitis virus (or viruses). The carrier rate for type C hepatitis virus in the volunteer donor population is said to be about 1.5%. Currently, there is no commercially available serologic test for type C hepatitis virus antigen or antibody. Many blood banks are trying to eliminate donor blood containing hepatitis C by use of certain tests that are not specific for hepatitis C but that are often abnormal in hepatitis C infection (surrogate tests). The combination of elevated alanine aminotransferase (ALT, formerly SGPT) that is usually abnormal in acute liver cell injury and presence of hepatitis B core antibody (which is associated with about a threefold increased incidence of type C hepatitis in addition to indicating type B hepatitis) is reported to result in elimination of about one third of donor blood carrying hepatitis C infection. About 5%–10% of transfusion-related hepatitis virus infections are due to hepatitis B. Mandatory blood bank screening of donor blood for hepatitis B surface antigen (HBsAg) in addition to attempts to eliminate high-risk carrier groups among donors by careful questioning and reliance on nonpaid volunteer donors has eliminated more than 90% of hepatitis B transfusion–related infections. Use of frozen RBC was originally thought to eliminate hepatitis B virus infectivity, but this has proven to be untrue, although the incidence of transmission may be somewhat reduced. Therefore, any type of blood or blood product can transmit hepatitis virus infection. In general, single-donor products are less likely to carry infection than pooled-donor products. Two percent to 12% of persons who test positive for HBsAg are also carriers of delta hepatitis virus (hepatitis D virus), a virus that requires a liver cell already infected by hepatitis B to replicate. Therefore, a small percentage of patients infected by hepatitis B virus develop superimposed hepatitis D virus. Serologic tests for hepatitis D virus are just becoming available. A very small number of transfusions carry hepatitis A virus.

Cytomegalic Inclusion Virus.—After hepatitis virus, the most frequent transfusion-related virus infection is cytomegalovirus (CMV). The carrier rate for CMV in the donor population is reported to be 6%–12%, whereas 35%–70% of donors have antibody to CMV. The percentage of infected persons who develop symptoms is not well documented, but most of those who have symptoms display an illness clinically resembling infectious mononucleosis ("heterophil-negative mononucleosis"). The disease is most serious when contracted by immunocompromised persons and premature infants of low birth weight. Serologic tests for CMV antibody are now available and are used by some institutions to screen donor blood intended for low birth weight newborns and some immunocompromised persons. Since CMV is carried by WBCs, washed RBCs and frozen RBCs are reported to have a lower incidence of CMV infection than standard packed RBCs.

Human Immunodeficiency Virus.—The third important virus group is the human immunodeficiency virus-I (HIV-I, formerly called human T-cell lymphotrophic virus-III [HTLV-III] or lymphadenopathy-associated virus [LAV]). This virus is the cause of *acquired immunodeficiency syndrome* (AIDS) and the various pre-AIDS conditions. Studies have indicated a 65%–70% rate of recipient infection (based on appearance of HIV-I antibody in recipients) from antibody-positive donor blood. Until 1986, about 2% of AIDS was due to transfusion of blood or blood products. Current mandatory donor blood screening tests for HIV-I antibody plus attempts to persuade high-risk persons not to donate are thought to have eliminated well over 95% of infected donor blood. Heat treatment of factor VIII concentrate also reduces the incidence of HIV-I transmission; this plus donor testing has virtually eliminated factor VIII concentrate infectivity by HIV-I. Unfortunately, heat treatment does not affect hepatitis virus infectivity. *Therapeutic immune globulin* is also free of HIV infectivity due to the way it is prepared, although the preparations may contain detectable antibody against HIV-I. This passively transferred antibody may be responsible for a false positive HIV-I antibody test result, which may persist for as long as 6 months, if the recipient is tested for HIV antibodies. Human T-cell leukemia virus-I (HTLV-I) that causes human T-cell leukemia and human T-cell leukemia virus-II (HTLV-II) that may be associated with hairy cell leukemia (chapter 7) can also be transmitted by transfusion. Transmission of HTLV-I could be a problem in donor blood from endemic areas, such as Japan and the Caribbean. Finally, other viruses, such as the Epstein-Barr virus, can also be transmitted by transfusion. Certain *parasites*, notably malaria, could be transmitted by infected donor blood, although this is very rare outside endemic areas.

OTHER TRANSFUSION PROBLEMS

Storage of Red Blood Cells.—After approximately two thirds of RBC shelf life, some of the RBCs lose vitality and become spherocytes. Since spherocytosis is a feature of certain isoimmune and autoimmune hemolytic anemias, transfusion of such blood prior to diagnostic investigation may cause confusion. Potassium concentration slowly rises during storage as it escapes from devitalized RBCs. After about two thirds of RBC shelf life, plasma potassium levels reach about 18 mEq/L, roughly four times normal. Although the hyperkalemia of stored RBCs seems to have little effect on most persons, even when many units are transfused, it may be undesirable if the patient already has an elevated serum potassium level, as seen in uremia or acute renal failure Ammonium levels of stored blood also increase and may reach values of 10–15 times normal toward the expiration date of the RBCs. Transfusion of large volumes of such blood may be dangerous in patients with severe liver disease. *Medications in donor blood* theoretically could be a problem to the recipient. This is rarely mentioned in the medical literature, possibly due to current use of packed RBCs rather than whole blood.

Massive Blood Transfusion

Massive blood transfusion is defined by the AABB as replacement of the patient's blood volume (equivalent to 8–10 units of whole blood in a 70-kg person) within 12 hours (some define the time period as 24 hours). Transfusion of such volumes presents special difficulties, depending on the substance being transfused and the rate of administration. By the end of a transfusion sufficient to replace the equivalent quantity of one blood volume, roughly one third of any substance originally in the patient's blood will remain (range 18%–40%), predominantly because of dilution with transfused material. The most common and serious complication of massive transfusion is bleeding; the most common identifiable cause is platelet related, with factor deficiency next most frequent. Massive transfusion is sometimes complicated by disseminated intravascular coagulation (reported in 5%–30% of severely traumatized patients).

Platelets.—Platelets devitalize rapidly on storage if they are not separated from RBCs. In fresh whole blood, platelets are about 60% effective at 24 hours and almost completely ineffective after 48 hours. Ordinary bank blood or packed RBCs, therefore, essentially have no functioning platelets, even though the platelet count may be normal. This may produce difficulty in massive transfusions using stored bank blood or packed RBCs, although there is usually no problem when administration takes place over longer periods of time. After one total blood volume replacement, the majority of patients still have platelet counts of roughly 100,000/cu mm or more due to the 35%–40% of original platelet count remaining plus some mobilization of platelets from the spleen and bone marrow. However, the platelet count may reach 50,000/cu mm or less with not all of these platelets being functional. Nevertheless, the 1986 Consensus Conference on Platelet Transfusion Therapy noted that most patients undergoing massive transfusion do not bleed because of dilutional thrombocytopenia alone and recommended that evidence of clinically abnormal bleeding or oozing plus thrombocytopenia be present before transfusing platelets instead of prophylactic administration of platelets.

Citrate anticoagulant may cause difficulty when large volumes of whole blood are given in very short periods of time. Citrate has calcium-binding activity that may lead to hypocalcemia and also has a potential depressant effect on the myocardium. Ionized calcium measurement is much more helpful to assess this possibility than total serum calcium. Fortunately, most patients are able to tolerate a large amount of citrate if liver function is adequate. One investigator states that the average person could receive one unit of whole blood every 5 minutes without requiring calcium supplements. At the other extreme, some have used 1 ampule (1 gm) of calcium gluconate for every five units of citrated whole blood. Calcium chloride has four times as much calcium as calcium gluconate, so that dosage using calcium chloride must be reduced proportionately. The majority of investigators currently deemphasize need for calcium supplements, and use of packed RBCs considerably reduces the amount of transfused citrate. *Temperature of transfused blood* is ordinarily not a problem. However, large amounts of rapidly administered cold blood increase the possibility of ventricular fibrillation. Ordinarily, blood can be allowed to warm in room air; if this is not possible, one can use a water bucket (30°C) for unopened blood containers or special warming devices (37°C) through which the blood passes via tubing while being administered. Transfusion of blood at ordinary speed does not require warming. *Coagulation factor deficiency* must be considered during massive transfusion. This involves primarily the labile factors V and VIII. Factor V has a storage half-life of about 10–14 days (range, 3–16 days), and levels in stored whole blood may be 30% (of normal) or even more in stored whole blood at 21 days. Factor VIII has a half-life of about 5–10 days (range, 3–16 days), and the level in stored whole blood is reported to be 15%–50% at 21 days. Lesser amounts would be present in packed RBCs due to the decreased amount of plasma. In either case, transfused material would probably contribute some factor V and VIII activity to residual patient activity. Whereas some have advocated transfusing 1 unit of fresh blood (or fresh frozen plasma or cryoprecipitate) for every 5 units or 10 units of stored whole blood during massive transfusion, a 1984 Consensus Development Conference on Fresh-Frozen Plasma stated that there is no evidence that the prophylactic use of fresh frozen plasma is necessary unless documented coagulation defects due to factor V or VIII deficiency are present. Coagulation defects are manifest by abnormal bleeding or oozing (not accounted for by failure to ligate damaged blood vessels). One relatively frequent contributing problem is concurrent disseminated intravascular coagulation due to tissue damage from trauma or tissue hypoxia from blood loss.

BIBLIOGRAPHY

Tegtmeier GE: The use of cytomegalovirus-screened blood in neonates. *Transfusion* 1988; 28:201.

McMican A: Neonatal transfusion therapy. *Lab Med* 1988; 19:353.

CDC-MMWR: Lack of transmission of human immunodeficiency virus through Rho(D) immune globulin (human). *JAMA* 1987; 258:3225.

Leslie GI, et al: Capillary and venous bilirubin values. *Am J Dis Child* 1987; 141:1199.

Aster RH, et al: Consensus Conference: Platelet transfusion therapy. *JAMA* 1987; 257:1777.

Bradshaw DA: Red blood cell antibody testing of obstetric patients. *Lab Med* 1987; 18:77.

Novak RW: Immediate transfusion reactions in the pediatric population. *Lab Med* 1987; 18:388.

Panzer S, et al: Haemolytic transfusion reactions due to HLA antibodies. *Lancet* 1987; 1:474.

Luban NLC, et al: Low incidence of acquired cytomegalovirus infection in neonates transfused with washed red blood cells. *Am J Dis Child* 1987; 141:416.

Wenk RE, et al: Significance of anti-c in hemolytic disease of the newborn. *Obstet Gynecol* 1986; 67:623.

Coffin CM: Current issues in transfusion therapy: 1. Risks of infection. *Postgrad Med* 1986; 80:219.

Caine ME, Mueller-Heubach E: Kell sensitization in pregnancy. *Am J Obstet Gynecol* 1986; 154:85.

Ness PM: The failure of postinjection Rh immune globulin titers to detect large fetal-maternal hemorrhages. *Am J Clin Pathol* 1986; 85:604.

Hoegsberg B: Surveillance of high-risk pregnancies. *J Med Technol* 1986; 3:486.

American College of Obstetrics and Gynecology: *Management of Isoimmunization in Pregnancy*. ACOG Technical Bulletin No 90, January 1986.

Stedman CM, et al: Rosette test in screening for excessive fetomaternal hemorrhage. *Am J Obstet Gynecol* 1986; 154:1363.

Tullis JL, et al: Consensus Conference: fresh-frozen plasma. *JAMA* 1985; 253:551.

Leitman SF, Holland PV: Irradiation of blood products. *Transfusion* 1985; 25:293.

Edinger SE: A closer look at fatal transfusion reactions. *Med Lab Observ* 1985; 17(4):41.

Popovsky MA, Moore SB: Diagnostic and pathogenetic considerations in transfusion-related acute lung injury. *Transfusion* 1985; 25:573.

Moore BPL: Does knowledge of Du status serve a useful purpose? *Vox Sang* 1984; 46(suppl 1):95.

Lamola AA, Fanaroff AA: Bilirubin fluorescence and prevention of kernicterus. *Diagn Med* 1984; 7(2):9.

Myhre BA, Van Antwerp R: Diagnosis of unexpected reactions to transfusion. *Lab Med* 1983; 14:153.

Caswell AK, Caswell M: Antenatal treatment to prevent Rh immunization. *Lab Med* 1983; 14:655.

Ritter DA, et al: A prospective study of free bilirubin and other risk factors in the development of kernicterus in premature infants. *Pediatrics* 1982; 69:260.

Lucey JF: Bilirubin and brain damage—a real mess. *Pediatrics* 1982; 69:381.

Stoerner JW: Neonatal jaundice. *Am Fam Physician* 1981; 24:226.

American College of Obstetrics and Gynecology: The *Selective Use of Rho(D) Immunoglobulin (RhIg)*. ACOG Technical Bulletin No 61, March 1981.

Guy LR: Transfusion patient identification and related problems. *Lab Med* 1981; 12:542.

Dufour DR, Monoghan WP: ABO hemolytic disease of the newborn. *Am J Clin Pathol* 1980; 73:369.

Moore SB, et al: Delayed hemolytic transfusion reactions. *Am J Clin Pathol* 1980; 74:94.

Rice L: Serum haptoglobin in hemolytic disease. *JAMA* 1980; 244:2607.
Kim MH, et al: Lack of predictive indices in kernicterus: A comparison of clinical and pathologic features in infants with and without kernicterus. *Pediatrics* 1980; 66:852.
Gitzelmann-Cumarasamy N, Kuenzlek CC: Bilirubin-binding tests: Living up to expectations? *Pediatrics* 1979; 64:375.

12 Urinalysis and Renal Disease

URINALYSIS

Urinalysis is an indispensable part of clinical pathology. It may uncover disease anywhere in the urinary tract. Also, it may afford a semiquantitative estimate of renal function and furnish clues to the etiology of dysfunction. Certain systemic diseases may produce quantitative or qualitative alterations of urine constituents or excretion of abnormal substances, quite apart from direct effects on the kidneys. Conversely, urinary tract disease may produce striking systemic symptoms.

The standard urinalysis profile includes appearance of the specimen, pH, specific gravity, protein semiquantitation, presence or absence of glucose and ketones, and microscopic examination of the centrifuged urinary sediment for white blood cells (WBCs), red blood cells (RBCs), and other abnormalities. (Table 12–1). These tests (not including microscopic examination) can be performed separately or together in various combinations on dipsticks available from several manufacturers. Some manufacturers have added one or more of the following tests to their dipsticks: hemoglobin, bile (conjugated bilirubin), urobilinogen, nitrite, leukocyte esterase, and specific gravity. Instruments that process and read the dipsticks are now available, thereby improving accuracy by eliminating some of the subjective element that is inherent in color changes read by human eye.

Appearance

The appearance of the specimen is usually reported only if it is abnormal.

Red:	Blood; porphyria; occasionally urates, phenophthalein, or dihydroxyanthraquinone (Dorbane) (laxative use)
Brown:	Blood (acid hematin); alkaptonuria (urine turns brownish on standing); melanin (may be brown and turn black on standing)
Dark orange:	Bile, pyridium (a urinary tract disinfectant)

pH

Normal urine pH is 5.0–6.0 (4.5–8.0); it is over 6.0 in alkalosis or, rarely, if the acidifying mechanism of the kidney fails (renal acidosis syndrome) or is poisoned (carbonic anhydrase inhibitors). Proteus infections typically will alkalinize. Finally, urine standing at room temperature will often slowly become alkaline due to bacterial growth. A pH determination is of minor importance except in a few circumstances.

Specific Gravity

Specific gravity will be discussed in greater length in chapter 13 (renal function). It is important for several reasons: (1) it is one parameter of renal tubular function; (2) inability to concentrate may accompany certain diseases with otherwise relatively normal tubular function, such as diabetes insipidus or, occasionally, severe hyperthyroidism and sickle cell anemia; and (3) it affects other urine tests; a

TABLE 12–1.
Most Important Conditions Screened for in Basic Urinalysis

Procedure or Urine Constituent	Significance
Specific gravity	Kidney function test
Color/appearance	Blood, pus
Albumin	Kidney disease
Sugar/acetone	Diabetes
Hemoglobin	Blood
Microscopic	
RBCs	Tumor, stone, glomerulonephritis
WBCs	Infection
Casts	Kidney disease
Crystals	Stones
Squamous epithelial cells	Index of contamination

concentrated specimen may give higher results for substances such as protein than a dilute specimen, although the amount of substance excreted per 24 hours may be the same in both cases. That is, the same amount of substance assayed in a small quantity of fluid (high specific gravity) may appear more than if present in a large dilute urine volume (low specific gravity).

Specific gravity is an estimate of relative density (for fluids, the proportion of dissolved solids in a defined volume of solvent) and can be measured in various ways. The oldest was by hydrometer (weighted flotation device), whose reproducibility was poor and which was relatively inaccurate. Most laboratories use some version of a refractometer (e.g., a total solids meter), which is fairly reproducible and accurate, but which is affected by moderate amounts of protein, glucose, or x-ray contrast media. More recently, dipstick specific gravity tests have become available based on changes in urine ion content that produce a pH change of the polyelectrolyte content of the reagent pad, which, in turn, induces color changes of an indicator (bromthymol blue). This method is read in increments of 0.005 units. Several evaluations suggest that the dipstick results will agree within ± 0.005 units of total solids meter values about 85% (range 72%–90%) of the time. This suggests that the dipstick method is somewhat less accurate than the total solids meter. Whether the dipstick method is useful depends on whether a difference of 0.004–0.005 from the total solids meter value is considered clinically acceptable. The dipstick is affected by moderate changes in pH or protein but not by glucose or x-ray contrast media.

Protein

In health the glomerular membrane prevents most of the relatively large protein molecules of the blood from escaping into the urine. A small amount does filter through, of which a small fraction is reabsorbed by the tubules, and the remainder (up to 0.1 gm/24 hours) is excreted. These amounts are normally not detected by routine clinical methods. One of the first responses of the kidney to a great variety of clinical situations is an alteration in the glomerular filtrate. To a lesser extent, a mere increase in glomerular filtration rate (GFR) may increase normal protein excretion. Since albumin has a relatively small molecular size, it tends to become the dominant constituent in proteinuria but rarely so completely as to justify the term "albuminuria" in a pure sense. Depending on the clinical situation, the constituents of proteinuria may or may not approach the constituents of plasma. Besides an excess of normal plasma proteins, at times abnormal proteins may appear in the urine. The most important of these is Bence Jones protein, which is excreted in up to 50% of patients with multiple myeloma.

Etiologies of Proteinuria.—To interpret proteinuria, one must know not only the major conditions responsible but also the reason for production of excess urine protein. A system such as the following one is very helpful in this respect; proteinuria is classified according to the relationship of its etiology to the kidney and also the mechanism involved.

A. Functional: not associated with easily demonstrable systemic or renal damage.
   1. Severe muscular exertion. This etiology is becoming more important with current popularity of sports and jogging.
   2. Pregnancy.
   3. Orthostatic proteinuria. (This term designates slight to mild proteinuria associated only with the upright position. The exact etiology is poorly understood, with usual explanations implicating local factors that cause renal passive congestion when the patient is in an upright position. Orthostatic pro-

teinuria is easily diagnosed by comparing a specimen of early morning urine, produced entirely while the patient is asleep, with one obtained later when the patient has been upright for some time. This is probably the most common cause of "functional" proteinuria; some reports indicate that it occurs in 15%–20% of healthy young men who have proteinuria on routine urinalysis.)

B. Organic: associated with demonstrable systemic disease or renal pathology.
   1. Prerenal proteinuria: not due to primary renal disease.
      a. Fever or a variety of toxic conditions. (This is the most common etiology for "organic" proteinuria and is quite frequent.)
      b. Venous congestion. (This is most often produced by chronic passive congestion due to heart failure. It is occasionally produced by intra-abdominal compression of the renal veins.)
      c. Renal hypoxia. Renal hypoxia may be produced by severe dehydration, shock, severe acidosis, acute cardiac decompensation, or severe anemias, all of which lead to a decrease in renal blood flow and sometimes hypoxic renal changes. Very severe hypoxia, especially if acute, may lead to renal tubular necrosis.
      d. Hypertension (moderate or severe chronic hypertension, malignant hypertension or eclampsia).
      e. Myxedema.
      f. Bence Jones protein.
   2. Renal proteinuria: primarily kidney disease.
      a. Glomerulonephritis.
      b. Nephrotic syndrome, primary or secondary.
      c. Destructive parenchymal lesions (tumor, infection, infarct).
   3. Postrenal proteinuria: protein added to the urine at some point farther down the urinary tract from the renal parenchyma.
      a. Infection of the renal pelvis or ureter.
      b. Cystitis.
      c. Urethritis or prostatitis.
      d. Contamination with vaginal secretions. This etiology may be suggested by presence of moderate or large numbers of squamous epithelial cells in the urine sediment.

Protein Tests Are Not Specific for Serum Protein.—Test results demonstrating protein detect filtered serum protein but may also result from test reaction with WBCs or RBCs, regardless of their origin, if they are present in sufficient number. However, intrinsic renal disease usually (not always) is associated with proteinuria whether abnormal cells are present or not. Thus, by testing the supernate of a centrifuged specimen for protein, one can tentatively assume that WBCs or RBCs originated mainly in the lower urinary tract if pyuria or hematuria occurs in the absence of proteinuria.

Urine Protein Test Methods.—There are several clinically acceptable methods for semiquantitative protein testing. The older methods are heat with acetic acid and sulfosalicylic acid (3%, 10%, or 20%). Sulfosalicylic acid (SSA) is slightly more sensitive than the heat–acetic acid method. Sulfosalicylic acid false positive reactions may occur, notably with tolbutamide (Orinase), urates, hemoglobin (RBCs or hemolysis), WBCs, massive penicillin doses, dextran, occasionally with salicylates, and with various radiopaque x-ray substances. Bence Jones protein also gives a positive reaction. Results are expressed as 1+ to 4+; this correlates very roughly with the amount of protein present (Table 12–2).

Kingsbury-Clark Procedure.—This is a quantitative sulfosalicylic acid method using a series of permanent standards, each representing a different but measured amount of protein. After sulfosalicylic acid is added to the un-

TABLE 12–2.
Relationship of Qualitative and Quantitative Urine Protein Results

Qualitative	Protein	Rough Quantitative Correlation (gm/L)
Light cloud	Trace	0.1–0.5
Medium cloud	1+	0.5–1.0
Heavy cloud	2+	3.0
Light coagulum	3+	5.0
Heavy coagulum	4+	≥ 10.0

known specimen, a precipitate is formed that is compared with the standards and reported as the amount in the particular standard that it matches.

Dipstick Methods.—Most laboratories now use dipstick methods, usually with multiple tests on the same paper strip. The sulfosalicylic acid method will detect as little as 10 mg/100 ml of protein, whereas the dipsticks are not reliable for less than 20–30 mg/100 ml. The dipsticks will react with hemoglobin but not with the other substances previously listed which might produce false positive results with sulfosalicylic acid. Dipstick behavior with Bence Jones protein is erratic; in many cases the results are positive, but a significant number do not react. Dipsticks are said to give false positive protein results when the urine has a very alkaline pH, although my experience has been that no change occurs even at pH 8.5 (a value that is very rarely exceeded). False negative results may occur if contact of the dipstick with urine is greatly prolonged, since this could wash out the buffer in the protein detection zone on the test strip. In addition, protein readings are only semiquantitative, and it is often difficult to obtain uniform results from the same specimens read by different individuals. This happens because the result depends on a color change corresponding to a change from one quantity (or level) of protein to the next; the color change may not always be clear cut, and interpretation of any color change is always partially subjective. There tends to be a fairly wide variation in results when specimens containing large amounts of protein are tested.

24-Hour Measurement.—Because individuals often vary in their interpretations, and also because the degree of urine concentration may greatly influence results on random urine specimens, it is sometimes useful to determine 24-hour urine protein excretion. A 24-hour specimen may also be affected by degree of concentration but to a lesser extent. However, 24-hour specimens also have their problems. One of these is incomplete specimen collection. Another is variation in results using different test methods or reagents, most of which have relatively poor reproducibility (coefficient of variation exceeding 10%) and react differently with different proteins. In some reports this occasionally led to very substantial differences in results of different methods on the same specimen.

Several studies indicate that the protein/creatinine ratio in single voided specimens produces an adequate estimation of normality or degree of abnormality compared with 24-hour urine specimens. Since the recumbent and the upright protein excretion rate is often different, first-morning urine specimens are not recommended for this test.

Microalbuminuria.—Recently, several studies have suggested that a latent period exists in renal disease associated with insulin-dependent diabetics. In this phase there is ongoing glomerular damage that is manifest by increased albumin excretion but in quantities too small to be detectable by standard laboratory protein tests, either dipstick or usual 24-hour procedures. One current definition of diabetic microalbuminuria is albumin excretion of 20–200 μg/minute (30–300 mg/24 hours) found in at least two of three specimens collected within 6 months. Dipsticks will begin detecting proteinuria slightly above the microalbuminuria range upper limit. Multiple samples are required because diabetics with or without microalbuminuria may have day-to-day variation in albumin excretion as high as 50%.

In summary, not all proteinuria is pathologic; even if so, it may be transient. Often the kidney is only indirectly involved, and occasionally protein may be added to the urine beyond the kidney. Individual interpretations of turbidity tests vary significantly and so do various assay methods for 24-hour urine protein.

Glucose

The most common and important glucosuria occurs in diabetes mellitus. The normal renal threshold is usually about 180 mg/100 ml (literature range 165–200 mg/100 ml) serum glucose level; above that, enough glucose is filtered to exceed the usual tubular transfer maximum for glucose reabsorption, and the surplus remains in the urine. However, individuals vary in their tubular transfer reabsorptive capacities. If the capacity happens to be low, the individual may spill glucose at lower blood levels than the average person ("renal glucosuria"). Certain uncommon conditions may elevate blood glucose levels in nondiabetic persons. A partial list of the more important conditions associated with glucosuria includes the following (discussed more fully in chapter 27):

1. Glucosuria without hyperglycemia
   a. Glucosuria of pregnancy (lactosuria may occur as well as glucosuria)
   b. Renal glucosuria
   c. Certain inborn errors of metabolism (Fanconi's syndrome)
   d. After certain nephrotoxic chemicals (carbon monoxide, lead, mercuric chloride)
2. Glucosuria with hyperglycemia
   a. Diabetes mellitus
   b. Alimentary glucosuria (hyperglycemia is very transient)
   c. Increased intracranial pressure (tumors, intracerebral hemorrhage, skull fracture)
   d. Certain endocrine diseases or hormone-producing tumors (Cushing's syndrome, pheochromocytoma)
   e. Hyperthyroidism (occasionally)
   f. Occasionally, transiently, after myocardial infarction
   g. After certain types of anesthesia, such as ether

The most commonly used tests for urine glucose are glucose oxidase enzyme paper dipsticks such as Clinistix, Tes-Tape, and the multiple-test strips, all of which are specific for glucose. Another widely used test is Clinitest, which, like the old Benedict's method (rarely used today), is based on copper sulfate reduction by reducing substances and is therefore not specific for glucose or even sugar. In several reported comparisons of these tests, Tes-Tape proved most sensitive but also gave occasional false positives. Clinistix gave few false positives but sometimes gave equivocal results or missed a few positive results that Tes-Tape detected. The copper reduction tests included about 10% positive results from reducing substances other than glucose. Clinitest is a copper reduction tablet test that seemed to have median sensitivity, whereas Benedict's method, which is a standard type of chemical procedure, was least sensitive, missing 10%–15% of tests positive by glucose oxidase, but with very few false positives apart from other reducing substances.

Dipstick Problems.—Although theoretically specific and relatively sensitive, the enzyme papers are not infallible. False positive results have been reported due to hydrogen peroxide and to hypochlorites (found in certain cleaning compounds). These substances give negative copper reduction test results. Large amounts of vitamin C may produce false negative results with the glucose oxidase methods but false positive results with reducing substance methods. False negative results using Clinistix (but not Tes-Tape) have been reported from homogentisic acid (alkaptonuria), levodopa, and large doses of aspirin. Also, the enzyme papers may unaccountably miss an occasional positive result that is detected by copper sulfate reduction techniques. As with urine protein dipsticks, studies have demonstrated considerable variation in test reports by different persons on the same specimens, especially at glucose levels that are borderline between two test strip color change levels.

Clinitest (copper reduction) false positive results are produced by sugars other than glucose (galactose, lactose) and by hemogentisic acid (alkaptonuria). Other potentially troublesome substances are *p*-aminosalicylic acid (PAS), methyldopa (Aldomet), heavy salicylate therapy (salicyluric acid excreted), and heavy concentrations of urates. Various beta-lactam antibiotics in large doses (especially the cephalosporins, but also the penicillins, monobactams, and carbapenems) may interfere with Clinitest interpretation by forming various colors. An important technical consideration is to keep Clinitest tablets and the enzyme papers free from moisture before use.

Change in Clinitest Methodology.—The original methodology for Clinitest used five drops of urine. When urine contains large amounts of sugar, the color change typical of a high concentration may be unstable and quickly change to another color, which could be misinterpreted as an end point produced by smaller amounts of sugar ("pass-through" phenomenon). Many laboratories now use a two-drop specimen, which avoids the pass-through effect. However, the color changes that represent different concentrations of reducing substances are not the same with five drops as with two drops. Knowledge of the method used is essential for correct interpretation by the patient or the physician.

Acetone and Diacetic Acid (Ketone Bodies)

Ketone bodies include β-hydroxybutyric acid (BHBA), diacetic (acetoacetic) acid (DAA), and acetone. Under normal conditions, anaerobic metabolism of glucose proceeds to eventual formation of a compound called acetyl–coenzyme A, or acetyl-CoA. It can also be produced by metabolism of fatty acids. Most acetyl-CoA is utilized in the tricarboxylic (citric acid) metabolic cycle. However, acetyl-CoA can also enter the pathway to ketone body formation in the liver. Diacetic acid is formed initially, with the great majority being metabolized to BHBA and a small amount spontaneously decarboxylated to acetone and carbon dioxide. The major (but not the only) impetus toward increased ketone formation is either carbohydrate restriction or impaired carbohydrate metabolism. Skeletal and cardiac muscle can utilize a limited amount of DAA and BHBA as an energy source when normal glucose-derived energy is insufficient; but after a certain point, metabolic capacity is exceeded and excess ketone bodies are excreted by the kidney. However, renal excretion rate is also limited, and when ketone formation exceeds muscle utilization and renal excretory capacity, ketone bodies accumulate in the plasma, a condition known as *ketosis*. Normal plasma ketone composition is about 78% BHBA, 20% DAA, and 2% acetone.

Technical Methods and Their Drawbacks.—Most chemical tests for ketones employ a nitroprusside reagent. Nitroprusside detects both DAA and acetone but not BHAA. The most commonly used product of this type is a tablet reagent formulation called Acetest. Acetest will detect concentrations of 5 mg/100 ml of DAA as well as react with acetone and can be used with serum, plasma, or urine. In addition, there is a dipstick method called Ketostix that is specific for DAA and detects 10 mg/100 ml (980 μmol/L). This method is also incorporated into certain multiple-test urine dipsticks from several manufacturers. Dipstick false positive results have been reported with levodopa. Since the concentration of DAA is several times that of acetone, and also because Acetest is only about one fifth as sensitive to acetone as it is to DAA, the dipstick tests that detect only DAA give equivalent results in urine to those of Acetest. However, the majority of literature references prefer Acetest when testing plasma or serum. The majority also recommend crushing the Acetest tablet for serum but not for urine.

Some case reports describe instances in which the dipstick test for ketones failed to detect ketones in the plasma of certain patients with diabetic ketoacidosis. Acetest tablets were able to detect the ketones. The manufacturer states that the ketone portion of multiple-test strip dipsticks is more sensitive to effects of moisture than the other test areas and that the dipstick container lid must be replaced and fastened immediately after a test strip is removed (which is an unrealistic expectation in many laboratories).

Interpretation of Test Results.—Standard chemical tests for ketone bodies do not detect the small amounts in normal plasma or urine. Detectable urine ketones with nondetectable plasma (or serum) ketones indicates mild or moderate overproduction of ketone bodies. A positive test result in both urine and plasma usually indicates severe excess of ketones. Presence of ketone bodies in urine (ketonuria) is fairly frequent. In one study, it was reported in 14%–28% of all hospital admission urines. Ketonuria is a classic finding in diabetic acidosis. However, ketonuria may also be found in starvation, in alcoholism, in many normal pregnancies at time of delivery, and especially in severe dehydration from many causes (vomiting, diarrhea, severe infections). In children, ketone bodies are prone to appear on what, by adult standards, would be relatively small provocation. A weakly positive urine test result for ketones is usually of little significance.

It must be emphasized that diabetes is practically the only disease in which ketonuria has real diagnostic importance. Slight to moderate degrees of ketonuria are fairly common in other conditions, as mentioned earlier, but are only incidental. Serum ketone results are usually negative. In my experience, trace, 1+, and 2+ (using a scale of 0–4+) urine ketone results are rarely accompanied by positive serum ketone results, and the same was true even for some patients with 3+ ketonuria. In diabetes the presence of large amounts of urine ketones is important confirmatory evidence of diabetic ketoacidosis or impending acidosis. In well-established diabetic ketoacidosis the serum or plasma acetone test result will usually be positive (exceptions are the rare cases of hyperosmolar coma or lactic acidosis). In fact, the quantity of plasma ketones, estimated by testing dilutions of plasma, provides some (although not an exact) indication of the severity of acidosis and the amount of insulin needed. In the urine, nitroprusside test results usually will be strongly positive. In most cases, there will be glucosuria as well as marked ketonuria. The major exception is renal insufficiency with oliguria due to severe renal disease, shock, or exceptionally severe acidosis with secondary renal shutdown, since some of these patients may be unable to filter the increased serum ketone bodies into the urine. The blood urea nitrogen (BUN) level is frequently elevated in diabetic acidosis; even so, there usually will be ketonuria. If there is any question, a plasma or serum ketone test should be done.

In summary, the urine ketone result in diabetic acidosis usually is very strongly positive and the plasma ketone result is positive. However, if symptoms of diabetic acidosis are present, lack of strongly positive urine ketone results does not rule out the diagnosis if renal failure is present.

Serum Ketone Quantitative Measurement.—Biochemical methods (usually enzymatic) are available to measure BHBA, which actually is the dominant ketone form in ketosis and provides a better estimation of severity in diabetic acidosis than DAA measurement. In early ketoacidosis, the BHBA level becomes elevated, whereas the DAA level is still normal. However, BHBA has not replaced DAA because of the ease, convenience, speed, and low cost of Acetest and the dipsticks.

Hemoglobin (Blood)

Characteristics of Test Methods.—Several biochemical procedures for detecting hemoglobin in urine are on the market. Some have a sensitivity of approximately 1:100,000, about that of the old benzidine method. A representative of this type is an orthotolidine reagent tablet method called Occultest. This is reported to detect fewer than five RBCs per high-power field in centrifuged urine sediment. Hematest is another tablet test with the same basic reagents but is adjusted to approximately 1:20,000 sensitivity, slightly more than the guaiac method. Experimentally, it will not reliably detect fewer than 200 RBCs per high-power field unless some of the cells have hemolyzed. It is much more sensitive to free hemoglobin, where it can detect amounts produced by hemolysis of only 25–30 RBCs per high-power field. It has been used for feces as well as urine, although at this sensitivity there is an appreciable number of false positives. A dipstick called Hemastix and the occult blood section of different multitest dipsticks are likewise based on orthotolidine but are more sensitive than the reagent tablets, detecting 0.04 mg/100 ml of hemoglobin, or, in my experience, more than two–three RBCs per high-power field of centrifuged urine sediment. There is a small but probably significant variation in sensitivity among the different dipsticks. The usefulness of these chemical tests is enhanced by their ability to detect hemoglobin even after some or all of the RBCs have disintegrated and are no longer visible microscopically. Red blood cell lysis is particularly likely to occur in alkaline or dilute urine. Failure to mix a specimen before testing could result in testing a supernate without RBCs and could yield a false negative dipstick reaction. Large doses of vitamin C interfere with the test chemical reaction and may produce a false negative result. One report indicates that providone-iodine (Betadine) can produce a false positive reaction. Contamination from vaginal secretions in the female may introduce RBCs into the specimen as an artifact. Myoglobin reacts as well as hemoglobin.

Biochemical Methods Versus Microscopic Examination.—There is disagreement in the literature as to whether the dipstick tests for hemoglobin could be used in place of microscopic examination (for RBCs) of the urine sediment. In my experience with one company's multitest dipstick, almost all patients with microscopic findings of two or more RBCs per high-power field were detected by the dipstick. However, testing with dipstick only would not reveal abnormal numbers of squamous epithelial cells, which would raise the question of possible contamination artifact. Also, detection of urine hemoglobin or hematuria would necessitate a microscopic sediment examination for RBC casts. Etiologies of hematuria are discussed later in the section on microscopic sediment examination.

Leukocyte Esterase (White Blood Cells)

A dipstick called Chemstrip-L that will detect WBCs in urine by means of hydrolysis of the reagent by esterase enzyme contained in the cytoplasm of neutrophils has been introduced. The same reagent has been incorporated into some of the multitest dipsticks. Reports indicate that the leukocyte esterase test will detect about 85%–95% (range, 73%–99%) of patients with abnormal numbers of WBCs in centrifuged urinary sediment. The test reportedly will also detect abnormal numbers of WBCs that have lysed due to alkaline urine or other factors. The leukocyte esterase test is about 80%–90% sensitive in detecting urinary tract infection (defined as 100,000 colony-forming units/ml) compared with urine culture. However, when performed with the nitrite test (discussed later), sensitivity vs. quantitative urine culture improves to about 85%–90% (range, 78%–100%). Several reports suggest false positive results due to *Trichomonas* organisms, but others suggest relatively little interference. In addition, leukocyte esterase will not differentiate urinary tract WBCs from WBCs added through contamination of the specimen (especially by vaginal secretions) during specimen collection.

Nitrite

Many bacteria produce an enzyme called *reductase* that can reduce urinary nitrates to nitrites. Some of the multitest dipsticks contain a reagent area that reacts with nitrite to produce a color, thus indirectly suggesting the presence of bacteria in certain quantity. Sensitivity of the nitrite test vs. quantitative urine culture is only about 50% (range, 35%–69%). However, it can enhance the sensitivity of the leukocyte esterase test to detect urinary tract infection.

Bile (Conjugated Bilirubin)

Conjugated bilirubin is not normally detected in urine but can appear secondary to biliary tract obstruction, either extrahepatic (common duct obstruction) or intrahepatic (cholestatic liver cell injury due to such conditions as active cirrhosis or hepatitis virus hepatitis). Typically, in hepatitis virus hepatitis the urine appears dark 2 or 3 days before the patient becomes icteric and clears swiftly once skin jaundice develops.

In pulmonary infarction, some elevation in the serum unconjugated bilirubin level may occur, but unconjugated bilirubin does not appear in urine.

Tests for conjugated bilirubin in urine include Fouchet's reagent, Ictotest tablets, or dipstick tests. The simple foam test (yellow foam after shaking) may be all that is necessary (false positive result may be produced by pyridium). Ictotest and the dipstick tests are based on the same chemical reaction and are fairly sensitive, detecting as little as 0.1 mg/100 ml. These tests are reasonably specific, but chlorpromazine may produce false positive results. If urine is allowed to stand for some time before testing, conjugated bilirubin decomposes and a false negative result may occur. Ictotest is somewhat less sensitive to this change than the dipsticks and therefore is a little less likely to become falsely negative.

Most requests for urine bile could be questioned, since the serum bilirubin level would provide more useful information (chapter 19).

Urobilinogen

Urobilinogen is produced from conjugated bilirubin by metabolic activity of bacteria in the intestine, followed by reabsorption into the bloodstream (chapter 19). Urine urobilinogen becomes increased from either a marked increase in production secondary to increase in serum unconjugated bilirubin (usually from hemolytic processes) or because of inability of damaged liver parenchymal cells to metabolize normal amounts of urobilinogen absorbed from the intestine (usually due to cirrhosis or severe hepatitis). The metabolic pathways involved are discussed in the chapter on liver function tests.

Tests for the presence of urobilinogen include both a standard chemistry method and a dipstick procedure, both based on Ehrlich's reagent. Either a random urine specimen or a 24-hour specimen can be used. The 24-hour specimen must contain a preservative.

For routine specimens, it is of great importance that the test be done within 30 minutes after voiding. Urobilinogen rapidly oxidizes in air to nondetectable urobilin, and without special preservative it will decrease significantly after 30 minutes. This unrecognized fact probably accounts for the test's poor reputation. If the procedure cannot be done relatively soon after voiding, it is better to get a 24-hour specimen with preservative.

Urine urobilinogen determination is rarely needed, since liver function or other tests provide more useful information.

Microscopic Examination of Urinary Sediment

Urine microscopic examination is routinely done on centrifuged urinary sediment. There is no widely accepted standardized procedure for this, and the varying degrees of sediment concentration that are produced make difficult any unquestioning interpretation of quantitative reports. However, it is fairly safe to say that normally so few cellular elements are excreted that most results of examination in normal uncontaminated specimens fall within normal clinical values no matter how much the specimen is centrifuged. The majority of sources (including my experience) use a reference range of 0–2 RBCs or 0–5 WBCs per high-power field and only an occasional cast. However, there is disagreement in the literature regarding the reference range for both WBCs and RBCs. Reference ranges for WBC can be found that vary from 1 WBC per high-power field to as many as 20 WBCs per high-power field. Red blood cell ranges are discussed in the section on hematuria investigation in chapter 13. Some commercial systems for preparation of the urine sediment that can improve reproducibility are available.

The main pathologic elements of urinary sediment include RBCs, WBCs, and casts. Less important elements are yeasts, crystals, or epithelial cells.

Red Blood Cells.—Gross urinary bleeding is usually associated with stones, acute glomerulonephritis, and tumor, although these conditions may (less often) be manifested only by microscopic hematuria. Tuberculosis traditionally has been listed as a fourth cause but is rare today. In several series, benign prostate hyperplasia and bladder or urethral infection were also frequent etiologies. There are conditions that frequently are associated with significant microscopic hematuria and occasionally approach gross bleeding. Some of the more important include bleeding and clotting disorders (e.g., purpura or anticoagulants), blood dyscrasias (including sickle cell anemia or leukemia), renal infarction, malignant hypertension, subacute bacterial endocarditis, collagen diseases (especially lupus and polyarteritis nodosa), Weil's disease, and certain lower urinary tract conditions such as cystitis, urethritis, and prostatitis. In the female, vaginal blood or leukocytes may contaminate ordinary voided specimens; finding significant numbers of squamous epithelial cells in the urinary sediment suggests such contamination. Yeast may simulate RBCs (discussed later).

Red blood cell casts are the most reliable way to localize the source of bleeding to the kidney. Some reports indicated that the presence of "dysmorphic RBCs" (distorted or shrunken RBCs) using ordinary microscopy, phase contrast, Wright's stain on a sediment smear, or a Papanicolaou cytology technique is also helpful in suggesting renal origin.

White Blood Cells.—White blood cells may originate anywhere in the urinary tract. Hematogenous spread of infection to the kidney usually first localizes in the renal cortex. Isolated cortical lesions may be relatively silent. Retrograde invasion from the bladder tends to involve calyces and medulla initially. Urinary tract obstruction is often a factor in retrograde pyelonephritis. Generally speaking, pyuria of renal origin is usually accompanied by significant proteinuria. Pyuria originating in the lower urinary tract may be associated with proteinuria, but it tends to be relatively slight.

Urinary tract infections tend to be accompanied by bacteriuria. Tuberculosis of the kidney, besides producing hematuria, characteristically is associated with pyuria without bacteriuria. An ordinary urine culture would not reveal tuberculosis organisms. White blood cell casts are definite evidence that urinary WBCs originate in the kidney (discussed later); WBCs in clumps are suggestive of renal origin but are not diagnostic.

Correlation of Pyuria With Urine Culture.—Although many physicians regard pyuria as a good screening test for urinary tract infection, false normal results are reported in approximately 25%–30% of patients (literature range 7%–87%) who have a positive quantitative urine culture result. White blood cell counting of uncentrifuged urine in a WBC counting chamber is reported to be more accurate than urine sediment, but very few laboratories use this technique. Abnormal numbers of WBCs are a reasonably good indicator of urinary tract infection, although reports indicate 2%–13% false positive results compared to urine culture. In females, one should take precautions to avoid artifactual increases in urine WBCs from contamination by vaginal or labial secretions. Several studies (including my own experience) have suggested female urine contamination rates as high as 30%. In any specimen it is important to perform the microscopic examination promptly (i.e., within 1 hour after voiding) or else use some method of preservation. White blood cells lyse in hypotonic or alkaline urine. Some studies reported that as many as 30%–50% of specimens containing abnormal numbers of WBCs were normal after 2–3 hours of standing at room temperature.

Casts.—Casts are protein conglomerates that outline the shape of the renal tubules in which they were formed. Factors involved in cast formation include:

1. pH: Protein casts tend to dissolve in alkaline medium.
2. Concentration: Casts tend to dissolve in considerably dilute medium. Concentration also has an important role in the formation of casts; a concentrated urine favors precipitation of protein.
3. Proteinuria: Protein is necessary for cast formation, and significant cylindruria (cast excretion) is most often accompanied by proteinuria. Proteinuria may be of varied etiology. The postrenal type is added beyond the kidneys and obviously cannot be involved in cast formation.
4. Stasis: Stasis is usually secondary to intratubular obstruction and thus allows time for protein precipitation within tubules.

Mechanisms of Cast Formation.—Mechanisms of cast formation are better understood if one considers the normal physiology of urine formation. The substance filtered at the glomerulus is essentially an ultrafiltrate of plasma. In the proximal tubules, up to 85% of filtered sodium and chloride is reabsorbed, with water passively accompanying these ions. In the thick ascending loop of Henle, sodium is actively reabsorbed; however, since the membrane here is impermeable to water, an excess of water (free water) remains. As water passes along the distal tubules, some may be reabsorbed with sodium ions, and in the collecting tubules, up to 5% of the glomerular filtrate is osmotically reabsorbed due to the relatively high osmolality of the renal interstitial cells. Water reabsorption in distal and collecting tubules is under the control of antidiuretic hormone. At this point, the urine reaches its maximum concentration and proceeds to the bladder relatively unchanged. Thus, cast formation takes place ordinarily in the distal and collecting tubules, where acidification takes place and concentration reaches its height.

Cast Types.—There are two main types of casts, cellular and hyaline, depending on their main constituents. Other types include fatty casts, broad casts, and hemoglobin casts.

Cellular Casts.—Red blood cells, WBCs, desquamated renal epithelial cells, or any combination of these may conglomerate together in a protein matrix. The cast is basically cellular in content (Fig 12–1).

As the cellular cast moves slowly down the nephron, the cells begin to disintegrate. Eventually, all that is left of the cells are relatively large fragments, chunks, or granules. The cellular cast has now become a coarsely granular cast. It is composed entirely of large irregular or coarse solid granules.

If disintegration is allowed to continue, the coarse granules break down to small granules, and a relatively homogeneous finely granular cast is formed.

The end stage of this process is the production of a homogeneous refractile material still in the shape of the tubule, known as a *waxy cast*. The waxy cast is translucent, without granules, and reflects light, which gives it a somewhat shiny, semisolid appearance. What stage of cast finally reaches the bladder depends on how long the cast takes to traverse the nephron and thus how long it remains in the kidney, where the forces of disintegration may work. A waxy cast thus indicates fairly severe stasis in the renal tubules.

Hyaline Casts.—Hyaline casts are composed almost exclusively of protein alone. They pass almost unchanged down the urinary tract. They are dull, nearly transparent, and reflect

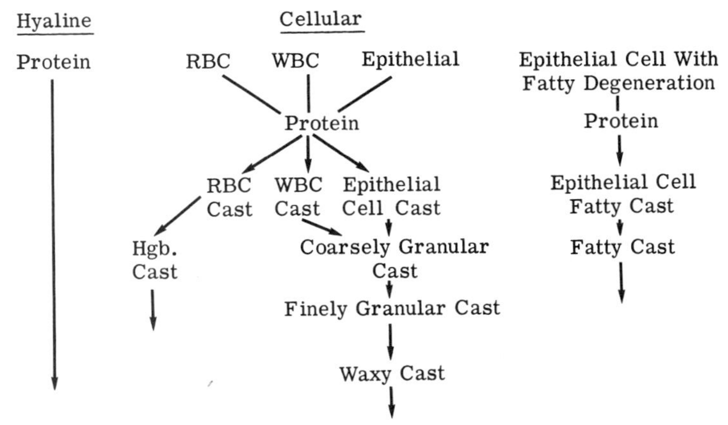

FIG 12–1.
Formation of casts.

light poorly compared with waxy casts. Thus, hyaline casts are often hard to see, and the microscope condenser usually must be turned down to give better contrast.

Sometimes cellular elements may be trapped within hyaline casts. If hyaline material still predominates, the result is considered a hyaline cast with cellular inclusions. Degenerative changes can take place similar to those of regular cellular casts, with the production of hyaline coarsely granular and hyaline finely granular casts.

Fatty Casts.—Fatty casts are a special type of cellular cast. In certain types of renal tubular damage, fatty degeneration of the tubular epithelial cells takes place. These cells desquamate and are incorporated into casts. The epithelial cells contain fatty droplets. As the cells degenerate, the fatty droplets remain and may even coalesce somewhat. The final result is a cast composed mainly of fatty droplets and protein. Sometimes either renal epithelial cells with fatty degeneration or the remnants thereof containing fat droplets are found floating free in the urine and are called *oval fat bodies*.

When oval fat bodies or fatty casts are present in significant number, the patient usually has a disease that is associated with the nephrotic syndrome, such as primary lipoid nephrosis or nephrosis secondary to Kimmelstiel-Wilson syndrome, systemic lupus, amyloid, subacute glomerulonephritis, the nephrotic stage of chronic glomerulonephritis, certain tubule poisons such as mercury, and rare hypersensitivity reactions such as those from insect bites. Oval fat bodies have essentially the same significance as fatty casts. Fat droplets have a Maltese cross appearance in polarized light but are recognized without polarized light. They can also be identified using fat stains such as Sudan IV.

Broad Casts.—When very severe stasis occurs regardless of the type of cast involved, cast formation may take place in the larger more distal collecting tubules, where large ducts drain several smaller collecting tubules. If this occurs, a broad cast is formed, several times wider than ordinary-sized casts. This is always indicative of severe localized tubule damage. These broad casts may be of any cast type, and due to their peculiar mode of formation they are sometimes spoken of as "renal failure casts." This is not entirely accurate, because the kidney may often recover from that particular episode and the problem sometimes involves only part of a kidney.

Hemoglobin Casts.—Hemoglobin casts are derived from RBC casts that degenerate into granular (rarely, even waxy) material but still have the peculiar orange-red color of hemoglobin. Not all casts derived from RBCs retain this color. Strongly acid urine changes the characteristic color of hemoglobin to the nonspecific gray-brown color of acid hematin. Also, one must differentiate the brown or yellow-brown coloring derived from bile or other urine pigments from the typical color of hemoglobin.

Significance.—The significance of casts in the urine varies according to the type of cast. Fatty casts, RBC casts, and WBC casts are always significant. The only general statement one can make about ordinary hyaline or granular casts is that their appearance in significant numbers has some correlation with the factors involved in cast formation—proteinuria, concentration, and stasis. Of these, the most general correlation is with stasis, although one cannot tell whether the stasis is generalized or merely localized. It is common for showers of casts to clear dramatically once the underlying cause of their formation is corrected. On the other hand, significant numbers of casts that persist for some time despite therapeutic efforts may suggest serious intrarenal derangement. In this respect, granular casts in the late stages of development will be seen. Generally speaking, hyaline casts alone are of little practical importance and are usually only an acute, mild, and temporary phenomenon. Thus, to have any meaning, the appearance of casts must be correlated with other findings and with the clinical situation. A few hyaline or granular casts in themselves have no importance.

Crystals.—Crystals are often overemphasized in importance. They may, however, be a clue to calculus formation and certain metabolic diseases. Crystals tend to be pH dependent:

Acid urine: uric acid, cystine, calcium oxalate.

Alkaline urine: phosphates, as triple phosphate (magnesium ammonium phosphate), which comprises many staghorn calculi. *Note:* Alkaline urine is most often produced by *(Proteus)* infection.

Amorphous (loose finely granular) crystals: If the pH is acid, the material is urate; if the pH is alkaline, it is phosphate. Rarely one might find sulfa crystals in acid urine, since sulfadiazine is still sometimes used. Most sulfa crystals resemble needle-like structures in bunches, but this appearance can be mimicked by certain nonpathologic crystals.

Epithelial Cells.—Squamous epithelial cells are useful as an index of possible contamination by vaginal secretions in females or by foreskin in uncircumcised males. I have found (unpublished study) that more than 10 squamous epithelial cells per low power (10 × objective) field provide an adequate guidepost for suspicion of contamination. However, contamination (especially bacteriologic contamination) might occur without abnormal numbers of squamous cells, and the presence of abnormal numbers of squamous cells does not mean that RBCs and WBCs are present only because of contamination. The squamous cells only alert one to a definite possibility of contamination and, if abnormalities are present, suggest the desirability of a carefully collected midstream specimen. Unfortunately, however, even specimens that supposedly are collected by careful midstream voiding technique may be contaminated, especially if the patient collects the specimen without expert assistance.

Miscellaneous Microscopic Sediment Findings.—***Trichomonas***—Female vaginal infection by the protozoan parasite *Trichomonas* is fairly common; it is often associated with mild proteinuria, WBCs, and epithelial cells in the urine sediment. The organism is frequently found in urine specimens, where diagnosis is greatly assisted by the organism's motility (so a fresh specimen is essential). When nonmotile, it resembles a large WBC or small tubular epithelial cell. Fluorescent antibody methods are now available for diagnosis and are more sensitive than ordinary urine sediment examination but are relatively expensive. *Trichomonas* is found occasionally in the male.

Spermatozoa.—Spermatozoa may appear in the urine of males and, occasionally, in that of females.

Yeast.—Yeast is a relatively common sediment finding; the most common is *Candida albicans (Monilia)*. Yeast cells are often misdiagnosed as RBCs. Differential points are budding (not always noticed without careful search), ovoid shape (not always pronounced), an appearance slightly more opaque and homogeneous than that of the RBC, and insolubility in both acid and alkali. If the cells are numerous and their identity is still in doubt, a chemical test for blood is recommended.

Pitfalls in Microscopic Examination of Urine Sediment.—The most common and most important mistake is failure to mix the specimen sufficiently before a portion of it is poured into a centrifuge tube for concentration of the sediment. Certain other points deserve reemphasis. If the specimen remains at room temperature for a long time, there may be disintegration of cellular elements, bacterial growth, and change toward an alkaline pH. If RBC or WBC casts are not reported, this does not mean that they are not present, since it usually takes careful and somewhat prolonged search to find them (especially RBC casts).

Other Urine Tests

Calcium.—Urine can be tested for calcium with Sulkowitch reagent; it is a semiquantitative method in which results are reported as 0–4+ (normal is 1+) or as negative, moderately positive, and strongly positive. Standard clinical chemistry quantitative methods have almost entirely replaced this test. Interpretation of urine calcium is discussed in chapter 24. Excessively concentrated or diluted urine may produce unreliable results, just as it does for protein.

Porphobilinogen.—Porphobilinogen is diagnostic of acute porphyria (episodes of abdominal crampy pain with vomiting and leukocytosis, chapter 20). Porphobilinogen is colorless and is easily identified by rapid screening tests, such as the Watson-Schwartz procedure.

Urinary Coproporphyrins.—Coproporphyrin type III excretion is increased in lead poisoning (chapter 34) and has been used as a relatively simple screening test for that condition. However, increased coproporphyrin III is not specific for lead poisoning.

Phenylpyruvic Acid.—Phenylpyruvic acid is excreted in phenylketonuria (chapter 33). A ferric chloride test is the classic means of detection. There is a dipstick method (Phenistix) for the diagnosis of phenylketonuria that depends on the reaction between ferric ions and phenylpyruvic acid, as does the classic ferric chloride test. It is more sensitive than ferric chloride, detecting as little as 8 mg/100 ml or trace amounts of phenylpyruvic acid in urine. False positive results occur if large amounts of ketone bodies are present. Reactions will take place with salicylates, PAS, and phenothiazine metabolites, but the color is said to be different from that given by phenylpyruvic acid. The urine screening tests have become less important since neonatal blood test screening has become mandatory in many areas. It takes approximately 3–6 weeks after birth before phenylpyruvic acid becomes detectable in urine, and by that time treatment is much less effective.

Points to Remember in Interpretation of Urinalysis Results

1. Laboratory reports usually err in omission rather than commission (except occasionally in RBCs vs. yeast). If technicians cannot identify something, they usually do not mention it at all.

2. Certain diagnostic findings, such as RBC casts, may not appear in every high-power (or even every low-power) field. If hematuria is present, one should look for RBC casts and, similarly, for WBC casts and other such structures in the appropriate sediment settings.

3. If laboratory personnel know what the physician is trying to find, they usually will give more than a routine glance. Otherwise, the pressure of routine work may result in examination that is not sufficient to detect important abnormalities.

4. In many laboratories, reports will include only items specifically requested, even when other abnormalities are grossly visible (e.g., bile).

5. Contamination of urine by vaginal secretions in the female may introduce RBCs, WBCs, or protein into the specimen as an artifact. The presence of more than 10 squamous epithelial cells per low-power field is a warning of possible contamination. Nevertheless, abnormalities should not be dismissed on the basis of possible contamination without careful and repeated attempts to obtain a noncontaminated specimen, because contamination may be superimposed on true abnormality. In some cases this problem may necessitate expert help in specimen collection.

One fact that should be stressed when commercial tests of any type are used is to follow all the directions exactly. Any dipstick or tablet method requires a certain length of time in contact with the specimen. When this is true, a quick dip-and-read technique, or, on the other hand, overly prolonged contact with the specimen, may lead to false results. Moisture may affect some of the test reagents, so the tops on reagent bottles should be replaced and tightened immediately after the dipsticks or tablets are taken out.

THE KIDNEY IN DISEASE

Primary glomerular renal disease for a long time was subdivided into glomerulonephritis (acute, subacute, chronic) and the nephrotic syndrome, based on clinical and light microscopic findings. With the advent of renal biopsy, electron microscopy, and immunoglobulin fluorescent staining of tissue sections, the clinical categories are being reclassified on the basis of ultrastructure and immunologic characteristics (see Table 36–6). Diseases in some of the immunohistopathologic subdivisions have different prognoses (and, in some cases, different responses to certain therapeutic agents) and therefore could logically be regarded as separate entities. Nevertheless, I have chosen to describe laboratory findings in terms of the original clinical syndromes, since this is the way most clinicians encounter primary renal disease. A morphologic classification of glomerular disease is given in Table 36–6.

Glomerulonephritis

Acute Glomerulonephritis.—Classic acute glomerulonephritis (AGN) corresponds to a subcategory of proliferative glomerulonephritis that is considered a hypersensitivity reaction, usually associated with concurrent or recent infection. The most common organism incriminated is the beta-hemolytic Lancefield group A *Streptococcus*. Only a relatively small number of specific group A strains are known to cause AGN (see Table 30–8) in contrast to the large number that initiate acute rheumatic fever.

Clinically, onset of the disease is frequently manifested by gross hematuria. The urine may be red or may be the color of coffee grounds (due to breakdown of hemoglobin to brown acid hematin). In mild cases, gross hematuria may be less evident, or the hematuria may be microscopic only. Varying degrees of peripheral edema, especially of the upper eyelids, are often present. Hypertension of varying degree is a frequent initial finding.

Laboratory features usually include an elevated erythrocyte sedimentation rate and frequently a mild to moderate normocytic-normochromic (or slightly hypochromic) anemia. There is mild to moderate proteinuria (0.5–3.0 gm/24 hours). The urinary sediment reflects varying degrees of hematuria, often with WBCs also present. Red blood cell casts are characteristic and are the most diagnostic laboratory finding. They may be present only intermittently, may be few in number, and may be degenerated enough to make recognition difficult. Although RBC casts are not specific for AGN, relatively few diseases are consistently associated with RBC casts. These conditions include AGN, subacute and occasionally chronic glomerulonephritis, subacute bacterial endocarditis, some of the collagen diseases (especially systemic lupus), and hemoglobinuric acute tubular necrosis.

Renal Function Tests.—Prolonged azotemia is not common in poststreptococcal AGN (5%–10% of cases), despite hypertension, although as many as 50% of affected persons have some BUN elevation initially. Renal function tests are said to be essentially normal in nearly 50% of patients; the rest have varying degrees of impairment for varying time intervals, and a small percentage show renal insufficiency with uremia. Urine concentrating ability is generally maintained for the first few days; in some patients, it may then be impaired for a considerable time. Function tests in general tend to reflect (although not exclusively) the primarily glomerular lesion found in AGN, manifested on light microscopy by increased glomerular cellularity and swelling and proliferation of capillary endothelial cells and on electron microscopy by subepithelial "humps."

Antistreptococcal Antibodies.—In addition to urinalysis, the antistreptolysin-O (ASL or ASO) titer may be helpful, since a significant titer (> 200 Todd units) suggests recent or relatively recent group A streptococcal infection. However, since up to 20% of AGN patients have ASO titers in the normal range, a normal ASO titer does not rule out the diagnosis, nor does a high titer guarantee that the condition is indeed AGN (the group A streptococcal infection may be unrelated to the renal disease). Measurement of other streptococcal enzyme antibodies, such as anti-ADN-B, in addition to ASO, will improve sensitivity of the test. Several commercial kits now have combined reagents active against several of the antistreptococcal antibodies. The third component (C3) of serum complement is nearly always depressed in streptococcal AGN and returns to normal in 6–8 weeks. Consistently normal early C3 levels are evidence against streptococcal etiology, and failure of the C3 level to return to normal in 8 weeks also suggests a different etiology.

Acute glomerulonephritis is a relatively benign disease in childhood, since mortality is only about 1%, and an even smaller percentage suffer permanent damage. In adults, the incidence of the disease is much lower, but 25%–50% of adult patients develop chronic renal disease.

Rapidly Progressive Glomerulonephritis.—Rapidly progressive glomerulonephritis may follow the acute stage of AGN but much more commonly appears without any previous clinical or serologic evidence of AGN. It is more common in older children and adults. The original term "subacute glomerulonephritis" was misleading; originally it referred to the duration of the clinical course, longer than that of AGN in the average patient but much shorter than that of chronic glomerulonephritis. Histologically, the glomeruli show epithelial cell proliferation with resultant filling in of the space between Bowman's capsule and the glomerular tuft (epithelial crescent). The urine sediment includes many casts of hyaline and epithelial series; RBCs and often WBCs are present in varying numbers, often with a few RBC casts. There is moderately severe to marked proteinuria, and both the degree of proteinuria and the urinary sediment may sometimes be indistinguishable from similar findings in the nephrotic syndrome, even with fatty casts present. Clinically, rapidly progressive glomerulonephritis behaves as a more severe form of AGN and generally leads to death in weeks or months. It is not the same process as the nephrotic episodes that may form part of chronic glomerulonephritis. In addition to urinary findings, anemia is usually present. Renal function tests demonstrate both glomerular and tubule destruction, although clinically there is usually little additional information gained by extensive renal function studies. Serum complement C3 is temporarily depressed in cases of poststreptococcal origin but otherwise is usually normal.

Chronic Glomerulonephritis.—Chronic glomerulonephritis infrequently is preceded by AGN, but usually there is no antecedent clinical illness or etiology. It most often runs a slowly progressive or intermittent course over many years. During the latent phases there may be very few urinary abnormalities, but RBCs are generally present in varying small numbers in the sediment. There is almost always proteinuria, generally of mild degree, and rather infrequent casts of the epithelial series. Disease progression is documented by a slowly decreasing ability to concentrate the urine, followed by deterioration in creatinine clearance. Intercurrent streptococcal upper respiratory tract infection or other infections may occasionally set off an acute exacerbation. There may be one or more episodes of the nephrotic syndrome, usually without much, if any, hematuria. The terminal or azotemic stage produces the clinical and laboratory picture of renal failure. Finely granular and waxy casts predominate, and broad casts are often present. There is moderate proteinuria.

Nephrotic Syndrome

The criteria for diagnosis of the nephrotic syndrome include high proteinuria (> 3.5 gm/24 hours), edema, hypercholesterolemia, and hypoalbuminemia. However, one or occasionally even more of these criteria may be absent. The level of proteinuria is said to be the most consistent criterion. In addition, patients with the nephrotic syndrome often have a characteristic serum protein electrophoretic pattern, consisting of greatly decreased albumin and considerably increased alpha-2 globulin. However, in some cases the pattern is not marked enough to be characteristic. The nephrotic syndrome is one of a relatively few diseases in which the serum cholesterol level may substantially contribute toward establishing the diagnosis, especially in borderline cases.

The nephrotic syndrome has nothing in common with the entity formerly called hemoglobinuric nephrosis (or lower nephron nephrosis), despite the unfortunate similarity in names. The term hemoglobinuric nephrosis has generally been discarded, since it is only a subdivision of acute tubular necrosis, due to renal tubule damage from hemoglobin derived from marked intravascular hemolysis. Even the term "nephrotic syndrome" as it is currently used is actually a misnomer and dates from the time when proteinuria was thought primarily to be due to a disorder of renal tubules. The word "nephrosis" was then used to characterize such a situation. It is now recognized that various glomerular lesions form the actual basis for proteinuria in the nephrotic syndrome, either of the primary or the secondary type. The nephrotic syndrome as a term is also confusing because it may be of two clinical types, described in the following section.

Primary (or Lipoid) Nephrosis.—Primary nephrosis is the idiopathic form and is usually found in childhood. The etiology of primary (idiopathic or lipoid) nephrosis is still not definitely settled. Renal biopsy has shown various glomerular abnormalities, classified most easily into basement membrane and focal sclerosis varieties. In most children the basement membrane changes may be so slight (null lesion) as to be certified only by electron microscopy (manifested by fusion of the footplates of epithelial cells applied to the basement membrane). The null lesion is associated with excellent response to steroids, a great tendency to relapse, and eventually relatively good prognosis. Focal sclerosis most often is steroid resistant and has a poor prognosis.

In lipoid nephrosis, the urine contains mostly protein. The sediment may contain relatively small numbers of fatty and granular casts, and there may be small numbers of RBCs. Greater hematuria or cylindruria suggests greater severity but not necessarily a worse prognosis. Renal function tests are normal in most patients; the remainder have various degrees of impairment.

Nephrotic Syndrome.—Although lipoid nephrosis may be found in adults, the nephrotic syndrome is more common and may be either idiopathic or secondary to a variety of diseases. The most common idiopathic lesions include a diffuse light microscope "wire loop" basement membrane thickening, which has been termed *membranous glomerulonephritis,* and a type that has been called *membranoproliferative.* Prognosis in these is worse than in childhood lipoid nephrosis.

The most common etiologies of secondary nephrotic syndrome are chronic glomerulonephritis, Kimmelstiel-Wilson syndrome, systemic lupus, amyloid and renal vein thrombosis. In the urine, fat is the most characteristic element, appearing in oval fat bodies and fatty casts. Also present are variable numbers of epithelial and hyaline series casts. Urine RBCs are variable, usually only few, but sometimes many. Significant hematuria suggests lupus, the presence of diabetes and hypertension suggests Kimmelstiel-Wilson syndrome, a history of previous proteinuria or hematuria suggests chronic glomerulonephritis, and the presence of chronic long-standing infection suggests an amyloid etiology. About 50% of cases are associated with chronic glomerulonephritis. Renal function tests in the nephrotic syndrome secondary to lupus, Kimmelstiel-Wilson syndrome, and amyloid generally show diffuse renal damage. The same is true of chronic glomerulonephritis in the later stages; however, if the nephrotic syndrome occurs relatively early in the course of this disease, test abnormalities may be minimal, reflected only in impaired concentrating ability. Histologically, renal glomeruli in the nephrotic syndrome exhibit lesions that vary according to the particular disease responsible.

Membranoproliferative glomerulonephritis occurs in older children and teenagers and displays some features of AGN as well as nephrotic syndrome. Hematuria and complement C3 decrease occur, but the C3 decrease usually is prolonged beyond 8 weeks (60% or more cases). However, C3 levels may fluctuate during the course of the disease.

Malignant Hypertension (Accelerated Arteriolar Nephrosclerosis)

Malignant hypertension is most common in middle age, with most patients aged 30–60 years. There is a tendency toward males and an increased incidence in blacks. The majority of patients have a history of preceding mild or benign hypertension, most often for 2–6 years, although the disease can begin abruptly. The syndrome may also be secondary to severe chronic renal disease of several varieties. Clinical features are markedly elevated systolic and diastolic blood pressures, papilledema, and evidence of renal damage. Laboratory tests show anemia to be present in most cases, even in relatively early stages. Urinalysis in the early stages most often shows a moderate proteinuria and hematuria, usually without RBC casts. The sediment thus mimics to some extent the sediment of AGN. Later the sediment may show more evidence of tubular damage. There usually develops a moderate to high proteinuria (which uncommonly may reach 5–10 gm/24 hours) accompanied by considerable microscopic hematuria and often many casts, including all those of the hyaline and epithelial series—even fatty casts occasionally. In the terminal stages, late granular or waxy casts and broad renal failure casts predominate. The disease produces rapid deterioration of renal function, and most cases terminate in azotemia. Nocturia and polyuria are common owing to the progressive renal damage. If congestive heart failure is superimposed, there may be a decreased urine volume plus loss of ability to concentrate urine.

Pyelonephritis (Renal Infection)

Acute pyelonephritis often elicits a characteristic syndrome (spiking high fever, costovertebral angle tenderness, dysuria, back pain, etc.). Proteinuria is mild, rarely exceeding 2 gm/24 hours. Pyuria (and often bacteriuria) develops. The presence of WBC casts is diagnostic, although they may have to be carefully searched for or may be absent. Urine culture may establish the diagnosis of urinary tract infection but cannot localize the area involved. Hematogenous spread of infection to the kidney tends to localize in the renal cortex and may give fewer initial urinary findings; retrograde ascending infection from the lower urinary tract reaches renal medulla areas first and shows early pyuria.

In chronic low-grade pyelonephritis, the urine may not be grossly pyuric, and sediment may be scanty. In some cases, urine cultures may contain fewer than 100,000 organisms/cu mm (100×10^9/L) or may even be negative. Very frequently, however, there is a significant increase in pus cells; they often, but not invariably, occur in clumps when the process is more severe. Casts other than the WBC type are usually few or absent in pyelonephritis until the late or terminal stages, and WBC casts themselves may be absent.

A urine specimen should be obtained for culture in all cases of suspected urinary tract infection to isolate the organism responsible and determine antibiotic sensitivity (chapter 14).

Tuberculosis is a special type of renal infection. It involves the kidney in possibly 25% of patients with chronic or severe pulmonary tuberculosis, although the incidence of clinical disease is much less. Hematuria is frequent; it may be gross or only microscopic. Pyuria is also common. Characteristically, pyuria is present without demonstrable bacteriuria (of ordinary bacterial varieties), but this is not reliable due to a considerable frequency of superinfection by ordinary bacteria in genitourinary tuberculosis. Dysuria is also present in many patients. If hematuria (with or without pyuria) is found in a patient with tuberculosis, genitourinary tract tuberculosis should be suspected. Urine cultures are said to be positive in about 7% of patients with significant degrees of active pulmonary tuberculosis. At least three specimens, one obtained each day for 3 days, should be secured, each one collected in a sterile container. A fresh early morning specimen has been recommended rather than 24-hour collections. Acid-fast urine smears are rarely helpful. If suspicion of renal tuberculosis is strong, intravenous pyelography should be done to assess the extent of involvement.

Renal papillary necrosis is a possible complication of acute pyelonephritis, particularly in diabetics.

Renal Papillary Necrosis (Necrotizing Papillitis)

As the name suggests, this condition results from necrosis of a focal area in one or more renal pyramids. Papillary necrosis is most frequently associated with infection but may occur without known cause. It is much more frequent in diabetics. A small minority of cases are associated with sickle cell hemoglobin diseases or phenacetin toxicity. The disease usually is of an acute nature, although some patients may have relatively minor symptoms or symptoms overshadowed by other complications or disease. The patients are usually severely ill and manifest pyuria, hematuria, and azotemia, especially when renal papillary necrosis is associated with infection. Drip-infusion intravenous (IV) pyelography is the diagnostic test of choice. Naturally, urine culture should be performed.

Renal Embolism and Thrombosis

Renal artery occlusion or embolism most often affects the smaller renal arteries or the arterioles. Such involvement produces renal infarction in that vessel's distribution, usually manifested by hematuria and proteinuria. Casts of the epithelial series may also appear. Renal infarction frequently produces elevation of serum lactic dehydrogenase (LDH), with the LDH-1 isoenzyme typically greater than LDH-2 (chapter 20). Aspartate aminotransferase (serum glutamic oxaloacetic transaminase) may also be increased but less frequently. Alkaline phosphatase is temporarily increased in some patients after 5–10 days (range 3–15 days), possibly related to the granulation tissue healing process.

Acute Tubular Necrosis

This syndrome may result from acute or sudden renal failure of any cause, most often secondary to hypotension, although intravascular hemolysis from blood transfusion reactions is probably the most famous etiology. Acute tubular necrosis begins with a period of oliguria or near anuria and manifests subsequent diuresis if recovery ensues. Urinalysis demonstrates considerable proteinuria with desquamated epithelial cells and epithelial hyaline casts. There are usually some RBCs (occasionally many) and often large numbers of broad and waxy casts (indicative of severe urinary stasis in the renal parenchyma). Hemoglobin casts are usually present in cases due to intravascular hemolysis. Specific gravity is characteristically fixed at 1.010 after the first hours, and the BUN level begins rising shortly after onset. In cases of acute tubular necrosis not due to intravascular hemolysis, the pathogenesis is that of generalized tubular necrosis, most often anoxic.

Congenital Renal Disease

Polycystic Kidney.—There are two clinical forms of polycystic kidney, one fatal in early infancy and the other (adult type) usually asymptomatic until the third or fourth decade. The urinary sediment is highly variable; microscopic intermittent hematuria is common, and gross hematuria may occasionally take place. Cysts may become infected and produce symptoms of pyelonephritis. In general, the rate of proteinuria is minimal or mild but may occasionally be higher. Symptoms may be those of hypertension (50%–60% of cases) or renal failure. If the condition does progress to renal failure, the urinary sediment is nonspecific, reflecting only the presence of end-stage kidneys of any etiology. Diagnosis may be suggested by family history and the presence of bilaterally palpable abdominal masses and is confirmed by radiologic procedures, such as IV pyelography. Ultrasound can also be useful.

Renal Developmental Anomalies.—This category includes horseshoe kidney, solitary cysts, reduplication of a ureter, renal ptosis, and so forth. There may be no urinary findings or, sometimes, a slight proteinuria. In children, urinary tract anomalies often predispose to repeated urinary tract infection. Recurrent urinary tract infection, especially in children, should always be investigated for the possibility of either urinary tract obstruction or anomalies. Diagnosis is by IV pyelography.

Renal Neoplasia

The most common sign of carcinoma anywhere in the urinary tract is hematuria, which is present in 60%–80% of patients with primary renal adenocarcinoma and (according to one report) in about 95% of bladder, ureter, and renal pelvis carcinoma. In renal cell carcinoma, hematuria is most often visible grossly and is intermittent. In persons over age 40 a neoplasm should be suspected if increased urine RBCs are not explained by other conditions known to produce hematuria. Even if such diseases are present, this does not rule out genitourinary carcinoma. The workup of a patient with hematuria is discussed in chapter 13. Methods for detecting renal cell carcinoma are described in chapter 32.

Lupus Erythematosus or Polyarteritis Nodosa

About two thirds of lupus patients have renal involvement. Generally, there is microscopic hematuria; otherwise there may be a varying picture. In the classic case of lupus (much less often in polyarteritis), one finds a "telescoped sediment," that is, a sediment containing the characteristic elements of all three stages of glomerulonephritis (acute, subacute, and chronic, manifest by fatty, late granular, and RBC casts). Usually, hematuria is predominant, especially in polyarteritis. In lupus, RBC casts are more commonly found. Up to one third of lupus patients develop the nephrotic syndrome. Complement C3 levels are frequently decreased in active lupus nephritis.

Embolic Glomerulonephritis

Embolic glomerulonephritis is most commonly associated with subacute bacterial endocarditis. Scattered small focal areas of necrosis are present in glomerular capillaries. There is some uncertainty whether the lesions are embolic, infectious, or allergic in origin. Since the glomerular lesions are sharply focal, there usually is not much pyuria. Hematuria usually is present and may be pronounced. If localized tubular stasis occurs in addition, RBC casts may appear, with resultant simulation of latent glomerulonephritis or AGN. The rate of proteinuria often remains relatively small, frequently not more than 1 gm/24 hours.

Diabetes

The kidney may be affected by several unrelated disorders, including (1) a high incidence of pyelonephritis, sometimes renal papillary necrosis; (2) a high incidence of arteriosclerosis with hypertension; and (3) Kimmelstiel-Wilson syndrome (intercapillary glomerulosclerosis). The nephrotic syndrome may occur in the late stages of the Kimmelstiel-Wilson syndrome. Otherwise, only varying degrees of proteinuria are manifest, perhaps with a few granular casts. Diabetic microalbuminuria, a stage that precedes overt diabetic renal disease, was discussed in the earlier section on urine protein.

Pregnancy

Several abnormal urinary findings are associated with pregnancy.

Benign Proteinuria.—Proteinuria may appear in up to 30% of otherwise normal pregnancies during labor but surpasses 100 mg/100 ml in only about 3% of these cases. It is unclear whether proteinuria must be considered pathologic if it occurs in uncomplicated pregnancy before labor. Some authorities believe that proteinuria is not found in normal pregnancy; others report an incidence of up to 20%, which is ascribed to abdominal venous compression.

Eclampsia.—This condition, also known as toxemia of pregnancy, denotes a syndrome of severe edema, proteinuria, hypertension, and convulsions associated with pregnancy. This syndrome without convulsions is called *preeclampsia*. In most cases, onset occurs either in the last trimester or during labor, although uncommonly the toxemic syndrome may develop after delivery. The etiology is unknown, despite the fact that delivery usually terminates the signs and symptoms. Pronounced proteinuria is the rule; the most severe cases may have oval fat bodies and fatty casts. Other laboratory abnormalities include principally an elevated serum uric acid level in 60%–70% of cases and a metabolic acidosis. The BUN level is usually normal. Diagnosis at present depends more on physical examination, including ophthalmoscopic observation of spasm in the retinal arteries and blood pressure changes, than on laboratory tests, except tests for proteinuria. Gradual onset of eclampsia may be confusing, since some degree of edema is common in pregnancy, and proteinuria (although only slight or mild) may appear during labor.

Glucosuria.—Glucosuria occurs in 5%–35% of pregnancies, mainly in the last trimester. Occasional reports state an even higher frequency. It is not completely clear whether this is due to increased glucose filtration resulting from an increased GFR, a decreased renal tubular transport maximum (reabsorptive) capacity for glucose, a combination of the two, or some other factor. Lactosuria may also occur in the last trimester and may be mistaken for glucosuria when using copper sulfate reducing tests for urine glucose.

Renal Function Tests.—The glomerular filtration rate is increased during pregnancy. Because of this, the BUN level may be somewhat decreased, and clearance tests are somewhat increased. Renal concentration may appear falsely decreased because of edema fluid excretion that takes place during sleep.

Infection.—Bacteriuria has been reported in 4%–7% of pregnant patients, whereas the incidence in nonpregnant healthy women is approximately 0.5%. It is believed that untreated bacteriuria strongly predisposes to postpartum pyelonephritis.

URINALYSIS IN MISCELLANEOUS DISEASES

Fever.—Fever is the most common cause of proteinuria (up to 75% of febrile patients). If severe, it may be associated with an increase in hyaline casts (etiology unknown, possibly dehydration).

Cystitis-Urethritis.—Cystitis and urethritis are lower urinary tract infections, often hard to differentiate from renal infection. Clumping of WBCs is suggestive of pyelonephritis but not absolutely specific, as WBC casts are. Necrotizing cystitis may cause hematuria. The two-glass urine test helps to differentiate urethritis from cystitis. After cleansing the genitalia, the patient voids about 10–20 ml into container number 1 and the remainder into container number 2. A significant increase in the WBC count of container number 1 over that of container number 2 suggests urethral origin.

Genitourinary Tract Obstruction.—Neuromuscular disorders of the bladder, congenital urethral strictures and valves, intrinsic or extrinsic ureteral mechanical compressions, and intraluminal calculi produce no specific urinary changes but predispose to stasis and infection. Obstruction, partial or complete, is a frequent etiology for recurrent genitourinary tract infections.

Amyloidosis.—Renal involvement usually leads to proteinuria. In a minority of cases, when the process severely affects the kidney, there may be high proteinuria and sediment typical of the nephrotic syndrome. The urinary sediment, however, is not specific, and RBC casts are not present. Renal amyloidosis is usually associated with chronic disease, such as longstanding osteomyelitis or infection, or multiple sclerosis.

Urinary Calculi.—Urinary calculi often cause hematuria of varying degree and, depending on the composition of the stone, may be associated with excess excretion of calcium, uric acid, cystine, phosphates, or urates in the urine, even when calculi are not clinically evident. Frequent complications are infections or obstruction, and infection may occur even in the absence of definite obstruction. Ureteral stone passage produces hematuria, often gross. Intravenous pyelography is the best means of diagnosis. Some types of calculi are radiopaque, and others may be localized by finding a site of ureteral obstruction.

Sickle Cell Anemia.—Hematuria frequently occurs due to kidney lesions produced by intracapillary RBC plugs, leading to congestion, small thromboses, and microinfarctions. Hematuria is also frequent at times of hematologic crises. Hematuria may be present even without crises in sickle cell disease or sickle cell variants. Sickle cell patients may lose urine-concentrating ability for unknown reasons. This happens even with sickle cell variants but is less common.

Chronic Passive Congestion.—One cause of renal congestion is inferior vena cava obstruction. It produces mild diffuse tubular atrophy and hyperemia, leads to proteinuria (usually mild to moderate) and hyaline casts, and sometimes also elicits epithelial casts and a few RBCs. Occasionally, but not commonly, severe chronic passive congestion (CPC) may simulate the nephrotic syndrome to some extent, including desquamated epithelial cells containing fat plus many casts of the epithelial series. In CPC of strictly cardiac origin without significant previous renal damage, there is decreased urine volume but usually retained urine-concentrating ability. No anemia is present unless it is due to some other systemic etiology.

Benign Arteriosclerosis.—Benign arteriosclerosis involves the renal parenchyma secondarily to decreased blood supply. In most cases in the earlier stages, there are few urinary findings, if any; later, there is often mild proteinuria (0.1–0.5 gm/24 hours) and a variable urine sediment, which may contain a few hyaline casts, epithelial cells, and perhaps occasional RBCs. If the condition eventually progresses to renal failure, there will be significant proteinuria and renal failure sediment with impaired renal function tests.

Weil's Disease.—Weil's disease is leptospiral infection (chapter 14) and clinically presents with hepatitis and hematuria. Characteristically, there are also high fever and severe muscle aching, and there may be associated symptoms of meningitis.

Infectious Mononucleosis.—Renal involvement with hematuria occurs in 5%–6% of cases.

Purpura and Hemorrhagic Diseases.—These diseases should be recognized as causes of hematuria, either by itself or in association with glomerular lesions. The Henoch-Schönlein syndrome (anaphylactoid purpura) is a rare condition featuring GI bleeding (Henoch) or skin purpura (Schönlein) that often is concurrent with hematuria and nephritis.

Hypersensitivities.—Hypersensitivities may lead to proteinuria (usually slight) with hematuria and perhaps a moderate increase in casts. Kidney involvement may occur due to hypersensitivity to mercurials, sulfas, or other substances.

Fat Embolism.—Fat embolism commonly occurs after trauma, especially fractures. Cerebral or respiratory symptoms develop the second or third day after injury, usually associated with a significant drop in hemoglobin values. Fat in the urine is found in 50% or more of patients and is a very valuable diagnostic test. Unfortunately, a physician's order for a test for fat in the urine will usually result in microscopic examination of the sediment. Whereas this is the correct procedure to detect fat in the nephrotic syndrome, in which fat is located in renal epithelial cells and casts, it is worthless for a diagnosis of fat embolism, in which free fat droplets must be identified. Since free fat tends to float, a simple procedure is to fill an Erlenmeyer (thin-neck) flask with urine up into the thin neck, agitate gently to allow fat to reach the surface, skim the surface with a bacteriologic loop, place the loop contents on a slide, and stain with a fat stain such as Sudan IV.

Hemochromatosis.—This condition is suggested by hepatomegaly, gray skin pigmentation, and proteinuria in a diabetic patient. Proteinuria may exceed 1 gm/24 hours, but sediment may be scanty and fat is absent. In severe cases yellow-brown coarse granules of hemosiderin are seen in cells, in casts, and lying free. Prussian blue (iron) stains in this material are positive. Distal convoluted tubules are the areas primarily involved. Since hemochromatosis does not invariably involve the kidney until late, a negative urine result does not rule out the diagnosis. False positive results (other types of urine siderosis) may occur in pernicious anemia, hemolytic jaundice, and in patients who have received many transfusions.

Thyroid Dysfunction.—***Myxedema***—Proteinuria is said to occur without other renal disease. Its incidence is uncertain, especially since some reports state that proteinuria is actually not common and usually persists after treatment.

Hyperthyroidism.—The kidney may lose its concentrating ability so that specific gravity may remain low even in dehydration; this is reversible with treatment and a return to a euthyroid condition. Glucosuria occurs in occasional patients.

BIBLIOGRAPHY

Lawrence VA, Kroenke K: The unproven utility of preoperative urinalysis. *Arch Intern Med* 1988; 148:1370.

Sawyer N: Nephrotic syndrome. *Intern Med Specialist* 1987; 8:135.

Gutman SI, Soloman RR: The clinical significance of dipstick-negative, culture-positive urines in a veterans population. *Am J Clin Pathol* 1987; 88:204.

Koch D, Feldbruegge DH: Optimized kinetic method for automated determination of beta-hydroxybutyrate. *Clin Chem* 1987; 33:1761.

Schwab SJ, et al: Quantitation of proteinuria by the use of protein-to-creatinine ratios in single urine samples. *Arch Intern Med* 1987; 147:943.

Rotblatt MD, Koda-Kimble MA: Review of drug interference with urine glucose tests. *Diabetes Care* 1987; 10:103.

Scheer WD: The detection of leukocyte esterase activity in urine with a new reagent strip. *Am J Clin Pathol* 1987; 87:86.

Thal SM, et al: Comparison of dysmorphic erythrocytes with other urinary sediment parameters of renal bleeding. *Am J Clin Pathol* 1986; 86:784.

Rosenstock J, Raskin P: Early diabetic nephropathy: assessment and potential ther-

apeutic interventions. *Diabetes Care* 1986; 9:529.
Thompson C: Hematuria: A clinical approach. *Am Fam Pract* 1986; 33:194.
Froom P, et al: The effect of age on the prevalence of asymptomatic microscopic hematuria. *Am J Clin Pathol* 1986; 86:656.
Benbassat J, et al: The importance of leukocyturia in young adults. *Arch Intern Med* 1985; 145:79.
Jackson JA, Conrad ME: Technical aspects of urine dipstick reagent areas. *Am Clin Prod Rev* 1985; 4(12):10.
Li PK: Beta-hydroxybutyrate. *Clin Chem Newslett* 1985; 11(2):13.
Poortmans JR: Postexercise proteinuria in humans. *JAMA* 1985; 253:236.
Shiba KS, et al: A cause of discrepancy between values for urinary protein as assayed by the Coomassie brilliant blue G-250 method and the sulfosalicylic acid method. *Clin Chem* 1985; 31:1215.
Ciulla AP, et al: Reagent strip method for specific gravity: An evaluation. *Lab Med* 1985; 16:38.
Jackson JA, Conrad ME: New instrumentation in urinalysis. *Pathologist* 1984; 38:652.
Stewart DW, et al: Evaluation of proteinuria. *Am Fam Pract* 1984; 29:218.
Loo SYT, et al: Urine screening strategy employing dipstick analysis and selective culture: An evaluation. *Am J Clin Pathol* 1984; 81:634.
Abuelo JG: Proteinuria: Diagnostic principles and procedures. *Ann Intern Med* 1983; 98:186.
Dilena BA, et al: Six methods for determining urinary protein compared. *Clin Chem* 1983; 29:553.
Brandt ZL, et al: Evaluation of determination of glucose in urine with some commercially available dipsticks and tablets. *Clin Chem* 1982; 28:1220.
McElderry LA: Six methods for urinary protein compared. *Clin Chem* 1982; 28:356.
Szwed JJ: Urinalysis and clinical renal disease. *Am J Med Technol* 1980; 46:720.
Cannon DC: The identification and pathogenesis of urine casts. *Lab Med* 1979; 10:8.

13 Renal Function Tests

Renal function testing and liver function testing share many of the same problems. In both the kidney and the liver a multiplicity of enzyme and transport systems coexist—some related, others both spatially and physiologically quite separate. Processes going on in one section of the nephron may or may not directly affect those in other segments. Like the liver, the kidney has not one but a great many functions that may or may not be affected in a given pathologic process. By measuring the capacity to perform these individual functions, one hopes to extract anatomical and physiologic information. Unfortunately, the tests available to the clinical laboratory are few and gross compared with the delicate network of systems at work. It is often difficult to isolate individual functions without complicated research setups, and it is even more difficult to differentiate between localized and generalized damage, between temporary and permanent malfunction, and between primary and secondary derangements. One can measure only what passes into and out of the kidney. What goes on inside is all-important but must be speculated on by indirect means. A tremendous handicap that results from this situation is the inability of function tests to reveal the etiology of dysfunction; the only information obtained is whether or not a certain degree of dysfunction is present and a rough estimate of its severity. Therefore, useful information can be obtained only through knowledge of the physiologic basis for each test and by careful correlation with other clinical and laboratory data.

Renal function tests fall into three general categories: (1) tests predominantly of glomerular function, (2) tests reflecting severe glomerular or tubular damage (or both), and (3) tests of predominantly tubular function.

TESTS PREDOMINANTLY OF GLOMERULAR FUNCTION

Clearance Tests

Clearance is a theoretical concept and is defined as the volume of plasma from which a measured amount of substance can be completely eliminated (cleared) into the urine per unit of time. This depends on the plasma concentration and excretory rate, which, in turn, involve the glomerular filtration rate (GFR) and renal plasma flow (RPF). Clearance tests in general are the best available means for estimating mild to moderate diffuse glomerular damage (e.g., acute glomerulonephritis [AGN]). Serum levels of urea or creatinine reveal only extensive renal disease. However, many extrarenal conditions (shock, hyponatremia, etc.) cause vasoconstriction and reduce the RPF and thus possibly reduce clearance values.

Urea Clearance

Urea is a nitrogen-containing waste product of protein metabolism synthesized in the liver from ammonia (derived predominantly from the metabolism of protein by intestinal bacteria) and from various amino acids (of which alanine is the most important). Urea is filtered at the glomerulus, but approximately 40% is reabsorbed in the tubules by passive back-diffusion. Thus, under usual conditions, urea clearance values parallel the true GFR at about 60% of it. However, two factors may adversely influence this situation. First, the test is dependent on rate of urine flow. At low levels (< 2 ml/minute), the values are very inaccurate, even with certain correction formulas. Second, levels of blood urea change to some extent during the day and vary according to diet and other conditions.

Creatinine Clearance

Creatinine is a metabolic product of creatine-phosphate dephosphorylation in muscle. It has a relatively (although not completely) constant hourly and daily production and is present at fairly stable blood levels. Excretion is by a combination of glomerular filtration (70%–80%) and tubular secretion. It usually parallels the true GFR by ± 10%. However, at low filtration rates (< 30% of normal), creatinine clearance values become increasingly inaccurate because the tubular secreted fraction becomes a larger proportion of total urinary creatinine. Creatinine clearance has an advantage over urea clearance because creatinine has a more constant production rate than urea. Since the serum value is part of the clearance formula, less fluctuation in the serum value permits larger urine time interval collections and more reproducible results. In addition, there is less tubular secretion of creatinine than urea. Theoretical and clinical considerations have shown creatinine clearance to be a better estimate of the GFR than urea clearance. Thus, creatinine clearance has replaced urea clearance in most laboratories.

Creatinine clearance has certain drawbacks. The reference limits (90–120 ml/minute) were established for young adults. The GFR has been shown to decrease with age; one report indicates a 4 ml/minute decrease for each decade after age 20. Several studies found creatinine clearances as low as 50 ml/minute in clinically healthy elderly persons, and one study found values between 40% and 70% of normal. Creatinine excretion also diminishes with age, although serum creatinine remains within population reference limits. Whether age-related normal values should be applied depends on whether these changes are regarded as physiologic (because they occur frequently in the population) or pathologic (because they are most likely due to renal arteriolar nephrosclerosis). Several nonrenal factors influence creatinine clearance. One major problem is shared by all clearance tests: the necessity for very accurately timed urine collections without any loss of urine excreted during the collection period. Incomplete urine collection will usually falsely decrease apparent clearance values. Another factor to be considered is serum creatinine dependence on muscle mass, which can vary considerably in different individuals. Also, decreased muscle mass (as seen in the elderly, chronic renal failure, or malnourished persons) can result in a greater decrease in apparent clearance values than in serum creatinine levels. Finally, there are laboratory variables. Certain substances (e.g., ketones) can interfere with biochemical assay of creatinine. Enzymatic methods for creatinine assay produce creatinine clearance values that reportedly can be as much as 30 ml/min higher than those derived from the standard biochemical Jaffe method. Using any method, day-to-day variation in assay of the same creatinine specimen produces differences in results of 15%–20% in most laboratories (representing ± 2 standard deviation from the mean value). To conclude, creatinine clearance is a useful estimate of the GFR, but there are problems in collection, measurement, and body physiology (normal or disease induced) that can produce inaccuracy.

The standard urine collection time for creatinine clearance is 24 hours. Several reports indicate that a 2-hour collection period provides results that correlate reasonably well with those of 24-hour collection. The 2-hour collection should be performed in the early morning with the patient fasting, since there is a postprandial increase in creatinine blood and urine levels of 10%–40%.

Some investigators believe that creatinine clearance results are more accurate if patient weight, surface area, age, or some combination of these variables is included in the clearance computation. One frequently used correction formula is the following:

$$\text{Corrected creatinine clearance} = \frac{\text{Measured creatinine clearance} \times 1.73}{\text{Patient surface area (sq m)}}$$

Various nomograms and formulas have been published based on serum creatinine levels and some of the variables just listed to predict creatinine clearance without requiring urine collection. However, all such formulas assume that patient renal function is stable. None has been widely accepted to date. The formula of Gault and Cockcroft seems reasonably simple and is reported to be fairly reliable:

$$\text{Creatinine clearance (ml/min) for men} = \frac{(140 - \text{age [yr]}) \times (\text{weight [kg]})}{72 \times \text{serum creatinine (mg/100 ml)}}$$

Clearance values for women determined by using this formula are 90% of those for men. All predictive formulas give some results that are at variance with measured clearances.

Creatinine clearance has been reported to be one of the most sensitive tests to warn of renal failure, since the clearance falls swiftly to low levels. However, many conditions produce a fall in creatinine clearance, and if the clearance is already decreased, a further fall would be difficult to interpret. The most useful information would be provided if the clearance were known to be normal or close to normal prior to testing. A major drawback is the nonspecificity of a clearance decrease, which cannot be used to differentiate between the etiologies of abnormality.

Creatinine clearance determinations are most commonly used in three situations: (1) in AGN, to follow the clinical course and as a parameter of therapeutic response; (2) to demonstrate the presence of acute, strictly glomerular disease in contrast to more diffuse chronic structural damage; and (3) as a measurement of overall renal functional impairment. In AGN, there frequently (but not always) is a decrease in the GFR due to primary glomerular involvement. When this is true, the clearance tests have been used to evaluate the length of time that bed rest and other therapy are necessary. However, the erythrocyte sedimentation rate (ESR) gives the same information in a manner that is cheaper, simpler, and probably more sensitive. Therefore, the ESR seems preferable in most cases. Concerning the second category, it is not so easy to demonstrate strictly glomerular disease because many diseases reduce renal blood flow and thus the GFR. Also, some patients with AGN may have some degree of tubular damage. One situation in which clearance tests may be used to diagnostic advantage is the rare case of a young person with sudden gross hematuria but without convincing clinical or laboratory evidence of AGN. Since one expects normal clearance values in a young person, a reduced creatinine clearance rate could be some evidence in favor of nephritis.

TESTS REFLECTING SEVERE GLOMERULAR DAMAGE, TUBULAR DAMAGE, OR BOTH

Blood Urea Nitrogen

Blood urea nitrogen (BUN) is actually measured in serum rather than whole blood and can be assayed in urine. Urea can be measured biochemically or enzymatically (with the specific enzyme urease). Few substances interfere seriously with either method. Two screening methods for BUN, called Urograph and Azostix, are commercially available. Evaluations to date indicate that both of these methods are useful as emergency or office screening procedures to separate normal persons (BUN level < 20 mg/100 ml [7 mmol/L]) from those with mild azotemia (20–50 mg/100 ml [7–18 mmol/L]) and those with considerable BUN elevation (> 50 mg/100 ml [18 mmol/L]). If accurate quantitation is desired, one of the standard quantitative BUN procedures should be done.

As noted previously, urea is produced in the liver and excreted by the kidneys. When the kidneys are not able to clear urea sufficiently, urea accumulates in the blood. If reasonable liver function is assumed, measurement of urea (BUN) thus provides an estimate of renal function. Elevation of BUN levels is also known as azotemia. However, elevated BUN levels are not specific for intrinsic kidney disease. Elevated BUN levels may occur from excessive quantities of urea presented to the kidney; from decreased renal blood flow, preventing adequate glomerular filtration; from intrinsic renal disease, which affects glomerular or tubular function; or from urinary obstruction, which results in back-pressure interference with urea removal. Therefore, in some types of azotemia the kidney is not structurally affected and the azotemia is transient. In other azotemic patients the primary cause is renal parenchymal damage, and whether the BUN elevation is reversible depends on whether the kidney is able to recover a sufficient degree of function. Blood urea nitrogen levels may be decreased below expected levels in severe liver disease (insufficient manufacture) and sometimes in late pregnancy.

Following is a classification of azotemia

based on etiology. It is subdivided into azotemia primarily due to increased urea or decreased blood flow (prerenal), intrinsic kidney disease, or postrenal obstruction.

PRERENAL AZOTEMIA

1. Traumatic shock (head injuries; postsurgical hypotension)
2. Hemorrhagic shock (varices, ulcer, postpartum hemorrhage, etc.)
3. Severe dehydration or electrolyte loss (severe vomiting, diarrhea, diabetic acidosis, Addison's disease)
4. Acute cardiac decompensation (especially after extensive myocardial infarction)
5. Overwhelming infections or toxemia
6. Excess intake of proteins or extensive protein breakdown (usually other factors are also involved, such as the normally subclinical functional loss from aging)

RENAL

1. Chronic diffuse bilateral kidney disease or bilateral severe kidney damage (e.g., chronic glomerulonephritis or bilateral chronic pyelonephritis)
2. Acute tubular necrosis (glomerular or tubular injury [or both] due to hypotension or shock with renal shutdown, traumatic or nontraumatic rhabdomyolysis, transfusion or allergic reactions, certain poisons, and precipitation of uric acid or sulfa crystals in renal tubules)
3. Severe acute glomerular damage (e.g., AGN)

POSTRENAL (OBSTRUCTION)

1. Ureteral or urethral obstruction by strictures, stones, external compression, pelvic tumors, and so forth.
2. Obstructing tumors of bladder; congenital defects in bladder or urethra
3. Prostatic obstruction (tumor or benign hypertrophy; a very common cause in elderly men)

Prerenal azotemia etiologies can be divided into two main categories: (1) decreased blood volume or renal circulation and (2) increased protein intake or endogenous protein catabolism.

In *azotemia due to excessive protein*, some of the more common clinical situations are high-protein tube feedings or gastrointestinal (GI) tract hemorrhage (where protein is absorbed from the GI tract); low-calorie diet (as in patients receiving intravenous [IV] fluids, leading to endogenous protein catabolism); and adrenocortical steroid therapy (since these substances have a catabolic action).

In *decreased renal blood flow*, etiologies include blood volume deficit, cardiac failure to pump sufficient blood, or toxic effects on blood vessels. It should be pointed out that decreased renal blood flow may produce prerenal azotemia without structural renal damage, but it may also produce severe acute renal damage (acute renal failure, also called *acute tubular necrosis*).

Primary renal disease may produce azotemia due to primarily glomerular or tubular destructive conditions or to diffuse parenchymal destruction. Rarely is there glomerular damage to the point of severe azotemia (5%–10% of AGN cases) without some effect on the tubules, and vice versa. Therefore, the BUN level must be correlated with other clinical findings before its significance can be interpreted. There is nothing etiologically distinctive about the terminal manifestations of chronic kidney disease, and it is most important to rule out treatable diseases that may simulate the uremic laboratory or clinical picture. Anuria (urine output < 100 ml/24 hours) always suggests urinary obstruction.

Terminal azotemia, sometimes to uremic levels, occurs in the last hours or days of a significant number of seriously ill patients with a variety of diseases, including cancer. Often no clinical or pathologic cause is found, even microscopically. Urine specific gravity may be relatively good.

Serum Creatinine

Serum creatinine is derived from muscle metabolism, as described earlier. Serum creatinine levels are dependent on body muscle mass; the greater the muscle mass, the higher the creatinine value, both in serum and urine. Creatinine values increase after meals, with the greatest increases (20%–50%) after meat ingestion. There is said to be a diurnal variation, with the lowest values about 7 A.M. and the peak about 7 P.M.; the late-afternoon values are reported to be about 20%–40% higher than in the morning. Some of the variation may be related to meals. Reference values for females are about 90% of those for males.

Normally, the BUN/serum creatinine ratio is approximately 10:1. Under standard conditions a 50% decrease in the GFR produces an approximate doubling of the BUN level or serum creatinine level, and the reverse occurs when the GFR is increased. However, these relationships can be altered by many factors, including those that increase or decrease either BUN or serum creatinine level without affecting the other. The serum creatinine level has much the same significance as the BUN level but tends to rise later. Significant creatinine elevations thus suggest chronicity without being diagnostic of it.

Laboratory Methodology.—Creatinine is most often assayed by a chemical method (Jaffe reaction) that includes about 20% noncreatinine substances. It has been reported that ketone bodies and certain cephalosporin antibiotics (cephalothin and cefoxitin) may give false elevation of creatinine assays in serum or urine using the Jaffe reaction. Several enzymatic methods for creatinine assay are now available that are specific for creatinine and produce creatinine values that are lower and creatinine clearance results that are higher than those derived from the Jaffe reaction.

Summary of Glomerular Function Studies

Clearance as a measurement of overall renal function impairment yields roughly the same information as that obtained from the phenolsulfonphthalein (PSP) test and has mostly replaced it in practice. Clearance tests are reliable in detecting mild to moderate diffuse renal disease, but they depend on completely collected specimens and accurate recording of the time the specimens were collected and presuppose adequate renal blood flow. If a patient is incontinent of urine, one must use either a short period of collection or a catheter or else some other test. Of course, if a Foley catheter is already in place, there is no problem. A clearance value between 60% and 80% of normal is usually taken to represent mild diffuse renal function impairment. Values between 40% and 60% of normal represent moderate decrease, and values between 20% and 40% of normal are considered severe renal function impairment, since about one half of the patients in this group also have an elevated BUN level. Most (but not all) of the causes of an increased BUN level also result in a considerable decrease in creatinine clearance. When the serum creatinine level is elevated in addition to the BUN level, a creatinine clearance rate less than 40 ml/minute (and usually < 25 ml/minute) can be predicted with reasonable assurance (Fig 13–1). Therefore, as long as the BUN level is significantly elevated (except in unusual cases when BUN elevation is due to increased protein load), and especially if azotemia is accompanied by an elevated serum creatinine level, clearance tests usually do not provide additional information.

The question sometimes arises whether both the BUN and the serum creatinine should be assayed to screen for decreased renal function. In 130 consecutive patients in our hospital whose admission BUN or creatinine were elevated, 47% had elevated levels of both, 38% had elevated BUN levels only, and 15% had an elevated creatinine level only.

In the classic case of chronic diffuse bilateral renal disease, the first demonstrable test abnormality is a decrease in urine-concentrating ability in the concentration test. As the disease progresses, the creatinine clearance becomes reduced. Then the specific gravity becomes fixed, and there is a considerable decrease in creatinine clearance. Finally, clearance becomes markedly decreased, and the BUN level starts to rise, followed shortly by the serum creatinine level.

The question sometimes is raised as to the degree of BUN increase that is possible in short periods of time. In one study, daily increase after onset of acute renal failure ranged from 10 to 50 mg/100 ml (3.5 to 18 mmol/L) during the first week, with the average daily increase being 25 mg/100 ml (9 mmol/L). After the first week, the amount of increase tended to be less.

TESTS OF PREDOMINANTLY TUBULAR FUNCTION

Several tests will be discussed within the

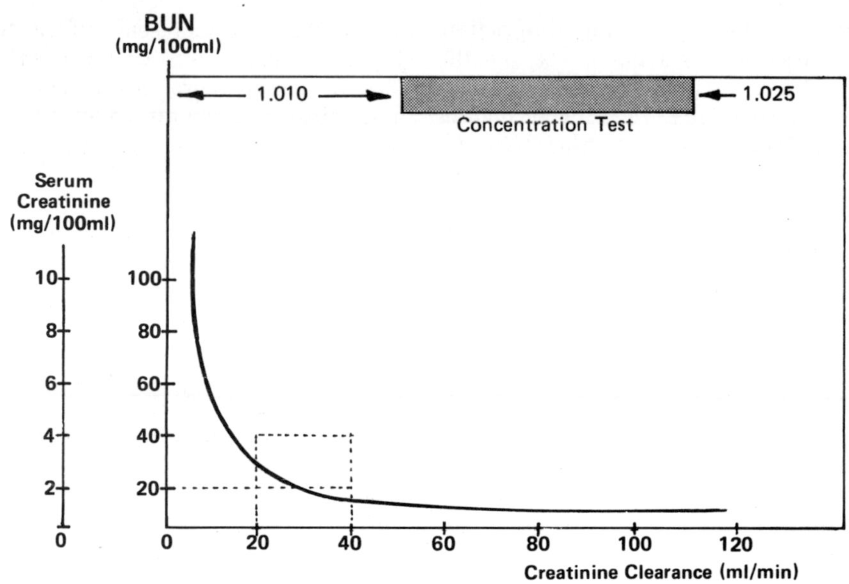

FIG 13–1.
Correlation of renal function test results. *Dotted box* represents clearance values found when blood urea nitrogen *(BUN)* or serum creatinine level begins to rise.

broad category of concentration and dilution. These include specific gravity, osmolality, urine excretion of electrolytes, and the free water clearance test.

Phenolsulfonphthalein Excretion

Phenolsulfonphthalein is excreted mainly by the renal tubules (chapter 35). In general, results give about the same clinical information as the creatinine clearance rate since glomerular and tubular dysfunction usually occur together in acute and chronic kidney damage. Creatinine clearance tests seem to have mostly replaced PSP tests in the relatively few situations in which this type of information is needed.

Specific Gravity

Specific gravity (defined and described in chapter 12) is important in the evaluation of chronic diffuse parenchymal disease (chronic glomerulonephritis, chronic pyelonephritis, etc.). As such conditions progress, tubular ability to concentrate urine is often affected relatively early and slowly decreases until the urine has the same specific gravity as the plasma ultrafiltrate—1.010. This usually, but not always, occurs in advance of final renal decompensation. For concentration tests to be accurate, the patient must be deprived of water over a long time period to exclude influence from previous ingestion. The usual test should run 16–17 hours. If forced fluids were given previously, a longer time may be necessary. This may be impossible in patients with cardiac disease, those with renal failure, aged persons, or those with electrolyte problems. Under these test conditions, the average person should have a urine specific gravity over 1.025, at least as high as 1.020. Concentration tests are also impaired in patients with diabetes insipidus, the diuretic phase of acute tubular necrosis, and occasionally in hyperthyroidism, severe salt-restricted diets, and sickle cell anemia. These conditions may result in failure to concentrate without the presence of irreversible renal tubular damage. Ten grams of protein per liter raises specific gravity by 0.003; 1% glucose raises specific gravity by 0.004. In addition, the radiopaque contrast media used for IV pyelograms (IVPs) considerably increase urine specific gravity; this effect may persist for 1–2 days. Proven ability to concentrate urine does not rule out many types of active kidney disease, nor does absence of ability to concentrate necessarily mean closely approaching renal failure. Adequate ability to concentrate is, however, decidedly against the diagnosis of chronic severe diffuse renal disease. A relatively early manifestation of chronic diffuse bilateral renal disease is impairment of concentrating ability (on a concentration test), which becomes manifest before changes in other function tests appear. (This refers to beginning impairment, not to fixation of specific gravity.)

Clinically, fixation of specific gravity is usually manifested by nocturia and a diminution of the day/night urine excretion ratio (normally 3:1 or 4:1) toward 1:1. Other causes must be considered: diabetes mellitus and insipidus, hyperparathyroidism, renal acidosis syndrome, early congestive heart failure, and occasionally hyperthyroidism. True nocturia or polyuria must be distinguished from urgency, incontinence, or enuresis.

One improvement on the standard concentration procedure is to substitute for water deprivation a single injection of vasopressin tannate (Pitressin Tannate in Oil). Five units of this long-acting preparation is given intramuscularly in the late afternoon, and urine collections for specific gravity are made in the early morning and two times thereafter at 3-hour intervals. One danger of this procedure is the possibility of water intoxication in certain patients, such as infants on a liquid diet.

Urine at refrigerator temperature may have a falsely decreased specific gravity. Urinometers of the floating bulb type exhibit a specific gravity change of 0.001 for each 3°C above or below the calibration temperature indicated for the instrument. A refractometer also may be affected outside the temperature range of 16°C–38°C.

Osmolality

Another way to obtain information about renal concentrating capability is to measure urine osmolality (sometimes incorrectly called osmolarity) instead of conventional specific gravity. Osmolality is a measure of the osmotic strength or number of osmotically active ions or particles present per unit of solution. Specific gravity is defined as the weight or density per unit volume of solution compared to water. Since the number of molecules present in a solution is a major determinant of its weight, it is obvious that there is a relationship between osmolality and specific gravity. Since the degree of ionic dissociation is very important in osmolality but not in specific gravity, values of the two for the same solution may not always correspond closely. The rationale for using urine osmolality is that specific gravity is a rather empirical observation and does not measure the actual ability of the kidney to concentrate electrolytes or other molecules relative to the plasma concentration; also, certain substances are of relatively large molecular weight and tend to disproportionately affect specific gravity. The quantity of water present may vary, even in concentration tests, and influence results.

Osmolality is defined in terms of milliosmoles (mOsm) per kilogram of solution and can be easily and accurately measured by determining the freezing point depression of a sample in a specially designed machine. (In biologic fluids, such as serum or urine, water makes up nearly all of the specimen weight; since water weighs 1 gm/ml, osmolality may be approximated clinically by values reported in terms of milliosmoles per liter rather than per kilogram.) Normal values for urine osmolality after 14-hour test dehydration are 800–1,300 mOsm/L. Most osmometers are accurate to less than 5 mOsm, so the answer thus has an aura of scientific exactness that is lacking in the relatively crude specific gravity method. Unfortunately, having a rather precise number and being able to use it clinically may be two different things. Without reference to the clinical situation, osmolality has as little meaning as specific gravity. In most situations, urine osmolality and specific gravity have approximately the same significance. Both vary and depend on the amount of water excreted with the urinary solids. In some cases, however, such as when the specific gravity is fixed at 1.010, urine osmolality after dehydration may still be greater than serum osmolality, which suggests that it is a more sensitive measurement. Also, urine osmolality does not need correction for glucosuria, proteinuria, or urine temperature. For example, 200 mg/100 ml of glucose increases urine osmolality about 11 mOsm/L. This magnitude of change would be insignificant in urine, since urine osmolality can vary in normal persons between 50 and 1,200 mOsm/L (depending on degree of hydration). However, adding the same 200 mg of glucose to blood could significantly increase serum osmolality, which normally varies between only 275 and 300 mOsm/L (chapter 24).

Intravenous Pyelogram (IVP)

Intravenous pyelogram is a radiologic

technique to outline the upper and lower urinary tract that uses iodinated contrast media, most of which are tubular secreted. To be seen radiographically, once secreted the contrast media must also be concentrated. Thus, incidental to delineating calyceal and urinary tract outlines and revealing postrenal obstruction, the IVP also affords some information about kidney concentrating ability or ability to excrete the dye—two tubular functions. Renal function is usually not sufficient for visualization when the BUN level is more than 50 mg/100 ml (18 mmol/L) using ordinary (standard) IVP technique. Drip-infusion IVP methods can be used with higher BUN levels, but they are not routine and usually must be specifically requested. Radioisotope techniques using the scintillation camera are frequently able to demonstrate the kidneys when IVP fails.

Electrolyte Excretion

Urine excretion of electrolytes may be utilized as a renal function test. Normally, the kidney is very efficient in reabsorbing urinary sodium that is filtered at the glomerulus. In severe diffuse bilateral renal damage (acute or chronic), renal ability to reabsorb sodium is impaired, and renal excretion of sodium becomes fixed between 30 and 90 mEq/L (mmol/L), whereas renal excretion of chloride is fixed between 30 and 100 mEq/L. A urine sodium or chloride concentration more than 15 mEq/L above or below these limits is evidence against acute tubular necrosis or renal failure because it suggests that some kidney tubule reabsorption or excretion ability is still present. There is considerable overlap between prerenal azotemia and acute tubular necrosis patients in the urine sodium region between 15 and 40 mEq/L. The urine sodium excretion must be less than 15 mEq/L to be reasonably diagnostic of prerenal azotemia. Values between 40 and 105 mEq/L are more difficult to interpret, since they may occur normally as well as in renal failure, depending on body sodium balance. If hyponatremia is present, evaluation is much easier. Hyponatremia prompts the kidney to reabsorb more sodium ions, normally dropping the urine sodium level to less than 15 mEq/L. In the presence of hyponatremia, urine sodium in the 40–90 mEq/L range strongly suggests renal failure. One major difficulty is the frequent use of diuretics in patients with possible renal problems, since diuretics change normal renal electrolyte patterns and may increase urine sodium excretion over what one would expect in hyponatremia. Urine sodium excretion, although it can be helpful, is no longer considered the most useful or reliable test to differentiate prerenal azotemia from renal failure.

Free Water Clearance

The free water clearance test is based on that part of renal tubule function that involves reabsorption of fluid and electrolytes with the formation of free water. This activity is one of the last kidney functions to be lost. When water reabsorption can no longer take place normally, free water excretion increases. The free water clearance test can be used to demonstrate renal concentrating ability by calculating the clearance of osmotically active particles (influenced by urine electrolyte and free water content) and relating it to the rate of urine flow to derive the fraction of excreted free water.

The reference range for the free water clearance test is −20 to −100. In either acute tubular necrosis or chronic renal failure the values are usually near zero or are positive (+). However, certain other conditions may produce similar values, including excretion of excess water in a person with a low serum osmolality and diuresis in patients with a normal serum osmolality induced by various factors such as diuretics. However, usually a positive free water clearance value will not persist longer than 24 hours in these conditions but will persist in patients with severe kidney damage. I have personally found the free water clearance to be the most helpful of the renal function tests in differentiating prerenal azotemia from renal failure. The major drawbacks are necessity for exactly timed urine collections and interference by diuretics.

Fraction of Excreted Sodium (FE_{Na}) or Filtered Fraction of Sodium

Several reports indicate that patients with prerenal azotemia tend to reabsorb more urine sodium after glomerular filtration than patients with severe intrinsic renal damage such as acute tubular necrosis or chronic renal failure. The formula used is:

$$FE_{Na} = \frac{\text{Urine Na} \times \text{serum creatinine}}{\text{Serum Na} \times \text{urine creatinine}} \times 100$$

The normal or prerenal azotemia level is said to be less than 2.0. Diuretics may inhibit sodium reabsorption and produce a falsely elevated value. Although there are several favorable reports about this test in the literature, in my limited personal experience I have not found this test to be as sensitive as the free water clearance.

Other Tests

A variety of research techniques not generally available can measure one or another of the many kidney functions, such as tubular secretion of various substances, glomerular filtration of nonreabsorbed materials (e.g., inulin), and renal blood flow by clearance of substances (e.g., p-aminohippuric acid) that are both filtered and secreted.

AZOTEMIA (ELEVATED BLOOD UREA NITROGEN LEVEL) AND RENAL FAILURE

Many use the term "uremia" as a synonym for azotemia, although uremia is a syndrome and should be defined in clinical terms. A BUN level of approximately 100 mg/100 ml is usually considered to separate the general category of acute reversible prerenal azotemias from the more prolonged acute episodes and chronic uremias. In general, this is an accurate distinction, but there is a small but important minority of cases that do not follow this rule. Thus, some uremics seem to stabilize at a lower BUN level until their terminal episode, whereas a few persons with acute transient azotemia may have a BUN level close to 100 mg/100 ml (36 mmol/L) and, rarely, more than 125 mg/100 ml (45 mmol/L), which rapidly falls to normal levels after treatment of the primary systemic condition. It must be admitted that easily correctable prerenal azotemia with an appreciably elevated BUN level is almost always superimposed on previous subclinical renal damage or function loss. Although the previous damage may not have been severe enough to cause symptoms, the functional reserve of these kidneys has been eliminated by aging changes, pyelonephritis, or similar conditions. The same is usually true for azotemia of mild levels (30–50 mg/100 ml [11–18 mmol/L]) occurring with dehydration, high protein intake, cardiac failure, and other important but not life-threatening situations. After the BUN level has returned to normal levels, a creatinine clearance determination will allow adequate evaluation of the patient's renal status.

The onset of oliguria always raises the question of possible renal failure. For a long time oliguria was considered a constant clinical sign of acute renal failure (also called acute tubular necrosis); however, it is now recognized that 30%–50% of patients with acute renal failure do not have oliguria (literature range, 20%–88%). Normal adult urine volume is 500–1,600 ml/24 hours (upper limit depends on fluid intake); a volume less than 400 ml/24 hours is considered to represent oliguria if all urine produced has actually been collected. Incomplete collection or leakage around a catheter may give a false impression of oliguria. Occasionally a patient develops oliguria and progressive azotemia, and it becomes necessary to differentiate between prerenal azotemia, which is correctable by improving that patient's circulation, and acute renal tubular necrosis. This problem most frequently occurs after a hypotensive episode or after surgery.

The differential diagnosis of azotemia includes prerenal azotemia, acute renal failure (acute tubular necrosis), and chronic renal failure. Two tests, filtered fraction of sodium and the free water clearance, under certain conditions, are usually capable of differentiating prerenal azotemia from renal failure. In general, if the serum creatinine level as well as the BUN level is elevated, this is more suggestive of renal failure than prerenal azotemia. However, this assumes that the BUN elevation is discovered very early after onset. Under most conditions the differentiation between prerenal azotemia and acute tubular necrosis by means of the serum creatinine level is not sufficiently reliable. A number of other tests have been proposed for the same purpose (chapter 35). These tests have been found useful by some investigators but not useful in a sufficient number of cases by others. Part of the difference of opinion is based on the test criteria each investigator uses to differentiate prerenal azotemia from acute tubular necrosis. In general, when the test criteria are structured simply to provide best statistical separation for all cases of prerenal azotemia and acute tubular necrosis, there is considerable overlap between the two groups. When the criteria are deliberately structured to separate out either the cases of prerenal azotemia or those of acute tubular necrosis and the diagnosis is made only on the remaining cases, the test becomes insufficiently sensitive. A good example is the test using urine excretion of sodium. If one uses the urine sodium cutoff point of less than 15 mEq/L (mmol/L), the test has excellent reliability in ruling out acute tubular necrosis. However, one investigator found that 67% of patients with acute tubular necrosis and 63% of patients with prerenal azotemia had urine sodium values between 15 and 40 mEq/L (mmol/L). Therefore, if one wishes to use less than 15 mEq/L (mmol/L) as a diagnostic limit to avoid the overlap, one excludes 63% of this investigator's prerenal azotemia cases, and the test becomes poorly sensitive for prerenal azotemia, despite excellent specificity created by ruling out nearly all cases of acute tubular necrosis.

Part of the problem is the fact that acute tubular necrosis may be oliguric or nonoliguric. Some test criteria that enable good separation of prerenal azotemia and oliguric acute tubular necrosis are not as good in distinguishing prerenal azotemia from nonoliguric acute tubular necrosis. If the test cutoff points are restructured to include both oliguric and nonoliguric acute tubular necrosis, the overall accuracy of the test may suffer.

In occasional cases, initial tests indicate that some renal function still remains, but the patient then develops acute tubular necrosis due to progression of the underlying disease or superimposition of some other factor.

Urinalysis may provide useful information in patients with acute tubular necrosis. Red blood cell (RBC) or hemoglobin casts suggest glomerulonephritis, subacute bacterial endocarditis, transfusion reaction, and collagen disease. Uric acid crystals may provide a clue to uric acid nephropathy. Strongly positive urine chemical tests for hemoglobin without significant microscopic RBC raises the possibility of myoglobin.

Differentiation of acute tubular necrosis and chronic renal failure is extremely difficult without clinical evidence of acute onset. If the patient does not have an elevated serum creatinine level when first investigated, or if the creatinine level is only mildly elevated and there is no anemia or other evidence of uremia, the evidence is more in favor of acute tubular necrosis than chronic renal failure. Even more difficulty exists when a patient develops acute tubular necrosis and the question is raised as to whether the patient's renal function is likely to recover. Radioisotope studies with a scintillation camera may be helpful. Bilateral poor uptake, poor cortex-pelvis transit, and decreased blood flow suggest chronic diffuse renal disease. Good cortex uptake, poor cortex-pelvis transit, and good blood flow are more indicative of acute tubular necrosis or prerenal azotemia. Isotope techniques can demonstrate postrenal obstruction and frequently can visualize the kidneys when the IVP cannot.

In a patient with uremia (chronic azotemia), there is no good way to determine prognosis by laboratory tests. The degree of azotemia does not correlate well with the clinical course in uremia except in a very general way.

Other Diagnostic Tests

Addis Count.—This procedure is used in suspected subclinical cases of chronic glomerulonephritis to demonstrate 12-hour abnormally increased rates of RBCs and cast excretion too small to exceed the normal range in ordinary random specimen microscopic examinations. If the random urine specimen already shows hematuria or pyuria, and if contamination can be ruled out by catheter or clean catch collection technique, the Addis count cannot do anything more than show the same abnormality. Addis counts are very rarely necessary with a good history and adequate workup.

Renal Biopsy.—This procedure is now widely used. It may be the only way to find which disease is present, but it should be reserved for patients whose treatment depends on exact diagnosis. The general category of most renal disease entities can be inferred using routine methods. Because of the random sample nature of renal biopsies, ordinary light microscopy more often than not shows only nonspecific changes reflecting the result rather than the etiology of the disease process, and frequently renal biopsies are requested only for academic rather than for practical diagnostic or therapeutic reasons. In children, electron microscopy and immunofluorescent techniques are more useful than light microscopy

THE PROBLEM OF PROTEINURIA

As discussed in chapter 12, proteinuria is not itself a renal function test but almost invariably accompanies serious renal damage. Its severity does not necessarily correlate with the amount of damaged renal parenchyma or the status of any one renal function or group of systems. Its presence and degree may, in association with other findings, aid in the diagnosis of certain syndromes or disease entities whose renal pathologic findings are known. Proteinuria may be secondary to benign or extrarenal etiologies or even to contamination of the specimen.

One question that continually arises is the significance of small degrees of proteinuria. The urine protein reference range lower limit is usually stated in textbooks to be 10 mg/100 ml (0.1 g/L). Generally speaking, values of up to 30 mg/100 ml are within normal range; 30–40 mg/100 ml may or may not be significantly abnormal. It should be noted that reference values in terms of total urinary protein output per 24 hours may be up to 100 mg/24 hours. Values stated in terms of milligrams per 24 hours may not coincide with values expressed in terms of milligrams per 100 ml due to varying quantities of diluent water. One exception to conventional reference values is diabetes mellitus, in which lesser degrees of albuminuria may reflect early renal damage and may suggest need for revised therapy (chapter 12). It must be stressed that duration of proteinuria is even more important than quantity, especially at low values. As an example, 60 mg/100 ml (0.6 g/L) or even more on an admission urine test may have minor or little importance if it subsequently disappears, whereas 40 mg/100 ml (0.4 g/L) may be significant if this level persists. This becomes clear by examining the list of possible causes of proteinuria (chapter 12). Intrinsic renal disease is usually associated with persistent proteinuria, whereas the proteinuria seen with many of the extrarenal types quickly disappears if the primary disease is successfully treated. However, this does not always hold true, and one must remember that a single disease may cause permanent damage to more than one organ. For example, arteriosclerosis or hypertension may reduce or destroy functioning kidney tissue by means of arteriolar nephrosclerosis, although cardiac symptoms due to heart damage may overshadow the renal picture.

A common situation is the patient who has asymptomatic proteinuria alone or in association with a disease in which it is not expected. The first step is to repeat the test after 2 or 3 days (in clinically healthy persons) or when the presenting disease is under control (in hospitalized patients) using an early morning specimen to avoid orthostatic proteinuria. This is important because orthostatic proteinuria is common; several reports indicate that it is the etiology in about 20% (range, 15%–70%) of healthy young men with proteinuria on routine urinalysis. If proteinuria persists and orthostatic proteinuria is ruled out, the microscopy report should be analyzed for any diagnostic hints. Care should be taken to prevent contamination of the urine specimen, especially in female patients. The presence and degree of hematuria or pyuria suggest a certain number of diseases. If either is present, there should be a careful search for RBC or WBC casts. A careful history may elicit information of previous proteinuria or hematuria, suggesting chronic glomerulonephritis, or previous kidney infection or calculi, which favors chronic pyelonephritis. Uremia due to chronic bilateral renal disease often has an associated hypertension. (Of course, hypertension may itself be the primary disease and cause extensive secondary renal damage.) In addition, a low-grade or moderate anemia, either normochromic or slightly hypochromic and without evidence of reticulocytosis or blood loss, is often found with severe chronic diffuse renal disease. The next step is to note any random specific gravities obtained. If one measurement is normal (i.e., > 1.020), renal function is probably adequate. If all are lower, one can proceed to a concentration or creatinine clearance test, since low random specific gravities may simply mean high water excretion rather than lack of urine-concentrating ability. If the creatinine clearance rate is mildly or moderately reduced, the patient most likely has only mild or possibly moderate functional loss. If the creatinine clearance rate is markedly abnormal and the BUN level is normal with no hypertension or anemia present, the patient most likely has severe diffuse bilateral renal abnormality but not completely end-stage disease. When the BUN level is elevated but the serum creatinine level is still within reference range, some test or tests, such as the free water clearance, could be done to differentiate prerenal azotemia from early renal failure (acute or chronic). When both the BUN and serum creatinine levels are elevated and there is no anemia or hypertension, the differential diagnosis of prerenal azotemia or renal failure must still be made, but prerenal azotemia becomes less likely. When the BUN and serum creatinine levels are significantly elevated and there is anemia and other evidence of uremia, the prognosis is generally very bad, although some patients with definite uremia may live for years with proper therapy. There are exceptions to the situations just outlined but not too many.

THE PROBLEM OF HEMATURIA

Major etiologies of hematuria and details of available tests were discussed in chapter 12. The problem of hematuria is somewhat different from that of proteinuria. About 4% (range, 1.2%–9%) of asymptomatic men under age 40 have microhematuria of two or more RBCs per high-power field compared with about 15% (range, 13%–19%) of clinically healthy men over age 40 years. A major consideration is not to overlook genitourinary system cancer. Hematuria is the most frequent symptom of bladder and renal carcinoma, being reported in about 80% (range, 65%–85%) of bladder carcinoma and about 60%–70% (range, 32%–80%) of renal carcinoma. Gross hematuria comprises the majority of hematuria in both bladder and renal carcinoma. About 98% of bladder carcinoma and about 96% of renal carcinoma (not including Wilms' tumor of childhood) occurs after age 40. Renal carcinoma is reported in about 1% (range, 0%–2.0%) of patients with hematuria of any type under age 40 years and in about 1.5%–2.0% (range, 0.4%–3.5%) in patients over age 40 years. Bladder carcinoma is reported in about 3% (range, 0.2%–8.0% of patients with hematuria under age 40 years and in about 7%–10% (range, 0.1%–15%) of patients over age 40 years. In younger patients, several investigators have found IgA glomerulonephritis in 35%–40% of patients with gross or considerable microscopic hematuria in whom renal biopsy was performed. Over age 40, gross hematuria is much more strongly associated with cancer (although less frequently, neoplasia may present with microscopic hematuria and sometimes may be discovered with a completely normal urinalysis). Therefore, in persons under age 40 years (and especially between age 10 and 30 years) with gross hematuria, the majority of investigators do not expect cancer and do not favor extensive workup unless hematuria persists or there are other symptoms that suggest cancer. However, this opinion is not unanimous. In persons over age 40 with gross hematuria, the standard response would be, as a minimum, an IVP and cystoscopy (if the IVP results were negative). In persons under age 40 years with microscopic hematuria, most investigators question the need for additional investigation unless other symptoms suggest cancer or hematuria persists. In patients over age 40 years with asymptomatic microscopic hematuria only, especially if there are relatively few RBCs, opinion is divided whether to test further, and how much. Presence of other symptoms greatly increases pressure for further tests. Substantial numbers of RBCs (> 10 RBCs per high-power field) also seem to influence opinions, although most studies have shown rather poor correlation in microhematuria between presence of cancer and the number of RBCs in the urine sediment. Also, it must not be forgotten that the patient may have hematuria due to carcinoma of the kidney or bladder and at the same time have other diseases, such as hypertension, which themselves are known causes of hematuria. Finding RBC casts means that the RBCs are from the kidney and that the problem is a medical disease rather than cancer.

Red blood cells or hemoglobin (from lysed RBCs) in the urine may appear because of contamination during specimen collection. Female vaginal secretions may contain RBCs, WBCs, or both. A significant number of squamous epithelial cells in urine sediment (arbitrarily defined as more than 10 squamous cells per low-power field) suggests possible contamination, and the study should be repeated using a midstream voided specimen. It may be necessary to assist the patient with expert personnel.

Additional tests relevant to this chapter are described in chapter 35.

BIBLIOGRAPHY

Davidman M, Schmitz P: Renal tubular acidosis. *Hosp Pract* 1988; 23:77.

Schoolwerth AC: Hematuria and Proteinuria: Their causes and consequences. *Hosp Pract* 1987; 22:45.

Silverberg E: Statistical and epidemiologic data on urologic cancer. *Cancer* 1987; 60(suppl):692.
Copley JB, Hasbargen JA: "Idiopathic" hematuria. *Arch Intern Med* 1987; 147:434.
Mohr DN, et al: Asymptomatic microhematuria and urologic disease: A population-based study. *JAMA* 1986; 256:224.
Apple F, et al: Creatinine clearance: Enzymatic vs Jaffe determinations of creatinine in plasma and urine. *Clin Chem* 1986; 32:388.
Porush JG: New concepts in acute renal failure. *Am Fam Pract* 1986; 33:109.
Thal SM: Comparison of dysmorphic erythrocytes with other urinary sediment parameters of renal bleeding. *Am J Clin Pathol* 1986; 86:784.
Thompson C: Hematuria: A clinical approach. *Am Fam Pract* 1986; 33:194.
Froom P, et al: The effect of age on the prevalence of asymptomatic microscopic hematuria. *Am J Clin Pathol* 1986; 86:656.
Levinsky NG: Acute kidney failure: Prerenal, renal, or postrenal? *Hosp Pract* 1985; 20:68G.
Stewart DW, et al: Evaluation of proteinuria. *Am Fam Pract* 1984; 29:218.
Hou SH, et al: Hospital-acquired renal insufficiency: A prospective study. *Am J Med* 1983; 74:243.
Abuelo JG: Proteinuria: Diagnostic principles and procedures. *Ann Intern Med* 1983; 98:186.
Jamison RL, Oliver RE: Disorders of urinary concentration and dilution. *Am J Med* 1982; 72:308.
Bauer JH, et al: Clinical appraisal of creatinine clearance as a measurement of glomerular filtration rate. *Am J Kidney Dis* 1982; 2:337.
Diamond JR, Yoburn DC: Nonoliguric renal failure. *Arch Intern Med* 1982; 142:1882.
Waltzer WC: Acute renal failure. *Am Fam Phys* 1982; 26:173.
Schrier RW: Acute renal failure. *JAMA* 1982; 247:2518.
Grylack L, et al: Nonoliguric renal failure in the newborn. *Am J Dis Child* 1982; 136:518.
Ellis EN, Arnold WC: Use of urinary indexes in renal failure in the newborn. *Am J Dis Child* 1982; 136:615.
Sawyer WT: A multicenter evaluation of variables affecting the predictability of creatinine clearance. *Am J Clin Pathol* 1982; 78:832.
Cogan MG: Disorders of proximal nephron function. *Am J Med* 1982; 72:275.
Sebastian A: Disorders of distal nephron function. *Am J Med* 1982; 72:289.
Swartz S: Solving antidiuretic hormone puzzles. *Patient Care* 1982; 16:114.
Sherman RA, Byun KJ: Nuclear medicine in acute and chronic renal failure. *Semin Nucl Med* 1982; 12:265.
Oken DE: On the differential diagnosis of acute renal failure. *Am J Med* 1981; 71:916.
Brown R, et al: Renal function in critically ill postoperative patients: Sequential assessment of creatinine, osmolar, and free water clearance. *Crit Care Med* 1980; 8:68.

14 Bacterial Infectious Diseases (Including *Chlamydia* and *Mycoplasma* Infections)

Proper therapy for infectious disease requires knowledge of the etiologic agent. This knowledge can be gained in two ways: directly, either by isolating and identifying the organism in culture or by some method (e.g., fluorescent antibody or nucleic acid probe) that permits specific visual detection of the organism in clinical material; or indirectly, by using serologic tests that demonstrate antibodies in the patient's blood against an organism. Certain problems arise in the interpretation of direct methods or serologic test results. If results of the direct method are positive, one must determine whether the organism reported has clinical significance. It may be a fortuitous contaminant, an ordinarily nonpathogenic species that has become infectious under the prevailing circumstances, or a recognized pathogen that is a normal inhabitant of the area and whose presence may be entirely harmless (see Table 36–11). If results of the direct method are negative, one must consider the possibility of having missed the diagnosis because the laboratory was not given a proper specimen, because the specimen was obtained at an unfavorable moment during the disease, or because of laboratory technical problems (and, if culture is involved, because special culture techniques or media might have been needed). Serologic tests that detect antibodies also have drawbacks in bacterial diseases, since it takes 7–10 days after infection (sometimes longer) to develop detectable antibodies, and it is often necessary to demonstrate either a very high titer or a fourfold rising titer of antibodies to differentiate recent from old infection. Therefore, to evaluate laboratory data, the clinical situation has at least as much importance as laboratory methodology. It seems desirable to provide a brief survey of the major infectious agents, the diseases and circumstances in which they are most often found, and the conditions under which the appearance of these organisms may be confusing. There is an element of classification because of the way laboratory reports are usually worded. Techniques of diagnosis in the area of infectious disease are discussed in this chapter in relation to specific organisms, specific clinical situations, or general laboratory methods.

DIRECT METHODS OF BACTERIAL DETECTION

Culture.—This is the classic definitive method for detection and identification and will be discussed later in more detail. The major drawback is time; it usually takes 1 full day to grow the organism and then part or all of 1 day to identify it. It may take an additional day to isolate it prior to identification if there is a mixture of organisms. Some organisms take longer than 1 day to grow. There is always a certain percentage of false negative results (sometimes a large percentage) due to various factors, both clinical and technical. Three major difficulties are suppressive effects of antibiotic therapy on bacterial growth (even though clinical cure is not achieved), inadequate or inappropriate specimens obtained or faulty specimen transport to the laboratory, and differences in the way any individual laboratory processes the specimen compared to a research laboratory.

Immunologic Methods.—Immunologic methods depend on antibody attachment to organisms of a specific bacterial species or to a cell component of the species (see Table 36–7,A). There is some type of readout system (e.g., latex agglutination, fluorescent dye, or chemical reaction color change) to show that antibody-antigen combination has occurred. These methods produce same-day results; the latex agglutination tests usually take less than 1 hour. Some of the immunologic methods are capable of accuracy that is equivalent to culture (e.g., fluorescent antibody method for *Corynebacterium diphtheriae*); others are less reliable, depending on the technique and the particular kit manufacturer. All antibodies do not behave the same, even under the same conditions.

Nucleic Acid Probe (DNA Probe).—Greatly simplified, this technique attempts to construct a nucleic acid sequence (the "probe") that matches a sequence in the DNA or RNA of the organism to be detected. This sequence or probe is incorporated (or grafted) into a larger nucleic acid molecule, usually a single strand of DNA (although a strand of RNA could be used) that can be tagged with an indicator system (radioisotope or biochemical reaction). Then the specimen to be tested is prepared for analysis. If the target molecule is DNA, since DNA usually exists as a double-stranded molecule, the target molecule DNA double strands are first separated into single strands by various means, and then the test DNA single strands containing the probe sequence are introduced. If the probe sequence matches a sequence in the target, the probe hybridizes with the target DNA (combines with the target single strand) to again form a double strand. If the target molecule is RNA, RNA exists in living cells in single-strand state, so that the DNA single-strand test molecule containing the RNA probe area can hybridize directly with an RNA single strand (instead of another DNA single strand) if the probe area matches a nucleic acid sequence in the target RNA strand. After incubation, nonhybridized (nonattached) test probe-carrying single strands are washed away and the indicator system is used to demonstrate whether any probe remains combined to target molecules. In some ways this technique is similar to direct immunologic detection methods. Advantages of nucleic acid probe systems are much greater sensitivity than current antibody systems, specificity that can be varied to the genus, species, or even strain level, theoretical possibility of use for any organism in any clinical specimen, and same-day results. The major disadvantage thus far is relatively high cost of the test when performed on a single specimen basis.

LABORATORY CLASSIFICATION OF BACTERIA

The most useful laboratory classification of bacteria involves a threefold distinction: the Gram stain characteristics (gram positive or gram negative), morphology (coccus or bacillus), and oxygen requirements for growth (aerobic or anaerobic). Species exist that are morphologic exceptions, such as spirochetes; others are intermediate in oxygen requirements; still others are identified by other techniques, such as the acid-fast stain. Reaction to Gram stain has long been correlated with bacterial sensitivity to certain classes of antibiotics. A classic example is the susceptibility of most gram-positive organisms to penicillin. Morphology, when used in conjunction with this primary reaction, greatly simplifies identification of large bacterial groups, and oxygen growth requirements narrow the possibilities still further. The interrelationship of these characteristics also helps to control laboratory error. For example, if cocci seem to be gram negative instead of gram positive, a laboratory recheck of the decolorization step in the Gram procedure is called for since nearly all cocci are gram positive. If the staining technique is verified, the possibility of a small bacillus (*Coccobacillus*) or a *Diplococcus* must be considered.

Gram-Positive Cocci

Streptococci

Streptococci are gram-positive cocci that, on Gram stain, typically occur in chains. Streptococci are subclassified in several ways. The three most useful classifications are by bacterial oxygen requirements, by colony appearance on blood agar, and by specific carbohydrate from the organism. Depending on clinical oxygen environment associated with disease, streptococci may be considered aerobic, microaerophilic, or anaerobic. Most streptococci are aerobic. The microaerophilic organisms sometimes cause a chronic resistant type of skin ulcer and occasionally are isolated in deep wound infections. The anaerobic streptococci are discussed later.

Streptococci are divided into three types by the appearance of the hemolysis that the streptococcal colonies produce on sheep blood agar—alpha, beta, and gamma. Alpha (hemolytic) streptococci are characterized by incomplete hemolysis surrounding the colony; this area usually has a greenish appearance on sheep blood agar, and streptococci producing green hemolysis are often called "viridans." The beta-hemolytic organisms produce a complete, clear (colorless) hemolysis. Gamma streptococci do not produce hemolysis on sheep blood agar. These differences have clinical value. Alpha streptococci of the viridans subgroup are one of the most frequent causes of subacute bacterial endocarditis. Beta streptococci are the causative agent of several different types of infection and syndromes, as will be discussed later, and account for the great majority of disease associated with streptococci with the exception of subacute bacterial endocarditis. Gamma streptococci are of lesser importance, but some of the organisms known as enterococci belong to this category.

The third classification is that of Lancefield, who discovered antibodies produced to a somatic carbohydrate of streptococcal organisms. Streptococci can be divided into groups according to the particular carbohydrate they possess on the basis of organism reaction to the different Lancefield antibodies (antisera). These groups are given a capital letter name ranging from A to G (in some classifications, even letters farther in the alphabet but excluding E). Lancefield grouping does not depend on the presence of hemolysis or the type of hemolysis; for example, streptococci of group A are all beta hemolytic but streptococci of group D can be either alpha or beta hemolytic or even gamma nonhemolytic. Lancefield grouping cannot be done on some streptococci that are not beta hemolytic with the exception of those from groups B and D. *Lancefield group A organisms*, as mentioned earlier, are always beta hemolytic, and colonies are definitively identified with group-specific antiserum. This requires culture of a specimen, isolation of several colonies of a beta hemolytic organism resembling *Streptococcus* by colony appearance or Gram stain, and testing a colony with the Lancefield antisera. However, Lancefield antisera are relatively expensive, and since group A organisms seem to have an unusually marked susceptibility to the antibiotic bacitracin, Lancefield grouping is very frequently replaced by a less expensive identification method based on demonstrating inhibition of growth around a disk impregnated with a standardized concentration of bacitracin in an agar culture containing a pure growth of the organism (the organism is first identified as a *Streptococcus* by Gram stain or biochemical tests). However, this method is only presumptive rather than definitive, since about 5% (range, 4%–10%) of hemolytic group A streptococci are not inhibited by bacitracin (these organisms would be incorrectly excluded from group A), whereas 8%–22% of beta hemolytic streptococci from groups other than A (e.g., B, C, D, and G) have been reported to be sensitive to bacitracin (and therefore would be incorrectly assigned to group A). Also, the bacitracin method takes 2 and sometimes even 3 days—1 day to culture the organism, 1 day to perform the disk susceptibility test, and sometimes another day to separate the organism colony from other bacterial colonies prior to the bacitracin test if the original culture grows several different organisms. Rapid immunologic identification tests from many manufacturers have now become commercially available for group A streptococci that directly test for the organisms in swab specimens without culture. Usually the organism is extracted from the swab chemically or enzymatically and then tested with antiserum against group A antigen. The rapid tests can be performed in about 10–15 minutes (range, 5–60 minutes, not counting setup time of perhaps 5–15 minutes). Compared to throat culture, average overall sensitivity of the new direct methods is about 87%–95% (range 61%–100%, including different results on the same manufacturer's kits by different investigators). Reported sensitivity is about 5%–10% higher if comparison culture specimens contain at least 10 organism colonies than if the culture density is less than 10 colonies. There is debate in the literature whether throat cultures with density of less than 10 colonies represent clinically significant infection. Some consider growth less than 10 colonies to represent a carrier state, but others disagree. Another point to remember is that rapid test sensitivity quoted in reports is not true clinical sensitivity, since rapid test sensitivity is usually less than culture sensitivity and culture sensitivity itself is rarely more than 95%. (It is probably less, since various changes in usual laboratory culture technical methodology for throat cultures have each been reported to increase culture sensitivity about 5%–10%, sometimes even more. In fact, one study on tonsillectomy patients found only 82% of preoperative throat cultures were positive when operative tonsillar tissue culture obtained group A streptococci.) Group A organisms may be further separated into subgroups (strains) by use of special antisera against surface antigens (M antigens). Strain typing is mostly useful in epidemiologic work, such as investigating outbreaks of acute glomerulonephritis, and is not helpful in most clinical situations. Group A streptococci produce certain enzymes, such as streptolysin-O, which can be detected by serologic tests (antistreptolysin-O titer, chapter 22). Antibodies against these enzymes do not appear until 7–10 days after onset of infection, so they are usually not helpful in diagnosing acute streptococcal infection. Their major usefulness is in the diagnosis of acute rheumatic fever and acute glomerulonephritis.

Lancefield group A streptococci are also known as *Streptococcus pyogenes*. Certain strains are associated with specific diseases, such as acute glomerulonephritis and acute rheumatic fever. Group A beta streptococci also produce various infections without any stain specificity. The most common is acute pharyngitis. Wound infections and localized skin cellulitis are relatively frequent. Other diseases that are much less common, although famous historically, include scarlet fever, erysipelas (vesicular cellulitis), and puerperal fever. There are even a few reports describing several patients with a condition resembling staphylococcal toxic shock syndrome.

Group A beta-hemolytic streptococci may be isolated from throat or nasopharyngeal cultures in 15%–20% (range, 11%–60%) of clinically normal children. Nevertheless, for clinical purposes they are not considered normal inhabitants of the throat or nasopharynx since the usual present-day culture or serologic methods, which are done in the acute stage of infection, cannot reliably differentiate between carrier state and true pathogen, and prompt therapy for group A streptococcal nasopharyngeal infection is thought to decrease the possibility of acute rheumatic fever or acute glomerulonephritis. The accuracy of group A streptococcal isolation from throat cultures can be enhanced in several ways. Anaerobic rather than aerobic incubation has been reported to increase sensitivity about 15% (range, 0%–35%). Obtaining specimens on two swabs instead of one is reported to increase yield approximately 10%. Use of special differential media (with certain antibiotics added) helps to suppress growth of other organisms (e.g., hemolytic *Hemophilus* species) that may simulate beta hemolytic streptococcal colonies. However, not all of these enhancement techniques produce the same reported additive effect if they are combined. Although group A streptococci are almost always sensitive to penicillin on in vitro antibiotic sensitivity tests, 10%–30% of adequately treated patients continue to harbor the organisms and are considered carriers.

Lancefield group B streptococci (also known as *Streptococcus agalactiae*) are one of the most common causes of neonatal septicemia and meningitis. *Escherichia coli* is the most frequent etiology of neonatal meningitis, but it has been reported that about one third of cases are due to group B streptococci. Neonatal group B streptococcal infection may occur in two clinical forms: early onset (before age 7 days, usually within 48 hours of birth), and late onset (after age 7 days). Septic neonates may have respiratory distress that mimics the noninfectious respiratory distress syndrome. The source of *Streptococcus* infection is the maternal genital tract, with 10%–20% (literature range 4.6%–36%) of mothers being culture positive. Premature onset of labor or premature rupture of the amniotic membranes places the infant into the high-risk category. Group B streptococci also may infect adults (although this is not frequent), with postpartum endometritis, infection after urinary tract or gynecologic operations, pneumonia, and soft tissue infections being the most common types. Many affected adults have some underlying disease or predisposing cause. Group B streptococci also produce mastitis in cows.

Culture is the major diagnostic test for group B streptococci. Besides culture, rapid latex agglutination slide tests for group B streptococcal antigen in body fluids are now available from several manufacturers. Although not many studies are published, reports indicate that these tests when performed on concentrated urine specimens detect 90%–100% of cases in culture-positive neonatal group B streptococcal bacteremia. Serum or unconcentrated urine are generally less successful.

Lancefield group C streptococci are primarily animal pathogens. However, these organisms may be found in the nasopharynx, vagina, and gastrointestinal (GI) tract of clinically normal persons and occasionally produce human disease, most commonly (but not limited to) pharyngitis and meningitis.

Lancefield group D streptococci contain several species, of which *Streptococcus faecalis* (one of the enterococci) and *Streptococcus bovis* (one of the nonenterococci) are the most important. Group D streptococci are responsible for approximately 20% (range, 8%–21%) of infectious endocarditis, typically that subgroup formerly called subacute bacterial endocarditis (SBE), and about 10% of urinary tract infections, as well as constituting the third most common cause of biliary tract infections. Group D streptococci are also associated with mixed wound infections, intra-abdominal infections and a wide variety of other conditions, although there is some controversy about their relative pathogenicity in these circumstances. The majority of serious group D infections are due to enterococci. Enterococci are certain species of group D streptococci that are found normally in the human intestinal tract and that have certain special laboratory characteristics. These include resistance to heating and growth in certain media such as bile-esculin and 6.5% sodium chloride. Some species of enterococci produce alpha hemolysis, some produce beta hemolysis, and some are (gamma) nonhemolytic. Besides their role in infectious endocarditis (10%–12% of cases, range, 6%–20%), enterococci assume importance because they frequently are involved in other nosocomial (hospital-acquired) infections, particularly urinary tract infections (about 10%, range 6%–16%) and because they are usually resistant to penicillin. Bacteremia due to nonenterococcal *S. bovis* has been very frequently associated with either benign or malignant colon neoplasms (about two thirds of cases, range 17%–95%). Recently it has been proposed that the enterococci should be removed from the streptococci and placed into a new genus called *Enterococcus*. The new genus would include *Enterococcus faecalis*, *Enterococcus faecium*, *Enterococcus durans*, and several others. *Streptococcus* group D would include *S. bovis* and *Streptococcus equinus*.

Lancefield group F streptococci (*Streptococcus anginosus* or *Streptococcus milleri*) form tiny colonies. Infection is uncommon, but they have been reported to cause bacteremia, dental abscesses, and abscesses in other body tissues, usually superimposed on preexisting abnormality.

Lancefield group G streptococci are among the normal flora in the nasopharynx (up to 23% of persons), skin, vagina, and GI tract. The most common serious infection is bacteremia, being isolated in 3.5% of all patients with bacteremia in one study. Many of these patients had serious underlying disease, especially cancer (21%–65% of patients in this study with group G bacteremia). Other infections are uncommon, but pharyngitis and arthritis are among the more important. *Other Lancefield groups* have occasionally been reported to produce human infection.

Viridans Streptococci.—The viridans group has been defined in several ways. The most common definition is streptococci that lack Lancefield antigens and produce alpha hemolysis on sheep blood agar. However, other investigators state that some viridans organisms are nonhemolytic, and still others say that some species can react with various Lancefield group antisera, although not with group B or D. Viridans streptococci are the most common cause of infectious endocarditis (that subgroup formerly known as SBE), being isolated in approximately 35%–40% of cases (range 30%–52%). They may also cause urinary tract infection, pneumonia, and wound infection. They are normal inhabitants of the mouth and may have a role in producing dental caries.

Streptococcus pneumoniae.—This organism is clinically known as pneumococcus and occasionally is called *Diplococcus pneumoniae* in the literature. Although *S. pneumoniae* is a member of the *Streptococcus genus*, most nonmicrobiologists usually think of pneumococcus as a separate entity from the other streptococci. Pneumococci are gram-positive diplococci that can be found in the throat of 30%–70% of apparently normal persons. They are still the most common cause of bacterial pneumonia, usually comprising at least 50% (range, 26%–78%) of community-acquired cases. They also produce many cases of middle ear infection in children and are an important cause of meningitis in older children, adolescents, and adults, most commonly in debilitated persons. Pneumococcal bacteremia develops in about 20% (range, 15%–25%) of patients with pneumococcal pneumonia, and pneumococcus is found in about 18% of all bacteremias, with the incidence being even higher in children. Splenectomy (or sickle cell anemia hyposplenism) is one well-known predisposing cause. The great majority of pneumococcal strains are very sensitive to penicillin, although about 2%–8% (range, 0%–18%, depending on the geographical area) of isolates are now relatively resistant or resistant. Pneumococci usually produce alpha (green) incomplete hemolysis on blood agar and thus mimic viridans streptococci. Morphologic differentiation from streptococci may be difficult, especially in cultures, since streptococci may appear singly or in pairs (instead of chains), and pneumococci often do not have the typical lancet shape or grouping in pairs. In the laboratory, differentiation is readily made because of the special sensitivity of pneumococci to a compound known as optochin. A disk impregnated with optochin is placed on the culture plate; inhibition of an alpha hemolytic coccus denotes pneumococci.

Besides diagnosis by culture, rapid slide latex agglutination tests for pneumococcal antigen are now available (developed for testing of cerebrospinal fluid [CSF] in patients with meningitis). Unfortunately, in the few reports available, detection of antigen in serum or unconcentrated urine has been less than 40%. Sensitivity in concentrated urine may be considerably better, but too little data are available.

Staphylococci

Staphylococci are gram-positive cocci that typically occur in clusters. Originally they were divided into three groups, depending on colony characteristics on blood agar: *Staphylococcus albus* (*Staphylococcus epidermidis*), with white colonies; *Staphylococcus aureus*, with yellow colonies; and *Staphylococcus citreus*, with pale green colonies. In that classification, *S. aureus* was by far the most important; it was generally hemolytic, and the pathogenic species were coagulase positive. The newer classification recognizes that coagulase activity (the ability to coagulate plasma) is a better indication of pathogenicity than colony color, since a significant number of coagulase-positive organisms are not yellow on blood agar. Therefore, all coagulase-positive staphylococci are now called *S. aureus*. Many microbiology laboratories still issue reports such as "*S. aureus* coagulase positive"; it is not necessary to include the coagulase result because *S. aureus* by definition is coagulase positive. Detection of heat-stable anti-DNA ("thermonuclease"), another enzyme produced by *S. aureus*, is generally considered to be the best confirmatory test for *S. aureus* should this be necessary. This test is nearly as sensitive and specific as coagulase but is more expensive and time consuming.

At this point, a few words should be said regarding coagulase tests. *Staphylococcus aureus* produces two types of coagulase, known as *bound coagulase* ("clumping factor") and *free coagulase*. The standard procedure is known as the *tube coagulase test*, based on the ability of free coagulase to clot plasma. This test requires 4 hours' incubation and sometimes as long as 24 hours to confirm nonreactive results or weak positive reactions. Bound coagulase alone was originally used in a slide coagulase test that required only 1–2 minutes but produced about 20% false negative results. More recently, rapid 15- to 60-second slide tests based on reagents that react with either bound coagulase, protein A (another substance produced by *S. aureus*), or both have been introduced. Evaluations have shown sensitivities of about 98%–99% (range, 94%–100%) for these tests. However, false positive results have been reported in a few percent of most such tests, although the majority of evaluations of each test have not reported false positive results. Also, at least one investigator has reported at least 1% (and sometimes more) false negative results with each test when used with methacillin-resistant *S. aureus*. The family Micrococcaceae contains several genera, including *Staphylococcus* and *Micrococcus*. Both of these genera are composed of organisms that are identical on Gram stain and have certain biochemical similarities. As noted above, those that are coagulase positive are placed in the *Staphylococcus* genus and designated *S. aureus*. Gram-positive cocci that resemble *S. aureus* morphologically but that are coagulase negative have not yet been subjected to a uniform method of reporting. Some laboratories call all of them "*S. epidermidis*" or "*coagulase-negative staphylococci*." Others differentiate organisms from the genus *Staphylococcus* and the genus *Micrococcus* on the basis of certain biochemical tests such as the ability of staphylococci to produce acid from glucose anaerobically. In general, non-*aureus* staphylococci, although much less pathogenic than *S. aureus*, are more pathogenic than micrococci. Some of the larger laboratories differentiate species of non-*aureus* staphylococci using certain tests. The species most commonly associated with human disease are *S. epidermidis* and *Staphylococcus saprophyticus*.

Staphylococci, as well as the enteric gram-negative rod organisms and some of the *Clostridia* gram-positive anaerobes (to be discussed later), are normal inhabitants of certain body areas. The habitat of staphylococci is the skin. Therefore, a diagnosis of staphylococcal infection should not be made solely on the basis of *S. aureus* isolation from an external wound; there should be evidence that *S. aureus* is actually causing clinical disease. Besides the skin, about one half of all adults outside the hospital carry *S. aureus* in the nasopharynx; this reportedly increases to 70%–80% if cultures are performed repeatedly on the same population over a long period. More than 50% of hospitalized persons have positive nasopharyngeal cultures. Exactly what factors induce these commensal organisms to cause clinical disease is not completely understood.

***Staphylococcus aureus*.**—*Staphylococcus aureus* is typically associated with purulent inflammation and characteristically produces abscesses. The most common site of infection is the skin, most frequently confined to minor lesions, such as pustules or possibly small carbuncles, but occasionally producing widespread impetigo in children and infants. The most frequent type of serious staphylococcal disease (other than childhood impetigo) is wound infection or infection associated with hospital diagnostic or therapeutic procedures.

In a small but important number of cases, *S. aureus* produces certain specific infections. Staphylococcal pneumonia may occur, especially in debilitated persons, or following a viral pneumonia. Meningitis and septicemia are also occasionally found, again, more commonly in debilitated persons or those with decreased resistance—often without any apparent portal of entry. *Staphylococcus aureus* produces about 20%–25% (range, 9%–33%) of infectious endocarditis (especially that subgroup that used to be called acute rather than subacute). *Staphylococcus aureus* causes a type of food poisoning different from that of the usual infectious agent; symptoms result from ingestion of bacterial toxins rather than from actual enteric infection by living organisms.

Staphylococcus aureus frequently produces an enzyme known as beta-lactamase, which makes the organism resistant to certain antibiotics that contain a beta-lactam ring structure such as penicillin G and ampicillin. *Staphylococcus aureus* resistant to methacillin (MRSA) is a particularly difficult problem and will be discussed later in the section on antibiotic sensitivity testing. The nationwide incidence of MRSA (as a percentage of all *S. aureus* isolates) is about 4%; for individual hospitals, the range is 0%–60%. *Staphylococcus epidermidis* in many areas of the country is frequently resistant to a considerable number of antibiotics, including methacillin.

***Toxic Shock Syndrome*.**—The toxic shock syndrome is a disease strongly linked to *S. aureus* infection. The syndrome has been seen in various age groups in both sexes but occurs predominantly in females of childbearing age. There is an association with use of vaginal tampons, but a considerable number of cases have occurred when tampons were not used. Many (but not all) cases occur during the menstrual period. At least 15% of cases are not related to menses or tampon use but instead are preceded by surgical wound infection or by infections of other types. Clinical criteria for the syndrome include temperature of 102°F (38.9°C) or greater, erythematous sunburn-like or macular rash with eventual skin peeling or desquamation (especially on the palms and soles), hypotension or shock, clinical or laboratory involvement of at least four organ systems, and no definite evidence of bacteremia.

Involvement of organ systems is evidenced by a combination of symptoms and laboratory data. The classic syndrome includes at least four of the following organ systems (the approximate incidence of laboratory abnormality reported in one study is listed after each test):

1. Gastrointestinal: Vomiting and watery diarrhea.
2. Central nervous system: Headache, confusion, and disorientation. Stiff neck may occur. Cerebrospinal fluid tests are usually normal.
3. Liver: Aspartate aminotransferase (SGOT, 75%) or alanine aminotransferase (SGPT, 50%) more than twice the upper limit of the reference range. Total bilirubin may also be increased (70%).
4. Kidney: Blood urea nitrogen (BUN, 68%) or serum creatinine (90%) levels more than twice the upper limit of the reference range. There may be increased numbers of urinary white blood cells (WBCs) (73%) with negative urine cultures. Oliguria may occur.
5. Mucous membranes: Conjunctivitis.
6. Hematologic: Hemoglobin level is usually normal (77%). The WBC count may be normal (52%) or increased (48%). Neutrophil percentage is usually increased (86%), and frequently there are increased band forms. Dohle bodies are often present. Schistocytes are present in some patients (48%). The platelet count is less than 100,000/cu mm in 42%, the activated partial thromboplastin time is elevated in 46%, and fibrin split products are frequently elevated; but the fibrinogen level is normal in 86% and the prothrombin time is normal in 93%.
7. Muscular: Myalgias; creatine phosphokinase level is more than twice the upper limit of the reference range (63%).

It is not clear how many of the laboratory abnormalities are due to the disease itself or are secondary to hypotension with tissue hypoxia.

Staphylococcus aureus has been cultured from the cervix or vagina in approximately 75% of toxic shock patients (literature range 67%–92%) as opposed to approximately 7% (literature range 0%–15%) of normal persons. Some series include culture data from the nasopharynx in addition to the cervix-vaginal region. This is more difficult to interpret since about 20% of normal persons carry *S. aureus* in their nasopharynx. Blood cultures are usually sterile. Toxic shock *S. aureus* is said to be usually nonhemolytic phage type 1, able to produce toxic shock toxin-1 (TSST-1) exotoxin, sensitive to erythromycin but resistant to penicillin. Currently, there is no readily available test to differentiate toxic shock from other entities with similar clinical or laboratory manifestations. It is possible to culture the organism and send an isolate to some reference laboratory able to test for production of TSST-1, but this would take several days.

Staphylococcus epidermidis.—*Staphylococcus epidermidis* is found in more abundance on the skin than *S. aureus* and is a relatively frequent contaminant in cultures from the skin area. It may also be a contaminant in blood cultures or other cultures when the material for culture is obtained by needle puncture of the skin. However, *S. epidermidis* may produce disease. Infections most frequently associated with *S. epidermidis* are related to indwelling catheters, vascular grafts, or joint prosthetic devices; bacteremia in patients who are immunosuppressed; and infection after eye surgery (endophthalmitis). It is the causal agent of infectious endocarditis in 2%–3% of all endocarditis cases (range, 1%–8%), more often in persons with an artificial heart valve (where it may comprise up to 40% of prosthetic valve endocarditis). *Staphylococcus epidermidis* is the most frequent cause of bacterial colonization or infection associated with indwelling vascular catheters and those used for hyperalimentation, where it is reported to cause about 20% of bacteremias and 40% of septicemias. Other catheter-related problem areas include CSF shunts (causing about 50% of infections, range, 44%–70%) and peritoneal dialysis catheters (about 50% of infections). *Staphylococcus epidermidis* is also reported to cause about 40% (range, 25%–70%) of orthopedic joint prosthesis infections. Since *S. epidermidis* is a common skin-dwelling organism, it is a frequent culture contaminant. When it is obtained from a blood culture, there is always a question regarding its significance. Some rules of thumb from the literature that would tend to suggest contamination are isolation from only one of a series of cultures, isolation from only one of two cultures drawn close together in time, and isolation from only one bottle of an aerobic and anaerobic two-bottle culture set inoculated from the same syringe. However, none of these conclusively proves that the organism is a contaminant. Whereas *S. aureus* is differentiated from other staphylococci by a positive coagulase test result, many laboratories do not perform tests to identify the exact species of coagulase-negative staphylococci but report them all as *S. epidermidis*. However, not all of these organisms are *S. epidermidis*. Also, at least one of the coagulase-negative nonepidermidis staphylococci, *S. saprophyticus*, has been implicated as the causal agent in about 20% of urinary tract infections occurring in young women. On the other hand, *S. epidermidis* is not considered to be a urinary tract pathogen in young women, at least by some investigators. Therefore, it might be better to use the term "coagulase-negative *Staphylococcus*" in culture reports if the laboratory does not speciate these organisms. *Staphylococcus epidermidis* is often resistant to many antibiotics, with 33%–66% reported to be resistant to methacillin.

Gram-Negative Diplococci

Gram-negative diplococci include several *Neisseria* species, such as meningococci and gonococci; and *Branhamella catarrhalis*. *Branhamella catarrhalis* (formerly *Neisseria catarrhalis*) is a member of the genus *Moraxella* but closely resembles neisseriae in many respects, including microscopic appearance. *Branhamella catarrhalis*, as well as some of the neisseriae, is normally found in the upper respiratory tract. Although usually nonpathogenic, it occasionally can produce pneumonia (especially in patients with chronic lung disease) and very uncommonly has caused bacteremia.

Meningococci

Meningococcal infection is still the most common type of meningitis, although the incidence varies with age (chapter 18). Meningococci are present in the nasopharynx of approximately 5% of clinically normal persons, and it takes special subculturing to differentiate these from nonpathogenic *Neisseria* species that are normal common inhabitants of the nasopharynx. In rare instances one of the (usually) nonpathogenic *Neisseria* species may be associated with serious disease, such as septicemia or meningitis.

Gonococci

Neisseria gonorrhoeae causes gonorrheal urethritis and initiates the majority of cases of acute salpingitis, so-called pelvic inflammatory disease (PID). Gonorrhea is not symptomatic in about 75%–80% (range, 60%–83%) of infected females and in about 10%–15% (range, 5%–42%) of infected males. Currently, about 2% of gonococcal strains are resistant to penicillin (range, 0%–6%, depending on the location in the United States. Rates of 10%–30% have been reported in parts of the Far East and Africa). A presumptive diagnosis of gonorrhea can often be made by a Gram-stained smear of discharge from the male urethra. Gonococci appear as bean-shaped gram-negative intracellular diplococci, located within the cytoplasm of polymorphonuclear neutrophils. Extracellular organisms are not considered reliable for diagnosis. Certain organisms in the *Acinetobacter* group (formerly *Mima polymorpha*) may have a similar morphologic appearance to the gonococcus; these bacteria are usually extracellular but can be intracellular. *Staphylococcus aureus* sometimes may have the appearance on Gram stain of a *Diplococcus*, although it is rounder than the typical gonococcal organisms and is gram positive rather than gram negative. Finally, rare urethral infections by *N. meningitidis* have been reported. Nevertheless, the consensus seems to be that diagnosis of gonorrhea can be made from a male urethral smear with reasonable confidence if there are definite gram-negative diplococci having characteristic

Neisseria morphology within neutrophils. In males, if a urethral exudate is present, a smear is usually all that is required. The patient can wait while the smear is processed, and if the smear is negative or equivocal, culture can be done. In females, although a Gram-stained smear can be prepared from the endocervix, the number of positive diagnoses from such a smear are much less frequent (approximately 50% of cases, literature range, 20%–70%). Cultures should therefore be done, both to supplement the smear as a screening technique and to provide definitive diagnosis. In females, the endocervical canal is the single best site for culture, detecting about 82%–92% of cases that would be uncovered by culture from multiple sites. About 30%–50% of patients have positive rectal cultures (swab cultures using an anoscope, taking care to avoid contamination with feces). Rectal culture adds an additional 5%–10% of cases to those detected by endocervical culture. Cultures repeated on specimens obtained 1 week later will uncover an additional 5%–10% of cases. In males, a rectal culture is positive much less frequently. However, in male homosexuals, rectal culture assumes more importance, with one study finding approximately 30% of cases positive only by rectal culture.

Certain technical points deserve mention. Gonococci should be cultured on special media, such as Thayer-Martin or NYC, rather than on the traditional less selective media like chocolate agar, and need a high carbon dioxide atmosphere for adequate growth. Speculum instruments should not be lubricated with material that could inhibit gonococcal growth (which includes most commercial lubricants). Specimens should be inoculated immediately into special transport media. There are several commercial transport systems available specifically for gonococci, most of them based on modified Thayer-Martin medium and incorporating some type of carbon dioxide source. Some authors state that the medium on which the specimen is to be inoculated should be warmed at least to room temperature before use, since gonococci may not grow if the medium is cold. However, others obtained similar results with cold or room temperature media. To make matters more confusing, some investigators report that vancomycin used in gonococcal selective media to prevent bacterial contaminant overgrowth may actually inhibit gonococcal growth if the gonococcal strain is sensitive to vancomycin (about 5%–10% of strains, range, 4%–30%). Due to the 24- to 48-hour delay in obtaining culture results and lack of adequate Gram stain sensitivity in female infection, additional rapid tests to detect gonococcal infection have been introduced. One of these is Gonozyme, an immunologic enzyme-linked immunosorbent assay (ELISA) procedure that takes 3 hours to perform. Sensitivity (compared to culture) in males is reported to be about 97% (range, 93%–100%, similar to Gram stain results) and about 93% (range, 74%–100%) in females. Disadvantages are that Gram stain is faster and less expensive in males, the test cannot be used for rectal or pharyngeal specimens due to crossreaction with other *Neisseria* species, there is an inability to determine if a positive result is a penicillin-resistant infection, and there are a significant number of false-negative results in females. At present, the test is not widely used. Gonorrhea precedes the majority of cases of acute and chronic salpingitis (PID). However, gonococci can be isolated from endocervical culture in only about 40%–50% of patients with proved PID (literature range, 5%–80%). *Chlamydia trachomatis* apparently is also an important initiator of PID—or at least associated with it in some way—with acute infection with *Chlamydia* being present in a substantial minority of patients, either alone or concurrently with gonorrhea (combined infection of the endocervix is reported in 25%–50% of cases). The organisms most frequently recovered from infected fallopian tubes or from tubo-ovarian abscesses include gonococci, group D streptococci, anaerobes such as *Bacteroides* or anaerobic streptococci, and gram-negative rods. Infection is often polymicrobial.

Nongonococcal Urethritis and the Acute Urethral Syndrome

In men, nongonococcal urethritis reportedly constitutes about 40% of urethritis cases, and some believe that it is more frequent than gonorrhea. The most common symptom is a urethral discharge. *Chlamydia trachomatis* is the most commonly reported organism, identified in 30%–50% of male nongonococcal urethritis patients. *Chlamydia* has also been found in some female patients with nongonococcal cervicitis, and *Chlamydia* may coexist with gonococci in other patients. *Ureaplasma urealyticum* (formerly called T mycoplasma) is frequently cultured in male nongonococcal urethritis, but its relationship to disease is not proved. Reiter's syndrome might also be mentioned as an occasional cause of nongonococcal urethritis. *Chlamydia* organisms have been found in some cases of Reiter's syndrome. In females, nongonococcal urethritis is usually called the *acute urethral syndrome*. Symptoms are most commonly acute dysuria and frequency, similar to those of acute cystitis. In females with these symptoms, about 50% have acute cystitis, and about 25%–30% (range, 15%–40%) are due to the acute urethral syndrome. Some of the remainder are due to vaginitis. Differentiation between acute cystitis and the acute urethral syndrome is made through urine culture. A urine culture with no growth or quantitative growth less than 100,000/cu mm suggests acute urethral syndrome. Diagnosis of urethral infection usually requires the following steps:

1. Symptoms of urethritis (urethral discharge or dysuria).
2. Objective evidence of urethritis. In men, a urethral Gram-stained smear demonstrating more than four segmented neutrophils per oil immersion field or (alternatively) 10 or more leukocytes per high-power field (some require 15 rather than 10) in the centrifuged sediment from the first portion (first 10–30 ml collected separately) of a clean-catch (midstream) voided urine specimen is required. In women, a urine culture without growth or growing an organism but quantitatively less than 100,000 (10^5) organisms/ml is required.
3. Exclusion of gonococcal etiology (urethral smear or culture in men, urethral culture in women). Culture or direct identification (e.g., fluorescent antibody or nucleic acid probe methods) would be needed to detect *Chlamydia* or *Mycoplasma* organisms.

Other Venereal Diseases

Other venereal diseases include lymphogranuloma venereum (caused by a subspecies of *C. trachomatis* different from the one that causes nongonococcal urethritis), syphilis, granuloma inguinale, trichomoniasis, chancroid, herpesvirus type 2, molluscum contagiosum, and condyloma acuminatum. Most of these will be discussed elsewhere.

Gardnerella vaginalis

This organism (also called *Corynebacterium vaginalis* and *Hemophilus vaginalis*) is a small bacillus or coccobacillus that gives variable results on Gram stain, most often gram negative, but sometimes gram positive. The organism has been implicated as the cause of most cases of "nonspecific vaginitis" (i.e., vaginitis not due to *Candida albicans* or *Trichomonas*). Clinical infection in women occurs only when estrogen levels are normal or increased, so postmenopausal women usually are not involved. *Gardnerella vaginalis* can also be cultured from the urethra of many male sexual partners of infected women, so the disease is postulated to be at least potentially sexually transmissible.

Clinically, there is a vaginal discharge that typically is malodorous (although this odor was present in only two thirds of cases in one report). Other than the discharge, there usually are few or no symptoms in the female and none in the male.

Diagnosis is usually made either from aspiration of vaginal discharge or from swab specimens of the vaginal wall (avoiding the cervix). The vaginal discharge specimens have a pH greater than 4.5, with 90% between 5.0 and 5.5 (normal pH is <4.5 except during menstruation, when the presence of blood raises the pH to 5.0 or more). Trichomonas parasitic infection may also produce a vaginal discharge with a pH greater than 4.5, whereas the pH in *Candida* infection usually is less than 4.5. Therefore, a discharge with a pH less than 4.5 is strong evidence against *Trichomonas* or *Gardnerella* infection, whereas a discharge with a pH greater than 5.0 suggests infection by these organisms. Addition of 10% sodium hydroxide to the specimen from *G. vaginalis* infection typically results in a fishy odor. A wet mount or Gram stain of discharge or swab material from the vaginal wall (avoiding the cervix) demonstrates clue cells in about 90% of *G. vaginalis* infections (literature ranges in the few studies available are 76%–98% for wet mount and 82%–100% for Gram stain). Clue cells are squamous epithelial cells with a granular appearance caused by adherence of many tiny *G. vaginalis* gram-negative bacteria. Wet mount may occasionally produce a false positive result, and Gram stain is said to be somewhat more liable to false positive errors by mistaking diphtheroids for *G. vaginalis*. Papanicolaou cytology stain can also be used. The organism can be cultured on special media or on the same Thayer-Martin medium with increased carbon dioxide that is used for the diagnosis of gonorrhea. However, isolation of *Gardnerella* is not diagnostic of vaginitis, since *Gardnerella* can be cultured from the vagina in 42%–50% of clinically normal women. In addition, there is substantial evidence that anaerobic bacteria are associated with symptomatic infection by *G. vaginalis*.

Several studies suggest that *Gardnerella* is responsible for urinary tract infection in some pregnant patients and some patients with chronic renal disease. Since *Gardnerella* does not grow on culture media routinely used for urine, urine culture in these patients would be negative. However, *Gardnerella* has been isolated with equal frequency in similar patients without clinical evidence of urinary tract infection.

Enteric Bacilli (Enterobacteriaceae)

Enteric bacilli form a large family of gram-negative rods (see Table 36–12). As their name implies, most are found primarily in the intestinal tract. These include species such as *Salmonella, Shigella, E. coli, Enterobacter, Klebsiella, Proteus*, and several others (see Table 36–12). Many are normal inhabitants and cause disease only if they escape to other locations or if certain pathogenic types overgrow; others are introduced from contaminated food or water. Salmonellae and shigellae are not normal gastrointestinal inhabitants and always indicate a source of infection from the environment.

Salmonella

These organisms cause several clinical syndromes. Typhoid fever is produced by *Salmonella typhi (Salmonella typhosa)*. The classic symptoms are a rising fever during the first week, a plateau at 103°F–104°F (39.4°C–40.0°C) for the second week, then a slow fall during the third week, plus GI symptoms and splenomegaly. Despite fever, the pulse rate tends to be slow (bradycardia). This picture is often not present in its entirety. Diarrhea occurs in 30%–60% of patients. There typically is mild leukopenia with lymphocytosis and monocytosis. However, in one series only 10% of patients had leukopenia and 7% had a WBC count more than 15,000/cu mm.

Laboratory Diagnosis.—During the first and second weeks of illness, blood cultures are the best means of diagnosis; thereafter, the incidence of positive specimens declines rapidly. During the latter part of the second week to the early part of the fourth week, stool cultures are the most valuable source of diagnosis. However, stool cultures may occasionally be positive in the first week; in carriers, positive stool cultures may persist for long periods. (About 3%–5% of typhoid patients become carriers—persons with chronic subclinical infection.) Urine cultures may be done during the third and fourth weeks but are not very effective. Even with maximum yield, blood cultures miss at least 20% of cases, stool cultures miss at least 25%, and urine cultures miss at least 75%. Repeated cultures increase the chance of diagnosis. Besides cultures, serologic tests may be performed. There are three major antigens in *S. typhi:* the H (flagellar), O (somatic), and Vi (capsule or envelope) antigens. Antibody titers against these antigens constitute the Widal test. Most authorities agree that of the three antibodies, only that against the O antigen is meaningful for diagnosis. Vaccination causes a marked increase in the anti-H antibodies; the level of anti-O antibodies rises to a lesser degree and returns much more quickly to normal. The Widal test (anti-O) antibodies begin to appear 7–10 days after onset of illness. The highest percentage of positive test results is reported to be in the third and fourth weeks. As with any serologic test, a fourfold (change of at least two dilution levels) rising titer is more significant than a single determination. There has been considerable controversy over the usefulness of the Widal test in the diagnosis of *Salmonella* infections. It seems to have definite but limited usefulness. Drawbacks to the Widal test include the following: (1) antibodies do not develop early in the illness and may be suppressed by antibiotic therapy; (2) antibody behavior is often variable and often does not correlate with the severity of the clinical picture; (3) an appreciable number of cases (15% or more) do not have a significantly elevated anti-O titer, especially if only one determination is done. Only about 50% (one study obtained only 22%) display a fourfold rise in titer. In some cases, therapy may suppress the response. A normal Widal titer is 0–1:40.

To summarize, in typhoid fever, blood cultures during the first and second weeks and stool cultures during the second, third, and fourth weeks are the diagnostic tests of choice. The Widal test may occasionally be helpful. Negative diagnostic test results do not exclude the diagnosis.

Paratyphoid fever (enteric fever) is produced by salmonellae other than *S. typhi*; the clinical picture is similar to typhoid fever but milder. *Salmonella typhimurium* and *Salmonella enteritidis* (formerly *Salmonella paratyphi*) are usually the most common causes in the United States. Diagnosis is similar to that for typhoid fever.

In the United States, ***Salmonella*** **gastroenteritis** is more frequent than typhoid fever or enteric fever. The gastroenteritis syndrome has a short incubation, features abdominal pain, nausea, and diarrhea, and is most commonly produced by *S. typhimurium*. There is usually leukocytosis with a minimal increase in neutrophils, in contrast to the leukopenia in textbook cases of typhoid fever. Blood cultures are said to be negative; stool cultures are usually positive.

Other *Salmonella* Diseases.—Septicemia may occasionally be found, and salmonellae may rarely cause focal infection in various organs, resulting in pneumonia, meningitis, and endocarditis. *Salmonella* osteomyelitis has been associated with sickle cell anemia. *Salmonella* bacteremia is relatively frequent in patients with systemic lupus erythematosis. *Salmonella* infections, including bacteremia, are also more frequent in the acquired immunodeficiency syndrome (AIDS) and in patients with leukemia or lymphoma.

Sources of *Salmonella* Infection.—*Salmonella typhi* is found only in humans, and infection is transmitted through fecal contamination of food and water. Other salmonellae infect poultry and animals. Nontyphoid salmonellosis is most commonly acquired from poultry and eggs. Contaminated meat and nonpasteurized or powdered milk have been an occasional problem.

Due to DNA hybridization and other research work, the genus *Salmonella* is being reorganized to include certain organisms, such as *Arizona*, that previously were not considered salmonellae. The organisms previously considered *Salmonella* species are now serotypes (serovars) of the subspecies *choleraesuis* from the species *Salmonella choleraesuis*. The other organisms, such as *Arizona*, form part of other subspecies of *S. choleraesuis*.

Shigella

The shigellae are also important sources of intestinal infection as well as the salmonellae. *Shigella* organisms cause so-called bacillary dysentery. Shigellae usually remain localized to the colon and do not enter the peripheral blood; blood cultures are therefore negative, in contrast to blood cultures in early *Salmonella* infection. Stool culture is the main diagnostic test. Besides salmonellae and shigellae, certain other bacteria (e.g., *Yersinia enterocolitica*, *Campylobacter jejuni*, *Clostridium difficile*, and enteropathogenic *E. coli*) may cause diarrhea from GI infection; these are discussed elsewhere.

Enterobacter *and* Klebsiella

These bacteria are normal GI tract inhabitants. Nomenclature has been particularly confusing in relation to these organisms. *Enterobacter* was formerly called *Aerobacter*. *Enterobacter* and *Klebsiella* react differently to certain test media but are similar enough that previous classifications included both in the same group. According to previous custom, if infection by these organisms was in the lungs it was called *Klebsiella*; if it was in the urinary tract, it was called *Aerobacter*. Current classification does not make this distinction. The species of *Klebsiella* called *Klebsiella pneumoniae* is the organism that produces so-called Friedländer's pneumonia, a resistant necrotizing pneumonia that often cavitates and that is characteristically found in alcoholics and debilitated patients. *Klebsiella pneumoniae* also is an important cause (about 10%) of both community-acquired and hospital-acquired urinary tract infection. The species of *Enterobacter* called *Enterobacter aerogenes* is an important agent (about 5%) in nosocomial urinary tract infections, is often resistant to therapy, and occasionally produces septicemia.

Present classification differentiates *Enterobacter* from *Klebsiella*. Sources of confusion include the family name Enterobacteriaceae, which is similar to the name of one component genus, *Enterobacter*. Enterobacteriaceae is a group of several tribes, each of which contains a genus or genera. One tribe, Klebsiellae, has a similar name to one of its three component genera, *Klebsiella*, and also includes the genus *Enterobacter*. A further source of difficulty is that the predominant species of *Klebsiella* is *K. pneumoniae*, which, despite its name, is found more frequently in the urinary tract than in the lungs.

Escherichia

Escherichia coli is the most common cause of community-acquired (about 70%) and of hospital-acquired urinary tract infection (about 50%). *Escherichia coli* is likewise the most common cause of gram-negative bacteremia or septicemia, both of community-acquired or hospital-acquired origin. The primary site of infection leading to bloodstream entry is most often the urinary tract, as happens with the majority of the gram-negative rod bacteria. This is more frequent with urinary tract obstruction. *Escherichia coli* is one of the most common causes of severe infection in the newborn, especially meningitis. *Escherichia coli* causes periodic outbreaks of epidemic diarrhea in newborns and infants. In the past it was thought that only certain strains of *E. coli* were responsible for diarrhea, and that serotyping (using antisera against the so-called enteropathogenic strains) was helpful in deciding whether or not *E. coli* was responsible for diarrhea by demonstrating or excluding the presence of the enteropathogenic subspecies (see Table 36–9). However, so many exceptions have been noted that serotyping is no longer advocated except as an epidemiologic tool to show that patients in an epidemic are infected by the same *E. coli* strain. Nevertheless, there is an uncommon condition caused by a specific strain of *E. coli* (0157:H7) called *hemorrhagic colitis*, manifested by severe diarrhea with bloody stools. *Escherichia coli* has been incriminated as an important cause of traveler's diarrhea, which may affect U.S. tourists in other countries. *Escherichia coli* is a normal inhabitant of the colon, so a stool culture growing *E. coli* does not prove that the organism is the causative agent of diarrhea.

Proteus

This is a group of gram-negative rods that assumes most importance as the cause of urinary tract infection in hospitalized patients (about 5%) but occasionally causes community-acquired cystitis and some cases of hospital-acquired bacteremia and other infections.

Yersinia

The genus *Yersinia*, which includes several organisms formerly located in the genus *Pasteurella*, contains three important species: *Yersinia pestis*, *Yersinia pseudotuberculosis*, and *Yersinia enterocolitica*. ***Yersinia pestis*** is the cause of plague, which was transmitted historically by rat fleas, followed in some cases by nasopharyngeal droplet dissemination from infected humans. Today, plague is not a serious menace in Western nations, although a few cases in rodents (including prairie dogs) are reported each year from the American West and Southwest, from which source the disease is occasionally transmitted to humans. There are three clinical forms: septicemic, bubonic, and pneumonic. The septicemic type is responsible for 5%–10% of cases and is associated with a bacteremic form of febrile illness that progresses to septicemia and shock. Diagnosis is made by blood culture. When lymph nodes are primarily involved, the condition is known as *bubonic plague*. This constitutes the great majority of plague cases. However, septicemia or pneumonia may develop. Only one group of lymph nodes is enlarged in the majority of cases. Diagnosis is made by blood culture (positive in about 80% of cases) or lymph node aspiration and culture (positive in about 80% of cases). Pneumonic plague has been uncommon in recent years and is rapidly fatal. Blood culture and sputum culture provide the diagnosis. *Yersinia pestis* grows on ordinary laboratory culture media.

Yersinia pseudotuberculosis is found in many wild and domestic animals and in various domestic fowl. Human infection is uncommon, or at least, is uncommonly recognized, and most often consists of mesenteric adenitis. There usually is abdominal pain, fever, and leukocytosis, a clinical picture that simulates acute appendicitis. Diagnosis is made by culture of affected lymph nodes (lymph nodes are likely to be placed in chemical fixative for microscopic examination, which makes culture impossible unless the surgeon orders a culture to be performed and directs personnel not to fix the specimen).

Yersinia enterocolitica is by far the most common pathogen of these three *Yersinia* species. *Yersinia enterocolitica* most often produces acute enteritis, with clinical features including headache, fever, malaise, crampy abdominal pain, and nonbloody diarrhea. The organism also can produce mesenteric adenitis and, rarely, intra-abdominal abscess or septicemia. Enteritis is more common in children and mesenteric adenitis in adolescents and adults. Diagnosis is made by stool culture in patients with enteritis and by lymph node culture in those with mesenteric adenitis. Culture is less reliable for *Y. enterocolitica* than for the other yersiniae, because the organism grows somewhat slowly and forms tiny pinpoint colonies on ordinary media used for gram-negative rods, which can easily be overlooked among normal stool organism colonies. The organism grows much better at room temperature (25°C) than at the usual incubation temperature of 37°C. Some investigators believe that "cold enrichment" is necessary (special media incubated at 4°C for several weeks). Therefore, *Y. enterocolitica* will usually be missed on routine culture unless the laboratory takes special precautions.

"Opportunistic" Enterobacteriaceae

There are a considerable number of species located in various genera of the Enterobacteriaceae that are less common pathogens. It was originally thought that these organisms were nonpathogenic or rarely pathogenic and that their importance was only in the necessity for differentiation from more pathogenic enteric organisms such as *Salmonella*. Now, however, it is recognized that these organisms produce disease, most often urinary tract infections but also septicemia and pulmonary infections, although the frequency of infection for any individual species is not high. Most of these organisms have been renamed and reclassified since initial studies were done. Some of the more important organisms include *Arizona*, *Providentia* (formerly *Proteus inconstans* and *Proteus rettgeri*), *Citrobacter* (formerly Bethesda group and *Escherichia freundii*), and *Serratia*. Infections caused by these organisms are often associated with decreased host resistance and with long-term bladder catheterization. *Serratia* is usually considered the most dangerous of these organisms. About 90% of *Serratia* infections involve the urinary tract, the great majority following urinary tract surgery or cystoscopy or associated with indwelling catheters. As many as 50% of *Serratia* urinary tract infections are asymptomatic. Bacteremia develops in about 10%. A few patients develop *Serratia* pneumonia, although respiratory tract colonization is much more frequent than pneumonia. The most common (but not the only) means of *Serratia* spread from patient to patient is the hands of hospital personnel.

Other Gram-Negative Organisms

Pseudomonas

These gram-negative rods are not classified with the Enterobacteriaceae, although they may be found normally in the GI tract. The most important is *Pseudomonas aeruginosa*. *Pseudomonas* is less common in community-acquired infection than with most of the major Enterobacteriaceae but becomes more frequent in hospital-acquired infections (about 10% of nosocomial infections). The conditions for which it is best known are urinary tract infection, septicemia, pneumonia (especially in patients with cystic fibrosis), extensive burn infection, malignant otitis externa, and infection associated with ocular contact lenses or physical therapy whirlpool tubs. *Pseudomonas aeruginosa* is also known for its resistance to many antibiotics and for its high mortality rate.

In the environment, *Pseudomonas* organisms live in water or on moist surfaces. In human disease, *Pseudomonas* has many attributes similar to "opportunistic fungi" in that infection is rare in healthy persons; and even in hospitalized persons, colonization is more common than infection. Infection is most often superimposed on serious underlying diseases such as hematologic or nonhematologic malignancy (especially during chemotherapy), severe burns, wounds, and foreign bodies (tracheostomy, catheter), or in immunocompromised patients. *Pseudomonas aeruginosa* is resistant to many of the standard antibiotics and therefore may become a secondary invader after antibiotic therapy for the original infection. This is most frequent in urinary tract infections. *Pseudomonas* may be found normally on the skin (as well as in the GI tract) and thus is a very important and frequent problem in severe burns. *Pseudomonas* septicemia is increasing as a complication or a terminal event in patients with malignancy or immunocompromised state. In some tertiary medical centers, *Pseudomonas* is reported involved in as many as 20% (range, 6%–25%) of bacteremic episodes.

Calymmatobacterium granulomatis (Donovania granulomatis)

Granuloma inguinale is a venereal disease caused by a gram-negative rod bacterium that has some antigenic similarity to the *Klebsiella* group. Infection is transmitted by sexual contact. After incubation, an elevated irregular flattened granulomatous lesion develops, usually in or around the medial aspect of the inguinal area or on the labia. The organism is difficult to culture and requires special media, so culture is not usually done. Diagnosis is accomplished by demonstration of the organisms in the form of characteristic Donovan bodies, found in the cytoplasm of histiocytes. The best technique is to take a punch biopsy of the lesion, crush the fresh tissue between two glass slides, and make several smears with the crushed tissue. These smears are air-dried and stained with Wright's stain. (It is possible to process a biopsy specimen in the routine manner and do special stains on tissue histologic sections, but this is not nearly as effective.) Granuloma inguinale is sometimes confused with lymphogranuloma venereum, a totally different disease, because of the similarity in names and because both are venereal diseases.

Haemophilus (Hemophilus)

This genus is one of three in the family Pasteurellaceae (the other two are *Pasteurella* and *Actinobacillus*). The genus *Haemophilus* contains several species, most of which are normal nasopharyngeal inhabitants, that on Gram stain are very small gram-negative rods ("coccobacilli"). The most important species is *H. influenzae*, which is the most common etiology of meningitis between the ages of 2 months and 5 years (about 70% of cases). *Haemophilus influenzae* occasionally produces a serious type of laryngitis (croup) in children known as acute epiglottitis and occasionally is associated with childhood bacteremia, septic arthritis, otitis media, sinusitis, and pneumonia. *Haemophilus influenzae* infection in adults is far less common than in early childhood, but the same types of diseases may occur. *Haemophilus influenzae* exists in both capsulated and noncapsulated forms. In early childhood, 90%–95% of cases of meningitis or bacteremia are caused by capsulated type B. Non-B encapsulated serotypes and nonencapsulated forms increase in frequency in localized pediatric infection and in adult infection. Currently, most typing of *Haemophilus* organisms is done with antibodies to the capsular antigens of *H. influenzae*. "Nontypable" *H. influenzae* means a noncapsulated strain and cannot be ignored, on this basis alone, as a cause for serious disease. Organisms in the genus *Haemophilus* require one or both substances called *X* and *V factors*. Therefore, the traditional *H. influenzae* culture plate contains blood agar (supplying the X factor) on which is a small area previously inoculated with *S. aureus* ("staph streak"), which supplies V factor ("satellite test"). However, other satisfactory culture and identification systems are now available. In addition to culture, latex agglutination tests are available to detect *H. influenzae* antigen in spinal fluid. These will be discussed in more detail in the chapter on CSF tests. In very limited studies involving patients with infections other than CSF, latex agglutination test results on urine were positive in 92%–100% of cases. *Haemophilus influenzae* is considered normal flora of the nasopharynx and also sputum (which acquires these organisms as it passes through the oropharynx). Heavy growth or predominance of a single "normal flora" organism increases the suspicion that it may be pathogenic.

Other members of the *Haemophilus* genus that deserve special mention are *H. aegyptius* (Koch-Weeks bacillus), which produces purulent conjunctivitis; and *H. ducreyi*, which is the etiologic agent of the venereal disease chancroid. *Haemophilus aphrophilus* is being reported more often in recent years as a pathogen.

Pasteurella

The most important organism in this genus is *Pasteurella multocida*. This is a small gram-negative bacillus found normally in the mouth of many (but not all) cats and dogs. Dog bites and either cat bites or cat scratches inoculate the organism, leading to cellulitis and occasionally to osteomyelitis or infection of prosthetic devices. The organism grows on ordinary laboratory media. Isolation and identification is made much easier if the laboratory knows that the specimen is from a dog- or cat-inflicted wound.

Bordatella

For a long time these organisms were included in the genus *Haemophilus*. The most important of this group is *Bordatella pertussis*, the etiologic agent of pertussis (whooping cough). *Bordatella pertussis* is best isolated from nasopharyngeal culture, preferably on the special Bordet-Gengou medium ("cough plate"). Nasopharyngeal swabs can also be tested directly for *B. pertussis* antigen using fluorescent antibody techniques, and some laboratories use this technique instead of culture. However, fluorescent antibody is only 50%–68% as sensitive as culture.

Campylobacter

There are several species within this genus, of which the most important is *Campylobacter fetus*. This is a gram-negative curved or spiral organism that originally was classified as a *Vibrio*. There are three subspecies (ssp.) of which two may infect humans. One of these is *Campylobacter fetus* ssp. *fetus* (formerly, ssp. *intestinalis*), which causes abortion in sheep and cattle and which can rarely infect humans. It produces disseminated disease without diarrhea, presenting as newborn or infant meningitis and childhood or adult septicemia. It also can produce thrombophlebitis. Patients usually are immunocompromised or have some debilitating disease such as alcoholism, cancer, or renal failure. Diagnosis is made by blood culture in septicemia and by spinal fluid culture in meningitis. Ordinary culture media can be used. The other *Campylobacter* organism, *Campylobacter fetus* ssp. *jejuni*, is much more common and infects cattle, dogs, and birds, in addition to humans. Poultry, especially turkeys, have been responsible for some epidemics. *Campylobacter fetus* ssp. *jejuni* produces enteric infection with diarrhea, which in some areas is responsible for as many cases as *Salmonella* and *Shigella* combined. Overall, both children and adults are affected in about equal proportion, although there is variance in different reports. Published studies indicate that *C. fetus* ssp. *jejuni* can be isolated from approximately 4%–8% of patients with diarrhea (literature range, 3%–32%).

Typical symptoms include a prodromal period of 12–24 hours with fever, headache, abdominal pain, and malaise, followed by diarrhea with crampy abdominal pain. Fever often disappears after onset of diarrhea. The diarrhea is sometimes grossly bloody, typically lasts 2–3 days, and usually is self-limited. In some patients it is more prolonged. The severity of illness varies considerably.

Laboratory Tests.—Helpful laboratory studies include tests for fecal blood and Gram stain of the feces for WBCs. About two thirds of patients demonstrate gross or occult stool blood (literature range, 60%–90%), and about the same number have segmented neutrophils in the stool. About two thirds of patients have peripheral blood leukocytosis. Fecal culture is the mainstay of diagnosis (blood cultures are usually negative in ssp. *jejuni* infection). However, routine stool culture will be negative, because the organism is microaerophilic and must be incubated 48–72 hours on special media in special gas mixtures. It grows best at 42°C but will grow at 37°C. Routine laboratories can perform the cultures, but it takes special effort and special techniques. The organism is extremely sensitive to drying. If specimens are sent to an outside laboratory, they should be inoculated into special transport media (not ordinary media) and sent with ice if more than 1 day's travel is necessary. Gram stain of the feces can demonstrate *Campylobacter* in about 50% of cases (range, 43%–65%). The organism is gram negative and has different shapes; most typically curved, S-shaped, and "gull winged." A few reports indicate that 1% aqueous basic fuchsin stain is more sensitive than Gram stain.

Another species, *Campylobacter pyloridis*, has been reported to be associated with chronic gastritis and with peptic ulcer, with infection rates being reported in up to 90% of duodenal ulcers and up to 70% of gastric ulcers. Although its exact role has not been proven, it is suspected that it alters the mucin that overlies gastric mucosa and thus predisposes the mucosa to inflammation and ulceration. Current tests for *C. pyloridis* are not ideal. The organism can be cultured on chocolate agar but is slow-growing and needs reduced oxygen tension. Also, the specimen must be obtained from a biopsy. It can be cultured in 10% or more persons without clinical symptoms, and culture is negative in 10% or more persons with peptic ulcer. The organism can be visualized in biopsy material using the Warthin-Starry silver stain. *Campylobacter pyloridis* produces large amounts of the enzyme urease, and this can be demonstrated in biopsy specimens in several ways. A breath test has also been devised using isotope-labeled urea.

Legionella

Members of this genus are tiny gram-negative rods that require special media for culture. They seem to be rather widely distributed and in some cases are linked to water habitats. Most are associated with respiratory tract infection. There are two basic types of clinical illness: an influenza-like form (sometimes called *Pontiac fever*), which is nonfatal; and a form classified as *atypical pneumonia*, which has been fatal in 10%–20% of cases. The predominant species is *Legionella pneumophilia*, which tends to cause pneumonia, but other species have been identified (e.g., *Legionella micdadei*, the etiology of *Pittsburgh pneumonia*; see Table 36–10). There is an increased incidence of *L. pneumophilia* infection in patients who are immunocompromised or have conditions associated with decreased resistance to infection. Spread of infection has most frequently been associated with water in cooling systems.

In the pneumonic form of illness, there typically is a prodromal stage of 1–10 days with influenza-like symptoms (headache, fatigue, myalgias, and sometimes chills). After this, pneumonia develops with high fever (>103° F; >39.4°C) in approximately 70% or more of cases, recurrent chills in about 70%, nonproductive or poorly productive cough in 50%–80%, pleuritic chest pain in 15%–40%, pleural effusion in 15%–40%, relative bradycardia in approximately 50%, toxic encephalopathy (confusion, disorientation) in 35% or more, and diarrhea in 20%–50%. Laboratory abnormalities include leukocytosis (10,000–30,000/cu mm) in 60%–80% of affected persons and mild liver function test elevations in approximately 30%–40%. Proteinuria occurs in about 40% of cases and microscopic hematuria in about 10%. In some series 50% or more of patients had hyponatremia and hypophosphatemia. Radiologically there is pneumonia, which begins unilaterally in 50%–70% of cases, and consists of patchy bronchopneumonia or small densities. This progresses to lobar pneumonia in up to two thirds of patients in some reports, which frequently becomes multilobar and which may become bilateral. Some patients have lobar pneumonia when they are first seen.

Diagnosis is made by culture on special media (not often available in routine laboratories). Although *Legionella* can be cultured from sputum, there frequently is little sputum produced, and there may be too much contamination by oropharyngeal bacteria. Yield is much better from transtracheal aspiration, bronchial washings, pleural fluid, and lung biopsies. Sensitivity of culture presently is about 70% (range, 15%–80%), and the procedure usually takes 3–5 days. Direct fluorescent antibody stain on smears prepared from respiratory tract material can be performed in 1–2 hours. However, sensitivity on these specimens is only about 50% (range, 20%–75%). Serologic testing, generally by fluorescent antibody methods, is still used, especially for epidemiologic investigation. A fourfold rise in titer to at least 1:128 is diagnostic, and a single titer of at least 1:256 is considered presumptive evidence when combined with appropriate symptoms. However, only about 50% of patients seroconvert by the second week of clinical illness, and it may take 4–6 weeks to obtain maximal rates of seroconversion. Ten percent to 20% of patients do not develop detectable antibodies. Nucleic acid (DNA) probe techniques are beginning to be introduced. The first of these to be reported is said to detect about 60% of cases when applied to respiratory material. However, DNA probe is expensive and is very expensive when only single specimens are processed.

Brucella

Three members of the *Brucella* genus produce an uncommon febrile disease known as "brucellosis," which sometimes must be considered in the differential diagnosis of fever of unknown origin. The *Brucella* organism is a gram-negative coccobacillus with three main species. One species infects cattle, the second one infects goats, and the third is found in swine. Classic brucellosis was most often transmitted to humans by infected milk or milk products. However, persons most likely to contact the infection today in the United States are workers in the meat-processing industry, especially those working with swine. Veterinarians and dairy farmers are also at risk. Clinical symptoms include fever, chills, and myalgia. About 25% of patients develop single-joint arthralgia. Lymph nodes are usually not enlarged. Splenomegaly occurs in about 20% of cases. Some patients develop pneumonia. White blood cell counts are usually normal or decreased. Blood culture is positive in 30%–50% of cases, but the organisms need added carbon dioxide and grow very slowly on ordinary culture media, so that under ordinary circumstances the brucellae may either not grow at all or the culture bottle is discarded as negative before growth is evident. Special media are available that will assist growth. A slide agglutination test is the most frequent method for diagnosis. Test results greater than 1:80 are suspicious for brucellosis. After recovery, antibody titer elevation lasts 1–2 years.

Francisella

Formerly included in the genus *Pasteurella*, the genus *Francisella* contains one medically important species, *Francisella tularensis*, which is the causative agent of tularemia. *Francisella tularensis* is a very small gram-negative aerobic coccobacillus that requires special media for adequate growth. The major reservoir for human infection in the United States is wild animals, predominantly wild rabbits, and in some cases deerflies or ticks. Most persons who contract the disease are those who handle raw wild rabbit meat. Tularemia may exist in several clinical forms, but the most common symptoms are painful single-area lymphadenopathy (ulceroglandular form, comprising 75%–80% of cases) and prolonged low-grade fever. Much less common is a septicemic form (5%–15% of cases). Pneumonia may occur in 15% or more of either the ulceroglandular or the septicemic forms, especially the septicemic type. Rabbit-associated infection is usually associated with a small ulcerated skin lesion at the place of entry on the hand and also with axillary adenopathy, whereas in tick-associated infection the ulcer is located on the trunk or lower extremities and the lymph nodes affected are most commonly in the inguinal area. About 15% of affected persons lack either the ulcer or both the ulcer and the adenopathy. White blood cell counts are normal in at least 50% of patients and slightly or mildly elevated in the remainder. The differential cell count is usually normal. Inconsistent elevation of one or more liver function test results is present in about one half of the patients.

Tularemia must occasionally be considered in the differential diagnosis of fever of unknown origin. The organisms will not grow on standard laboratory culture media. Special media can be obtained and culture performed from lymph node aspiration, but this is rarely done due to an unusually high rate of laboratory technologist infection from the specimens. The standard diagnostic test is a slide agglutination procedure. Titers are said to be negative during the first week of illness and begin to rise at some time during the second week, become maximal in 4–8 weeks, and remain elevated for several years. A fourfold rising titer is necessary to prove acute infection. There is considerable disagreement regarding a single titer level that could be considered presumptive evidence of infection; 1:160 seems to be the least controversial value.

Cat-Scratch Disease

This condition is caused by a small bacillus that stains faintly gram negative and which has only recently been cultured on special media. About 80% of patients affected are children (about 90% are less than 18 years old and about 70% are less than 10 years old). About 85% (range, 83%–90%) have a history of contact with cats, most of which (about 80%) are less than 1 year old. Cat inoculation via scratch, bite, or lick is followed in 4–14 days (range, 3–50 days) by development of a primary inoculation site pustule or papule in 54%–93% of patients. The primary lesion persists 1–3 weeks but can persist up to 1–3 months. Regional lymphadenopathy develops in 1–3 weeks after appearance of the primary site lesion; the nodes are unilateral in about 90% (range, 85%–95%) of patients and are tender in about 80%. Cat-scratch disease is possibly the most common cause of chronic lymphadenopathy in children. The node or nodes are located in the head and neck area in about 25% of cases; the axilla (occasionally the epitrochlear area) in about 45%, and the groin in about 20%. They generally regress in size in 2–4 months but can persist longer. Adenopathy is accompanied by fever and malaise in about 35% of patients (range, 30%–59%), but the fever is usually (90%) less than 102°F (38.9°C). The lymph nodes suppurate in 10%–30% of cases and may drain in 10%–20% of cases. *Parinaud's oculoglandular syndrome* (unilateral conjunctivitis with regional lymphadenitis) is present in 4%–6% of patients. The lymph nodes often raise the clinical question of mycobacterial infection and sometimes of malignant lymphoma. Biopsy specimens display a characteristic lesion consisting of focal granulomatous collections of lymphocytes and of histiocytes with scanty cytoplasm surrounding a central area containing segmented neutrophils. The lesions may be single or can be stellate (branching) due to coalescence of the original lesions. The same histologic pattern can be found in tularemia and in lymphogranuloma venereum. It is extremely difficult to find the organisms by Gram stain, and more success is obtained with the Warthin-Starry silver stain. Interestingly, the more commonly used silver stain methods such as methenamine silver are not useful. Even with Warthin-Starry, the organisms may be difficult to find or may be absent. The best areas are the center of suppurative granulomas. A skin test has been described using antigen derived from lymph node pus, but the antigen is not readily available.

Vibrios

Vibrios are gram-negative small curved rods. The most important species is *Vibrio cholerae,* which produces cholera. The *V. cholerae* species is subdivided into many serotypes, of which only one, the 01 strain, is associated with epidemic cholera. Classic cholera results in severe watery diarrhea, which can lead to death from loss of fluid and electrolytes. However, there are more mild cases than severe ones. Humans usually become infected by drinking contaminated water or eating shellfish from contaminated water. Diagnosis is made by stool culture. The organism is very sensitive to drying, and if swabs are used, they must be placed in transport media as soon as the specimen is obtained.

Gram-Positive Rods

Listeria monocytogenes

Listeria monocytogenes is a short gram-positive rod. Although most gram-positive rods of medical importance are anaerobes, *Listeria* is an aerobic (rather than anaerobic) organism. It is found widely in soil, sewage, and various animals, as well as in the feces of about 15% (range, 2%–60%) of asymptomatic adults. Infection in children and adults is most often from contaminated food (salads, milk, cheese) or unpasteurized milk. In newborns, infection may occur from the mother's vagina. Most cases are found in neonates, the elderly, and immunocompromised persons. Infection is especially associated with renal transplants, leukemia or lymphoma, and pregnancy. The most common infection at nearly all ages is meningitis (about 80% of *Listeria* cases). Next most common is bacteremia (which is the type of *Listeria* infection found in pregnancy). *Listeria* occasionally has been reported to cause stillbirth and may produce septicemia in newborns (especially in premature infants). Culture of the mother's lochia has been suggested as an aid in diagnosis, as well as blood cultures from the infant. On Gram stain the organism may be mistaken for diphtheroids, streptococci, or improperly stained *H. influenzae. Listeria* may cause meningitis in early infancy, usually after the first week of life. In *Listeria meningitis,* CSF Gram stain is said to be negative in about one half of the patients and misinterpreted in some of the others. About one third of patients have predominance of lymphocytes or mononuclears rather than neutrophils. Cerebrospinal fluid glucose may be normal in some patients. Cerebrospinal fluid culture is the most reliable method of diagnosis.

Anaerobic Bacteria

The three major sources of anaerobic organisms are the dental and mouth area, the lower intestinal tract (ileum and colon), and the female external genital tract (vagina and vulva area). Anaerobes comprise about 95% of the bacterial flora of the colon and outnumber aerobes in the mouth and vagina. From the mouth the organisms can reach the lungs and brain; from the vagina they may involve the remainder of the female genital tract; diseases of the lower intestinal tract may release anaerobes into the abdominal cavity; and all of these locations may be the source of organisms found in the bloodstream. In addition, anaerobic bacteria are frequently associated with chronic infection, such as bronchiectasis, abscess, or chronic osteomyelitis. Infections with anaerobes frequently are mixed infections which also contain aerobes. The types of infection most frequently associated with anaerobes are listed in Table 14–1.

Anaerobic infections usually center on three groups of organisms: *Clostridia* species, *Bacteroides* species, and the anaerobic streptococci.

Clostridia

These gram-positive anaerobic rods include several important organisms. ***Clostridium perfringens*** (*Clostridium welchii*) is the

TABLE 14–1.

Types of Infection Most Frequently Associated With Anaerobes (Alone or as a Mixed Infection)

Dental or mouth area infection
Chronic sinus infection
Bite wounds
Bronchiectasis and aspiration pneumonia
Gynecologic intra-abdominal and extra-abdominal infection
Abscess of any area other than skin; including brain, abdominal and thoracic cavities, and any organ
Infections associated with the intestinal tract, especially the colon (diverticulitis, appendicitis, bowel perforation, etc.)
Deep tissue infection or necrosis
Biliary tract infection
Chronic osteomyelitis

usual cause of gas gangrene. It is a normal inhabitant of the GI tract and reportedly can be isolated from the skin in about 20% of patients and from the vagina and female genitalia in about 5%. Therefore, just as with *S. aureus,* a culture report of *C. perfringens* isolated from an external wound does not necessarily mean that the organism is producing clinical infection. When isolated from abdominal or biliary tract infections, *C. perfringens* most often is part of a polymicrobial infection and, although serious, is not quite as alarming as isolation from a deep tissue wound. *Clostridium perfringens* occasionally is a cause of "food poisoning" (discussed later).

Clostridium tetani causes tetanus. The organism can be found in the human GI tract but is more common in animals. Spores are widely distributed in soil. Clinical disease is produced by release of bacterial exotoxin after local infection in a manner analogous to diphtheria. Puncture type wounds are notorious for high risk of *C. tetani* infection. The incubation time is 3–14 days in most patients, a few cases being reported as early as 24 hours after exposure. Cultures for *C. tetani* are said to be positive in less than 50% of patients. ***Clostridium difficile*** is the most frequent proven cause of antibiotic-associated diarrhea. In the 1950s and early 1960s, broad-spectrum oral antibiotics were frequently used, and *S. aureus* was thought to be the major cause of antibiotic-associated enteritis. Beginning in the late 1960s parenteral antibiotics became much more common in hospitals, and *C. difficile* was eventually proven to be the major etiology. *Clostridium difficile* enteritis usually occurs during or after therapy with antibiotics, although some patients have not received antibiotics. One report indicated a possible association with diarrhea induced by cancer chemotherapeutic agents. The condition may consist only of varying degrees of diarrhea; may progress to inflammation of portions of the colon mucosa; and in the more severe form (known as pseudomembraneous colitis) there is inflammation and partial destruction of varying areas of the colon mucosa, with formation of a pseudomembrane of fibrin, necrotic cells, and segmented neutrophils on the surface of the remnants of the affected mucosa. Some patients develop intestinal perforation and sepsis.

Diagnosis of *C. difficile* colitis is not always easy. Only about 25%–30% (range, 20%–33%) of diarrhea occurring with antibiotic therapy is due to *C. difficile,* with most of the remainder not associated with currently known infectious agents. Sigmoidoscopy or colonoscopy can be done to document pseudomembrane formation, but this procedure runs the risk of perforation; and even in pseudomembraneous enterocolitis (PMC), pseudomembranes can be demonstrated in only about 50% (range, 40%–80%) of patients. The patient stools in PMC typically contain WBCs and often contain red blood cells, but gross blood is uncommon. However, WBCs on Gram stain actually are present in only about 45%–50% of cases. For several years, culture was the usual means of diagnosis. Today, this is not often done. *Clostridium difficile* can be cultured, with reliable results, only on special media, so diagnosis usually is made through detection of *C. difficile* cytotoxin. Stool specimens must be frozen and sent to a reference laboratory with dry ice. The specimen container must be sealed tightly since the carbon dioxide from the dry ice can inactivate the toxin. Another problem is the fact that *C. difficile* can be found in the stool of some clinically healthy persons, including 30%–40% (range, 11%–63%) of clinically healthy neonates, 10%–15% of children, 3% (range, 0%–10%) of adults, 20% (range, 11%–36%) of hospitalized persons without diarrhea and not taking antibiotics, and about 30% (range, 20%–46%) of patients taking antibiotics but without diarrhea. Even in patients with endoscopy-proven PMC, stool culture is positive for *C. difficile* in only about 90% (range, 75%–95%) of cases. Most laboratories today rely more on tests to detect *C. difficile* toxin, which has been shown to correlate much better with *C. difficile* clinical infection than does stool culture. There are several *C. difficile* toxins, of which the best characterized are called *toxins A* and *B*. Toxin B is a cytotoxin that must be detected by a tissue culture system with an incubation period of 48 hours. In endoscopy-proven PMC, toxin B sensitivity is reported to be about 90% (range, 64%–100%). Results may be positive in some patients with positive *C. difficile* cultures who are clinically normal, especially in infants. Toxin A is an enterotoxin, which currently is assayed with a biologic system, the rabbit ileal loop test. This method is not practical for most laboratories. There is a simple latex agglutination system available from Marion laboratories that can provide same-day results. This system was originally thought to detect toxin A but subsequently was found to be detecting some other toxin or antigen (currently unknown type) from *C. difficile*. Nevertheless, in several limited studies this test gave results equivalent to those of the cytotoxicity test (about 90% positive in patients with proven PMC) with roughly equal specificity.

Clostridium botulinus produces botulism. Botulism is a severe food poisoning due to ingestion of preformed botulinal endotoxin (a powerful neurotoxin) contained in the contaminated food, rather than actual infection of the patient by the organism. *Clostridium botulinum* spores are widespread, but they can germinate only in anaerobic conditions at a fairly high pH (> 4.6). These conditions are met in canned foods that have not been sufficiently heated during the canning process. Therefore, *C. botulinum* is usually associated with canned food, especially home canned. Vegetables are the most frequently involved home-canned food, but any variety of canned food may become contaminated. Fortunately, the disease is not common. Although the endotoxin is preformed, symptoms most often appear 12–36 hours after ingestion (in adult patients) and commonly include nausea, vomiting, and abdominal cramps (about 50% of patients), constipation (75%), cranial nerve signs of dysphagia, dysarthria, and dry mouth (80%–90%), upper or lower extremity weakness (70%), and diplopia or other eye abnormalities (90%). There is no fever or diarrhea. Differential diagnosis in adults includes Guillain-Barré syndrome, drug reaction (especially phenothiazines), myasthenia gravis, cerebrovascular accident, chemical poisoning (mercury, arsenic, etc.), diphtheria, and tick bite paralysis (Landry's ascending paralysis). Botulism may also occur in infants, usually between ages 3 and 26 weeks (median age 10 weeks). The classic syndrome is onset of constipation followed by 4–5 days of progressive feeding difficulty, ptosis, muscle hypotonia, and possibly respiratory distress. Mildly affected infants may have varying degrees of "failure to thrive" with feeding difficulty and mild muscle weakness, whereas severely affected infants may have severe respiratory distress. Some cases of *sudden infant death syndrome* (SIDS) have been ascribed to infant botulism, whereas some infants and older children (investigated during studies initiated by botulism cases) were found to harbor *C. botulinum* organisms without symptoms. Honey was incriminated in some cases as the source of infection but was not used in the majority of cases.

Standard laboratory tests, including those on the CSF, are usually normal in botulism. Electromyography (EMG) may be helpful in differentiating adult botulism from certain other neurologic diseases, but the typical EMG findings are neither specific nor always present. The diagnosis is confirmed by stool culture and demonstration of *C. botulinum* toxin, neither of which can be done in the ordinary laboratory. In addition, food suspected of contamination should always be tested. Patient vomitus and gastric contents have also been tested. The basic specimens in adult botulism are stool (25 gm or more) and serum (at least 5 ml). For diagnosis of infant botulism a stool specimen is required, but infant serum rarely contains *C. botulinum* toxin and therefore infant serum specimens are not necessary. The specimens should be kept refrigerated, since the toxin is heat labile, and sent to a reference laboratory with a coolant (for short distances) or dry ice (for more than 1-day transit). There are several *C. botulinum* serotypes, but most cases are caused by types A and B, with type A predominating.

Bacteroides

Bacteroides are the most frequent organisms found in anaerobic infections. They comprise several species of gram-negative rods normally found in the mouth, the intestine, and the female genital tract. Isolation of these organisms often raises the question of their significance or pathogenicity. It seems well established that bacteroides occasionally cause serious infection, which frequently results in abscess or gangrene. The most commonly associated clinical situations include septic abortion, aspiration pneumonia, focal lesions of the GI tract (e.g., carcinoma or appendicitis), and pelvic abscess in the female.

Anaerobic Streptococci

Anaerobic streptococci are frequently associated with *Bacteroides* infection but may themselves produce disease. They are normally present in the mouth and GI tract. Septic abortion and superinfection of lesions in the perirectal area seem to be the most commonly associated factors. Anaerobic streptococci are also part of the fusiform bacteria-spirochetal synergistic disease known as *Vincent's angina*.

Laboratory Diagnosis of Anaerobic Infections

Anaerobic specimens cannot be processed by the laboratory as easily as those from aerobic infections. Anaerobic bacteria in general do not grow as readily as common aerobic bacteria, and prereduced media or other special media are often needed. Achieving and maintaining anaerobic culture conditions are not a simple matter. However, by far the greatest problem is the specimen received by the laboratory. If the specimen is not properly maintained in an anaerobic environment en route to the laboratory, the best and most elaborate facilities will be of little help. For abscesses or any fluid material, the preferred collection technique is to aspirate the material with a sterile syringe and needle, then expel the residual air from the needle by pushing the syringe plunger slightly, and then immediately cap the needle point with a sterile cork or other solid sterile material. The syringe must be transported immediately to the laboratory. If there is no liquid content, a swab that forms part of one of the special commercially available anaerobic transport systems should be used. Directions for creating the anaerobic environment should be followed exactly. A less satisfactory procedure is to inoculate a tube of thioglycollate medium immediately after the specimen is obtained and immediately recap the tube.

Spirochetal Diseases

Only four members of this large group of diseases will be mentioned. **Vincent's angina** is an infection of the mouth caused by an interesting synergistic group of organisms, including anaerobic streptococci, a fusiform gram-negative bacillus, and a spirochete. Gram-stained smears demonstrating all three organisms are usually sufficient for diagnosis. **Syphilis** is a very important disease and is discussed separately in chapter 31. **Leptospirosis** is caused by several species of *Leptospira* organisms found most often in rats but sometimes present in some farm animals and in some cats and dogs (presumably from rat-transmitted infection). Transmission is most often through accidental contact with water contaminated by infected rat urine. Those most at risk are sewer workers and slaughterhouse employees, but farmers and campers sometimes come into contact with contaminated water. There is an incubation period of 4–20 days, then abrupt onset of fever, often accompanied by chills, headache, malaise, and conjunctivitis. Muscle pain is present in 50% of cases. The fever typically lasts 4–9 days. White blood cell count can be normal or elevated. Urinalysis often contains protein and some WBCs. Serum bilirubin is usually normal, but about 10% of cases have mild elevation. Alanine aminotransferase is elevated in about 50% of cases, usually to less than five times normal. About 50% of patients experience a recurrence of fever about 1 week (range, 2–10 days) after the end of the first febrile period. Patients are more likely to demonstrate signs of hepatitis in this phase and may develop symptoms of meningitis. The most severe form of leptospirosis is called Weil's disease and occurs in about 5% of infections. The most striking findings are a combination of hepatitis and glomerulonephritis, clinically manifested by jaundice with hematuria. Therefore, the disease is sometimes considered in the differential diagnosis of jaundice of unknown etiology. Symptoms of meningitis occasionally predominate. Laboratory findings include leukocytosis with a shift to the left. A mild normocytic-normochromic anemia usually develops by the second week. Platelet counts are normal. After jaundice develops, liver function test results are similar to those in viral hepatitis. After onset of kidney involvement, the BUN level is often elevated, and hematuria is present with proteinuria. Cerebrospinal fluid examination shows normal glucose levels but increased cell count, which varies according to the severity of the case; initially, these are mainly neutrophils, but later, lymphocytes predominate. Cultures on ordinary bacterial media are negative.

Diagnosis often requires isolating the organisms or demonstrating specific antibodies in the serum. During the first week (days 1–8), spirochetes may be found in the blood by darkfield examination in about 8% of cases and can be cultured from the blood in many more. Instead of ordinary blood cultures, one–three drops of blood are inoculated into a special culture medium (Fletcher's), since larger quantities of blood inhibit the growth of leptospires. The CSF may be cultured toward the end of the first week. During the second week the blood results quickly become negative. During the third week (days 14–21) the spirochetes may often be recovered from the urine of patients with nephritis. Animal inoculation is the most successful method. Antibodies start to appear at about day 7 and are present in most cases by day 12. Antibodies persist for months and years after cure. A titer of 1:300 is considered diagnostic, although without a rising titer, past infection cannot be ruled out completely. If a significant titer has not developed by day 21, it is very rare for it to do so later. In summary, blood cultures during the first week and serologic tests during the second and third weeks are the diagnostic methods of choice.

Lyme disease is caused by the spirochete *Borrelia burgdorferi* by means of several tick vectors, the principal one being the deer tick *Ixodes dammini*. The three major affected areas in the United States are the northeastern states (New Jersey to Connecticut), the far western states, and the upper midwestern states. However, cases have been reported elsewhere and also in Canada, Europe, and Australia. After the initial tick bite, about 1 week later (range, 3–68 days) a reddish macular expanding lesion with central clearing ("erythema chronicum migrans") develops on the skin at the inoculation site often followed by similar skin lesions in some other areas. This is usually accompanied by low-grade fever, weakness, fatigue, and regional lymphadenopathy. Migratory arthralgias and myalgia are frequently present. About 10% of patients develop anicteric hepatitis. Central nervous system or peripheral nervous system abnormalities (most often, aseptic meningitis) occur about 4 weeks after the tick bite in about 20% of patients (range, 11%–35%). About 10% of patients develop transitory ECG abnormalities or myocardial inflammation, usually about 5 weeks after the tick bite. About 40% (range, 26%–60%) of patients develop recurrent arthritis. This is the most famous manifestation of Lyme disease and involves one or more joints, most commonly the knee, beginning about 6 weeks after the tick bite.

Laboratory test abnormalities include elevated erythrocyte sedimentation rate in about 50% of cases. Peripheral blood WBCs are elevated in only about 10%. Fluid aspirated from arthritic joints is similar to that from patients with rheumatoid arthritis. Culture or tissue biopsy examination for spirochetes using special stains can be done but have generally had poor success. Currently, the most helpful procedures are serologic tests. Immunoglobulin M antibodies peak about 3–6 weeks after tick exposure, whereas IgG antibodies peak at about 8–16 weeks. The most commonly used tests are immunofluorescent and ELISA methods. False positive results can be obtained in patients with other spirochetal diseases, such as syphilis, but this is usually not a problem. Both of the test methods give about the same results, although some investigators have a more favorable opinion of one or the other. In the early stage of the disease (first 4 weeks after exposure), the tests are positive in about 40% of patients; in the latter part of the early stage coincident with systemic symptoms, about 65% are positive; and in the later (arthritic) stage, about 90%–95% (range, 80%–97%) are positive. Although development of the characteristic skin lesion should be strongly suggestive of the diagnosis, only 20%–30% of patients recall such a lesion.

Tuberculosis and Mycobacterial Disease

Tuberculosis is caused by *Mycobacterium tuberculosis*, a rod-shaped bacterium that requires special media for culture and that has the peculiarity of "acid-fastness" (resistance to decolorization by strong acidic decolorizing chemicals such as acid alcohol after being stained by certain stains such as carbol fuchsin). Tuberculosis is still very important and common despite advances in drug therapy. The disease usually begins in the chest due to inhalation of airborne infectious material. This material is carried to some localized area of the lung alveoli and provokes a host response of granulomatous inflammation around the material (the "Ghon complex"). It is thought that in many cases there is also a silent hematogenous spread of the organisms. In most cases the host is able to contain and eventually destroy the organisms in the chest and those reaching other locations. Those in the lungs seem better able to survive than those deposited elsewhere. In some cases the organisms remain dormant, and the infection can be reactivated at a later date; in some cases the initial infection spreads; and in some cases reinfection takes place. If infection in the lungs progresses to clinical disease, the most important symptoms are cough, fever, and hemoptysis. (The most important diseases to rule out are lung carcinoma and bronchiectasis.) The kidney is involved in a small percentage of advanced cases, with the main symptom being hematuria (chapter 12). A small number of patients develop widespread extrapulmonary disease, known as *miliary tuberculosis*. The laboratory findings in tuberculosis depend to some extent on the stage and severity of the disease.

Chest X-ray Films

Chest x-ray films often provide the first suggestion of tuberculosis and are a valuable parameter of severity, activity, and response to therapy. Depending on the situation, there are a variety of possible roentgenographic findings. These may include one or more of the following:

1. Enlargement of hilar lymph nodes.
2. Localized pulmonary infiltrates. These occur characteristically in an upper apical location or, less commonly, in the superior segment of the lower lobes. Cavitation of lesions may occur.
3. Miliary spread (small punctate lesions widely distributed). This pattern is not common and may be missed on routine chest x-ray films.
4. Unilateral pleural effusion. The most common causes are tuberculosis, carcinoma, and congestive heart failure. Tuberculosis has been reported to cause 60%–80% of so-called idiopathic pleural effusions, although this percentage varies greatly depending on the patient's geographic location and other factors.

Sputum Smear

Sputum smears provide a rapid presumptive diagnosis in pulmonary tuberculosis. The smear is usually stained by one of the acid-fast (acid-fast bacillus, or AFB) procedures (usually the Ziehl-Neelsen method). Fluorescent staining methods are also available, and many believe they are more sensitive. The more advanced the infection, the more likely it is to yield a positive smear. Therefore, the rate of positive findings is low in early, minimal, or healing tuberculosis. Also, the smear may be normal in a substantial minority of advanced cases. Culture is more reliable for detection of tuberculosis (and also is necessary for confirmation of the diagnosis), for differentiation of *M. tuberculosis* from the "atypical" mycobacteria, and for sensitivity studies of antituberculous drugs. According to the literature, false negative smears (smear negative but culture positive) have been reported in an average of 50% of cases (literature range, 22%–70%). Some of these false negative results may be due to laboratory technique problems and differences in smear staining methods. A high centrifugation speed when concentrating the specimen is said to increase the yield of positive smears. False positive smears (positive smear but negative culture) have been reported, averaging about 1%–5% of positive smears (literature range, 0.5%–55%). Some of these were apparently due to contamination of water used in the smear-staining procedure by saprophytic mycobacteria. Control slides are necessary to prevent this. Some authorities believe that only one–two acid-fast organisms/300 oil immersion fields should be considered negative (although indicative of need for further specimens). Smears may sometimes be positive for up to 2 months when cultures are negative if the patient is on antituberculous drug therapy (this would not be considered a genuine false positive, since the drugs inhibit mycobacterial growth or the organisms may be nonviable). After 2 months, persistence of positive smears raises the question of treatment failure. Temporary persistence of positive smears with negative cultures is more likely to occur in severe cavitary disease (in one series, this occurred in 20% of cases). Sputum specimens should be collected (for culture and smear of the concentrated specimen) once daily for at least 3 days. If the smear is definitively positive, further smears are not necessary. Also, a definitively positive smear means high probability that culture of the specimens already collected will obtain positive results, and it is not necessary to collect more than three specimens or to proceed to more complicated diagnostic procedures. If smears are negative, one must consider the possibility that the culture may also be negative, and cultures take from 3 to 8 weeks to demonstrate growth. Therefore, other procedures may be considered for diagnosis so as not to lose so much time.

Nucleic Acid Probe

Nucleic acid (DNA) probe methods are now becoming available that permit direct nonsmear detection of mycobacteria in clinical specimens. The first such test available (Gen-Probe, Inc.) is reported by the manufacturer to be 85% sensitive compared with culture using sputum specimens. Ten percent of specimens were positive by probe but negative by culture, which may represent additional true positives that could not be confirmed. A DNA probe is also available specifically for *M. tuberculosis*. Same-day results can be obtained. Disadvantages of this first-generation method are need for considerable technologist time and certain special equipment. Compared with culture, the general *Mycobacterium* screen probe will not differentiate *M. tuberculosis* from other mycobacteria, whereas the specific *M. tuberculosis* probe will not detect the other mycobacteria. Neither probe would provide therapeutic drug sensitivity information. The major drawback regarding its use as replacement for the acid-fast smear is the relatively high cost of the probe method, very high if only one specimen at a time is processed.

Culture

Sputum culture is preferred for pulmonary tuberculosis (gastric aspiration may be done if adequate sputum specimens cannot be obtained); urine culture is preferred for renal involvement; and bone marrow culture is preferred in miliary tuberculosis. Reports indicate that an early morning specimen, either of sputum or urine, produces almost as many positive results as a 24-hour specimen and has much less problem with contamination. Special mycobacteria culture media are needed. The necessity for adequate sputum culture specimens, regardless of the concentrated smear findings, should be reemphasized. Several reports indicate that aerosol techniques produce a significantly greater yield of positive cultures than ordinary sputum collection. The aerosol mixture irritates the bronchial tree and stimulates sputum production. At any rate, it is necessary to get a "deep cough" specimen; saliva alone, although not completely useless, is much less likely to reveal infection and is much more likely to be contaminated. If sputum cultures are negative or if the patient is unable to produce an adequate sputum sample, gastric aspiration may be used. Gastric contents are suitable only for culture; nontuberculous acid-fast organisms may be found normally in the stomach and cannot be distinguished from *M. tuberculosis* on AFB smear. If renal tuberculosis is suspected, urine culture should be done (chapter 12). However, renal tuberculosis is uncommon; and even with urine specimens obtained on 3 consecutive days, only about 30% of cases are positive.

Cultures should be grown in high carbon dioxide atmosphere, since this is reported to increase the number of positive cultures by at least 10%. Inoculation on several varieties of media increases the number of positive results by 5%–10%. The 4% sodium hydroxide traditionally used to digest and decontaminate sputum prior to concentration also kills some mycobacteria. Use of weaker digestion agents increases culture yield, but troublesome overgrowth by other bacteria may also increase.

Culture should be done on all tissue specimens when tuberculosis is suspected. Acid-fast stains on tissue slides reveal tuberculosis organisms in only 30%–40% of cases that are positive by culture.

Skin Test (Mantoux Test)

This test is performed with purified protein derivative (PPD) or old tuberculin (Table 14–2). A positive result is represented by an area of induration at least 10 mm in diameter by 48 hours. A positive skin test is a manifestation of hypersensitivity to the tubercle bacillus. This reaction usually develops about 6 weeks after infection, although it may take several months. A positive reaction means previous contact and infection with tuberculosis;

TABLE 14–2.

Comparison of Tuberculosis Skin Tests*

TUs	1†	10	250†
Micrograms of PPD	0.02	0.2	5.0
"Strength" of PPD	1st	Intermediate	2d
OT equivalent	1:10,000	1:1,000	1:100
Milligrams of OT	0.01	0.1	1.0

*OT = old tuberculin; TUs = tuberculin units.
†Some experts do not ever use 1 TU or 250 TU.

the positive reaction does not itself indicate whether the disease is currently active or inactive. However, in children under 3 years of age it usually means active tuberculosis infection. Apparently, once positive, the reaction persists for many years or for life, although there is evidence that a significant number of persons revert to negative reactions if the infection is completely cured early enough. In a few cases of infection the test never becomes positive. The Mantoux test may revert to negative or fail to become positive in the following circumstances:

1. In about 20% of seriously ill patients, due to malnutrition (severe protein deficiency).
2. In newborns and occasionally in old age.
3. In some persons with viral infections, or within 1 month after receiving live virus vaccination.
4. In 50% or more of patients with miliary tuberculosis.
5. In a high percentage of patients with overwhelming pulmonary tuberculosis.
6. In a considerable number of patients who are on steroid therapy or immunosuppressive therapy.
7. In many persons who also have sarcoidosis or Hodgkin's disease.
8. In some persons with chronic lymphocytic leukemia or malignant lymphoma.
9. In some patients with chronic renal failure or severe illness of various types.
10. In some persons with old infection ("waning" of reactivity).
11. When there is artifact due to improper skin test technique (e.g., subcutaneous rather than intradermal injection).

In cachectic patients and those with protein malnutrition, treatment with an adequate protein diet can restore Mantoux test reactivity to most patients after about 2 weeks. In patients after age 50 with *M. tuberculosis* infection, especially those with old previous infection, the PPD skin test sometimes may slowly decrease in reactivity and eventually become negative. (How often this occurs is controversial; the best estimate seems to be 8%–10%, but studies range from 0.1%–21%, possibly influenced by the elapsed time period since infection and time intervals between testing.) If another skin test is performed, the new skin test itself stimulates body reaction and may restore reactivity ("booster phenomenon"). This phenomenon could simulate a new infection if previous infection were not known, since the next time a skin test is performed the physician would see only conversion of a negative to a positive reaction. Restoration of skin reactivity can take place in only 1 week, so that retesting 1 week after the first negative reaction can usually show whether or not there is potential for the booster reaction. (The 1-week interval would in most cases not be long enough for true conversion in persons with their first infection.) Repeated skin tests will not cause a nonexposed person to develop a positive reaction. Some investigators recommend skin testing with antigens used to demonstrate the presence of skin test anergy (e.g., *Candida* or *Trichophyton* antigen) if the Mantoux test is repeatedly negative in a person with substantial suspicion of mycobacterial infection.

The standard procedure for skin testing is to begin with an intermediate strength PPD (or the equivalent). If the person has serious infection, some clinics recommend starting with a first-strength dose to avoid necrosis at the injection site. A significant minority of patients with tuberculosis (9%–17%) fail to react to intermediate strength PPD; a second-strength dose is then indicated.

Miliary Tuberculosis

Miliary tuberculosis (TB) is clinically active TB that is widely disseminated in the body by hematogenous spread. Clinical symptoms are often nonspecific, such as fever, weakness, and malaise. There frequently is an associated condition, such as alcoholism, intravenous (IV) drug abuse, or malignancy, that decreases immunologic defenses. About 20% have a negative tuberculin skin test reaction. About 35% do not show a miliary pattern on chest x-ray film. If routine clinical and culture methods fail, biopsy of bone marrow or liver may be useful. Liver biopsy has a fairly good positive yield (up to 80%), considering that a needle biopsy specimen is such a tiny random sample of a huge organ. However, it is usually difficult to demonstrate acid-fast organisms on liver biopsy even when tubercles are found, and without organisms the diagnosis is not absolutely certain. Bone marrow aspiration is probably the best procedure in such cases. Bone marrow yields much better results for mycobacterial culture than for demonstration of tubercles. Routine marrow (Wright-stained) smears are worthless for histologic diagnosis in TB. Aspirated material may be allowed to clot in the syringe, then formalin-fixed and processed as a regular biopsy specimen for histologic study. Before clotting, some of the aspirate is inoculated into a suitable TB culture medium. It should be emphasized that bone marrow aspiration or liver biopsy is not indicated in pulmonary tuberculosis (since this disease is relatively localized), only in miliary TB.

Renal Tuberculosis

Renal TB is almost always bilateral and presumably results from nonhealing infection produced during the transient bacteremia of the lung primary stage. There is usually a latent period of many years before clinical infection becomes evident. The estimated incidence of eventual active renal infection is about 2%–5%, but this probably represents incidence in high-risk groups. About 25% (range, 20%–75%) of patients are said to have a normal chest x-ray film. About 14% (range, 12%–15%) of patients are reported to have a negative purified protein derivative (PPD) skin test result. Even the intravenous pyelogram results (IVP) are normal in about 25% (range, 14%–39%) of cases. Most patients do not have systemic symptoms, such as fever. The erythrocyte sedimentation rate was elevated in 23% of patients in one report. Only 20%–56% have urinary tract symptoms. Gross hematuria is the classic finding in renal TB but is present in only about 20% of patients. Pyuria (with negative urine culture) and microscopic hematuria are more frequent, occurring in about 65%–85% of cases. Some patients have a positive urine culture with some ordinary pathogen in addition to renal TB. Urine culture for TB was mentioned previously; 30%–80% of patients have positive cultures when three 24–hour or early morning specimens are collected (true culture sensitivity is probably less than 80%, since the diagnosis could easily be missed with negative cultures).

NONTUBERCULOUS MYCOBACTERIA

There are other mycobacteria besides *Mycobacterium tuberculosis*, some of which are frequently pathogenic for humans and some of which rarely cause human infection. The nontuberculous mycobacteria were originally called "atypical mycobacteria." The first useful classification was that of Runyon, who subdivided the nontuberculous mycobacteria into four groups, depending on growth speed and colony characteristics (Table 14–3). These groups have some clinical value as rough guides to the type of organism present while awaiting more definitive identification and speciation. It is desirable to place the organisms in the correct species, since some members (species) of any of the Runyon groups may not be pathogenic very often or may differ in degree of pathogenicity. *Mycobacterium intracellulare* or *Mycobacterium avium-intracellulare* complex (formerly known as the Battey *Mycobacterium*), a member of Runyon group III, and *Mycobacterium kansasii*, from Runyon group I, together cause the majority of significant nontuberculous mycobacterial infections in about equal proportions. These organisms produce a disease similar to pulmonary tuberculosis (although often milder or more indolent) that is much more frequent in adults. *Mycobacterium avium-intracellulare* infections are very frequent in persons with acquired immunodeficiency syndrome (AIDS) or AIDS-related conditions. The mycobacterial infection frequently becomes bacteremic or disseminated due to compromise of the immune system by the human immunodeficiency virus, type I (HIV I) causing AIDS. Runyon group II organisms are more frequent in children and clinically tend to cause cervical lymphadenopathy. Diagnosis of the nontuberculous mycobacteria is essentially the same as for *M. tuberculosis*. Skin tests (old tuberculin or PPD) for *M. tuberculosis* will also cross-react with the nontuberculous my-

TABLE 14–3.

Classification of the Atypical Mycobacteria

Group I	Photochromogens	(*Mycobacterium kansasii* and others)
Group II	Scotochromogens	(*Mycobacterium scrofulaceum* and others)
Group III	Nonphotochromogens	(*Mycobacterium intracellulare* [*avium-intracellulare complex*] and others)
Group IV	Rapid growers	(*Mycobacterium fortuitum* and others)

cobacteria. In general, the nontuberculous mycobacteria tend to produce less reaction to standard tuberculin skin tests than *M. tuberculosis*. In fact, several studies claim that the majority of positive intermediate-strength tuberculin skin test results that produce a reaction of less than 10 mm diameter are due to nontuberculous mycobacterial infection rather than tuberculosis. Skin test antigens are available for each of the nontuberculous mycobacterial groups, although some reports challenge the specificity of these preparations. The main clinical importance of these nontuberculous organisms is resistance that many have toward one or more of the standard antituberculous chemotherapeutic agents.

OTHER BACTERIA OF MEDICAL IMPORTANCE

Corynebacteria

These organisms are gram-positive aerobic rods of varying length, frequently arranged on smear in sheafs (palisades) or Chinese letter–type configurations. The most important member of this genus is ***Corynebacterium diphtheriae***, which causes diphtheria. Infection usually becomes established in the pharynx. *Corynebacterium diphtheriae* produces a toxin that affects the heart and peripheral nerves. There is also necrosis of the infected epithelium, with formation of a pseudomembrane of fibrin, necrotic cells, and neutrophils. The disease is now uncommon, but cases appear from time to time, some of them fatal. Contrary to usual belief, the laboratory cannot make the diagnosis from Gram-stained smears. Heat-fixed smears stained with methylene blue are better, but, although helpful in demonstrating organisms resembling diphtheria, they still are not reliable enough for definite morphologic diagnosis. Nonpathogenic diphtheroids are normal nasopharyngeal inhabitants and may look very much like *C. diphtheriae*. To be certain, one must culture the organisms on special Loeffler's media and do virulence (toxin production) studies. Nevertheless, direct Gram-stained and methylene blue smears are of value, since other causes of pharyngeal inflammation and pseudomembrane formation, such as fungus and Vincent's angina, can be demonstrated. Therefore, two or three pharyngeal swabs should be obtained, if possible, for smears and for cultures. About 20% of cases will be missed if specimens for culture are not obtained from the nasopharynx as well as the pharynx.

Certain nondiphtheritic species of *Corynebacterium* are called **diphtheroids.** These are normal skin and nasopharyngeal inhabitants and appear rather frequently in cultures as contaminants. However, on occasion diphtheroids may produce endocarditis or urinary tract infection, usually in persons with decreased resistance to infection. Various aerobic and anaerobic gram-positive rods such as *Propionibacterium, Lactobacillus,* and *Listeria,* morphologically resemble corynebacteria on Gram stain and are frequently included together in the name diphtheroids without being further identified.

Chlamydiae

Chlamydiae (formerly called bedsoniae) are tiny coccobacillary organisms classified as bacteria because they have a cell wall, are capable of protein synthesis, contain both DNA and RNA, and can reproduce by fission. On the other hand, they have some features of a virus in that they are obligate cell parasites, they cannot synthesize adenosine triphosphate (ATP), and must depend on host cell metabolic processes for energy, and they cannot be grown on artificial laboratory media, only in living cells.

There are two species of *Chlamydia*. One is *Chlamydia psittaci*, the etiologic agent of psitticosis in birds and humans. The other is *Chlamydia trachomatis*. *Chlamydia trachomatis* includes several serotypes that can be placed into three groups. One group causes lymphogranuloma venereum, a venereal disease. A second group causes the eye disease known as trachoma, and the third group produces genital tract and certain other infections, the genital infections being different from lymphogranuloma venereum.

Psitticosis.—*Chlamydia psittaci* produces psitticosis in humans through contact with infected birds, most often parakeets, or as an occupational disease from infected turkeys in the poultry-processing industry. Only a few cases are reported each year in the United States. There are two types of clinical illness: a respiratory type resembling "atypical" pneumonia and a much less common typhoid-like illness. The respiratory type is characterized by headache, chills, fever, and nonproductive or poorly productive cough. There may be myalgias, arthralgias, gastrointestinal (GI) tract symptoms, bradycardia, and changes in mental status. Splenomegaly is found in many patients. The white blood cell (WBC) count is normal or slightly decreased. There are various patterns of lung infiltrates on chest x-ray film, although the most typical are patchy lower lobe infiltrates radiating from the hilar areas. Diagnosis can be made by culture, although this is rarely done since tissue culture is required. Diagnosis is usually made by serologic testing of acute- and convalescent-stage serum.

Lymphogranuloma Venereum.—*Chlamydia trachomatis* produces a distinctive venereal disease known as lymphogranuloma venereum, which is transmitted through sexual intercourse. After an incubation period, the inguinal lymph nodes become swollen and tender in males; in females, the lymphatic drainage is usually to the intra-abdominal, perirectal, and pelvic lymph nodes. In a considerable number of cases, the perirectal nodes develop abscesses, and the nearby wall of the rectum is involved, eventually leading to scar tissue and constriction of the rectum. In either male or female, in the acute stage of lymphatic involvement there may be fever, malaise, headache, and sometimes joint aching, but all of these may be absent. In the majority of cases the main findings are acute inguinal node enlargement in the male and chronic rectal stricture in the female.

Laboratory Findings and Diagnosis.—Laboratory findings in active disease include mild anemia, moderate leukocytosis, and serum protein hypoalbuminemia and hypergammaglobulinemia. On serum protein electrophoresis the gamma-globulin fraction is often considerably elevated without the homogeneous sharp spikelike configuration of monoclonal protein. Similar polyclonal configurations can be found in granulomatous diseases such as TB or sarcoidosis, in some patients with cirrhosis, and in some patients with rheumatoid-collagen disease.

Laboratory diagnosis is usually made through a complement fixation (CF) serologic test. The CF reaction becomes positive about 1 month after infection and remains elevated for years. There is also a microimmunofluorescence serologic test that is said to be more sensitive than CF. Acute and convalescent serum specimens should be obtained to demonstrate a rising titer. Relatively low positive CF titers (up to 1:64) may occur in persons with genital tract infections due to serotypes or strains of *C. trachomatis* that do not cause lymphogranuloma venereum. Also, the test cross-reacts with psittacosis, although this is usually not a problem. It is possible to aspirate affected lymph nodes for culture (although tissue culture is required) and for smears with Giemsa stain or immunofluorescent stains, although reports indicate that positive results are obtained in less than one third of the cases. At one time a skin test known as the Frei test was the mainstay of diagnosis, but the antigen is no longer commercially available. Lymph node biopsy shows a characteristic histologic pattern, which, however, is also seen in tularemia and cat-scratch fever. Lymphogranuloma venereum is associated with a relatively high incidence of syphilis serology biologic false positive reactions. This may be difficult to interpret, because syphilis must be suspected in any patient with venereal disease, and early syphilis can produce inguinal lymph node enlargement similar to that caused by lymphogranuloma venereum.

Chlamydial Urethritis and Endocervicitis.—*Chlamydia trachomatis* also produces urethral and genital infections that differ clinically from lymphogranuloma venereum and are associated with different organism serotypes. *Chlamydia trachomatis* is reported to cause about 50% (range, 30%–60%) of nongonococcal urethritis in men. Several studies of clinically normal sexually active men not at high risk for venereal disease report asymptomatic chlamydial infection rates of about 10% (range, 5%–26%). About one third of male urethral chlamydial infection is asymptomatic. In some geographic areas or patient populations the incidence of nongonococcal urethritis is two–three times that of gonorrhea. Patients with gonococcal infection also have chlamydial infection in 20%–30% of cases; and about 70% of cases of postgonococcal urethritis have been attributed to *Chlamydia*. The urethral discharge in nongonococcal urethritis is usually less purulent than the discharge produced by gonorrhea. *Chlamydia trachomatis* has been found in 40%–50% (range, 6%–69%) of patients with Reiter's syndrome. Finally, male sexual consorts of women who have chlamydial cervicitis or chlamydial pelvic inflammatory disease (PID) are themselves infected by *Chlamydia* in 25%–50% of cases.

Chlamydiae can infect the female urethra and also the endocervix. Exact incidence in the normal population is unknown, but it has been cultured from the endocervix in about 10% (range, 2%–30%) of asymptomatic women not thought to have venereal disease, 8%–26% of girls attending adolescent clinics, 6%–23% of women attending contraception clinics, and in 20%–30% (or more) of women seen in venereal disease clinics. Up to two thirds of female cervical infection by *Chlamydia* are asymptomatic. Patients with PID have a 20%–30% rate of chlamydial recovery from the endocervix and from the fallopian tubes or pelvic abscesses. About 40% of gonococcal infections also have chlamydial infection. *Chlamydia* is also reported to be a major cause for culture-negative female dysuria with frequent urination (acute urethral syndrome), described earlier in this chapter. Finally, female sexual consorts of men who have proven chlamydial urethritis are themselves infected by *Chlamydia* in up to 70% of cases. If the male consort has gonorrhea, female infection rate for *Chlamydia* is about 35%; if the male has nongonococcal urethritis, the female will have chlamydial infection in 30%–40% of cases.

Diagnosis.—Diagnosis of *C. trachomatis* urethritis or cervicitis has been attempted in several ways. Culture (McCoy cell tissue culture) is still considered the gold standard. In males, a thin nasopharyngeal-type calcium alginate swab is inserted 3–4 cm into the urethra. In females, *Chlamydia* infects only the columnar and squamocolumnar cervical cells, so that endocervical specimens produce maximum isolation rates, whereas vaginal specimens are not recommended. Gently cleaning the endocervical canal with a swab before taking the specimen is reported to decrease cell culture contamination and increase positive results. Obtaining two swabs instead of one is reported to increase positive yield as much as 45%. Immediately after the specimen is obtained, special transport media should be inoculated with the swabs. A recently available specimen collection brush (Cytobrush) is claimed to considerably increase the number of columnar cells and thereby increase satisfactory cultures or direct smears. Sensitivity of culture is estimated to be about 80%–90%. Recently, several manufacturers have marketed kits for direct fluorescent antibody (FA) detection of *Chlamydia* organisms within infected cells, using the same specimens obtained for culture applied directly to a slide or microtiter wells. This permits same-day results without many of the technical problems of tissue culture. Only two of these (FA) systems have had reasonably adequate evaluation. Their sensitivity has averaged about 80%–85% (for one of these, the range has been 60%–96%) compared to culture (since culture sensitivity is not 100%, true sensitivity of the FA methods is less than the stated figures). Specificity has averaged 97%–98%. Two other kits have manufacturer's claims of 96% sensitivity compared to culture. Some investigators recommend that the direct tests not be used on low-prevalence (< 10% incidence) populations, since in that patient group, although the percentage of false positive test results is low, in terms of the number of patients the false positive results become too high. In addition, the percentage of false positive and negative results using FA methods would probably be higher in ordinary laboratories compared to research laboratories.

Other Chlamydial Infections

About 5%–10% (range, 2%–25%) of pregnant women have *Chlamydia* infestation of the cervix. Fifty percent to 60% of infants born to these infected mothers acquire *Chlamydia* infection or colonization during birth. Of these, about 30%–40% (range, 18%–50%) develop chlamydial conjunctivitis, with onset about 1–3 weeks after birth; and about 10%–15% (range, 3%–20%) develop chlamydial pneumonia, with onset about 4–12 weeks after birth. According to some reports, chlamydial infection causes 25%–80% of infant conjunctivitis and about 30% of infant pneumonia. Diagnosis can be made by culture or FA methods from swab material obtained from the posterior nasopharynx, similar to specimens for pertussis. Special transport media are necessary for culture specimens. In possible chlamydial conjunctivitis, culture specimens can be obtained or smears can be made from conjunctival scrapings. Purulent material should be wiped off before scrapings or cultures are obtained since the organisms are found in conjunctival epithelial cells and not in the inflammatory cells of the exudate. Giemsa-stained smears have been used for many years but are difficult to interpret and detect only about 25%–40%.

Trachoma.—Finally, *C. trachomatis* produces trachoma, a serious eye disease that is endemic to North Africa, the Middle East, and Southeast Asia. The conjunctiva is infected and becomes scarred. The cornea is eventually invaded by granulation tissue and is destroyed. Diagnosis usually is made from Giemsa-stained smears of conjunctival scrapings. The infected cells contain cytoplasmic inclusion bodies. However, results of only about one half of the cases are positive. Immunofluorescent techniques applied to the smears produce positive results in about 85% of cases. McCoy cell culture detects about 95% of cases.

Mycoplasmas

Mycoplasmas are similar to bacteria in most respects and can be grown on artificial media. However, they lack a cell wall and are smaller than bacteria. There are several genera in the Mycoplasmataceae family. One of these is *Ureaplasma*, which contains a species, *Ureaplasma urealyticum* (formerly known as T mycoplasma) that has been cultured from the urethra of both sexes and the genital organs of females in a substantial number of clinically normal persons. The incidence of positive cultures is increased (50%–70% of cases) in persons seen in venereal disease clinics. It is thought that *U. urealyticum* is an important cause of nongonococcal urethritis in men.

Another genus has the name of *Mycoplasma* and contains two species associated with human disease, *Mycoplasma hominis* and *Mycoplasma pneumoniae*. *Mycoplasma hominis*, like *U. urealyticum*, is a normal inhabitant of the male and female urethra and female genital organs. In addition, it is found in the oropharynx of both sexes. The role of *M. hominis* in nongonococcal urethritis is not clear, but it currently is not thought to produce many cases, if any. There is more evidence for occasional involvement in female PID.

Mycoplasma pneumoniae.—*Mycoplasma pneumoniae* (formerly called Eaton agent, pleuropneumonia-like organism) is the etiologic agent of a lower respiratory tract infection formerly called *primary atypical pneumonia*. Some investigators report that *Mycoplasma* caused 20%–25% of all cases of community-acquired pneumonia in their area. Older children and young adults are most likely to be affected. Most cases appear as an upper respiratory infection of varying severity. If pneumonia develops, it is usually preceded by headache, fever, and malaise. Sore throat or chills occur in 30%–50% of patients, and GI symptoms or earache in a lesser number. After 2–4 days there is onset of a nonproductive or poorly productive cough. Chest x-ray typically shows lower lobe mottled infiltrates that are most pronounced in the hilar region and that are most often unilateral. However, in some cases other abnormalities develop. Despite the symptoms and chest x-ray findings there is characteristically little abnormality on physical examination.

Laboratory Findings and Diagnosis.—White blood cell counts are usually normal, although about 25% of affected persons have mild leukocytosis (between 10,000 and 15,000/cu mm; 10–15 × 10^9/L). An unusually severe case may produce more abnormal results. Several modalities are available for diagnosis. **Culture** can be done using sputum or nasopharyngeal swabs. *Mycoplasma pneumoniae* is very sensitive to drying, so the swab must be placed immediately in a special transport medium. Special culture media is required, and most laboratories must send the specimen to a reference laboratory. Such specimens should be frozen and transported with dry ice. Growth takes about 2 weeks (range, 1–3 weeks). In one university laboratory, isolation rates ranged from 0%–43% at various times, so that culture does not seem very helpful. **Cold agglutinins** are elevated in 50%–60% of patients. Cold agglutinins are antibodies that are able to agglutinate type O human blood cells at refrigerator temperatures but not at room temperature. They are found in other diseases and thus are nonspecific; but in adults with an acute respiratory syndrome, their presence in significant titer is usually associated with mycoplasmal pneumonia. Cold agglutinin titers elevated more than 1:32 are abnormal and can be found during the second week of illness, reaching a peak in the third or fourth week. A rising titer is more significant than a single determination.

Serologic tests are the most common method of diagnosis. Mycoplasmal CF test results are abnormal in 55%–70% of cases. Antibody becomes detectable during the second week of illness and peaks in the fourth week. Immunofluorescent methods for antibody detection are replacing the cumbersome and time-consuming CF technique. Immunofluorescent methods that can detect either IgM or IgG antimycoplasmal antibodies are available. The presence of IgM antibodies, especially if present in high titer, usually means acute or recent infection. Immunoglobulin G antibodies rise later than IgM antibodies and persist much longer. However, since a negative IgM result could be obtained before antibodies have appeared, and since a low IgM titer could mean either beginning or ending of the IgM response, it is still useful to obtain two serum specimens with a 1-week interval between the first and the second. This is also helpful with IgG antibodies, since low levels of mycoplasmal IgG antibodies are frequent in the general population. Finally, one company has recently marketed a nucleic acid (DNA) probe method for *Mycoplasma* that can be applied directly to throat swab specimens, can be performed the same day, and is claimed to give 100% correlation with culture. Drawbacks are high cost (very high if only one patient specimen is processed at a time), plus possible low sensitivity if detection rates are no better than culture.

Actinomyces

The genus *Actinomyces* contains several species, of which *Actinomyces israelii* is the most important. This is a gram-positive filamentous branching bacterium that segments into reproductive bacillary fragments. The organism prefers anaerobic conditions with increased carbon dioxide, but some strains are microaerophilic. *Actinomyces israelii* produces actinomycosis, a chronic internal abscess-forming infection that characteristically develops sinus tracts to the skin. There typically is a purulent exudate containing small yellow granules, called *sulfur granules,* which are masses of actinomycetes. Actinomycetes are normal inhabitants of the human oropharynx. Most infections occur in the neck and chest, but infection may occur elsewhere. Several reports indicate a linkage between pelvic infection by *A. israelii* (which ordinarily is not common) and intrauterine contraceptive devices (IUDs). It has been reported that 5%–10% of asymptomatic IUD users and 40% of IUD users with pelvic infection demonstrate *A. israelii* on vaginal smear. Culture has not been very successful in isolating the organisms, at least not culture of vaginal specimens. Sulfur granules are rare in vaginal smears. Fluorescent antibody studies on vaginal smears have been more reliable than Papanicolaou cytology smears, although some cytology experts have a high success rate.

Laboratory diagnosis of nonvaginal actinomycosis consists of Gram stain and acid-fast stain on smears of purulent material containing sulfur granules. The granules should be crushed and smeared. Gram-positive filaments without spores could be either actinomycetes or *Nocardia* asteroides. *Nocardia* is acid fast, whereas *Actinomyces* is not. When material for smear or culture is obtained, special precautions should be taken to avoid contamination by normal oropharyngeal or skin bacteria, which may include nonpathogenic *Actinomyces* species. *Actinomyces israelii* can be cultured under anaerobic conditions using ordinary anaerobic media. If thioglycollate is used, it should be the enriched type and should be incubated in an increased carbon dioxide atmosphere. Rarely, staphylococci or *Pseudomonas* bacteria may produce infection with formation of sulfur granules, a condition known as *botryomycosis.*

Actinomyces was originally thought to be a fungus, and actinomycosis has many clinical characteristics of a deep fungal infection. Actinomycosis is often included in the differential diagnosis of fungal diseases.

Nocardia

The genus *Nocardia* has similarities to *Actinomyces,* since the members of both genera are gram-positive filamentous branching bacteria that segment into reproductive bacillary fragments. However, *Nocardia* is aerobic rather than anaerobic, is weakly acid-fast, and usually does not form sulfur granules. The organisms are saprophytes and are found in soil, grasses, grains, straw, and decaying organic matter. The major pathogenic species (80%–90% of *Nocardia* infections) is *Nocardia asteroides.* The human infections produced are primary skin lesions (mycetomas), very uncommon in the United States, and visceral infections. Of the visceral infections, the lungs are involved in 60%–80% of cases, and the brain is affected in 20%–40%. In the lung, the most common disease produced is focal pneumonia, which often progresses to abscess formation (frequently multiple). However, various x-ray findings have been reported. Pulmonary nocardiosis frequently resembles TB. Occasionally the infection becomes disseminated. There is no preexisting disease in about 25%–35% of cases (range, 15%–71%). About 25% are associated with malignancy (range, 0%–48%). Some series found association with some type of immunosuppression in 50% or more (chronic infection, TB, steroids, diabetes, AIDS, etc.). *Nocardia braziliensis* is the most common cause of the chronic focal skin and subcutaneous infection known as *mycetoma*.

Culture is the usual method of diagnosis. The organism grows on various media. However, colonies may take 3 days or more to appear so that cultures on ordinary bacteria media may be discarded before being detected. If cultures are placed on mycobacterial culture media, *Nocardia* may be mistaken for a rapid-growing nontuberculous *Mycobacterium*. The weak acid-fast stain reaction may reinforce this impression.

BACTERIA ASSOCIATED WITH CONTAMINATION OF SPECIMENS

Certain bacteria that ordinarily are nonpathogenic (such as normal inhabitants of certain areas; see Table 36–11) frequently appear in cultures and are traditionally considered contaminants, presumably introduced by faulty culture technique. The major species are *Staphylococcus epidermidis* and the diphtheroids. Occasionally there are others, such as *Bacillus subtilis*. However, under certain circumstances, especially when the patient is immunocompromised, these organisms may produce disease. Three or more species of bacteria appearing in culture from ordinarily sterile areas (e.g., blood, spinal fluid, body cavity fluid, urine without a long-term indwelling catheter) suggest contamination. However, true polymicrobial infections may occur.

Bacterial Species Omitted.—Discussion of bacterial infections in this chapter has been limited to the common organisms in clinical practice and a few that enter the differential diagnosis of certain common situations, such as hepatitis or fever of unknown origin. Many others have been omitted, such as *Hemophilus ducreyi*, which produces the venereal disease chancroid, and *Borrelia spirilis*, which causes relapsing fever. In general, most are diagnosed through culture of appropriate specimens. The reader is referred to standard textbooks on microbiology for additional information on these organisms.

GENERAL ISOLATION AND IDENTIFICATION TECHNIQUES

It is useful to know certain technical information involved with isolation and identification of bacteria. This information may improve physician understanding of the microbiology laboratory, to the mutual benefit of physician and laboratory.

If a culture is ordered, it usually takes at least 48 hours, and often longer, for definitive diagnosis—1 day to culture the organism and 1 day to identify it. Sometimes an additional day must be used to isolate the organism if it is present in a mixed culture. One additional day may be needed for antibiotic sensitivities. A technologist uses knowledge of the site and source of culture material in deciding what media or techniques (e.g., anaerobic conditions) to use for isolation. Some organisms are normal inhabitants of certain body areas but pathogens in other areas, so an experienced technologist knows to some extent what to subculture from a mixture of organisms growing in a specific location and also what special media to use for the pathogens usual in that anatomical location. This knowledge can easily save 1 day's time. Information that a certain specific organism is suspected may save even more time by permitting original inoculation of the culture material into special test media. Even if definitive isolation is not yet accomplished, the technologist can often provide useful information or even a presumptive diagnosis. For example, among the enteric gram-negative rods, *Escherichia coli*, *Enterobacter*, and *Klebsiella* ferment lactose, whereas most of the other pathogens do not. Therefore, a lactose fermenter cannot be *Salmonella* or *Shigella*. *Pseudomonas*, in addition, does not ferment glucose, whereas most of the other pathogens do. Some organisms have a fairly characteristic appearance on isolation media. For example, it may be possible to make a rapid presumptive diagnosis for some of the gram-positive aerobic bacteria based on their appearance on original blood agar culture plates combined with their Gram stain morphology.

OBTAINING A SPECIMEN FOR CULTURE

After material has been taken for culture, three steps should be followed. First, the specimen must be taken to the laboratory as soon as possible, since many organisms die on prolonged exposure to air or drying. This is especially true for swab preparations. Swab kits are available that contain a carrier medium into which the specimen is placed. This is a great help in preserving most bacteria, but the medium is not ideal for all organisms. For example, gonococci or anaerobes must have special transport systems. Anaerobic specimens require special precautions when the specimen is obtained and during transport to the laboratory. Second, the source of the culture should be written on the request sheet. This tells the laboratory what normal flora organisms are to be expected and provides some information on the pathogens that should be looked for and thus what media should be used. Finally, if a specific organism is suspected, this information should also be written on the request, so that if special culture methods are required, the requisite techniques will be anticipated and used.

URINE CULTURE

Contamination of urine specimens by vaginal or labial bacteria is a serious problem. The most reliable way to obtain the specimen, especially in young children, is by suprapubic puncture and aspiration of the bladder with a needle and syringe. However, this technique has never become popular. Catheterization is another way to solve the difficulty, but approximately 2% of patients are reported to develop urinary tract infection following a single catheterization. A midstream "clean-catch" voided specimen is the third best procedure. The urinary opening is cleansed. The labia are held apart in the female and the foreskin pulled back in the male. The first portion of urine is allowed to pass uncollected, then the sterile container is quickly introduced into the urine stream to catch the specimen.

Quantitative urine cultures have now replaced simple cultures, since it has been generally accepted that a titer of 100,000 (10^5) or more organisms/ml has excellent correlation with clinical infection, whereas a titer of less than 1,000 (10^3) organisms/ml is usually not significant. However, there are certain important reservations and exceptions to this commonly accepted statement. The original studies that established this concept were performed on nonsymptomatic women using clean-catch urine collection. In addition, it was found that a single urine specimen collected this way that contained more than 100,000 organisms/ml had only an 80% chance of representing true infection (i.e., there was a 20% chance that the specimen was contaminated). Two consecutive urine specimens containing more than 100,000 organisms/ml had a 95% chance of indicating true infection. If the patient is receiving antibiotics or if the specimen is obtained by catheterization, many authorities accept a colony count of 1,000 or more organisms/ml as significant. If the specimen is obtained by suprapubic puncture or by cystoscopy, any growth at all is considered significant. If the patient has symptoms of urinary tract infection (fever, chills, flank pain, and pyuria), many authorities are willing to accept a clean-catch specimen colony count of 1,000 or more organisms/ml as significant even if the patient is not taking antibiotics. Not all patients with symptoms of urinary tract infection have colony counts over 1,000 organisms, because some females who have dysuria and frequency have urethritis (acute urethral syndrome, discussed earlier) rather than cystitis. About 20%–30% of these cases of urethritis are due to *Chlamydia trachomatis,* which does not grow on standard urine culture media. There is also the possibility that some cases could be chlamydial in origin but that the urine culture becomes contaminated with other bacteria, which leads to a false impression of cystitis. Finally, in some cases of pyelonephritis there are few or intermittent symptoms, and the urine cultures may be consistently negative, intermittently positive, or contain relatively low numbers of organisms. If there is a strong suspicion of pyelonephritis, repeat cultures may be necessary if the initial culture is negative or equivocal.

Use of the quantitative (titer) technique with a cutoff level of 100,000 organisms/ml is supposed to compensate for small degrees of unavoidable contamination, but contamination can easily be severe enough to give a positive result. Various studies using midstream specimens have shown a surprisingly high rate of contamination in the female. In my experience, a microscopic examination of centrifuged specimen sediment in which more than 10 squamous epithelial cells per low-power field (10 × ocular, 10 × objective) are demonstrated suggests possible contamination. Three or more species of bacteria isolated from the same urine specimen also suggests contamination if the patient is not on long-term indwelling catheter drainage. All available information emphasizes that good technique in collecting the specimen is essential. Also essential is getting the specimen to the laboratory as soon as possible after collection. Urine is an excellent culture medium, and specimens that stand for more than 1 hour at room temperature permit bacterial incubation and proliferation to the point that quantitative counts are not reliable. If delivery to the laboratory must be delayed, the specimen should be refrigerated. The specimen can be preserved up to 12 hours in a refrigerator (4°C).

Quantitative urine culture has two other drawbacks. Culture involves trained technical personnel and relatively expensive media, thus curtailing use for mass screening to detect urinary tract infection. Culture takes 24 hours to determine bacterial quantity and another 24–48 hours to identify the organism, thus delaying treatment in suspected infection.

Screening Tests For Bacteriuria

Because of the delay inherent in culture methods, several screening tests for rapid detection of significant degrees of bacteriuria have been introduced. If organisms are seen on Gram stain of uncentrifuged urine, reports indicate about 93% (range, 88%–95%) probability of a positive (100,000 organisms/ml) quantitative culture. The same is said to be true of direct examination of unstained centrifuged urine sediment. Gram-stained centrifuged sediment apparently gives too many false positive results. Gram-stained uncentrifuged urine and unstained urine sediment examination are said to give relatively few false positive results. Microscopic examination of centrifuged urine sediment to detect pyuria (increased number of WBCs) is widely used to screen for urinary tract infection. However, pyuria is found in only about 70%–80% (range, 13%–93%) of patients with positive urine cultures, and about 30% (range, 2%–40%) of patients with pyuria do not have a positive urine culture. Leukocyte esterase dipsticks have been used as a substitute for microscopic examination. They are positive in about 80%–90% (range, 72%–98%) of patients with a positive culture. Some urine test dipsticks have both the leukocyte esterase and a biochemical nitrite test; if results of both are positive, this detects 85%–90% (range, 78%–100%) of positive results from culture. Several chemical methods have been advocated. The most successful include the triphenyl tetrazolium chloride (TTC) test, the Greiss nitrate test (previously mentioned), and the catalase test. Best results have been reported with the TTC test. Nevertheless, reports vary as to its accuracy, with a range of 70%–90% correlation with quantitative culture, including both false positive and false negative results. The Greiss nitrate test detects about 55% (range, 35%–69%) of cases with a positive culture. The catalase test is even less reliable. Finally, there are several other bacteriuria screening systems now available, and more keep appearing. The Marion Laboratories Bac-T-Screen filters the urine, trapping any bacteria on the filter, which is then stained to reveal presence of bacteria. Sensitivity (compared to culture) is reported to be about 93% (range, 88%–99%). However, false positive results are about 29% (range, 16%–55%). Two companies market tests using firefly luciferase (bioluminescence) that reacts with bacterial ATP. Three companies market automated screening instruments, two detecting turbidity produced by bacterial growth (Autobac and MS-2 systems) and one (AMS system) scanning a multiwell card containing various test media. Results from all of these systems are similar to those of the Bac-T-Screen. The advantages of these systems are that negative test results suggest that culture would not be necessary. Results are available the same day. Drawbacks are that positive test results by any of these methods must be followed by quantitative culture (except possibly the AMS system). False positive test results are relatively frequent, and negative test results do not completely rule out urinary tract infection (especially since the sensitivity figures quoted earlier are for 100,000 organisms/ml, and detection rates become less if bacterial numbers are less).

Drawbacks of Urine Quantitative Culture

In summary, although quantitative culture with a cutoff titer value of 100,000 organisms/ml is widely considered the most reliable index of urinary tract infection, there are several major limitations:

1. Using a titer of 100,000 organisms/ml as the cutoff point for a positive culture decision eliminates specimens with low-grade contamination but does not identify those with greater degrees of contamination.
2. The cutoff point of 100,000 organisms/ml does not apply to catheterized or suprapubic aspiration specimens and may be misleading if used to interpret them.
3. There are circumstances in which fewer than 100,000 organisms/ml may be significant in clean-catch specimens.
4. A positive culture does not reveal which area of the urinary tract is involved.
5. Tuberculosis of the urinary tract, anaerobic infections, and chlamydial infections of the urethra give negative culture results on ordinary culture media.
6. Bacteremia from many causes, even if transient, involves organisms that are filtered by the kidney and may produce a temporarily positive quantitative culture result.
7. Some cases of urinary tract infection may give negative cultures at various times. In several studies, a sizable minority of patients required repeated cultures before one became positive. This may be due to the location of the infection in the kidney and to its degree of activity.

Therefore, two cautions are required when one is interpreting a urine culture report. If the results suggest that urinary tract infection is present, the physician must be certain that the specimen was properly collected, especially in the female. If the result is negative, this does not rule out chronic pyelonephritis. The problem of pyelonephritis and bacteriuria is also discussed in chapter 12.

Kits with agar-coated slides that not only yield quantitative urine culture results but also act as a culture medium for the organisms are now available. These are reported to have 90%–98% accuracy in various university hospital laboratories when compared with standard quantitative culture methods. The average is about 95% reliability. There is some question whether office laboratories can approach this figure and what provision would be made to identify the organisms.

SPUTUM CULTURE

The usefulness of sputum culture is controversial. This method of diagnosis has evoked the same spectrum of emotions and suffers from most of the same potential drawbacks as Gram stain of sputum. Various studies have demonstrated that either sputum or bronchoscopic specimens are frequently contaminated by upper respiratory tract bacteria. Some of the contaminants, such as *Staphylococcus aureus, Streptococcus pneumoniae, Haemophilus influenzae,* enteric gram-negative bacteria, and *Candida* organisms, are potential lower respiratory tract pathogens. In addition, bronchoscopy may introduce local anesthetic into the specimen. Transtracheal aspiration (insertion of a needle into the trachea) or direct needle aspiration of the lung has been shown to produce relatively uncontaminated specimens. However, these techniques have potential complications. Although there is general agreement on the possibility of contamination, there is difference of opinion in the literature on the possibility that sputum culture may sometimes fail to detect the bacteria responsible for pneumonia. The importance of a specimen from the lower respiratory tract rather than the mouth or nasopharynx must be reemphasized, especially in seriously ill, uncooperative, or mentally clouded patients. As mentioned previously, a "pure culture" or marked predominance of one organism enhances suspicion of pathogenicity.

Several studies have found that the number of squamous epithelial cells in sputum provides a useful index for degree of oropharyngeal contamination; the greater the number of squamous epithelial cells per low-power field (10 × microscope objective), the more likely to have significant degrees of contamination. There is some disagreement in the literature between 10 or 25 squamous epithelial cells per low-power field as the criterion cutoff number. Significant contamination strongly suggests that a new specimen should be collected with special attention given to obtaining true lower respiratory tract material with a minimum of oral contamination. Some investigators also quantitate the number of segmented neutrophils (WBCs) per low-power field; more than 25 suggests acute inflammation (however, this alone does not differentiate upper from lower respiratory tract origin).

GRAM STAIN

Gram staining provides a presumptive diagnosis and some indication of the organism involved without waiting for culture results. On occasion, Gram stain may reveal organisms that (for technical reasons) do not grow when cultured. Best information comes from areas that are normally sterile. Gram staining is considered a routine procedure for cerebrospinal fluid in possible meningitis, for urethral smears in possible venereal disease, and for material from abscesses or effusions. (This is especially true when anaerobes may be present. These may fail to grow, since "anaerobic" culture is often suboptimal, but the organisms might be seen on a Gram stain.) In certain other types of specimens, such as urine or stool, a Gram stain need not be done routinely but should be performed in special circumstances, such as on stool specimens when pseudomembranous enterocolitis is suspected or on urine specimens if quantitative culture is not available.

The Gram stain is controversial in several other areas. The most important example is sputum. One can find opinions in the literature on the usefulness of a sputum Gram stain ranging from "essential" to "worthless and misleading." One major problem is contamination by normal organisms from the mouth and nasopharynx. Certain pathogens, such as pneumococci or *S. aureus*, may be located in the upper respiratory tract of many clinically normal persons, and these may gain entry into the sputum. Similarly, upper respiratory tract colonization by enteric gram-negative organisms is relatively frequent in alcoholics and in patients who have been hospitalized for more than a few days. Another difficulty is occasional discovery of opportunist organisms in the lower respiratory tract, organisms not normally present but not apparently causing disease. Another problem is the morphologic similarity of pneumococci and streptococci, among others. Finally, and most important, the sputum sample may, in fact, be only saliva.

There are certain maneuvers that may help to circumvent some of these drawbacks. The number of organisms may provide a clue to their significance. Marked predominance or heavy growth of one organism suggests true abnormality. Many polymorphonuclear leukocytes is some evidence in favor of acute infection. Significant quantities of squamous epithelial cells (> 10 per low-power field) usually means oral contamination. The patient should be instructed how to produce a deep cough and, if possible, should be observed while he or she produces the specimen. In some cases aerosol therapy may be helpful.

MISCELLANEOUS CULTURE PROBLEMS

One controversial area in microbiology is the reliability of blood cultures drawn from an indwelling vascular catheter. Another is usefulness of catheter tip culture in diagnosis of bacteremia etiology. In general, investigators have encountered higher rates of contamination when drawing culture specimens from vascular catheters, due to colonization of the catheter tip or other areas of the apparatus, such as the stopcock or reservoir. Likewise, interpretation of a positive culture of a catheter tip is frequently difficult, since even if the same organism is isolated from the blood and from the catheter tip, the tip could be secondarily colonized from a bacteremia originating from some other source. Another problem area is surface cultures from decubitus ulcers and similar chronic open wounds. These generally yield a mixed flora. The Public Health Service Communicable Disease Center believes that little clinically relevant information will be obtained from chronic open surface lesions. If for some reason a culture is necessary, they recommend culture of a tissue biopsy from the base of the lesion rather than a surface swab culture.

FEBRILE AGGLUTININS

Febrile agglutinins are serologic tests for a group of unrelated infectious diseases that are sometimes responsible for so-called fever of unknown origin. They include typhoid and enteric (*Salmonella*) fever, certain rickettsial diseases, brucellosis, and tularemia. Since organisms causing these diseases are potential causes of fever of unknown origin, and since relatively simple slide agglutination serologic techniques are available for each, most laboratories automatically include the same selection of tests when febrile agglutinins are ordered. Typhoid or enteric (paratyphoid) fever may be caused by certain serotypes of the *Salmonella* species. The more common salmonellae are separated into groups on the basis of antigens prepared from these organisms; these antigens are used to detect antibodies in the patient's serum (Widal test). The groups are given a letter designation; for example, *Salmonella typhi* is included in *Salmonella* D (see Table 36–13). The Widal agglutination test involves antibodies produced to the somatic (O) and flagellar (H) antigens of *Salmonella* organisms. These antibodies appear approximately 7–10 days after onset of illness. Peak titers are reached between the 3rd and 4th weeks. In nonvaccinated individuals or most of those vaccinated more than 1 year previously, titers of 1:40 for the H antigen and 1:80 for the O antigen are suspicious; titers of 1:80 for the H antigen and 1:160 for the O antigen are definitely significant. However, recent (<1 year) vaccination may cause a greatly increased titer of either the O or the H antigen or both. The O antigen is more significant for diagnosis than the H antigen.

Most investigators today seriously question the usefulness of the Widal agglutination tests for typhoid or paratyphoid. Only about 65% (range, 58%–82%) of typhoid patients eventually reach a definitely abnormal titer of 1:160. False-positive elevations may occur due to cross-reaction with other *Salmonella* organisms in group D, are relatively frequent (20% in one series) in narcotics addicts, and possibly may occur due to cross-reaction in other conditions. Correlation of titers between laboratories on the same specimens have been rather poor. False negative results may be due to antibiotic therapy, inconsistent antibody formation in previously vaccinated persons, or specimens obtained before peak titer was reached.

Antibody-antigen agglutination tests for brucellosis and tularemia are also included. Again, titers of 1:80 are suspicious, and 1:160 are definitely abnormal. Antibodies appear 2–3 weeks after onset of the illness. Similar slide agglutination tests for rickettsia (Weil-Felix reaction) complete the febrile agglutinin battery. Interpretation of Weil-Felix results is discussed in chapter 16.

It is necessary to emphasize that negative febrile agglutinin test results or low titers do not rule out the diagnosis in any of these diseases. On the other hand, a single titer of 1:160 or more raises the suspicion of infection but is not conclusive. Only a fourfold rising titer can definitely confirm the diagnosis and prove acute infection. Unfortunately, for a variety of reasons, the fourfold rising titer is not easy to obtain (only 22% of typhoid patients in one series). Also, serologic tests obviously are not helpful in the early stage of the disease.

GENERAL CONCEPTS IN BACTERIAL INFECTION

The main systemic signs and symptoms of severe bacterial infection are fever and weakness. The most characteristic laboratory finding is leukocytosis, with an increase in number and immaturity of the neutrophils. However, in overwhelming infection, sometimes leukocytosis may be minimal or even absent, and occasionally fever may be minimal or may not be present. This is not frequent but happens more often in infants and the elderly. It also happens more frequently in debilitated persons, especially those with other severe diseases that may impair the ability of the body to respond normally to infection. Overwhelming infection may be focal, such as massive pneumonia, or generalized, such as septicemia.

SEPTICEMIA AND BACTEREMIA

The concept of septicemia should probably be separated from that of bacteremia, although in many studies the two are not clearly separated. In bacteremia, a few bacteria from a focal area of infection escape from time to time into the peripheral blood. However, the main focus remains localized, and symptoms are primarily those that are caused by infection in the particular organ or tissues involved. Bacteremia may occur without infection following certain procedures, such as dental extraction (18%–85%), periodontal surgery (32%–88%), tooth brushing (0%–26%), bronchoscopy (15%), tonsillectomy (28%–38%), upper GI endoscopy (8%–12%), sigmoidoscopy (0%–10%), urethral dilatation (18%–33%), cystoscopy (0%–17%), and prostate transurethral resection (12%–46%). In one representative series, *E. coli* was isolated in about 20% of patients with bacteremia; *S. aureus*, 10%; and *Klebsiella*, pneumococcus, *Streptococcus viridans*, *Bacteroides*, and *Pseudomonas*, about 6% each. The percentage of *S. epidermidis* isolates varies greatly (3%–34%), probably depending on how many were considered contaminants. Polymicrobial bacteremia is reported in about 7% of cases (range, 0.7%–17%). In septicemia there is widespread and relatively continuous peripheral blood involvement. The characteristic symptoms are systemic, such as marked weakness and shock or near shock. Shock has been reported in 16%–44% of patients with gram-negative bacteremia. These symptoms are usually accompanied by high fever and leukocytosis. However, septic patients may be afebrile in about 10% (range, 4%–18%) of cases. Leukocytosis is reported in about 60%–65% of patients (range, 42%–76%), bands are increased in about 70%–75% (range, 62%–84%), and total neutrophils are increased in about 75% (range, 66%–92%). Any bacteria may cause septicemia. More than one half of the cases are due to gram-negative rod organisms, with *E. coli* being the most frequent. *Staphylococcus aureus* probably is next most common. The portal of entry of the gram-negative organisms is usually from previous urinary tract infection. Many cases of septicemia follow surgery or instrumentation. The source of *Staphylococcus* septicemia is often very difficult to trace, even at autopsy. However, pneumonia and skin infections (sometimes very small) are the most frequent findings.

Diagnosis.—Blood cultures are the mainstay of septicemia diagnosis. Strict aseptic technique must be used when cultures are obtained, since contamination from skin bacteria may give false or confusing results. In cases of bacteremia or in septicemia with spiking fever, the best time to draw blood cultures is just before or at the rise in temperature. Three cultures, one drawn every 3 hours, are a reasonable compromise among the widely diverging recommendations in the literature.

Antibiotics and Blood Cultures.—Blood should be drawn for culture before antibiotic therapy is begun, although a substantial number of cultures are positive despite antibiotics. Certain antibiotic removal devices are commercially available that can be of considerable help in these patients. It is essential that the culture request contains the information that antibiotics have been given, unless they have been stopped for more than 1 week. If penicillin has been used, some laboratories add the antipenicillin enzyme penicillinase to the culture medium. However, others believe that penicillinase is of little value and might actually be a potential source of contamination.

INFECTIVE ENDOCARDITIS

Endocarditis is infection of one or more heart valves, although infection of mural thrombi is usually included. The disease used to be separated into two types, acute and subacute. The acute type was most often caused by *S. aureus*, usually affected a normal heart valve, and had a relatively short severe course. Other bacteria less frequently associated with acute endocarditis were *Streptococcus pyogenes*, *Streptococcus pneumoniae*, and *Neisseria gonorrheae*. The subacute type was most often caused by streptococci of the viridans group with the enterococci next in frequency, usually involved previously abnormal heart valves, and had a relatively protracted course of varying severity. However, there is considerable overlap of clinical symptoms and severity of disease between the acute and subacute groups, and infections that would fit into the acute group may occur on previously abnormal heart valves. Therefore, many experts now include both types of endocarditis within one term, infective endocarditis.

Predisposing Conditions.—Certain conditions predispose to infection of normal heart valves. Some examples are IV injection of drugs by drug abusers, indwelling vascular catheters or other devices, major surgical operations, and factors that decrease immunologic resistance. Conditions that create abnormal heart valves are congenital heart disease, rheumatic fever, atherosclerotic valve lesions, prosthetic heart valves, mitral valve prolapse, and nonbacterial valve thrombi. In addition to the same conditions that predispose to infection of normal valves, dental operations and urinary tract manipulation frequently precede development of infection on already abnormal valves.

Organisms Associated With Endocarditis.—Almost every pathogenic (and many relatively nonpathogenic) bacterium has been reported to cause infective endocarditis. Streptococci are the most frequent organisms (about 60%, range 50%–83%), with viridans group streptococci accounting for about 35% of all cases (range, 30%–52%); group D streptococci about 20%, and enterococci about 12% (range, 5%–20%). *Staphylococcus aureus* is isolated in about 20%–25% (range, 9%–33%) of cases. Coagulase-negative staphylococci are seen more frequently in association with intravascular catheters. When the patient has decreased resistance to infection (Table 14–4), fungi and bacteria that ordinarily are considered uncommonly pathogenic or nonpathogenic may become involved.

Clinical Findings.—Infective endocarditis falls about halfway between bacteremia and septicemia. Bacteria grow in localized areas on damaged heart valves and seed the peripheral blood; this may be infrequent, intermittent, or relatively continuous, with gradations between the two extremes. Classic signs and symptoms include fever, heart murmurs, petechial hemorrhages in the conjunctivae, small "splinter hemorrhages" in the fingernail beds, and splenomegaly. Hematuria is very frequent, and red blood cell (RBC) casts are a common and very suggestive finding. There often (but not always) is a normocytic and normochromic anemia. Leukocytosis is often present, but it too may be absent. Signs and symptoms are variable among individual patients, and the diagnostic problem is often that of a fever of unknown origin.

Diagnosis of infective endocarditis and identification of the organism involved are made through blood cultures. The clinical picture, evidence of abnormal heart valves, and the organism that is isolated (e.g., *S. viridans*) are major considerations in differentiating endocarditis from bacteremia and septicemia. However, in spite of the fact that viridans and group D streptococci together cause about 50%–60% of infective endocarditis, a few investigators state that when these organisms are isolated from blood culture, they are actually contaminants (or are not responsible for clinically significant disease) in 75% or more of the isolates. Blood culture methods used for diagnosis of infective endocarditis are the same as those used for septicemia.

TABLE 14–4.
Conditions Associated With Increased Rate of Infection or Infection by Unusual or Resistant Organisms

GENERAL CONDITIONS
Human immunodeficiency virus infection (e.g., AIDS)
Diabetes mellitus (poorly controlled)
Uremia
Alcoholism
Trauma (severe)
Burns (extensive or severe)
Malnutrition
Very young or very old age
THERAPY ASSOCIATED
Adrenocorticosteroid therapy
Immunosuppressant therapy
Chemotherapy of tumors
Antibiotic therapy (inappropriate or broad-spectrum)
MALIGNANCY
Myeloma
Leukemia and lymphomas
Widespread nonhematologic malignancies
INSTRUMENTATION
Indwelling urinary catheters
Indwelling vascular catheters

Blood Cultures.—Blood culture methods used for diagnosis of infective endocarditis are the same as those used for septicemia. When one obtains material for blood culture, not only must proper aseptic techniques be followed, but extra precautions must be taken to avoid contamination by skin bacteria. Iodine or an iodophore such as povidone-iodine complex (Betadine) should be used, if possible, because it has the most efficient bactericidal effect of the common antiseptics available. The iodophore must remain on the skin a minimum of 1 minute, then it is removed by alcohol. Alcohol requires at least 2 minutes contact time to be effective. Several reports emphasize the need for adequate quantities of blood per bottle (at least 5 ml and preferably 10 ml) to maximize bacterial recovery rate. The optimum specimen quantity depends on the amount of diluting medium and the presence or absence of certain additives, such as sodium polyanetholsulfonate (Liquoid). Repeated blood cultures are even more necessary in possible endocarditis than in diagnosis of septicemia because of the often intermittent nature of the blood involvement; avoidance of culture contamination becomes even more important. About 15% of patients (literature range, 2.5%–64%) do not have positive blood cultures. Uremia is especially apt to be associated with negative cultures.

False Negative Blood Cultures.—Some possible reasons for false negative blood cultures include recent antibiotic therapy, insufficient blood obtained for the amount of culture media, use of culture media unsuitable for anaerobes or for bacteria with special growth requirements, slowly growing organisms not detected during usual examination periods, various technical laboratory problems (specimens not obtained at optimal times), and combinations of these factors. One of the most important problems is insufficient blood specimen, especially when the number of organisms is small. Most investigators consider a 1:10 ratio of blood to culture medium to be optimal, and some insist on a minimum of 10 ml of blood (in adults) instead of the usual 5 ml. As noted previously, the optimal amount of specimen depends on the amount of diluting medium and the type of culture medium and system. There have been many blood culture systems advocated: use of many different media, vented and unvented containers, different anticoagulants and additives, hypertonic glucose media, filter or radioisotope detection equipment, and so forth. Interestingly, no system has consistently detected all bacteria all of the time. When two or more culture systems are compared, each system almost invariably detects a certain percentage of organisms that the others miss although some systems provide overall better results than others.

Nutritionally Deficient Streptococci.—Occasional patients are infected by streptococci that grow in blood culture media but not on media used to subculture and identify the organisms. This could lead to a false impression of a negative culture. These streptococci are nutritionally deficient (not all in the same nutrient) and will grow on subculture media that is supplemented with the nutrients (e.g., pyridoxine) that they need. They usually grow as satellites around colonies of staphylococci, much as *H. influenzae* does.

INFECTIOUS DIARRHEA DUE TO BACTERIAL AGENTS

Diarrhea caused by *Clostridium difficile* related to antibiotic therapy was discussed previously. Many cases of diarrhea produced by bacterial infection are also part of the spectrum of "food poisoning." *Clostridium botulinum* generates a preformed neurotoxin and in adults is associated with improperly canned food. Usually there is no diarrhea. The organism was discussed earlier with the clostridia. *Staphylococcus aureus* also generates a preformed toxin after it is allowed to grow in certain foods (typically custards, creams, potato salad, and ham, usually when allowed to remain warm). Symptoms most often occur less than 7 hours after ingestion of the food (average, 3 hours) and consist of nausea, vomiting, abdominal cramps, and diarrhea.

Clostridium perfringens occasionally may contaminate food, typically meat or gravy, that has been cooked and then allowed to cool slowly. Symptoms are due to exotoxin formed within the intestine, occur about 12 hours after eating, and consist of simultaneous abdominal cramps and diarrhea without fever or vomiting. *Bacillus cereus* uncommonly causes food poisoning, usually in fried rice that is kept warm. *Bacillus cereus* forms an endotoxin that can either be preformed (such as *C. botulinum* or S. aureus) or produced as the bacteria multiply after being ingested by the patient (such as *C. perfringens*). Diarrhea without vomiting is the major symptom. *Vibrio parahaemolyticus* is ingested with raw or poorly cooked fish or shellfish. The organism may invade tissue or may produce an exotoxin. Average onset of symptoms is 12–24 hours after ingestion. Symptoms are vomiting, nausea, cramps, diarrhea, chill, and fever.

Other Bacteria Associated with Diarrhea.—Several bacterial species cause infectious diarrhea but are not ordinarily considered to be agents of food poisoning because of their relatively long incubation periods. These include *Salmonella, Shigella, Yersinia enterocolitica, Campylobacter fetus* ssp. *jejuni, E. coli, Vibrio cholerae*, and possibly *V. parahaemo-*

lyticus. Other bacteria less often involved that should be mentioned are *Aeromonas hydrophila* and *Plesiomonas shigelloides.* Recent reports suggest the possibility that *Bacteroides fragilis* may cause diarrhea. Most of the bacteria listed are associated with contaminated water. Several of them, such as *E. coli,* may be transmitted via contaminated food or water. *Escherichia coli* may invade tissue or may produce an exotoxin. Symptoms occur 10–12 hours after contact and consist of vomiting, nausea, cramps, diarrhea, chills, and fever. *Salmonella* or *Shigella* gastroenteritis is due to tissue infection by the organisms, although *Shigella* is capable of toxin production. *Shigella* dysentery symptoms ordinarily occur 36–48 hours after infection, but the time is variable. *Salmonella* gastroenteritis (due to species other than *Salmonella typhi*) is most frequently associated with ingestion of poultry, eggs and egg products, powdered milk, and fresh pork. Symptoms most often manifest in 8–48 hours, with an average onset at 24 hours. Symptoms of both *Shigella* and *Salmonella* gastroenteritis are similar to those of *E. coli. Salmonella* dysentery should be differentiated from typhoid and paratyphoid fever, which have considerably longer incubations and different emphasis in symptoms.

Nonbacterial Causes of Diarrhea.—There are other causes for food poisoning that do not involve bacterial agents. Some of these are ingestion of toxins from certain fish (e.g., ciguatera or scombroid fishes) or shellfish, and the Chinese restaurant syndrome (due to excess monosodium glutamate seasoning. However, at least one report disputes this etiology). Other causes for nonbacterial infectious diarrhea include viral infection (especially by rotavirus) and infection by the parasite *Giardia lamblia.* Ulcerative colitis and other conditions may also have to be considered.

Differential Diagnosis.—Some differential points include incubation time and presence of fever, vomiting, or diarrhea. Incubation time less than 7 hours without fever suggests *S. aureus* or ingestion of the preformed toxin of B. cereus. Both of these usually are associated with vomiting, but *S. aureus* is more likely to cause diarrhea (about 75% of cases) than *B. cereus* (<40% of cases). Incubation of about 12 hours favors *C. perfringens* and *B. cereus* without preformed toxin; in both disorders toxin is formed after the organism is ingested rather than before. Symptoms of both are predominantly abdominal cramps and diarrhea, usually without fever or vomiting. Presence of neurologic symptoms suggests *C. botulinum* or chemical poisoning (mushrooms or fish toxins).

Laboratory diagnosis includes stool culture and culture of possibly contaminated food or water. Diagnosis of *C. botulinum* or *C. difficile* infections usually requires demonstration of toxin, which was discussed earlier in the section on clostridia. Gram stain of the stool may be helpful in some patients. Patients with infection by bacteria that invade the mucosa of the GI tract tend to have WBCs in the stools, whereas those whose effect is produced by toxin usually do not. However, this is only a general rule. Many WBCs in the stool are typical of *Shigella, Campylobacter,* or *C. difficile* infection, although it also frequently occurs with *Salmonella* gastroenteritis, *E. coli, Y. enterocolitica,* or *V. parahaemolyticus.* Grossly visible blood in the stools is frequently found with *Campylobacter,* but gross blood may occasionally appear with severe infection by the other enteroinvasive bacteria, and microscopic blood is fairly frequent. Diagnosis of *S. aureus* or *C. perfringens* contamination usually necessitates culture of the affected food, since these organisms are considered normal stool flora.

PNEUMONIA

The word pneumonia means inflammation of the lung. Although this could result from noninfectious sources (e.g., a chemical inflammation secondary to aspiration), the great majority of cases are due to bacterial or nonbacterial infectious agents. Almost any bacterium, many species of fungi, and many viruses could be associated with pneumonia under some circumstances. Except for the newborn, in the early pediatric age group viruses are the most common etiology, followed by *Staphylococcus* infections. In older children and young adults, viruses still markedly predominate, but pneumococci become more prevalent. In middle-aged and older adults, pneumococci assume considerable importance, although viruses still are more frequent numerically. *Mycoplasma pneumoniae* is a very important cause of pneumonia in older children, young adults, and middle-aged adults but may appear at any age. In debilitated persons, alcoholics, persons with depressed immunologic defenses, and the elderly, pneumococci are still very important, but other bacteria become much more common, especially *Staphylococcus* and *Klebsiella*. Staphylococcal pneumonia is particularly likely to occur following a viral pneumonia, such as influenza. *Legionella* infections are assuming more importance in adults and the elderly, although their true incidence is not known because diagnostic tests are still cumbersome.

The most important nonbacterial agents producing lung infection are the respiratory-syncytial virus, influenza virus, the *Aspergillus* fungus, and an organism classified as a parasite, *Pneumocystis carinii*. Diseases caused by viruses, fungi, and parasites are discussed in other chapters.

INTRA-ABDOMINAL ABSCESS

Intra-abdominal abscess is a recurrent problem that deserves attention. Some use the term "subphrenic" synonymously with intra-abdominal, although most use the term subphrenic to refer only to abscess just below the diaphragm. The most common etiologies are postoperative complications of biliary tract or peptic ulcer surgery, penetrating abdominal trauma, and perforated appendix. Some 80%–90% of cases occur intraperitoneally. The spaces above and below the liver are the most common locations. About 25% of abscesses are located on the left side. The percentage of multiple abscesses ranges from 5%–40%. *Bacteroides, E. coli, S. aureus*, and streptococci are the most frequent organisms.

X-ray film shows pleural effusion in about 60%–80% of cases (range, 43%–89%), elevated diaphragm in about 70% (range, 34%–82%), and gas in the abscess in about 25%–50% (range, 9%–61%). Atelectasis and pneumonia are frequent in the closest lung base.

Computerized tomography (CT), gallium radioisotope scanning, and B-mode gray scale ultrasound may assist in diagnosis and localization of intra-abdominal abscess. Of these, CT is probably the most sensitive, with approximately 90%–93% success rate (literature range, 82%–99%). Gallium 67 scanning has about 85% overall sensitivity (literature range, 75%–95%). The great advantage of gallium is total body scan capability with detection of inflammatory lesions located anyplace in the body (e.g., dental abscess, acute cholecystitis, or arthritis and osteomyelitis) rather than only intra-abdominal infection when the scan is ordered for suspicion of intra-abdominal abscess. There are major disadvantages, however. Gallium is excreted in the feces beginning about 12 hours after injection, so that bowel cleansing by laxatives and enemas (similar to barium enema preparation) is necessary and may have to be repeated. Scanning is usually performed 48 hours after injection, and the scan may have to be repeated if residual isotope is detected in the colon. This means that the study may take several days to complete. A certain percentage of various tumors may concentrate gallium and simulate abscess. There is normal uptake of isotope by the skeleton, liver, and spleen. B-mode gray scale ultrasound also has about 85% accuracy in detection of abdominal abscess and is less expensive than CT or gallium scanning. However, ultrasound in general gives better results in examining relatively small areas than in screening the entire abdomen. Ribs and air within the intestines may interfere.

NOSOCOMIAL INFECTIONS

A nosocomial infection is one that is acquired in a hospital. This subject is extremely important but cannot be covered in detail in a book that concentrates on laboratory tests. The most common cause of nosocomial infection is the indwelling urinary catheter. Some other important factors are surgery, long-term indwelling vascular catheters or equipment, conditions that depress patient resistance to infection, malnutrition, severe trauma or burns, overuse of antibiotics, and instrumentation of the urinary tract or other areas.

ANTIBIOTIC SENSITIVITY PROCEDURES

Disk Diffusion Method

Antibiotic sensitivity testing is usually done using either the tube dilution or the agar diffusion (sometimes called "disk sensitivity") technique. Of these, agar diffusion is by far the more common, and the Kirby-Bauer modification of this technique is the standard procedure. The Kirby-Bauer method involves (1) isolating a bacterial colony from its original growth medium, (2) allowing the bacteria to grow in a broth medium to a predetermined visual density, (3) covering the entirety of a Mueller-Hinton agar plate with the bacterial isolate, (4) placing antibiotic sensitivity disks at intervals on the surface, (5) incubating for 18–20 hours, (6) examining for clear areas around individual disks representing bacterial growth inhibition by the antibiotic-impregnated disk, and (7) measuring the diameter of these inhibition zones. Results are reported as resistant, sensitive, or intermediate, depending on previously established values for zone size based on tube dilution studies most often furnished by the disk manufacturer. Consistent results depend on strict adherence to good technique at each step, as well as the quality of the antibiotic disks and agar used. Variation in potency of antibiotic disks from different shipments and disk or agar deterioration during storage necessitate a good quality control program. The Kirby-Bauer technique has limitations. To be accurate, it can be used only when the bacterium to be tested is aerobic and grows rapidly (produces colonies within 24 hours) on the agar growth medium. Thus, it can be used for the Enterobacteriaciae, *Pseudomonas* organisms, staphylococci, and streptococci. The Kirby-Bauer method can also be used with *H. influenzae, N. gonorrheae,* and *S. pneumoniae,* but a different agar medium is necessary.

Most organisms, fortunately, may be classified as sensitive or resistant. Intermediate sensitivity is a controversial area. In general, many believe that intermediate zones should be considered resistant, although certain organisms, such as enterococci, may be exceptions. If the particular antibiotic with the intermediate degree of inhibition is important in therapy of the patient, the sensitivity test should be repeated to rule out technical problems. It might also be useful to have the sensitivity test performed by the tube dilution method, if available. Another subject of dispute is the need for sensitivity testing in those bacteria that almost always are sensitive to certain antibiotics. These organisms include group A aerobic streptococci, pneumococci, *Neisseria* organisms, and *Corynebacterium diphtheriae.* A few resistant or partially resistant strains of pneumococci (about 3%; range, 0%–35%) are being reported, and resistant gonococci (about 2%; range, 0%–6%) are beginning to appear in various areas. At present, many laboratories do not perform sensitivity studies routinely on these bacteria. An occasional laboratory problem is requests by physicians to include additional sensitivity disks in sensitivity panels. Only a limited number of disks can be spaced on a sensitivity agar plate, so that an additional disk either means that another antibiotic must be deleted or else an additional plate must be used at extra expense. In many cases the extra antibiotic requested has a similar sensitivity spectrum to one already on the panel. Laboratories frequently include only one representative of an antibiotic family in sensitivity test panels because sensitivity differences among antibiotic family members (e.g., the various tetracycline derivatives) are usually very minor.

Serial Dilution Method.—The other major test procedure is serial dilution (sometimes called "tube dilution"). A standardized concentration of the bacterium to be tested is placed in tubes or microtiter plate wells containing liquid culture medium. Serial dilutions of the antibiotic to be tested are added to consecutive tubes containing the bacterial suspension and the tubes are incubated, usually for 24 hours. The bacterial suspension is cloudy, and any tube in which the bacteria are sufficiently inhibited will become clear due to absence of bacterial multiplication. The last dilution tube (i.e., the tube with the highest degree of antibiotic dilution) that is clear (i.e., still shows acceptable bacterial inhibition) is reported as the minimal inhibitory concentration (MIC). This is defined as the smallest concentration of antibiotic that will inhibit bacterial growth. Therefore, the higher the antibiotic dilution before bacterial growth overcomes the effect of the antibiotic, the smaller the amount (concentration) of antibiotic necessary to inhibit the organism. The MIC is actually reported in terms of the antibiotic concentration per milliliter of solution that is necessary to inhibit the bacteria (e.g., an MIC of 15 means a level or concentration of 15 μg of the antibiotic/ml of solution). To determine if the organism is sensitive or resistant to the antibiotic, one compares the MIC with the achievable blood level of antibiotic, which varies according to size of dose, frequency of dosage, route of administration, and so forth. If the maximal achievable blood level of the antibiotic is less than the minimal concentration of the antibiotic necessary to inhibit the organism (the MIC), the antibiotic presumably will not be effective (or, to consider it in another way, the organism is resistant). In general, this means that the lower the MIC value, the more sensitive the organism is likely to be toward the antibiotic. The same tube dilution procedure is carried out for each antibiotic to be tested with each organism. As a general rule, an adequate serum antibiotic level should be at least two–four times the MIC to compensate for some of the clinical and laboratory variables.

Disk Method vs. Dilution Method.—There are certain advantages and disadvantages to each antibiotic sensitivity technique. The disk method is cheaper and easier than tube dilution if both are done manually. Semiautomated and fully automated equipment is available for tube dilution, but the cost of the equipment usually restricts this to larger or high-volume laboratories. The disk diffusion method can be used only for certain common, rapidly growing organisms. Tube dilution can be used with more organisms than disk diffusion, but many cannot be tested with either technique. Neither technique can be used for anaerobes, under usual conditions. The disks employed in the Kirby-Bauer disk sensitivity method contain antibiotic concentration based on serum antibiotic levels achieved with usual drug doses. In certain body tissues or body fluids such as urine, the concentration of the antibiotic may be considerably more or less than the serum concentration, and the disk sensitivity result may therefore be misleading. For example, the urine concentration of some antibiotics may be much greater than the serum concentration. Thus, the organism may not be inhibited by the disk (serum) antibiotic concentration but may actually be inhibited at the higher antibiotic concentration in urine. In this case, a disk sensitivity result showing the organism to be sensitive is correct, but a disk result showing the organism to be resistant may not be correct. The opposite could be true if infection took place in a location where the antibiotic concentration was considerably less than the level in serum. Another problem, of course, is that the disk sensitivity method uses a single concentration of antibiotic. The organism might be inhibited at a lower concentration than the disk contains. Even more important, the actual concentration of that antibiotic in the serum of any individual patient may be quite different from the disk concentration for a variety of reasons (differences in dosage, absorption, degradation, excretion rate, etc.).

The tube dilution method shares some of the drawbacks of the disk diffusion method, the principal difficulty being that neither method takes into account the actual antibiotic concentration in patient serum or in the area of infection, these concentrations being unknown. However, the tube dilution method does have the advantage in that it roughly indicates the actual antibiotic concentration necessary to inhibit the organism. As noted previously, if one can learn the theoretical antibiotic concentration from a given dosage at the expected site of infection (in micrograms per milliliter), one can compare this with the level needed to inhibit the organism (the MIC, also reported in micrograms per milliliter) and have a better estimate of probable therapeutic effectiveness. However, this does not guarantee that the actual concentration of antibiotic at the site of infection is the same as the theoretical or experimental concentration. It is also possible to test the effects of antibiotic combinations using the tube dilution method; this is not possible with the Kirby-Bauer method. Finally, it is possible to obtain the minimal bactericidal concentration (MBC) using a modification of the tube dilution method. The MBC is the smallest concentration of the antibiotic necessary to kill at least 99.9% of the bacteria. This may or may not require a higher concentration of antibiotic than the MIC and might be useful information if the patient's theoretical or actual antibiotic blood level is higher than that required by the MIC but the patient is not responding to therapy.

Bacterial Resistance: Beta-Lactamase.—Certain antibiotics, notably penicillin and the cephalosporins, have a certain structural area containing a nitrogen atom known as a beta-lactam ring. A group of bacterial enzymes (of which penicillinase was the first to be recognized) can split the beta-lactam ring and destroy the antibacterial activity of the molecule. These bacterial enzymes are now collectively called beta-lactamase. Certain tests have been devised to demonstrate bacterial production of beta-lactamase. There is considerable variation in the technical details of these tests and some variation in accuracy. Most, however, can be done in less than 1 hour and are reasonably accurate, possibly more so when indicating a positive reaction. A positive beta-lactamase test result suggests that the organism should be considered resistant to penicillin, ampicillin, and the first- and second-generation cephalosporins until results of antibiotic sensitivity studies are available. The test is particularly important in *H. influenzae* type B infection; up to 20%–30% (range, 6%–38%, depending on geographical location) have been reported to produce beta-lactamase. *Staphylococcus aureus* is even more likely to produce beta-lactamase, so much so that resistance to penicillin is usually taken for granted pending sensitivity study results. *Staphylococcus epidermidis* and *N. gonorrheae* may produce beta-lactamase but are usually not tested for this except under special circumstances.

Methacillin-resistant *S. aureus* (MRSA) is not only a therapeutic problem but also presents difficulties in susceptibility testing. Standard susceptibility protocols will not demonstrate methacillin resistance in a significant minority of these organisms. There are certain changes in temperature and length of incubation, salt content of the media, and density of the bacterial inoculum that will provide the greatest rate of detection. Many laboratories do not use some or any of these recommended changes. Some antibiotics, such as certain cephalosporins, may sometimes appear to be effective against MRSA by in vitro sensitivity tests, whereas they will usually not be effective if given to the patient.

SERUM BACTERIOSTATIC OR BACTERIOCIDAL CONCENTRATION (SCHLICHTER TEST)

In patients with bacterial endocarditis whose symptoms persist despite treatment, it is important to know whether antibiotic therapy really is effective in vivo. Also, some antibiotics, such as gentamycin, have a therapeutic range close to the toxic range. Blood levels of some antibiotics can be measured using various methods. This will provide some assurance that antibiotic blood levels have been reached that ordinarily should be effective. However, this does not guarantee that the organisms are in fact being sufficiently inhibited or killed. For estimate of in vivo effectiveness, a Schlichter test may be performed. A patient blood specimen is obtained 15 minutes after IV infusion of the antibiotic (1 hour after an intramuscular dose). This represents the peak antibiotic level. If a trough level is desired, the specimen is drawn just before the next antibiotic dose is to be given. A standard suspension of the organisms previously cultured from the patient is placed in serial dilutions of patient serum and incubated overnight. If the lowest serum dilutions (i.e., those tubes with the least dilution of the antibiotic) do not inhibit growth of the organism, therapy is probably not effective. There is some dispute on which dilution level to use as the peak value cutoff for therapeutic effectiveness; Schlichter accepted 1:2, but currently the majority of investigators require 1:8. In fact, for a test that is widely used and relied on, there is a surprising amount of disagreement about many critical technical aspects, including whether to obtain peak or trough level or both and what their optimal values are; whether to make the patient serum dilutions with saline, Mueller-Hinton broth, nonantibiotic-containing serum, or a mixture of these; what criteria should define the bacteriocidal endpoint; and so forth. For this reason some investigators doubt the value of the test.

ANTIBIOTIC REMOVAL

One of the major frustrations in microbiology is the interference to bacterial growth caused by previous administration of antibiotics. Culture growth inhibition may occur even if the organism is not sensitive to the antibiotic. Several antibiotic removal devices are now available, based on membrane filtration or resin adsorption. These are useful for liquid specimens such as spinal fluid, body cavity fluid, or blood. Most, although not all, of the early evaluations have found these devices to be very helpful.

Additional tests relevant to this chapter are discussed in chapter 35.

BIBLIOGRAPHY

Haslett TM, et al: Microbiology of indwelling central intravenous catheters. *J Clin Microbiol* 1988; 26:696.

Gleckman R, et al: Sputum Gram stain assessment in community-acquired bacteremic pneumonia. *J Clin Microbiol* 1988; 26:846.

Stamm WE: Diagnosis of *Chlamydia trachomatis* genitourinary infections. *Ann Intern Med* 1988; 710.

Johnson RC: Lyme borreliosis. *Lab Mgmt* 1988; 26:34.

Lyerly DM, et al: *Clostridium difficile:* Its disease and toxins. *Clin Microbiol Rev* 1988; 1:1.

Winn WC: Legionnaires disease. *Clin Microbiol Rev* 1988; 1:60.

Stratton CW: Serum bactericidal test. *Clin Microbiol Rev* 1988; 1:19.

Dickison L, Kwasnik I: Current strategies in the laboratory detection of methicillin-resistant *Staphylococcus aureus*. *Med Lab Prod* 1988; 3:22.

Sitges-Serra A, Linares J: Limitations of semiquantitative method for catheter culture. *J Clin Microbiol* 1988; 26:1074.

Hsu CCS, et al: High rate of methacillin resistance of *Staphylococcus aureus* isolated from hospitalized nursing home patients. *Arch Intern Med* 1988; 148:569.

Dooley CP, Cohen H: The clinical significance of campylobacter pylori. *Ann Intern Med* 1988; 108:70.

Ruoff KL: An update on streptococcal taxonomy. *Clin Microbiol Newsletter* 1988; 10:1.

Rauws EAJ: *Campylobacter pyloridis*-associated chronic active antral gastritis. *Gastroenterology* 1988; 94:33.

Ditchek A, et al: The changing epidemiology of endocarditis. *Intern Med Specialist* 1987; 8:130.

Harrell R, Bates JH: Clinical recognition and treatment of tularemia. *Intern Med Specialist* 1987; 8:115.

Males BM, et al: Laboratory indices of clinical peritonitis: Total leukocyte count, microscopy, and microbiologic culture of peritoneal dialysis effluent. *J Clin Microbiol* 1987; 25:2367.

Wilkins EGL: Liquoid in blood cultures. *Ann Intern Med* 1987; 106:912.

Woolfrey BF: Evaluation of *Hemophilus* type B systemic isolates for beta-lactamase and non-beta-lactamase mediated ampicillin resistance and for susceptibility to other antimicrobial agents. *Am J Clin Pathol* 1987; 88:361.

Caputo GM, et al: Native valve endocarditis due to coagulase-negative staphylococci. *Am J Med* 1987; 83:619.

Myers LL, et al: Isolation of enterotoxigenic *Bacteroides fragilis* from humans with diarrhea. *J Clin Microbiol* 1987; 25:2330.

Cunha BC: The toxigenic diarrheas. *Intern Med Specialist* 1987; 8:92.

MacDonald KL, et al: Toxic shock syndrome. *JAMA* 1987; 257:1053.

Spencer JAD: Perinatal listeriosis. *Br Med J* 1987; 295:349.

Stead WW, To T: The significance of the tuberculin skin test in elderly persons. *Ann Intern Med* 1987; 107:837.

Mizrachi HH, Valenstein PN: Randomized trial interpreting sputum quality in a clinical laboratory. *J Clin Microbiol* 1987; 25:2327.

Leport C, et al: Incidence of colonic lesions in *Streptococcus bovis* and enterococcal endocarditis. *Lancet* 1987; 1:748.

Lentino JR, Lucks DA.: Nonvalue of sputum culture in the management of lower respiratory tract infections. *J Clin Microbiol* 1987; 25:758.

Crowe HM, Levitz RE: Invasive *Haemophilus influenzae* disease in adults. *Arch Intern Med* 1987; 147:241.

Rowe LD: Oropharyngeal colonization with bacterial pathogens in the elderly. *Intern Med Specialist* 1987; 8:203.

Terpenning MS, et al: Infective endocarditis: Clinical features in young and elderly patients. *Am J Med* 1987; 83:626.

Hatheway CL, McCroskey LM: Examination of feces and serum for diagnosis of infant botulism in 336 patients. *J Clin Microbiol* 1987; 25:2334.

Yannelli B, Cunha BA: Nosocomial *Serratia marcescens* infection. *J Nosocomial Infect* 1987; 4(2):26.

Thisyakorn U, et al: Typhoid and paratyphoid fever in 192 hospitalized children in Thailand. *Am J Dis Child* 1987; 141:862.

Klotz SA, Penn RL: Acid-fast staining of urine and gastric contents is an excellent indicator of mycobacterial disease. *Am Rev Respir Dis* 1987; 136:1197.

Facklam RR: Specificity study of kits for detection of group A streptococci directly from throat swabs. *J Clin Microbiol* 1987; 25:504.

Centor RM, et al: Throat cultures and rapid tests for diagnosis of group A streptococcal pharyngitis. *Ann Intern Med* 1986; 105:892.

Washington JA, Ilstrup DM: Blood cultures: Issues and controversies. *Rev Infect Dis* 1986; 8:792.

Martin R: DNA probes: Molecular technology for the clinical microbiology laboratory. *J Med Technol* 1986; 3:395.

Kohne DE: Application of DNA probe tests to the diagnosis of infectious disease. *Am*

Clin Prod Rev 1986; 5(11):20.
Rolston KVI: Group G streptococcal infections. *Arch Intern Med* 1986; 146:857.
Nicotra B, et al: *Branhamella catarrhalis* as a lower respiratory tract pathogen in patients with chronic lung disease. *Arch Intern Med* 1986; 146:890.
Woolfrey BF: Significance of *Gardnerella vaginalis* in urine cultures. *Am J Clin Pathol* 1986; 86:324.
Stamm WE: Diagnosis of *Neisseria gonorrhoeae* and *Chlamydia trachomatis* infections using antigen detection methods. *Diagn Microbiol Infect Dis* 1986; 4:93S.
Kohler RB: Antigen detection for the rapid diagnosis of *Mycoplasma* and *Legionella* pneumonia. *Diagn Microbiol Infect Dis* 1986; 4:47S.
White A, Kohler RB: Pneumonia: When to suspect Legionnaires' disease. *Mod Med* 1986; 54:118.
Jaggers RL, et al: Significance of clostridial isolates in abdominal sepsis. *Surg Gynecol Obstet* 1986; 163:310.
Welty TK: Plague. *Am Fam Pract* 1986; 33:159.
Peterson LR, et al: Detection of *Clostridium difficile* toxins A (enterotoxin) and B (cytotoxin) in clinical specimens. *Am J Clin Pathol* 1986; 86:208.
Jevon TR, et al: A point-source epidemic of leptospirosis. *Postgrad Med* 1986; 80:121.
Dammin GJ: Lyme disease: Its transmission and diagnostic features. *Lab Mgmt* 1986; 24:33.
Pruessner HT, et al: Diagnosis and treatment of chlamydial infections. *Am Fam Pract* 1986; 34:81.
Decker MD, et al: The detection of penicillin-resistant pneumococci. *Am J Clin Pathol* 1985; 84:357.
Hook EW, Holmes KK: Gonococcal infections. *Ann Intern Med* 1985; 102:229.
Bronken TP: A solid-phase enzyme immunoassay in detection of cervical gonorrhea in a low-prevalence population. *J Fam Pract* 1985; 20:43.
Archer GL: Coagulase-negative staphylococci in blood cultures: The clinician's dilemma. *Infect Control* 1985; 6:477.
Evans ME: Tularemia: A 30-year experience with 88 cases. *Medicine* (Baltimore) 1985; 64:251.
Lorber B: Diagnosis and management of listeriosis. *Intern Med Specialist* 1985; 6:68.
Carithers HA: Cat-scratch disease. *Am J Dis Child* 1985; 139:1124.
Isaac-Renton JL: Microscopic evaluation of sputum specimens submitted for *Mycobacterium tuberculosis* culture. *Am J Clin Pathol* 1985; 84:361.
Zuerlein TJ, Smith PW: The diagnostic utility of the febrile agglutinin tests. *JAMA* 1985; 254:1211.
Rubin SJ: Species identification and clinical significance of viridans streptococci. *Lab Med* 1984; 15:171.
Doern GV: Coagulase-negative staphylococci: Clinical significance and laboratory identification. *Lab Med* 1984; 15:25.
Esposito AL: Community-acquired bacteremic pneumococcal pneumonia. *Arch Intern Med* 1984; 144:945.
Farmer JJ III, et al: The *Salmonella-Arizona* group of Enterobacteriaceae: Nomenclature, classification, and reporting. *Clin Microbiol Newslett* 1984; 6(9):1.
Sodeman RM, Colmer J: Microbiology of the respiratory tract. *Lab Med* 1983; 14:96.
Meadows JC: The acute urethral syndrome: Diagnosis, management, and prophylaxis. *Cont Ed Fam Pract* 1983; 17:1112.
Orbegoso CM: New anaerobic bacteriologic syndromes. *Lab Med* 1982; 13:628.
Finegold SM: Pathogenic anaerobes. *Arch Intern Med* 1982; 142:1988.
Snider DE: The tuberculin skin test. *Am Rev Respir Dis* 1982; 125:108.
Manos JP: Group B streptococcal infection in the neonate. *Ann Clin Lab Sci* 1982; 12:239.
Kaye D: Enterococci. *Arch Intern Med* 1982; 142:2006.
Agarwal AK: Culture-negative infective endocarditis. *Postgrad Med* 1982; 72:123.
Nordbring F: *Pseudomonas*. *Arch Intern Med* 1982; 142:2010.
Forgacs P: The gallium scan and inflammatory lesions. *Arch Intern Med* 1982; 142:231.
Binford CH, et al: Leprosy. *JAMA* 1982; 247:2283.
Mufson MA: Pneumococcal infections. *JAMA* 1981; 246:1942.
Chesney PJ, et al: Clinical manifestations of toxic shock syndrome. *JAMA* 1981; 246:741.
Hughes JM, et al: Clinical features of types A and B food-borne botulism. *Ann Intern Med* 1981; 95:442.
Young LS: Infection in the compromised host. *Hosp Pract* 1981; 16:73.
Wise RI: Brucellosis in the United States. *JAMA* 1980; 244:2318.
Brook I, Finegold SM: Bacteriology of chronic otitis media. *JAMA* 1979; 241:487.
Wolensky E: Nontuberculous mycobacteria and associated diseases. *Am Rev Respir Dis* 1979; 119:107.

15 Mycotic Infections

SYSTEMIC MYCOSES

Certain fungi, known as the *deep* or *systemic fungi*, are characterized by involvement of visceral organs or penetrating types of infection. Besides true fungi, actinomycetes and nocardiae are bacteria that produce disease resembling deep fungal infection in many ways. These are discussed in the chapter on bacterial infections. The systemic fungi include *Blastomyces dermatitidis* (blastomycosis), *Coccidioides immitis* (coccidioidomycosis), *Cryptococcus neoformans* (cryptococcosis), *Histoplasma capsulatum* (histoplasmosis), and *Sporothrix schenckii* (sporotrichosis). Certain *Candida* species (especially *Candida albicans* and *Candida tropicalis*), *Aspergillus* species (*Aspergillus fumigatus* and *Aspergillus flavus*), and certain zygomycetes (rhizopus species and mucor species) may, on occasion, produce infection that would qualify as a systemic mycosis. *Blastomyces, Coccidioides, Histoplasma,* and *Sporothrix* organisms are considered diphasic (dimorphic) fungi, since they grow as a mycelial phase in culture but in a yeast (budding) phase within tissue infections.

Diagnosis of Fungal Infections

The diagnosis of mycotic infection can be assisted in several ways:

1. Wet mount of scraping, exudate, fresh swab smear, or other specimen such as sputum. This is usually done with 10% sodium hydroxide. India ink or nigrosin preparations are used for cryptococcosis. The advantages of wet mounting are same-day results and, in some instances, reasonably accurate diagnosis. Disadvantages are that few laboratory personnel are expert in this technique, and consequently there are frequent false positive and negative results. A recent aid to wet-mount examination are naturally fluorescing compounds, such as Calcofluor white, that bind nonspecifically to fungus cell walls and can outline the organism when it is viewed with the proper filters under a fluorescent microscope. Unfortunately, false negative results are frequent regardless of technique because the specimen may not contain organisms. Also, in most cases (except possibly cryptococcosis) the most the technique can offer is recognition that a mycotic infection may be present without reliable identification of what the organism is, or its species. Speciation may be important because some species are more likely to be true pathogens in certain body areas than other species. When material such as sputum is examined, there is often a problem in deciding whether an organism is causing infection, is colonizing the area without actual infection, or is a contaminant.

2. Stained smear of a clinical specimen. Gram stain or Papanicolaou stain can be used. Wright's stain or Giemsa stain is used for histoplasmosis. The advantages of the stained smear are same-day results and a permanent preparation that may be a little easier to interpret than a wet-mount preparation. However, others find the wet preparation easier to examine. The disadvantages are the same as those of the wet-mount preparation.

3. Tissue biopsy with demonstration of the organism by special stains, such as periodic acid–Schiff or methenamine silver. The yield from this procedure depends on whether the biopsy specimen contains organisms, the number of organisms present, and whether the organism is suspected so that the special stains are actually used.

4. Culture of a lesion. This permits definite isolation of an organism with speciation. The yield depends on whether the proper specimen is obtained, whether the organism is still alive by the time it reaches the laboratory, whether proper culture media are used, and the experience of the technologists. Because of the locations involved in deep mycotic infections, it may be difficult to secure a specimen or obtain material from the correct area. The organisms usually take several days to grow.

5. Serologic tests. The major advantage is that specimens for other types of tests may not be available or the results may be negative. The disadvantages are the usual need for two specimens ("acute" and "convalescent") and the long time period involved, the second specimen being obtained 1–2 weeks after the first to see if there is a rising titer. This means 2–3 weeks' delay, possibly even more, since the specimens usually must be sent to a reference laboratory. There are usually a significant percentage of false negative results (sometimes a large percentage), and there may be a certain number of false positive and nondiagnostic results as well.

6. Skin tests. The advantage is a result in 24–48 hours. The disadvantages include the time period needed to develop antibodies, false positive or negative test results, and the problem of differentiating a positive result due to old infection from one due to recent or active infection. In addition, the skin test in some cases may induce abnormality in the serologic tests, so a rising titer does not have its usual significance.

Blastomycosis

Blastomycosis may involve primarily the skin or the visceral organs. Granulomatous lesions are produced that are somewhat similar histologically to the early lesions of tuberculosis. Skin test results are unreliable, reportedly being positive in only about 50% of cases. Complement fixation (CF) tests also detect fewer than 50% of cases and produce false positive results in *Histoplasma* infections. Immunodiffusion tests are more specific for blastomycosis and are reported to detect about 80% of active cases. These procedures usually must be sent to a reference laboratory, since the number of requests for these tests in most institutions is quite small.

Coccidioidomycosis

Coccidioidomycosis is most often contracted in the San Joaquin Valley of California but occasionally appears elsewhere in the Southwest. It has a predilection for the lungs and hilar lymph nodes but occasionally may become systemic to varying degrees. Clinical symptoms are most often pulmonary, manifested usually by mild or moderate respiratory symptoms and sometimes by fever of unknown origin. Rarely, overwhelming infection much like miliary tuberculosis develops. Diagnosis is usually made through either biopsy or serologic tests. The most sensitive tests are tube precipitin (results of which become positive 1–3 weeks after onset of infection, with about 80% of cases positive by 2 weeks), latex agglutination (slightly more sensitive than tube precipitin, but with 6%–10% false positive results), and immunodiffusion. The tube precipitin test usually reverts to negative by 6 months after onset of infection. A CF test is also widely used, especially for spinal fluid specimens. In cerebrospinal fluid (CSF) specimens it detects more than 90% of active coccidioidomycosis infections, whereas the tube precipitin test is not reliable on spinal fluid. These tests usually must be sent to a reference laboratory unless the laboratory receiving the request is located in an area where coccidioidomycosis is endemic. The coccidioidomycosis skin test is very useful, being equally as sensitive as the serologic tests. It does not produce an antibody response that would interfere with the other tests.

Cryptococcosis

Cryptococcosis (torulosis) is a fungal disease with a marked predilection for lung and brain. Pigeon feces seems to be the major known source of human exposure. Persons with illnesses that are associated with decreased immunologic resistance, such as acquired immunodeficiency syndrome (AIDS), Hodgkin's disease, and acute leukemia, or those undergoing therapy with steroids or immunosuppressive agents are particularly susceptible. Pulmonary infection is apparently more common than central nervous system (CNS) infection but is often subclinical. Pulmonary infection radiologically can present in much the same way as tuberculosis and histoplasmosis, such as pneumonia or focal nodules, or occasionally as miliary lesions. Central nervous system disease typically occurs without respiratory disease and typically is very slowly progressive but may occasionally be either asymptomatic or severe and acute. In CNS disease, headache is found in about 75% of cases and fever in about 35%. Peripheral blood complete blood cell count and erythrocyte sedimentation rate are most often normal in respiratory and CNS cryptococcosis. Laboratory findings in CNS disease are described in chapter 18. Diagnosis can be made through culture of sputum or CSF, by histologic examination of biopsy specimens (special stains for fungi are required), by microscopic examination of CSF using an india ink or nigrosin preparation to show the characteristic organism thick capsule (chapter 18), and by serologic tests. Serologic tests that detect either antigen or antibody are available. Antibody is usually not present in the CSF; and in serum, antibody appearance is inconsistent in the early acute phase of the illness. In addition, some of the antibody-detection systems cross-react with histoplasmosis antibody. *Cryptococcus* antigen detection systems do not react when the patient is infected by other fungi.

The most widely used serologic test is the slide latex agglutination procedure, which detects antigen. In localized pulmonary cryptococcosis, the latex agglutination test can be used on serum, but it detects fewer than 30% of cases. In patients with cryptococcal meningitis, the latex test can be used on either serum or CSF specimens. When used on CSF specimens, it detects about 85%–90% of culture-positive cases of cryptococcal meningitis (range, 75%–100%) vs. 40%–50% for india ink. Testing both serum and CSF increases the number of culture-positive cases. Rheumatoid factor may produce a false positive reaction, so patient serum must be heat inactivated, and a control for rheumatoid factor and nonspecific agglutinins must be used when either serum or CSF is tested. It should be mentioned that a few investigators have not obtained as good results on CSF specimens as most others have. Some of the test evaluations on CSF reported in the literature are difficult to interpret, however, since kits by different manufacturers apparently produce different results, and some investigators used their own reagents. As noted previously, the latex test may be nonreactive in low-grade chronic infections. The half-life of cryptococcal polysaccharide antigen is about 48 hours, so that once positive, the results of a test detecting antigen may remain positive for several days even if therapy is adequate. Besides latex agglutination, a CF test is also available. This is said to be more specific than the latex procedure, although not as sensitive (results being positive in about 65% of cases involving the CNS). Enzyme-linked immunosorbent assay (ELISA) tests more sensitive than the latex tests have been reported. Neither the CF nor the ELISA test is widely available since most laboratories use the latex test.

Histoplasmosis

Histoplasmosis is the most common of the systemic fungal infections. It is most often encountered in the Mississippi Valley and Ohio Valley areas but may appear elsewhere. Certain birds, especially chickens and starlings, are the most frequent vectors in the United States. In endemic areas, 60% or more of infected persons are asymptomatic. The remainder have a variety of illness patterns, ranging from mild or severe, acute or chronic pulmonary forms, to disseminated infection.

Histoplasmosis begins with a small primary focus of lung infection much like the early lesion of pulmonary tuberculosis. Thereafter, the lesion may heal or progress or reinfection may occur. Mild acute pulmonary infection with influenza-like symptoms may develop. The illness lasts only a few days, and skin test results, cultures, and chest x-ray films are usually normal. More severe acute pulmonary involvement produces a syndrome resembling primary atypical pneumonia. Chest x-ray films may show hilar adenopathy and single or multiple pulmonary infiltrates. Results of histoplasmin skin tests and CF or latex agglutination tests are negative during the first 2–3 weeks of illness but then become positive. Sputum culture is sometimes positive but not often. Chronic pulmonary histoplasmosis resembles chronic pulmonary tuberculosis clinically. Cavitation sometimes develops. Results of skin tests and CF tests usually are positive by the time the disease is chronic. Sputum is the most accessible material for culture, although results are reportedly negative in 50%–60% of cases. In clinically inactive pulmonary disease, such as coin lesions, sputum culture is usually negative. Even if the organism is present in the specimen, it takes 3–4 weeks for growth and identification. Histoplasmosis is a localized pulmonary disease in the great majority of patients, so there is usually little help from cultures obtained outside the pulmonary area. In the small group that does have disseminated histoplasmosis, either acute or chronic, there is a range of symptoms from a febrile disease with lymphadenopathy and hepatosplenomegaly to a rapidly fatal illness closely resembling miliary tuberculosis. In disseminated (miliary) histoplasmosis, standard blood cultures are positive in 40%–70% of patients. Bone marrow aspiration is the diagnostic method of choice; it is useful both for cultures and for histologic diagnosis of the organisms within macrophages on Wright-stained smear or fungus stain on a marrow clot section. Occasionally lymph node biopsy may be helpful. If it is performed, a culture should also be taken from the node before it is placed in fixative. Bone marrow aspiration and liver or lymph node biopsy are not helpful in the usual forms of histoplasmosis, which are localized to the lungs.

The most commonly used diagnostic test in histoplasmosis is the CF test. Titers of 1:16 are considered suspicious, and 1:32 or more are strongly suggestive of histoplasmosis. Two types of CF test are available, based on mycelial antigen and yeast phase antigen. The test based on yeast phase antigen is considerably more sensitive than that based on mycelial antigen. Neither test result is likely to be positive in the early phase of acute infection. Later on (about 3–4 weeks after infection), results of the yeast antigen CF test become positive in 70%–85% of cases. Some additional cases may be detected with the mycelial CF antigen. About 3.5%–12% of clinically normal persons demonstrate positive results, usually (but not always) in titers less than 1:16. Thirty-five percent to 50% of patients with positive CF test results in the literature could not be confirmed as having true histoplasmosis infections. How many of these positive results were due to previous old infection or localized active infection without proof is not known. Because of the false positive and negative results, a fourfold (two-dilution level) rise in titer is much more significant than a single result, whether the single result is positive or negative. The CF test result may be negative in 30%–50% of patients with acute disseminated (miliary) histoplasmosis and when the patient has depressed immunologic defenses or is being treated with steroids.

Latex agglutination tests are also available and are reported to be a little more sensitive than the CF tests. However, there are conflicting reports on their reliability, with one investigator unable to confirm 90% of the cases with positive results and other studies being more favorable. Differences in reagents may be a factor.

Besides serologic tests, a skin test is available. Results of the skin test become positive about 2–3 weeks after infection and remain positive for life in 90% of persons. The skin test result is falsely negative in about 50% of patients with disseminated (miliary) histoplasmosis and is said to be negative in about 10% of patients with cavitary histoplasmosis. A (single) skin test result is difficult to interpret, whether it is positive (because of past exposure) or negative (because it may be too early for reaction to develop, or reaction may be suppressed by miliary disease, depressed immunologic status, or steroid therapy). Also, about 15% of patients develop a positive CF test result because of the skin test. The histoplasmin skin test reacts in about 30% of patients who actually have blastomycosis and in about 40% of those with coccidioidomycosis. For these reasons, routine use of the histoplasmin skin test is not recommended.

In serious localized infection or widespread dissemination of the deep fungi, there is often a normocytic-normochromic or slightly hypochromic anemia. The anemia is usually mild or moderate in localized infection.

Sporotrichosis

Sporotrichosis is caused by *S. schenckii*, which lives in soil and decaying plant material. Most of those who contract the disease are gardeners, florists, or farmers. The fungus is acquired through a scratch or puncture wound. The lymphocutaneous form constitutes two thirds to three fourths of all cases. A small ulcerated papule develops at the site of inoculation and similar lesions appear along lymphoid channels draining the original lesion area. Lymph nodes are not involved. The classic case is a person who does gardening and has contact with roses who develops a small ulceration on one arm followed by others in a linear ascending distribution. In children it is found as frequently on the body or face as on the extremities. Other than the lesions the patient usually has few symptoms.

The major diagnostic tests are culture of the lesions, biopsy, and serologic tests. The latex agglutination test, tube agglutination, and immunofluorescent test on serum are the most sensitive (±90% detection rate). Complement fixation tests detect approximately 65% of cases.

OPPORTUNISTIC FUNGI

Other fungi may, under certain circumstances, produce visceral or systemic infection. The most common of these conditions are candidiasis, aspergillosis, and mucormycosis. Persons predisposed to infection include aged persons, cachectic or debilitated patients, persons with diseases such as AIDS or leukemia that affect the body's immunologic mechanisms, and, most commonly, persons under treatment with certain drugs that impair the same immunologic mechanisms. Such drugs include many types of antileukemic or anticancer chemotherapeutic agents and sometimes adrenocortical steroids if use has been heavy or prolonged. Occasionally, overgrowth of *Candida* may be caused by prolonged oral antibiotic therapy that destroys normal gastrointestinal tract bacterial flora. *Candida fungemia* may be associated with indwelling intravenous (IV) catheters. Diagnosis in many of these patients is difficult, since the original underlying disease usually overshadows advent of the fungal infection. If the patient has a condition that predisposes to infection by fungi, culture of a fungus from an area where it is normally absent should not be disregarded as mere contamination but should be investigated further.

Candida Infections

Candida organisms may be present as either normal nasopharyngeal area or gastrointestinal tract inhabitants (20%–40% of persons), as colonization without infection (10%–15% of vaginal cultures in asymptomatic women, with a range of 0%–50%), as superficial infection (e.g., the oral cavity or the vaginal area), or as deep or disseminated infection. Some species are more often pathogenic than others. Of these, *C. albicans* is by far (up to 90%) the most frequent and important. Serious *C. albicans* infections are associated with diabetes, extensive surgery, AIDS and other conditions (e.g., leukemia and lymphoma) producing decreased immunologic resistance, chemotherapy or immunosuppressive therapy, and also following antibiotic therapy. Localized skin, oral mucous membrane (thrush), or vaginal infection by *C. albicans (Monilia)* is a fairly common fungus problem, associated with the same conditions as the more serious infections. Other *Candida* species of importance are *C. tropicalis* and *C. parapsilosis*. *Candida tropicalis* infections are next in frequency to those of *C. albicans*. *Candida tropicalis* is most frequently associated with fungemia due to colonized venous catheters or with hyperalimentation. *Candida parapsilosis* is most frequently associated with narcotic addiction and with hyperalimentation catheters.

Diagnosis consists of wet-mount or stained slide preparations from accessible areas (which provide a presumptive diagnosis only), culture, and serologic tests. A potassium hydroxide (KOH) wet preparation detects *Candida* in about 60%–70% of vaginal KOH preparations (40%–85% of all KOH cases, depending on number of organisms present, compared to culture). One report found that nonmicrobiologists could detect only about 20%. Use of fluorescent stains such as Calcofluor white could increase detection rates. A new slide latex agglutination test for *Candida* antigen in vaginal specimens has recently become available, with manufacturer claims of 80% sensitivity. Papanicolaou-stained slides are reported to detect about 50% of vaginal candidiasis.

Various serologic tests for antibody are available. The latex agglutination procedure is the easiest to perform. It has a reported sensitivity of 81%–94%. Counterimmunoelectrophoresis (CIE) is a little less sensitive (78%–88%). Immunosuppressed patients tend to have lower detection rates. At present, none of the commonly used serologic tests will reliably differentiate between superficial infection (or colonization) and deep infection, and neither will cultures from accessible specimen sites. Isolation of *Candida* from both blood and urine culture, however, is very suggestive of disseminated candidiasis.

Torulopsis glabrata is a species from the genus *Torula* that clinically resembles *Candida* in many respects. In some hospitals it may surpass *C. tropicalis* in frequency and is isolated under essentially the same conditions (associated with IV catheters, antibiotic therapy, Foley catheters, and extensive surgery). Pathogenicity is considered to be less than that of *Candida*, so that isolation may or may not be clinically significant.

Aspergillus

Aspergillus is a fungus with branching septated (bamboo-like) hyphae present normally in soil and different vegetation. In medicine, *A. fumigatus* is most frequently isolated, followed by *A. flavus* and *Aspergillus niger*. The organism spreads through dust or airborne spores; therefore, human entry involves the respiratory tract. There is widespread exposure in the environment; but with the exception of some individuals with allergy, persons with normal immune systems usually do not develop *Aspergillus*-related disease. About 5%–10% of hospitalized patients have nasopharyngeal colonization. *Aspergillus*-related medical problems may occur in several forms:

1. Reactive allergic disease. This is caused by allergy to inhaled *Aspergillus* organisms without *Aspergillus* colonization or infection.
2. Allergic bronchopulmonary aspergillosis. This is usually associated with preexisting asthma and is a type of hypersensitivity lung disease. After inhalation, *Aspergillus* produces a localized small infection of the respiratory tract that is a source of antigen to an already sensitized person. Affected patients all have a history of asthma that becomes much worse. There frequently are low-grade fever and chest x-ray abnormalities of various types. However, the chest film may be normal.
3. Aspergilloma. This is a "fungus ball" type of localized infection within cystic spaces of the lung due to preexisting chronic lung disease. About 85% are located in the upper portions of the lungs. Chronic tuberculosis is the most frequent precursor (25%–72% of aspergilloma cases). An aspergilloma may be asymptomatic or may result in hemoptysis (50%–80% of cases). Cough and sputum production is also common.
4. "Invasive" aspergillosis. This may be localized, usually in the lung, or disseminated. Invasive aspergillosis is usually associated with patients with leukemia or lymphoma, patients with solid tumors undergoing chemotherapy, or patients who are immunosuppressed. The patients frequently have neutropenia. The same group of patients have a markedly increased incidence of *Candida* infection.

The lungs and skull sinuses are frequently involved infection sites. Contaminated air conditioning systems or air ducts have often been implicated as the source of *Aspergillus* infection. Diagnosis requires the same procedures that were described for candidiasis. Demonstration of *Aspergillus* in sputum is more alarming than finding *Candida*. However, colonization rather than infection may be present. In one series of patients, one third of those with *Aspergillus* in the sputum failed to yield evidence of *Aspergillus* infection. *Aspergillus fumigatus* and *A. flavus* are much more likely to be respiratory tract pathogens than the other species of *Aspergillus*. On the other hand, in invasive pulmonary aspergillosis, only 13%–34% produced sputum that grew *Aspergillus*. Biopsy of lesions with culture or tissue examination are the best ways to make a definitive diagnosis. *Aspergillus* typically invades blood vessel walls in tissue specimens. If biopsy material is obtained, special stains are usually needed to find and identify the organism. Various serologic test procedures have been reported, but the ones most commonly used are CIE or some type of agar gel diffusion. These tests detect about 90%–95% of well-established *Aspergillus* infections. False positive results have been reported in about 3% of the general population and in up to 25% of patients with asthma. *Aspergillus fumagatus*–specific IgE antibody detected by ELISA or radioimmunoassay methods is reported to be present in about 85% of patients with allergic bronchopulmonary aspergillosis but less than 20% of those with aspergilloma or *Aspergillus*-associated asthma. A skin test for *Aspergillus* that gives results similar to those of the serologic tests, including the false positive reactions, is available.

In patients with aspergilloma, helpful laboratory findings include eosinophils in sputum and a peripheral blood eosinophilia. In classic cases the sputum contains golden brown plugs that contain *Aspergillus* hyphae. In one series, *Aspergillus* hyphae were seen microscopically in 40%, and sputum culture was positive in about 55%. Fiberoptic bronchoscopy is reported to increase the isolation rate (55%–100%). Results of skin tests and serologic tests are usually positive, as noted previously, but results of these tests may be positive without evidence of aspergillosis in persons with asthma.

Mucormycosis

Mucormycosis (Zygomycosis) is usually caused by saprophytic bread mold fungi with nonseptate hyphae of the genus *Mucor* or *Rhizopus*. Infection is characteristically associated with diabetic ketoacidosis and is also more common in patients with leukemia or lymphoma and immunocompromised persons. Infection is most common in the nasopharynx region and paranasal sinuses. There may be spread to the brain or blood-borne dissemination. Diagnosis is through culture and biopsy.

FUNGAL CULTURES

When fungal culture is indicated, the laboratory must be notified, because bacterial culture media are not generally suitable for fungi. All-purpose mycotic culture media, such as Sabouraud's agar under aerobic conditions are satisfactory for most of the systemic fungi.

DERMATOPHYTES

The dermatophytes include a number of fungi that attack the nails and skin. A presumptive etiologic diagnosis may be made by examining scrapings of the affected area microscopically in a wet mount of 10% KOH. Calcofluor white or similar fluorescent methods enhance detection. Definitive diagnosis is by culture, usually on an all-purpose medium such as Sabouraud's agar, although some special media are available. Additional tests relevant to this chapter are described in chapter 35.

BIBLIOGRAPHY

Thaler M, et al: Hepatic candidiasis in cancer patients. *Ann Intern Med* 1988; 108:88.

Paya CV: Laboratory methods for the diagnosis of disseminated histoplasmosis: Clinical importance of the lysis-centrifugation blood culture technique. *Mayo Clin Proc* 1987; 62:480.

Weems JJ: *Candida parapsilosis* fungemia associated with parenteral nutrition and contaminated blood pressure transducers. *J Clin Microbiol* 1987; 25:1029.

Cross AS: Nosocomial aspergillosis: An increasing problem. *J Nosocom Infect* 1987; 4(2):6.

Green LK: Fluorescent compounds that nonspecifically stain fungi. *Lab Med* 1987; 18:456.

Brummund W, et al: *Aspergillus fumigatus*–specific antibodies in allergic bronchopulmonary aspergillosis and aspergilloma. *J Clin Microbiol* 1987; 25:5.

Watts JC, Chandler FW: Primary pulmonary sporotrichosis. *Arch Pathol Lab Med* 1987; 111:215.

Yu VL, et al: Significance of isolation of *Aspergillus* from the respiratory tract in diagnosis of invasive pulmonary aspergillosis. *Am J Med* 1986; 81:249.

Elder BL, Roberets GD: Rapid methods for the diagnosis of fungal infections. *Lab Med* 1986; 17:591.

Oakley LA: Bread mold infection in diabetes. *Postgrad Med* 1986; 80:93.

Diamond R: The immunologic diagnosis of cryptococcosis. *Lab Mgmt* 1985; 23(7):35.

Schmid GP, Larsen SA: Candidiasis: When yeasts are pathogenic. *Diagn Med* 1985; 8:34.

Jones JM: The immunobiology of candidiasis and aspergillosis. *Lab Mgmt* 1985; 23(3):53.

Dar MA, et al: Thoracic aspergillosis (part I). *Cleve Clin Q* 1984; 51:615.

Saubolle MA: Clinical significance and laboratory identification of yeasts. *Lab Med* 1984; 15:98.

George RB, Penn RL: Blastomycosis: More common than you thought? *J Respir Dis* 1984; 5:95.

Barbee R: Coccidioidomycosis: No longer a regional problem. *J Respir Dis* 1983; 4:78.

Philip A: Some infrequently isolated fungi in a clinical laboratory. *Lab Med* 1983; 14:158.

Wheat J, et al: The diagnostic laboratory tests for histoplasmosis. *Ann Intern Med* 1982; 97:680.

16 Viral and Rickettsial Infectious Diseases

VIRAL DISEASES

Viral diseases form a large heterogeneous group. A general classification of the most important viruses is presented in Table 16–1.

Viral Upper Respiratory Tract Diseases

Respiratory disease may take several forms, and the predominant etiologies are different in different age groups. Incidence statistics also vary depending on the geographic area and the population selected. Of the known viruses, rhinoviruses are predominantly associated with acute upper respiratory tract disease (including the common cold) in adults, whereas in children, rhinovirus, adenovirus, parainfluenza virus, and the enteroviruses are important. Acute bronchitis in children is most often due to respiratory syncytial virus and parainfluenza virus. In croup, parainfluenza is said to be the most important virus.

Viral Pneumonia

Respiratory syncytial virus is the predominant cause of pneumonia in infants and young children, beginning at age 1 month with a peak incidence at about age 6 months, followed by adenovirus or parainfluenza virus. In older children or adults, bacterial pneumonia (most often due to *Pneumococcus* or *Mycoplasma pneumoniae*) is more common than viral pneumonia. Among viral agents known to cause pneumonia in adults, the most common is probably influenza. In any study, a large minority of cases do not yield a specific etiologic agent.

Viral Meningitis

Viruses are an important cause of meningitis, especially in children. They typically produce the laboratory picture of aseptic meningitis: the classic cerebrospinal fluid (CSF) findings are variable, but often include mildly increased protein levels, increased cell counts with mononuclear cells predominating, normal glucose levels, and no organisms found on culture. It should be remembered, however, that tuberculous meningitis gives similar findings, except for a decreased CSF glucose level, and likewise shows a sterile culture on ordinary bacterial culture media. Some patients with mumps meningoencephalitis may have decreased CSF glucose levels in addition to CSF lymphocytosis. Enteroviruses are the largest etiologic group causing aseptic meningitis. Among the enteric viruses, poliomyelitis used to be the most common organism, but with widespread polio vaccination programs, echovirus and coxsackievirus have replaced polio in terms of frequency.

After the enteroviruses, mumps is the most important. A small but significant number of patients with mumps develop clinical signs of meningitis, and a large number show CSF changes without demonstrating enough clinical symptoms to warrant a diagnosis and workup for meningitis. Changes in CSF or the clinical picture of meningitis may occur in patients without parotid swelling or other evi-

TABLE 16–1.
Classification of Viruses

Taxonomic Classification	
RNA Viruses	
Arenavirus	Lassa fever; lymphocytic choriomeningitis
Calicivirus	Norwalk virus
Orthomyxovirus	Influenza
Paramyxovirus	Measles (rubeola); mumps, parainfluenza, respiratory syncytial virus; Newcastle disease; canine distemper
Picornavirus	Enterovirus (coxsackie; enteric cytopathic human orphan [ECHO]; poliomyelitis; rhinovirus; hepatitis A virus (HAV)
Reovirus	Reovirus ("respiratory enteric orphan virus" of common cold); and rotavirus
Togavirus	Arbovirus ("Arthropod-borne virus")— (dengue, equine encephalitis, St. Louis encephalitis, yellow fever); and rubella
Rhabdovirus	Rabies
Retrovirus	Oncoviruses; HIVs; HTLVs; lentiviruses
DNA Viruses	
Adenovirus	Acute upper respiratory tract infections
Hepadnavirus	Hepatitis B virus (HBV)
Herpesvirus	Cytomegalic inclusion virus; Epstein-Barr (E-B) virus; herpes simplex virus (HSV); herpes zoster–varicella
Papovirus	Papillomavirus (wart virus)
Parvovirus	B-19 virus
Poxvirus	Vaccinia; variola; molluscum contagiosum

Clinical Classification (Characteristic Organ Systems Involved Clinically)	
Central nervous system	Liver
Arbovirus	Hepatitis viruses
Enterovirus	Yellow fever
Rabies	Squamous epithelium
Lentiviruses	Papillomavirus
Gastrointestinal system	Poxvirus
Rotavirus	Salivary glands
Norwalk virus	Cytomegalic inclusion virus
Enterovirus	Mumps
Respiratory tract	Lymphocytes
Adenovirus	Human immunodeficiency viruses (HIVs)
Myxovirus	Human T-cell leukemia viruses (HTLVs)
Reovirus	E-B virus
Rhinovirus	

dence of mumps. Lymphocytic choriomeningitis and leptospirosis are uncommon etiologies for aseptic meningitis.

Encephalitis is a syndrome that frequently has CSF alterations similar to those of meningitis. The two cannot always be separated, but the main difference is clinical; encephalitis features depression of consciousness (lethargy, coma) over a prolonged period, whereas meningitis usually is a more acute illness with manifestations including fever, headache, vomiting, lethargy, stiff neck, and possibly convulsions. In severe bacterial infection, encephalitis may follow meningitis. Encephalitis is most often caused by viruses, of which the more common are mumps, herpes simplex type I (HSV-I), measles, and the arboviruses. Sometimes encephalitis is a complication of vaccination.

Viral Gastroenteritis

Viruses are likely to be blamed for diarrhea that cannot be explained otherwise. In most cases, definitive evidence is lacking because enteric virus is present in a significant number of apparently healthy children. Bacterial infection should always be carefully ruled out. Two clinical types of viral gastroenteritis have been described. One type usually occurs in epidemics, more often in older children and in adults, with clinical signs of an acute self-limited gastroenteritis of 1–2 days' duration. The most commonly associated etiology is the Norwalk-type group of viruses. The other type of illness is sporadic and affects mostly infants and younger children. There is severe diarrhea, usually accompanied by fever and vomiting, which lasts for 5–8 days. Rotavirus is the most frequently isolated virus in these patients. About 10% of gastroenteritis in infants less than 2 years old is said to be caused by adenovirus types 40 and 41.

Viral Infections in Pregnancy

By far the most dangerous viral disease during pregnancy is rubella. Statistics are variable, but they suggest about a 15%–25% risk of fetal malformation when rubella infection occurs in the first trimester (literature range, 10%–90%). The earlier in pregnancy that maternal infection occurs, the greater the risk that the fetus will be infected. However, not all infected fetuses develop congenital malformation. When the fetus is infected early in the first trimester, besides risk of congenital malformation, as many as 5%–15% of fetuses may die in utero. Risk of fetal malformation in second trimester infections is about 5%. After the fourth month of pregnancy, there is no longer any danger to the fetus. Cytomegalovirus (CMV) infection is more frequent than rubella, but CMV has a lower malformation rate. Cytomegalovirus damage is more severe in the first two trimesters. Other viruses may cause congenital malformations, but evidence is somewhat inconclusive as to exact incidence and effects. Herpes simplex and the hepatitis viruses are in this group.

Diagnosis of Viral Diseases

Culture.—Until the 1980s, except in a relatively few cases the only available laboratory methods were culture and serologic tests for antibodies. There have been significant advances in culture techniques in the past few years, but most virus culture still is difficult and expensive. Culture is performed using living cell preparations or in living tissues. This fact in itself rules out mass production testing. Partly for this reason, facilities for culture are limited and are available mainly at sizable medical centers, regional reference laboratories, or large public health laboratories. In addition, culture and identification of the virus takes several days. Finally, cultural isolation of certain viruses does not absolutely prove that the virus is causing actual patient disease, since many viruses are quite prevalent in the general clinically healthy population. In these instances, confirmation of recent infection is helpful, such as presence of IgM antibodies or a fourfold rising titer of antibodies.

Antigen Detection.—In the 1980s, several other diagnostic techniques that can detect viral antigen have appeared. These include electron microscopy, fluorescent antibody (FA) methods, enzyme-linked immunoassay (ELISA), latex agglutination (LA) methods, and, even more recently, nucleic acid (DNA) probes (chapter 14). These methods can provide same-day results. However, many of them are relatively expensive, especially the DNA probes, particularly when only one patient specimen is tested at a time. Except in large-volume reference laboratories, most institutions do not receive a large number of orders for virus tests in general, and with the possible exception of rubella, HBV, HIV type I (formerly HTLV type III [HTLV-III]), E-B virus, and possibly rotovirus, laboratories usually receive very few requests for diagnosis of any one particular virus. This makes it difficult for the average laboratory to keep reagents for testing many different viruses, and without having the advantage of testing many specimens at the same time, costs (and therefore, prices) are much higher.

Antibody Detection.—In addition to culture and tests for viral antigen, serologic tests for antibody are available for most viruses. There are many techniques, including complement fixation (CF), hemagglutination (HA or HAI), radioimmunoassay (RIA), enzyme-linked immunoassay (ELISA), FA, and latex agglutination (LA). Some of these methods can be adapted to detect either antigen or antibody. Although they are considerably less exacting than culture, most techniques other than LA are still tedious and time consuming. Therefore, these tests are not immediately available except at reference laboratories. Serologic tests have the additional disadvantage that antibodies usually take 1–2 weeks to develop after onset of illness, and unless a significantly (fourfold or two-tube) rising titer is demonstrated, they do not differentiate past from recent infection by the viral agent in question. One serum specimen is obtained as early in the disease as possible ("acute" stage) and a second sample is obtained 2–3 weeks later ("convalescent" stage). Blood should be collected in sterile tubes or Vacutainer tubes and serum processed aseptically to avoid bacterial contamination. Hemolyzed serum is not acceptable. To help prevent hemolysis, serum should be separated from blood clot as soon as possible. The serum should be frozen as soon as possible after collection to minimize bacterial growth and sent still frozen (packed in dry ice) to the virus laboratory. Here a variety of serologic tests can be done to demonstrate specific antibodies to the various organisms. A fourfold rise in titer from acute to convalescent stage of the disease is considered diagnostic. If only a single specimen is taken, an elevated titer could be due to previous infection rather than to currently active disease. A single negative test result is likewise difficult to interpret, since the specimen might have been obtained too early (before antibody rise occurred) or in the case of short-lived antibodies such as IgM, a previously elevated antibody value may have decreased to nondetectable levels.

There is one notable exception to the rule of acute and convalescent serologic specimens. In some circumstances, it is desirable to learn whether a person has an antibody titer to a particular virus that is sufficient to prevent onset of the disease. This is especially true for a woman in early pregnancy who might be exposed to rubella. A single significant antibody titer to rubella suggests immunity to the virus.

Two types of antibodies are produced in most, but not all, bacterial or viral infections. A macroglobulin (IgM) type appears first, usually shortly before or just after onset of clinical illness; reaches a peak titer about 1–2 weeks after clinical symptoms begin; and then falls to normal levels within a few weeks (usually in less than 6 months). A gamma-globulin (IgG) type appears 1 or more weeks after detection of IgM antibody. The IgG antibody reaches a peak 1–3 weeks (sometimes longer) after the peak of the IgM antibody. The IgG antibody typically persists much longer than the IgM antibody (several years or even for life). Therefore, presence of the IgM antibody usually indicates recent acute infection. Presence of the IgG antibody usually requires that a rising titer be obtained to diagnose acute infection (although in some diseases there are circumstances that alter this requirement), since without a rising titer one does not know whether the IgG antibody elevation is due to recent or to old infection.

Viral Test Specimens

The type of specimen needed for viral culture depends on the type of illness. In aseptic meningitis, a CSF specimen should be obtained. In addition, stool culture for virus should be done, since enteroviruses are frequent causes of meningitis. In enterovirus meningitis, stool culture is 2–3 times more effective than CSF culture.

In any kind of meningitis with negative spinal fluid cultures, or severe respiratory tract infection of unknown etiology, it is a good idea to freeze a specimen of serum as early in the disease as possible. Later on, if desired, another specimen can be drawn and the two sent for virus studies. As noted, serum specimens are generally drawn 2 weeks apart.

In suspected cases of (nonbacterial) encephalitis, whole blood should be collected for virus culture during the first 2 days of illness. During this short time there is a chance of demonstrating arbovirus viremia. This procedure is not useful in aseptic meningitis. Spinal fluid should also be sent for virus culture. Although the yield is relatively small in arbovirus infections, the specimen results sometimes are positive, and culture also helps to rule out other organisms, such as enterovirus. In upper respiratory tract illness, throat or nasopharyngeal swabs are preferred. These should be placed in trypticase broth (a standard bacterial medium). Swabs not preserved in some type of medium such as trypticase or Hank's solution are usually not satisfactory, since they dry out quickly, and most viruses are killed by drying. Throat washings or gargle material can be used but are difficult to obtain properly. In viral pneumonia, sputum or throat swabs are needed. If throat swabs are used, they should be placed in acceptable transport solutions. Whether throat swab or sputum is used, the specimen must be frozen immediately and sent to the virus laboratory packed in dry ice. In addition, a sputum specimen (or throat swab) should be obtained for *Mycoplasma* culture (chapter 14).

In possible viral gastroenteritis, the most logical specimen is stool. At present, rotavirus and Norwalk viruses cannot be cultured from stool, but stool can be examined for Norwalk virus by immune electron microscopy and for rotovirus antigen by RIA, ELISA, or slide LA. Serologic tests on serum can be used for diagnosis of rotavirus infection, but only a few laboratories are able to do this. Whenever a stool culture for virus is needed, actual stool specimens are preferred to rectal swabs, since there is a better chance of isolating an organism from the larger sample. Stool samples should be collected as soon as possible—according to the U.S. Centers for Disease Control (CDC), no later than 48 hours after onset of symptoms (to ensure the best chance of success). The stool specimen should be refrigerated not frozen; and if sent to an outside laboratory, the specimen should be shipped the day of collection (if possible), and kept cool with dry ice. However, it is better to mail any virus specimens early in the week to avoid arrival on weekends. An insulated container helps prolong effects of the dry ice.

An adequate clinical history with pertinent physical and laboratory findings should accompany any virus specimen, whether for culture or serologic studies. As a minimum, the date of clinical illness onset, collection date of each specimen, and clinical diagnosis must be included. The most likely organism should be indicated. This information helps the virus laboratory to decide what initial procedures to use. For example, some tissue culture cell types are better adapted than others for certain viruses. Considerable time and effort can be saved and a meaningful interpretation of results can be provided.

Certain viruses deserve individual discussion. The method of diagnosis or type of specimen required for some of these organisms is different from the usual procedure, whereas in other cases it is desirable to emphasize certain aspects of the clinical illness that suggest the diagnosis.

Rubella

Rubella (German measles) is a very common infection of childhood, although primary infection can occur in adults. The major clinical importance of rubella is maternal infection during pregnancy, which may produce the *congenital rubella syndrome* in the fetus. The congenital rubella syndrome includes one or more of the following: congenital heart disease, cataracts, deafness, and cerebral damage. Diagnosis is made by documenting active rubella infection in the mother during early pregnancy and by proving infection of the infant shortly after birth. Rubella antibody tests are used to determine (1) if a woman is susceptible to rubella infection (and, therefore, should be immunized to prevent infection during pregnancy), (2) to prove that a woman is immune (and therefore, does not have to be immunized or be concerned about rubella infection), (3) to determine if possible or actual exposure to rubella infection during pregnancy actually produced maternal infection, and (4) to determine if an infant has been infected. For a number of years, the hemagglutination inhibition (HI) and complement fixation (CF) serologic tests formed the backbone of diagnosis. Rubella has an incubation period of about 2 weeks (range, 10–21 days), followed by development of the skin rash (Fig 16–1). Hemagglutination inhibition–reacting antibodies appear during the first week after onset of a rash; they are sometimes detectable after only 2–3 days. Peak levels are reached near the beginning of the second week after onset of the rash. Afterward the titer slowly falls, but an elevated titer persists for many years or for life. Although the standard HI test detects both IgM and IgG antibodies, the HI time sequence just described is similar to that of rubella IgG antibodies. Complement fixation–reacting or immunofluorescent-demonstrable antibodies develop in the more conventional time of 7–14 days after onset of the rash, reach a peak about 14–21 days after the rash and usually disappear in a few years. Serologic tests for rubella IgM antibody are available. Immunoglobulin M antibody titer begins to rise about the time of onset of the rash, peaks about 1 week after onset of the rash, and becomes nondetectable about 4–5 weeks after onset of the rash (range 21 days–3 months). Therefore, the rubella IgM and IgG antibody rise and peak are relatively close together, in contrast to serologic behavior in most other viral diseases, in which IgG usually follows IgM by at least 1 week. Some IgM procedures, but not others, may be affected by IgM produced against nonrubella antigen (e.g., rheumatoid factor). If so, this might lead to a false positive result. Besides primary infection, rubella reinfection can occur. If this happens there is often a rise in IgG antibody, but IgM antibody is not produced. Reinfection of the mother during pregnancy is not dangerous to the fetus, in marked contrast to primary infection. Although the HI test became the standard for rubella testing, there were a significant number of technical problems and significant variation in results between laboratories. In the 1980s it has been mostly replaced by other techniques such as ELISA, and, especially, LA. The ELISA method or similar methods generally detect about 94%–97% of nonneonatal patients with well-established rubella compared with HI and can be modified to detect either IgM or IgG, whereas most LA kits detect 97%–99% and are easier, quicker, and less expensive but detect only the IgG response. The LA test is most often used as a screen for immunity to rubella infection; if so, it is carried out on a single 1:8 serum dilution and reported as positive (immune) or negative (the 1:8 dilution is the HI titer level that has become accepted as demonstrable of an immune IgG antibody response). If multiple serum dilutions are tested, the antibody responses detected by LA are similar in time sequence to the IgG response of HI.

Absence of HI IgG (1:8 level) or LA antibody indicates susceptibility to rubella since elevated IgG levels usually persist for many years, whereas titers of other antibodies return to normal. Presence of LA antibody means either past or recent infection. In a person who is clinically well, this means immunity to subsequent infection. In a person with clinically suspected rubella, an immediate serum specimen and a second one drawn 2 weeks later should be obtained, the standard procedure for all serologic tests. A fourfold rise in titer confirms very recent (active) infection. However, if the first serum specimen was not obtained until several days after onset of a rash, the LA antibody titer peak may already have been reached, and no further increase may occur. If tests for rubella IgM antibody are available, presence of this antibody means recent acute infection. Absence of IgM antibody in a single specimen, however, does not completely rule out acute or recent infection, since the specimen could have been obtained either before antibody rise or after antibody fall. If IgM antibody tests are not available, a significant two-tube dilution or fourfold rise in titer of CF or fluorescent antibody may be demonstrable, since these antibodies develop later than LA. However, if both the LA and CF antibodies are at their peak, it is impossible with this information alone to differentiate between recent infection and infection occurring months or even years previously. Height of titers by itself is not reliable in differentiating acute from old infection; only a sufficient change in titer can provide this information.

Infants with congenital rubella infection can produce both IgM and IgG antibody before birth, beginning in the late second trimester. In addition, the fetus acquires passively transferred maternal IgG antibody, whether or not the mother acquired the infection during pregnancy, so that neonatal serum IgG antibodies could represent either old or current maternal infection. Therefore, neonatal serum IgG antibodies might originate from the infant, the mother, or both. By age 6–8 months, maternal antibody in the child has disappeared, and persistence of IgM or IgG antibody past this time indicates congenital or neonatal infection. For some reason, however, at least 20% of children with congenital rubella lose their HI titer by age 5 years. Congenital rubella can also be diagnosed by detection of specific rubella IgM antibody in the blood of the newborn. If the

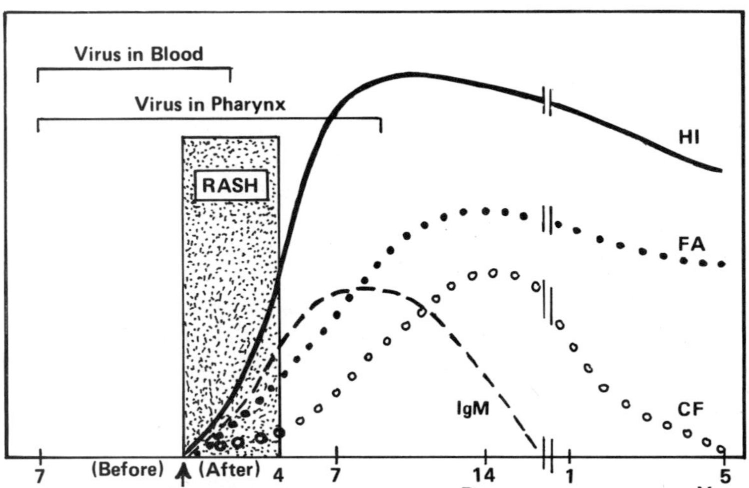

FIG 16–1.
Serologic tests in rubella infection.

specimen is drawn before 10 days of life (the incubation period of rubella acquired during or just after birth before postnatal antibody has a chance to rise), specific rubella IgM antibody is diagnostic of intrauterine infection. If the specimen is obtained later, this antibody may be highly suggestive of congenital rubella but is not absolutely diagnostic, since there could be a small chance that infection was acquired after delivery.

The ELISA and LA tests are, in general, more reliable than the HI test in the average laboratory. However, false positive or negative results may occur for various reasons, just as they may occur with any test in any laboratory. If the patient is pregnant and test results may lead to some action, it may be advisable to split each sample, keeping part of each frozen, if the specimens are sent to an outside laboratory, in case a recheck is desired. If the tests are performed in-house, immediate redraw of a specimen that suggests active maternal infection might be useful. Because of technical factors, most laboratories list a specific titer below which the antibody level is not considered significant. This depends to some extent on the test being used. The cutoff titer level most frequently is 1:8 or 1:10. This fact is mentioned because theoretically any antibody titer ought to be significant in terms of indicating previous infection. However, in actual practice, antibody levels below the cutoff value are considered negative since it is not certain how much artifact is involved in very low titers.

Summary of Rubella Test Results

To test for immunity to rubella in a pregnant or nonpregnant woman, an LA test (or other standard rubella test) is obtained. If the result is negative, the woman is susceptible to infection. A positive test result means immunity; and in a nonpregnant woman and in many pregnant women, this is usually enough information. However, a positive test result could either be due to past infection or recent infection. If there is some reason to rule out recent infection in a pregnant or nonpregnant woman, a rubella IgM titer could be obtained. An alternative could be a titer of the original specimen plus another specimen for titer in 2 weeks. To determine whether recent infection took place, the time relationship of two critical events—date of exposure or date of rash—is extremely important regarding what test to use and when to obtain the test specimen or specimens. To determine the presence or absence of immunity only, such timing is not important.

If a pregnant woman has been exposed to someone with rubella, and the question is whether infection has been acquired, serum should be obtained immediately for rubella antibody titer. A significant titer obtained less than 10 days after exposure usually means immunity because of previous disease (the incubation period of rubella is 10–21 days). If the result is negative or a borderline low titer, a second specimen should be obtained 3–4 weeks later to detect a rising titer (to permit sufficient time for antibody to be produced if infection did occur). If exposure was more than 10 days previously and the LA titer is borderline or elevated, a second specimen should be obtained 2–3 weeks later to detect a possible rising titer. Alternatively, a rubella IgM antibody test could be obtained about 3 weeks after exposure. Significantly elevated IgM proves recent primary infection.

If a person develops a rash, and the question is whether it was due to rubella, two specimens for rubella antibody titer should be drawn, one immediately and the other 2 weeks later. Alternatively, a rubella IgM antibody test could be obtained 7 days after the rash onset. The information on rubella test diagnosis is presented again in chapter 35 in a different format.

Measles

Measles (rubeola) is still important, even though widespread vaccination has begun. The two main complications are encephalitis and pneumonia. Fortunately, encephalitis is rare, the incidence being 0.01%–0.2%. Due to the great frequency of the disease, however, the total number of cases is appreciable. About one third of those with encephalitis die, one third recover completely, and the remainder survive but show moderate to severe residua. Measles encephalitis is considered postinfectious because it develops 4–21 days after the onset of rash. Measles involves lymphoid tissue and respiratory epithelium early in the illness. Therefore, pneumonia is fairly frequent. Most cases of pneumonia are due to superimposed bacterial infection (staphylococci, pneumococci, streptococci), but some are caused directly by the rubeola virus. For diagnosis, culture and serologic tests are available. Culture depends on the stage of disease. For a period of 1 week ending with the first appearance of the rash, blood, nasopharyngeal swabs, or urine provide adequate specimens. After appearance of the rash, urine culture is possible up to 4 days. Beyond this, culture is not useful, and serologic tests must be employed using acute and convalescent serum specimens. Measles HI–detectable antibodies appear about the end of the first week after appearance of the rash and peak about 2 weeks later. Measles IgM antibody appears less than 1 week following rash onset, peaks about 10–14 days after rash onset, and becomes undetectable at about 30 days. Interpretation is similar to that of rubella tests. However, one report indicates about 30% false negative IgM results even 3 weeks after disease onset.

Mumps

Mumps is a disseminated virus infection, although the main clinical feature is salivary gland enlargement. Evidence of nonsalivary gland involvement is most commonly seen in adults. In men, orchitis (usually unilateral) is reported in about 20% of cases. Adult women occasionally develop oophoritis. Persons of any age may be affected by meningoencephalitis, the most serious complication of mumps. This is reported in 0.5%–10% of patients. Many persons with CSF changes are asymptomatic. Females are affected five times more frequently than males. Complications of mumps may appear before, during, or after parotitis, sometimes even without clinical parotitis. Diagnosis is made by culture or serologic tests. Saliva is probably best for culture; mouth swabs or CSF can be used. Serologic tests require acute and convalescent serum specimens.

Respiratory Syncytial Virus

Respiratory syncytial virus (RSV) is the most common cause of severe lower respiratory illness of infants and young children, causing 5%–40% of pneumonias and 60%–90% of bronchiolitis episodes. Peak incidence is at 2–3 months of age. About 30%–50% of children have been infected by 12 months of age and about 95% by age 5 years. However, no significant clinical immunity is produced; repeat infections may occur, and persons of any age may develop acute infection. The most common clinical illness is upper respiratory tract infection similar to the common cold. The virus is spread through airborne droplets. The incubation period is 2–8 days. Diagnosis can be made by culture, by tests for antigen, and by tests for antibody. The best specimen for culture is nasal washings; the next best is nasopharyngeal swab. In either case, the specimen should include cells from the nasopharyngeal epithelium, since they contain the virus. Swab specimens should be placed immediately into a transport medium, and any specimen should be placed into wet ice. However, culture is expensive, time consuming (4–14 days), and usually must be sent to a reference laboratory with wet ice. The virus survives only about 4 days at 4°C and dies quickly at ordinary freezer temperatures or at high temperatures. Culture (under optimal conditions) is still considered the "gold standard" for diagnosis. However, some investigators report less than optimum results (69%–83% sensitivity), especially with mailed-in specimens. Antibody detection methods include CF, immunofluorescence, and ELISA. Antibody detection methods have several drawbacks: the fact that sensitivity is often less than 50% in infants less than 3 months old; the need for acute and convalescent specimens unless sufficiently elevated IgM titers are present; and the necessity in most cases to send the serum specimens to a reference laboratory. Methods for antigen detection in patient specimens are also available, including fluorescent antibody and ELISA, with same-day results. Nasopharyngeal aspirates are reported to provide the best specimens. Compared to culture, sensitivity of these methods are about 70%–90% (range, 41%–99%). Antigen detection methods may be positive on some specimens that are negative by culture, especially with mailed-in specimens. Antigen detection is rapidly replacing culture and antibody detection for diagnosis of RSV infection. However, the sensitivity of different manufacturers' kits may differ considerably.

Rotavirus

Rotavirus is the most frequent cause for infectious diarrhea of infants and young children. Symptoms include diarrhea, fever, and vomiting. Peak infection rates in the United

States are in winter months but are equally distributed in tropical areas. One investigator found that rotavirus produced 23% of childhood gastroenteritis in his geographic area. Another estimated that rotavirus caused 50% of pediatric hospitalizations for diarrhea in the winter. Rotavirus, however, can be isolated from the stool of some clinically healthy young children, especially in day-care centers or nurseries (about 10% in one study). Same-day diagnosis can be obtained from stool specimens using ELISA or LA antigen-detection methods. Sensitivity of the various kits available is about 90% (range, 61%–100%), compared to electron microscopy of the stool. There is a significant difference in sensitivity between some of the kits.

Hepatitis Viruses

There are at least four antigenically distinct members of the group called hepatitis virus. Originally only two were recognized.

Hepatitis A Virus

Hepatitis A virus was originally called "infectious hepatitis," or "short-incubation hepatitis," and has an incubation period of 2–6 weeks. It is highly contagious. During infection it is excreted in the stool and is usually transmitted via fecal-oral routes, especially by contaminated water or food. However, infection can spread from person to person. Clinical illness is usually not severe, and fatality is rare. There usually is complete recovery in 1–3 weeks without a carrier state. Occasional patients may have more prolonged illness lasting as long as 1 year. Also, cases of severe hepatitis with a high fatality rate have been reported. There is increased incidence of HAV infection in children, and epidemics occur within institutions for mentally retarded children, day-care centers, and orphanages. Occasional epidemics occur in adults, usually associated with eating contaminated food or shellfish from contaminated water. About 40%–60% of adults in the United States who have been tested have antibody against HAV. More than 50% of acute HAV infections are subclinical.

Hepatitis B Virus (HBV)

Hepatitis B virus was originally called "serum hepatitis," or "long-incubation hepatitis," and has an incubation period of 5 weeks–6 months. Hepatitis B virus is found in blood and body secretions. Infection was originally thought to be limited to parenteral inoculation (blood transfusion or injection with a contaminated needle). Although this is still the major source of infection, the virus may be contracted by inoculation of infected blood, saliva, or semen through a small break in the skin or a mucous membrane (e.g., the rectum) or by sexual intercourse. The virus seems less infectious through nonparenteral transmission than is HAV. Hepatitis B virus infection has a wide range of severity and is fatal in about 1% (range, 1%–3%) of patients. In general, only about 30%–40% of patients with acute HBV develop clinically apparent acute hepatitis; the remainder are subclinical infections. Nonicteric hepatitis is even more frequent in HAV. There is an increased incidence in persons receiving two units or more of blood, in male homosexuals, in drug abuse patients, in renal dialysis patients or dialysis unit personnel, in renal transplant patients, and in persons with leukemia or lymphoma. Hospital personnel are also at risk for HBV infection, most often due to accidental needle stick after drawing blood from an infected patient. It is reported that the risk of contracting HBV infection from a contaminated needle stick is 6%–30%. There is disagreement regarding risk of HBV spread in day-care centers. In the past few years, blood bank screening for donor HBV surface antigen (HB_sAg) has markedly reduced transmission by blood or blood products. Mothers who are HBV carriers frequently transmit HBV infection to their infants during the birth process (70%–90% of cases, especially when the mother is positive for both HBV surface antigen and the HBV e antigen. Without therapy, 80%–90% of infected infants become chronic carriers of HB_sAg. These infants are said to have a 25% risk of fatal cirrhosis or hepatoma. A combination of HBV vaccine and HBV immune globulin administered to the newborn can reduce risk of the chronic carrier state by 85%–95%.

Some 5%–15% of HBV infections become chronic, either as the carrier state or as chronic hepatitis. Although various definitions of these terms can be found in the literature, the *carrier state* is usually defined as persistence of HB_sAg for more than 6 months but with normal liver function tests and normal microscopic findings on liver biopsy. Chronic hepatitis can be divided into *chronic persistent hepatitis* (abnormal liver function tests plus relatively normal liver biopsy findings) and *chronic active hepatitis* (abnormal liver function tests plus abnormal findings on liver biopsy). The abnormalities on liver biopsy may exist in a spectrum of severity and may progress to cirrhosis. About 15%–20% of chronic HBV infections exist in the asymptomatic carrier state; of the remainder, about two-thirds are chronic persistent hepatitis and about one-third are chronic active hepatitis.

Non-A, Non-B Hepatitis Virus

Non-A, non-B (NANB) hepatitis virus is sometimes called "hepatitis C." It typically has an incubation period similar to that of HBV, although a short incubation type has also been reported. Transmission is similar to that for HBV. The NANB hepatitis now accounts for about 80%–90% of posttransfusion hepatitis cases when blood comes from volunteer donors whose serologic test results for HBV are negative. The NANB hepatitis virus is also reported to cause 12%–25% of cases of sporadic hepatitis (hepatitis not related to parenteral inoculation or sexual transmission). The clinical illness produced is also similar to HBV but tends to be a little less severe. However, progression to chronic hepatitis is more frequent than in HBV and is reported to occur in 40%–50% (literature range, 20%–62%) of apparent posttransfusion cases and 6%–7% of sporadic cases.

Hepatitis D Virus

Hepatitis D virus (HDV) is also called "delta hepatitis." It is a partially defective virus that requires the outer envelope of the HBV (which contains the HBV surface antigen) to replicate and produce clinical disease. Therefore, a person must have HBV present, either as clinical infection or as a carrier, to acquire HDV infection. When HBV infection is over, HDV infection will also disappear. Hepatitis D virus infection is acquired by the same routes as HBV infection. In the United States, infection is predominantly, but not entirely, spread through blood or blood products. The highest incidence is in drug addicts. There are three types of clinical infection. In the first type, HBV and HDV infection are transmitted at the same time. Clinically, this resembles an HBV infection that is more severe than the average. In the second type, acute HDV infection is superimposed on preexisting chronic HBV disease. Clinically, this resembles either an acute exacerbation of the preexisting HBV disease (if the HBV infection had previously been symptomatic), or it may appear to be onset of hepatitis without previous infection (if the initial HBV infection had been subclinical). There is increased incidence of progression to cirrhosis. In the third type, there is chronic HDV infection in addition to chronic HBV infection. Liver function test abnormalities are similar in HAV, HBV, NANB, and HDV infections and are discussed in chapter 19.

Diagnosis of Hepatitis A Virus Infection

Viremia and stool virus excretion begin 1–2 weeks after exposure. Viremia terminates just before or at the beginning of clinical symptoms, whereas virus excretion in the stool usually ceases within 1–4 days after onset of symptoms (however, it may cease before onset of symptoms or not until 2 weeks after development of symptoms). Serologic testing currently is the best method for diagnosis. Both RIA and ELISA methods have been used. Tests for HAV antigen are not yet commercially available. When they do become available, the major problem will be the disappearance of antigen before or shortly after onset of clinical symptoms. Two types of antibody to HAV antigen are produced. One is a macroglobulin (IgM), which appears about 3–4 weeks after exposure (range, 15–60 days), or just before the beginning of the AST increase (range, 10 days before to 7 days after the beginning of the AST increase). Peak values are reached approximately 1 week after the rise begins, with return to normal (nondetectable) in about 2 months (range, 1–5 months or 1–2 weeks after clinical symptoms subside to about 4 months after symptoms subside). However, in a few cases detectable IgM antibody has remained as long as 12–14 months. The second type of antibody is IgG, which appears about 2 weeks after the beginning of the IgM increase (between the middle stages of clinical symptoms and early convalescence), reaches a peak about 1–2 months after it begins to rise, and then slowly falls to lower titer levels, remaining detectable for more than 10 years (Fig 16–2).

If the IgM antibody is elevated but the IgG antibody is not, this proves acute HAV infection. If the IgM antibody is nondetectable and the IgG antibody is elevated, this could mean residual elevation from old HAV infection or a recent infection in the convalescent stage. If

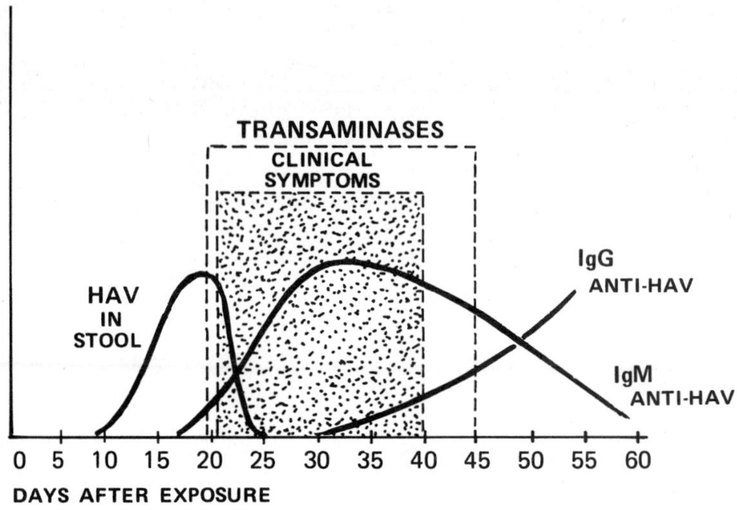

FIG 16–2.
Serologic tests in HAV infection.

clinical symptoms began less than 1 week before the specimen was obtained, an old HAV infection is more likely. If the test for IgM antibody is not done and the IgG antibody is elevated, this could mean either a recent infection or residual elevation from a previous infection. A rising titer is necessary to diagnose recent infection using the IgG antibody alone. If the test for IgM antibody is not done and the IgG test is nonreactive, it could mean either no infection by HAV or that the specimen was drawn before the IgG antibody titer began to rise. Whether another specimen should be drawn 2 weeks later to rule out a rising titer depends on the length of time that elapsed since clinical symptoms began or ended. Therefore, interpretation of HAV antibody test results depends on when the specimen was obtained relative to onset of clinical symptoms and which antibody or antibodies are being assayed.

Diagnosis of Hepatitis B Virus Infection

Studies have shown that the intact HBV molecule (Dane particle) has a double shell structure that contains several different antigens or antigenic material. There is an outer envelope that incorporates the HB_sAg (formerly known as the Australia antigen, or HAA antigen). There is an inner core that contains an HBV core antigen (HB_cAg). Also within the core is a structure consisting of double-stranded viral DNA, as well as the material called HB_eAg and an enzyme known as DNA polymerase. Antibodies are produced to the surface antigen (the antibody HB_sAb), to the core antigen (HB_cAb), and to the e antigen (HB_eAb). Serologic tests are currently available to detect each of the three antigen-antibody systems. The characteristics of these tests can be summarized as follows:

1. HB_sAg. The surface antigen test is the first serologic procedure to become abnormal, rising soon after infection and before onset of clinical symptoms, peaking during the week before to the week after onset of symptoms (usually shortly before onset of jaundice), and then falling rapidly to normal in most cases by the time jaundice subsides. It may become undetectable even before onset of jaundice (5%–15% of cases), but more often it persists for 1–6 weeks (average, 2–3 weeks). Therefore, detectable HB_sAg means active infection by HBV. Surface antigen is more likely to be undetectable in persons with subclinical infection and typically disappears before antibody to surface antigen appears (but not always; coexistence at some point in time is reported in 2%–25% of cases).

Some 5%–15% of HBV infections become chronic either as the carrier state or as chronic hepatitis. The carrier state usually has detectable HB_sAg by definition. About 20%–60% of patients with chronic persistent hepatitis and 9%–60% of patients with chronic active hepatitis have detectable HB_sAg levels.

Various test systems have been devised to detect HB_sAg. Sensitivity in patients with HB_sAg is variable: counterimmunoelectrophoresis detects about 40%; reverse passive hemagglutination about 70%, and RIA more than 85% (see Table 36–14). Interpretation of HB_sAg results thus must take into account (1) the knowledge that less than one half of the cases of hepatitis virus are due to HBV and, therefore, are potentially detectable by HB_sAg; (2) the type of test used; and (3) how early in the clinical course the specimen was obtained.

Antigenic subgroups of HB_sAg exist; the most important to date are adw, ayw, adr, and ayr, but others are being discovered. These are thought to indicate possible subgroups (strains) of HBV.

2. HB_cAb. No test is currently available for hepatitis B core antigen. Tests are available for HBV core antibody (HB_cAb, both the IgM and the IgG type). In most patients HB_cAb-IgM starts to rise about 2 weeks after appearance of HB_sAg (about 4 weeks before onset of clinical symptoms), peaks about 1 week after onset of symptoms, and becomes nondetectable about 6–8 months later (range, 2 weeks–2 years). In one study, HB_cAb-IgM persisted for more than 1 year in about 15% of patients. In patients who become chronic HBV carriers, HB_cAb-IgM is usually not detectable. In those who go on to chronic HBV disease, there is disagreement whether HB_cAb-IgM is detectable; with some investigators stating it is usually absent and one report finding that about one third of cases had detectable HB_cAb-IgM (most often relatively low level and sometimes present only intermittently). About 3–4 weeks after the appearance of HB_sAg (1–2 weeks after the appearance of HB_cAb-IgM) HB_cAb-IgG rises, roughly coinciding with the onset of clinical symptoms but before jaundice is evident. It peaks in about 1–2 weeks after onset of symptoms (often roughly coincident with jaundice), then declines very slowly but remains elevated to some degree for many years. Thus, HB_cAb-IgG becomes elevated while HB_sAg is still present, remains elevated when HB_sAg becomes nondetectable, continues in its elevation until a rise in HB_sAb develops, and then very slowly decreases over many years, usually remaining detectable for life.

In many persons with HBV there is a time lag or gap in time of variable length between disappearance of the HBV surface antigen and appearance of the surface antibody. This has been called the "core window," because the core IgG antibody is elevated during this time and represents the only HBV marker elevated in acute infection that is consistently detectable (the core IgM antibody is also present during part or all of the acute infection and also during part or all of the core window, but may become nondetectable during the window period, depending on when the patient specimen was obtained and the time span of the core window). The core window typically is 2–8 weeks in length but varies from 1 week (or less) to more than a year. Elevation of HB_cAb-IgG in itself does not mean that one has discovered the core window; a test for HB_sAg (and, if nondetectable, a test for HB_sAb) must be performed because both HB_sAg and HB_sAb must be absent. The core antibody nearly always is present in chronic hepatitis when surface antigen is detectable unless the patient is severely immunosuppressed.

The major clinical difference between IgM and IgG antibody is that the presence of IgM antibody usually means recent infection, whereas with IgG antibody one cannot differentiate between recent and old infection without being able to obtain a fourfold rising titer. Besides suggesting recent HBV infection, the presence of HB_cAb-IgM may be useful to differentiate between acute HBV infection (HB_cAb-IgM present and usually HB_sAg present) and acute NANB or delta hepatitis virus infection superimposed on the HBV carrier state (HB_sAg present but HB_cAb-IgM absent). There are some tests for HBV antibody that detect both IgM and IgG antibodies and do not distinguish between them. These tests behave essentially like those for IgG antibody.

3. HB_sAb. The appearance of antibody to HB_sAg occurs after about 2–6 weeks following disappearance of HB_sAg (range, 1 week to >1 year) and signifies the end of acute infection and immunity to future infection. Hepatitis B virus surface antibody usually persists for years. However, some patients have been reported to lose detectable HB_sAb in less than 6 years (2%–33% in three studies, most in < 2 years). Also, in about 10% (range, 5%–15%) of HBV acute infections, detectable HB_sAb never develops after the HB_sAg marker disappears. In patients with symptoms of acute or chronic hepatitis who lose their HB_sAb reactivity, if the initial patient blood specimen is obtained after HB_sAg

and HB_sAb has disappeared, an incorrect diagnosis of NANB hepatitis virus might be made unless an HB_cAb test is obtained. However, HBV core antibody (IgG type) is usually present when HB_sAg is elevated; in addition, it overlaps the core window between disappearance of HB_sAg and appearance of HB_sAb, and it remains elevated indefinitely with or without long-term elevation of HB_sAb. Finally, an elevation of HB_sAb does not indicate whether HBV infection was recent or old; a fourfold rising titer indicates recent infection, but a stable titer is not helpful.

Various studies have reported that 2%–25% of patients with HBV infection may have detectable HB_sAg and HB_sAb concurrently. In one study, on 16 months follow-up, about 55% were unchanged, about 25% lost the HB_sAg, and about 15% lost the HB_sAb (Table 16–2, Table 16–3, and Fig 16–3).

4. HB_eAg. The e antigen is usually not employed for diagnostic purposes but as an index of infectivity. It has been reported that the presence of e antigen means several times greater potential for infection than the risk if the e antigen is absent (although HBV infection can occur with no detectable e antigen). Hepatitis B virus e antigen is considered a marker for continued replication of the HBV and correlates with the presence of DNA polymerase, another marker of virus activity. Hepatitis B virus e antigen begins to rise about 3–5 days after detection of HB_sAg. It returns to normal (nondetectable) levels about 2–4 weeks before HB_sAg disappears in about 70% of cases and within 1 week before or after disappearance of HB_sAg in about 20% of patients. Hepatitis B virus e antigen accompanies HB_sAg in most patients who become chronic excreters of HB_sAg, although one report indicates that about 40% of patients eventually convert the e antigen to e antibody with subsequent coexistence of HB_sAg and HB_eAb. One report suggests that chronic persistence of HB_eAg with HB_sAg suggests chronic hepatitis rather than a simple carrier state.

5. HB_eAb. Antibody to the e antigen appears either coincidentally with or within 1–2 weeks after disappearance of the e antigen. Since disappearance of the e antigen occurs shortly before disappearance of the surface antigen, detection of e antibody means that the acute state

TABLE 16–3.

Interpretation of Hepatitis B Serologic Tests

I. HB_sAg positive, HB_cAb negative*
   About 5% (range, 0%–17%) of patients with early stage HBV acute infection (HB_cAb rises later)

II. HB_sAg positive, HB_cAb positive, HB_sAb negative
   a. Most of the clinical symptom stage
   b. Chronic HBV carriers without evidence of liver disease ("asymptomatic carriers")
   c. Chronic HBV hepatitis (chronic persistent type or chronic active type)

III. Hb_sAg negative, HB_cAb positive,* HB_sAb negative
   a. Late clinical symptom stage or early convalescence stage (core window)
   b. Chronic HBV infection with HB_sAg below detection levels with current tests
   c. Old previous HBV infection

IV. HB_sAg negative, HB_cAb positive, HB_sAb positive
   a. Late convalescence to complete recovery
   b. Old infection

*HB_cAb = combined IgM + IgG. In some cases (e.g., category III), selective Hb_cAb-IgM assay is useful to differentiate recent and old infection.

TABLE 16–2.

Summary of Major Diagnostic Tests for Hepatitis B Infection

HB_sAg
- Appearance: 2–6 wk after exposure (range, 6 days–6 mo)
- Peak: 1–2 wk before to 1–2 wk after onset of symptoms
- Becomes nondetectable: 1–3 mo after peak (range, 1 wk–5 mo)

HB_cAb-IgM
- Appearance: About 2 wk after HB_sAg (range, 0–6 wk)
- Peak: About 1 wk after onset of symptoms
- Becomes nondetectable: 3–6 mo (range, 2 wk–2 yr)

HB_cAb (HB_cAb-IgM + IgG)
- Appearance: 3–4 wk after HB_sAg (range, 2–10 wk)
- Peak: 3–4 wk after first detection
- Becomes nondetectable: Slow decline to lower titer levels over many years

HB_sAb
- Appearance: 2–6 wk after disappearance of HB_sAg (range, HB_sAg still present to >1 yr after HB_sAg is gone)
- Peak: 2–8 wk after appearance
- Becomes nondetectable: About 15% (range, 2%–33%) of patients lose HB_sAb in <6 years; remainder show decline to low titers over many years

of HBV infection is over or nearly over and that infectivity is much less. Hepatitis B virus e antibody titers reach their peak in the core window time segment between disappearance of HB_sAg and appearance of HB_sAb. Hepatitis B virus e antibody may persist for several years but usually returns to a nondetectable state before HB_sAb or HB_cAb.

6. HDV. Delta virus antigen is detectable only for 1–4 days before elevation of transaminase enzymes or appearance of symptoms. The antigen can be detected by certain research tests, but these tests are not commercially available. Tests for HDV antibody, both IgM and IgG, are now becoming available. In simultaneous acute infection by HBV and HDV, both HDV-IgM and HDV-IgG antibody rise shortly after HB_cAb-IgM and HB_cAb-IgG antibody begins to rise in the acute clinical phase, peak toward the end of clinical infection, and become nondetectable during the core window phase. Therefore, in the acute clinical phase, HB_cAb-IgM and HDV-IgM antibody are detectable at the same time. When HDV acute infection is superimposed on HBV chronic infection or carrier state, HDV-IgM and HDV-IgG antibody rise, followed by decline of HDV-IgM antibody and persistance of HDV-IgG antibody. Therefore, when acute HDV infection superimposes on chronic HBV infection, HDV-IgM antibody is present but HB_cAb-IgM is not (since HBV is in the chronic or carrier state, HB_sAg and HB_cAg-IgG are elevated but HB_cAg-IgM has previously returned to normal). Symptoms of acute viral hepatitis with presence of HB_sAg and HB_cAb-IgG but not HB_cAb-IgM suggests the diagnosis of possible superimposed HDV (another possibility could be superimposed acute NANB hepatitis virus). When HDV and HBV carrier state coexist, HB_sAg, HB_cAb-IgG, and HB_eAb are present; HDV-IgG is present in high titer and HDV-IgM is present in low titer.

Nucleic Acid (DNA) Probe.—Recently, a nucleic acid probe method (discussed earlier) has become commercially available to detect HBV DNA material circulating in serum. Detection of circulating viral DNA is an indication of actual virus replication and infectivity. As yet, no evaluations of this kit have been published.

Chronic Hepatitis B Virus Infection

Three serologic patterns have been described in chronic HBV infection (infection persisting > 6 months). The first pattern consists of elevated levels of HB_sAg, HB_cAb, and HB_eAg. The second consists of elevated levels of HB_sAg, HB_cAb, and HB_eAb. The third (and least frequent) consists of an elevated HB_cAb level only. The third pattern is seen with some asymptomatic carriers (however, this pattern could also be seen with healed HBV infection many years previously and no currently active

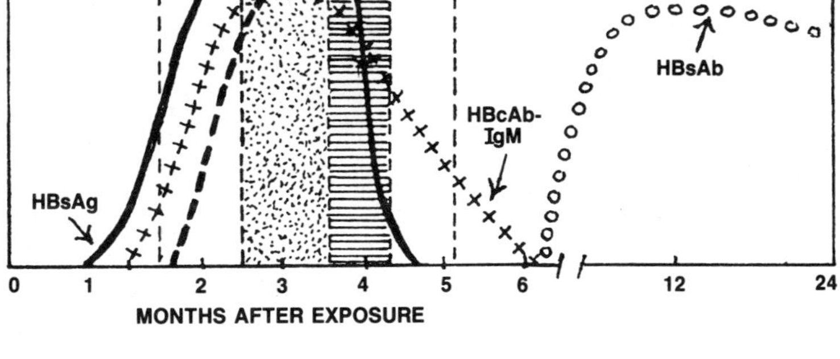

FIG 16–3.
Serologic tests in HBV infection. $^*HB_cAb = HB_cAb\text{-IgM} + HB_cAb\text{-IgG}$ (combined).

infection). In all three patterns, HB_sAb is not elevated.

Blood Bank Screening for Hepatitis B Virus

The major impetus for hepatitis testing was the hope that transfusion-related hepatitis could be eliminated by testing all donor blood for evidence of hepatitis virus infection. Prior to mandatory donor hepatitis testing, the incidence of posttransfusion hepatitis was recorded as high as 33%. After all donor blood was tested for HB_sAg using RIA methods (or tests of equivalent sensitivity) and after excluding high-risk donor population groups, the incidence of posttransfusion hepatitis is reported to be 5% or less. However, some studies have suggested that the majority of this improvement was obtained by donor population selection rather than HB_sAg testing. Eighty percent to 90% of posttransfusion hepatitis cases are now due to NANB hepatitis virus. It has been suggested that screening of donor blood with the enzyme ALT (which is sensitive to acute liver cell injury) plus HB_cAb (because of frequent coexistence of HBV and NANB hepatitis virus infection) could reduce donor blood risk of NANB hepatitis virus by about one-third. The risk of posttransfusion hepatitis due to HAV is considered to be negligible.

The HB_sAg has been found in some cases of polyarteritis nodosa, membranous or membranoproliferative glomerulonephritis, and serum sickness, the latter occurring as the initial phase of hepatitis clinical illness. Some type of autoimmune mechanism is believed to be responsible.

Although many use "viral hepatitis" as a synonym for infection by hepatitis viruses A, B, NANB, and D, a wide range of viruses may infect hepatic cells with varying frequency and severity. The most common (but not the only) examples are infectious mononucleosis (E-B virus), and the cytomegalic inclusion virus.

Cytomegalic Inclusion Virus Disease

Cytomegalic inclusion virus, or CMV, is a very common infectious agent. About 30%–60% of the population have anti-CMV antibodies, and even more in some population subgroups. Infection is acquired through contact with body secretions and excretions, with virus present in saliva, blood, cervical secretions, semen, urine, and breast milk. It initially produces a viremia but can then go into a latent state with or without later reactivation. After infection there is an incubation period of 40–60 days (range, 4–12 weeks). Thereafter, clinical illness develops, manifested by shedding of the virus with or without clinical symptoms. The majority of infected persons remain asymptomatic, but in those who develop clinical disease, a variety of manifestations may be produced, depending on the age of the patient, the presence of underlying diseases that might alter the patient's immunologic response to the virus, or the visceral organs affected.

About 1%–2% (range, 0.7%–4.0%) of pregnant women develop primary CMV infection; of these, fetal infection is thought to occur in 30%–50% of cases. About 5%–15% have CMV reactivation during pregnancy, with fetal infection occurring in about 10%. There are some reports that congenital (in utero) infection is more likely to occur in the second and third trimesters but that severe injury to the fetus is more likely to occur when infection takes place in the first or second trimester. There is also some evidence that primary CMV maternal infection is more dangerous to the fetus than a recurrent infection during pregnancy. Overall, congenital intrauterine CMV infection is reported in 0.2%–2.2% of infants, of which about 5%–10% develop clinical symptoms. In the newborn, CMV disease may appear in two forms:

1. A subacute form with predominantly cerebral symptoms, manifested by the picture of cerebral palsy or mental retardation. This is the classic form acquired in utero.
2. An acute form with various combinations of hepatosplenomegaly, thrombocytopenia, hepatitis with jaundice, and cerebral symptoms, such as convulsions. There usually is anemia, and there may be nucleated red blood cells (RBCs) and an increase in immature neutrophils (predominantly bands) on peripheral blood smear.

Noncongenital infection in the newborn may take place during or after birth. It has been reported that 3%–28% of pregnant women have cervical infection by CMV, this presumably being the source of infection during birth. The infant can also become infected through breast milk. The great majority of these infants are asymptomatic, but some develop various aspects of the acute congenital CMV syndrome, which may include pneumonia. Infants, especially when premature or seriously ill, who acquire CMV infection through blood transfusion are more likely to have severe disease. In young nontransfused children less than age 6 months, some may develop pneumonia as the predominating or only manifestation of CMV infection. In young children in general, infection is common, with reported infection rate of 10%–15% by age 1 year and about 35% (range 20%–80%) by age 10 years. Infection is most commonly acquired from other children. Infection is especially common in day-care centers and similar institutions. The great majority of affected children are clinically asymtomatic, but in those with symptoms, probably the most common manifestation is a virus-like febrile illness (often mild), frequently accompanied by laboratory evidence of a mild hepatitis. In older children, incidence of infection is much less. In adults, the majority (but not all) of primary infections are thought to be related to sexual intercourse. In older children and adults those patients with symptoms usually have a clinical picture resembling infectious mononucleosis (IM) in nearly all respects except for negative serologic test results for IM. It has been estimated that 10%–25% of heterophil-negative IM-like illnesses are due to CMV. Cytomegalovirus infection is unusually frequent in renal transplant and cardiac transplant patients (38%–96% of cases). It is also frequent in immunosuppressed persons, patients on steroid therapy, and patients with leukemia or lymphoma. In these patients there is predominantly lung or liver involvement that usually is overshadowed by the preexisting nonviral disease. Cytomegalovirus is the predominant cause for the mononucleosis-like postperfusion (posttransfusion) syndrome that may occur 3–7 weeks after multiple-unit blood transfusion or bypass surgery. Studies have estimated that about 7% of single unit transfusions produce CMV infection and about 20% (range 3%–38%) of multiple-unit transfusions. More than 90% of homosexual males are said to have CMV antibody, and severe infection occurs with increased frequency in the AIDS syndrome and other conditions associated with HIV-I infection.

Laboratory Abnormalities in Cytomegalovirus Infection.—In symptomatic adult CMV infection, splenomegaly is reported in about 35% of cases (range, 22%–40%), adenopathy in about 15% (range, 5%–28%), anemia in 13%–67%, leukocytosis in 4%, elevated percentage of bands in 20%, absolute lymphocytosis in 50%–60%, 20% or more of the lymphocytes atypical in 30%–40% (range, 20%–100%), thrombocytopenia in 10%–15%, erythrocyte sedimentation rate elevation in 66%, positive rheumatoid factor test result in 35% (range, 27%–50%), and abnormal antinuclear antibody level in about 20% (range, 4%–40%). In one study, about one half of the patients had a mild hemolytic anemia that was Coombs positive in about 30%. In the same study, serum lactic dehydrogenase (LDH) was elevated in 90% of all patients. More than 90% of patients demonstrate atypical lymphocytes in their peripheral blood smear at some time; in the great majority more than 20% of total lymphocytes are atypical (similar to findings in IM), but there may be less than 20% (of total lymphocytes) affected and in some cases none may be found. Liver function tests are said to be elevated in more than 95% of patients. Aspartate aminotransferase is elevated in 88%–95% of cases, with less than 5% over 10 times upper reference limit and about 20% over 5 times upper limit. Alkaline phosphatase (ALP) is elevated in 50%–64% with about 3% over five times upper reference limit and about 9% over three times upper limit. γ-Glutamyltransferase (GGT) level is elevated in about 75% with about 12% over five times upper reference limit and about 30% over three times upper limit. Lactic dehydrogenase level also is usually abnormal. Total bilirubin value is rarely more than 2.0 mg/100 ml. In general, abnormal enzyme levels display only about one half the degree of elevation seen in patients with IM (which themselves are only mild to moderate), but there is a considerable degree of overlap. Peak elevations are reported to occur about 5–4 days after onset of illness for bilirubin, AST, and ALP and between 7–21 days for GGT. Enzyme elevations usually return to normal by 90 days after onset of clinical illness. γ-Glutamyltransferase abnormality is often the last to disappear and occasionally may persist to some degree for several months.

Laboratory Diagnosis of Cytomegalovirus Infection.—The most definitive method for diagnosis of CMV infection is virus culture, but serologic tests are also used, and other procedures may sometimes be helpful. In the newborn, periventricular cerebral calcification is demonstrable by x-ray film in about 25%; this is highly suggestive, although the same pattern may be found in congenital toxoplasmosis.

Cytomegalovirus Inclusion Body Cytology.—In newborns or young children, characteristic CMV inclusion bodies may be demonstrated within renal epithelial cells on stained smears of the urinary sediment in about 60% of cases; this may be an intermittent finding and may require specimens on several days. A fresh specimen is preferable to a 24-hour collection, since the cells tend to disintegrate on standing. Virus culture is unquestionably better than search for urine cells with cytomegalic inclusion bodies. In older children and adults the kidney is not often severely affected, so urine specimens for CMV inclusion bodies usually are not helpful.

Virus Culture.—Virus culture shows active production of virus and, therefore, active infection but cannot differentiate between primary infection, reinfection, or reactivation of latent infection. Urine, sputum, or mouth swab culture for the virus is the method of choice. Fresh specimens are essential. For urine, an early morning specimen is preferable. For best results, any specimen must reach the virus culture laboratory within 1–2 days. The specimen should not be frozen, because freezing progressively inactivates the virus. This is in contrast to most other viruses, for which quick freezing is the procedure of choice for preserving specimens. The specimen should be refrigerated without actual freezing. In this way it may be preserved up to 1 week. It should be sent to the virus laboratory packed in ordinary ice (not dry ice) and, if possible, in an insulated container. Isolation of the CMV may take several weeks. Both urine and throat swab specimen results may be positive for CMV several weeks or months after the end of acute illness. Cytomegalovirus may also be cultured from blood (leukocyte layer) but only during the acute phase of illness.

Serologic Tests.—Conversion of a negative to a significantly reactive test or a fourfold rising titer in specimens taken 1–2 weeks apart are the best ways to demonstrate primary infection. Complement fixation used to be the standard technique but is technically cumbersome, takes 2 days to perform, and is able to demonstrate a fourfold rising titer in only 50% or less patients with acute CMV infection. Therefore, it is being replaced by faster and more sensitive fluorescent procedures, ELISA, indirect hemagglutination, and LA methods. These tests detect IgG antibody. Since CMV antibody is common in the general population, and since antibody levels persist for years, acute and convalescent specimens are necessary to demonstrate active infection. One difficulty with these tests applied to neonatal specimens is maternal IgG antibody to CMV, which may appear in the fetus or newborn serum. Procedures are available that detect IgM antibody alone. IgM antibody persists in the blood for only a relatively short time (1–6 months, occasionally as long as 1 year). Also, IgM antibody does not cross the placenta. Theoretically, the presence of IgM antibody should mean acute or recent infection. Unfortunately, CMV-IgM tests have several drawbacks. Besides acute infection, reinfection and reactivation can also induce a CMV-IgM response. Other sources of IgM, such as rheumatoid factor, can produce false abnormality in CMV-IgM tests. Rheumatoid factor may be present in 27%–60% of patients with CMV infection, both neonates and adults. In addition, acute Epstein-Barr virus infection (which resembles CMV infection clinically) also produces IgM antibody that may react in the CMV—IgM tests. Finally, it is reported that 10%–50% of infants with symptomatic CMV disease have no detectable CMV–IgM antibody. Among other tests for CMV infection, a few investigators have reported CMV early nuclear antigen tests to be useful in diagnosis of neonatal CMV infection. A few reports suggest that testing for rheumatoid factor provides good results in screening cord blood for congenital CMV infection.

Detection of Cytomegalovirus Antigen.—Recently, nucleic acid (DNA) probe methods have been used to detect CMV virus in bronchial lavage and urine specimens. Electron microscopy has also been used. Both methods are very expensive, especially electron microscopy.

Epstein-Barr Virus (Infectious Mononucleosis)

The Epstein-Barr (E-B) virus is a member

of the herpesvirus group and one of the most widespread virus infections. It is thought to be spread from person to person, most likely through saliva, with the majority of infections occurring in early childhood with few or no clinical symptoms. The E-B virus infects B lymphocytes. In common with the other herpes viruses, once infection takes place the virus becomes dormant but can be reactivated later into clinical disease. Reactivation is said to occur in 15%–20% of healthy persons and in up to 85% in some groups of immunosuppressed patients. Epstein-Barr virus infection is associated with several illnesses. The most common is the infectious mononucleosis (IM) syndrome associated with heterophil antibodies. Preadolescent children and some adults may develop a subclinical infection or infection with minimal symptoms. Children less than age 4 frequently do not produce heterophil antibodies. There is another syndrome known as chronic mononucleosis, also without heterophil antibodies, although this entity is somewhat controversial. The E-B virus is also thought to be associated with a peculiar type of malignant lymphoma called *Burkitt's lymphoma.*

Infectious Mononucleosis

Infectious mononucleosis patients are most often young adults, but a significant number are children, and some are older adults. When IM is part of a primary infection, the incubation period is 3–7 weeks. The most common features are fever, pharyngitis, and adenopathy, with lymph node enlargement being the most frequent. It may be localized or generalized. The posterior cervical nodes are the most commonly enlarged. Soft palate petechiae are found in 10%–30% of the cases. Jaundice is found in approximately 5% of patients in large series. Uncommon symptoms are skin rashes and supraorbital edema. The spleen is mildly enlarged in about 50% of patients (range, 40%–75%).

Laboratory Findings.—Patients usually show normal hemoglobin values and platelet counts, although mild thrombocytopenia is reported in 15%–35% of patients. Incidentally, normal hemoglobin values help in differentiation from lymphoma and leukemia, which the clinical symptoms may resemble, because these two are usually associated with anemia. There is leukocytosis, usually by the second week or by the time lymphadenopathy is well established. However, during the first week there may be leukopenia. The peripheral blood differential (WBC) white blood cell count is characteristic and includes two of the three criteria for diagnosis (serologic tests being the third). This will be discussed later. About 85%–90% (range, 80%–100%) of patients with IM have laboratory evidence of hepatic involvement. Aspartate aminotransferase (AST) is elevated at some time in about 85% of cases (literature range, 79%–97%). The AST is more than ten times upper reference limit in 5%–10% of patients (literature range, 4%—22%), more than five times upper limit in about 40%, and more than three times in about 60%. Alkaline phosphatase (ALP) is elevated in about 70% of cases (literature range, 38%–94%). It is more than five times upper reference limit in about 13% and more than three times upper limit in about 50%. Lactic dehydrogenase (LDH) is also elevated in more than 80% of cases. Total bilirubin value is less than 2.0 mg/100 ml (34 μmol/L) in 80%–85% of cases. γ-Glutamyltransferase (GGT) is reported to be elevated in about 90% of cases. It is elevated more than 10 times upper reference limit in about 2% of cases, more than five times upper limit in about 15% of cases, and more than three times upper limit in about 50% of cases. Peak values are reported to occur 5–14 days after onset of illness for AST, bilirubin, and ALP and between 7 and 21 days for GGT. The AST and ALP levels return to normal in nearly all patients by 90 days, but some degree of GGT elevation is reported occasionally to persist up to 12 months.

Laboratory Diagnosis of Epstein-Barr Infection

Peripheral Blood Smear.—Infectious mononucleosis usually produces a lymphocytosis, with lymphocytes making up more than 50% of the total WBCs. Lymphocytosis is said to begin about 7 days after onset of clinical illness, peaks during the second or third week, and lasts for an additional 2–6 weeks. A significant number of these lymphocytes must be atypical to diagnose IM. The majority of investigators use 20% or more atypical lymphocytes (of total lymphocytes) as one of the criteria for diagnosis of IM, but some use 10% or more. These atypical lymphocytes are of three main types: type I has vacuolated or foamy blue cytoplasm and a rounded nucleus; type II has an elongated flattened nucleus and large amounts of pale cytoplasm with sharply defined irregular borders; and type III has an immature irregular nucleus, which may have a nucleolus or show folding. All three types are larger than normal mature lymphocytes, and their nuclei are somewhat less dense. These atypical lymphocytes are not specific for IM and may be found in small to moderate numbers in a variety of viral diseases, especially CMV and hepatitis virus acute infection. Some call these cells virocytes. However, they may also be present in toxoplasmosis. In addition, an appearance similar to that of the type II variety may be created artificially by crushing and flattening normal lymphocytes near the thin edge of the blood smear. Infectious mononucleosis cells are sometimes confused with those of acute leukemia or disseminated lymphoma, although in the majority of cases there is no problem.

Although most reports state or imply that nearly all patients with IM satisfy the criteria for lymphocytosis and percent atypical lymphocytes, one study found only 55% of patients had a lymphocytosis and only 45% had more than 10% atypical lymphocytes on peripheral smear when the patients were first seen.

Serologic Tests.—Two types of serologic tests for diagnosis of IM are available. The classic procedure is the heterophil agglutination tube test (Paul-Bunnell test). Rapid heterophil antibody slide agglutination tests have also been devised. Slide tests now are the usual procedure done in most laboratories. However, since the basic principles, interpretation, and drawbacks of the slide tests are the same as those of the older Paul-Bunnell tube test, there are some advantages in discussing the Paul-Bunnell procedure in detail.

Heterophil antibodies are IgM-type antibodies that are reasonably (although not completely) suggestive of IM since they are seldom found in other disorders. They begin to appear in the first week of clinical illness (in one study, 40% of patients), reach a peak in the second week (60% of patients positive) or third (sometimes the fourth) week (85%–90% positive; range, 75%–100%), then begin to decline in titer during the fourth or fifth week, most often becoming undetectable 8–12 weeks after beginning of clinical illness. However in some cases some elevation is present as long as 1–2 years (20%–75% of patients). In children less than 2 years old, only 10%–30% develop heterophil antibodies; about 50%–75% of those 2–4 years old develop heterophil antibodies. One report states that these antibodies are rarely elevated in Japanese patients of any age. Once elevated and returned to undetectable level, heterophil antibodies usually will not reelevate in reactivated IM, although there are some reports of mild heterophil responses to other viruses. The test for heterophil antibodies is known as the Paul-Bunnell test and is based on the discovery that the heterophil antibody produced in IM would agglutinate sheep RBCs. Dilutions are set up for 1:7, 1:14, 1:28, 1:112, and so on serially, and the last tube dilution to show agglutination is reported as the titer. Normally, the titer is less than 1:112 and most often is almost or completely negative. The Paul-Bunnell test is also known as the "presumptive test," because later it was found that certain antibodies different from those of IM would also attack sheep RBCs. This is true of antibodies produced to the Forssman antigen found naturally in humans and certain other animals. Thus, if the Paul-Bunnell test is elevated, one does not know if this represents IM heterophil antibody or a nonspecific Forssman antibody. Fortunately, Forssman antibodies are usually not produced in high titers, and this fact may help in many cases. Eventually, the differential absorption test (Davidsohn differential test) was developed.

Guinea pig kidney is a good source of Forssman antigen. Therefore, if a serum containing Forssman antibody is allowed to come in contact with guinea pig kidney material, the Forssman antibody will combine with the kidney antigen and be removed from the serum when the serum is taken off. The serum will then show either a very low or a negative titer, whereas before it was strongly positive. The IM heterophil antibody is not significantly absorbed by guinea pig kidney but is nearly completely absorbed by beef RBCs, which do not significantly affect the Forssman antibody. The only other antigen that may be involved is that produced in serum sickness, and this will absorb both with beef RBCs and guinea pig kidney. In the absorption test, there must be at least a three-tube decrease in titer for absorption to be considered significant. In other words, true IM antibody will not drop more than three tube dilutions when treated with guinea pig kidney, whereas Forssman antibody will. The height of the titer after absorption has no diagnostic value. However, the original presumptive test must have at least a 1:28 titer to permit the differential to be done at all. As noted previously, the Paul-Bunnell (heterophil antibody) test titer usually begins to decrease in the fourth or fifth week but can remain elevated for several weeks or months after clinical symptoms have disappeared. The level of Paul-Bunnell titer does not correlate well with the clinical course of IM. Titer is useful only in making a diagnosis and should not be relied on to follow the clinical course of the disease or to assess results of therapy.

In suspected mononucleosis, the presumptive test should be done first; if necessary, it can be followed by a differential absorption procedure. The Paul-Bunnell and differential test results are usually positive by 3 weeks after onset of symptoms. Most test results are positive during the second week, although the Paul-Bunnell titer may not yet have risen to its full height. Many cases have such high presumptive titers that a differential is not necessary. Some never reach 1:112, and it is in these patients and those with only moderate titer elevation that the differential absorption is most helpful.

"Spot" tests in which the Paul-Bunnell and differential absorption tests are converted to a rapid slide procedure without titration have been devised. Citrate-preserved horse RBCs are used instead of sheep RBCs to increase test sensitivity. The antigen-antibody reactions and absorptions are demonstrated visually by adding drops of reagents to areas on a slide or piece of paper rather than by titration in test tubes. If properly done, most investigators indicate that the method is as sensitive and nearly as specific as the classic procedure. However, at least one report indicates that false positives may occur in a few patients with malignant lymphoma when this particular technique is used.

A rapid modification of the heterophil procedure called Mono-Test uses formalin-fixed RBCs without differential absorption. The Mono-Test has been reported to have almost the same specificity as the differential absorption technique. Burkitt's lymphoma may produce a false positive reaction.

Heterophil-Negative Infectious Mononucleosis.—False positive differential absorption results have been reported but are extremely rare. Since elevated titer from IM may persist for months, it is possible that even the few reported cases of false positive results had subclinical mononucleosis sometime earlier. On the other hand, there are reports describing outbreaks of a disease that clinically was identical to IM with typical blood changes but with negative Paul-Bunnell test results in many or even all cases. A similar situation has been reported following blood transfusions. This was especially common after open heart or other types of surgery using extracorporeal blood-oxygenation equipment and was called the "postperfusion," or "postpump," syndrome. The etiologic agent in the majority of the transfusion or postperfusion cases has been found to be the cytomegalovirus. Some other agents beside CMV that may produce clinical and peripheral smear findings raising the question of IM include toxoplasmosis, other viruses (hepatitis virus, rubella, adenovirus, etc.), *Listeria monocytogenes*, rickettsiae, drug reaction (serum sickness), and lymphocytic lymphoma. However, some cases are due to reactivated E-B disease without heterophil antibody response.

Diagnosis of Infectious Mononucleosis.—When all three criteria for IM are satisfied, there is no problem in differential diagnosis. When the results of Paul-Bunnell test or differential absorption test are positive, most authors believe that the diagnosis can be made, although there are reports that viral infections occurring after IM can cause anamnestic false positive heterophil reelevations. When the clinical picture is suggestive of IM but results of the Paul-Bunnell test, differential absorption procedure, or the spot test are negative, at least one follow-up specimen should be obtained in 14 days, since about 20%–30% of IM patients have negative heterophil test results when first seen. Although the usual time of antibody appearance is 7–10 days, it may take as long as 21 days and, uncommonly, up to 30 days. About 5% (literature range, 2%–20%) of patients over age 5 years and 25% or more under age 5 years never produce detectable heterophil antibody. If the clinical picture is typical and the blood picture is very characteristic (regarding both number and type of lymphocytes), many believe that the diagnosis of IM can be considered probable but not established. This may be influenced by the expense and time lapse needed for serologic or culture investigation of CMV and the various other possible infectious etiologies. Parenthetically, many articles in the literature give only the results of the presumptive test; as mentioned, one can have a presumptive test within normal range (which is < 1:112) and still have a positive differential absorption (if the titer is at least 1:28). Heterophil antibodies usually subside in 8–12 weeks, but in 20% the titers are still elevated 1 year later.

In summary, the three criteria for the diagnosis of IM are:

1. Lymphocytes comprising more than 50% of total WBC count.
2. Atypical lymphocytes comprising more than 20% of the total lymphocytes.
3. Significantly elevated Paul-Bunnell test or differential absorption test result. A positive Mono-Test or spot test result satisfies this criterion.

Serologic Tests for Epstein-Barr Virus.— The other type of serologic test for IM consists of antibodies against various parts of the E-B virus (see chapter 35). The most important of these is antibody against the viral capsid (outer envelope) antigen (VCA). The initial VCA antibody is an IgM type, the level of which rises during the first 2–3 weeks after infection (about 1–2 weeks before onset of symptoms) and falls to nondetectable levels during the next 8–12 weeks. However, about 20% of cases still have detectable VCA-IgM levels 1 year after onset of illness, although at low titer. In one study, 94% of cases had elevated VCA-IgM levels at the time the patient was first seen by a physician. The major drawback to the VCA-IgM assay is false positive results due to cross-reaction with other IgM antibodies, especially rheumatoid factor. Also, in some patients the initial blood specimen is drawn late enough in the illness that the VCA-IgM titer had already become undetectable. Because of these problems, there is some controversy regarding reliability of this test in diagnosis of IM. A VCA-IgG antibody appears about 1 week after the VCA-IgM antibody, peaks in another week or less, stays at a plateau for several weeks, and then falls slowly during several months before reaching stable titer levels that persist for years or for life. Titers of 1:320 or more are considered strongly suggestive of recent infection, although some investigators are not willing to make a definitive diagnosis on the basis of a single value for a single antibody. Titers of 1:20–1:160 usually persist for years, and a titer of this magnitude could thus represent either an early rising titer or a persistent old titer. In several reports, about 80% (range, 25%–91%) had elevated peak VCA-IgG titers when first seen by a physician and the remainder developed a titer of 1:320 or a fourfold rising titer 2 weeks later. Only about 20% developed a fourfold titer increase. In summary, a fourfold rise in VCA-IgG titer is considered diagnostic of recent E-B virus infection, although this does not happen often. Some would consider a VCA-IgG titer of 1:320, and possibly, an elevated VCA-IgM titer, as diagnostic or strongly suggestive, but this is more controversial.

There are other E-B antibodies besides the VCA. One of these is the antibody against *E-B nuclear antigen (EBNA)*. This antibody rises during convalescence, reaches a plateau in 3–12 months, and persists for life. Anti-EBNA may sometimes be helpful, since it is a late-rising permanent antibody, and therefore elevation of VCA-IgG levels with absent EBNA would suggest acute infection. Finally, there is antibody to *E-B early antigen (EA)* complex. There are two varieties, EA diffuse component (EA-D) and EA restricted component (EA-R). Of these, EA-D is more helpful. This antibody is produced in about 66%–85% of patients with IM; it appears shortly after VCA-IgG but the level returns to normal during convalescence. The EA-D level often becomes reelevated in IM reactivation. Therefore, presence of EA-D antibody suggests recent E-B infection, whether primary or reactivation. However, some reports indicate that it may remain detectable for several months in some patients with IM and also that it may not become detectable in many patients with subclinical E-B infection.

The *chronic mononucleosis syndrome* was mentioned earlier. The major symptom is chronic fatigue, with minor components of low-grade fever, adenopathy, myalgia, and sore throat. The typical E-B serologic profile in those patients considered to have chronic E-B infection is negative heterophil test result and VCA-IgM titer, markedly elevated VCA-IgG titer, and somewhat elevated EBNA and EA-D titers. Some investigators accept negative or low titers of EBNA and EA-D if the other laboratory findings are strongly suggestive. Some investigators do not accept the concept of a chronic mononucleosis syndrome and do not believe that the evidence for E-B infection is strong enough to be considered the cause.

Serologic tests for E-B virus are relatively expensive and are available predominantly in university centers and large reference laboratories. Such tests are not needed to diagnose IM in the great majority of cases. The E-B virus tests are useful in persistently heterophil-negative patients, in problem cases or in patients with atypical clinical symptoms when serologic confirmation of heterophil results is desirable, and for epidemiologic investigations. If the initial heterophil test is nonreactive or equivocal, it is desirable to freeze the remainder of the serum in case E-B virus tests are needed later.

Herpes Simplex

Herpes simplex virus infection is characterized by a primary infection, often asymptomatic, after which the virus remains dormant in the dorsal root ganglia of peripheral nerves for varying periods of time. Primary infection usually requires a person without preexisting HSV antibody. However, a person can have antibody against one strain of HSV (from previous infection) and become infected by a different strain (reinfection as opposed to reactivation or recurrence of preexisting disease). Primary infection or reinfection is usually acquired from close contact with an infected person; the mouth, in cases of nongenital infection, and sexual intercourse in cases of genital infection. However, transmission can occur through body secretions. There are two closely related but distinct types of HSVs that share some antigens but not others. Herpes simplex virus type I typically produces nongenital infections of various types such as lesions of the mouth, blisters on the mucous membrane border of the lips ("canker sores," or "cold sores"), keratitis (corneal ulcers of the eye), focal lesions of the fingers ("Whitlow"), and meningoencephalitis (most frequently involving the temporal lobes of the brain). Occasional immunocompromised patients develop disseminated HSV-I disease. At one time about 90% of the population was found to have antibodies against HSV-I, but more recently this incidence is said to have fallen to about 25%–50%. Herpes simplex virus type II (HSV-II) produces blistering lesions (vesicles) on the genitalia of males and females and is considered a venereal disease. In one report from a venereal disease clinic, the incidence of HSV-II infection was about 45% as high as gonorrhea (5% of total patients). However, about 5%–15% of patients with genital herpes have HSV-I isolated rather than HSV-II, and one report indicates that up to 20% of labial or facial lesions are due to HSV-II rather than HSV-I. There is a statistical association between HSV-II infection and carcinoma of the cervix, but as yet there is not a proved causal relationship. There has been more emphasis recently on genital herpes than on other areas of herpes infection. In primary HSV-II genital infection that is symptomatic, the incubation period is about 5–7 days (range, 1–45 days). About one half of the patients (range, 39%–68%) develop systemic symptoms (e.g., fever, malaise, myalgia, and headache), including a subset of about 25% (range, 13%–36%) of all patients who experience a mild self-limited episode of aseptic meningitis (which has a marked difference in severity and prognosis from the severe brain infection of HSV-I). Extragenital lesions on skin or mucous membranes occur in about 25% of patients (range, 10%–30%), most often in the general area of the groin. A few patients develop lesions on one or more fingers, and herpes ocular keratitis sometimes occurs. About 20% are reported to show evidence of pharyngeal involvement, and about 50% have urethral involvement. Herpes simplex virus can be cultured from the cervix in 80%–90% of female patients. About 80% of all patients develop tender inguinal adenopathy in the second or third week.

Recurrent infection differs considerably from primary infection. Only about 5%–10% of patients experience systemic symptoms. Extragenital lesions appear in about 5%. Cervical culture is reported to detect HSV in less than 15%.

Neonatal HSV infection is associated with active maternal HSV genital infection and is usually (but not always) acquired during birth rather than by transmission through the placenta. About 1% of pregnant women are estimated to have either overt or nonapparent HSV-II infection. However, asymptomatic cervical or vulvar infection has itself been reported in about 1% (range, 0.5%–8.0%) of women. In genital HSV infection during pregnancy only about 40% of infected women have typical lesions, and about 40% do not have visible lesions. It is estimated that if primary HSV infection is present at delivery, there is a 40%–60% chance of overt neonatal HSV-II infection. If this occurs, there is serious or fatal disease in 50% or more of those infants. If recurrent HSV is present, there is only about a 5% chance of infant infection. It is also reported that 70%–80% of neonatally infected infants are born to mothers who are asymptomatic at the time of delivery.

Diagnosis of Herpes Simplex Infection

Culture.—Culture is still the most reliable and sensitive method for HSV diagnosis. Material for culture must be inoculated into special transport media. Although some authorities advocate freezing the specimen, others report that refrigerator temperature is better for virus in transport media. Culture sensitivity depends on several factors. Some types of cells used for culture give better results than others. Specimens taken from vesicular lesions may be considerably (50%–100%) more sensitive than material taken from ulcerative lesions, which, in turn, provide better results than crusted lesions. The earlier a lesion is cultured after it appears, the more likely it will yield a positive result. A lesion from a primary infection is more likely to be positive than a lesion due to reinfection or recurrence. When urine or other secretions are cultured, the results from patients with primary infections are much more likely to be positive, since they shed virus much longer than patients with reinfection or recurrent disease. Culture in asymptomatic patients is much less likely to be positive than in patients with lesions. In addition to problems with sensitivity, specimens (in most hospitals) must be sent to a reference laboratory, and once there, it takes several days to obtain a result. Nevertheless, culture is still the gold standard in HSV diagnosis.

Antigen Detection.—Several methods are available to detect HSV antigen; most differentiate between HSV-I and HSV-II or claim to be specific for one or the other. Most have the advantage of same-day or overnight results. Some depend on abbreviated culture followed by use of specific antibody to HSV. Others (such as fluorescent antibody or latex agglutination) employ specific antibody directly on clinical specimens. The newest entry into this field is the nucleic acid (DNA) probe technique. To date, all methods have failed to consistently detect 95% or more patients who have positive results by standard culture and, in general, independent evaluations have not consistently upheld manufacturer's claims. Some have achieved sensitivity in the 85%–95% range compared to culture; others have not. In general, the type of clinical specimen and the time frame in which the specimen was obtained that imposed sensitivity limitations on culture likewise affect methods that detect HSV antigen. Also, there have been problems in cross-reaction between HSV-I and HSV-II, especially in fluorescent antibody methods.

Direct Smear Methods.—The most rapid diagnosis is made through stained smears from scrapings obtained from a lesion. A sterile scalpel blade is used to unroof a vesicle and material from gentle scraping of the base of the lesion is smeared on a slide. Either Giemsa or Papanicolaou stains can be used. For Giemsa, the smear is air-dried; for Papanicolaou, the smear is immediately fixed in cytology fixative. The slide preparation is sometimes called a *Tzanck test*. The technologist looks for multinucleated epithelial cells with enlarged atypical nuclei. Papanicolaou stain also can show intranuclear inclusions. Sensitivity of the Tzanck test is reported to be 37%–75%, with average sensitivity probably about 45%–50%. It is probably less with persons who are inexperienced in obtaining specimens and interpreting the smears. Sensitivity is higher from vesicle scrapings than from other specimens. Fluorescent antibody tests have been applied to the smears, which increases positive results to about two thirds of cases.

Serologic Tests for Antibody.—Antibody detection has also been somewhat disappointing. Acute and convalescent specimens must be obtained 2 weeks apart. A fourfold rise in titer is needed to prove recent onset of infection; this is most likely to be found in HSV-II disease and during the time of primary infection (60%–70% of cases). Only about 5% of patients with recurrent HSV demonstate a fourfold rise in titer. There may also be problems with interpretation due to the high rate of positive results in the general population and because of cross-reaction between HSV-I and HSV-II antibodies.

Other Tests.—In culture-proved HSV-I encephalitis, one study reported that radionuclide brain scan revealed a focal lesion or lesions in the temporal lobe in 50% of cases, computerized tomography scan displayed some type of abnormality in 59%, and EEG was abnormal in 81%. However, these procedures or their results cannot prove that the etiology is herpes infection. Spinal fluid tests show elevated CSF protein levels in about 80% of cases, increased WBC count in 97% (with about 75% of all cases between 50 and 500 WBCs/cu mm), and normal glucose levels in 95% of cases. Another study found a normal cell count and protein level in 10% of cases on first spinal tap. Increase in WBC count is predominantly lymphocytic, although segmented neutrophils may be present in varying percentage (occasionally substantial) in the early stages. At present, brain biopsy with culture of the specimen is the most accurate method of diagnosis. However, there is controversy about biopsy of such a vital organ. Culture of brain biopsy specimens is said to detect up to 95% of patients with HSV-I encephalitis. Microscopic examination of the biopsy specimens is only about 50% sensitive. Clinical assessment alone is not sufficiently accurate: in one series of patients who underwent brain biopsy for suspected herpes, about 45% did not disclose herpes and about 10% were found to have treatable diseases other than herpes. Cerebrospinal fluid culture was positive in only about 5% of patients whose brain biopsy results were culture positive. In one large series, serologic tests suggested that 30% of patients had primary HSV infection and 70% had recurrent infection.

Human Immunodeficiency Virus Group

The HIVs are retroviruses; their genetic information (genome) is composed of RNA rather than the usual DNA. To reproduce, the virus uses an enzyme known as reverse transcriptase to produce a DNA copy of its genetic RNA and incorporates this material into the host cell genetic material. Some of the copied viral genome also exists in the host cell without being incorporated into host chromosomes. Thus, the host cell nucleus reproduces the virus as well as itself. The HIVs have an unusual property, similar to the herpesvirus group, that active reproduction and infection can coexist with presence of antibodies against the virus. In most other virus infections, appearance of specific antibody marks the end of the infection and confers partial or complete protection against subsequent infection by that virus. The HIVs attack a subgroup of T lymphocytes known as helper (inducer) T cells (sometimes called T 4 cells, after one of the antibody systems used to identify them in the peripheral blood). Helper T cells are important in cell-mediated immunity (delayed hypersensitivity), which is the immunologic mechanism classically defending against chronic lower virulence infections such as tuberculosis, fungus, and parasites. Monocytes, macrophages, and possibly Langerhans cells also become infected.

The first HIV to be discovered was isolated from patients with the acquired immunodeficiency syndrome (AIDS) by three different groups of investigators who each gave the virus a different name (human T-cell lymphotropic virus type III, or HTLV-III; lymphadenopathy-associated virus, or LAV; and AIDS-associated retrovirus, or ARV). Later, it became evident that all three were strains of the same virus. The current terminology for this virus is human immunodeficiency virus type I (HIV-I). This virus is present endemically in Central Africa. A related virus that produces a syndrome similar to AIDS is found in West Africa and has been named HIV-II (originally called HTLV-IV). The HIV viruses are related to a similar virus found in African green monkeys. They are also related, but less closely, to certain animal viruses called lenteviruses ("slow viruses"), of which the most well known is the visna virus of sheep. Besides the HIV virus group that injures or destroys helper T cells, there is another group of viruses that affects T cells but that causes excessive T-cell proliferation rather than destruction. This group has retained the name of HTLV and includes HTLV-I (which causes human T-cell leukemia) and HTLV-II (which may be associated with hairy cell leukemia). Similarly to the HIV viruses, the HTLV virus group is related to a monkey T-cell leukemia virus and more distantly to a T-cell leukemia virus of cattle.

Clinical Findings

Human immunodeficiency virus I can be

isolated from many body fluids (including blood or blood products, semen, cervical secretions, saliva, tears, cerebrospinal fluid, breast milk, urine, and various tissues including the cornea). However, HIV-I is transmitted in predominantly three ways: by sexual intercourse (heterosexual or male homosexual), by transfusion or inoculation of infected blood or blood products, and by mother to fetus through the placenta. After exposure, there is an incubation period that typically lasts 2–6 weeks (range, 6 days–8 weeks, but sometimes lasting several months or years). This is often followed by an acute viral-type illness resembling IM or CMV infection that usually lasts 2–3 weeks (range, 3 days–several weeks). Symptoms usually include fever, sore throat, and lymphadenopathy; often include skin rash, myalgias, diarrhea, vomiting, and aseptic meningitis; and sometimes include thrombocytopenia. Some patients never develop the initial acute febrile illness or any clinical infection; they may recover completely from the initial exposure (although this is probably uncommon) or may become an asymptomatic carrier. Those who develop the initial acute illness exhibit a wide spectrum of possible outcomes. After recovery they may become asymptomatic carriers; may have defective immunologic responses without clinical disease; may develop persistent generalized lymphadenopathy (PGL); may develop a variety of non-life-threatening fungal, bacterial, or viral infections (e.g., oral *Candida*) as part of the so-called AIDS-related complex (ARC); or may develop the AIDS syndrome. This initial acute illness is sometimes referred to in the literature as "seroconversion-associated," which is confusing, since actual seroconversion (appearance of detectable antibodies) usually does not take place until after onset of initial acute illness (if the patient develops this initial illness).

The AIDS syndrome is the most severe manifestation of HIV-I infection, defined briefly as serologic evidence of HIV antigen or antibody plus certain opportunistic infections or Kaposi's sarcoma (a malignant tumor of fibroblasts and capillary-sized blood vessels) in a patient who is immunocompromised without known cause. The most frequent opportunistic organism producing active infection in AIDS is *pneumocystis carinii* (about 60% of cases; range, 35%–80%); other common agents include *Cryptococcus neoformans* (4%–13% of cases), *Candida albicans* esophagitis (14%–25%), "atypical" mycobacteria of the *Mycobacterium avium-intracellulare* complex (22%–30%), and protozoans such as *Toxoplasma* (3%–12%) and *Cryptosporidium* (4%–13%). Other organisms with evidence of frequent past or recent infection include CMV (66%–94%) and HSV (4%–98%, the lower figures being active infection). Incidence of Kaposi's sarcoma varies according to risk group; in male homosexuals with AIDS the incidence is about 35% (range, 25%–50%) in clinical studies and 30%–75% in autopsy studies, but in drug abusers and hemophiliacs it is found in less than 5%. A substantial number of patients develop varying degrees of mental disorder with or without neurologic abnormalities, which may precede other evidence of AIDS. In one series, 66% of these patients had elevated CSF protein levels (42–189 mg/100 ml; 0.42–1.89 g/L); 20% had a small degree of mononuclear cell count elevation (4–51 WBCs); and three of seven patients tested had oligoclonal bands detected in their CSF. Cerebral abnormalities were found in two thirds of the patients with AIDS who were autopsied.

In the United States, about 70% of AIDS patients have been male homosexuals, usually those who had multiple sex partners. About 15% are drug addicts using intravenous injection, about 3% are persons receiving many transfusions of blood or blood products, about 1%–2% are persons infected heterosexually, and the remainder are other categories. However, incidence of heterosexual infection (as opposed to current incidence of AIDS, a late-stage development of HIV-I infection) is becoming more frequent. Infection has been reported after a single heterosexual encounter, although more commonly it takes more than one episode. After an infected person develops detectable antibody, the current approximate calculated progression to AIDS per year is about 2.5% for asymptomatic patients, 3.5% for PGL patients, and 8.5% for ARC patients. Progression to AIDS is highest among infected male homosexuals (4%–10%/year) and low among transfusion-infected hemophiliacs. About 50%–60% of infected mothers transmit the virus to the fetus during pregnancy. A few infants appear to become infected during delivery or possibly afterward.

Laboratory Findings

In the few small studies that contain hematologic data, anemia was present in about 80% (range, 45%–95%), leukopenia in about 65% (range, 40%–76%), thrombocytopenia in about 25%–30% (range, 20%–59%), and pancytopenia in 17%–41%. Lymphocytopenia was reported in about 70%–80% (range, 30%–83%).

Diagnosis of Human Immunodeficiency Virus I Infection

Culture.—Human immunodeficiency virus I can be isolated from concentrated peripheral blood lymphocytes and less frequently from body fluids. Isolation rates in already seropositive patients average about 50%–60% (range, 8%–100%). Culture is difficult, is expensive, takes several days, is available only at a relatively few laboratories, and is positive more often in early stages of infection than in later stages. Culture may be the only method that can confirm infection in the first 2–3 weeks after exposure.

Antigen Detection.—Viral antigen may become detectable as soon as 2 weeks after infection (in one report it was detected 4 days after a transplant operation). Antigenemia lasts roughly 3–5 months. In several reports, antigen could be detected from a few days to as many as 6–9 months before first-generation ELISA antibody test results became positive. Several methods have been used, including RIA, fluorescent antibody, and ELISA. Thus far, these are first-generation methods, and sensitivity has varied considerably between kits of different manufacturers. One DNA probe kit has recently become commercially available. Eventually antigen detection should most likely be the method of choice to detect infection in the first few weeks after exposure.

Antibody Detection.—Seroconversion occurs on the average about 6–10 weeks after infective exposure (range, 12 days–5 years). Two types of antibodies are produced, IgM and IgG. Immunoglobulin M antibodies are detectable first, and several studies report IgM antibody present in some patients 1–10 weeks before IgG antibody (using first-generation IgG ELISA methods). However, one recent study using a new second-generation IgG ELISA found little difference. Commercial ELISA IgM, second-generation IgG, and LA methods are now being tested. Many of these use antibody against one (sometimes more) selected protein components of HIV-I obtained through recombinant DNA techniques (see Confirmatory Methods section). However, almost all current information is based on first-generation ELISA methods, which are based on crude extracts of the whole virus. There are a considerable number of such methods commercially available, but even the first was introduced in only mid-1985. These tests detect antibody in 94%–99.5% of patients with confirmed AIDS, depending on the particular assay and the investigator. Positive tests in random blood donors have averaged about 0.9% (range, 0.2%–2.56%). However, in some (not all) of these first-generation kits only about 25%–35% (range, 17%–44%) of initially positive ELISA test results on random blood donors remain reactive when retested with the same kit. Of those whose results were repeatedly positive, only about 20%–35% (range, 15%–62%) were positive on confirmatory tests. This means that only about 10%–15% (range, 3%–22%) of the initial positive results on random blood donors from these particular kits eventually were confirmed positive. Some manufacturer's kits were shown to be more sensitive than others, and some produced more false positive results than others. Some of this discrepancy is explained on the basis of different appearance times or quantity present of different viral antigens being detected by the different kit antibodies being used. There is also controversy whether reactivity against only a single antibody of a certain type (e.g., the core proteins gag p15/p17 or the envelope glycoproteins gp 120/160) is sufficient to consider the test truly reactive and thus indicative of HIV-I infection in the absence of reactivity against antibodies to more than the single protein. When this happens, it is often considered a false positive or an "indeterminant" reaction, although its significance has not yet been definitely established. In addition to these controversies, definite false negative results and false positive results may occur. Previously mentioned have been false negative results due to variable time periods before antibody is produced and variation in virus antigens detected by different kit antibodies. Two sources of false negative results in most kits are about 2%–4% (range, 0%–7%) of nonreactive results in patients with terminal AIDS. Most of these patients had previously detectable antibody. Also, about 10%–25% of neonates and children infected in utero may fail to produce antibodies. According to one report, IgM antibody is not produced or is poorly produced in pregnancy-acquired HIV-I infection. Immunoglobulin G antibody is not helpful for the first 3 months of life because it may be acquired from the mother through the placenta. False negative and positive results can be due to technical and clerical errors. False positive results in some kits may be due to patient antibodies against certain HLA antigens (most often, DR4) in antigenic material from infected H9 cells used in the kits to capture the patient antibodies. Antigenic material from different cell lines may not have this problem. Some kits, but not others, have an increased incidence of false positive results in active alcoholic cirrhosis, renal failure, and autoimmune diseases. Gamma globulin used for HBV prophylaxis may contain antibody against HIV-I, although the gamma globulin is noninfectious due to certain steps in its manufacture. This passively transferred antibody may be detectable for as long as 3 months.

Confirmatory Antibody Detection Methods.—Until 1988 these tests consisted of Western blot and immunofluorescent methods. Western blot is an immunochromatographic technique in which virus material from cell culture is separated into its major component proteins by electrophoresis, transferred ("blotted") onto a chromatography support medium, and exposed to patient serum. Antibody in patient serum, if present, attaches to whatever virus component proteins it recognizes. Then the preparation is stained to display visually what protein areas had reacted. Not all the virus proteins are considered specific for HIV-I. There is some controversy as to what specific proteins must be present for the results to be considered definitely positive. This affects sensitivity of the test. The two most specific proteins are the virus envelope glycoprotein gp41 and the group-specific antigen (gag) core protein p24 (the numbers refer to molecular weight). However, other proteins, particularly a precursor envelope protein called gp160 (from which gp41 is derived), often appears before either of the more specific proteins. Western blot in general has been shown to detect antibody earlier than most of the first-generation ELISA tests but not as early as IgM or antigen-detection methods. Unfortunately, Western blot is somewhat time consuming and takes 2 days to complete, and reliable results are considerably technique dependent. False negative and false positive results have been reported, although the exact incidence is currently unknown, due to lack of quality control surveys. The test is currently available only in large medical centers and reference laboratories. Immunofluorescence procedures are also available and are claimed to produce results equivalent to Western blot. Immunofluorescence is easier to perform and produces same-day results. However, a minority of investigators found Western blot to be more reliable. Both of these techniques are generally considered suitable to confirm screening test results. The Western blot, however, is currently considered the gold standard. There is also a radioimmunoprecipitation technique that has also been used as a confirmatory procedure. This method is slightly more sensitive than Western blot. However, it is technically difficult and currently is used only in research laboratories.

Recently, tests have become available based on genetically engineered HIV proteins, most often gp160, gp120, gp41, and p24. One kit (HIVAGEN) consists of separate ELISA tests for antibody against several of these antigens, thus becoming, in effect, a sort of ELISA version of the Western blot.

Tests for Immunologic Status.—As noted previously, HIV-I selectively infects T-lymphocyte helper cells (also called inducer, Leu3, or OKT4 cells), which eventually leads to defective immune function. Suppressor T cells (OKT8 cells) are normal or become increased. Eighty percent to 95% of AIDS patients have a decreased absolute number of helper T cells (< 400/cu mm) and a reversed (inverted) helper T cell/supressor T cell ratio, with a T4/T8 ratio less than 1.0. One possible cause of false T4 decrease is the recent report that about 20% of blacks have helper T cells that fail to react with the OKT4 antibody but do react with the Leu3 and certain other helper T-cell antibodies. A lesser but substantial number of AIDS patients display more nonspecific immune system abnormalities, such as lymphocytopenia (< 1,500/cu mm) and nonreactivity to skin test challenge by standard delayed sensitivity antigens such as *Candida*, mumps, or *Trichophyton*. Tests of immune function usually do not become abnormal until relatively late stages of HIV-I infection. These tests are not tests for HIV infection, nor are they diagnostic of AIDS.

Beta-2 Microglobulin.—Beta-2 microglobulin (B2M) is a small polypeptide that forms the light chain of HLA molecules present on the surface of many nucleated cells, including lymphocytes. It is released into serum by cell destruction or membrane turnover and is filtered by the renal glomerulus, after which it is more than 99% reabsorbed and metabolized by the renal tubules. Since lymphocytes are a source of B2M production, B2M levels can be a nonspecific marker for lymphocyte proliferation or turnover, as seen in immunologic stimulation or lymphoproliferative disorders. Since it is excreted by the kidney, it has been used to estimate renal function. Since T-helper lymphocytes are affected in HIV infection, B2M is reported to be elevated in about 85%–90% (range, 68%–100%) of patients with AIDS or ARC, 45% of patients with PGL, in smaller numbers of other persons with HIV infection but few or no symptoms, and in varying numbers of clinically healthy male homosexuals (20%–44% in two studies). Some investigators have used B2M as a marker for progression to AIDS, but this is controversial since some patients in clinically early stages of HIV infection had elevated B2M levels but remained stable for years. Beta-2 microglobulin can be assayed by RIA, EIA, or immunodiffusion.

Beta-2 microglobulin may also become elevated in persons with poor renal function; in various lymphomas and leukemias, especially (but not exclusively) those of B-cell origin; in myeloma; in nonlymphoid malignancies; in IM and certain other viral infections; in various chronic inflammatory diseases; and in autoimmune disorders.

Summary of Human Immunodeficiency Virus I Tests.—In summary, ELISA tests for HIV-I antibody are used as a general screen to detect persons infected with HIV-I. Western blot (or equivalent) tests help establish presence of infection. Culture, tests for HIV-I antigen, and possibly ELISA-IgM antibody tests, may detect infection earlier than the ELISA screening tests. Tests for decreased immunologic function are useful to help confirm a clinical impression of advanced-stage PGL, ARC, and AIDS.

Rabies

Human disease from rabies virus infection is very uncommon in the United States. The number of human cases in the United States is usually less than five per year, and only 9 were reported from 1980 to 1987. However, there are always questions about the disease, and several thousand cases of animal rabies are confirmed each year (6,405 in 1980). In 1980, skunks accounted for about 60% of cases; bats about 11%, raccoons about 6%, cattle about 6%, dogs about 4%, cats about 3%, and foxes about 3%. At present, wildlife rabies is most common in skunks; followed by raccoons, bats, and foxes in order of decreasing numbers. Actually most animal bites are from caged rodent pets such as rabbits, gerbils, or mice. This is not a problem since rodents (including squirrels) very rarely are infected by the rabies virus even when wild. Interestingly, of the 9 human rabies cases mentioned above, 6 did not give a history of bat or other animal contact when they were hospitalized.

The standard procedure for suspected rabies in domestic dogs or cats is to quarantine the animal under observation of a veterinarian for 10 days. The incubation period in humans is 1–3 months (although inoculation through facial bites may have an incubation as short as 10 days), which provides enough time for diagnosis of the animal before beginning treatment in the person who was bitten. Animal rabies will produce symptoms in the animal within 10 days in nearly all cases.

For wild animals, if the animal was defending itself normally, it might be captured and quarantined. If it was thought to be exhibiting abnormal behavior, the animal is usually killed and the head is sent for rabies examination of the brain. The head (or brain) should be kept at refrigerator temperature (not frozen) and sent to a reference laboratory (usually a public health laboratory) as soon as possible. If the specimen will be received within 1 day, it should be sent refrigerated with ordinary ice; if it is to be stored longer than 1 day, dry ice should be used.

Diagnosis.—Laboratory diagnosis consists of stained impression smears of the brain, mouse inoculation, and serologic tests. Impression smears from Ammon's horn of the hippocampal area in the temporal lobe stained with Seller's stain is the traditional method for diagnosis. The smears are examined microscopically for Negri body inclusions in neurons. Use of Seller's stain has approximately 65% sensitivity, with sensitivity reported to be somewhat greater than this in dogs (75%–80%) and somewhat less in skunks and bats. Fluorescent antibody stains on the smears have more than 95% sensitivity. Mouse inoculation with fresh brain extracts also has more than 95% sensitivity. Saliva from animals or humans can be used for mouse inoculation, but the sensitivity is not as great as brain testing. All specimens should be taken with sterile instruments, which should be immediately decontaminated by autoclaving after use. Serologic tests for diagnosis in humans (if the person has not been immunized against rabies) are also available. This requires two specimens drawn at least 1 week apart.

Reye's Syndrome

Reye's syndrome usually begins a few days after onset of a viral illness, which is the reason for including it with the viruses. The disease predominantly affects children and young adolescents, with a peak incidence between ages 5 and 15 years. Onset of the disease is manifested by symptoms of encephalitis (e.g., confusion, lethargy, or aggressive behavior), without focal neurologic signs, that accompany or follow onset of protracted or recurrent vomiting. Temperature is usually normal. There is laboratory evidence of liver cell injury, with AST or ALT more than three times the upper limit of the reference range. Serum total bilirubin is usually normal, and clinical jaundice is rare. Nevertheless, the prothrombin time is usually elevated, and blood ammonia level is frequently elevated. Routine CSF test results are usually normal. Creatine phosphokinase level is markedly abnormal, and phosphorus level is decreased, indicating muscle involvement. Fatty liver is frequently found on biopsy or autopsy. Although exact etiology is not known, influenza A and B, especially B, have been associated with the majority of cases, with chickenpox next most frequent and other viruses also implicated on occasion. There is also an association with aspirin use during a viral infection.

Conditions that may simulate Reye's syndrome and that can be ruled out by assay of serum levels or other tests include salicylate or acetaminophen overdose, valproic acid toxicity, encephalitis from other causes (e.g., HSV) with superimposed creatine phosphokinase elevation due to intramuscular injection, denatured alcohol poisoning, and acute lead poisoning. Certain rare inborn errors of metabolism (e.g., deficiency of ornithine transcarbamylase) may be manifested by symptoms that suggest Reye's syndrome.

RICKETTSIAL DISEASES

The rickettsiae to some extent resemble small bacteria but are not stained with Gram stain and cannot be cultured on artificial media. These organisms are spread only by insect vectors that have fed on blood from a patient with the disease, not from personal contact with a patient. Blood cultures can sometimes isolate and identify rickettsiae, especially in Rocky Mountain spotted fever. The blood specimens should be frozen and sent to the laboratory packed in dry ice. Since artificial culture media are not available, chick embryo or live animal inoculation must be done. Very few laboratories will perform rickettsial culture. Therefore, serologic tests or other procedures by far overshadow culture as diagnostic aids. The most commonly used procedure is the Weil-Felix reaction. This test takes advantage of the fact that certain rickettsial diseases produce antibodies that also react (or cross-react) with antigen contained in certain strains of *Proteus* bacteria. These *Proteus* groups are called OX-19 and OX-K. Titers of 1:80 are suspicious, and titers of 1:160 are definitely significant. Antibodies appear 7–10 days after onset of illness. Rickettsial diseases that may be diagnosed by means of the Weil-Felix reaction are the following:

Disease	*Proteus* Strain	Vector	Organism
Epidemic typhus	OX-19	Body louse	*R. prowazekii*
Endemic (murine) typhus	OX-19	Rat flea	*R. mooseri*
Scrub typhus	OX-K	Mite	*R. tsutsugamushi*
Rocky Mountain spotted fever	OX-19	Tick	*R. akari*

Unfortunately, there are serious limitations to the Weil-Felix test. First, there are a fairly large number of borderline false positive results as well as occasional outright false positives. Since the Weil-Felix reaction depends on *Proteus* antigen, urinary tract infection by *Proteus* should be ruled out if the Weil-Felix test result is positive. Second, about two thirds of patients with Rocky Mountain spotted fever or Brill's disease (recrudescent typhus) have false negative reactions. In these two diseases, other serologic tests (e.g., the microimmunofluorescence procedure) are preferred to the Weil-Felix test.

Rocky Mountain Spotted Fever.—Rocky Mountain spotted fever occurs in spring and summer, predominantly in the eastern two thirds of the United States (the area east of the Rocky Mountains). The disease is transmitted through the bite of an infected tick, with an incubation period of 3–12 days. Fever, severe frontal headache, severe myalgias, and a macular or maculopapular skin rash that develops on the third to fifth day and eventually develops a petechial component are the most characteristic clinical findings, with the rash typically involving the palms and soles. Nausea, vomiting, and diarrhea are reported in about 60% of patients and abdominal pain is reported in about 35%. The WBC count is usually normal, but thrombocytopenia is said to be common. In severe cases disseminated intravascular coagulation may develop. Serologic tests include the Weil-Felix test, CF test, microimmunofluorescence (MIF) test, LA test, and tissue biopsy with immunofluorescent staining. The Weil-Felix test has very poor sensitivity and is not specific, and the antibody does not develop until some time between 7–21 days after infective contact (compared with incubation period of 3–12 days). Complement fixation is more specific but detects 50% or fewer cases and is very laborious to perform, the antibody does not appear until 14–21 days after infection, and antibody elevations persist for years. Antibodies detected by the MIF and LA tests begin to appear 7–10 days after onset of illness. These tests are reported to detect considerably more than one half of Rocky Mountain spotted fever cases but are available only in reference laboratories or public health laboratories. The MIF test is currently considered the gold standard. Latex agglutination is reported to detect about 80%–85% of patients detected by MIF. Skin biopsy of a lesion with immunofluorescent antirickettsial antibody studies on the tissue can also be done (chapter 35), but the degree of sensitivity is controversial (50%–70%) and the test is not widely available.

Additional tests relevant to this chapter are discussed in chapter 35.

BIBLIOGRAPHY

Schwartz JS, et al: Human immunodeficiency virus test evaluation, performance, and use. *JAMA* 1988; 259:2574.

Jackson JB, Balfour HH: Practical diagnostic testing for human immunodeficiency virus. *Clin Microbiol Rev* 1988; 1:124.

Khan NC, et al: Isolation of human immunodeficiency virus type I from clinical samples obtained from AIDS patients. *Am Clin Prod Rev* 1988; 7:12.

Jacobson MA, Mills J: Serious cytomegalovirus disease in the acquired immunodeficiency syndrome (AIDS). *Ann Intern Med* 1988; 108:585.

Tindell B, et al: Characterization of the acute clinical illness associated with human immunodeficiency virus infection. *Arch Intern Med* 1988; 148:945.

Tribe DE, et al: Antibodies reactive with human immunodeficiency virus gag-coded antigens (gag reactive only) are a major cause of enzyme-linked immunosorbent assay reactivity in a blood donor population. *J Clin Microbiol* 1988; 26:641.

Thomas EE, et al: Evaluation of seven immunoassays for detection of rotavirus in pediatric blood samples. *J Clin Microbiol* 1988; 26:1189.

Holmes GP, et al: Chronic fatigue syndrome: A working case definition. *Ann Intern Med* 1988; 108:387.

Straus SE, et al: Varicella-zoster virus infections. *Ann Intern Med* 1988; 108:221.

Caussy D, et al: Evaluation of methods for detecting human papillomavirus deoxyribonucleotide sequences in clinical specimens. *J Clin Microbiol* 1988; 26:236.

Welliver RC: Detection, pathogenesis, and therapy of respiratory syncytial virus infections. *Clin Microbiol Rev* 1988; 1:27.

Sienko DG, et al: Q fever. *Arch Intern Med* 1988; 148:609.

Govidarajan S: Delta hepatitis: What have we learned in the last decade? *Lab Mgmt* 1988; 26(4):36.

Kane MA, et al: Routine prenatal screening

for hepatitis B surface antigen. *JAMA* 1988; 259:408.

Hofbauer JM, et al: Comparison of Western Blot (immunoblot) based on recombinant-derived p41 with conventional tests for serodiagnosis of human immunodeficiency virus infections. *J Clin Microbiol* 1988; 26:116.

Frontiera M, Myers AM: Peripheral blood and bone marrow abnormalities in the acquired immunodeficiency syndrome. *West J Med* 1987; 147:157.

Bryan JA: The serologic diagnosis of viral infection. *Arch Pathol Lab Med* 1987; 111:1015.

Saah AJ, et al: Detection of early antibodies in human immunodeficiency virus infection by enzyme-linked immunosorbent assay, western blot, and radioimmunoprecipitation. *J Clin Microbiol* 1987; 25:1605.

Riddle T, et al: Rabies: A dignostic review. *Lab Mgmt* 1987; 25(9):43.

Dickison L, Tilton RC: Respiratory syncytial virus: Cell culture and newer identification methods. *Lab Mgmt* 1987; 25(5):27.

Smith TF: Rapid methods for the diagnosis of viral infections. *Lab Med* 1987; 18:16.

Zito DR, et al: Hepatitis B virus serology. *Am J Clin Pathol* 1987; 88:229.

Halstead DC, et al: Evaluation of a rapid latex slide agglutination test for herpes simplex virus as a specimen screen and culture identification method. *J Clin Microbiol* 1987; 25:96.

Pochedly C: Laboratory testing for infectious mononucleosis. *Postgrad Med* 1987; 81:335.

Lennette ET, Henle W: Epstein-Barr virus infections: Clinical and serologic features. *Lab Mgmt* 1987; 25(6):23.

Buchwald D, et al: Frequency of "chronic active Epstein-Barr virus infection" in a general medical practice. *JAMA* 1087; 257:2303.

Gaines H, et al: Antibody response in primary human immunodeficiency virus infection. *Lancet* 1987; 1:1249.

Janda WM: AIDS and HIV: Recent findings and future directions. *Clin Microbiol Newslett* 1987; 9:9.

MMWR: Revision of the CDC surveillance case definition for acquired immunodeficiency syndrome. *JAMA* 1987; 258:1143.

Gocke DJ: Hepatitis A revisited. *Ann Intern Med* 1986; 105:960.

Burkes RL, et al: Serum beta-2 microglobulin levels in homosexual men with AIDS and with persistent, generalized lymphadenopathy. *Cancer* 1986; 57:2190.

Murray BJ: The hepatitis B carrier state. *Am Fam Phys* 1986; 33:127.

Navia BA, et al: The AIDS dementia complex. *Ann Neurol* 1986; 19:517.

Toon PG, et al: Human papillomavirus infection of the uterine cervix of women without cytological signs of neoplasia. *Br Med J* 1986; 293:1261.

Kessler HA, Pottage JC: Viral hepatitis: Aspects of nosocomial transmission and control. *J Nosocom Infect* 1986; 3:(2).

Koziol DE: Antibody to hepatitis B core antigen as a paradoxical marker for non-A, non-B hepatitis agents in donated blood. *Ann Intern Med* 1986; 104:488.

Lindsay KL. et al: Diagnostic usefulness of testing for anti-HBc IgM in acute hepatitis B. *Hepatology* 1986; 6:1325.

Tsang T-K, et al: Clinical significance of concurrent hepatitis B surface antigen and antibody positivity. *Diagn Dis Sci* 1986; 31:620.

Horwitz CA, et al: Clinical and laboratory evaluation of cytomegalovirus-induced mononucleosis in previously healthy individuals. *Medicine* (Baltimore) 1986; 65:124.

Corey L: Laboratory diagnosis of herpes simplex virus infections. *Diagn Microbiol Infect Dis* 1986; 4:111S.

Swinker ML: Clinical aspects of genital herpes. *Am Fam Pract* 1986; 34:127.

Rand KH: False positive indirect fluorescent antibody (IFA) tests for antibody to herpes simplex virus 1. *Am J Clin Pathol* 1986; 86:765.

Castro KG: The acquired immunodeficiency syndrome: Epidemiology and risk factors for transmission. *Med Clin North Am* 1986; 70:635.

Anderson KC, et al: Transfusion-acquired human immunodeficiency virus infection among immunocompromised persons. *Ann Intern Med* 1986; 105:519.

Cohen JI, Corey GR: Cytomegalovirus infection in the normal host. *Medicine* (Baltimore) 1985; 64:100.

Alford CA: Cytomegalovirus infection. *Ala J Med Sci* 1985; 22:169.

Armstrong D, et al: Treatment of infections in patients with the acquired immunodeficiency syndrome. *Ann Intern Med* 1985; 103:738.

Rainey PM: Rotavirus: Rapid detection may not mean infection. *Pathologist* 1984; 38:497.

Zolla-Pazner S, et al: Quantitation of beta-2-microglobulin and other immune characteristics in a prospective study of men at risk for acquired immune deficiency syndrome. *JAMA* 1984; 251:2951.

Schiff ER, De Medina MD: Delta agent: Another hepatitis virus. *Diagn Med* 1984; 8(3):17.

Aarnaes S, de la Maza LM: Isolation and identification of viruses from clinical specimens. *Am J Med Technol* 1983; 49:141.

Hoofnagle JH: Type A and type B hepatitis. *Lab Med* 1983; 14:705.

Hechemy KE: Evaluation of latex–*Rickettsia rickettsii* test for Rocky Mountain spotted fever in 11 laboratories. *J Clin Microbiol* 1983; 18:938.

Czaja AJ, Davis GL: Hepatitis non-A, non-B. *Mayo Clin Proc* 1982; 57:639.

NIH Consensus Conference: Diagnosis and treatment of Reye's syndrome. *JAMA* 1981; 246:2441.

Horwitz CA, et al: Hepatic function in mononucleosis induced by Epstein-Barr virus and cytomegalovirus. *Clin Chem* 1980; 26:243.

17 Medical Parasitology

TOXOPLASMOSIS

Toxoplasmosis is caused by a protozoan organism, *Toxoplasma gondii*. About 30%–50% (range, 20%–70%) of the U.S. population is reported to have serologic evidence of past infection. The disease is transmitted via raw or poorly cooked meat and possibly, in some cases, by oocysts in feces of infected cats. Once ingested, the organisms encyst in various tissues, particularly in muscle, and remain dormant for many years or for the life of the host. Initial infection may or may not be accompanied by clinical disease. There is a congenital form of clinical disease and an acquired form. The congenital form of toxoplasmosis occurs when *T. gondii* organisms are transmitted to the fetus through the placenta when the mother acquires active *Toxoplasma* infection near the time of conception or during pregnancy (infection several weeks or more before conception will not injure the fetus). About 90% of mothers acutely infected during pregnancy are asymptomatic. Congenital toxoplasmosis is manifested most often by chorioretinitis (usually bilateral), which may not become manifest until years afterward. Other frequent findings include brain damage (mental retardation, microcephalus or hydrocephalus, and convulsions) and intracerebral calcifications on x-ray film. Cerebrospinal fluid (CSF) is abnormal in about two thirds of patients, showing xanthochromia, mononuclear pleocytosis, and elevated protein levels (i.e., the findings usually associated with aseptic meningitis). Less frequently there is an acute neonatal disease with fever, hepatosplenomegaly, and cerebral symptoms that is clinically similar to bacterial septicemia. The more severe acute and chronic clinical disorders are more common when the mother is infected early in pregnancy, whereas infection later in pregnancy is more likely to result in symptoms (e.g., mental retardation) that are not manifest until after the neonatal period. Acquired toxoplasmosis is usually seen in older children or adults. The most common manifestations are either asymptomatic lymphadenopathy or a viral-type illness with lymphadenopathy, low-grade fever, malaise, and possibly other symptoms. There may (or may not) be some atypical lymphocytes, and the clinical picture may suggest "heterophil-negative" infectious mononucleosis, cytomegalovirus infection, other viral infections, or even malignant lymphoma. Another type of acquired infection is associated with deficient immunologic defense mechanisms, due to either immunologic suppression therapy or a disease such as leukemia or acquired immunodeficiency syndrome (AIDS). This is actually a reactivation of previous latent *Toxoplasma* infestation. Cerebral infection is often the most prominent manifestation.

Diagnosis

Diagnosis requires isolation of the organisms or serologic tests for antibody formation. Culture has proved to be very difficult, and most laboratories are not equipped to do it. Lymph node biopsy frequently can suggest the diagnosis by showing small groups of histiocytes that involve germinal centers, although the pattern is not specific enough for definitive diagnosis. Histologic slides rarely show organisms in lymph nodes.

Serologic tests form the backbone of diagnosis. The indirect fluorescent antibody (IFA) procedure is the most commonly used present-day serologic procedure. The IFA test detects the same antibody as the Sabin-Feldman dye test, which was the original standard test for toxoplasmosis. The dye test, however, required working with live *Toxoplasma* organisms. The IFA procedure can be used to detect either IgM or IgG antibody.

The IFA-IgM antibody titer begins to rise about 7 days after infection, reaches a peak in 1–3 weeks, and becomes nondetectable after approximately 4–5 months. However, it may revert to nonreactive in as little as 3 weeks or as long as 2 years. Immunoglobulin G antibody in the presence of rheumatoid factor or antinuclear antibody may produce false positive results. False positive results may also be found on tests of some newborns with other congenital infections. If the IgG can be separated from the IgM, the false positive reaction can be eliminated.

The IFA-IgG antibody titer begins to rise about 4–7 days after the IgM antibody, reaches a peak 1–3 weeks later, and begins to fall slowly in about 6 months. Low titers usually persist for many years. Antinuclear antibody may produce false positive results.

Rise in titer of either IgM or IgG antibody to *Toxoplasma* is rapid, with considerable elevation occurring during 1 week. Therefore, a low titer of IgM or IgG usually means old rather than recent infection in patients with maternal or congenital infection. However, when ocular infection is seen as an isolated finding in older children or adults, titers frequently are not high because the initial infection was congenital. Therefore, it may be difficult to tell whether the ocular disease is due to toxoplasmosis or to something else. This is made more difficult because exposure to *Toxoplasma* infection is very common. Surveys have shown elevated IgG or Sabin-Feldman dye titers in 20%–70% of the various populations studied.

An indirect hemagglutination (IHA) test that detects only IgG antibody is used in some laboratories. It is used mainly to see if a newly pregnant woman has antibody against *Toxoplasma*, thus suggesting immunity to infection. A complement fixation (CF) test that detects IgG antibodies has also been used, although mostly in reference laboratories. The CF level rises about 1 week after the IFA-IgG antibody titer, reaches a peak at about the same time, and declines to a nondetectable state in 6–8 months. It is not affected by rheumatoid factor or antinuclear antibodies. The CF test is used mainly in persons with a high IFA-IgG titer to help differentiate between relatively recent infection (in which the CF test result is positive) and a less recent infection (in which the CF test result is negative). However, the CF test is not always helpful clinically. If the result is negative, there is a problem with interpretation because it is not as sensitive as the other tests. If the result is positive, one knows only that acute infection began at least 3 weeks previously, but it could have begun several weeks before that.

Enzyme-linked immunosorbent assay (ELISA) methods detecting IgM, IgG, or both, as well as other methods such as latex agglutination (LA) have been reported. Initial reports have been very favorable; but most of the ELISA data are based on homemade reagents, and there has not been a sufficient number of studies of other methods.

Interpretation of Toxoplasma *Serologic Results*

If a woman is pregnant and it is desirable to know if she is immune to *Toxoplasma* infection, a negative titer means that she is susceptible to infection. A low titer of IgG (<1:1000) or the presence of IHA antibodies usually means that she had the disease at some time in the past and is immune. Since there is a small chance that a very early infection could be present and the titer is just beginning to rise, an IFA-IgM test can then be done. If the IFA-IgM antibody titer is greatly elevated but the IFA-IgG antibody titer is still low, this indicates early acute infection with the IgG antibody just starting to rise. Alternatively, an additional specimen may be drawn 7–10 days later and retested for IFA-IgG antibody. A fourfold rising titer indicates acute infection. A stable low titer means no recent infection. If the original specimen contains a high titer of IFA-IgG or IHA antibodies, the problem is difficult. The infection could be either acute or recent (within 1–2 years) but not acute. Only the acute infection is dangerous to the fetus. A high IgM titer is suggestive of recent infection, but in some cases it may persist for several weeks or months, falsely suggesting a more recent infection. On the other hand, it may fall rapidly and thus can be negative in association with a high IFA-IgG titer, even though acute infection began only a few weeks before.

In a newborn with possible congenital toxoplasmosis, most investigators believe that an elevated IgM level would support the diagnosis (although other infections can also produce IgM response). The IFA-IgG titer may be considerably elevated; but IgG antibody can cross the placenta; thus, maternal IgG antibody can appear in the fetal circulation if the mother has an elevated titer from either old or recent infestation. Therefore, to make a diagnosis of congenital toxoplasmosis, it is necessary to demonstrate a rising IgG titer in the infant. If no active infant infection is present and antibody is only passively acquired from the mother, the infant IgG titer, instead of rising, should fall by the sixth week as the maternally acquired antibody is eliminated.

MALARIA

Malaria is a widespread cause of serious infection in Asia and Africa and may be acquired by travelers or military personnel. The usual diagnostic tests are examinations of thick and thin peripheral blood smears. It has been recommended that smears be collected just after episodes of chills and also 10 hours later.

Babesiosis is an uncommon red blood cell infestation in the United States originally found on Nantucket island in New England. The organism responsible is a protozoan from the genus *Babesia,* which infects several species of animals (especially rodents) and has a tick vector. In humans, the infection is either asymptomatic or is manifested by a mild or moderate febrile illness, usually self-limited, which may be accompanied by mild hemolytic anemia. Splenectomized persons, however, develop severe illness. Diagnosis necessitates the same tests used in malaria.

GASTROINTESTINAL PARASITES

Ascaris, hookworm, *Strongyloides,* the tapeworms, and the protozoans *Giardia lamblia* and *Entamoeba histolytica* form the majority of gastrointestinal parasites that have clinical significance in the United States. Diagnosis usually depends on examination of the feces for larvae or eggs. In most situations (except for amebiasis), three routine stool specimens, collected one every other day and sent for "ova and parasites" is adequate. According to one report from a specialized parasitology laboratory, a single specimen obtained after use of magnesium sulfate cathartic detected about 80% of the most important parasites that were eventually detected using multiple specimens. The average laboratory would probably not obtain this degree of proficiency.

Stool Examination for Ova and Parasites

There are three standard methods of fecal examination for ova and parasites: direct examination, concentration methods followed by direct examination, and permanent stained slides prepared after concentration. Concentration techniques are useful on all types of stool specimens but especially on formed stools or soft stools. Concentration techniques detect larvae, ova, and protozoan cysts. Direct wet mounts can also be performed on all types of stools and also can detect larvae, ova, and protozoan cysts, but will not detect them as frequently as concentration techniques (in one study, only half as often). However, direct wet mount occasionally will detect some ova and protozoan cysts missed by concentration techniques. Permanent stained slide preparations are designed to detect protozoan cysts and trophozoites rather than ova or larvae, and should be performed on all very soft or liquid stools. Stained slides in addition to concentration plus direct examination are essential for optimal detection of *E. histolytica* and *G. lamblia*. In several reports, concentration techniques yielded about 50%–60% positive results for these two protozoans (literature range, 45%–74%), whereas stained smears yielded about 75%–85% positive results (literature range, 59%–95%). In another study, nonfixed direct wet mounts detected only 5% of trophozoites, whereas permanent stain detected about 60%. In the average laboratory, the sensitivity of a single stool specimen without a cathartic is probably about 50% and may be less, since many laboratories do not prepare stained slides routinely.

Entamoeba histolytica

This etiologic agent of amebiasis is acquired by ingestion of ameba cysts from contaminated food or water. Waterborne invasion is frequently associated with a water supply in close proximity to sewer material. Clinically, there are several forms of acute amebiasis: a severe acute colitis that may resemble severe ulcerative colitis (sometimes with blood and mucus in the stool) or shigellosis; chronic diarrhea similar to milder ulcerative colitis; intermittent mild diarrhea; asymptomatic carriers; and even a group with constipation. Acutely ill patients are usually afebrile and have normal white blood cell counts and hemoglobin values; although patients with severe amebic colitis or hepatic abscess frequently have low-grade fever, leukocytosis between 10,000 and 20,000/cu mm, and mild anemia. *Entamoeba histolytica* usually does not produce eosinophilia.

Stool Examination.—*Entamoeba histolytica* is more difficult to diagnose than most of the common intestinal parasites and requires special precautions. If the stool specimen is soft or liquid, it may contain trophozoites and should be sent to the laboratory immediately (with the time of collection noted) or placed into a special fixative, because trophozoites are fragile and quickly degenerate. Well-formed stools usually contain protozoan cysts rather than trophozoites and may be either temporarily refrigerated or placed into fixative. For collection procedure, three specimens, one specimen collected every other day, are more reliable than a single specimen. If results of the stool specimens on three alternate days are all negative, and if strong clinical suspicion is still present, a saline purge should be used. After a saline purge (e.g., Fleet Phosphosoda), the patient should pass liquid stools within a few hours. Oily laxatives (e.g., mineral oil or magnesia) make the stools useless for examination. Enema specimens are not advisable because they are too dilute to be of much value, and, in addition, the trophozoites may be destroyed. Barium, if present, also makes the preparation unfit to read. If stool specimens for amebae must be sent by mail, they should be placed in a preservative (one part specimen to three parts of 10% formalin). If possible, a second portion preserved in a special polyvinyl alcohol fixative (PVA) (in the same proportions) should be included along with the formalin-fixed portion. Formalin preserves ameba cysts and also eggs and larvae of other parasites. Polyvinyl alcohol fixative is used to make permanent stained preparations of protozoan trophozoites and cysts, which is not possible after formalin fixation (there is some disagreement about preservation of cysts with PVA). Stained slides considerably increase the chances of finding protozoan trophozoites and cysts and provide better cytologic detail for identification purposes.

Serologic Tests.—Serologic tests for amebiasis are available in reference laboratories. The most widely used procedures are gel diffusion, IHA, and slide LA. In patients with intestinal amebiasis, these tests detect about 10% of those who are asymptomatic *E. histolytica* carriers, less than 50% of those with mild amebic diarrhea, and about 85%–90% of those with invasive amebiasis. The IHA and LA tests are slightly more sensitive than gel diffusion. Thus, results of the more severe cases are more likely to be positive. The IHA and LA antibody levels persist for several years, so a positive test result does not necessarily mean active infection. Gel diffusion antibodies may become undetectable in 6 months, although some have reported persistent elevation for 1–2 years. An ELISA method for antigen detection in stool has been reported and is claimed to detect about 95% of patients. However, this needs adequate verification.

Extraintestinal Amebiasis

The preceding discussion was concerned with the usual type of amebiasis–amebiasis localized to the colon. Visceral amebiasis is not common. Liver involvement with abscess formation is seen in a majority of these cases. Clinical **hepatic amebiasis** is always associated with chronic rather than acute ameba infestation. Only 30%–50% of patients provide a history of diarrhea. Only about 25% of patients have amebae detectable in the stool. Patients with classic hepatic amebiasis have hepatomegaly, right upper quadrant pain, elevation of the right hemidiaphragm, leukocytosis as high as 20,000/cu mm (20×10^9/L), and fever. Surprisingly, the alkaline phosphatase level is normal in more than one half of patients. Liver scan is often very helpful, both for detection and localization of a lesion. Results of the various serologic tests for amebiasis are positive in 90%–95% of cases.

Amebic encephalitis is a rare condition produced by free-living amebae of the *Acanthamoeba* and *Naegleria* species. *Naegleria* infection takes place in normal individuals, usually with a recent history of swimming in rivers, fresh-water lakes, or fresh-water swimming pools. *Acanthamoeba* infections occur in persons with decreased immunologic defenses, frequently without any history of swimming. *Acanthamoeba keratitis* is also being reported due to contamination of contact lenses. Diagnosis can be made through phase contrast examination of spinal fluid or permanent slides of centrifuged spinal fluid stained by Wright's stain or trichrome stain. Centrifugation or refrigeration decreases motility of the organisms, which would hinder phase contrast examination but not permanent stained slide examination. Gram-stained smears are not recommended. Calcofluor white stain used for detection of fungus is reported to detect *Acanthamoeba* cysts as well (but not trophozoites).

Giardia lamblia

This protozoan lives in the duodenum and proximal jejunum and is said to be the most frequent intestinal parasite in the United States. An estimated 3%–7% of U.S. adults may have the disease. The organism is usually transmitted through fecal (sewage) contamination of water. Chloridation will not kill *Giardia,* but iodine will. Some reports suggest a high incidence in male homosexuals. Acute infection is manifested by foul-smelling watery diarrhea, usually accompanied by greasy floating stools, considerable intestinal gas, and epigastric pain. The symptoms may last 3–4 days or 1–3 weeks or may become chronic. In severe cases, steatorrhea and intestinal malabsorption have been reported.

Diagnosis.—Diagnosis is made through the same type of stool examinations discussed under amebiasis. Overall detection rate of stool microscopy (direct examination plus stained slide) is usually considered to be 50%–70%. Cathartics do not increase detection rates. Permanent stain techniques detect about one-third more cases than wet mounts. Cyst excretion in the stool may be irregular; although three specimens (each of the three collected on different days) are usually sufficient, more may be necessary. The first specimen detects about 75% of cases diagnosed through multiple specimens. Duodenal aspiration has been found to detect more infections (about 80% of cases) than repeated stool specimens. A commercial company has a string apparatus (Entero-Test) that can be swallowed instead of resorting to duodenal aspiration.

Serologic Tests.—ELISA tests for antibody and for antigen detection in stool have been reported but to date are available only in a few laboratories. A commercial indirect immunofluorescence test is also available, and the manufacturer claims 97% sensitivity. To date, no independent evaluations have been published.

Pneumocystis carinii

This organism is thought to be a sporozoan parasite, with some similarities to *Toxoplasma*. Clinical infection is very frequent in patients who are immunocompromised and is rare otherwise. About 60% of patients with AIDS develop pneumocystis disease (range, 35%–80%). Infections present as pneumonia that rapidly becomes bilateral, with an x-ray pattern of the interstitial type with or without an alveolar component. At present, tissue culture is necessary for culture diagnosis. Counterimmunoelectrophoresis and immunofluorescent serologic tests have been described, but they are not yet generally available. Currently, the most practical means of diagnosis are special stains performed on material from one of the following sources: lung transbronchial biopsies, with about 85% detected (range, 35%–98%); bronchial lavage, about 90% detected (range, 71%–100%); bronchial brushing, about 40% detected (range, 12%–53%); aerosol-induced sputum, about 57% detected (range, 55%–79%); open lung biopsy, about 65% detected, and lung needle aspiration. Ordinary (noninduced) sputum is not considered an adequate source material. There are advocates for rapid staining techniques using touch preparations and stains such as toluidine blue O and also for the much more time-consuming silver stains such as methenamine silver. Each stain has been reported to detect as many as 75%–85% of cases. However, such statistics depend to a considerable extent on how the specimen was obtained and the experience of the institution. In general, toluidine blue O stain takes significantly more experience to interpret than silver stains. Both of these methods stain *Pneumocystis* cyst walls. Gram stain, Giemsa, or Wright's stain used on smears can demonstrate *Pneumocystis* trophozoites within cysts; the cyst wall does not stain. Trophozoite detection requires considerable experience and is much more time-consuming and less sensitive (in most laboratories) than cyst wall stains. Yeast cells are about the same size as *Pneumocystis* cysts, and also stain with cyst wall stain. Differentiation between yeast and *Pneumocystis* cysts may sometimes be difficult, especially if there are only a few organisms. Monoclonal antibody methods for detection of *Pneumocystis* antigen are now being reported and should be commercially available in the near future. This should become the most accurate detection method.

Cryptosporidium

Cryptosporidium is another sporozoan organism with some similarities to *Toxoplasma*. Originally found in cattle with diarrhea, *Cryptosporidium* was next reported to cause diarrhea in humans who were immunocompromised, particularly those with AIDS. Then, it was discovered that *Cryptosporidium*-associated diarrhea occurred in nonimmunocompromised persons, most often children, with a frequency in Western countries of 0.6%–7.3% of patients with diarrhea. This incidence is similar to that of *Giardia* and the major bacterial gastrointestinal pathogens. The organism is rarely found in humans without diarrhea. The types found in cattle and humans live predominantly in the small intestine, from which oocysts pass in the feces to act as sources of infection. Transmission is most frequently through contaminated water, although person-to-person spread has been reported in families, hospital personnel, and day-care centers. The average incubation period is said to be about 7 days. In nonimmunocompromised persons, illness and oocyst shedding are nearly always finished by 31 days after exposure. The most severe and persistent infections occur in human immunodeficiency virus I infections, particularly in AIDS and AIDS-related illnesses (about 6% of patients; range, 3%–28%). These patients have long-standing watery diarrhea, anorexia, abdominal pain, weight loss, and low-grade fever.

Diagnosis.—Diagnosis is most commonly made through stool examination. Although the organism can be seen in standard concentrated stool preparations, they are hard to identify, are about the same size as yeast cells (4–6 μm) and are most often overlooked. Permanent stained slide preparations stained with a special modification of the mycobacterial acid-fast stain has been the most successful approach. In two quality control studies, detection rates varied between 75%–90%. Also, various non-cryptosporidial objects or organisms in stool specimens may appear acid-fast, requiring observer experience for accurate results. A fluorescent antibody method for use on prepared slides is now available and is claimed to be more sensitive than modified acid-fast bacillus staining.

Schistosoma mansoni

Schistosoma mansoni is sometimes encountered in the United States because it is endemic in Puerto Rico. Routine stools for parasite ova are often not sufficient, because the adult lays its eggs in the venous system, and the ova must penetrate the intestinal mucosa to appear in the stool. In difficult cases, proctoscopic rectal biopsy with a fresh unstained crush preparation of the biopsy specimen has been advocated. Serologic tests have been developed; the tests most commonly mentioned in the literature are CF and immunofluorescence. There is some disagreement on how much help the tests can provide. The major problem is differentiation between past exposure and current active infection.

Pinworm (*Enterobius vermicularis* or *Oxyuris vermicularis*)

Infestation with pinworms is fairly common in children. The female worm lays her eggs at night around the anal region. The best diagnostic procedure, therefore, is some method to swab the anal region thoroughly with an adhesive substance such as transparent celluloid tape (Scotch tape). The sticky surface with the eggs can then be directly applied to a glass slide and later examined microscopically for the characteristic pinworm ova. Such slides can also be sent through the mail, if necessary. Swabs lightly coated with vaseline are also useful to obtain specimens. The best time for obtaining the parasite ova is early in the morning, before the child gets up. Stool samples are less satisfactory for diagnosis of enterobiasis. Since the worms do not lay eggs every night, repeated specimens may be necessary.

Hookworm

Hookworm is a problem in some areas of the southern United States and occasionally may be the cause of an iron-deficiency anemia in children. Routine stool examination for ova and parasites is usually adequate for diagnosis.

Tapeworm

The fish tapeworm *Diphyllobothrium latum (Dibothriocephalus latus)* is only rarely a problem in the United States. The organisms are ingested with raw pike fish from the Great Lakes area. Usually very few symptoms are produced, but occasionally the syndrome of megaloblastic anemia may result from ingestion of dietary vitamin B12 by the parasite. Diagnosis consists of stool examination for ova or detached tapeworm proglottid segments. The beef tapeworm (*Taenia saginata*) and the pork tapeworm (*Taenia solium*) also are diagnosed by stool examination for ova or proglottids.

Tapeworm infestation in a human ordinarily occurs when the intermediate host (animal or fish) ingests tapeworm eggs or prolarvae, the egg (or prolarva) evolves to a larval form within the intermediate host, the person eats flesh from the intermediate host that contains the larva, and the larva develops into an adult worm in the lumen of the individual's intestine. If someone ingests ova or prolarva rather than the larva, larvae may develop within the person's intestine, proceed through the intestinal wall, and reach the bloodstream, whence they are capable of producing abnormality in various organs or tissues.

The most publicized tapeworm larval diseases are **Echinococcus** or hydatid cyst infection (*Echinococcus granulosus*, the larva of the dog tapeworm), **cysticercus cellulosa** (infection by the larva of *T. solium*, the swine tapeworm), and **sparganosis** (infection by the larva of a dog or cat tapeworm of the *Spirometra* genus related to the fish tapeworm *D. latum*). No good laboratory method for diagnosis of sparganosis is available. Enzyme immunoassays have been reported for IgM and IgG antibodies to cysticercosis, but these are available only in some reference laboratories. The laboratory may be helpful in *Echinococcus* (hydatid) disease, although this condition is rare in the United States. The primary host is the dog. The dog sheds ova in the feces, and material contaminated by dog feces is ingested by humans or sheep (or other animals) who act as intermediate hosts. Larvae emerge from the ova, penetrate the intestinal wall, and travel to the liver. Cystic structures (hydatid cysts) containing brood capsules filled with scolices grow in the liver (75% of cases) but may appear in the lungs or other locations. Diagnostic aids include imaging procedures such as the radioisotope liver scan, ultrasound, or computerized tomography; a skin test known as the Casoni test; a hemagglutination test; and immunofluorescent procedures. Results of the Casoni test and the hemagglutination tests are said to be positive in 90% of those patients with hepatic lesions but abnormal in less than one half of patients with cysts elsewhere. False positive results in the Casoni test are said to occur with some frequency. Therefore the Casoni test has mostly been replaced by serologic tests, such as immunofluorescence and enzyme immunoassay. These are available in reference laboratories.

Trichinella spiralis

The larvae of this small roundworm are usually ingested with raw or insufficiently cooked pork or insufficiently cooked meat products contaminated by infected pork. During the first week after ingestion, symptoms consist of nausea and diarrhea; these may be minimal or absent. About 7–8 days after ingestion there is onset of severe muscle pain, which sometimes begins in the face. Bilateral periorbital edema often develops. Eosinophilia may begin as early as 10 days after ingestion and, with muscle pain and periorbital edema, forms a very suggestive triad. Eosinophilia is present in about 90% of patients and reaches its peak during the third week. Most patients have a slight or mild leukocytosis. Most patients display elevation of creatine phosphokinase (CPK) enzyme of varying degree due to involvement of skeletal muscle. Hypoalbuminemia is also frequent. The most helpful laboratory procedures are bentonite flocculation or LA slide tests. Enzyme immunoassay (ELISA) is also available. The bentonite flocculation test is considered a little more sensitive than LA. It takes about 3 weeks after infection for results to become positive; peak titers develop in about 2 months, and titers remain elevated for several years. Reports indicate 90%–95% sensitivity by the time of maximum titers. The LA slide test detects about 20%–30% of cases by day 7 after onset of symptoms and 80%–90% in 4–5 weeks. False positive results have been recorded in polyarteritis nodosa (also in tuberculosis, typhoid, and infectious mononucleosis, but these are not ordinarily considered in the differential diagnosis).

Muscle biopsy is occasionally useful. It is considered best to wait until at least 3 weeks after infection to do this procedure in order to allow the larvae time to encyst. A painful area of a skeletal muscle has been recommended as the preferred site for biopsy.

Trichomonas vaginalis

This motile flagellated protozoan infests the vagina and labial area in the female and the prostate and urethra of the male. Estrogen effect on vaginal epithelial cells is a predisposing factor toward infestation in females, so that trichomoniasis is uncommon before puberty or after menopause. The infection is usually transmitted during sexual intercourse, although some cases are not. Symptoms in the female most often consist of vaginal discharge, with the differential diagnosis including infection by *Trichomonas, Gardnerella vaginalis,* and *Candida albicans*. The disease is usually asymptomatic in males. Also, 25%–50% of culture-positive female patients are asymptomatic, although there is some question as to whether these are true infections or the equivalent of bacterial colonization without infection.

Culture has been considered the "gold standard" for diagnosis. However, culture needs special media and may take several days. Also, some reports indicate that culture sensitivity is 86%–97%. One report found that only 60% of male urethral cultures were positive. A wet preparation collected by swab from the posterior vaginal fornix and placed into a drop of 0.9% saline is the most simple and rapid method of diagnosis. The specimen should not be taken from the endocervix, since this area is rarely involved. If the wet preparation cannot be made and read immediately, the swab can be inoculated into a standard bacteriologic transport medium. The wet preparation detects about 50%–60% (range, 37%–80%) of patients and correlates much better with symptomatic infection than does culture. The organism can also be detected with stained smears using either Wright's stain or Papanicolaou stain. Sensitivity of the Papanicolaou smear compared to culture is about 60% (range, 50%–70%), in addition to a considerable false positive rate in some laboratories. The diagnosis sometimes is made by accident from microscopic examination of urine sediment during a urinalysis if the organisms are still motile. Nonmotile *Trichomonas* organisms round up and become very difficult to differentiate from WBCs or small epithelial cells in urine or wet-mount preparations. If the organisms appear in the urine of female patients, the urine probably was contaminated by vaginal or labial contact. Fluorescent immunoassay kits that can be applied to prepared slides are now commercially available. One such kit was reported to detect about 80% of cases that were positive by culture. Even better results have been claimed from an enzyme-immunoassay method applied directly to prepared slides, but confirmation of these results is necessary.

Strongyloides stercoralis

Strongyloides is a small roundworm that infects the small intestine. Many cases are asymptomatic, but some infections produce diarrhea. In immunocompromised persons, especially those with AIDS, infection may spread to organs or tissues outside the intestine and become fatal. About 70%–80% of infected persons are said to have eosinophilia, but immunocompromised persons often have normal numbers of eosinophils. Diagnosis is usually made through stool examination, which contains rhabditiform larvae rather than ova. Single stool examinations are said to be positive in only 30%–40% of cases, so that two more specimens on different days should be done if results of the first are negative. Enzyme immunoassay for antibodies is available in some reference laboratories.

BIBLIOGRAPHY

Lossick JG: The diagnosis of vaginal trichomoniasis. *JAMA* 1988; 259:1230.

Pinals RS: Fever, eosinophilia, and periorbital edema. *Hosp Pract* 1988; 23(2A):55.

Kovacs JA, et al: Diagnosis of Pneumocystis carinii pneumonia: improved detection in sputum with use of monoclonal antibodies. *N Engl J Med* 1988; 318:589.

Watson B, et al: Direct wet mounts versus concentration for routine parasitological examination. *Am J Clin Pathol* 1988; 89:389.

Markell EK, Udkow MP: Association of *Blastocystis hominis* with human disease. *J Clin Microbiol* 1988; 26:609.

Wilson M, et al: Evaluation of commercial serodiagnostic kits for toxoplasmosis. *J Clin Microbiol* 1987; 25:2262.

Nieburg RK, Gong H: Diagnosis of *Pneumocystis carinii* pneumonia by bronchoalveolar lavage in patients with the acquired immunodeficiency syndrome. *Am Clin Prod Rev* 1987; 6(11):28.

Ramsey MK: Toxoplasmosis: Epidemiologic and diagnostic considerations. *Lab Mgmt* 1987; 25(8):43.

Fritsche TR, Bergeron DL: *Acanthamoeba* keratitis. *Clin Microbiol Newslett* 1987; 9:109.

Berk SL et al: Clinical and epidemiologic features of strongyloidiasis. *Arch Intern Med* 1987; 147:1257.

Binstock PB, et al: Cerebral cysticercosis in a 22-month-old infant. *Am J Clin Pathol* 1987; 88:655.

Janoff EN, Reller LB: *Cryptosporidium* species, a protean protozoan. *J Clin Microbiol* 1987; 25:967.

Morris PD, Katerndahl DA: Human toxocariasis. *Postgrad Med* 1987; 81:263.

Wilhelmus KR et al: Rapid diagnosis of *Acanthamoeba* keratitis using Calcofluor white. *Arch Ophthal* 1986; 104:1309.

Jones JE: String test for diagnosing giardiasis. *Am Fam Pract* 1986; 34:123.

Mones JM et al: Diagnostic procedures for detection of *Pneumocystis carinii* pneumonia. *Chest* 1986; 89:522.

Thomasen JL, et al: Trichomoniasis. *Clin Microbiol Newsletter* 1986; 8:9.

Wattal C et al: Comparative evaluation of enzyme-linked immunosorbent assay for the diagnosis of pulmonary echinococcosis. *J Clin Microbiol* 1986; 24:41.

Kochar AS: Human pulmonary dirofilariasis. *Am J Clin Pathol* 1985; 84:19.

Genta RM: *Strongyloides stercoralis*. *Pathologist* 1985; 39(12):21.

Thompson RB et al: Intestinal parasites: The necessity of examining multiple stool specimens. *Mayo Clin Proc* 1984; 59:641.

Amin NM: Giardiasis. *Hosp Med* 1984; 20(5):39.

Jones JE: Fleas. *Am Fam Pract* 1984; 29:143.

Wong B: Parasitic diseases in immunocompromised hosts. *Am J Med* 1984; 76:479.

Harrington BJ, Gaydos JM: Low pH acridine orange stain for trichomonads. *Lab Med* 1984; 15:180.

Schmid GP, Larsen SA: Finding the elusive *T. vaginalis*. *Diagn Med* 1984; 7(10):38.

Amin NM, Unger JR: Toxoplasmosis. *Fam Pract Recert* 1983; 5:118.

Seabolt JP: *Babesia*: Challenge for the medical technologist. *Lab Med* 1982; 13:547.

Campbell CC, Chin W: Diagnosing and monitoring malaria. *Diagn Med* 1981; 4:46.

Patterson M et al: Serologic testing for amoebiasis. *Gastroenterology* 1980; 78:136.

Marsden PD: Leishmaniasis. *N Engl J Med* 1979; 300:350.

18 Cerebrospinal Fluid Examination

BASIC CEREBROSPINAL FLUID TESTS

Pressure

Reference values for cerebrospinal fluid (CSF) pressure are 100–200 mm H_2O. Elevations are due to increased intracranial pressure. The two most common causes of elevated CSF pressure are meningitis and subarachnoid hemorrhage. Brain tumor and brain abscess will cause increased intracranial pressure in most cases but only after a variable period of days or even weeks. An increase is present in many cases of lead encephalopathy. The CSF pressure varies directly with venous pressure but has no constant relationship to arterial pressure. The Queckenstedt sign makes clinical use of this information; increased venous pressure via jugular vein compression increases CSF pressure at the lumbar region, whereas a subarachnoid obstruction above the lumbar area prevents this effect.

Appearance

Normal CSF is clear and colorless. It may be pink or red if many red blood cells (RBCs) are present or white and cloudy if there are many white blood cells (WBCs) or an especially high protein content. Usually there must be more than 400 WBCs/cu mm (0.4×10^9/L) before the CSF becomes cloudy. When blood has been present in the CSF for more than 4 hours (literature range, 2–48 hours), xanthochromia (yellow color) may occur due to hemoglobin pigment from lysed RBCs. Protein levels of more than 150 mg/100 ml (1.5 g/L) may produce a faint yellowish color that can simulate xanthochromia of RBC origin. Severe jaundice may also produce coloration that simulates xanthochromia.

Glucose

Reference values are 45 mg/100 ml (2.5 mmol/L) or higher ("true glucose" methods). Values of 40–45 mg/100 ml are equivocal, although in normal persons it is rare to find values below 45 mg/100 ml. The CSF glucose level is about 60% of the serum glucose value (literature range, 50%–80%). In newborns, the usual CSF level is about 80% of the serum glucose level. It takes between 0.5 and 2 hours for maximum change to occur in CSF values after a change in serum values.

The most important change in the CSF glucose level is a decrease. The classic etiologies for CSF glucose decrease are meningitis from standard bacteria, tuberculosis, and fungi. Occasionally in very early infection the initial CSF glucose value may be normal, although later it begins to decrease. A frequent impression from textbooks is that one should expect a decreased CSF glucose value in nearly all patients with acute bacterial meningitis. Actually, studies have shown that only 60%–80% of children with acute bacterial meningitis have CSF glucose levels below the reference range. Studies on patients of various ages have shown decreased glucose levels in 50%–90% of cases. A major problem is the effect of blood glucose levels on CSF glucose levels. Since elevated blood glucose levels may mask a decrease in CSF values, it is helpful to determine the blood glucose level at the same time that the CSF specimen is obtained, especially in diabetics or if intravenous (IV) glucose therapy is being given. On the other hand, a low CSF glucose level may be due to peripheral blood hypoglycemia, especially if the CSF cell count is normal. Other conditions that may produce a decrease in CSF glucose level are extensive involvement of meninges by metastatic carcinoma and in some cases of subarachnoid hemorrhage, probably due to release of glycolytic enzymes from the RBCs. In leptospiral meningitis and in primary amebic meningoencephalitis, the CSF glucose level is decreased in some patients but not in others. In most other central nervous system (CNS) diseases, including viral meningitis, encephalitis, brain abscess, syphilis, and brain tumor, CSF glucose levels typically are normal when bacterial infection of the meninges is not present. However, decreased levels are sometimes found in aseptic meningitis or in meningoencephalitis due to mumps, enteroviruses, lymphocytic choriomeningitis, and in both herpes simplex virus types I and II CNS infections. For example, one investigator reports that 10% of their cases of meningitis due to enterovirus had decreased CSF glucose.

Protein

The normal protein concentration of CSF is usually considered to be 15–45 mg/100 ml (0.15–0.45 g/L) (literature range, 9–90 mg/100 ml; 0.09–0.9 g/L). There is considerable discrepancy in the literature regarding the upper reference limit, which is most often listed as 40, 45, and 50 mg/100 ml. In newborns, CSF protein reference values are 75–150 mg/100 ml (literature range for upper limit, 140–200 mg/100 ml). Values slowly decline, reaching adult levels by 6 months of age. Over age 60 years, some persons increase the upper reference limit to 60 mg/100 ml (0.6 g/L). As a general but not invariable rule, an increased protein concentration is roughly proportional to the degree of leukocytosis in the CSF. The protein concentration is also increased by the presence of blood. There are, however, certain diseases in which a mild to moderate protein concentration increase may be seen with relatively slight leukocytosis; these include cerebral trauma, brain or spinal cord tumor, brain abscess, cerebral infarct or hemorrhage (CVA), CNS sarcoidosis, systemic lupus, lead encephalopathy, uremia, myxedema, multiple sclerosis (MS), variable numbers of hereditary neuropathy cases, and chronic CNS infections. Diabetics with peripheral neuropathy frequently have elevated CSF protein levels without known cause. Blood in the CSF introduces approximately 1 mg of protein/1,000 RBCs. However, when the RBCs begin to lyse, the protein level may appear disproportionate to the number of RBCs. In acute bacterial meningitis, the CSF protein is elevated in about 94% of cases (literature range, 74%–99%).

A marked protein elevation without a corresponding CSF cell increase is known as "albuminocytologic dissociation." This has usually been associated with the Guillain-Barré syndrome (acute idiopathic polyneuritis) or with temporal (giant cell) arteritis. Actually, about 20% of patients with the Guillain-Barré syndrome have normal CSF protein levels, and less than 25% have CSF protein levels of 200 mg/100 ml (2.0 g/L) or more.

Protein may be measured in the laboratory quantitatively by any of several methods. A popular semiquantitative bedside method is Pandy's test, in which CSF is added to a few drops of saturated phenol agent. This agent reacts with all protein, but apparently much more with globulin. Chronic infections or similar conditions such as (tertiary) syphilis or MS tend to accentuate globulin elevation and thus may give positive Pandy test results even though the total CSF protein level may not be greatly increased. Contamination by blood will often give false positive test results.

The technical method used can influence results. The three most common methods are sulfosalicylic acid, anazolene sodium (Coomassie Blue dye), and trichloracetic acid. Sulfosalicylic acid and Coomassie Blue are more influenced by the ratio of albumin to globulin than is trichloracetic acid.

In some CNS diseases there is a disproportionate increase in gamma-globulin levels compared with albumin or total protein levels. Several investigators have noted that increased CSF gamma globulin levels occur in approximately 70%–85% (literature range, 50%–88%) of patients with MS, whereas total protein levels are elevated in only about 25% of the patients (range, 13%–34%). Various other acute and chronic diseases of the brain may elevate CSF gamma-globulin levels, and this fraction may also be affected by serum hyperglobulinemia. The latter artifact may be excluded by comparing gamma-globulin quantity in serum and CSF.

The colloidal gold test also depends on changes in CSF globulins and at one time was considered very helpful in the diagnosis of MS and syphilitic tabes dorsalis. However, the colloidal gold procedure has very poor sensitivity (only 25% of MS patients display the classic first zone pattern) and poor specificity and is considered obsolete. When measurement of CSF protein fractions is ordered, the current standard procedure is some method of immunoglobulin quantitation.

Cell Count

Normally, CSF contains up to five cells/cu mm, almost all of which are lymphocytes. In newborns, the reference limits are 0–30 cells/cu mm, with the majority being segmented neutrophils. As a general rule, any conditions that affect the meninges will cause CSF leukocytosis; the degree of leukocytosis will depend on the type of irritation, its duration, and its intensity. Usually, the highest WBC counts are found in severe acute meningeal infections. The classic variety is the acute bacterial infection. It is important to remember that in a few cases if the patient is seen very early, leukocytosis may be minimal or even absent, just as the CSF glucose level may be normal. Although most investigators state or imply that 100% of patients with acute bacterial infection have elevated cell counts on initial lumbar puncture, in one study, 3% of patients had a WBC count less than six WBCs/cu mm, and there have been several reports of one or more isolated cases. Usually, in a few hours a repeat lumbar puncture reveals steadily increasing WBC counts. Therefore, normal initial counts are not frequent but may occur and can be very misleading. Another general rule is that in bacterial infections, polymorphonuclear neutrophils usually are the predominating cell type; whereas in viral infections, chronic nervous system diseases, and tertiary syphilis, lymphocytes or mononuclears ordinarily predominate (Table 18–1). However, there are important exceptions. One study reported that about one third of patients with usual bacterial pathogens but with CSF WBC counts less than 1,000/cu mm (1.0×10^9/L) had a predominance of lymphocytes on initial lumbar puncture (the only patient with a WBC count over 1,000 who had lymphocytosis had a *Listeria* infection). Another exception is tuberculous meningitis, which is both a bacterial and a chronic type of infection. In this case, the cells are predominantly lymphocytes (although frequently combined with some increase in neutrophils). A third exception is unusual nonviral organisms, such as *Listeria monocytogenes* (most often seen in neonates or in elderly persons or those who are immunocompromised), fungus, and spirochetes (leptospirosis and syphilis). *Listeria* meningitis may have lymphocytic predominance in some cases and neutrophilic predominance in others. On the other hand, coxsackievirus and echovirus infections may have a predominance of neutrophils in the early stages; in most of these patients, the CSF subsequently shifts to lymphocytosis. Uremia is said to produce a mild lymphocytosis in about 25% of patients. Partial treatment of bacterial meningitis may cause a shift in cell type toward lymphocytosis.

After therapy is started, WBC values usually decrease. However, in some cases more than 50 WBCs/cu mm may persist at least 48 hours and sometimes longer than 2 weeks following adequate therapy. This tends to be more common with *Haemophilus influenzae* infection but may also occur with pneumococcal infection. Fungal infections are more commonly associated with persistently elevated neutrophils than bacterial infections, even though fungi typically have CSF lymphocytosis rather than neutrophilia. *Nocardia* meningitis or brain abscess, however, is one bacterial infection that does tend to show persistent neutrophilia more often than other bacteria.

In cases of subarachnoid hemorrhage or traumatic spinal fluid taps, approximately 1 WBC is added for every 700 RBCs (literature range, 1 WBC/500–1,000 RBCs). This disagreement in values makes formulas unreliable that attempt to differentiate traumatic tap artifact from true WBC increase. Also, the presence of subarachnoid blood itself may sometimes cause meningeal irritation, producing a mild to moderate increase in polymorphonuclear leukocytes after several hours that occasionally may be greater than 500 WBCs/cu mm. A similar phenomenon occurs in occasional patients with intracerebral hematoma. Another exception is the so-called aseptic meningeal reaction that is secondary either to a nearby infection or some-

TABLE 18–1.
Patterns of Cerebrospinal Fluid Abnormality: Cell Type and Glucose Level

Polymorphonuclear: low glucose
Acute bacterial meningitis
Polymorphonuclear: low or normal glucose
Some cases of early phase acute bacterial meningitis
Primary amebic (*Naegleria* species) meningoencephalitis
Early phase Leptospira meningitis
Polymorphonuclear: normal glucose
Brain abscess
Early phase coxsackievirus and echovirus meningitis
Acute bacterial meningitis with IV glucose therapy
Lymphocytic: low glucose
Tuberculosis meningitis
Cryptococcal *(Torula)* meningitis
Mumps meningoencephalitis (some cases)
Meningeal carcinomatosis (some cases)
Meningeal sarcoidosis (some cases)
Lymphocytic: normal glucose
Viral meningitis
Viral encephalitis
Postinfectious encephalitis
Lead encephalopathy
CNS syphilis
Brain tumor (occasionally)
Leptospira meningitis (after the early phase)

times to acute localized brain destruction. In these cases, which are not common, there may be a wide range of WBC values, with neutrophils often predominating. When this occurs, however, the CSF glucose level should be normal, since the meninges are not directly infected. Aseptic meningitis is not the same as aseptic meningeal reaction. Aseptic meningitis is due to direct involvement of the meninges by nonbacterial organisms. Viruses cause most cases, but organisms such as amebae sometimes may cause meningitis. Bacterial CSF cultures are negative. The CSF glucose level is usually normal. Protein concentration is usually but not always increased. The WBC count is elevated to a varying degree; the predominant type of cell depends on the etiology. True aseptic meningitis also has to be differentiated from bacterial organisms that do not grow on ordinary culture media (anaerobes, leptospira, mycobacteria, bacteria inhibited by previous or current antibiotic therapy, etc.).

Neonatal CSF Reference Range Differences From Childhood and Adult Values

Neonates have different CSF reference ranges for protein, glucose, and cell count. Cell counts 1–7 days after birth average about 5–20/cu mm (range, 0–32 cu mm), with about 60% being segmented neutrophils. Glucose is about 75%–80% of the blood glucose level. Protein values are 20–150 mg/100 ml (0.2–1.5 g/L) during days 1 to 30; 20–100 mg/100 ml (0.2–1.0 g/L) during days 30 to 90; and 15–50 (0.15–0.5 g/L) during the time period 3 to 6 months. Therefore, neonatal values are elevated when compared with childhood and adult values, and some degree of protein elevation persists for as long as 6 months. This phenomenon could cause problems in separating normal from abnormal results in some patients.

SYPHILIS TESTS

Syphilis is discussed in chapter 31. Nevertheless, some of that discussion will be repeated here for the sake of continuity. Results of the standard serologic tests for syphilis (STS), such as the Venereal Disease Research Laboratory (VDRL) test, are nearly always positive in the blood in the secondary and latent stages and in about 75% of cases in the tertiary stage. The fluorescent treponemal antibody–absorbed test (FTA-ABS) or the microhemagglutination (MHA) test are more specific for syphilis than the VDRL and are reactive in the blood of nearly all syphilitic patients in the last half of the primary stage and in the secondary, latent, and tertiary stages. In CSF there currently is much confusion about sensitivity, specificity, and usefulness of these tests. Some difficulties are created by the small number of cases reported in different series, the effect of previous treatment (if any), the difficulty of establishing the diagnosis of CNS syphilis independently of the CSF tests being evaluated, the difficulty of proving whether CNS syphilis is active or inactive, and the problem of spinal fluid contamination by blood, which could produce false positive results if the contaminating blood contained serum antibodies.

Under these circumstances, increased CSF WBC counts and protein concentrations are better guides to actual CNS syphilitic activity than the CSF serology. One recent report indicates that an elevated IgG index (discussed later) helps suggest active infection. Positive serologic test results alone, either in the blood or the CSF, do not mean that the disease is currently active. Results of CSF serologic tests are usually negative in patients with so-called biologic false positive blood reactions. Overall, the VDRL when applied to CSF is estimated to detect 10%–50% of CNS syphilis cases. The three most important forms of CNS syphilis are general paresis, tabes dorsalis, and vascular neurosyphilis. According to the older literature, in general paresis, the STS on spinal fluid almost always yields positive results in untreated cases. In tabes dorsalis, the VDRL test result on spinal fluid is said to be reactive in most early untreated cases, but negative results may appear in up to 50% of late, or so-called burnt-out, cases. In vascular neurosyphilis, there are reactive results in approximately 50% of cases. More recent studies have suggested that the spinal fluid VDRL will be reactive in less than one half of the cases that eventually are diagnosed as neurosyphilis. They also indicate that the FTA-ABS test performed on spinal fluid is somewhat more sensitive than the VDRL test, but there is no agreement on the clinical significance of a reactive FTA-ABS test and nonreactive VDRL test on spinal fluid.

Culture

The diagnosis of acute bacterial meningitis often depends on the isolation of the organisms in the spinal fluid. In children, there is some regularity of the types of infection most commonly found. In infants under the age of 1–2 months, group B streptococci are most frequent, closely followed by *Escherichia coli*. *Listeria* monocytogenes is often listed as third, followed by other enteric gram-negative bacteria. In children from age 3 months to 5 or 6 years, *H. influenzae* is the most common organism; *Meningococcus* is second, and *Pneumococcus* is third. In older children and adolescents, *Meningococcus* is first and *Pneumococcus* second. In adults, *Meningococcus* and *Pneumococcus* are still dominant, but *Pneumococcus* is more prevalent in some reports. Staphylococci are the etiology in about 4%–7% of cases, most often associated with CNS operations (e.g., shunt procedures), septicemia, or endocarditis. In old age, pneumococci generally are more common pathogens than meningococci, with gram-negative bacilli in third place. However, there can be infection by nearly any type of organism, including *Listeria* and fungi. Also, in patients who are debilitated or have underlying serious diseases such as leukemia or carcinoma, *Listeria* and fungi are not uncommon. In many cases, a centrifuged spinal fluid sediment can be smeared and Gram stained so that the organisms can be seen. A (bacterial) culture should be done in all cases where bacterial meningitis is suspected or is even remotely possible. Special provision should be made for spinal fluid to reach the laboratory as quickly as possible; and if any particular organism is suspected, the laboratory should be informed so that special media can be used if necessary. For example, meningococci grow best in a high carbon dioxide atmosphere, and *H. influenzae* should be planted on media provided with a *Staphylococcus* streak. Culture is said to detect about 85% (range, 54%–100%) of cases. In one series there was thought to be about 5% false positive culture results due to contamination. Previous or concurrent antibiotic therapy is reported to decrease culture detection rates by about 30% and Gram stain detection rates by about 20%.

Gram Stain

Gram stain of the sediment from a centrifuged CSF specimen should be performed in all cases of suspected meningitis. Gram stain yields about 70% positive results (literature range, 50%–90%) in culture-proved acute bacterial meningitis cases. There is some controversy over whether Gram staining need be done if the CSF cell count is normal. In the great majority of such cases bacteriologic findings are normal. However, occasional cases have been reported of bacterial meningitis without an elevated cell count, most commonly in debilitated or immunosuppressed patients. It may also occur very early in the initial stages of the disease. Gram stain yields unquestioned benefits in terms of early diagnosis and assistance in choice of therapy. However, a negative Gram stain result does not rule out acute bacterial meningitis, and some false positive results occur. The majority of false positive results are due to misinterpretation of precipitated stain or debris on the slide. In some cases the presence of bacteria is correctly reported, but the type of organism may be incorrectly identified due to overdecolorization of the organisms or insufficient familiarity with morphologic variations of bacteria.

LATEX AGGLUTINATION TESTS FOR BACTERIAL ANTIGENS

Recently, rapid slide latex agglutination (LA) tests have become available for detection of pneumococcal, meningococcal, *H. influenzae* type B, and streptococcal group B bacterial antigen in CSF or in (concentrated) urine. Until the 1980s, CSF bacterial antigen detection was done by counterimmunoelectrophoresis (CIE). This method had an overall sensitivity of about 60%–70% (range, 32%–94%). The LA kits are considerably faster, easier, and have increased detection rates (about 85%–90%; range, 60%–100%). There is some variation in sensitivity between different manufacturers' kits. This is especially true for antibodies against meningococci. The major reason is that several different strains of meningococci may produce infection, and it is necessary to have an antibody against each one that it is desired to detect. The most common strains are type B (about 47% of cases; range, 28%–50%), type C (about 30%; range, 23%–63%), type Y (about 10%), type W135 (about 10%) and type A (about 3%). Some kits do not include antibodies against all of these strains. Besides not reaching 100% sensitivity, the LA kits are relatively expensive per patient (in part due to the multiple tests included in each kit to detect the different organisms). Besides LA, there is a commercially available kit based on a coagglutination method. This kit has an overall sensitivity about intermediate between CIE and LA, with similar results to LA for *H. influenzae,* and less sensitivity for pneumococci and meningococci.

Cerebrospinal Fluid Lactate

A number of published reports have evaluated CSF lactic acid assay in various diseases. In general, patients with acute bacterial, tuberculous, and fungal meningitis have elevated CSF lactate values, whereas normal persons and those with viral ("aseptic") meningitis do not. Sensitivity of the test for acute bacterial meningitis is about 93%–95% (range, 66%–100%). Most reports indicate clear-cut separation between bacterial and viral infection values (in the sense that the values in viral meningitis are not elevated), but several investigators found that some patients with viral meningitis have elevated CSF lactate levels (about 20% of cases in these reports). However, in all instances of viral meningitis the elevation was less than twice the reference range upper limits. One advantage of CSF lactate is that it may remain elevated 2–3 days after the start of antibiotic therapy. However, values in some cases of treated or partially treated bacterial infection do return to normal relatively early.

Xanthochromia has been reported to nonspecifically increase CSF lactate levels, although one report states that blood itself does not. Central nervous system tissue destruction from various causes (including brain tumor, head trauma, CVAs, and intracerebral hemorrhage, cerebral hypoxia, and seizures), may also produce elevated CSF lactate levels.

Because CSF lactate is not specific for bacterial infection, because it is not elevated in all cases of bacterial meningitis, and because there is some uncertainty as to whether lactate elevation excludes the possibility of viral meningitis, the true usefulness of the test is not clear. The availability of LA slide tests further complicates the picture. However, CSF lactate assay could be useful in patients with symptoms of meningitis if CSF Gram stain results are negative and LA test results (if available) are also negative. Such patients could have tuberculous or fungal meningitis, partially treated bacterial meningitis, or meningitis due to other organisms. Increased CSF lactic acid levels, especially if more than twice the upper reference limit, could suggest that further investigation is essential. A normal lactate level is not reliable in excluding bacterial meningitis.

Reference range for CSF lactate is usually based on specimens from children or adults. One investigator found that neonates 0–2 days old had mean values nearly 60% higher than those obtained after 10 days of life, whereas neonates aged 2–10 days had about 25% higher levels than after age 10 days.

COMPUTERIZED TOMOGRAPHY, MAGNETIC RESONANCE IMAGING, AND RADIONUCLIDE BRAIN SCANNING

Computerized tomography (CT) and magnetic resonance imaging (MRI) are now important aids in screening for abnormality in the CNS (chapter 35). Both can visualize the ventricular system as well as detect mass lesions both within CNS tissue and outside. In addition, the nature of the lesion can frequently be deduced from density characteristics. Both CT and MRI technology have been changing rapidly, and assessment of their capabilities relate to data currently available. Detection of brain tumors is to some extent influenced by location and type of tumor as well as by technical factors such as use of IV contrast media. Reports indicate CT abnormality in approximately 90%–95% of patients with mass lesions or areas of tissue destruction. Statistics from CT and MRI are not always comparable to radionuclide brain scans, since data from the scans vary according to the number of head positions employed, the isotope preparation used, the time between administration of isotope and scanning, and whether a blood flow study was included. In general, CT is about 10%–15% more sensitive than brain scan in cerebral tumor or about 5%–10% more sensitive when brain scanning is performed with optimal technique. It is somewhat more reliable than brain scanning in detecting posterior fossa lesions. Magnetic resonance imaging is about 5% more sensitive than CT. In chronic subdural hematoma, detection with CT is about equal to that achieved when brain scanning is combined with cerebral blood flow study. In acute subdural or epidural hematoma, CT is significantly better than radionuclide brain scanning. An important advantage over radionuclide techniques in either acute or chronic subdural hematoma is that CT can frequently permit a more exact diagnosis, whereas abnormalities found by radionuclide techniques are often not specific. Magnetic resonance imaging is reported to be equal to or slightly better than CT. In cerebral infarct, all three techniques are affected by the time interval after onset. During the first week, CT is somewhat more sensitive than MRI or radionuclide scanning without blood flow study but still detects only 50%–60% of infarcts. The sensitivity of all techniques increases to the 80% range by 3–4 weeks. Intracerebral hematoma is much better seen on CT than brain scan regardless of the time interval and better than MRI in the early stages. None of the three techniques are perfect. In most of the various focal lesion categories, a certain percentage are detected by one technique but not the other, although CT and MRI are generally superior to radionuclide scans. When Hakim's syndrome (normal pressure hydrocephalus) is a possibility, CT or MRI can rule out the disorder by displaying normal ventricular size. If ventricular dilation is seen, cerebral atrophy may be inferred in some cases, but in many the differentiation between atrophy and normal pressure hydrocephalus cannot be made with adequate certainty.

Overall advantages of CT over standard radionuclide procedures are ability to visualize the ventricular system, a relatively small but definite increase in detection rate for brain tumors, more specificity in the appearance of many lesions, and better delineation of CNS anatomy. Advantages over MRI are lower cost, better results in early CVA or early hemorrhage, and ability to detect calcifications and show details of bone (which is seen poorly on MRI). Advantages of radionuclide procedures are elimination of the need for x-ray contrast media (which many CT patients must receive), lower cost for equipment and lower charge to the patient, and ability to inspect major blood vessels via blood flow studies. Advantages of MRI are absence of any radiation, slightly and sometimes significantly better detection rate of many lesions compared to CT, better tissue detail, much better visualization of the spinal cord, and in some cases ability to suggest a more exact diagnosis. The major disadvantages are considerably higher cost, slower imaging time, and in some cases, problems with patients who have cardiac pacemakers or internal metal objects.

CEREBROSPINAL FLUID FINDINGS IN SELECTED BRAIN DISEASES

Mycobacterial Meningitis

Mycobacterial meningitis is commoner in children between the ages of 6 months and 5 years and in the elderly. Chest x-ray film is reported to show hilar adenopathy in 50%–90% of children, but normal chest findings are more common in adults (in one series, about 50% of adults had normal chest x-ray findings). Purified protein derivative skin test result is negative in 5%–50% of patients. Mild to moderate anemia is frequent. The erythrocyte sedimentation rate is elevated in 80% of patients. Cerebrospinal fluid findings typically show moderate WBC elevation (usually < 500/cu mm and almost always < 1,000), with the majority being lymphocytes. However, there frequently are a significant number of neutrophils and sometimes, in the early stages, a majority of neutrophils. Protein level is usually mildly or moderately elevated (in one series, 76% had elevated protein levels on admission). Glucose level is decreased in 50%–85% of patients on admission. Normal cell count, protein level, and glucose level on admission is extremely rare, although this happened in 3 of 21 patients in one report. Diagnosis is based on acid-fast smear, culture, exclusion of other etiologies, evidence of tuberculosis elsewhere, and clinical suspicion. Acid-fast smears on CSF are positive in about 20%–40% of cases (range, 10%–91%), and CSF culture is positive in only 45%–90% of cases.

Cryptococcal Meningitis

Cryptococcus neoformans is the most common fungus producing CNS infection and is an important, although not numerically frequent, etiology of meningitis. The organism is discussed in detail in chapter 15. About 70% of cryptococcal meningitis cases are male, and the majority are of middle age. About one-half are associated with malignancy or other severe diseases or with immunodeficiency (either from underlying disease or from therapy). Meningitis due to *Cryptococcus* is said to produce an elevated cell count in about 95% of cases (range, 90%–97%). The count is usually less than 300/cu mm and in the majority of cases is less than 150/cu mm. In one series, the CSF cell count was less than 100/cu mm in about 60% of patients. More than one half of the cells are lymphocytes. Protein levels are elevated in about 90% of cases. The CSF glucose level is decreased in 50%–75% of cases.

The LA slide test for cryptococcal antigen in CSF is the best rapid diagnostic test. It is reported to detect about 85%–90% of cases (literature range, 71%–100%). There is a slightly increased detection rate if both CSF and serum are tested. Serum testing alone detects about 50% of cases (range, 18%–71%). The LA test is discussed in detail in chapter 15. The older procedure for detection of *Cryptococcus* in CSF was a wet mount using india ink or nigrosin. *Cryptococcus neoformans* has a thick gelatinous capsule that gives the appearance of a clear zone or halo around the organism against the dark background of india ink particles. However, only about 50% (range, 40%–79%) of cases can be detected by india ink preparations, and some of these may require repeated examinations. In addition, experience is needed to avoid false positive and negative results. India ink has been replaced by the LA test.

Although LA tests for cryptococcal antigen are reasonably sensitive, culture of CSF is still considered essential. In some cases, culture may reveal organisms when the CSF cell count, protein levels, and glucose levels are all normal. Culture detects about 80% of patients on initial lumbar puncture (range, 72%–90%). Fungi require different culture media for optimum growth than the standard bacterial media, so the laboratory should be notified if fungi are suspected. In some patients, cryptococcal antigen latex studies on CSF have been positive when cultures were negative, and in a few cases, cultures were positive when the LA test result was negative.

Central Nervous System Infection by Other Fungi

Candida is said to be the most common fungal infection of the CNS. About one half of the patients with *Candida* CNS infection have a lymphocytic pleocytosis, and about one half show a predominance of neutrophils. Some reports have indicated a surprisingly high rate of CNS involvement in the systemic mycoses (blastomycosis, 3%–10%; histoplasmosis, up to 50%; coccidioidomycosis, up to 50%). These fungi most often produce a lymphocytic pleocytosis, but neutrophils may predominate. Cerebrospinal fluid glucose levels are typically reduced but may be normal.

Viral and Aseptic Meningitis

Viral meningitis is one component of a syndrome known as aseptic meningitis. The aseptic meningitis syndrome is now usually defined as meningitis with normal CSF glucose levels, normal or elevated protein levels, and elevated cell count with a majority of the cells being lymphocytes. A less common definition is nonbacterial meningitis; a definition no longer used is meningitis with a negative bacterial culture. The CSF findings of aseptic meningitis may be caused by a wide variety of agents, including different viruses, mycobacteria, *Listeria*, syphilis, *Leptospira*, *Toxoplasma*, fungi, meningeal carcinomatosis, and meningeal reaction to nearby inflammatory or destructive processes. However, viral meningitis is the most common and typical of the conditions that produce this syndrome. The commonest virus group associated with meningitis is enterovirus, which includes ECHO (enteric cytopathic human orphan) virus and coxsackievirus and comprises 50%–80% of viral meningitis patients; the second most common (10%–20%) is mumps. Other viruses include herpes simplex, arbovirus group, herpes zoster–varicella, and lymphocytic choriomeningitis. Although not usually listed, human immunodeficiency virus I (HIV-I) (or acquired immunodeficiency syndrome [AIDS]) may be, or may become, one of the most frequent etiologies. There are several reasons for describing the aseptic meningitis syndrome and specifically mentioning viral meningitis. First, it is useful to know what etiologies to expect with this pattern of CSF results. Second, this pattern is not specific for viral etiology. Third, a significant number of patients infected by many of these etiologies do not present with textbook aseptic meningitis findings. This is most true for the type of predominating cell in early enterovirus, mumps, and arbovirus infections and for initially decreased glucose levels in enterovirus, mumps, herpes simplex, and lymphocytic choriomeningitis. Reports estimate that 20%–75% of patients with viral meningitis have neutrophil predominance in the first CSF specimen obtained. For example, one investigator found that about 50% of enteroviral meningitis patients had more than 10% neutrophils on the first CSF specimen, and about 25% had neutrophils predominating; about 66% had normal protein levels; and about 10% had decreased glucose. Most reports indicate that repeat lumbar puncture in 8–12 hours frequently shows change from neutrophil to lymphocyte predominance, with conversion of the remainder taking place in 24–48 hours.

Differential diagnosis of aseptic meningitis syndrome etiologies generally involves differentiating virus etiology from mycobacterial and cryptococcal infection. Cerebrospinal fluid culture can be done for all the usual virus possibilities, but viral specimens usually must be sent to a reference laboratory, and the results are not available for several days or even longer. It has been recommended that CSF specimens either be processed in less than 24 hours or be frozen at −70°C to preserve infectivity. Many viruses lose infectivity when frozen at the usual temperature of −20°C. Serologic tests are also available but require acute and convalescent serum specimens and thus take even longer than culture. Diagnosis of herpes simplex infection is discussed in chapter 16. As noted there, herpes simplex type I has a predilection for involvement of the temporal lobe of the brain. *Cryptococcus* and mycobacterial tests have been discussed earlier in this chapter. Cerebrospinal fluid lactate (lactic acid) has been advocated to separate viral from nonviral etiology but, as discussed earlier, is not always helpful and thus is still somewhat controversial.

Human Immunodeficiency Virus Meningitis

As noted in chapter 16, the HIV-I (AIDS) virus may produce a mild aseptic meningitis lasting 2–3 weeks as the first clinical manifestation of infection. The exact incidence is unknown, but it is probably greater than the 2%–5% estimated in one report. The majority of patients do not manifest this stage but develop more advanced disease at some time in the future. Later in the disease, more than 30%–70% of patients develop symptoms of CNS infection. Some of these cases are due to superimposed infection by other organisms (*Toxoplasma*, *Cryptococcus*) rather than HIV alone. Human immunodeficiency virus infection of the brain is most often manifested by dementia, but more than 15% develop progressive focal leukoencephalopathy. There is relatively little information about CSF findings in this disorder. In one report, 27% had elevated protein levels and 14% had elevated WBC count, with all cell counts being less than 25/cu mm and with 80%–100% of the cells being mononuclear. The brain abnormalities are best shown by CT or MRI.

Brain Abscess

Brain abscess is most commonly due to direct extension of infection from infected middle ear, mastoid sinus, or paranasal sinuses; traumatic injuries, or infected prostheses. There can also be more distant spread from the lungs or from infected emboli. There is increased incidence in immunosuppressed patients. The most frequent organisms cultured are various streptococci, *Bacteroides*, gram-negative organisms, and *Staphylococcus aureus*. Mixed infections are present in 30%–60% of cases. Apparently the CSF findings in brain abscess are not significantly influenced by the causative organism or the location of the lesion. About 10% of patients are said to have normal CSF test results. The remainder usually have a picture compatible with aseptic meningitis. The spinal fluid is most often clear, and about 70% of patients are said to have increased pressure. Protein levels are normal in nearly 25% of patients, in about 55% the values are between 45 and 100 mg/100 ml (0.45–1.0 g/L), and in the remaining 20% the values are more than 100 mg/100 ml. The CSF glucose level is normal. Cell counts are variable; about 30% are between 5 and 25, about 25% are between 25 and 100, and about 25% are between 100 and 500/cu mm. Lymphocytes generally predominate, but a significant percentage (5%–25%) of polymorphonuclear neutrophils are said to be nearly always present. In occasional cases, an abscess breaks through to the subarachnoid space and results in purulent meningitis. Computerized tomography or MRI is very helpful in demonstrating intracerebral abscesses. Radionuclide brain scans are useful if CT is not available.

Brain Tumor

In primary cortical brain tumor, the CSF usually is clear and colorless, although xanthochromia may be present. Spinal fluid pressure is elevated in 70% of patients. Seventy percent show increased protein levels, with about one half of these more than 100 mg/100 ml (1.0 g/L). Cerebrospinal fluid glucose levels are normal. The majority (70%) of brain tumor patients have normal cell counts. Of the remainder, about two-thirds have counts less than 25/cu mm consisting mostly of lymphocytes. In the few patients with high cell counts, there may be appreciable numbers of neutrophils, and the spinal fluid pattern then resembles that of brain abscess. Other methods of diagnosis are discussed in chapter 32. Most metastatic tumors have CSF findings similar to primary neoplasms.

In occasional instances, metastatic carcinoma may spread widely over the meninges. In such cases, the findings are similar to those of tuberculous meningitis (elevated cell count, lymphocytes predominating; elevated protein concentration, and decreased glucose level). Cell blocks and cytologic smears of spinal fluid sediment are helpful for diagnosis. Cytology of CSF yields malignant cells in 55%–83%. Malignant lymphoma may involve the meninges in 5%–30% of cases. Cytology is said to be positive in 60%–80% of cases. Acute lymphocytic leukemia in childhood is reported to involve the meninges at some time in up to 50% of cases. Cerebrospinal fluid cytology is not helpful in the majority of metastatic carcinomas to the brain, which most often do not involve the meninges. However, some investigators detected as many as 20%–40% of cases. In primary tumors of the brain, the meninges are uncommonly involved, so that CSF cytology detects fewer than 10% of cases.

Computerized tomography or MRI is the most helpful procedure for demonstrating either primary or metastatic brain tumors. As noted previously, detection rate is reported to be approximately 90%–95% for primary intracerebral tumors. Radionuclide brain scans are useful if CT is not available; sensitivity is 5%–10% less than that of CT, and nonuniformity of technical details make results more variable from different institutions.

Subdural Hematoma

The classic subdural hematoma develops after trauma, but in one series 20% did not have a history of trauma. In that same series, 60% of patients were alcoholics, 30% of patients had no lateralizing signs, and one third of the patients had multiple hematomas (with 21% having bilateral subdural hematomas and 14% having additional hematomas elsewhere within the brain or brain coverings).

Cerebrospinal fluid findings vary depending on whether the hematoma is recent or several days old. In recent subdurals (within 7 days of injury), the CSF is usually blood tinged or xanthochromic, due to concurrent cerebral contusion from the injury or leakage of RBC breakdown products. In late cases the CSF is most often clear. Protein levels are elevated in most of the acute cases, usually in the range of 50–150 mg/100 ml (0.5–1.5 g/L), and in about 50% of the chronic cases. After several weeks the CSF protein level is usually normal. Cell counts may be slightly elevated in acute or subacute cases (usually < 25 WBCs/cu mm) and are usually normal in patients seen later.

The classic CSF triad of elevated protein level, relatively normal cell count, and xanthochromia is present in only about 50% of the subacute and chronic cases, with the percentage decreasing as the time from injury increases. Computerized tomography or MRI is the best means of demonstrating the lesion. Computerized tomography is probably better in the first week.

Cerebral Thrombosis

In one series of fatal cerebral thrombosis, 90% had clear CSF and most of the remaining 10% had xanthochromia. White blood cell counts were usually normal; about 15% had a small increase in cell count (usually < 50/cu mm). Cerebrospinal fluid protein level was normal in 50% of cases and usually less than 100 mg/100 ml in the remainder. Computerized tomography or MRI is the best method of demonstrating the lesion. Computerized tomography is better in the first week.

Subarachnoid Hemorrhage

In hemorrhage involving the subarachnoid space, the findings depend on the time interval following hemorrhage when the patient is examined. It takes about 4 hours (literature range, 2–48 hours) to develop xanthochromia. Therefore, CSF obtained very early may have a colorless supernatant. Initially, the WBC count and protein level are proportional to the amount of CSF blood (about 1 WBC/700 RBCs and 1 mg protein/1,000 RBCs). Later, the WBC count may rise, sometimes to levels greater than 1,000/cu mm, with predominance of segmented neutrophils. This may raise the question of intracranial infection. This rise is usually attributed to meningeal irritation by the blood. Protein also is initially correlated to RBC count but later may rise out of proportion to the number of RBCs as the WBCs increase and the RBCs lyse and disappear. Usually by 3 weeks after onset, xanthochromia has disappeared and both protein and cell count have returned to normal.

Intracerebral Hemorrhage

Cerebrospinal fluid findings depend on how close the hematoma is to the subarachnoid space. If penetration to the brain surface occurs, the CSF resembles that of subarachnoid hemorrhage; if situated relatively far from the brain surface, the CSF will be relatively normal. About 20% (literature range, 15%–25%) of cases are said to have clear CSF; the remainder are xanthochromic or contain blood. Cell count and protein values reflect the presence of spinal fluid blood and the closeness of the hematoma to the meninges. With bloody fluid, protein and cell count initially reflect the RBC count; after 12 or more hours, protein level and cell count may rise disproportionately to the number of RBCs, sometimes to moderately high levels (similar to effects of subarachnoid hemorrhage). Computerized tomography and MRI are the best methods for diagnosis, with CT better than MRI in the first week.

Multiple Sclerosis

Multiple sclerosis is a chronic demyelinating disease that has a reputation for recurrent illness of unpredictable length and severity. A multifocal demyelinating process in cerebral hemisphere white matter results in various combinations of weakness, ataxia, vision difficulties, and parasthesias, frequently ending in paralysis. Thus, the clinical symptoms, especially early in the disease, can be mimicked by a considerable number of other conditions.

Cerebrospinal Fluid Laboratory Findings.—Routine CSF test findings are nonspecific, and when abnormality is present, the standard CNS test results are similar to those of aseptic meningitis. The CSF total protein is increased in about 25% of cases (literature range, 13%–63%). The cell count is increased in about 30% of cases (literature range, 25%–45%), with the increase usually being mononuclear in type and relatively small in degree.

The CSF gamma-globulin (IgG) level is increased in 60%–80% of cases (literature range, 20%–88%). Technical methods such as radial immunodiffusion produce more accurate results than electrophoresis. Problems have been recognized in interpretation of CSF gamma-globulin values because elevated serum gamma-globulin levels can diffuse into the CSF and affect values there. Many investigators analyze a specimen of serum as well as of CSF to see if the serum gamma-globulin level is increased.

Several ratios have been devised to correct for or point toward peripheral blood protein contamination. The most widely used is the CSF IgG/albumin ratio. Albumin is synthesized in the liver but not in the CNS and therefore can be used to some degree as a marker for serum protein diffusion into the CSF or introduction into the CSF through a traumatic lumbar puncture or intracerebral hemorrhage. The IgG/albumin ratio is based on the theory that if serum leaks or is deposited into spinal fluid, albumin and IgG will be present in roughly the same proportion that they have in serum; whereas a disproportionate elevation of IgG relative to albumin suggests actual production of the IgG within the CNS. The normal CSF IgG/albumin ratio is less than 25% (literature range, 22%–28%). About 70% of MS patients have elevated IgG/albumin ratios (literature range, 59%–90%). The IgG/albumin ratio is a little more specific for MS than increase of IgG by itself. However, many conditions produce increased IgG within the CNS, such as chronic CNS infections, brain tissue destruction, CNS vasculitis, systemic lupus erythematosus and primary Sjögren's syndrome involving the CNS, and various demyelinating diseases.

Another way to estimate CNS production of IgG is the IgG index, which is (CSF IgG level/CSF albumin level) ÷ (serum IgG level/serum albumin level). This index is reported to be abnormal in about 85% (range, 60%–94%) of definite MS patients. A third method for estimating CNS IgG production is the IgG synthesis rate formula of Tourtellote. Sensitivity of this method is about 85% (range, 70%–96%). Consensus seems to be that the IgG index is slightly more sensitive and reproducible than the IgG synthesis rate. Both can be influenced by altered blood-brain barrier permeability or presence of blood in the CSF as well as the various conditions other than MS that induce CNS production of IgG antibody.

Another useful test is based on the observation that patients with MS demonstrate several narrow bands ("oligoclonal bands") in the gamma area when their spinal fluid is subjected to certain types of electrophoresis (polyacrylamide gel, high-resolution agarose, or immunofixation; ordinary cellulose acetate electrophoresis will not demonstrate the oligoclonal bands). Oligoclonal banding is present in 85%–90% of MS patients (literature range, 65%–100%. Some of this variation is due to different methods used). Similar narrow bands may be found in subacute sclerosing panencephalitis, destructive CNS lesions, CNS vasculitis, lupus or primary Sjögren's syndrome involving the CNS, diabetes mellitus, and the Guillain-Barré syndrome. A similar but not identical phenomenon has been reported in some patients with aseptic meningitis.

Antibodies have been produced against myelin components, and a radioassay for myelin basic protein (MBP) is available in some reference laboratories. Myelin basic protein level is reported to be increased in 70%–80% of patients with active MS (literature range, 62%–93%), depending to some extent on the status of active demyelination. Incidence is less if the disease is not active or if steroid therapy is being given. The various demyelinating conditions other than MS also produce abnormal MBP assay results. The MBP level may also be increased in destructive CNS lesions such as a CVA, in some patients with the Guillain-Barré syndrome, and in some patients with CNS lupus erythematosus.

Summary.—Of the various laboratory tests for MS, the two most widely used are the spinal fluid IgG index and presence of oligoclonal bands. Of these, the best single test is probably oligoclonal banding. Computerized tomography and MRI can often demonstrate focal demyelinized areas in the CNS, with CT reported to show abnormality in 40%–60% of patients with definite MS and MRI positive findings in about 90% (range, 80%–100%). Neither CT nor MRI is currently able to differentiate MS with certainty from other CNS demyelinizing diseases.

Lead Encephalopathy

Lead poisoning is discussed elsewhere (chapter 34). Lead encephalopathy occurs mainly in children (adults are more likely to develop peripheral neuropathy), and it is more common in acute than in chronic poisoning. Clinical signs and symptoms include visual disturbances, delirium, convulsions, severe headaches, hypertension, and sometimes papilledema. Cerebrospinal fluid usually displays increased pressure. The cell count varies from normal to several thousand; the majority of patients have mild to moderate pleocytosis. Mononuclears usually predominate, but polymorphonuclears may occasionally be high, especially in patients with the more elevated cell counts. The CSF protein level may be normal or increased; the glucose level is normal. These findings may suggest a variety of conditions, such as meningitis or meningoencephalitis due to virus or fungus, or early bacterial meningitis.

Cerebrospinal Fluid Artifacts

During or after a lumbar puncture the question frequently arises whether blood has been introduced into the spinal fluid by the spinal needle, resulting in a traumatic tap. There are several useful differential points. Xanthochromia, if present, suggests previous bleeding. However, a nonxanthochromic supernatant fluid does not rule out the diagnosis, since xanthochromia may be absent even when subarachnoid bleeding has occurred many hours before. A second differential point utilizes the fact that the standard method for collecting CSF involves catching the specimen in three consecutively numbered tubes. If blood was introduced by a traumatic tap, more blood should appear in the first tube, less in the second, and even less in the third, as the bleeding decreases. Previous CSF bleeding should distribute the RBCs equally throughout the spinal fluid and characteristically shows approximately equal numbers of RBCs in each of the three tubes. Therefore, RBC counts can, if necessary, be requested for all three tubes. However, sometimes traumatic taps, if severe, can yield roughly equal numbers of RBCs in each tube. As noted previously, blood in the CSF may falsely alter the various chemical tests.

Additional tests relevant to this chapter are described in chapter 35.

BIBLIOGRAPHY

Hische EAH, et al: Cerebrospinal fluid IgG and IgM indexes as indicators of active neurosyphilis. *Clin Chem* 1988; 34:665.

Davenport RD, Karen DF: Oligoclonal bands in cerebrospinal fluids: Significance of corresponding bands in serum for diagnosis of multiple sclerosis. *Clin Chem* 1988; 34:764.

Grant I, et al: Evidence for early central nervous system involvement in the acquired immunodeficiency syndrome (AIDS) and other human immunodeficiency virus (HIV) infections. *Ann Intern Med* 1987; 107:828.

Berger JR, et al: Progressive multifocal leukoencephalopathy associated with human immunodeficiency virus infection. *Ann Intern Med* 1987; 107:78.

Mayefsky JH, Roghmann KJ: Determination of leukocytosis in traumatic spinal tap specimens. *Am J Med* 1987; 82:1175.

Wildin S, Chonmaitree T: The importance of the virology laboratory in the diagnosis and management of viral meningitis. *Am J Dis Child* 1987; 141:454.

Stewart JM, et al: Magnetic resonance imaging and clinical relationships in multiple sclerosis. *Mayo Clin Proc* 1987; 62:174.

Maravilla KR: MRI gives direct insight into the vagaries of MS. *Diagn Imaging* 1986; 8(8):82.

Marton KI, Gean AD: The diagnostic spinal tap. *Ann Intern Med* 1986; 104:880.

Gerbaut L, Macart M: Is standardization more important than methodology for assay of total protein in cerebrospinal fluid? *Clin Chem* 1986; 32:353.

Wasilauskas BL, Hampton KD: Adult meningitis caused by *Hemophilus influenzae* serotype f, biotype I. *Arch Pathol Lab Med* 1986; 110:437.

Nelson N, et al: The diagnostic and predictive value of cerebrospinal fluid lactate in children with meningitis. *Acta Paediatr Scand* 1986; 75:52.

Dans PE, et al: Inappropriate use of the cerebrospinal fluid Venereal Disease Research Laboratory (VDRL) test to exclude neurosyphilis. *Ann Intern Med* 1986; 104:86.

Powers WJ: Cerebrospinal fluid lymphocytosis in acute bacterial meningitis. *Am J Med* 1985; 79:216.

Rubin RH, Hooper DC: Central nervous system infection in the compromised host. *Med Clin North Am* 1985; 69:281.

Schlech WF, et al: Bacterial meningitis in the United States, 1978 through 1981. *JAMA* 1985; 253:1749.

LeFrock JL: Gram-negative bacillary meningitis. *Med Clin North Am* 1985; 69:243.

Sabetta JR, Andriole VT: Cryptococcal infection of the central nervous system. *Med Clin North Am* 1985; 69:333.

Tourtellotte WW, et al: The basis of intra-blood-brain-barrier IgG synthesis. *Ann Neurol* 1985; 17:21.

Ho DD, Hirsch MS: Acute viral encephalitis. *Med Clin North Am* 1985; 69:415.

Molavi A, LeFrock JL: Tuberculous meningitis. *Med Clin North Am* 1985; 69:315.

Kaplan K: Brain abscess. *Med Clin North Am* 1985; 69:345.
Ratzan KR: Viral meningitis. *Med Clin North Am* 1985; 69:399.
Peacock JE, et al: Persistent neutrophilic meningitis. (Baltimore) *Medicine* 1984; 63:379.
Tilton RC, et al: Comparative evaluation of three commercial products and counterimmunoelectrophoresis for the detection of antigens in cerebrospinal fluid. *J Clin Microbiol* 1984; 20:231.
Oslon DA, Hoeprich PD: Analysis of bacterial isolates from cerebrospinal fluid. *J Clin Microbiol* 1984; 19:144.
Crowson TW, et al: Overutilization of cultures of CSF for mycobacteria. *JAMA* 1984; 251:70.
Gorse GJ. et al: Bacterial meningitis in the elderly. *Arch Intern Med* 1984; 144:1603.
Smith KBF, Matz R: Cerebrospinal fluid pleocytosis following hemorrhagic cerebral infarction. *Am J Med Sci* 1983; 286:37.
Jordan GW, et al: Questionable reliability of CSF lactate in diagnosis of meningitis. *Arch Intern Med* 1983; 143:85.
Black PM: Normal-pressure hydrocephalus. *Postgrad Med* 1982; 71:57.
Bell WE, McGuire GA: Suppurative central nervous system infections in the neonate. *Semin Perinatol* 1982; 6:1.
Hart RG, Sherman DG: The diagnosis of multiple sclerosis. *JAMA* 1982; 247:498.
Fishbein DB: Bacterial meningitis in the absence of CSF pleocytosis. *Arch Intern Med* 1981; 141:1369.
Galaid EI, et al: Meningococcal disease in New York City, 1973 to 1978. *JAMA* 1980; 244:2167.
Ward PCJ: Cerebrospinal fluid data: 2. Interpretation in intracranial malignancy and multiple sclerosis. *Postgrad Med* 1980; 68:190.
Fishman RA: *Cerebrospinal Fluid in Disease of the Nervous System*. Philadelphia, W.B. Saunders Co., 1980.
Geiseler PJ, et al: Community-acquired purulent meningitis. *Rev Infect Dis* 1980; 2:725.
Connolly KD: Lumbar puncture, meningitis, and persisting pleocytosis. *Arch Dis Child* 1979; 54:792.

19 Liver and Biliary Tract Tests

LABORATORY TESTS

Serum Bilirubin

Bilirubin is formed from breakdown of hemoglobin molecules by the reticuloendothelial system. Newly formed (unconjugated) bilirubin circulates in blood bound nonpermanently to serum albumin and is carried to the liver, where it is extracted by hepatic parenchymal cells, conjugated first with one and then with a second glucuronide molecule to form bilirubin diglucuronide, and then excreted in the bile. The bile passes through the common bile duct into the duodenal segment of the small intestine. It has been well documented that when a certain diazo compound discovered by van den Bergh is added to conjugated bilirubin, there will be color development maximal within 1 minute. This fast-reacting bilirubin fraction consists of bilirubin monoglucoronide, bilirubin diglucoronide, and a third fraction consisting of conjugated bilirubin bound permanently and covalently to albumin, called "delta bilirubin." If alcohol is then added, additional color development takes place for up to 30 minutes. This second component, which precipitates with alcohol, corresponds to unconjugated bilirubin. Actually color continues to develop slowly up to 15 minutes after the simple van den Bergh reaction maximal at 1 minute, and this extra fraction used to be known as the "delayed," or "biphasic reaction." It has since been shown that a considerable proportion of the substance involved is really unconjugated bilirubin. Since unconjugated bilirubin is measured more completely by the 30-minute alcohol precipitation technique, most laboratories do not report the biphasic reaction. The 1-minute van den Bergh color reaction is also called the "direct reaction" and the conjugated bilirubin it measures is known as "direct-acting bilirubin," whereas the 30-minute alcohol measurement of unconjugated bilirubin is called the "indirect reaction" and its substrate is "indirect bilirubin." Reference values are less than 1.5 mg/100 ml (25 μmol/L) for total bilirubin and less than 0.5 mg/100 ml (8.5 μmol/L) for 1-minute bilirubin.

Visible bile staining of tissue is called "jaundice." Three major causes predominate: hemolysis, extrahepatic biliary tract obstruction, and intrahepatic biliary tract obstruction.

Hemolysis causes increased breakdown of red blood cells (RBCs) and thus increased formation of unconjugated bilirubin. If hemolysis is severe enough, more unconjugated bilirubin may be present in the plasma than the liver can extract. Therefore, the level of total bilirubin will rise, with most of the rise due to the unconjugated fraction. The conjugated fraction remains normal or is only slightly elevated and rarely becomes greater than 1.2 mg/100 ml (20 μmol/L) (unless a nonhemolytic problem is superimposed). Hemolysis may result from congenital hemolytic anemia (e.g., sickle cell anemia or other hemoglobinopathies), from drug-induced causes, from autoimmune disease, and from transfusion reactions. An increased unconjugated bilirubin level may sometimes result from absorption of hemoglobin from extravascular hematomas or from pulmonary infarction. The unconjugated bilirubin level may also be increased in various other conditions. The reason is often obscure. In one study of patients with unconjugated bilirubin, the most common associated diseases (collectively 60% of the total cases) included cholecystitis, cardiac disease (only 50% having overt congestive failure), acute or chronic infection, gastrointestinal (GI) tract disease (mostly ulcerative or inflammatory), and cancer.

Extrahepatic biliary tract obstruction is caused by common bile duct obstruction, usually due to a stone or to carcinoma from the head of the pancreas. The height of the total serum bilirubin level depends on whether the obstruction is complete or only partial and how long the obstruction has existed. Also, in the majority of cases the bilirubin level stabilizes at less than 20 mg/100 ml even when there is complete common bile duct obstruction. Extrahepatic biliary tract obstruction initially produces an increase in conjugated bilirubin without affecting the unconjugated bilirubin, since obstruction of the common bile duct prevents excretion of already conjugated bilirubin into the duodenum. However, after several days, some of the conjugated bilirubin in the blood breaks down to unconjugated bilirubin. Eventually the ratio of conjugated to unconjugated bilirubin approaches 1:1. The amount of time necessary for this change in the composition of the serum bilirubin is quite variable, but there is some correlation with the amount of time that has elapsed since onset of obstruction. In addition, prolonged intrahepatic bile stasis ("cholestasis") due to extrahepatic obstruction of the bile drainage system often produces some degree of secondary liver cell damage, which also helps to change the ratio of conjugated to unconjugated bilirubin.

Intrahepatic biliary tract obstruction is usually caused by liver cell injury. The injured cells may obstruct small biliary channels between liver cell groups. Some bilirubin may be released from damaged cells. Liver cell injury may be produced by a wide variety of etiologies, such as alcohol- or drug-induced liver injury, acute or chronic hepatitis virus hepatitis, certain other viruses such as Epstein-Barr (infectious mononucleosis) or cytomegalovirus, active cirrhosis, liver passive congestion, primary or metastatic liver tumor, severe bacterial infection, and biliary cirrhosis. When serum bilirubin is increased due to liver cell damage, both conjugated and unconjugated bilirubin fractions may increase in varying proportions. The unconjugated fraction may be increased because of inability of the damaged cells to conjugate normal amounts of unconjugated serum bilirubin. The conjugated fraction increase usually results from intrahepatic cholestasis secondary to bile sinusoid blockage by damaged hepatic cells.

Effect of Renal Function on Serum Unconjugated Bilirubin.—Conjugated bilirubin in serum is excreted in urine until the renal threshold of 29 mg/100 ml (495 μmol/L) is exceeded. Nonconjugated bilirubin is not excreted by the kidneys. Renal function, as estimated by the serum creatinine level, has some effect on the serum conjugated bilirubin level. Although there is not exact correlation, a general trend has been reported toward rising serum conjugated bilirubin as the serum creatinine rises (if the serum creatinine changes are due to renal disease). Since conjugated bilirubin is excreted into the intestine through the biliary duct system, the influence of renal function would be seen only if abnormal quantities of conjugated bilirubin were present in patient serum.

Other Etiologies of Jaundice.—Carcinoma may be manifested either by predominantly conjugated hyperbilirubinemia (if the common bile duct is obstructed) or by a variable mixture of conjugated and unconjugated bilirubinemia (if the tumor is intrahepatic). Intrahepatic tumor can obstruct intrahepatic bile ducts or destroy liver cells by compression from expanding tumor masses or by invasion and replacement of liver tissue. Total bilirubin is increased in about 45% of patients with liver metastases, with the incidence of hyperbilirubinemia reported to be about 70% for metastatic biliary tract and pancreatic carcinoma, about 50% for breast and lung carcinoma, about 35% for colon and gastric carcinoma, and about 10% for other tumors. In pancreatic, colon, and gastric metastatic tumor, total bilirubin may exceed 10 mg/100 ml in 10% or more patients. Drugs may produce bilirubin elevation of variable type and degree (see Table 36–2, XIV). Some drugs exert predominantly cholestatic (obstructive) effects, others induce hepatocellular injury, and still others have components of both cholestasis and hepatic cell injury. There are a large number of conditions that may produce elevated serum bilirubin levels with or without visible jaundice. Septicemia is one etiology that is often not mentioned but that should not be forgotten. One report noted that in patients less than age 30 years, viral infections of the liver accounted for 80% of cases with jaundice. In age group 30–60 years, viral infections accounted for 30%; alcoholic liver disease accounted for 30%, and gallstones or cancer accounted for about 10% each. Over age 60, cancer accounted for 45% of cases; gallstones accounted for 25%, and alcoholic liver disease and medications accounted for about 10% each.

Urine Bilirubin and Urobilinogen

These tests follow much the same pattern as conjugated and unconjugated bilirubin. After bile reaches the duodenum, intestinal bacteria convert most of the bilirubin to urobilinogen. Much urobilinogen is lost in the feces, but part is absorbed into the bloodstream. Once in the blood, most of the urobilinogen goes through the liver and is extracted by hepatic cells. Then it is excreted in the bile and once again reaches the duodenum. Not all the blood-borne urobilinogen reaches the liver; some is removed by the kidneys and excreted in urine. Normally, there is less than 1 Ehrlich unit, or no positive result at greater than a 1:20 urine dilution.

Conjugated bilirubin, like urobilinogen, is partially excreted by the kidney if the serum level is elevated. Unconjugated bilirubin cannot pass the glomerular filter, so it does not appear in urine. However, when the serum unconjugated bilirubin level is high, more conjugated bilirubin is produced and excreted into the bile ducts; consequently, more urobilinogen is produced in the intestine. Additional urobilinogen is reabsorbed into the bloodstream and a portion of this appears in the urine, so that increased urine urobilinogen is found when increased unconjugated bilirubin is present. When increased serum unconjugated bilirubin is due only to increased RBC destruction, the serum conjugated bilirubin level is close to normal, because the liver excretes most of the conjugated bilirubin it produces into the bile ducts. Since the serum conjugated bilirubin level is normal in jaundice due to hemolytic anemia, the urine does not contain increased conjugated bilirubin.

When complete biliary obstruction occurs, no bile can reach the duodenum and no urobilinogen can be formed. The stool normally gets its color from bilirubin breakdown pigments, so that in complete obstruction the stools lose their color and become gray-white (so-called clay color). The conjugated bilirubin in the obstructed bile duct backs up into the liver, and some of it escapes (regurgitates) into the bloodstream. Serum conjugated bilirubin levels increase, and when these levels are sufficiently high, tests for urine conjugated bilirubin give positive results. In cases of severe hepatocellular damage, urobilinogen is formed by the intestine and absorbed into the bloodstream as usual. The damaged liver cells cannot extract it adequately, however, and thus increased amounts are excreted in urine. In addition, there may be conjugated bilirubin in the urine secondary to leakage into the blood from damaged liver cells. Incidentally, urine bilirubin is often called bile, which is technically incorrect, since conjugated bilirubin is only one component of bile. However, custom and convenience make the term widely used.

In summary, there is an increased urine conjugated bilirubin level when the serum conjugated bilirubin level is elevated but usually not until the serum conjugated bilirubin exceeds the reference range upper limit for total serum bilirubin. It is rarely necessary to order urine bilirubin determinations, since the serum bilirubin level provides more information. Increased urine urobilinogen may occur due to increased breakdown of blood RBCs or due to severe liver cell damage. Urine urobilinogen determination rarely adds useful information to other tests in conditions that produce increased urobilinogen excretion. In addition, there is the problem of inaccuracy due to urine concentration or dilution.

Alkaline Phosphatase

Alkaline phosphatase (ALP) is a group of closely related enzymes with maximal activity when the pH is about 10. Alkaline phosphatase is found in many tissues, with highest concentrations in liver and biliary tract epithelium, bone, intestinal mucosa, and placenta. Liver and bone are the two tissues most commonly responsible for ALP elevation. Alkaline phosphatase is composed of several isoenzymes, and each of the major sources of ALP contains a different isoenzyme. Reference range values are about 1.5–2.0 times higher in children than in adults due to active bone growth. Even higher levels occur during the adolescent "growth spurt," which occurs in girls aged 8–12 years and boys aged 10–14 years. Peak reference values for adolescents are reported to be three–five times adult values, although occasional persons are said to have values as high as seven times adult upper reference range. Three times adult reference range is more typical in my experience. Adult values were reported in girls by age 16 and in boys at approximately age 20.

Alkaline Phosphatase of Liver Origin

In liver, ALP is formed by liver cells and biliary tract mucosal cells. It is excreted into bile through a different mechanism from that controlling bilirubin excretion. Although ALP of liver origin can be increased in serum during any type of active liver disease, the serum level is especially sensitive to biliary tract obstruction, whether intrahepatic or extrahepatic, whether mild or severe, or whether localized in a small area of the liver or more extensive. As a general rule, the degree of ALP elevation reflects the severity of obstruction and the amount of biliary tissue involved. Unfortunately, there is considerable variation in behavior of ALP among individual patients.

Common etiologies for ALP elevation are listed in Table 19–1. The three liver conditions most frequently associated with ALP elevation are extrahepatic (common bile duct) biliary tract obstruction, intrahepatic biliary tract obstruction due to acute liver cell injury, and liver space-occupying lesions (tumor, abscess, granulomas). Common bile duct obstruction, metastatic tumor to the liver, and the uncommon condition of primary biliary cirrhosis are the most frequent etiologies for persistent ALP elevation more than three times upper reference limit. However, metastatic tumor may be present with lesser degrees of elevation or with no elevation. On the other hand, acute liver cell injury occasionally may produce ALP elevation more than three times upper reference limit. In one or more reports, ALP elevation five times upper reference limit or more occurred in 5% of patients with hepatitis virus hepatitis, 13%–20% of those with infectious mononucleosis, and 5% of persons with active alcoholic cirrhosis. Drug-induced liver dysfunction is another consideration.

TABLE 19–1.
Most Common Causes for Alkaline Phosphatase Elevation

Liver and biliary tract origin
Extrahepatic bile duct obstruction
Intrahepatic biliary obstruction
Liver cell acute injury
Liver passive congestion
Drug-induced liver cell dysfunction
Space-occupying lesions
Sepsis
Bone origin (osteoblast hyperactivity)
Physiologic (rapid) bone growth
Metastatic tumor with osteoblastic reaction
Fracture healing
Capillary endothelial origin
Granulation tissue formation (active)
Placental origin
Pregnancy
Some parenteral albumin preparations
Other
Thyrotoxicosis

In metastatic carcinoma to the liver, ALP levels are elevated in about 75%–80% of cases (literature range, 42%–100%). Alkaline phosphatase levels are also elevated in hepatoma, liver abscess, liver granulomas, and other active liver space-occupying lesions. The frequency of ALP elevation is not as well documented in these conditions as in metastatic tumor but apparently is similar. In extrahepatic biliary tract (common bile duct) obstruction or in primary biliary cirrhosis, ALP levels are elevated in nearly 100% of patients except in some cases of incomplete or intermittent obstruction. Values are usually greater than three times the upper reference range limit, and in the most typical cases exceed five times the upper limit. Elevation less than three times the upper limit is some evidence against complete extrahepatic obstruction. In patients with jaundice due to intrahepatic obstruction (most often severe active cirrhosis or hepatitis virus hepatitis), ALP levels are usually elevated and can exhibit a wide range of values. Most often the levels are less than three times the upper reference limit, but 5%–10% of patients have a greater degree of elevation. In nonjaundiced patients with active liver cell damage, ALP levels are elevated in about one half of the cases, usually less than three times the upper reference limit. Inactive cirrhosis or uncomplicated mild fatty liver usually does not result in ALP elevation. Fifteen percent to 20% of patients with infectious mononucleosis have ALP values greater then three times normal, even though liver biopsy shows relatively mild liver changes. Alkaline phosphatase levels are elevated in about 10%–20% of patients with liver passive congestion, with values usually less than twice normal. It may be higher in a few patients.

Alkaline Phosphatase of Bone Origin

Sources other than the liver can elevate serum ALP levels either alone or concurrently with liver source ALP elevation. Bone is by far the most frequent extrahepatic source. Osteoblasts in bone produce large amounts of ALP, and greatly increased osteoblastic activity hinders usefulness of ALP determination as a liver function test. Normal bone growth of childhood and adolescence, healing fractures, Paget's disease of bone, hyperparathyroidism, rickets and osteomalacia, and osteoblastic metastatic carcinoma to bone (chapter 32) all consistently produce elevated values. In a patient with jaundice, however, one can surmise that at least a portion of an ALP elevation is due to liver disease. When doubt exists as to the origin of the increased ALP values, several alternatives are available. One possibility is use of another enzyme that provides similar information to ALP in liver disease but is more specific for liver origin. Enzymes that have been widely used for this purpose are leucine aminopeptidase (LAP, chapter 35), 5′-nucleotidase (5-NT, chapter 35) and γ-glutamyltransferase (GGT). Of these, LAP was the first to be introduced, but it is significantly less sensitive than ALP. The methodology of 5-NT is probably a little too difficult for reliable results in the average laboratory; also, according to at least one report, about 10% of patients with bone disease may display slight elevation. The GGT has equal or greater sensitivity as ALP in obstructive liver disease and greater sensitivity in hepatocellular damage. Various reports in the literature state that the GGT level is not elevated in bone disease. However, some data in these reports suggest that γ-glutamyl transferase (GGT) nevertheless may occasionally be mildly elevated in bone disease. Another method for differentiating tissue origin of ALP is isoenzyme separation of specific ALP bone and liver fractions by the use of heat, chemical, enzymatic, or electrophoretic techniques. Of these, electrophoresis is the most difficult but probably the most reliable.

Other Sources of Alkaline Phosphatase Elevation

The level of alkaline phosphatase of placental origin begins to rise at about the end of the first trimester of pregnancy and can reach values up to three times the upper reference limit in the third trimester. Elevated values may persist as long as four weeks postpartum. Certain persons whose blood belongs to group B or O and secrete ABH substance (see Chapter 9) are reported to show an increase of ALP (of intestinal isoenzyme origin) about 2 hours after a fatty meal. Alkaline phosphatase levels may become elevated following therapeutic administration of albumin, since some companies use placental tissue as the source for their albumin. Alkaline phosphatase levels can become elevated 7–14 days after severe tissue damage or infarction due to ALP produced by fibroblasts and endothelial cells proliferating in new granulation tissue. Alkaline phosphatase levels are reported elevated in 42%–89% of patients with hyperthyroidism. Certain medications that may affect the liver (see Table 36–2; XIV) may sometimes be associated with ALP elevation. The most frequent of these is phenytoin (Dilantin). Alkaline phosphatase levels are elevated in about 40%–50% (range, 22%–63%) of patients taking phenytoin, with values in most cases not exceeding twice the upper reference limit. Finally, elevation of ALP has been reported in a few patients with sepsis.

Serum Aspartate Aminotransferase

Serum aspartate aminotransferase (AST; formerly SGOT) is an enzyme found in several organs and tissues, including liver, heart, skeletal muscle, and RBCs. Common etiologies for AST elevation are listed in Table 19–2. Aspartate aminotransferase elevation from nonhepatic sources is discussed elsewhere.

Aspartate aminotransferase elevation originating from the liver is due to some degree of acute liver cell injury. Following onset of acute hepatocellular damage from any etiology, AST is released from damaged cells. The serum level becomes elevated in approximately 8 hours, reaches a peak in 24–36 hours, and returns to normal in 3–6 days if the episode is short lived. In mild injury, serum levels may be only transiently and minimally elevated or may even remain within reference limits. In acute hepatitis virus hepatitis, AST levels frequently become elevated more than 10 times the upper reference range limit (about 75% of patients in one study and 100% in another) and typically rise more than 20 times the upper limit (about 45% of patients in the first study and 90% in the second). In fact, a serum AST more than 20 times normal usually includes acute hepatitis virus infection in the differential diagnosis. However, 1–2 weeks later the values fall toward normal, so that a test sample drawn in the subsiding phase may show moderate or possibly only mild abnormality. In extrahepatic obstruction there usually is no elevation unless secondary parenchymal acute damage is present; when elevations occur, they are usually only mild to moderate (< 10 times the upper reference limit). However, when extrahepatic obstruction occurs acutely, AST values may quickly rise to values more than 10 times normal, then fall swiftly after about 72 hours. In cirrhosis, whether the AST level is abnormal and (if abnormal) the degree of abnormality seems to depend on the degree of active hepatic cell injury taking place. Inactive cirrhosis usually is associated with normal AST levels. In active alcoholic cirrhosis, AST elevation is most often mild to moderate, with 95% of AST values less than 10 times normal. In active chronic hepatitis virus hepatitis, AST values are also usually less than 10 times normal. However, one group reported that about 15% of their patients presented at some time with values more than 10 times normal. However, some of these patients could have superimposed acute infection by non-A, non-B or delta hepatitis virus. In liver passive congestion, AST levels are elevated in 5%–33% of patients. About 80% of these patients have AST elevations less than three times normal. In severe acute congestive failure, liver hypoxia may be severe, and one study estimated that about 50% of these patients have AST elevation. In some of these patients AST levels may be higher than three times normal and occasionally may even exceed 20 times normal (about 1% of patients with substantial degrees of congestive failure). In some cases AST elevation due to acute myocardial infarction adds to AST arising from the liver. In infectious mononucleosis, AST levels are elevated in 88%–95% of patients, but only about 5% of elevations are greater than 10 times normal and about 2% are more than 20 times normal.

TABLE 19–2.

Some Etiologies for Aspartate Aminotransferase Elevation

Heart
Acute myocardial infarct
Pericarditis (active: some cases)
Liver
Hepatitis virus, Epstein-Barr, or cytomegalovirus infection
Active cirrhosis
Liver passive congestion or hypoxia
Alcohol or drug-induced liver dysfunction
Space-occupying lesions (active)
Fatty liver (severe)
Extrahepatic biliary obstruction
Skeletal muscle
Acute skeletal muscle injury
Myositis
Muscular dystrophy (active)
Recent surgery
Kidney
Acute injury or damage
Other
Intestinal infarction
Shock
Cholecystitis
Acute pancreatitis

There is a large group of common diseases with mild or moderate AST elevation (defined arbitrarily as elevated less than 10 times the upper reference limit); these include acute hepatitis in the subsiding or recovery phases, chronic hepatitis, active cirrhosis or alcoholic liver disease, liver passive congestion, drug-induced liver injury, metastatic liver tumor, long-standing extrahepatic bile duct obstruction, infectious mononucleosis, and cytomegalovirus infection (88%–95% of patients, only about 2% more than 10 times normal). As mentioned earlier, in a few patients with active cirrhosis, liver congestion, infectious mononucleosis, and drug-induced liver injury, the AST may attain levels more than 20 times upper reference limit that are suggestive of acute hepatitis virus infection. Aspartate aminotransferase levels are elevated in approximately 50% of patients with liver metastases, with most elevations less than five times the upper reference limit.

In active alcoholic cirrhosis, liver congestion, and metastatic tumor to the liver, the AST level usually is significantly (and frequently considerably) higher than the alanine aminotransferase (ALT; formerly SGPT) level, with an AST/ALT ratio greater than 1.0. Ratios less than 1.0 (ALT equal to or greater than AST) are the typical finding in acute hepatitis virus hepatitis and infectious mononucleosis. However, about one third of patients with acute hepatitis infection and some patients with infectious mononucleosis have a ratio greater than 1.0, and ratios either greater than or less than 1.0 may occur in patients with AST elevation due to extrahepatic obstruction. The ratio tends to be more variable and less helpful when the AST value is greater than 10 times the upper reference limit. Some prefer to use an AST/ALT ratio of 1.5 or 2.0 rather than 1.0 as the cutoff point (i.e., an AST value more than twice the ALT value is more suggestive of alcoholic active cirrhosis than hepatitis virus hepatitis, especially if the AST value is less than 10 times normal). Although most agree that active alcoholic liver disease usually yields AST values significantly higher than ALT, there is disagreement in the literature on the usefulness of the ratio (especially the 1.0 value) for diagnosis of individual patients.

Aspartate aminotransferase is found in other tissues besides liver, and this nonspecificity is a frequent problem. Some conditions in which the AST level is frequently elevated include acute myocardial infarction, skeletal muscle acute injury or inflammatory diseases, severe trauma, extensive burns, renal infarcts, hypothyroidism, and alcoholic patients with delerium tremens.

Serum Alanine Aminotransferase

Alanine aminotransferase (ALT) is an enzyme found predominantly in liver but with a moderate-sized component in kidney and small quantities in heart and skeletal muscle. In general, most ALT elevations are due to liver disease, although large amounts of tissue damage in the other organs mentioned may also affect serum levels. Alanine aminotransferase levels are elevated to approximately the same degree and frequency as AST in hepatitis virus hepatitis, infectious mononucleosis, and drug-induced acute liver cell injury. Alanine aminotransferase levels are elevated less frequently than AST and usually to a lesser degree in acute alcoholic liver disease or active cirrhosis, liver passive congestion, long-standing extrahepatic bile duct obstruction, and metastatic tumor to the liver. Alanine aminotransferase has been used predominantly to help confirm liver origin of an AST increase (although there are some limitations in ALT specificity) and occasionally as an aid in the differential diagnosis of liver disease by means of the AST/ALT ratio.

Lactic Dehydrogenase

Lactic dehydrogenase (LDH) is found in heart, skeletal muscle, and RBCs, with lesser quantities in lung, lymphoid tissue, liver, and kidney. A considerable number of malignant tumors are associated with LDH elevation in varying numbers of patients. The LDH level has not been very helpful as a liver function test. For unknown reasons, it is a relatively insensitive marker of hepatic cell injury, with values usually remaining less than three times the upper reference limit even in acute hepatitis virus hepatitis. However, occasional patients with hepatitis virus hepatitis, infectious mononucleosis, and severe liver damage from other causes may have values greater than three times the upper limits. Metastatic liver tumor sometimes is associated with very high LDH values, presumably due to the widespread tumor.

Tumor may be associated with increased LDH values even without liver involvement. Elevation is most frequently reported with leukemias and lymphomas, although LDH abnormality has been reported in varying numbers of patients with a wide variety of solid tumors. Other conditions that frequently produce LDH elevation include hemolytic or megaloblastic anemia, laboratory artifact hemolysis, acute myocardial infarction, renal infarcts, skeletal muscle damage, pulmonary infarct, infectious mononucleosis and cytomegalovirus infection, lymphoproliferative disorders, and shock or multiorgan hypoxia or congestion. Nonspecificity of LDH elevation is thus another reason for neglect of total serum LDH determination as a liver function test.

Lactic dehydrogenase can be fractionated into five isoenzymes using various methods. The electrophoretically slowest moving fraction (fraction 5) is found predominantly in liver and skeletal muscle. Compared to total LDH, the LDH-5 fraction is considerably more sensitive to acute hepatocellular damage, roughly as sensitive as the AST level, and is more specific. Degree of elevation is generally less than that of AST.

γ-Glutamyl Transferase

γ-Glutamyl transferase (GGT; formerly γ-glutamyltranspeptidase) is located mainly in liver cells, to a lesser extent in kidney, and in much smaller quantities in biliary tract epithelium, intestine, heart, brain, pancreas, and spleen. Some GGT activity seems to reside in capillary endothelial cells. The serum GGT level is increased in the newborn but declines to adult levels by age 3 months. By far the most common cause of serum GGT elevation is active liver disease. GGT is affected by both acute liver cell damage and biliary tract obstruction. In biliary tract obstruction and space-occupying lesions of the liver, GGT was found by some investigators to have the same sensitivity as ALP (with a few cases of metastatic tumor to liver abnormal by GGT but not by ALP and vice versa) and is reported to be more sensitive than ALP by other investigators. Overall sensitivity for metastatic liver tumor is said to be about 88% (literature range, 45%–100%) compared to about 80% for ALP. In acute liver cell injury, GGT levels are elevated with approximately the same frequency as the AST. Therefore, GGT has overall better sensitivity than either ALP or AST in liver disease. γ-Glutamyl transferase levels are elevated in about 90% of patients with infectious mononucleosis (Epstein-Barr virus) and about 75% with cytomegalovirus infection, presumably due to liver involvement from these viruses.

γ-Glutamyl transferase levels are not significantly affected by "normal" alcoholic beverage intake in most cases. In heavy drinkers and chronic alcoholics, GGT levels are reported to be elevated in about 70%–75% of patients (literature range, 63%–80%). Determining the GGT level has been advocated as a screening procedure for alcoholism.

γ-Glutamyl transferase levels may become elevated in several conditions other than liver disease. These include drugs that stimulate ("induce") liver microsomal activity, such as phenytoin (about 70% of cases; range, 58%–90%) and phenobarbital-type hypnotics (see Table 36–2, XVII), brain tumors (57% of cases), hyperthyroidism (0%–62% of cases), diabetes mellitus (24%–57%), acute pancreatitis (71%–100%), and acute cholecystitis. About 50%–85% of epileptics are reported to have elevated GGT levels, but some of the elevations could be due to anticonvulsant medication such as phenytoin. About 5%–30% of patients with acute myocardial infarction develop elevated GGT levels. This is usually attributed to proliferation of capillaries and fibroblasts in granulation tissue. The increase is usually reported 7–14 days after infarction. However, a few investigators found the elevation soon after infarction, and it is unclear how many cases are actually due to liver passive congestion rather than infarct healing. The GGT level may be transiently increased by extensive reparative processes anywhere in the body.

γ-Glutamyl transferase levels are usually not increased in bone disease, childhood or adolescence, and pregnancy, three nonhepatic conditions that are associated with increased ALP levels. γ-Glutamyl transferase has therefore been used to help differentiate liver from nonliver origin when ALP levels are increased. However, the possible nonhepatic sources for GGT must be kept in mind.

Prothrombin Time

In certain situations the prothrombin time (PT; chapter 8) can be a useful liver test. The liver synthesizes prothrombin but needs vitamin K to do so. Vitamin K is a fat-soluble vitamin that is present in most adequate diets and is also synthesized by intestinal bacteria; in either case, it is absorbed from the small bowel in combination with dietary fat molecules. Consequently, interference with vitamin K metabolism can take place because of (1) lack of vitamin K due to dietary deficiency, destruction of intestinal bacteria, or defective intestinal absorption due to lack of bile salts or through primary small bowel malabsorption; (2) inadequate utilization secondary to destruction of liver parenchyma; or (3) drug-induced, due to coumarin anticoagulants or certain cephalosporin antibiotics. Normally, the body has considerable tissue stores of vitamin K, so that it usually takes several weeks to get significant prothrombin deficiency on the basis of inadequate vitamin K alone. However, as noted in the discussion of PT in chapter 8, low vitamin K intake because of anorexia or prolonged IV feeding can be potentiated by antibiotics, other medications, or poor absorption. Nevertheless, the usual cause of prothrombin abnormality is liver disease. In most cases it takes very severe liver disease, more often chronic but sometimes acute, before prothrombin levels become significantly abnormal. In the usual case of viral hepatitis, the PT is either normal or only slightly increased. In massive acute hepatocellular necrosis the PT may be significantly elevated, but it seems to take a few days to occur. In mild or moderate degrees of cirrhosis the PT is usually normal. In severe end-stage cirrhosis the PT is often elevated. The test most often used to differentiate PT elevation due to liver cell damage from other conditions that affect vitamin K supply or metabolism is to administer an intravenous or intramuscular dose of vitamin K and then repeat the PT time 24–48 hours later. Prothrombin time elevation due to liver cell damage usually does not respond to parenteral vitamin K therapy, whereas the PT will return to reference range in other conditions affecting vitamin K. In metastatic carcinoma the PT is usually normal unless biliary tract obstruction is present.

Certain conditions not involving liver disease or vitamin K absorption can affect the PT. Anticoagulant therapy with coumarin drugs or heparin is discussed in chapter 8. Heparin flushes, blood with a very high hematocrit, and severe hyperlipemia (when photo-optical readout devices are used) can produce artifactually elevated PT results. Various medications can affect the PT time (see Table 36–2, V).

Serum Bile Acids

Bile acids are water-soluble components of bile that are derived from cholesterol metabolism by liver cells. Two primary bile acids are formed: cholic acid and chenodeoxycholic acid. Both are conjugated with glycine or taurine molecules and excreted from liver cells into bile in a manner similar but not identical to bilirubin excretion. The conjugated bile acids are stored in the gallbladder with bile and released into the duodenum, where they help to absorb fat and fat-soluble material. About 95% of the bile acids are reabsorbed from the jejunum and ileum and taken through the portal vein back to the liver, where they are reextracted by liver cells and put back into the bile. Cholic acid is reabsorbed only in the terminal ileum. A small proportion of circulating bile acids is excreted by the kidneys and a small proportion reaches the colon, where it undergoes some additional changes before being reabsorbed and taken back to the liver.

At least two cycles of bile acid metabolism occur in the 2 hours following a meal. Normally, 2-hour postprandial bile acid levels are increased two–three times fasting levels. Even so, the values are relatively low.

Due to the metabolic pathways of bile acids, diseases affecting hepatic blood flow, liver cell function (bile acid synthesis), bile duct patency, gallbladder function, and intestinal reabsorption can all affect serum bile acid levels. However, intestinal malabsorption is uncommon and usually does not simulate liver disease. Although gallbladder disease (cholecystitis or cholelithiasis) can occasionally mimic liver disease and may be associated with common bile duct obstruction, most cases of primary gallbladder disease can be differentiated from primary liver disease. Therefore, bile acid abnormality is relatively specific for liver or biliary tract disease. Both cholic acid and chenodeoxycholic acid can be measured by immunoassay techniques. Cholic acid assay is more readily available at the present time. The assays are not widely available but can be obtained in university centers or large reference laboratories. Because values fluctuate during the day and are affected by food, specimens should be obtained at the same time of day (usually in the early morning) and the same relationship to meals.

Bile acid assay is said to be the most sensitive test available to detect liver or biliary tract dysfunction. The 2-hour postprandial level is more sensitive than the fasting level, which itself is more sensitive than any one of the standard liver function tests. In most reports serum bile acid, even using a fasting specimen, was 10%–20% more sensitive than any other single liver function test in various types of liver and biliary tract conditions. There are only a few investigators who report otherwise. Bile acids are frequently abnormal in inactive cirrhosis when all other biochemical liver tests are normal and are frequently abnormal in resolving hepatitis when other tests have subsided below the upper limits of their reference ranges. Bile acid assay has mostly replaced bromsulphalein (BSP) and indocyanine green (Cardio-Green) for this purpose. A normal bile acid assay, especially the 2-hour postprandial value, is excellent evidence against the presence of significant liver or biliary tract disease. There have not been sufficient studies to establish the exact sensitivity of bile acid assay in early metastatic tumor to the liver. The major advantages of bile acid assay, therefore, are its sensitivity in most types of liver and biliary tract disease and its relative specificity for the liver and biliary tract. One report indicates that bile acids may be elevated by phenytoin or isoniazid therapy.

Bile acid assay might also be useful to prove liver origin of abnormal liver function test results in those cases where tests like GGTP are equivocal or are affected by nonhepatic conditions that could produce falsely elevated values. Bile acid assay could theoretically be used to differentiate jaundice due to hemolysis from that due to liver disease but is rarely necessary for this purpose. Bile acid assay has been suggested as a test for intestinal malabsorption, but few reports are available on this subject.

The major drawback of bile acid assay is lack of ability to differentiate among the various types of liver or biliary tract disease. Bile acid assay cannot differentiate between intrahepatic and extrahepatic biliary tract obstruction. Nearly anything that produces liver or biliary tract abnormality can affect the bile acid values. Although some conditions produce statistically different degrees of abnormality than other conditions, there is too much overlap when applied to individual patients for the test to be of much help in differential diagnosis. However, there are a few exceptions. Bile acid assay may be useful in the differential diagnosis of congenital defects in bilirubin metabolism (e. g., Gilbert's syndrome and Dubin-Johnson syndrome; chapter 35). In neonatal biliary obstruction, there are some reports that oral administration of cholestyramine, an anion exchange resin that binds the bile acids, can aid in differentiating neonatal hepatitis with patent common bile duct from common duct atresia by lowering serum bile acid values if the duct is patent.

In summary, bile acid assay is useful (1) to screen for liver disease when other liver function tests are normal or give equivocal results; (2) in some cases, to help differentiate between hepatic and nonhepatic etiology of other liver test abnormalities); (3) in some cases, to follow patients with liver disease when other tests have returned to normal; and (4) to help differentiate certain congenital diseases of bilirubin metabolism.

Serum Proteins

Serum albumin levels decrease to variable degrees in many severe acute and chronic disorders. Albumin is synthesized in the liver, so most acute or chronic destructive liver diseases of at least moderate severity also result in decreased serum albumin levels. In addition, there may be other serum protein changes. In cirrhosis of moderate to severe degree, there is a decreased albumin level and usually a "diffuse" ("polyclonal") gamma-globulin elevation, sometimes fairly marked. About 50% of patient with well-established cirrhosis have a characteristic serum protein electrophoretic pattern with gamma-globulin elevation that incorporates the beta area (so-called beta-gamma bridging). However, about 35% of cirrhotic patients show only various degrees of gamma elevation without any beta bridging, and about 10% have normal gamma levels. Hepatitis may also be associated with moderate elevation of the gamma globulins. Biliary obstruction eventually causes elevated beta-globulin levels, since beta globulins carry cholesterol.

Blood Ammonia

One function of the liver is the synthesis of urea from various sources of ammonia, most of which come from protein-splitting bacteria in the GI tract. In cirrhosis, there is extensive liver cell destruction and fibrous tissue replacement of areas between nodules of irregularly regenerating liver cells. This architectural distortion also distorts the hepatic venous blood supply and leads to shunting into the systemic venous system, a phenomenon often manifested by esophageal varices. Thus, two conditions should exist for normal liver breakdown of ammonia: (1) enough functioning liver cells must be present and (2) enough ammonia must reach these liver cells. With normal hepatic blood flow, blood ammonia elevation occurs only in severe liver failure. With altered blood flow in cirrhosis, less severe decompensation is needed to produce elevated blood ammonia levels. Nevertheless, the blood ammonia is not directly dependent on the severity of cirrhosis but only on the presence of hepatic failure.

Hepatic failure produces a syndrome known as "prehepatic coma" (hepatic encephalopathy), which progresses to actual hepatic coma. Clinical symptoms of prehepatic coma include mental disturbances of various types, characteristic changes on the electroencephalogram, and a peculiar flapping intention tremor of the distal extremities. However, each element of this triad may be produced by other causes, and one or more may be lacking in some patients. The ensuing hepatic coma may also be simulated by the hyponatremia or hypokalemia that cirrhotic patients often manifest or by GI bleeding, among other causes. Cerebrospinal fluid glutamate levels are currently the most reliable indicator of hepatic encephalopathy. However, this requires spinal fluid, and in addition, the test is often not available except in large medical centers or reference laboratories. Of more readily available laboratory tests, the blood ammonia level shows the best correlation with hepatic encephalopathy or coma. However, the blood ammonia level is not elevated in all of these patients, so that a normal blood ammonia level does not rule out the diagnosis. Arterial ammonia levels are more reliable than venous ones since venous ammonia may increase to variable degree compared to arterial values. Red blood cells contain about three times the ammonium content of plasma, so that hemolysis may affect results. Muscular exertion can increase venous ammonia. Plasma is preferred to serum since ammonia can be generated during clotting. Patient cigarette smoking within one hour of venipuncture may produce significant elevation of ammonia. One investigator reported transient ammonia elevation at 0.5–3 hours and again at 3.5–6 hours after a meal containing protein in some normal persons, with the effect being magnified in persons with liver disease.

Blood ammonia has been proposed as an aid in the differential diagnosis of massive upper GI tract bleeding, since elevated values suggest severe liver disease and thus esophageal varices as the cause of the bleeding. However, since cirrhotics may also have acute gastritis or peptic ulcer, this use of the blood ammonia level has not been widely accepted. At present, the blood ammonia is used mainly as an aid in diagnosis of hepatic encephalopathy or coma, since elevated values suggest liver failure as the cause of the symptoms. Otherwise, ammonia determination is not a useful liver function test, since elevations usually do not occur until hepatic failure.

Cell Component Autoantibodies

Antibodies that react against specific structures in cells, can be demonstrated by immunofluorescent technique. **Antimitochondrial antibodies** are found in 80%–100 biliary cirrhosis patients and may aid in the diagnosis of this uncommon disease. False positive results have been reported in some patients with drug-induced cholestasis and chronic active hepatitis, as well as in a relatively small number of patients with extrahepatic obstruction, acute infectious hepatitis, rheumatoid arthritis, and other conditions. **Anti–smooth muscle antibodies** were reported in 45%–70% of patients with chronic active ("lupoid") hepatitis but have also been found in biliary cirrhosis and, less frequently, in other liver diseases (except alcoholic cirrhosis). An immunofluorescence expert is needed to set up and interpret these procedures. Liver biopsy is still needed.

Fetoprotein Test

Fetal liver produces an alpha-1 globulin called "alpha fetoprotein" (AFP), which becomes the dominant fetal serum protein in the first trimester, reaching a peak at 12 weeks, then declining to 1% of the peak at birth. By age 1 year, a much greater decrease has occurred. Primary liver cell carcinomas (hepatomas) were found to produce a similar protein; therefore, a test for hepatoma could be devised using antibodies against AFP antigen. Original techniques, such as immunodiffusion, were relatively insensitive and could not detect normal quantities of AFP in adult serum. Extensive studies using immunodiffusion in several countries revealed that 30%–40% of hepatoma patients who were white had positive test results, whereas the rate among Chinese and blacks with hepatoma was 60%–75%. Men seemed to have a higher positive rate than women. Besides hepatoma, embryonal cell carcinoma and teratomas of the testes had an appreciable positivity rate. Reports of false positive results with other conditions included several cases of gastric carcinoma with liver metastases and a few cases of pregnancy in the second trimester. Subsequently, when much more sensitive radioimmunoassay techniques were devised, small quantities of AFP were detected in normal adult individuals. Radioimmunoassay has increased the abnormality rate in hepatoma somewhat, especially in white patients, whereas elevations accompanying other conditions are also more frequent. For example, according to one report, AFP levels were increased in approximately 75% of hepatoma cases, 75% of embryonal carcinomas or teratomas of the testes, 20% of pancreatic or gastric carcinomas, and 5% of colon and lung carcinomas. Others have found AFP elevations by immunoassay methods in 90% or more of hepatomas (literature range, 69%–100%) and in 0%–5% of various nonneoplastic liver diseases. The most frequent nonneoplastic elevations occurred in conditions associated with active necrosis of liver cells, such as hepatitis and active alcoholic cirrhosis. An AFP level of 500 mg/ml was suggested by several investigators as a cutoff point in differentiating hepatoma from nonneoplastic liver disease. Almost all of the nonneoplastic disease (except some cases of hepatitis virus hepatitis) were less than 500 ng/ml, whereas 50% or more patients with hepatoma had values higher than this.

Radionuclide Liver Scan

If a radioactive colloidal preparation is injected intravenously, it is picked up by the reticuloendothelial system. The Kupffer cells of the liver take up most of the radioactive material in normal circumstances, with a small amount being deposited in the spleen and bone marrow. If a sensitive radioactive counting device is placed over the liver, a two-dimensional image or map can be obtained of the distribution of radioactivity. A similar procedure can be done with thyroid and kidney using radioactive material that these organs normally take up (e.g., iodine in the case of the thyroid). Certain diseases may be suggested on liver scan if the proper circumstances are present:

1. Space-occupying lesions, such as tumor or abscess, are often visualized as discrete filling defects if they are more than 2 cm in diameter.
2. Cirrhosis typically has a diffusely nonuniform appearance accompanied by spenomegaly, but the cirrhotic process usually must be well established before scan abnormality (other than hepatomegaly) is seen. The most typical picture is obtained in far-advanced cases, but the scan appearance may differ somewhat even in these patients.
3. Fatty liver has an isotope distribution like that of cirrhosis, but only if severe.
4. Liver scanning may be useful to differentiate abdominal masses from an enlarged liver.

Undoubtedly, more sensitive equipment will become available and, perhaps, better radioactive isotopes. At present, useful as the liver scan may be, it is often difficult to distinguish among cirrhosis, fatty liver, and disseminated metastatic carcinoma with nodules less than 2 cm in diameter. Liver scan is reported to detect metastatic carcinoma in 80%–85% of patients tested (literature range, 57%–97%) and to suggest a false positive diagnosis in 5%–10% of patients without cancer. The majority of these false positive studies are in patients with cirrhosis.

Computerized Tomography and Ultrasound

Ultrasound has been reported to detect metastatic liver tumor in approximately 85%–90% of patients (literature range, 63%–96%, with some of the lower figures being earlier ones). Computerized tomography (CT) has a sensitivity of 90%–95%. Radionuclide scans detect a few more patients with diffuse liver abnormality than CT or ultrasound. However, CT and ultrasound can differentiate cysts from solid lesions in the liver, which both look the same on radionuclide scanning. Computerized tomography can also detect abnormalities outside the liver as incidental findings to a liver study. Ribs may interfere with ultrasound examination of the liver dome area, and gas in the hepatic flexure of the colon can interfere in the lower area of the liver. Magnetic resonance imaging (MRI) has about the same detection rate as CT but is much more expensive and at times has some problems with liver motion due to relatively slow scan speed.

Computerized tomography and ultrasound are important aids in differentiating extrahepatic from intrahepatic biliary tract obstruction through visualization of the diameter of the intrahepatic and common bile ducts. In complete extrahepatic obstruction, after a few days the common bile duct becomes dilated; in most cases the intrahepatic ducts eventually also become dilated. In intrahepatic obstruction the common bile duct is not dilated. Ultrasound has a sensitivity of about 93% (literature range, 77%–100%), and CT is reported to have a sensitivity of about 94% (literature range, 85%–98%). There have also been considerable advances in the ability of ultrasound and CT to demonstrate the approximate location of obstruction in the biliary system as well as making an overall diagnosis of obstruction. Gas in the intestine may interfere with ultrasound in a few cases.

In general, most investigators believe that ultrasound is the procedure of choice in possible biliary tract obstruction; those few cases that are equivocal or technically inadequate with ultrasound can be studied by CT or to some other technique such as percutaneous transhepatic cholangiography.

Percutaneous Transhepatic Cholangiography

Percutaneous transhepatic cholangiography consists of inserting a cannula into one of the intrahepatic bile ducts through a long biopsy needle and injecting x-ray contrast material directly into the duct. This procedure outlines the biliary duct system and both confirms biliary tract obstruction by demonstrating a dilated duct system and also pinpoints the location of the obstruction. The technique is not easy and requires considerable experience; more than 25% of attempts fail (most often in patients with intrahepatic obstruction due to liver cell damage). There is a definite risk (although very small) of producing bile peritonitis, which occasionally has been fatal. Preparation for surgical intervention should be made in advance in case this complication does develop.

Endoscopic Retrograde Choledochopancreatography

Endoscopic retrograde choledochopancreatography entails passing a special endoscopic tube system into the duodenum, entering the pancreatic duct or the common bile duct with the end of a cannula, and injecting x-ray contrast material. The procedure is used predominantly for diagnosis of pancreatic disease, but it may occasionally be helpful in equivocal cases of biliary tract obstruction. Cannulating the common bile duct is not easy, and best results are obtained by very experienced endoscopists.

Liver Biopsy

This procedure has been greatly simplified, and its morbidity and mortality markedly reduced, by the introduction of small-caliber biopsy needles such as the Menghini. Nevertheless, there is a small but definite risk. Contraindications to biopsy include a PT in the anticoagulant range or a platelet count less than 50,000/cu mm. Liver biopsy is especially useful in the following circumstances:

1. To differentiate among the many etiologies of liver function test abnormality when the clinical picture and laboratory test pattern are not diagnostic. This most often happens when the AST level is less than 10 or 20 times the upper reference limit and the ALP level is less than 3 times the upper limit. In cases of possible obstructive jaundice, extrahepatic obstruction should be ruled out first by some modality such as ultrasound.
2. To prove the diagnosis of metastatic or primary hepatic carcinoma in a patient who would otherwise be operable or who does not have a known primary lesion (in a patient with an inoperable known primary lesion, such a procedure would be academic).
3. In hepatomegaly of unknown origin whose etiology cannot be determined otherwise.
4. In a relatively few selected patients who have systemic diseases affecting the liver, such as miliary tuberculosis, in whom the diagnosis cannot be established by other means.

A discussion of liver biopsy should be concluded with a few words of caution. Two disadvantages are soon recognized by anyone who deals with a large number of liver specimens. First, the procedure is a needle biopsy, which means that a very small fragment of tissue, often partially destroyed, is taken in a random sample manner from a large organ. Localized disease is easily missed. Detection rate of liver metastases is about 50%–70% with blind biopsy and about 85% (range, 67%–96%) using ultrasound guidance. Second, many diseases produce nonspecific changes that may be spotty, may be healing, or may be minimal. Even with an autopsy specimen it may be difficult to make a definite diagnosis in many situations, including the etiology of many cases of cirrhosis. The pathologist should be supplied with the pertinent history, physical findings, and laboratory data; sometimes these have as much value for interpretation of the microscopic findings as the histologic changes themselves.

In summary, liver biopsy is often indicated in difficult cases but do not expect it to be infallible or even invariably helpful. The best time for biopsy is as early as possible after onset of symptoms. The longer that biopsy is delayed, the more chance that diagnostic features of the acute phase have disappeared or are obscured by transition to healing.

LABORATORY FINDINGS IN COMMON LIVER DISEASES

Having discussed various individual liver function tests, we may find it useful to summarize the typical laboratory abnormalities associated with certain common liver diseases.

Acute Hepatitis Virus Hepatitis

After an incubation period, acute viral hepatitis most often begins with some combination of GI tract symptoms, fever, chills, and malaise, lasting 4–7 days. During this phase there is no clinical jaundice. Leukopenia with a relative lymphocytosis is common, and there may be a few atypical lymphocytes. Hemoglobin values and platelet counts usually are normal. Liver function tests reflect acute hepatocellular damage, with AST and ALT values more than 10 times the upper reference limit and usually more than 20 times the upper limit. Alkaline phosphatase is usually elevated; values typically are less than three times the upper reference limit, but some patients may have elevation even higher than five times the upper limit. Serum bilirubin values begin climbing toward the end of this initial phase. The next development is visible jaundice; during this period, clinical symptoms tend to subside. The serum bilirubin level continues to rise for a time, then slowly falls. Both conjugated and unconjugated fractions are increased. The ALP level often begins to fall shortly after clinical icterus begins. The AST level begins to decrease about 1–2 weeks after it reached its peak. A convalescent phase eventually ensues, with return of all test values to normal, beginning with the ALP. Some patients continue to manifest a low-grade hepatitis (chronic persistent or chronic active), reflected by variable and intermittent AST abnormalities (usually mild or moderate in degree) with or without ALP elevation. The majority of patients (75%–80%) never develop jaundice during viral hepatitis; this condition is known as "anicteric hepatitis." In such situations, function tests reveal mild to moderate acute hepatocellular damage with a minimal obstructive component. Types of hepatitis virus and diagnosis with serologic tests are discussed in chapter 16.

The textbook picture of AST more than 20 times the upper reference limit and ALP less than 3 times the upper limit is strongly suggestive of hepatitis virus hepatitis. Other liver disorders that may be associated with an AST over 20 times the upper reference limit include a small minority of patients with drug-induced liver injury, active alcoholic cirrhosis, infectious mononucleosis, and severe liver passive congestion, as well as a few patients with early "atypical" biliary obstruction. The icteric phase of viral hepatitis may be brief and the patient may not be seen until the early convalescent phase, or the patient may have a mild anicteric episode. If so, the AST level may have decreased to less than 20 times the upper reference limit, and the differential diagnosis includes a wide variety of conditions, such as subsiding hepatitis, chronic hepatitis, alcoholic and active cirrhosis, infectious mononucleosis or cytomegalovirus infection, liver congestion, drug-induced liver dysfunction, liver space-occupying lesions, and severe fatty liver.

Chronic hepatitis is usually associated with AST values less than 20 times the upper reference limit and usually less than 10 times the upper limit. However, one study reported that about 15% of persons with the category of chronic hepatitis known as "chronic active hepatitis" had AST values at some time greater than 20 times the upper reference limit.

Biliary Obstruction

Obstruction may be complete or incomplete, extrahepatic or intrahepatic. Extrahepatic obstruction is most often produced by gallstones in the common bile duct or by carcinoma of the head of the pancreas. Intrahepatic obstruction is most often found in the obstructive phase of acute hepatocellular damage, as seen in "active" alcoholic cirrhosis, hepatitis virus hepatitis, in liver reaction to certain drugs such as chlorpromazine (Thorazine), and in occasional patients with other conditions such as metastatic carcinoma. In one series, 12% of patients with liver metastases had a total bilirubin level more than 10 mg/100 ml

(170 μmol/L). Serum bilirubin levels may become markedly elevated with either intrahepatic or extrahepatic obstruction. Although extrahepatic obstruction typically is associated with considerable bilirubin elevation, bilirubin values may be only mildly elevated in the early phases of obstruction, in persons with incomplete or intermittent obstruction, and in some persons with common duct obstruction by stones. In addition, occasional patients with intrahepatic cholestasis have considerably elevated serum bilirubin levels. Thus, the degree of bilirubinemia is not a completely reliable diagnostic point. Patients with extrahepatic obstruction typically have ALP elevation more than three times the upper reference limit, normal or minimally elevated AST levels, and moderately or considerably elevated total bilirubin levels, with 75% or more consisting of the conjugated fraction. In contrast, intrahepatic obstruction due to hepatocellular injury usually is associated with a considerably elevated AST level and a conjugated bilirubin/nonconjugated bilirubin ratio close to 1:1. Unfortunately, as time goes on, the serum bilirubin level in extrahepatic obstruction demonstrates a progressive decline in the conjugated bilirubin/nonconjugated bilirubin ratio, until a ratio not far from 1:1 is reached. Also, the AST level may increase somewhat as liver cells are damaged by distended biliary ductules. Therefore, differentiation of longstanding extrahepatic obstruction from intrahepatic obstruction may not always be easy. Metastatic tumor to the liver has the typical laboratory picture of extrahepatic obstruction without jaundice. Occasionally, however, it is accompanied by jaundice. Finally, some drugs such as chlorpromazine, anabolic steroids, or oral contraceptives may occasionally produce liver dysfunction that has a predominantly cholestatic-type biochemical pattern.

If extrahepatic obstruction is a possibility, it can be investigated with ultrasound on the biliary tract. If results of the ultrasound study are normal or equivocal and extrahepatic obstruction is strongly suspected, one of the other studies discussed previously can be attempted.

Primary Biliary Cirrhosis

Primary biliary cirrhosis is an uncommon type of biliary obstruction that should be briefly mentioned. It occurs predominantly in young or middle-aged women and typically is a slow process. On liver biopsy there is inflammation and destruction of small bile ducts within liver portal areas. Clinically there is pruritis with or without mild jaundice. Steatorrhea is sometimes present. Biochemically, there is an ALP increase more than three times the upper reference limit, increased serum cholesterol level, and normal or minimally increased AST levels. Serum antimitochondrial antibodies are elevated in 90% or more patients. Diagnosis is made on the basis of the clinical and biochemical pattern plus the presence of antimitochondrial antibodies. Liver biopsy may be necessary to differentiate the disease from chronic hepatitis, liver tumor, drug-induced cholestasis, or some other conditions associated with cholangitis.

Fatty Liver

Fatty liver is a common cause of hepatomegaly of unknown etiology. In uncomplicated fatty liver, function tests are variable. There may be no abnormality at all. Alkaline phosphatase levels in one series were elevated in nearly 48% of patients but usually were less than twice normal. An elevated AST level is found in 40% of patients, usually less than five times normal, and more often with severe degrees of fatty metamorphosis. The serum bilirubin level may be elevated in 35% of patients, but most have minimal abnormality, usually less than twice normal and without jaundice. Severe fatty liver may present clinically with jaundice, but this is very uncommon.

Cirrhosis

Cirrhosis exhibits a wide spectrum of test results, depending on whether the disease is active or inactive and on the degree of hepatocellular destruction. In patients with early or moderate degrees of inactive cirrhosis, there are usually no abnormalities in bilirubin or enzyme tests results. Bile acid assay may be abnormal. In more pronounced degrees of inactive cirrhosis there may be minimal or mild elevations of AST, serum gamma-globulin, ALP, and serum bilirubin levels, although no definite pattern can be stated. In advanced cases the PT begins to rise, and mild abnormalities on other liver function tests are more frequent.

In "active" cirrhosis (florid cirrhosis or alcoholic hepatitis), liver function tests show evidence of mild to moderate acute hepatocellular damage. Serum bilirubin may be normal or elevated; if elevated, it is usually elevated only to a mild extent, but occasionally it may rise quite high. Alkaline phosphatase levels are often less than three times normal, although occasionally they may be higher; and AST levels usually are less than 10 times normal. Active cirrhosis may have a clinical and chemical pattern simulating the minimal changes of advanced fatty liver, the moderate abnormalities of chronic hepatitis, the marked abnormalities of acute hepatitis with intrahepatic cholestasis, or the picture of obstruction with secondary liver damage. A history of chronic alcoholism, physical findings of spider angiomata and splenomegaly, AST level disproportionately elevated compared to ALT level, and GGT level disproportionately elevated compared to AST level help point toward cirrhosis. Liver biopsy is the best diagnostic test.

In childhood cirrhosis, the possibility of Wilson's disease (chapter 33) should be considered. Primary biliary cirrhosis would be likely in a 30- to 50-year-old woman with pruritus, slow onset of jaundice, protracted clinical course, liver biopsy showing bile duct destruction, and an abnormal antimitochondrial antibody test.

Metastatic Carcinoma

Metastatic tumor to the liver may be completely occult or may produce a clinical or laboratory picture compatible with hepatomegaly of unknown origin, normal liver with elevated ALP levels simulating bone disease, active cirrhosis, or obstructive jaundice. The liver is a frequent target for metastases, some of the most common primary sites being lung, breast, prostate, and both the upper and lower GI tract. Earlier reports frequently stated that metastases to a cirrhotic liver were rare, but later studies have disproved this. By far the most frequently noted abnormality is hepatic enlargement. About 25% of patients with metastatic tumor to the liver become jaundiced, and another 25% have elevated bilirubin levels (usually with the conjugated fraction predominating) without clinically evident jaundice. Occasional patients develop jaundice with relatively little hepatic tissue replacement. In about 10% of patients the bilirubin levels are high enough (> 10 mg/100 ml; 170 μmol/L) to simulate obstruction of the common bile duct. A significant minority of patients with tumor in the liver may have physical findings compatible with portal hypertension or cirrhosis.

In 50%–60% of patients with metastatic carcinoma to the liver, the serum bilirubin level is normal, whereas ALP levels are elevated in about 80% of patients (range 42%–100%). Therefore, ALP levels are frequently elevated in nonjaundiced patients with liver metastases, and ALP elevation may occur in some instances when only a relatively few tumor nodules are present. The most typical pattern for metastatic carcinoma to the liver is a normal bilirubin level, normal AST level and elevated ALP level of liver origin. If the serum bilirubin level is elevated, the typical metastatic tumor pattern becomes less typical or is obscured, because many of these patients develop mildly abnormal AST values suggestive of mild acute hepatocellular damage in addition to the elevated ALP level. Diagnosis is much more difficult when liver function test results other than ALP (or GGT) are abnormal since these other test results can be elevated (at least temporarily) from any of a considerable variety of etiologies. Unfortunately, only about one third (or less) of metastatic tumor cases have elevated ALP (or GGT) levels and normal AST levels. Finally, whether or not a patient has elevated bilirubin, ALP may be elevated due to nonhepatic etiology (i.e., phenytoin therapy, sepsis).

As mentioned previously, a liver scan (radionuclide, CT, or ultrasound) is very useful. Liver biopsy is usually necessary for definite diagnosis. Biopsy sometimes may demonstrate tumor when other tests are normal, equivocal, or conflicting, or when the biopsy is performed because of some other preliminary diagnosis.

Laboratory Test Patterns in Liver Disease

This section will review several typical patterns of laboratory values found in liver disease, with their differential diagnosis:

1. Aspartate aminotransferase value greater than 20 times the upper reference limit.

If the AST increase is due to liver disease rather than heart or skeletal muscle injury, this suggests acute hepatitis virus hepatitis. Less common etiologies are severe liver passive congestion, active cirrhosis, drug-induced liver injury, chronic active hepatitis, and infectious mononucleosis. Atypical early biliary tract extrahepatic obstruction could also be mentioned.

2. Alkaline phosphatase value elevated more than 4 times the upper limit; AST value elevated less than 10 times the upper limit.

If the ALP is derived from liver rather than bone, this suggests extrahepatic biliary tract obstruction. Serum bilirubin level would be expected to be more than 5 mg/100 ml. Other possible causes are cholestatic drug jaundice, metastatic liver tumor, and occasional cases of intrahepatic obstruction of various etiologies.

3. Alkaline phosphatase value elevated less than 3 times the upper limit; AST value elevated less than 10 times the upper limit.

This pattern is the most common one seen in patients with liver disease and can be associated with a wide variety of etiologies, including subsiding hepatitis virus hepatitis, chronic hepatitis, infectious mononucleosis, active cirrhosis, alcohol or drug-induced liver injury or dysfunction, severe fatty liver, and liver space-occupying lesions.

4. Alkaline phosphatase value elevated; AST value not elevated.

If the ALP elevation is due to liver rather than bone and if other nonhepatic causes (such as phenytoin therapy) for the elevated ALP value can be eliminated, this suggests a space-occupying lesion or lesions in the liver.

COMMENTS ON SELECTION OF LIVER FUNCTION TESTS

A few comments on the use of liver function tests are indicated. It is not necessary to order every test available and keep repeating them all, even those that give essentially the same information. For example, the ALT is sometimes useful in addition to the AST either to establish the origin of an increased AST value (because ALT is more specific for liver disease) or to obtain the AST/ALT ratio when this ratio might be helpful. However, once the results are available, it is rarely necessary to repeat the ALT because it ordinarily does not provide additional assistance to the AST in following the course of the patient's illness, nor will repetition add much additional useful information to assist diagnosis. The same is true of an elevated ALP level and the use of ALP test substitutes that are more specific for liver disease (GGT, LAP, 5-NT; chapter 35). Whichever additional enzyme of this group is used, a normal result suggests that bone rather than liver is the source of the increased ALP level, and the ALP level alone can be followed without repeating the other enzyme. If the AST level is moderately or markedly elevated and there are obvious signs of liver disease such as jaundice, it would be useless in most cases to assay GGT, LAP, or 5-NT even once, since all of them are likely to be elevated regardless of the cause of the liver disease and regardless of bone contribution to ALP. Therefore, rather than enzyme differentiation, many prefer ALP isoenzyme fractionation, which has the added benefit that concurrent elevation of both bone and liver fractions can be demonstrated. For this purpose, isoenzyme electrophoresis is more reliable.

Serum cholesterol determination is not a very helpful liver function test, although an elevated cholesterol level might add a little additional weight to the diagnosis of extrahepatic biliary tract obstruction or biliary cirrhosis. A urine bilirubin determination ("bile") is not necessary if the serum conjugated bilirubin value is known. Serum protein electrophoresis may help to suggest cirrhosis, but it is not a sensitive screening test, and the pattern most suggestive of cirrhosis is not frequent. The PT as a liver function test is useful only in two situations: (1) an elevated PT not corrected by parenteral vitamin K suggests far-advanced liver destruction, and (2) an elevated PT that is corrected by vitamin K is some evidence for longstanding extrahepatic obstruction in a patient with jaundice. If all test results are normal and inactive cirrhosis is suspected, serum bile acid assay might be useful. The most frequent use for liver scan is to demonstrate metastatic carcinoma to the liver. Ultrasound (or CT scan)—and, in some cases, percutaneous transhepatic cholangiography—are helpful in differentiating extrahepatic from intrahepatic biliary tract obstruction. Liver biopsy can frequently provide a definitive diagnosis, thereby shortening the patient's stay in the hospital and making lengthy repetition of laboratory tests or other procedures unnecessary. The earlier a biopsy is obtained, the more chance one has to see clear-cut diagnostic changes.

An initial liver test "profile" might include serum bilirubin, AST, and ALP determinations. If the serum bilirubin level is elevated, it could be separated into conjugated and unconjugated fractions. If the serum bilirubin level is not elevated determining the GGT may be useful, both to help confirm liver origin for other test abnormalities or to suggest alcoholism if it is elevated out of proportion to the other tests. The PT may be useful if other tests are abnormal to provide a rough idea of the severity of disease. In some cases the results of the initial screening tests permit one to proceed immediately to diagnostic procedures. An AST value more than 20 times normal suggests hepatitis virus hepatitis, and specimens can be obtained for serologic tests diagnostic of acute hepatitis A and B infection (e.g., hepatitis B virus surface antigen, hepatitis B virus core antibody–IgM, and hepatitis A virus–IgM; chapter 16). A high bilirubin level or other evidence suggesting biliary tract obstruction can be investigated with biliary tract ultrasound or similar studies. A normal bilirubin level with significantly elevated ALP level not due to bone disease raises the question of metastatic tumor and may warrant a liver scan. If liver screening test results are abnormal but do not point toward any single diagnosis, a liver biopsy might be considered. Liver function tests could be repeated in 2–3 days to see if a significant change takes place, but frequent repetition of the tests and long delays usually do not provide much help in establishing a diagnosis. Also, there are a significant number of exceptions to any of the so-called diagnostic or typical liver function test patterns.

EXTRAHEPATIC BILIARY TRACT

The major subdivisions of the biliary tract are the intrahepatic bile ducts, the common bile duct, and the gallbladder. The major diseases of the extrahepatic biliary system are gallbladder inflammation (cholecystitis, acute or chronic), gallbladder stones, and obstruction to the common bile duct by stones or tumor. Obstruction to intrahepatic bile channels can occur as a result of acute hepatocellular damage, but this aspect was noted in the discussion of liver function tests and will not be repeated here.

Acute cholecystitis usually presents with upper abdominal pain, most often accompanied by fever and a leukocytosis. Occasionally, difficulty in diagnosis may be produced by a right lower lobe pneumonia or peptic ulcer, and cholecystitis occasionally results in ST and T wave electrocardiographic changes that might point toward myocardial disease. Acute cholecystitis is very frequently associated with gallbladder calculi, and 90%–95% have a stone in the cystic duct. Some degree of increased bilirubin level is found in 25%–30% of patients, with a range in the literature of 6%–50%. Bilirubinemia may occur even in patients without stones. Acute cholecystitis without stones is said to be most common in elderly persons and in patients who are postoperative. Aspartate aminotransferase may be elevated in nearly 75% of acute cholecystitis patients; this is more likely if jaundice is present. In one study, about 20% of patients had AST levels more than 6 times normal, and 5% had levels more than 10 times normal. Of these, some had jaundice and some did not. Alkaline phosphatase levels are elevated in about 30% of patients with acute cholecystitis. Cholecystitis patients sometimes have an elevated serum amylase level, usually less than two times normal limits. About 15% of patients are said to have some degree of concurrent acute pancreatitis.

In our own hospital, of 25 consecutive surgical patients with microscopically proven acute cholecystitis, admission levels of total bilirubin, AST (SGOT), and ALP were all normal in 56% of the patients. Interestingly, all three tests were normal in some patients who had severe tissue abnormality. Total bilirubin, AST, and ALP were all elevated in 12% of the 25 patients. AST was elevated in 36% of the 25 patients, with about half the values less than twice the upper reference range limit and the highest value 7.5 times the upper limit. AST was the only value elevated in 16% of the 25 patients. ALP was elevated in 28% of the 25 patients; the highest value was three times the upper reference limit. The ALP was the only value elevated in 8% of the 25 patients. AST and ALP were elevated with normal total bilirubin in 8% of the 25 patients.

About 20% of patients with acute cholecystitis are reported to have common duct stones. In one series, about 40% of patients with common duct stones did not become jaundiced, and about 20% had an elevated bilirubin level less than 3 mg/100 ml. Common duct stones usually occur in association with gallbladder calculi but occasionally are present alone. In one study, 17% of patients with common duct stones had a normal ALP level; in 29%, the ALP level was elevated to less than twice normal; 11% had values between two and three times normal; and 42% were more than three times normal.

In uncomplicated obstructive jaundice due to common duct stones or tumor, AST and LDH values are usually normal. Nevertheless, when acute obstruction occurs, in some instances AST levels may become temporarily elevated very early after the onset of obstruction (sometimes with AST levels more than 10 times normal) in the absence of demonstrable hepatocellular damage. The striking AST elevation may lead to a misdiagnosis of hepatitis. Several reports indicate that LDH levels are also considerably elevated in these patients, usually five times the upper limits of normal. Since LDH levels are usually less than twice normal in hepatitis virus hepatitis (although occasional exceptions occur), higher LDH values point toward the "atypical obstruction" enzyme pattern. Both AST and LDH values usually fall steadily after 2–3 days.

Radiologic Procedures

Diagnosis of stones in the gallbladder or common bile duct rests mainly with the radiologist. On plain films of the abdomen, 20%–25% of gallbladder stones are said to be visible. Oral cholecystography consists of oral administration of a radiopaque contrast medium that is absorbed by intestinal mucosa and secreted by liver cells into the bile. When bile enters the common duct, it takes a certain amount of pressure to force open the ampulla of Vater. During the time this pressure is building up, bile enters the cystic duct into the gallbladder where water is reabsorbed, concentrating the bile. This process allows concentration of the contrast medium as well as the bile and, therefore, outlines the interior of the gallbladder and delineates any stones of sufficent size. An average of 70% of patients with gallbladder calculi may be identified by oral cholecystography. Repeated examination (using a double dose of contrast medium or alternative techniques) is necessary if the original study does not show any gallbladder function. In most of the remaining patients with gallbladder calculi, oral cholecystography reveals a poorly functioning or a nonfunctioning gallbladder. Less than 5% of patients with gallbladder stones are said to have a completely normal oral cholecystogram. (More than 50% of patients with cholecystitis and gallbladder tumor have abnormal oral cholecystograms.)

There are certain limitations to the oral method. Although false negative examination results (gallbladder calculi and a normal test result) are relatively few, false positive results (nonfunctioning gallbladder but no gallbladder disease) have been reported in some studies in more than 10% of cases. In addition, neither oral cholecystography nor plain films of the abdomen are very useful in detecting stones in the common bile duct. Visualization of the common bile duct by the oral method is frequently poor, whether stones are present or not.

Intravenous cholecystography supplements the oral procedure in some respects. Nearly 50% of common duct stones may be identified. Intravenous injection of the contrast medium is frequently able to outline the common duct and major intrahepatic bile ducts. However, IV cholecystography is being replaced by other techniques such as ultrasound, because limitations of the IV technique include poor reliability in demonstrating gallbladder calculi (since there are an appreciable number of both false positive and false negative results) and a considerable incidence of patient reaction to the contrast medium (although newer techniques, such as drip infusion, have markedly reduced the danger of reaction).

A limitation to both the oral and the IV procedure is that both depend on a patent intrahepatic and extrahepatic biliary system. If the serum bilirubin level is more than 2 mg/100 ml (34 μmol/L) (and the increase is not due to hemolytic anemia), neither oral nor IV cholangiography is usually satisfactory.

Ultrasound is another very useful modality in the diagnosis of cholecystitis. Sensitivity is about the same as that of oral cholecystography (94%–95%; literature range, 89%–96%). However, ultrasound gives fewer false positive results < 5%). Ultrasound visualizes more stones than oral cholecystography, which is an advantage in deciding whether or not to perform surgery. For example, one study showed that ultrasound detected twice as many calculus-containing gallbladders in patients with nonfunctioning gallbladders than oral cholecystography. In addition, ultrasound can be performed the same day that the diagnosis is first suspected and is not affected by some factors that make oral cholecystography difficult or impossible (e. g., a severely ill patient, severe diarrhea or vomiting, jaundice, pregnancy, and sensitivity to x-ray contrast media). Therefore, some physicians use ultrasound as the first or primary procedure in possible cholecystitis. Others perform single-dose oral cholecystography first, and if the gallbladder does not visualize but no stones are found on first examination, ultrasound is performed.

Computed tomography was discussed earlier. It is generally not ordered in acute cholecystitis unless there is suspicion of additional problems in the gallbladder area or in the abdomen.

Biliary tract radionuclide scanning is becoming available in larger centers using technetium-labeled iminodiacetic acid (IDA) complexes such as diisopropyl-IDA (DISIDA), which are extracted by the liver and excreted in bile. Normally the gallbladder, common bile duct, and isotope within the duodenum can be visualized. In acute cholecystitis there is cystic duct obstruction, and the gallbladder does not visualize on scan. This technique is said to have a sensitivity of 95%–98% with less than 5% false positive results. Many consider it the current procedure of choice in acute cholecystitis. Standard gray-scale ultrasound is not quite as good in detecting acute cholecystitis as it is in detecting chronic cholecystitis, although real-time ultrasound sensitivity is said to be 95% accurate or better. The ability of ultrasound to visualize stones is an advantage, but radionuclide scanning has an advantage in patients with acute acalculous cholecystitis. Radionuclide scan diagnosis of chronic cholecystitis is not nearly as accurate as detection of acute cholecystitis, and the technique usually does not visualize stones. Because the common duct can be visualized even when the serum bilirubin level is elevated, DISIDA scanning can also be useful in early or acute extrahepatic obstruction. In early or acute common duct obstruction the common duct may not yet be sufficiently dilated to produce abnormal ultrasound sonograms or abnormal CT scans. However, in long-standing obstruction, hepatic parenchymal cells are injured and cannot extract the IDA compounds from the blood sufficiently well to consistently fill the common duct. If symptoms persist or if there is a suggestion of complications, DISIDA scanning is useful after biliary tract operations.

One report indicates a significant number of false positive results (gallbladder nonvisualization) in patients who have alcoholic liver disease and in patients on total parenteral nutrition therapy.

Additional tests relevant to this chapter are discussed in chapter 35.

BIBLIOGRAPHY

Yasmineh WG, et al: Conjugated hyperbilirubinemia and renal function in bone marrow transplant recipients. *Arch Pathol Lab Med* 1988; 112:245.

Stahl TJ et al: Partial biliary obstruction caused by chronic pancreatitis. *Ann Surg* 1988; 207:26.

Zimmerman HJ, Deschner KW: Differential diagnosis of jaundice. *Hosp Pract* 1987; 22:99.

Patwardhan RV, et al: Serum transaminase levels and cholescintigraphic abnormalities in acute biliary tract obstruction. *Arch Intern Med* 1987; 147:1249.

Lott JA: New concepts in serum bilirubin measurement. *Lab Mgmt* 1987; 25(4):41.

Riely CA, et al: Acute fatty liver of pregnancy. *Ann Intern Med* 1987; 106:703.

Kubo SH et al: Liver function abnormalities in chronic heart failure. *Arch Intern Med* 1987; 147:1227.

Silberstein EB: No single imaging method best for hepatic lesions. *Diagn Imag* 1986; 8:212.

Behr W, Barnert J: Quantification of bone alkaline phosphatase in serum by precipitation with wheat-germ lectin. *Clin Chem* 1986; 32:1960.

Anciaux ML, et al: Biochemical features of choledocholithiasis. *Dig Dis Sci* 1986; 31:444.

Greenfield SM et al: Serum bile acid assays for liver disease: When and how to use them. *Dig Dis Sci* 1986; 31:785.

Fornage BD, et al: Ultrasound-guided fine-needle aspiration biopsy of the liver. *Applied Radiol* 1986; 15:65.

Kaplowitz N, et al: Drug induced hepatotoxicity. *Ann Intern Med* 1986; 104:826.

Lee AW, et al: Technetium-99m BIDA biliary scintigraphy in the evaluation of the jaundiced patient. *J Nucl Med* 1986; 27:1407.

Silberstein EB, et al: Comparative efficacy of radionuclide, ultrasound, and computed tomographic liver imaging for hepatic metastases. *Curr Concepts Diagn Nucl Med* 1985; 2(3):3.

Fortman CS, et al: Serum 5-nucleotidase in patients receiving anti-epileptic drugs. *Am J Clin Pathol* 1985; 84:197.

Benjamin DR: The isolated high alkaline phosphatase value. *Pathologist* 1984; 38:812.

Rosalki SB: More on transient hyperphosphatasemia of infancy. *Clin Chem* 1983; 29:723.

Craig RM, Clayman CB: The use and abuse of endoscopic retrograde cholangiopancreatography. *JAMA* 1983; 249:783.

Crowe J, et al: Early features of primary biliary cirrhosis. *Am J Gastroenterol* 1985; 80:466.

Stenson WF: Pyogenic liver abscess. *Arch Intern Med* 1983; 143:126.

Van Blankenstein M et al: Endogenous bile acid tolerance test for liver function. *Dig Dis* 1983; 28:137.

Pappas SC, Jones EA: Methods for assessing hepatic encephalopathy. *Sem in Liver Dis* 1983; 3:298.

Siegel JH, Yatto RP: Approach to cholestasis: An update. *Arch. Intern Med* 1982; 142:1877.

Frietas JE: Cholescintigraphy in acute and chronic cholecystitis. *Semin Nucl Med* 1982; 12:18.

Davis GL, et al: Prognostic and therapeutic implications of extreme serum aminotransferase elevation in chronic active hepatitis. *Mayo Clin Proc* 1982; 57:303.

Batsakis JG: Serum alkaline phosphatase. *Diagn Med* 1982; 5:25.

Shaw LM: GGT. *Diagn Med* 1982; 5:59.

Shuman WP, et al: PIPIDA scintigraphy for cholestasis: False positive in alcoholism and total parenteral nutrition. *AJR* 1982; 138:1.

Grey CF, et al: Endoscopic retrograde cholangiopancreatography. Am J Surg 1982; 144:109.

Thomas MJ, et al: Usefulness of diagnostic tests for biliary obstruction. *Am J Surg.* 1982; 144:102.

Berk RN, et al: The radiologic diagnosis of gallbladder disease. *Radiology* 1981; 141:49.

Monroe PS, Baker AL: Alcoholic hepatitis. *Postgrad Med* 1981; 69:32.

Stoerner JW: Neonatal jaundice. *Am Fam Phys* 1981; 24:226.

Beinart C et al: Obstruction without dilation. *JAMA* 1981; 245:353.

Glasgow AM: Clinical applications of blood ammonia determinations. *Lab Med* 1981; 12:151.

Hollander IJ: Nonhemolytic hyperbilirubinemias. *Ann Clin Lab* Sci 1980; 10:204.

Rhone DP, et al: Tissue sources of elevated serum alkaline phosphatase activity in hyperthyroid patients. *Am J Clin Path* 1980; 74:381.

Fang MH, et al: Marked elevation in serum alkaline phosphatase activity as a manifestation of systemic infection. *Gastroenterology* 1980; 78:592.

Brill AB, et al: Radioisotopic methods in diagnosis and assessment of liver metastases. *Curr Concepts Cancer* 1979; 119.

Cohen JA, Kaplan MM: The SGOT/SGPT ratio: An indicator of alcoholic liver disease. *Dig Dis Sci* 1979; 24:835.

Abdi W, et al.: Sampling variability on percutaneous liver biopsy. *Arch Intern Med* 1979; 139:667.

20 Cardiac, Pulmonary, and Miscellaneous Diagnostic Procedures

ACUTE MYOCARDIAL INFARCTION

Clinical signs and symptoms are extremely important in both suspicion and diagnosis of myocardial infarction (MI). The type of pain, its distribution, and its response to nitroglycerin may be very characteristic. However, it may not be easy to differentiate the pain of angina from that of acute infarct; in addition, 10%–25% (literature range, 1%–60%) of acute MIs have been reported to occur without chest pain. This is said to be more frequent in diabetics. Even when diagnosis is virtually certain on clinical grounds alone, the physician often will want laboratory confirmation, and this becomes more important when symptoms are atypical or minimal.

Tests in Acute Myocardial Infarction

ECG, WBC Count, and ESR

An electrocardiogram (ECG) is the most useful direct test available. Approximately 50% of acute MIs show unequivocal changes on the first ECG. Another 30% have abnormalities that might be due to acute infarct but that are not diagnostic, because the more specific changes are masked or obscured by certain major conduction irregularities such as bundle-branch block or by previous digitalis therapy. About 20% do not show significant ECG changes, and this occasionally happens even in patients who otherwise have a typical clinical and laboratory picture. Ordinary general laboratory tests cannot be used to diagnose acute infarction, although certain tests affected by tissue damage give abnormal results in the majority of patients. In classic cases a polymorphonuclear leukocytosis in the range of 10,000–20,000/cu mm ($10–20 \times 10^9$/L) begins 12–24 hours after onset of symptoms. Leukocytosis generally lasts between 1 and 2 weeks, depending on the extent of tissue necrosis. Leukocytosis is accompanied by a moderately elevated temperature and an increased erythrocyte sedimentation rate (ESR). The ESR abnormality persists longer than the leukocytosis, remaining elevated sometimes as long as 3–4 weeks.

Aspartate Aminotransferase (AST)

Certain enzymes are present in cardiac muscle that are released when tissue necrosis occurs. Serum aspartate aminotransferase (AST, formerly oxaloacetic transaminase, or SGOT) is elevated at some time in 90%–95% of acute MI patients (literature range, 87%–97%). These statistics for sensitivity of the AST in acute MI are based on multiple sequential AST determinations and are therefore not valid for any single determination. Aspartate transaminase levels become elevated 8–12 hours after infarction, reach a peak 24–48 hours after infarction, and fall to normal within 3–8 days. The AST blood levels correlate very roughly with the extent of infarct and may be only transiently and minimally abnormal.

Besides myocardial injury, the AST level may become elevated due to acute damage to parenchymal cells of the liver, skeletal muscle, kidney, and pancreas (see Table 19–2). Abnormality due to liver cell injury is especially common (e.g., liver congestion, active cirrhosis, and acute or chronic hepatitis), but an increased AST level will occur with sufficient degrees of skeletal muscle injury (including trauma or extensive surgical damage) and is also found fairly frequently in acute pancreatitis. In some of these situations, myocardial infarct may have to be considered in the differential diagnosis of the patient's symptoms. Chronic hypokalemia may elevate both AST and creatine phosphokinase (CPK) levels; morphine and meperidine (Demerol) may temporarily raise AST levels, and AST elevations have been reported in occasional patients receiving warfarin sodium (Coumadin) anticoagulant therapy and in some patients taking large doses of salicylates.

The major drawbacks of the AST in diagnosis of acute MI are the many conditions (especially liver congestion) that can produce AST elevation.

Lactic Dehydrogenase

Lactic dehydrogenase (LDH) values refer to total serum LDH. Total LDH levels are elevated at some time in 92%–95% (literature range, 82%–100%) of patients with acute MI. Statistics for sensitivity in acute MI refer to multiple sequential LDH specimens and are therefore not valid for any single determination. In acute MI, LDH levels become elevated 24–48 hours after MI, reach a peak 48–72 hours after MI, and slowly falls to normal in 5–10 days. Thus, LDH values tend to parallel AST values at about double the time interval. Total LDH is slightly more sensitive than AST in acute MI and is reported to be elevated even in small infarcts that showed no AST abnormality.

Lactic dehydrogenase is found in cardiac muscle, skeletal muscle, liver, red blood cells (RBCs), lung, and kidney. In acute liver cell damage, the total LDH value is not as sensitive as the AST value. In mild acute or chronic passive congestion of the liver, the LDH level is frequently normal or only minimally increased. In moderate or severe congestion, LDH values range from mild to substantial degrees of elevation.

Since LDH fraction 1 (discussed later) is contained in RBCs as well as cardiac muscle, LDH is greatly influenced by accidental hemolysis in serum and thus must be collected and transported with care. Heart valve prostheses may produce enough low-grade hemolysis to affect LDH, and LDH levels are also abnormal in many patients with megaloblastic and moderate or severe hemolytic anemias. Skeletal muscle contains LDH, so total LDH (or even hydroxybutyric acid dehydrogenase [HBD]) values are not reliable in the first week after extensive surgery. LDH levels may be elevated in 60%–80% of patients with pulmonary embolism (reports vary from 30%–100%) possibly due to pulmonary tissue damage or to hemorrhage.

Finally, LDH becomes elevated in some patients with malignant neoplasms and leukemia, and in some patients with uremia.

The major drawback of total LDH, similar to AST, is the many conditions that can elevate LDH values.

Lactic Dehydrogenase Isoenzymes.— Total LDH is actually a group of enzymes. The individual enzymes (isoenzymes) that make up total LDH have different concentrations in different tissues. Therefore, the tissue responsible for an elevated total LDH value may often be identified by fractionation (separation) and measurement of individual isoenzymes. In addition, since the population normal range for total LDH is rather wide, abnormal elevation of one isoenzyme may occur without lifting total LDH out of the total LDH normal range.

Five main fractions (isoenzymes) of LDH are measured. With use of the standard international nomenclature (early U.S. investigators used opposite terminology), fraction 1 is found mainly in RBCs and in heart and kidney, fraction 3 comes from lung, and fraction 5 is located predominantly in liver and to a lesser extent in skeletal muscle. Skeletal muscle contains some percentage of all the fractions, although fraction 5 predominates. Various methods of isoenzyme separation are available. The two most commonly used are heat and electrophoresis. Heating to 60°C for 30 minutes destroys most activity except that of fractions 1 and 2, the heat-stable fractions. With electrophoresis, the fast-moving fractions are 1 and 2 (heart), whereas the slowest-migrating fraction is 5 (liver). Electrophoresis has the advantage that one can see the relative contribution of all five fractions.

The relative specificity of LDH isoenzymes is very useful because of the large number of

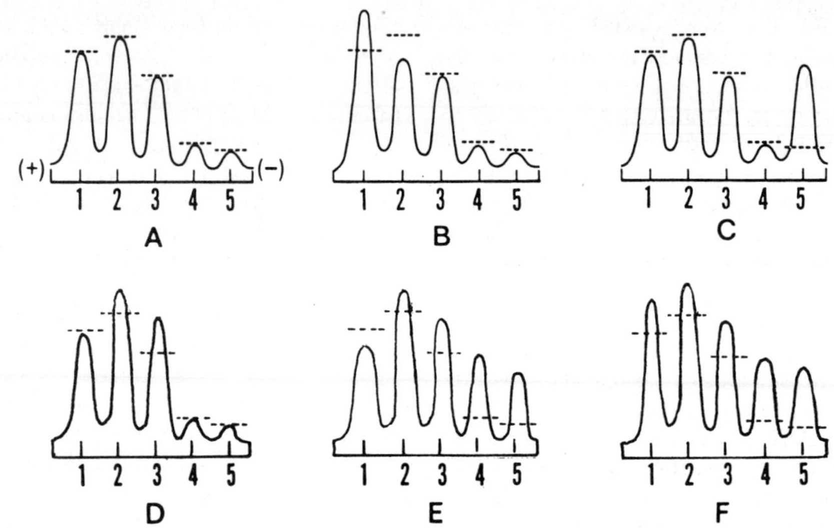

FIG 20–1.
Representative LDH isoenzyme patterns with most frequent etiologies. **A**, normal. **B**, fraction 1 increased with fraction 1 greater than fraction 2: acute MI; artifactual hemolysis; hemolytic or megaloblastic anemia; renal cortex infarct. **C**, fraction 5 increased: acute hepatocellular injury (hepatitis, passive congestion, active cirrhosis, etc.); acute skeletal muscle injury. **D**, fractions 2 and 3 elevated: pulmonary hypoxia (pulmonary embolization, cardiac failure, extensive pneumonia, etc.); pulmonary congestion, viral pulmonary infection. **E**, fractions 2 through 5 elevated: lung plus liver abnormality (pulmonary hypoxia and/or congestion plus liver congestion, infectious mononucleosis or cytomegalovirus infection, lymphoproliferative disorders). **F**, all fractions elevated, relatively normal relationships preserved between the fractions (fraction 5 sometimes elevated disproportionately): multiorgan hypoxia and/or congestion (with or without acute MI); malignancy; occasionally in other disorders (trauma, infection/inflammation, active cirrhosis, chronic obstructive pulmonary disease, uremia, etc.)

diseases that affect standard heart enzyme tests. For example, one study of patients in hemorrhagic shock with no evidence of heart disease found an elevated AST level in 70%, an elevated total LDH level in 52%, and an elevated alanine aminotransferase (ALT) (formerly serum glutamate pyruvate transaminase) level in 37%. Lactic dehydrogenase enzyme fractionation offers a way to diagnose MI when liver damage is suspected of contributing to total LDH increase. In liver damage without MI, fraction 1 is usually normal, and most of the increase is due to fraction 5.

Several characteristic LDH isoenzyme patterns are illustrated in Figure 20–1. However, not all patients with the diseases listed necessarily have the "appropriate" isoenzyme configuration; the frequency with which the pattern occurs depends on the particular disease and the circumstances. Multiorgan disease can be a problem since it may produce combinations of the various patterns. For example, in acute MI the typical pattern is elevation of LDH-1 values with LDH-1 values greater than LDH-2. However, acute MI can lead to pulmonary congestion or hypoxia, with elevation of LDH-2 and LDH-3 values, and may also produce liver congestion or hypoxia, with elevation of LDH-4 and LDH-5 values. Acute MI can also produce multiorgan hypoxia or shock. In shock all LDH fractions tend to be elevated, and in severe cases the various fractions tend to move toward equal height. In malignancy, there may be midzone elevation only, elevation of only fraction 4 and 5, or elevation of all fractions. In my experience, the most common pattern in malignancy is elevation of all fractions with normal relationships preserved between the fractions.

The LDH isoenzymes may be of help in evaluating postsurgical chest pain. Skeletal muscle mostly contains fraction 5 but also some fraction 1, so total LDH, HBD, or fraction 1 elevations are not reliable during the first week after extensive surgery. However, a normal LDH-1 value in samples obtained both at 24 and 48 hours after onset of symptoms is considerable evidence against acute MI, and an elevation of the LDH-1 value with the LDH-1 value greater than LDH-2 is evidence for acute MI. Creatine phosphokinase isoenzyme levels, if available, are of greater assistance than LDH isoenzyme levels in the first 24 hours.

Immunoassay methods are now available for measurement of LDH-1 alone. Measurement of LDH-1 has been claimed to be superior to the LDH-1/LDH-2 ratio in diagnosis of acute MI. The typical reversal of the LDH-1/LDH-2 ratio is found in only 80%–85% of patients (literature range, 61%–95%) with acute MI. In some cases, reversal of the ratio is prevented (masked) by an increase of LDH-2 values due to pulmonary hypoxia occurring concurrently with the increase of LDH-1 values due to MI. An elevated LDH-1 fraction as demonstrated on immunoassay is more sensitive (detection rate about 95%; literature range, 86%–100%) than reversal of the LDH-1/LDH-2 ratio in acute MI. However, in my experience and that of others, LDH-1 values can be increased in myocardial hypoxia without any definite evidence of acute MI (e.g., in hypovolemic shock). In addition, the LDH-1 value by immunoassay is increased by all the noncardiac conditions that reverse the LDH-1/LDH-2 ratio (hemolytic or megaloblastic anemia, renal cortex infarct). Thus, the increase in sensitivity gained by LDH-1 immunoassay in acute MI must be weighed against the possible loss of specificity (increase in LDH-1 values not due to acute MI, Table 20–1). Lactic dehydrogenase isoenzyme fractionation by electrophoresis also demonstrates increased LDH-1 values even when the LDH-1/LDH-2 ratio is not reversed.

Most LDH fractions are stable for several days at refrigerator temperature. If the specimen is frozen, LDH-5 rapidly decreases.

TABLE 20–1.

Causes of Lactic Dehydrogenase Fraction 1 Elevation

Acute MI
Cardiac muscle hypoxia without definite acute MI
Blood specimen hemolysis
Hemolytic anemia
Megaloblastic anemia
Renal cortex infarct
LDH isomorphic isoenzyme pattern
Multiorgan hypoxia
Neoplasia
Other conditions (less common)

Hydroxybutyric Acid Dehydrogenase

Hydroxybutyric acid dehydrogenase (HBD) has been used as a substitute for LDH-1 (heart) isoenzyme measurement. Actually, HBD is total LDH that is forced to act on an α-ketobutyric acid substrate instead of pyruvic or lactic acid. Under these conditions, LDH-1 and LDH-2 show relatively greater activity than LDH-5, so that HBD therefore indirectly measures LDH-1 (heart) activity. However, if the LDH-5 (liver) value is elevated sufficiently, it will also produce measurable HBD effect. Therefore, HBD is not as specific as electrophoresis or heat fractionation in separating heart from liver isoenzymes. Nevertheless, since HBD assay is easier to perform (and therefore cheaper) than LDH isoenzyme assay, some follow the practice of using a more specific isoenzyme method if in doubt about LDH heart vs. liver contribution. Once there is proof that the heart fraction is elevated, they follow subsequent activity levels with HBD.

Creatine Phosphokinase

Creatine phosphokinase is found in heart muscle, skeletal muscle, and brain. It is elevated at some time in about 90%–93% (literature range, 65%–100%) of patients with acute MI. In acute MI, CPK behaves similarly to AST. However, acute liver cell damage, which frequently causes an abnormal AST value, has no effect on CPK. This is an advantage, since the situation often arises in which an elevated AST (or LDH) level might be due to severe hepatic passive congestion from heart failure rather than from acute MI.

Use of CPK measurements in diagnosing primary diseases of skeletal muscle is discussed elsewhere (chapter 33). A considerable number of conditions associated with acute muscle injury or severe muscle exertion affect CPK values. Thus, CPK values are usually elevated in muscle trauma, myositis, muscular dystrophy, after surgery, postpartum, after moderately severe exercise (e.g., long-distance running), and in delirium tremens or convulsions. Increased serum values have been reported in about 80% of patients with hypothyroidism (literature range, 20%–100%) and in patients with severe hypokalemia, due to changes induced in skeletal muscle. In addition, elevations have also been reported in some patients with tachyarrhythmias (mostly ventricular) for unknown reasons. Creatine phosphokinase elevation can be due to effects of alcohol on muscle. For example, one study found that CPK levels became abnormal after 24–48 hours in the majority of persons following heavy drinking episodes as well as in most patients with delirium tremens. Levels of CPK are said to be normal in chronic alcoholics without heavy intake.

Creatine phosphokinase levels are frequently elevated after intramuscular injection. Since therapeutic injections are common, this probably constitutes the most frequent cause of CPK elevation. Specimens must be drawn before injection or at least within 1 hour after injection. Trauma to muscle makes the CPK level unreliable for a few days postoperatively.

Although CPK is present in brain tissue as well as muscle, reports differ to some extent as to the effect of central nervous system (CNS) disease on serum CPK levels. According to one report, CPK levels may be elevated in a wide variety of conditions that affect the brain, including bacterial meningitis, encephalitis, cerebrovascular accident, hepatic coma, uremic coma, and grand mal epileptic attacks. Elevation is not always present, and when it is present, the degree of elevation varies considerably. Elevations in some patients in acute phases of certain psychiatric diseases, notably schizophrenia have been reported; the cause is not known.

Normal CPK values for black males are double those for white males; values for black and white females are nearly equal in most (but not all) reports.

The major drawbacks of total CPK are (1) the relatively short time period after onset of infarction during which the CPK value is elevated and (2) false positive elevations due to skeletal muscle injury (especially intramuscular injections).

Creatine Phosphokinase Isoenzyme Measurement.—Total CPK can be separated into three major fractions (isoenzymes): CPK-BB (CPK-1), found predominantly in brain and lung; CPK-MM (CPK-3), found in skeletal muscle; and the hybrid CPK-MB (CPK-2), found predominantly in cardiac muscle. Creatine phosphokinase isoenzyme assays are now available in most hospital laboratories. Isoenzymes offer a way to detect myocardial damage that minimizes skeletal muscle contribution to CPK values.

Creatine Phosphokinase MM Fractions.—Elevation of the MM fraction is usually due to skeletal muscle abnormality, including that induced by moderately severe or severe exercise, convulsions, inflammation, trauma, intramuscular injection, or muscular dystrophy. Some conditions producing less obvious effects on muscle, such as hypothyroidism and hypokalemia, may also produce CPK-MM increase.

Creatine Phosphokinase MB Fraction.—The CPK-MB level begins to rise 3–6 hours after onset of acute MI, reaches a peak in 12–24 hours, and returns to normal in 24–48 hours (sometimes earlier). There is a rough correlation between the size of the infarct and the degree of elevation. Since small infarcts may not elevate the MB fraction dramatically, it is important to time the collection of specimens so as not to miss the peak values. Some recommend four specimens, one obtained every 6 hours after onset of symptoms. However, three specimens, one obtained every 12 hours (one on admission, one at 12 and one at 24 hours after admission), seems a more reasonable compromise.

There is some dispute as to whether ischemia without actual infarct will elevate either total CPK or CPK-MB levels. The controversy revolves around the fact that currently there is no way to rule out the possibility that a small infarct may have occurred in a patient who clinically is thought to have only ischemia.

In equivocal cases it is helpful to obtain LDH isoenzyme determinations as well as CPK-MB, both to enhance diagnostic specificity and because specimens for CPK-MB may have been obtained too late to detect elevation. If a CPK isoenzyme sample is obtained immediately, at 12 hours, and at 24 hours; and LDH isoenzyme determinations are performed at 24 and 48 hours, 95% or more acute MIs detectible by these tests will be documented. Of course, if one of the CPK-MB determinations is strongly positive, it might not be necessary to obtain further samples. The time course of LDH, CPK, and other enzyme titers in acute MI is given in Table 20–2. Figure 20–2 shows the relative increases and decreases in graphic form.

The question sometimes arises whether both CPK-MB and LDH isoenzyme fractionation should be done. At our hospital, CPK-MB assay is performed immediately and then 12

TABLE 20–2.
Laboratory Tests in Acute Myocardial Infarction*

	Titer		
	Begins to Rise	Peak	Returns to Normal
CPK	4–6 hr (2–8 hr)	24 hr (12–36 hr)	3–4 days (1.5–10 days)
CPK-MB	4 hr (2–12 hr)	18 hr (12–24 hr)	2 days (1.2–3 days)
AST	8 hr (2–36 hr)	24–48 hr (24–48 hr)	4 days (3–7 days)
LDH	24 hr (12–48 hr)	3 days (2–4 days)	8–9 days (7–18 days)
LDH-1 (or HBD)	24 hr (12–48 hr)	3 days (1–5 days)	12 days (7–16 days)

*Figures in parentheses indicate ranges found in the literature.

and 24 hours later; and LDH isoenzyme study is performed at 24 and 48 hours (both using electrophoresis). In 50 consecutive patients with either CPK-MB elevated or LDH-1 elevated, with LDH-1 greater than LDH-2, CPK-MB was first elevated in the initial sample in 28%; first elevated in the 12-hour sample in 50%; in the 24-hour specimen in 4%; and in none of the specimens in 18%. The LDH-1/LDH-2 ratio was reversed in the 24-hour specimen in 70%; in the 48-hour specimen in 18%; and in neither specimen in 12%. Therefore, with the commonly used protocol, 12% of patients would have been missed relying on LDH isoenzyme studies alone and 18% with CPK-MB alone.

CPK-MB Fraction and Skeletal Muscle.—Although CPK-MB is found mainly in cardiac muscle (25%–40% of total myocardial CPK), skeletal muscle CPK contains a small amount of CPK-MB (3%–5%). Skeletal muscle contains two types of muscle fibers: type 1 predominates

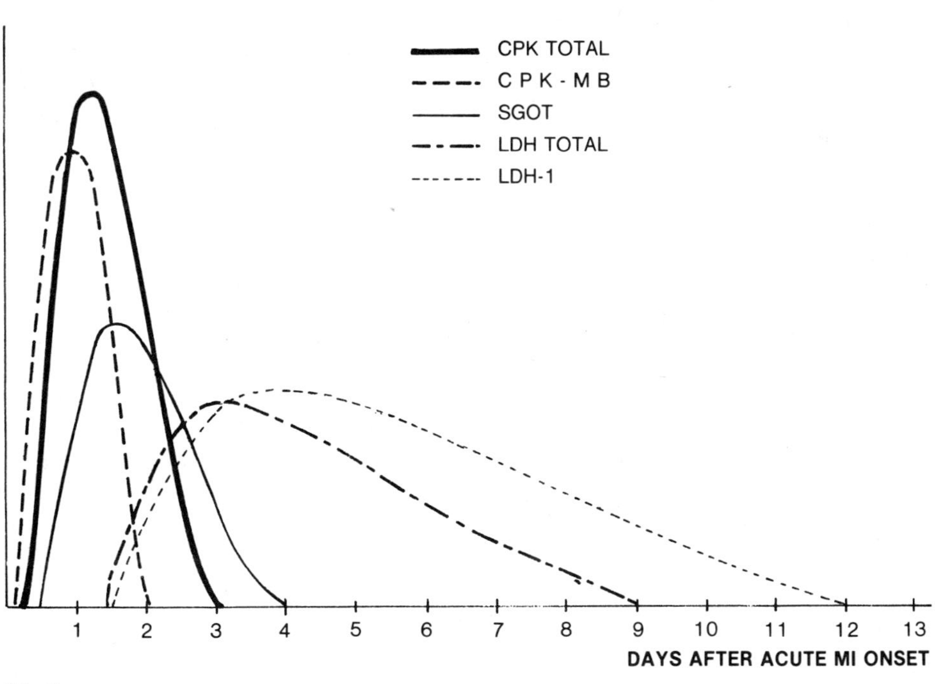

FIG 20–2.
Laboratory tests in acute MI.

in muscles such as the gastrocnemius; total CPK of type 1 fibers only contains about 1% CPK-MB (range, 0%–4%) in addition to CPK-MM. Type 2 fibers predominate in the soleus muscle and comprise 40% of the fibers in such muscles as the quadriceps. The total CPK of type 2 fibers contains 2%–10% CPK-MB in addition to CPK-MM. In Duchenne's muscular dystrophy, especially in the earlier stages, serum levels of CPK-MB may be increased, presumably due to skeletal muscle type 2 involvement, with CPK-MM levels increased to a much greater degree. An increase in CPK-MB value may also occur in some patients with gangrene or severe ischemia of the extremities. In addition, patients with acute myositis of various types, long-distance runners, idiopathic myoglobinemia, Reye's syndrome, and Rocky Mountain spotted fever frequently display some degree of CPK-MB elevation.

When acute skeletal muscle hypoxia or other injury of sufficient degree elevates CPK-MB levels above the upper limit of the reference range in terms of CPK-MB units, CPK-MM levels are usually increased at the same time and to a greater degree. Because of the CPK-MM increase, the CPK-MB level (although it may be increased) usually remains less than 5% of total CPK. Therefore, when the CPK-MB value is increased, it is very helpful to know the total CPK value in order to calculate the percentage of CPK relative to total CPK. If the CPK-MB level in terms of units is not increased, the percentage of CPK-MB is not useful and may be misleading (e.g., if normal CPK-MB levels are 0–10 units and normal total CPK levels are 0–40 units, a CPK-MB level of 2 units is 20% of a total CPK value of 10 units, even though both values are well within reference range).

CPK-MB Fraction in Defibrillation, Coronary Angiography, and Coronary Angioplasty.—In patients undergoing defibrillation or cardiac resuscitation, the CPK-MB value is usually normal unless actual myocardial injury (e.g., contusion) takes place. At least one report indicates that the CPK-MB value is normal in most patients with myocarditis, pericarditis, and subacute bacterial endocarditis, even when LDH isoenzymes display a "cardiac" pattern. Coronary angiography and even coronary angioplasty are likewise reported to be associated with normal MB values unless some degree of myocardial infarction is occurring. In open heart surgery, such as coronary artery revascularization, a CPK-MB isoenzyme elevation raises the question of MI, even though operative manipulation of the heart takes place. Nearly 15% of such patients (ranging from 1%–37%) have displayed CPK-MB elevation just prior to operation. Others have CPK-MB increase during institution of cardiopulmonary bypass or during anesthesia induction before actual cardiac surgery begins.

Elevation of Total CPK Values vs. CPK-MB Fraction Values.—Some laboratories do not perform CPK-MB assay unless the total CPK value is elevated. However, reports indicate that about 10% of acute MI patients (literature range 0%–16%) demonstrate elevated CPK-MB levels with the total CPK value remaining within reference range limits. This is especially common in persons with relatively small muscle mass, whose preinfarct normal total CPK value is apt to be in the lower part of the population reference range.

Creatine Phosphokinase BB Fraction.—Elevation of the CPK-BB value is not common. It is occasionally elevated after pulmonary embolization, and one report indicated that it may occasionally be increased in some patients who undergo cardiopulmonary resuscitation or in some patients in shock. It has also been reported in a few patients with some types of cancer (more often widespread and most frequently in prostate and lung small-cell carcinoma) but not sufficiently often to be useful as a screening test. In brain disorders, where one theoretically would expect release of CPK-BB, the actual isoenzyme detected in serum is usually CPK-MM. In some patients (especially those with chronic renal disease) an unusually accentuated albumin may be mistaken for CPK-BB on electrophoresis, since albumin migrates between MB and BB.

Creatine Phosphokinase MB Fraction Technical Problems and Pseudo-MB Substances.—Creatine phosphokinase isoenzyme fractionation can be performed in several ways. The most commonly used techniques are column chromatography, electrophoresis, and immunoinhibition. The accuracy of column chromatography depends to some extent on the method used. The major disadvantage is the tendency in some kits for some MM isoenzyme to carry over into the MB fraction if the value of the MM fraction is greatly increased. In addition, some patients have a variant of BB isoenzyme called "macro-CK" (or "macro-CK type 1") in which BB isoenzyme becomes complexed to gamma globulin, with the resulting complex migrating electrophoretically between MM and MB instead of in the usual BB location on the opposite (anodal) side of MB from MM. Macro-CK is carried into the MB elution fraction in ordinary CPK isoenzyme column methods and, if it is present, can falsely increase apparent MB values. Macro-CK is reported present in about 1% of all CPK-MB isoenzyme studies (literature range, 0.2%–1.8%), and in one report it accounted for about 8% of elevated CPK-MB results. Another CPK-MB method is electrophoresis. Electrophoresis is reasonably sensitive, although there is some variation among different methods. Electrophoresis is more specific than column chromatography (and immunoinhibition methods, discussed later) since the various isoenzyme fractions can be inspected visually, and therefore atypically migrating CPK variants such as macro-CK can be detected. However, macro-CK may be falsely included with CPK-MB even with electrophoresis when automatic electrophoretic fraction quantitation devices are used or the technologist does not inspect the pattern carefully before manually quantitating the major isoenzyme fractions. Immunoinhibition methods are becoming widely used. Most kits currently available are based on elimination of the M subunit and measurement of the B subunit. This measures both MB and BB together. The rationale for this is the infrequency of elevated BB values. However, macro-CK is detected and produces falsely elevated MB results. Several immunoassay methods that are not affected by macro-CK are now available, and it is helpful to ask the laboratory whether their method will be affected.

Other variant CPK isoenzymes besides macro-CK have been reported. The best characterized one is a macromolecular CPK isoenzyme variant derived from mitochondria (mitochondrial CK, or Macro-CK type 2), which electrophoretically migrates cathodal to MM (on the other side of MM from MB). In the few reports in which data are provided, 0.8%–2.6% of patients who had CPK-MB studies done had mitochondrial CK present. It was present more often in patients with cancer than in those with other conditions and tended to be associated with a poor prognosis. In addition to CPK isoenzyme variants, there is an enzyme called "adenylate kinase," present in RBCs as well as certain other tissues, which electrophoretically migrates in the same area as mitochondrial CK. Specimens with visible degrees of RBC hemolysis may contain increased adenylate kinase, which, in turn, may falsely increase (apparent) CPK-MB results unless there is some way to detect the problem. Hemolysis, whether artifactual or due to hemolytic or megaloblastic anemia, may also elevate LDH-1 isoenzyme values, which adds to the potential for misdiagnosis of acute MI.

Radionuclide Heart Scan

Heart scanning can now be performed in two ways. Scan for acute MI is done with technetium pyrophosphate or certain other radiopharmaceuticals. These agents localize in acutely damaged myocardium, producing a focal area of increased radioactivity. The scan is not reliable less than 24 hours after onset of infarct and returns to normal by 6–7 days after infarct. Best results are obtained with transmural infarcts and with locations in the anterior and lateral walls of the left ventricle. Subendocardial infarcts, especially small ones, are much more likely to be missed. Another consideration is the necessity of transporting the patient to the scanner, unless the institution is one of the few that have a portable unit. Combined use of CPK and LDH isoenzyme determinations has lessened scan necessity in diagnosis. Heart scanning may, however, assist in the diagnosis of acute MI that occurs during or after cardiac surgery, when enzyme or isoenzyme diagnosis is not reliable. Some additional areas of difficulty in myocardial scanning include the fact that size of the scan abnormality cannot at present be reliably correlated with infarct size. Ventricular aneurysms may concentrate the phosphate radiopharmaceuticals in a manner suggesting infarct, and this unexplained capability may persist for years.

Heart scanning can also be done by using radioactive elements, such as thallium, that localize in viable myocardium. Scars and infarcts are seen as areas without uptake. Areas of ischemia (if sufficiently large) also may be detected by scanning before and after exercise.

The optimal scan time for acute MI is within 6 hours after onset of chest pain. After 24 hours, reports indicate that as many as 25% of patients may not demonstrate a lesion. Therefore, optimal scan times for thallium and for pyrophosphate are quite different.

PULMONARY EMBOLISM

Pulmonary emboli are often difficult both to diagnose and to confirm. Sudden dyspnea is the most common symptom; but clinically there may be any combination of chest pain, dyspnea, and possibly hemoptysis. Diseases that must be also considered are acute MI and pneumonia. Pulmonary embolism is often associated with chronic congestive heart failure, cor pulmonale, postoperative complications of major surgery, and fractures of the pelvis or lower extremities, all situations in which MI itself is more likely. The classic x-ray finding of a wedge-shaped lung shadow is often absent or late in developing, because not all cases of embolism develop actual pulmonary infarction, even when the embolus is large.

Laboratory tests in pulmonary embolism have not been very helpful. Initial reports of a characteristic test triad (elevated total bilirubin and LDH values with normal AST) proved disappointing, because only 20%–25% of patients display this combination. Reports that LDH values are elevated in 80% of patients are probably optimistic. In addition, LDH values may be elevated in MI or liver passive congestion, conditions that could mimic or be associated with embolism. Theoretically, LDH isoenzyme fractionation should help, since the classic isoenzyme pattern of pulmonary embolism is a fraction 3 increase. Unfortunately this technique also has proved disappointing, since a variety of patterns have been found in embolization (some due to complication of embolization, such as liver congestion), and fraction 3 may be normal. Total CPK initially was advocated to differentiate embolization (normal CPK) from MI (elevated CPK value), but later reports indicate that the total CPK value may become elevated in some patients with embolism. The CPK isoenzymes, however, are reliable in confirming MI, and a normal CPK-MB value plus normal LDH-1/LDH-2 ratio (obtained at proper times) is also reliable in ruling out MI.

Arterial oxygen saturation has been proposed as a screening test for pulmonary embolism, since most patients with embolism develop arterial oxygen saturation values less than 80 mm Hg. However, 10%–15% of patients with pulmonary embolization have oxygen saturation greater than 80 mm Hg, and 5%–6% have values greater than 90%. Conversely, many patients have chronic lung disease or other reasons for decreased oxygen saturation; so that in many patients one would need a previous normal test result to interpret the value after a possible embolism.

The most useful screening procedure for pulmonary embolism is the lung scan. Serum albumin is tagged with a radioisotope, and the tagged albumin molecules are treated in such a way as to cause aggregation into larger molecular groups (50–100 μm). This material is injected into a vein, passes through the right side of the heart, and is sent into the pulmonary artery. The molecules then are trapped in small arterioles of the pulmonary artery circulation, so that a radiation detector scan of the lungs shows a diffuse radioactive uptake throughout both lungs from these trapped radioactive molecules. A scan is a visual chart of the radioactivity counts over a specified area that are received by the radiation detector. The isotope solution is too dilute to cause any difficulty by its partial occlusion of the pulmonary circulation; only a small percentage of the arterioles are affected, and the albumin is metabolized in 3–4 hours. If a part of the pulmonary artery circulation is already occluded by a thrombus, the isotope does not reach that part of the lung, and the portion of lung affected does not show any uptake on the scan (abnormal scan).

The lung scan becomes abnormal immediately after total occlusion of the pulmonary artery or any branches of the pulmonary artery that are of significant size. There does not have to be actual pulmonary infarction, since the scan results do not depend on tissue necrosis, only on mechanical vessel occlusion. However, in conditions that temporarily or permanently occlude or cut down lung vascularity, there will be varying degrees of abnormality on lung scan; these conditions include cysts, abscesses, many cases of carcinoma, scars, and a considerable number of pneumonias, especially when necrotizing. However, many of these conditions may be at least tentatively ruled out by comparison of the scan results with a chest x-ray film. A chest x-ray film should therefore be obtained with the lung scan.

Asthma in the acute phase may also produce focal perfusion defects due to bronchial obstruction. These disappear after treatment and therefore can mimic emboli. Congestive heart failure or pulmonary edema frequently causes multiple perfusion abnormalities on the lung scan. This is a major problem in the elderly, since dyspnea is one of the symptoms associated with embolization or may be a source of confusion when emphysema and emboli coexist. Emphysema abnormality can be differentiated from that of embolization by a follow-up lung scan after 6–8 days. Defects due to emphysema persist unaltered, whereas those due to emboli tend to change configuration. The repeat study could be performed earlier but with increased risk of insufficient time lapse to permit diagnostic changes.

The lung scan, like the chest x-ray, is nonspecific; that is, a variety of conditions produce abnormality. Certain findings increase the probability of embolization and serial studies provide the best information. In some cases, a xenon ventilation study (chapter 35) may help differentiate emboli from other etiologies of perfusion defect; but when congestive heart failure is present, when the defect is small, and when embolization is superimposed on severe emphysema, the xenon study may not be reliable. Pulmonary artery angiography provides a more definitive answer than the lung scan; but it is a relatively complicated invasive procedure, entails some risk, and may miss small peripheral clots. The lung scan, therefore, is more useful than angiography as a screening procedure. A normal lung scan effectively rules out pulmonary embolization. A minimum of four lung scan views (anterior, posterior, and both lateral projections) is required to constitute an adequate perfusion lung scan study.

SARCOIDOSIS

This disease, of as yet unknown etiology, is manifested by noncaseating granulomatous lesions in many organ systems, most commonly in the lungs and thoracic lymph nodes. The disease is much more common in blacks. Laboratory studies may suggest or support the diagnosis. Anemia is not frequent but appears in about 5% of cases. Splenomegaly is present in 10%–30% of cases. Leukopenia is found in approximately 30%. Eosinophilia is reported in 10%–60%, averaging 25% of cases. Thrombocytopenia is very uncommon, reported in less than 2% of patients in several large series. Serum protein abnormalities are common, with polyclonal hyperglobulinemia in nearly 50% of patients and with albumin levels frequently decreased. Hypercalcemia is reported in about 20% of cases, with a range in the literature of 2%–55%. Uncommonly, primary hyperparathyroidism and sarcoidosis coexist. Alkaline phosphatase (ALP) levels are elevated in nearly 35% of cases, which probably reflects either liver or bone involvement.

The major diagnostic tests that have been used include the Kveim skin test, biopsy (usually of lymph nodes), and assay of angiotensin-converting enzyme (ACE).

The Kveim test consists of intradermal inoculation of an antigen composed of human sarcoidal tissue. A positive reaction is indicated by development of a papule in 4–6 weeks, which, on biopsy, yields the typical noncaseating granulomas of sarcoidosis. The test is highly reliable, yielding less than 3% false positives. The main difficulty is inadequate supplies of sufficiently potent antigen. For this reason, few laboratories are equipped to do the Kveim test. Between 40% and 80% of cases give positive results, depending on the particular lot of antigen and the duration of disease. In chronic sarcoidosis (duration more than 6 months after onset of illness), the patient is less likely to have a positive result on the Kveim test. Steroid treatment depresses the Kveim reaction and may produce a negative test result. The value of the Kveim test is especially great when no enlarged lymph nodes are available for biopsy, when granulomas obtained from biopsy are nonspecific, or when diagnosis on an outpatient basis is necessary. One report has challenged the specificity of the Kveim test, suggesting that a positive test is related more to chronic lymphadenopathy than to any specific disease.

Biopsy is the most widely used diagnostic procedure at present. Peripheral lymph nodes are involved in 60%–95% of cases, although often they are small. The liver is said to show involvement in 75% of cases, although it is palpable in 20% or less. Difficulties with biopsy stem primarily from the fact that the granuloma of sarcoidosis, although characteristic, is nonspecific. Other diseases that sometimes or often produce a similar histologic pattern are early miliary tuberculosis, histoplasmosis, some fungal diseases, some pneumoconioses, and the so-called pseudosarcoid reaction sometimes found in lymph nodes draining areas of carcinoma.

Angiotensin-converting enzyme (ACE) is found in lung epithelial cells and converts angiotensin I (derived from inactive plasma angiotensinogen in a reaction catalyzed by renin) to the vasoconstrictor angiotensin II. It has been found that serum ACE values are elevated in approximately 75%–80% of patients with active sarcoidosis (literature range, 45%–86%). Sensitivity is much less in patients with inactive sarcoidosis (11% in one report) or in patients undergoing therapy. Unfortunately, 5%–10% of ACE elevations are not due to sarcoidosis (literature range, 1%–33%). The highest incidence of ACE abnormality in diseases other than sarcoidosis is seen in Gaucher's disease, leprosy, active histoplasmosis, and alcoholic cirrhosis. Other conditions include tuberculosis, non-Hodgkin's lymphoma, Hodgkin's disease, scleroderma, hyperthyroidism, myeloma, pulmonary embolization, nonalcoholic cirrhosis, and idiopathic pulmonary fibrosis. Usually patients with these diseases (and normal persons) have a less than 5% incidence of elevated ACE values. However, either normal or increased ACE levels must be interpreted with caution. Angiotensin-converting enzyme levels are useful to follow a patient's response to therapy. Certain conditions such as adult respiratory distress syndrome, diabetes, hypothyroidism, and any severe illness may decrease ACE levels.

ERYTHROCYTE SEDIMENTATION RATE

The erythrocyte sedimentation rate (ESR) is determined by filling a calibrated tube of standard diameter with anticoagulated whole blood and measuring the rate of RBC sedimentation during a specified period, usually 1 hour. When the RBCs settle toward the bottom of the tube, they leave an increasingly large zone of clear plasma, which is the area measured. Most changes in RBC sedimentation rate are caused by alterations in plasma proteins, mainly fibrinogen, with a much smaller contribution from alpha-2 globulins. Fibrinogen increases 12–24 hours after onset of an acute inflammatory process or acute tissue injury. Many conditions cause abnormally great RBC sedimentation (rate of fall in the tube system). These include acute and chronic infection, tissue necrosis and infarction, well-established malignancy, rheumatoid-collagen diseases, abnormal serum proteins, and certain physiologic stress situations such as pregnancy or marked obesity. The ESR is frequently increased in patients with chronic renal failure, with or without dialysis. In one study, 75% had Westergren ESRs more than 30 mm/hour, and some had marked elevations. Marked elevation of the Westergren ESR (defined as a value > 100 mm/hour) was reported in one study to be caused by infectious diseases, neoplasia, noninfectious inflammatory conditions, and chronic renal disease. This degree of ESR abnormality was found in about 4% of patients who had ESR determined. Erythrocyte sedimentation rate determination has three major uses: (1) as an aid in detection and diagnosis of inflammatory conditions or to help exclude the possibility of such conditions; (2) as a means of following the activity, clinical course, or therapy of diseases with an inflammatory component, such as rheumatoid arthritis, acute rheumatic fever or acute glomerulonephritis; and (3) to demonstrate or confirm the presence of occult organic disease, either when the patient has symptoms but no definite physical or laboratory evidence of organic disease or when the patient is completely asymptomatic.

The ESR has three main limitations: (1) it is a very nonspecific test, (2) it is sometimes normal in diseases where usually it is abnormal, and (3) technical factors may considerably influence the results. The tubes must be absolutely vertical; even small degrees of tilt have great effect on degree of sedimentation. Most types of anemia falsely increase the ESR as determined by the Wintrobe method. The Wintrobe method may be "corrected" for anemia by using a nomogram, but this is not accurate. The Westergren method has a widespread reputation for being immune to the effects of anemia, but studies have shown that anemia does have a significant effect on the Westergren method (although not quite as much as the Wintrobe method). Although no well-accepted method is available to correct the Westergren ESR for effect of anemia, one report included a formula that is easy to use and provides a reasonable degree of correction: Corrected (Westergren) ESR = ESR − [(Std. Ht − Actual Ht) × 1.75], where Std. Ht (standard hematocrit) is 45 for males and 42 for females.

Besides anemia and changes in fibrinogen and alpha-2 globulins, other factors affect the ESR. Changes in serum proteins that alter plasma viscosity influence RBC sedimentation. A classic example is the marked increase in ESR seen with the abnormal globulins of myeloma. Certain diseases such as sickle cell anemia and polycythemia falsely decrease the ESR. The majority (but not all) investigators report that normal values are age related; at least 10 mm/hour should be added to young adult values after age 60. Some use a formula for Westergren values: for men, age in years ÷ 2; for women, (age in years +10) ÷ 2.

Zeta Sedimentation Rate

Blood in vertical capillary tubes is subjected to low-speed centrifugation in a special Zeta sedimentation rate (ZSR) centrifuge that alternates directions of spin for several cycles. The RBCs are thrown against the capillary wall in a zigzag pattern; the end point is measurement of the packed cell mass similarly to a hematocrit, with the result then being compared with the ordinary hematocrit of the specimen. The ZSR is not affected by anemia but is affected by most of the other conditions that alter the ESR. Since the ZSR requires a special centrifuge, the procedure is not available in most laboratories.

C-Reactive Protein

C-reactive protein (CRP) is a glycoprotein produced during acute inflammation or tissue destruction. The protein gets its name from its ability to react (or cross-react) with *Pneumococcus* somatic C-polysaccharide and precipitate it. The CRP level is not influenced by anemia or plasma protein changes. It begins to rise about 4–6 hours after onset of inflammation and has a half-life of 5–7 hours, less than one-fourth that of most other proteins that react to acute inflammation. For many years the standard technique was a slide or tube precipitation method, with the degree of reaction estimated visually and reported semiquantitatively. The test never enjoyed the same popularity as the ESR because the result was not quantitative and the end point was difficult to standardize due to subjective visual estimations. Recently, new methods such as rate reaction nephelometry and fluorescent immunoassay have enabled true quantitative CRP measurement. C-reactive protein determination using the new quantitative methods offers several important advantages over the ESR, including lack of interference by anemia or serum protein changes, fewer technical problems, and greater sensitivity to acute inflammation because of shorter half-life of the protein being measured. Many now consider quantitative CRP measurements the procedure of choice to detect and monitor acute inflammation and acute tissue destruction. Erythrocyte sedimentation rate determination is preferred, however, in chronic inflammation. There is some evidence that CRP levels are useful in evaluation of postoperative recovery. Normally, CRP reaches a peak value 48–72 hours after surgery and then begins to fall, entering the reference range 5–7 days after operation. Failure to decrease significantly after 3 days postoperatively or a decrease followed by an increase suggests postoperative infection or tissue necrosis. For maximal information and easier interpretation of the data, a preoperative CRP level should be obtained with serial postoperative CRP determinations.

General clinical indications for CRP are essentially the same as those listed for the ESR.

FAT EMBOLIZATION

Fat embolization is most often associated with severe bone trauma, but may also occur in fatty liver, diabetes, and other conditions. Symptoms may be immediate or delayed. If they are immediate, shock is frequent. Delayed symptoms occur 2–3 days after injury, and pulmonary or cerebral manifestations are most prominent. Frequent signs are fever, tachycardia, tachypnea, upper body petechiae (50% of patients), and decreased hemoglobin values. Laboratory diagnosis includes urine examination for free fat (special technique, chapter 12), results of which are positive in 50% of cases during the first 3 days; and serum lipase, results of which are elevated in nearly 50% of patients from about day 3 to day 7. Fat in sputum is unreliable; there are many false positive and negative results. Chest x-ray films sometimes demonstrate diffuse tiny infiltrates, occasionally coalescing, described in the literature as having a "snowstorm" appearance. Some patients have a laboratory picture suggestive of disseminated intravascular coagulation. One report has indicated that diagnosis by cryostat frozen section of peripheral blood clot is sensitive and specific, but adequate confirmation of this method is not yet available. The most sensitive test for fat embolism is said to be a decrease in arterial PO_2, frequently to levels less than 60%. However, patients with chronic lung disease may already have decreased PO_2.

SELECTED TESTS OF INTEREST IN PEDIATRICS

Neonatal Immunoglobulin Levels.—Maternal IgG can cross the placenta, but IgA or IgM cannot. Chronic infections involving the fetus, such as congenital syphilis, toxoplasmosis, rubella, and cytomegalic inclusion disease, induce IgM production by the fetus. Increased IgM levels in cord blood at birth or in neonatal blood during the first few days of life suggest chronic intrauterine infection. Infection near term or subsequent to birth results in an IgM increase beginning 6–7 days postpartum. Unfortunately, there are pitfalls when such data are interpreted. Many cord blood samples become contaminated with maternal blood, thus falsely raising IgM values. Normal values are controversial; 20 mg/dl is the most widely accepted upper limit. Various techniques have different reliabilities and sensitivities. Finally, some investigators state that fewer than 40% of rubella or cytomegalovirus infections during pregnancy produce elevated IgM levels before birth.

Agammaglobulinemia.—This condition may lead to frequent infections. Electrophoresis displays decreased gamma globulin levels, which can be confirmed by quantitative measurement of IgG, IgA, and IgM. There are several methods available to quantitatively measure IgG, IgA, and IgM such as radial immunodiffusion, immunonephelometry, and immunoassay. Immunoelectrophoresis provides only semiquantitative estimations of the immunoglobulins and should not be requested if quantitative values for IgG, IgA, or IgM are desired.

Nitroblue Tetrazolium Test.—Chronic granulomatous disease of childhood is a rare sex-linked disorder of the white blood cells (WBCs) that is manifested by repeated infections and that ends in death before puberty. Polymorphonuclear leukocytes are able to attack high-virulence organisms, such as streptococci and pneumococci, which do not produce the enzyme catalase, but are unable to destroy staphylococci and certain organisms of lower virulence such as the gram-negative rods, which are catalase producers. Normal blood granulocytes are able to phagocytize yellow nitroblue tetrazolium (NBT) dye particles and then precipitate and convert (reduce) this substance to a dark blue. The test is reported as the percentage of granulocytes containing blue dye particles. Monocytes also ingest NBT, but they are not counted when performing the test. Granulocytes from patients with chronic granulomatous disease are able to phagocytize but not convert the dye particles, so that the NBT result will be very low or zero, and the NBT test is used to screen for this disorder. Because neutrophils increase their phagocytic activity during acute bacterial infection, the nitroblue tetrazolium test has been used to separate persons with bacterial infection from persons with leukocytosis of other etiologies. In general, acute bacterial infection increases the NBT count, whereas viral or tuberculous infections do not. It has also been advocated as a screening test for infection when the WBC count is normal and as a means to differentiate bacterial and viral infection in febrile patients. Except for chronic granulomatous disease there is a great divergence of opinion in the literature on the merits of the NBT test, apportioned about equally between those who find it useful and those who believe that it is not reliable because of unacceptable degrees of overlap among patients in various diagnostic categories. Many modifications of the original technique have been proposed that add to the confusion, including variations in anticoagulants, incubation temperature, smear thickness, method of calculating data, and use of phagocytosis "stimulants," all of which may affect test results.

Some conditions other than bacterial infection that may elevate the NBT score (false positives) include normal infants aged less than 2 months, echovirus infection, malignant lymphomas (especially Hodgkin's disease), hem-

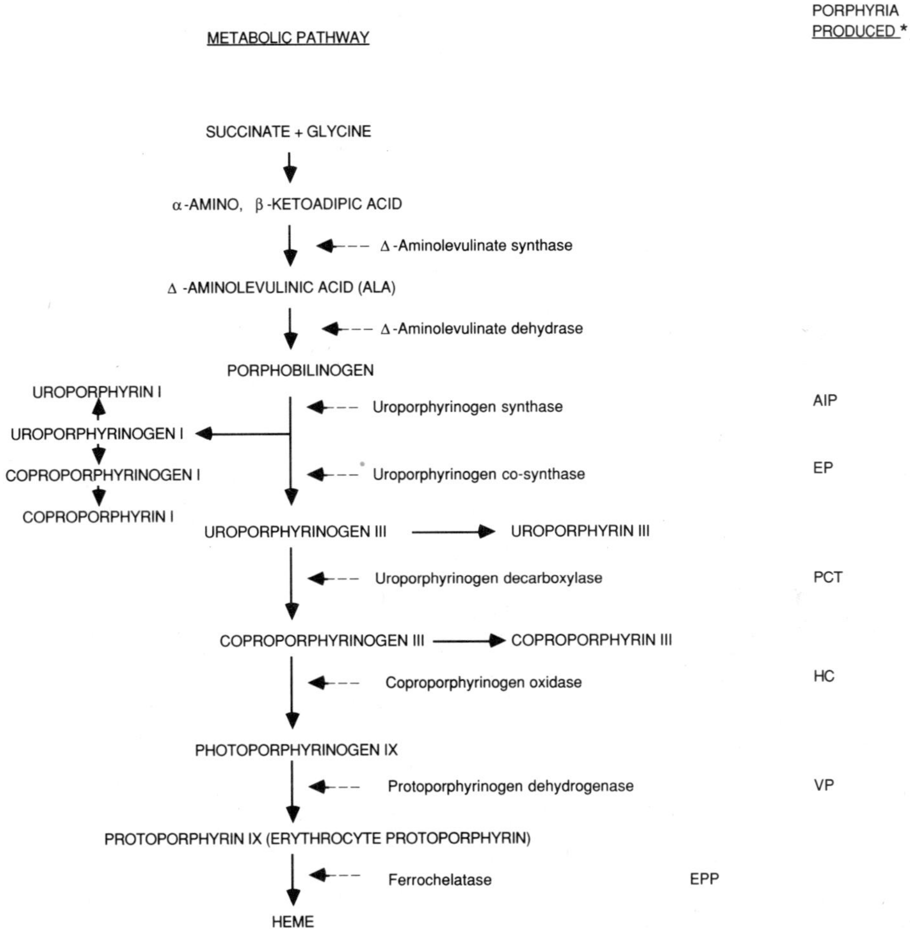

FIG 20–3.
Porphyrin synthesis. * = porphyria category resulting from specific enzyme deficiency.

ophilia A, malaria, certain parasitic infestations, *Candida albicans* and *Nocardia* infections, and possibly the use of oral contraceptives. Certain conditions may (to varying degree) induce normal scores in the presence of bacterial infection (false negatives); these include antibiotic therapy, localized infection, systemic lupus erythematosus, sickle cell anemia, diabetes mellitus, agammaglobulinemia, and certain anti-inflammatory medications (corticosteroids, phenylbutazone).

PORPHYRIAS

In porphyric diseases, the main similarity is the abnormal secretion of substances that are precursors of the porphyrin compound heme (of hemoglobin). The known pathways of porphyrin synthesis begin with glycine and succinate, which are combined to eventually form a compound known as δ-aminolevulinic acid (ALA). This goes on to produce a substance known as "porphobilinogen," composed of a single pyrrole ring. Four of these rings are joined to form the tetrapyrrole compound proporphyrinogen; this is the precursor of protoporphyrin, which, in turn, is the precursor of heme (Fig 20–3). The tetrapyrrole compounds exist in eight isomers, depending on where certain side groups are located. The only isomeric forms that are clinically important are I and III. Normally, very small amounts of porphyrin degradation products appear in the feces or in the urine; these are called "coproporphyrins" or "uroporphyrins" (their names refer to where they were first discovered, but both may appear in either urine or feces).

The porphyrias have been classified in several ways, none of which is entirely satisfactory. The most common system includes erythropoietic porphyria (EP), hepatic porphyria, porphyria cutanea tarda (PCT), and acquired (toxic) porphyria (Table 20–3). Erythropoietic porphyria is a small group of rare congenital diseases characterized clinically by skin photosensitivity without vesicle formation, pink discoloration of the teeth that fluoresces under ultraviolet light, and sometimes mild hemolytic anemia. If erythropoietic porphyria is suspected, the best diagnostic test is measurement of erythrocyte porphyrin.

Hereditary hepatic porphyria may be subdivided into three types: acute intermittent porphyria (AIP) (Swedish genetic porphyria), variegate porphyria (VP) (South African genetic porphyria), and hereditary coproporphyria (HC). All three are inherited as autosomal dominants, and all three may be associated with episodes of acute porphyric attacks, although such attacks are more widely publicized in association with AIP. All three subdivisions manifest increases in the enzyme ALA-synthetase, which catalyzes formation of ALA from its precursors. Acute intermittent porphyria is characterized by a decrease of 50% or more in the enzyme uroporphyrinogen-I-synthetase (abbreviated URO-I-S and also known as "porphobilinogen deaminase"), which catalyzes the formation of uroporphyrinogen I from porphobilinogen. Levels of URO-I-S are said to be normal in VP and HC. Acute intermittent porphyria is not associated with photosensitivity, whereas skin lesions due to photosensitivity are common in VP and also occur in HC. Parenthetically, these skin lesions resemble those of PCT, and some of these patients were probably included in the PCT group in some early classifications. In VP and HC, increased amounts of protoporphyrin are excreted in the feces, whereas this does not happen in AIP. Although AIP, VP, and HC have increased amounts of coproporphyrin in the feces, HC patients excrete much larger amounts of fecal coproporphyrin III than does AIP or VP. Porphyrin excretion patterns in the various porphyrias are summarized in Table 20–4.

Acute Intermittent Porphyria

Uroporphyrinogen-I-synthetase is said to be decreased in all patients with AIP. However, about 5%–10% of AIP patients have values within the reference range, so that some over-

TABLE 20–3.
Classification of the Porphyrias

	Heredity	Photosensitivity and/or Skin Involvement	Onset	Acute Symptoms: Abdominal Pain or Psychologic Symptoms
Erythropoietic				
Erythropoietic porphyria (EP)	Recessive	Yes	Infancy	No
Erythropoietic protoporphyria (EPP)	Dominant	Yes	Infancy	No
Hepatic				
Acute intermittent porphyria (AIP)	Dominant	No	Adolescence	Yes
Variegate porphyria (VP)	Dominant	Variable	Young adult	Variable
Hereditary coproporphyria (HC)	Dominant	Variable	Young adult	Yes
Porphyria cutanea tarda (PCT)	Familial = dominant Sporadic = renal dialysis	Yes	All ages (peak in middle age)	No
Erythropoietic and hepatic				
Hepatoerythropoietic porphyria (HEP)	Recessive	Yes	Childhood	No
Acquired (toxic)				
Drug-induced	N/A	Yes	Variable	No
Lead	N/A	No	Variable	Yes

TABLE 20–4.
Prophyrin Excretion in the Porphyrias*

	Urine	Feces	RBCs
EP	Great increase in UP level Small increase in CP level	Small increase in CP and PP levels	Considerable increase in PP level Mild increase in CP level
EPP	Normal UP and CP levels	Small increase in CP level Moderate increase in PP level	Considerable increase in PP level
AIP	Considerable increase in PBG level Moderate increase in ALA level Mild increase in UP level Smaller increase in CP level	Normal CP and PP levels	
VP	Increased PBG and ALA levels only during attacks Mild increase in CP level Smaller increase in UP level	Considerable increase in PP level Smaller increase in CP level	
HC	Mild increase in PBG and ALA levels Moderate increase CP, smaller increase in UP level	Great increase in CP level Mild increase in PP level	
PCT	Considerable increase in UP level Smaller increase in CP level	Mild increase in CP level Smaller increase in PP level	
Lead poisoning	Increase in ALA level Mild increase in CP level		Increase in PP level
Organochemical toxicity	Same as PCT	Same as PCT	

*UP = uroporphyrin; CP = coproporphyrin; PP = protoporphyrin; PBG = porphobilinogen.

lap occurs. Uroporphyrinogen-I-synthetase is also said to be decreased in relatives of patients with AIP, again with some overlap at the borderline areas of the reference range. At least one kindred with a condition closely resembling AIP has been reported with normal URO-I-S levels, but the significance of this is not clear. There may be some laboratory variation in results, and equivocal results may have to be repeated. Blood samples should be stored frozen and kept frozen during transit to the laboratory to avoid artifactual decrease in enzyme activity. Therefore, falsely low URO-I-S values may be obtained through improper specimen handling. Hemolytic anemia or reticulocytosis greater than 5% may produce an increase in URO-I-S activity. Assay for URO-I-S is available mostly in university medical centers and large reference laboratories.

The acute porphyric attacks consist of colicky abdominal pain, vomiting, and constipation (> 80% of patients); and mental symptoms (10%–30% of patients) such as confusion, psychotic behavior, and occasionally even convulsions. About one half of the patients display hypertension and some type of muscle motor weakness. The attacks are frequently accompanied by leukocytosis. These attacks may be precipitated by certain medications (especially by barbiturates; see chapter 36), by estrogens, and by carbohydrate deprivation (dieting or starvation). The attacks usually do not occur until adolescence or adulthood. Porphobilinogen is nearly always present in the urine during the clinical attacks and is an almost pathognomonic finding, but the duration of excretion is highly variable. It may occasionally disappear if not searched for initially. Between attacks, some patients excrete detectable porphobilinogen and others do not. Urine ALA levels are usually increased during acute attacks but not as markedly as porphobilinogen. During remission, ALA levels also may become normal. Patients with AIP may also have hyponatremia and sometimes have falsely elevated thyroxine (T_4) results due to elevated thyroxine-binding protein levels.

Porphobilinogen is usually detected by color reaction with Ehrlich's reagent and confirmed by demonstrating that the color is not removed by chloroform (Watson-Schwartz test). Since false positive results may occur, it is essential to confirm a positive test by butanol (butyl alcohol) extraction. Porphobilinogen will not be extracted by butanol, whereas butanol will remove most of the other Ehrlich-positive, chloroform-negative substances. Therefore, porphobilinogen is not removed by either chloroform or butanol. A positive result on the porphobilinogen test is the key to diagnosis of symptomatic acute porphyria; some investigators believe that analysis and quantitation of urinary porphyrins or ALA are useful only if the Watson-Schwartz test results are equivocal. However, the majority believe that a positive qualitative test result for porphobilinogen should be confirmed by quantitative chemical techniques (available in reference laboratories) due to experience with false positive Watson-Schwartz test results in various laboratories. They also advise quantitative analysis of porphyrins in urine and feces to differentiate the various types of porphyria. Glucose administration may considerably decrease porphobilinogen excretion.

Some investigators prefer the Hoesch test to the modified Watson-Schwartz procedure. The Hoesch test also uses Ehrlich's reagent but is less complicated and is said to be more specific for porphobilinogen (although the possibility of drug-induced false reactions has not been adequately investigated).

Porphyria cutanea tarda is a chronic type of porphyria. There usually is some degree of photosensitivity, but it does not develop until after puberty. There often is some degree of liver disease. No porphobilinogen is excreted and acute porphyric attacks do not occur.

Toxic porphyria may be produced by a variety of chemicals, but the most common is lead. Lead poisoning produces abnormal excretion of coproporphyrin III but not of uroporphyrin III. ALA excretion is also increased.

TESTS FOR ALLERGY

The atopic diseases were originally defined as sensitization based on hereditary predisposition (thus differentiating affected persons from nonaffected persons exposed to the same commonly found antigens) and characterized by immediate urticarial skin reaction to offending antigen and by the Prausnitz-Küstner reaction. Prausnitz and Küstner demonstrated in 1921 that serum from a sensitized person, when injected into the skin of a nonsensitized person, would produce a cutaneous reaction on challenge with appropriate antigen (cutaneous passive transfer). The serum factor responsible was known as reagin (skin-sensitizing antibody). In 1966, reagin was found to be IgE, which has subsequently been shown to trigger immediate local hypersensitivity reactions by causing release of histamines and vasoactive substances from mast cells, which, in turn, produce local anaphylaxis in skin or mucous membranes. The IgE system thus mediates atopic dermatitis, allergic rhinitis, and many cases of asthma. In patients with rhinitis, nasal itching is the most suggestive symptom of IgE-associated allergy. Allergens may come from the environment (pollens, foods, allergenic dust, molds), certain chronic infections (fungus, parasites), medications (penicillin), or industrial sources (cosmetics, chemicals). Sometimes there is a strong hereditary component; sometimes none is discernible. Discovery that IgE is the key substance in these reactions has led to measurement of serum IgE levels as a test for presence of atopic allergy sensitization.

Total Immunoglobulin E Levels

Serum total IgE levels are currently measured by some type of immunoassay technique. The most common method is a paper-based radioimmunosorbent test procedure. Values are age dependent until adulthood. Considerably elevated values are characteristically found in persons with allergic disorders, such as atopic dermatitis and allergic asthma, and also in certain parasitic infections and *Aspergillus*-associated asthma (chapter 15). Values above reference range, however, may be found in some clinically nonallergic persons and therefore are not specific for allergy. On the other hand, many patients with allergy have total IgE levels within normal population range. It has been reported, however, that total IgE values less than 20 international units/ml suggest small probability of detectable specific IgE. Besides IgE, there is some evidence that IgG4 antibodies may have some role in atopic disorders.

Specific Immunoglobulin E Levels

Specific serum IgE (IgE directed against specific antigens) can be measured rather than total IgE. This is being employed to investigate etiology of asthma and atopic dermatitis. The current system is called the **radioallergosorbent test** (RAST). Specific antigen is bound to a carrier substance and allowed to react with specific IgE antibody. The amount of IgE antibody bound is estimated by adding radioactive anti-IgE antibody and quantitating the amount of labeled anti-IgE attached to the IgE-antigen complex. The type of antigen, the degree and duration of stimulation, and current exposure to antigen all influence IgE levels to any particular antigen at any point in time. Studies thus far indicate that RAST has an 80%–85% correlation with results of skin testing using the subcutaneous injection method (range, 35%–100%, depending on the investigator and the antigen used). It seems a little less sensitive than the intradermal skin test method, but some claim that it predicts the results of therapy better (in other words, it is possibly more specific). Since only a limited number of antigens are available for use in the RAST system, each antigen to be tested for must be listed by the physician. Some advise obtaining a serum total IgE assay in addition to RAST; if results of the RAST panel are negative and the serum IgE level is high, this raises the question of allergy to antigens not included in the RAST panel. Total serum IgE values can be normal, however, even if the findings of one or more antigens on the RAST panel are positive. There is some cross-reaction between certain antigens in the RAST system. The RAST profile is more expensive than skin testing with the same antigens. However, the skin test is uncomfortable, and in a few hyperallergic patients it may even produce anaphylactic shock. Modifications of the RAST technique that are more simple and easy to perform are being introduced, and a dipstick method with a limited number of selected antigens is now commercially available.

Eosinophilia

Peripheral blood eosinophilia is frequently present in persons with active allergic disorders, although a rather large minority of these patients do not display abnormal skin tests. Correlation is said to be better in persons less than 50 years old. Unfortunately, there are many possible causes for peripheral blood eosinophilia (see chapter 6), which makes interpretation more difficult. Presence of more than an occasional eosinophil in sputum suggests an allergic pulmonary condition.

In some patients with nasopharyngeal symptoms, a nasal smear for eosinophils may be helpful. The specimen can be collected with a calcium alginate swab and thin smears prepared on glass slides, which are air-dried and stained (preferably) with Hansel's stain or with Wright's stain. If more than a few eosinophils are present but not neutrophils, this suggests allergy without infection. If neutrophils outnumber eosinophils, this is considered nondiagnostic (neither confirming nor excluding allergy).

LABORATORY TESTS IN PSYCHIATRY

Until recently, the laboratory had relatively little to offer in psychiatry. Laboratory tests were used mainly to diagnose or exclude organic illness. For example, in one study about 5% of patients with dementia had organic diseases such as hyponatremia, hypothyroidism, hypoglycemia, and hypercalcemia; about 4% were caused by alcohol; and about 10% were due to toxic effects of drugs. A few psychiatric drug blood level assays were available, of which lithium was the most important (see chapter 34). In the 1970s, important work was done suggesting that the neuroendocrine system is involved in some way with certain major psychiatric illnesses. Thus far, melancholia (endogenous psychiatric depression or primary depression) is the illness in which neuroendocrine abnormality has been most extensively documented. It was found that many such patients had abnormal cortisol blood levels that were very similar to those seen in Cushing's syndrome (as described in the chapter on adrenal function) without having the typical signs and symptoms of Cushing's syndrome. There often was blunting or abolition of normal cortisol circadian rhythm, elevated urine-free cortisol excretion levels, and resistance to normally expected suppression of cortisol blood levels after a low dose of dexamethasone.

Because of these observations, the low-dose overnight dexamethasone test, used to screen for Cushing's syndrome, has been modified to screen for melancholia. One milligram of oral dexamethasone is given at 11 P.M., and blood is drawn for cortisol assay on the following day at 4 P.M. and 11 P.M. Normally, serum cortisol levels should be suppressed to less than 5 μg/100 ml (138 nmol/L) in both specimens. An abnormal result consists of failure to suppress in at least one of the two specimens (about 20% of melancholia patients demonstrate normal suppression in the 4 P.M. specimen but no suppression in the 11 P.M. specimen; and about the same number of patients fail to suppress in the 4 P.M. specimen but have normal suppression in the 11 P.M. sample). The psychiatric dexamethasone test is different from the dexamethasone test for Cushing's syndrome, because in the Cushing protocol a single specimen is drawn at 8 A.M. in the morning after dexamethasone.

The Cushing's disease protocol is reported to detect only about 25% of patients with melancholia, in contrast to the modified two-specimen psychiatric protocol, which is reported to detect up to 58%. Various investigators using various doses of dexamethasone, and collection times have reported a detection rate of about 45% (literature range, 24%–100%). False positive rates using the two-specimen protocol are reported to be less than 5%. Since some patients with Cushing's syndrome may exhibit symptoms of psychiatric depression, differentiation of melancholia from Cushing's syndrome becomes necessary if test results show nonsuppression of serum cortisol. The patient is given appropriate antidepressant therapy and the test is repeated. If the test result becomes normal, Cushing's syndrome is virtually excluded.

Various conditions not associated with either Cushing's syndrome or melancholia can affect cortisol secretion patterns. Conditions that must be excluded to obtain a reliable result include severe major organic illness of any type, recent electroshock therapy, trauma, severe weight loss, malnutrition, alcoholic withdrawal, pregnancy, Addison's disease, and pituitary deficiency. Certain medications such as phenobarbital, phenytoin (Dilantin), steroid therapy, or estrogens (see Table 36–16) may produce falsely abnormal results.

At present, there is considerable controversy regarding the usefulness of the modified low-dose dexamethasone test for melancholia, since the test has a sensitivity no greater than 50% and significant potential for false-positive results.

Besides the overnight modified low-dose dexamethasone test, the thyrotropin-releasing hormone (TRH) test (chapter 28) has been reported to be abnormal in about 60% of patients with primary (unipolar) depression. Abnormality consists of a blunted (decreased) thyrotropin-stimulating hormone response to administration of TRH, similar to the result obtained in hyperthyroidism or hypopituitarism. Various factors that affect the TRH test are discussed in chapter 28. However, occasional patients with melancholia have hypothyroidism, which produces an exaggerated response in the TRH test rather than a blunted (decreased) response.

One investigator found that about 30% of patients with melancholia had abnormal results on both the TRH and the modified dexamethasone tests. About 30% of the patients had abnormal TRH results but normal dexamethasone responses, and about 20% had abnormal dexamethasone responses but normal TRH responses. The TRH test has not been investigated as extensively as the modified dexamethasone test.

A more controversial area is measurement of 3-methoxy-4-hydroxyphenylglycol (MHPG) in patients with depression. One theory links depression to a functional deficiency of norepinephrine in the CNS. 3-Methoxy-4-hydroxyphenylglycol is a major metabolite of norepinephrine (chapter 29, Fig 29–5). It is thought that a significant part of urinary MHPG is derived from CNS sources (20%–63% in different studies). Some studies indicated that depressed patients had lower urinary (24-hour) excretion of MHPG than other patients, and that patients in the manic phase of bipolar (manic-depressive) illness had increased MHPG levels. There was also some evidence that depressed patients with subnormal urinary MHPG levels responded better to tricyclic antidepressants such as imipramine than did patients with normal urine MHPG levels. However, these findings have been somewhat controversial and have not been universally accepted.

LABORATORY TESTS IN NEUROLOGY

Most laboratory tests concerned with diagnosis or function of the central nervous system are discussed in the chapter on cerebrospinal fluid. The major condition affecting the peripheral nervous system which involves the laboratory is myasthenia gravis.

Myasthenia Gravis

Myasthenia gravis (MG) is manifested primarily by muscle weakness. Clinically, there is especially frequent involvement of cranial nerves, most commonly manifested by diplopia and ptosis. In more serious cases there is difficulty in swallowing. Peripheral nerve involvement tends to affect proximal muscles more severely than distal ones. In the most severe cases there is paralysis of chest respiratory muscles. The disease affects only the eyes in about 20% of cases. Whenever muscles are involved, the degree of muscle weakness may fluctuate over short or long periods of time. The basic problem is located at the neuromuscular junction area of striated muscle. In normal persons, acetylcholine is released at nerve terminals on the proximal side of the neuromuscular junction, and the acetylcholine crosses the nerve-muscle junction and acts on acetylcholine receptor sites in the muscle membrane to set off muscle contraction. In patients with MG, acetylcholine receptor antibodies are present that interfere with the binding of acetylcholine to the receptor sites. The classic test for MG used to be a "therapeutic trial" of drugs such as edrophonium (Tensilon). Assays are now available in reference laboratories for serum acetylcholine receptor antibodies. Current assays are positive in 85%–90% of acute MG patients. The test is less sensitive in congenital MG and MG localized to the eyes; also, test results may become negative with therapy. Definitely elevated levels of acetylcholine receptor antibody are fairly specific for MG, with only a few conditions known to produce false positive results (such as D-penicillamine therapy for rheumatoid arthritis).

It is of interest that about 10% (range, 8.5%–15%) of MG patients have an associated thymoma, and about 50%–60% have hyperplasia of the thymus. Antistriated muscle (antistriational) antibodies have been reported in about 95%–99% of patients with MG plus thymoma and about 30% of patients with thymoma but without MG. Since the incidence of MG in patients with thymoma is about 35% (range, 7%–59%), the test results would be expected to be elevated in about 55% of all thymoma patients. Unfortunately, the test results are also elevated in about 25% of MG patients without thymoma. Therefore, absence of this antibody in a patient with MG is strong evidence against thymoma, but presence of antistriated muscle antibody does not prove that the patient has a thymoma.

Additional tests relevant to this chapter are discussed in chapter 35.

BIBLIOGRAPHY

Hull RD, et al: Pulmonary embolism in outpatients with pleuritic chest pain. *Arch Intern Med* 1988; 148:838.

Nierenberg AA, Feinstein AR: How to evaluate a diagnostic marker test: Lessons from the rise and fall of dexamethasone suppression test. *JAMA* 1988; 259:1699.

Muller JE, et al: Myocardial infarct extension: Occurrence, outcome, and risk factors in the multicenter investigation of limitation of infarct size. *Ann Intern Med* 1988; 108:1.

AMA Council on Scientific Affairs: In vitro testing for allergy. Report II. *JAMA* 1987; 258:1639.

APA Task Force on Laboratory Tests in Psychiatry: The dexamethasone suppression test: An overview of its current status in psychiatry. *Am J Psychiatry* 1987; 144:1253.

Khaw BA, et al: Acute myocardial infarct imaging with indium-111-labeled monoclonal antimyosin Fab. *J Nucl Med* 1987; 28:1671.

Tsapogas MJ: Pulmonary embolism. *Ala J Med Sci* 1987; 24:405.

Mustard RA, et al: Postoperative C-reactive protein detects septic complications. *Arch Surg* 1987; 122:69.

Hoffman DR: Insect-venom allergy: Patho-

physiology and laboratory evaluation. *Lab Mgmt* 1987; 25(8):25.
Schifferli JA, et al: Macro-creatine kinase type 1. *Arch Path Lab Med* 1986; 110:425.
Hong RA, et al: Elevated CK-MB with normal total creatine kinase in suspected myocardial infarction. *Am Heart J* 1986; 111:1041.
Pierce GF, et al: Increased creatine kinase MB in the absence of acute myocardial infarction. *Clin Chem* 1986; 32:2044.
Tinetti ME, et al: Use of the erythrocyte sedimentation rate in chronically ill, elderly patients with a decline in health status. *Am J Med* 1986; 80:844.
Sox HC, et al: The erythrocyte sedimentation rate. *Ann Intern Med* 1986; 104:515.
Shusterman N, et al: The erythrocyte sedimentation rate and chronic renal failure. *Ann Intern Med* 1986; 105:801.
Sekula SA, et al: The porphyrias. *Am Fam Pract* 1986; 33:219.
Hindmarsh JT: The porphyrias: Recent advances. *Clin Chem* 1986; 32:1255.
Lin RY: Serum sickness syndrome. *Am Fam Pract* 1986; 33:157.
Zimmerman M, et al: The validity of the dexamethasone suppression test as a marker for endogenous depression. *Arch Gen Psychiatry* 1986; 43:347.
Lehrer M, Gold MS: Psychiatric laboratory tests: A growing role. *Drug Ther* 1986; 16:124.
Larson EB, et al: Diagnostic tests in the evaluation of dementia. *Arch Intern Med* 1986; 146:1917.
Stein W, et al: Macro creatine kinase type 2: Results of a prospective study in hospitalized patients. *Clin Chem* 1985; 31:1959.
Aalberse RC, et al: IgG4 antibodies in atopic allergy. *Lab Mgmt* 1985; 23(7):19.
Pesce MA: The CK and LD macroenzymes. *Lab Mgmt* 1984; 22(11):29.
Feinberg NV, et al: Serum creatine kinase MB isoenzyme in chronic muscle disease. *Clin Chem* 1984; 30:575.
Smallridge RC: Angiotensin converting enzyme: findings and prospects. *Lab Mgmt* 1984; 22(12):53.
Ramos CE, Tapia RH: C-reactive protein. *Lab Med* 1984; 15:737.
De Leon Jones F, et al: MHPG excretion and red-cell lithium transport in diagnostic psychiatry. *Lab Mgmt* 1983; 21(5):17.
Studdy PR, et al: Angiotensin-converting enzyme and its clinical significance—a review. *J Clin Pathol* 1983; 36:938.
Seybold ME: Myasthenia Gravis. *JAMA* 1983; 250:2516.
Koslow SH, et al: CSF and urinary biogenic amines and metabolites in depression and mania. *Arch Gen Psychiatry* 1983; 40:999.
Heller GV, et al: Implications of increased myocardial isoenzyme level in the presence of normal serum creatine kinase activity. *Am J Cardiol* 1983; 51:24.
Fisher ML, et al: Serum creatine kinase in the diagnosis of acute myocardial infarction: Optimal sampling frequency. *JAMA* 1983; 149:393.
Ali M, et al: Immunochemical CK-MB assay for myocardial infarction. *Am J Clin Pathol* 1982; 77:573.
Bais R, Edwards JB: Creatine Kinase. *CRC Crit Rev Clin Lab Sci* 1982; 16:291.
Johnston CC, Bolton EC: Cardiac enzymes. *Ann Emerg Med* 1982; 11:27.
Bissell DM: Laboratory evaluation in porphyria. *Semin Liver Dis* 1982; 2:100.
Weidner N: Laboratory diagnosis of acute myocardial infarction: Usefulness of determination of lactate dehydrogenase (LDH)-1 level and of ratio of LDH-1 to total LDH. *Arch Pathol Lab Med* 1982; 106:375.
Dillon MC, et al: Diagnostic problem in acute myocardial infarction: CK-MB in the absence of abnormally elevated total creatine kinase levels. *Arch Intern Med* 1982; 142:33.
Tow DE, Bianco JA: Imaging acute myocardial infarction: Practical considerations. *Appl Radiol NM* 1982; 11:90.
Miller RE: The nasal smear for eosinophils. *Am J Dis Child* 1982; 136:1009.
Cheely R, et al: The role of noninvasive tests versus pulmonary angiography in the diagnosis of pulmonary embolism. *Am J Med* 1981; 70:17.
Gerson MC: Applications of thallium-201 myocardial perfusion imaging in acute myocardial infarction. *Cardiovasc Rev Rep* 1981; 2:801.
Carroll BJ, et al: A specific laboratory test for the diagnosis of melancholia. *Arch Gen Psychiatry* 1981; 38:15.
Sharland DE: Erythrocyte sedimentation rate: The normal range in the elderly. *J Am Geriatr Soc* 1980; 28:346.
Spry CJF: Eosinophilia and allergic reactions to drugs. *Clin Haematol* 1980; 9:521.
Burrows B: Epidemiologic observations on eosinophilia and its relation to respiratory disorders. *Am Rev Respir Dis* 1980; 122:709.
Peter JB: When nerves short-circuit. *Diagn Med* 1980; 3(3):54.
Baillie EE: CK isoenzymes: Part 1. Clinical aspects. *Lab Med* 1979; 10:271.

Marmor A, et al: Creatine kinase isoenzyme MB (CK-MB) in acute coronary ischemia. *Am Heart J* 1979; 97:574.

Gossling HR, Donohue TA: The fat embolism syndrome. *JAMA* 1979; 241:2740.

Jacobs DS, et al: Clinical significance of the isomorphic pattern of the isoenzymes of serum lactate dehydrogenase. *Ann Clin Lab Sci* 1977; 7:411.

Saleem A, et al: Comparison of Zeta sedimentation ratio with Westergren sedimentation rate. *Ann Clin Lab Sci* 1977; 7:357.

21 Serum Proteins

Serum protein is composed of albumin and globulin, either nonbound or acting as carrier proteins. The word "globulin" is an old chemical fractionation term that refers to the nonalbumin portion of serum protein; it was subsequently found that this portion includes a heterologous group of proteins such as glycoproteins, lipoproteins, and immunoglobulins. Most globulin molecules are considerably larger than albumin, although the total quantity of albumin is normally two to three times the level of globulin. Albumin seems most active in maintaining the serum oncotic pressure, where it normally has about four times as much importance as globulin, accounting for about 80% of the plasma oncotic pressure. Albumin also acts as a transport protein for some drugs and a few other substances. The globulins have more varied assignments than albumin and form the main transport system for various substances as well as constituting the antibody system, the clotting proteins, complement, and certain special-duty substances such as the "acute reaction" proteins. Most serum albumin is produced by the liver. Some of the globulins are produced by the liver, some by the reticuloendothelial system, and some by other tissues or by poorly understood mechanisms.

Plasma contains fibrinogen in addition to the ordinary serum proteins.

SERUM PROTEIN ASSAY METHODS

There are many widely used procedures for fractionating the serum proteins. "Salting out" by differential chemical solubility yields rough separation into albumin and globulin. Cohn devised a more complicated chemical fractionation method by which certain parts of the protein spectrum may be separated from one another in a large-scale industrial-type procedure. Albumin is most often assayed by a chemical method (biuret) that reacts with nitrogen atoms, or with a dye (such as bromcresol green or bromcresol purple) that preferentially binds to albumin. The ultracentrifuge has been used to study some of the subgroups of the globulins. This is possible because the sedimentation rate at high speeds depends on the molecular size and shape, the type of solvent used to suspend the protein, and the force of centrifugation. The velocity of any particular class of globulins under standard conditions depends primarily on molecular size and is known as the "Svedberg number"; the most common classes of globulins are designated as 7S, 19S, and 22S. Electrophoresis separates molecules by the electrical charge of certain structural atomic configurations and is able to subdivide the globulins, but only into groups rather than into individual proteins. Serum protein nomenclature derived from electrophoresis subgroups the serum globulins into alpha, beta, and gamma, corresponding to electrophoretic mobility. Using antibodies against antigens on the protein molecule, immunoassay (including radial immunodiffusion, Laurell "rocket" electroimmunodiffusion, immunonephelometry, immunofluorometry, and radioimmunoassay, among others) is another technique for measuring serum proteins that is assuming great importance. Immunoassay techniques quantitate individual proteins rather than protein groups and in general produce reliable results with excellent sensitivity and specificity. Immunoelectrophoresis or similar techniques such as immunofixation goes one step beyond immunoassay and separates some of the individual globulin molecules into structural components or into subclasses. Immunoelectrophoresis also can detect abnormal proteins that either differ structurally from normal proteins or are produced with different proportions of structural components.

Laboratory Application of Serum Protein Assay Methods

Chemical methods are primarily useful to detect hyperglobulinemia and hypoalbuminemia. Chemical methods are poorly sensitive for hypoglobulinemia and not particularly sensitive even for hyperglobulinemia, due to the wide population reference range, differences among various chemical methods, and the unpredictable influence of all the various globulin molecules on the total result. Electrophoresis is also used as a screening test and in addition to partial separation of the globulins can suggest certain diagnoses or diagnostic possibilities by means of certain patterns of change in the electrophoretic fractions. Immunoassay permits accurate quantitation of various individual serum proteins and thus can either provide a diagnosis (e.g., alpha-1 antitrypsin deficiency) or suggest diagnostic possibilities (e.g., hypogammaglobulinemia or increased transferrin). Immunoelectrophoresis is used to detect abnormal proteins (such as those found in myeloma) and protein components such as the free light chains of Bence Jones protein. However, immunoelectrophoresis cannot quantitate these proteins with acceptable accuracy.

Different assay methods do not produce identical values for all protein fractions. For example, the serum albumin value by electrophoresis may be about 0.5 gm/100 ml less than the value determined by the usual chemical method. This is fortunately not often very important as long as the same laboratory performs the tests on the same patient and provides its own reference range. Since even modifications of the same method can produce slightly but significantly different results, reference values should be obtained by the individual laboratory for its own particular procedure.

Serum Protein Electrophoresis

Electrophoresis is still the most commonly used screening test for serum protein abnormalities except for measurement of albumin only. Before electrophoresis was readily available, the albumin/globulin ratio was widely used; this was determined with a chemical method and should no longer be ordered, since electrophoresis not only provides the same information but also pinpoints areas where globulin abnormalities may be found. Various electrophoretic methods produce some differences within the same basic framework of results due to differences in technical factors and the type of electrophoretic migrating field material used. Some of the standard materials include filter paper, cellulose acetate film, agarose gel, and polyacrylamide gel. Each method has advantages and disadvantages in terms of laboratory ease of performance, cost, or sensitivity to certain protein fractions. However, all are capable of identifying the areas where major serum protein shifts take place, which sometimes have as much diagnostic importance as the shifts themselves.

Serum protein electrophoresis ordinarily displays bands corresponding to albumin, alpha-1 and alpha-2 globulins, beta globulins, and gamma globulins. A special instrument (densitometer) translates the quantity of protein or density of these bands into a linear pattern (Fig 21–1), which is a rough visual approximation of the amount of substance present. The main problem with this method is the difficulty in separating some of the serum components. It has been found that by using potato starch in a gel-like state, the separation of some of these fractions can be sharpened, especially the separation of some of the abnormal hemoglobins. Polyacrylamide gel has also been used. However, these procedures are technically somewhat more difficult than the other techniques, so that filter paper, cellulose acetate, and agarose gel remain the routine clinical laboratory methods of choice. On filter paper, cellulose acetate, or agarose, the alpha-2 fraction migrates faster toward the anode than the beta fraction. On starch or polyacrylamide gel, the reverse occurs.

Proteins Visualized by Serum Protein Electrophoresis: Acute Reaction Proteins.—Certain reasonably predictable changes take place in plasma protein levels in response to acute illness, including acute inflammation, trauma, necrosis, infarction, burns, and chemical injury. The same changes may occur in focal episodes associated with malignant tumors (possibly due to infarction of a portion of the tumor). The acute reaction protein pattern has

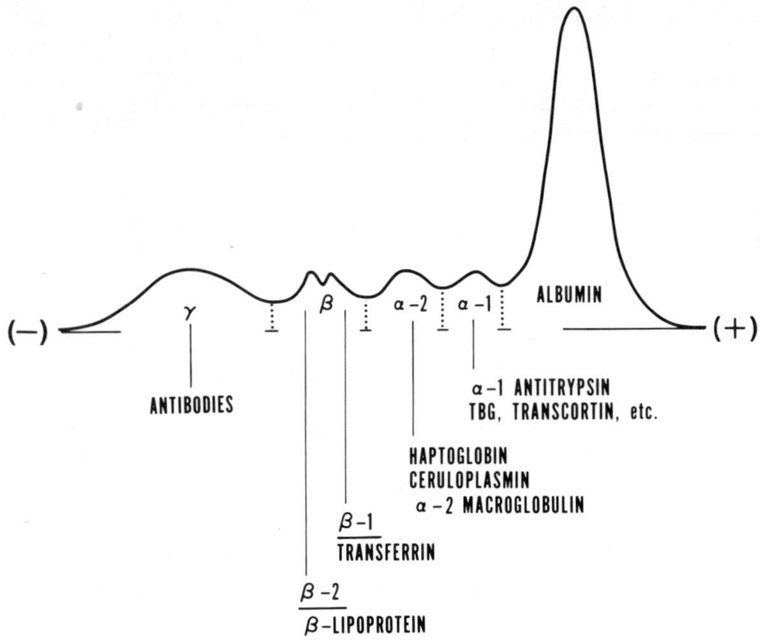

FIG 21–1.
Some important components of serum protein fractions.

also been called "acute inflammatory response pattern," "acute stress pattern," and "acute-phase protein pattern." The protein changes involved are increases in fibrinogen, alpha-1 antitrypsin, haptoglobin, ceruloplasmin, C-reactive protein (CRP), C3 portion of complement, and alpha-1 acid glycoprotein (orosomucoid) levels. There frequently is an associated decrease in albumin and transferrin levels. Of those proteins that are increased, the greatest effect is produced by haptoglobin, alpha-1 antitrypsin, CRP, and fibrinogen. C-reactive protein increase begins approximately 4–6 hours after onset of the acute episode, with alterations of the other proteins occurring 12–36 hours after onset. C-reactive protein is located in the beta-gamma interface area on electrophoresis, and a distinct peak is not usually seen. Fibrinogen is normally not present in serum (unless the blood has not completely clotted), so ordinarily it is not detected on serum electrophoresis. Haptoglobin migrates in the alpha-2 region, with the result that alpha-2 elevation is the most common abnormality associated with acute reaction. An alpha-1 elevation due to alpha-1 antitrypsin increase is seen less frequently but can be present. Albumin is often decreased under acute reaction conditions, presumably due to decreased liver synthesis, for which there often is no good explanation. Albumin is not always decreased; due to the wide reference range, a substantial reduction could occur in a person whose normal level is toward the upper end of the reference range, with the final level remaining within the lower reference range despite the reduction. A decrease in transferrin levels is usually not seen on electrophoresis but is manifested by a decrease in the total iron-binding capacity. In summary, the typical electrophoretic change of acute reaction is increased alpha-2 globulin, frequently associated with decreased albumin and sometimes with increased alpha-1 globulin. Acute reaction frequently is accompanied by a polymorphonuclear leukocytosis and usually by an increase in CRP test values (especially when using immunoassay methods) and an increased erythrocyte sedimentation rate (ESR).

Serum Albumin.—Elevation of serum albumin is very unusual other than in dehydration. Most changes involve diminution, although the normal range is somewhat large, and small decreases are thus hidden unless the individual patient's normal levels are known. In pregnancy, albumin levels decrease progressively until delivery and do not return to normal until about 8 weeks postpartum. In infants, adult levels are reached at about age 1 year. Thereafter, serum protein levels are relatively stable except for a gradual decrease after age 70. Malnutrition leads to decreased albumin levels, presumably from lack of essential amino acids, but also possibly from impaired liver manufacture and unknown causes. Impaired synthesis may itself be a cause of decreased albumin levels, since it is found in most forms of clinical liver disease. In chronic cachectic or wasting diseases, such as tuberculosis or carcinoma, the albumin level is often decreased, but it is not clear whether this is due to impaired synthesis or to other factors. Chronic infections seem to have much the same effect as the cachectic diseases.

Serum albumin may be directly lost from the bloodstream by hemorrhage, burns, exudates, or leakage into the gastrointestinal (GI) tract in various protein-losing enteropathies. In the nephrotic syndrome there is a marked decrease in the serum albumin level from direct loss into the urine. Albumin frequently decreases rather quickly in many severe acute illnesses or injuries, beginning at about 12–36 hours, with the average maximal albumin decrease being reached in about 5 days. This is part of the acute reaction pattern described earlier and seems to have a different mechanism from hypoalbuminemia due to protein loss or to malnutrition. Finally, there is a rare genetic cause for low serum albumin levels known as "familial idiopathic dysproteinemia," in which the albumin level is greatly decreased while all the globulin fractions are elevated and seem to take over most of the functions of albumin.

Alpha-1 Globulins.—The alpha-1 globulin area on electrophoresis is almost 90% alpha-1 antitrypsin. The other 10% includes alpha-1 acid glycoprotein, alpha-fetoprotein, and certain carrier proteins such as cortisol-binding protein (transcortin) and thyroxine-binding globulin (which is actually located more toward the area between alpha-1 and alpha-2). Alpha-1 globulin is increased to some extent (usually not great) in pregnancy and by estrogen administration and in some patients with the acute reaction protein pattern. Alpha-1 globulin is absent or nearly so in alpha-1 antitrypsin deficiency, a hereditary disorder that predisposes to development of emphysema. Serum protein electrophoresis detects homozygous alpha-1 antitrypsin deficiency but frequently displays a normal alpha-1 peak in those who are heterozygous. Immunoassay is needed to detect heterozygotes or to confirm electrophoretic findings.

Alpha-2 Globulins.—Alpha-2 globulins include haptoglobin, alpha-2 macroglobulin, and ceruloplasmin. This electrophoretic area is seldom depressed; diminution of one component is usually masked by the other components within the reference range. Haptoglobin values are decreased in severe liver disease, in patients on estrogen therapy, in megaloblastic anemia, and also whenever free hemoglobin appears in the blood, as occurs in red blood cell (RBC) hemolysis or even from resorption of a large hematoma located outside the vascular system. Haptoglobin levels are increased by adrenocorticosteroid therapy. Ceruloplasmin levels are decreased in Wilson's disease, malnutrition, nephrotic syndrome, and protein-losing enteropathy. Ceruloplasmin levels are increased by estrogen therapy. Both haptoglobin and ceruloplasmin levels are increased, resulting in alpha-2 elevation, in the many disorders that produce the acute reaction pattern.

In subacute and severe chronic illnesses the acute reaction pattern may exist in a lesser degree or may disappear. The alpha-2 increase usually diminishes and may return to normal. Albumin levels may return to normal, but an albumin decrease frequently persists or may even become more pronounced. Gamma-globulin levels may begin to increase.

There are certain diseases other than acute injury that often produce alpha-2 increase. In the nephrotic syndrome there is classically a marked alpha-2 peak, which may sometimes be accompanied by a beta-globulin elevation. In addition there is greatly decreased albumin. In hyperthyroidism, far-advanced diabetes, and adrenal insufficiency, there is reportedly a slightly to moderately elevated alpha-2 globulin level in some cases.

Beta Globulins.—The beta-globulin zone contains transferrin, beta-lipoprotein, and several components of complement. Free hemoglobin in serum produces a peak in the beta area, and fibrinogen from incompletely clotted blood migrates in the slow beta region.

A decrease in the beta-globulin level is not

very common. Transferrin is frequently decreased in protein malnutrition. Beta globulin increase may occur in many conditions. Probably the most common source is a nonfasting specimen. An increase in transferrin levels produced by chronic iron deficiency anemia and by pregnancy in the third trimester lead to a beta increase of varying degree that occasionally has a homogeneous spikelike configuration simulating a monoclonal peak. In conditions in which serum cholesterol levels are elevated, the beta-globulin levels are also likely to be increased; these include hypothyroidism, biliary cirrhosis, nephrosis, and some cases of diabetes. In liver disease, there is some variability. The beta-globulin level is usually, but not always, elevated in obstructive jaundice. It may be elevated to some extent in many cases of hepatitis but not as often as in obstructive jaundice. It is often elevated in cirrhosis; when so, it is often partially incorporated into the gamma globulin and occasionally does not even appear as a separate peak. This will be discussed later. Finally, beta elevation may occasionally be seen in certain other diseases, including malignant hypertension, Cushing's disease, polyarteritis nodosa, and sometimes carcinoma. These changes are probably due to increase in complement. A double peak in the beta area is a frequent and normal finding when the cellulose acetate method is used. Electrophoresis on polyacrylamide gel produces reversal of the alpha-2 and beta area positions compared to paper or cellulose acetate electrophoresis (i.e., the beta area on paper becomes alpha-2 on polyacrylamide gel).

Gamma Globulins.—The gamma region is predominantly composed of antibodies of the IgG type. Immunoglobulin A, IgM, IgD, and IgE antibodies underlie the beta-gamma junction area. The gamma globulin zone is decreased in hypogammaglobulinemia and agammaglobulinemia, which may be either primary or secondary. The secondary type sometimes may be found in patients on long-term steroid treatment, in the nephrotic syndrome, in occasional patients with overwhelming infection, and in a moderate number of patients with chronic lymphocytic leukemia, lymphocytic lymphoma, or multiple myeloma of the light chain type.

Many diseases produce an increase in the gamma-globulin level. Many types of infections are followed by an increased gamma-globulin level that reflects antibody production, although the increase is often not sufficient to demonstrate a clear-cut elevation above reference range, especially if the infection is mild or acute. Chronic infections typically produce antibody responses that are prolonged and substantial enough to increase gamma-globulin values above reference limits. Granulomatous diseases such as tuberculosis, sarcoidosis, lymphogranuloma venereum, and tertiary syphilis are also chronic diseases and frequently result in marked gamma increase by the time they become well established. Rheumatoid-collagen diseases, notably rheumatoid arthritis and lupus erythematosis, have electrophoretic gamma values that range from normal to considerably increased. Gamma levels are usually elevated while the disease is active if activity has persisted for several months. Gamma-globulin levels may be increased in some patients with Hodgkin's disease, malignant lymphoma, and chronic lymphocytic leukemia, although in other patients they may be decreased or normal. Multiple myeloma and Waldenström's macroglobulinemia characteristically demonstrate a homogeneous spikelike peak in a focal region of the gamma area, which may or may not result in the value for the total gamma area being increased. Liver diseases form a substantial group of etiologies for gamma elevation. In hepatitis there is classically a relatively mild separate increase in both beta- and gamma-globulin levels with a decrease in albumin level, but this does not always occur. About 90% of patients with well-established cirrhosis show some degree of gamma elevation. The gamma elevation is of considerable degree in about 30% of patients and of slight to moderate degree in about 60%. There is no electrophoretic gamma elevation in about 10% of patients with histologically well-established cirrhosis. The most suggestive pattern is a broad-based gamma-globulin elevation plus a fusion of beta and gamma globulin without the usual separation of the two peaks. However, only about 20% of cirrhotics display complete beta-gamma fusion with about 33% more showing partial fusion. In obstructive jaundice, alpha-2, beta, and gamma levels may all become elevated to some degree.

Typical Electrophoretic Patterns.—In this section several typical electrophoretic patterns are presented with diseases in which they are most commonly found (Fig 21–2). It must be strongly emphasized that no pattern is pathognomonic of any single disease and that there is considerable variation in the shape and height of the electrophoretic peaks in individual patients that may obscure a pattern. In addition, the patterns will not always appear when they should be expected and in some cases may be altered when two diseases are present together (e.g., acute infection in a patient with cirrhosis).

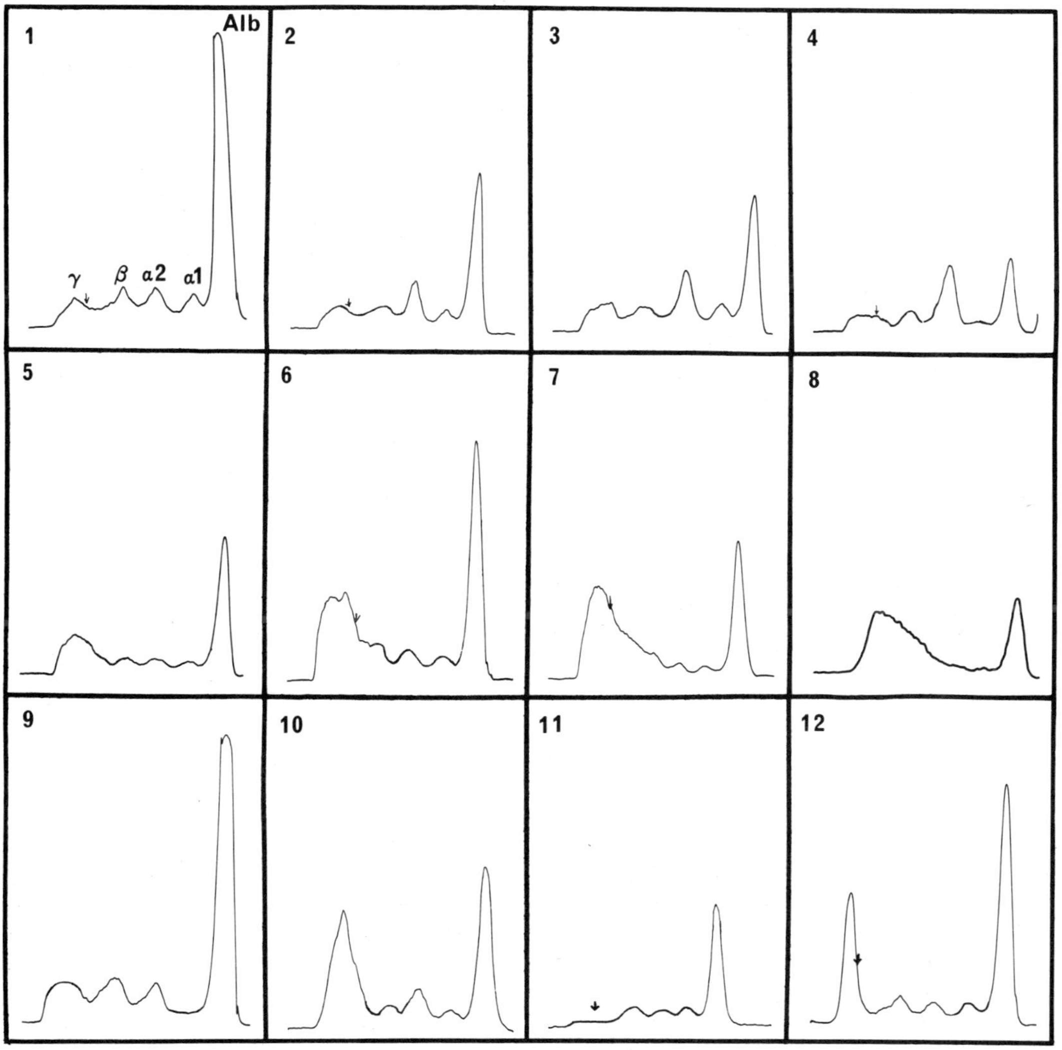

FIG 21–2.

Typical serum protein electrophoretic patterns. *1*, normal (*arrow* near gamma region indicates serum application point); *2*, acute reaction pattern; *3*, acute reaction or nephrotic syndrome; *4*, nephrotic syndrome; *5*, chronic inflammation, cirrhosis, granulomatous diseases, rheumatoid-collagen group; *6*, same as *5*, but gamma elevation is more pronounced. There is also partial (but not complete) beta-gamma fusion; *7*, suggestive of cirrhosis but could be found in the granulomatous diseases or the rheumatoid-collagen group; *8*, characteristic pattern of cirrhosis; *9*, alpha-1 antitrypsin deficiency with mild gamma elevation suggesting concurrent chronic disease; *10*, same as *5*, but the gamma elevation is marked. The configuration of the gamma peak superficially mimics that of myeloma, but is more broad-based. There are superimposed acute reaction changes; *11*, hypogammaglobulinemia or light-chain myeloma; *12*, myeloma, Waldenstrom's macroglobulinemia, idiopathic or secondary monoclonal gammopathy.

One electrophoretic configuration is called *the acute reaction pattern.* It consists of decreased albumin level and elevated alpha-2 globulin level and is found in acute infections in the early stages; some cases of myocardial infarct and tissue necrosis; some cases of severe burns, surgery, and other stress conditions; and in some of the rheumatoid diseases with acute onset. A second pattern consists of a slightly or moderately decreased albumin level, a slightly or moderately elevated gamma-globulin, and a slightly elevated or normal alpha-2 globulin level. This is the *chronic inflammatory pattern* and is found in chronic infections of various types, the granulomatous diseases, cirrhosis, and rheumatoid-collagen diseases. There may, of course, be various stages of transition between this chronic pattern and previously described acute one. A third pattern is typically found in *the nephrotic syndrome.* There is a greatly decreased albumin level and a considerably increased alpha-2 level with or without an increase in the beta-globulin level. This differs from the acute stress pattern in that the alpha-2 elevation of the nephrotic syndrome is usually either slightly or moderately greater than that seen in acute reaction, whereas the albumin fraction in the nephrotic syndrome has a definitely greater decrease (sometimes to extremely low levels) than the albumin fraction of acute reaction.

A fourth pattern represents *changes suggestive of far-advanced cirrhosis.* It consists of a decreased albumin level with a moderately or considerably increased gamma-globulin level and variable degrees of incorporation of the beta peak into the gamma. The more pronounced the beta-gamma bridging becomes, the more suggestive the pattern is for cirrhosis. However, complete incorporation of the beta peak into the gamma region is actually uncommon, since it is found in only about 20% of well-established cases of cirrhosis. About 10% of cirrhotic patients have no gamma elevation at all, about 25% have mild to moderate gamma elevation without any beta-gamma bridging, about 8% have marked gamma elevation without any bridging, and about 33% have mild to moderate gamma elevation with mild to moderate beta-gamma bridging but without complete loss of the beta peak. Surprisingly, the electrophoretic pattern correlates poorly with degree of liver function abnormality. Correlation is not consistent even with microscopic findings at autopsy, although there is a tendency for more pronounced electrophoretic changes to be associated with more advanced microscopic abnormality.

A fifth pattern consists of a *polyclonal gamma-globulin elevation,* that is, a greatly increased gamma-globulin level that involves the entire gamma zone rather than a focal area and does not have a thin spikelike appearance. There may or may not be some degree of beta-gamma bridging, but the beta peak does not totally disappear. This pattern is most often seen in some cases of cirrhosis, in patients with chronic infection, in granulomatous diseases such as sarcoidosis or far-advanced pulmonary tuberculosis, in subacute bacterial endocarditis, and in certain of the collagen diseases such as systemic lupus or polyarteritis nodosa.

A sixth pattern consists of *hypogammaglobulinemia,* defined electrophoretically as decreased gamma-globulin level, usually without very marked changes in other globulin zones. This configuration is suggestive of the light chain variant of multiple myeloma (about 20% of myeloma cases) in which Bence Jones protein is excreted into the urine without a serum myeloma protein being evident with ordinary electrophoretic techniques. Patients with a substantial degree of hypogammaglobulinemia from other causes have the same electrophoretic picture.

Finally, there is the so-called *monoclonal gammopathy spike* (M protein and paraprotein are synonyms). This is located in the gamma area (much less frequently in the beta and rarely in the alpha-2) and consists of a high, relatively thin spike configuration that is more homogeneous and needle shaped than the other gamma or beta elevations discussed earlier. The majority of persons with the monoclonal spike on serum electrophoresis have myeloma. However, a sizable minority do not, and these cases are divided among Waldenström's macroglobulinemia, secondary monoclonal gammopathies, and idiopathic monoclonal gammopathy (discussed later).

Certain conditions may produce globulin peaks that simulate a small or medium-sized monoclonal peak rather closely. A configuration of this sort in the alpha-2 area may occur in the nephrotic syndrome or in conditions that produce the acute reaction pattern (the alpha-2 elevation in both cases is due to elevated haptoglobin levels). A small monoclonal-type

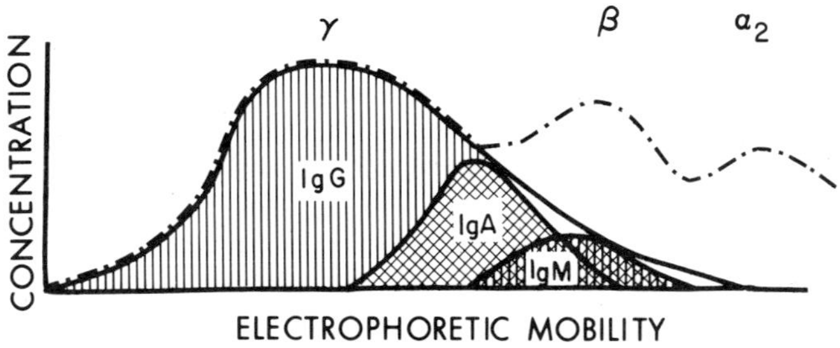

FIG 21–3
Diagrammatic relationship of immunoglobulins to the standard cellulose acetate serum protein electrophoretic pattern.

peak in the beta area may be seen in the third trimester of normal pregnancy or in some patients with chronic iron deficiency anemia (both due to increased transferrin levels). Similar beta region peaks may be caused by the presence of fibrinogen from incompletely clotted blood or by serum free hemoglobin. In the gamma area, somewhat similar peaks (but usually not as slender and needle like) may be found in rare patients with chronic disease, most often of the granulomatous type.

IMMUNOGLOBULINS

Gamma globulins (called immunoglobulins, or Igs, in current immunologic terminology) are not a homogeneous group. There are three main subdivisions: IgG, which migrates in the gamma region on electrophoresis; IgA, which migrates in the pregamma region or in the area between gamma and beta; and IgM, which migrates in the prebeta or beta region (Fig 21–3). There are two additional groups called IgD and IgE. Immunoglobulin G comprises about 75% of serum immunoglobulins and has a normal 7S molecular weight. Immunoglobulin G constitutes the majority of the antibodies, especially the warm-temperature incomplete type. Immunoglobulin M accounts for 5%–7% of total immunoglobulins and is a macroglobulin (19S group). The IgM class includes the earliest antibodies produced against infectious organisms (later followed by IgG antibodies), cold agglutinins, ABO blood group isoagglutinins, and rheumatoid factor. Immunoglobulin A constitutes about 15% of immunoglobulins. Although most are 7S, some molecules are larger. It is found primarily in secretions, such as saliva, tears, gastrointestinal secretions from stomach and accessory organs, and secretions from the respiratory tract. Selective deficiency of IgA (the other immunoglobulins being normal) is the most common primary immunodeficiency, and is associated with frequent upper respiratory and GI infections. There is also increased frequency of autoimmune disease. Phenytoin (Dilantin) is reported to decrease IgA levels to some extent in 20%–85% of patients on long-term therapy. In one report, about 15% of patients had IgA levels below reference range, and about 4% had very low levels. Immunoglobulin D is a normal 7S molecular weight molecule that makes up less than 1% of the immunoglobulins; its function is not known. Immunoglobulin E also has a 7S weight and occurs with less than 1% frequency. It is elevated in certain allergic conditions, especially atopic disorders (see chapter 20), and it is associated with reaginic antibody.

The normal immunoglobulin molecule is composed of two heavy chains (each chain of 50,000-dalton molecular weight) and two light chains (each of 20,000-dalton molecular weight) connected by disulfide bridges. Immunoglobulin M is a pentomeric arrangement of five complete immunoglobulin units.

MULTIPLE MYELOMA

Multiple myeloma is a malignancy of plasma cells that, in turn, are derived from B-type lymphocytes. The neoplastic plasma cells involve bone marrow and frequently produce multisystem disease. Patients are usually age 40 or older, with a peak incidence occurring in age group 60–65 years. About two thirds of the patients are male (literature range 54%–72%). Clinically, the most common symptom is bone pain, reported in about 70%. Pathologic fractures are common. Infections are more common in myeloma (10%–52% of cases) than in the general population. The classic infecting organisms are encapsulated bacteria such as pneumoccoci and, much less frequently, *Haemophilus influenzae*; some reports indicate that gram-negative infections are becoming more frequent. Recurrent infections are relatively frequent. Weight loss, weakness, and various GI symptoms are found in 35%–65% of cases. Neurologic symptoms are present in 30%–50% of cases. Some are due to nerve root or spinal cord compression by myelomatous infiltrates; some to amyloid deposition, and some to peripheral neuropathy. Hepatomegaly is present in about 20% of cases (literature range, 10%–38%) and splenomegaly in about 10% (literature range, 5%–15%). When patients over age 40 are seen because of bone pain, recurrent infection or unexplained nonpulmonary infection, or fracture, myeloma should be considered.

Laboratory Abnormalities

Standard Laboratory Test Findings.—Anemia is found in 60%–80% of patients. It is generally moderate in degree (although sometimes severe) and is usually of the normocytic-normochromic type. Red blood cell rouleaux formation (RBCs adhering together like a stack of coins due to the presence of abnormal protein) in peripheral blood smears is a clue to possible myeloma and can be found in 60%–85% of cases. Frequency of rouleaux detection depends to some extent on the degree of abnormality and also on the experience and interest of the examiner. Total white blood cell count is usually normal except during episodes of infection, with leukopenia reported in 15%–20% of cases. Although myeloma plasma cells infiltrate the bone marrow at some time during the course of the disease, ordinarily this does not result in peripheral blood plasmacytosis. In 1%–2% of patients there are more than 5% plasma cells in the peripheral blood, and some of these patients have been considered to have plasma cell leukemia. Occasional patients display some degree of myeloid cell immaturity. Thrombocytopenia is found in approximately 10% of patients.

Among other laboratory test results that may be abnormal, the ESR is usually moderately to markedly elevated (90% of patients in a large Mayo Clinic series). Hypercalcemia occurs in about 30% (literature range, 20%–50%). Azotemia is reported in 40%–55% of patients, and proteinuria is detected in 60%–90%. Hyperglobulinemia is present in approximately 60% of patients (literature range, 50%–80%) and hypogammaglobulinemia in about 10%. Serum albumin is decreased in about 50% of patients. The alkaline phosphatase level is most often normal unless a fracture is present, but reports of alkaline phosphatase abnormality in the literature range from 0%–48%. Amyloid is found in 5%–10% of cases and cryoglobulins in approximately 5%. Uric acid levels are increased in about 40% of patients.

X-Ray Findings.—X-ray examination displays abnormality in 80%–85% of patients. The most typical finding is the "punched-out" osteolytic lesion, most commonly in the skull, vertebral spine, and pelvis. Between 6% and 25% of patients demonstrate diffuse osteoporosis as the only abnormality; the rest have various combinations of focal osteolytic lesions, osteoporosis, and pathologic fractures. Results of radionuclide bone scan are not as frequently abnormal in myeloma as in metastatic tumor involving bone.

Bone Marrow Diagnosis.—Diagnosis of myeloma is made through bone marrow aspiration. The bone marrow of myeloma patients usually contains more than 20% plasma cells (however, criteria listed in the literature range from 5%–30%, sometimes based on presence or absence of other abnormalities such as bone lesions). If the plasma cell percentage is less than 20%, a considerable number of the plasma cells must be immature to make the diagnosis, because other diseases may be associated with an increase in mature marrow plasma cells. Ordinarily, a benign plasmacytic marrow reaction produces a plasma cell percentage less than 10%, but in some cases this figure may reach 20% and, rarely, even higher. Bone marrow aspiration is usually diagnostic by the time symptoms appear. However, about 15% of patients have less than 20% plasma cells in the marrow aspirate, and about 8% have less than 20% plus no evidence of plasma cell immaturity. Since marrow infiltration may have an irregular distribution in some patients, a repeat aspiration may be necessary. In some cases a cytologic diagnosis cannot be made until a later date. In occasional patients a bone marrow biopsy specimen may show changes suggestive of myeloma when the marrow smear is not diagnostic.

Abnormal Proteins (Immunoglobulins).— About 75%–80% of myeloma patients have plasma cell secretion of abnormal monoclonal serum protein with a molecular weight (160,000 daltons or 7S) typical of a normal complete immunoglobulin molecule. Of all patients with monoclonal protein, about two thirds have myeloma. Of those myeloma patients with normal weight serum monoclonal protein, roughly 70% have monoclonal protein categorized as IgG, about 25% have IgA, and fewer than 2% have IgD or IgE.

In addition to normal weight serum monoclonal protein, many patients excrete an abnormal, incomplete, low weight protein known as Bence Jones protein. Bence Jones protein is composed only of immunoglobulin light chains and therefore has a low molecular weight (40,000 daltons,or 3.5S). Unlike normal weight monoclonal proteins, it is able to pass the glomerular filter into the urine. In most cases it is cleared rapidly from plasma; therefore, even when Bence Jones proteinuria is marked, this substance usually is not demonstrable in serum by ordinary electrophoretic techniques and frequently not even by immunoelectrophoresis. About 70%–80% of myeloma patients show Bence Jones protein on urine electrophoresis, whereas urine Bence Jones protein can be detected only in about 50% of patients using the old heat test. About 50%–60% have a normal weight serum monoclonal protein in addition to Bence Jones protein in the urine, and about 20% (literature range 10%–26%) have Bence Jones protein in the urine as the only protein abnormality ("light chain" myeloma). Light chain myeloma is frequently associated with hypogammaglobulinemia on standard serum protein electrophoresis. Clinically, there tends to be a somewhat greater incidence of azotemia, hypercalcemia, and lytic bone lesions than in ordinary myeloma.

The classic method of detecting Bence Jones protein is by a carefully done heat coagulability test, in which the protein appears on heating to 60°C and disappears on boiling, only to reappear if the urine is cooled. As mentioned in chapter 12, with a few exceptions the sulfosalicylic acid test result for urine protein is positive with Bence Jones protein, but dipsticks frequently give negative results. Since various technical and human factors make the heat method unreliable, urine electrophoresis is the best method for demonstrating Bence Jones protein. In a large Mayo Clinic series, 49% of myeloma patients revealed urine Bence Jones protein by heat test, whereas 75% had a Bence Jones peak in nonconcentrated urine on electrophoresis. On urine electrophoresis, Bence Jones protein appears as a single homogeneous spike similar to that of monoclonal protein in serum. The normal weight monoclonal serum proteins of myeloma usually do not appear in the urine. In many cases it is necessary to concentrate the urine (5–100 times) to detect small quantities of Bence Jones protein. Urine immunoelectrophoresis is about 5% more sensitive than standard urine protein electrophoresis.

Bence Jones protein is excreted in urine by approximately 70% (literature range, 54%–80%) of myeloma patients, about 30% (0%–78%) of patients with Waldenström's macroglobulinemia, about 20% (15%–62%) of patients with monoclonal gammapathy associated with lymphoproliferative malignancy, and about 10% (0%–24%) of patients with so-called benign (secondary and idiopathic) monoclonal gammopathy. In general, patients with benign monoclonal gammopathy and Bence Jones protein excrete only small amounts of Bence Jones protein (≤60 mg/L). Only 2%–3% (0%–6%) of these patients excrete greater quantities. Patients with malignant gammopathies and Bence Jones proteinuria tend to excrete quantities greater than 60 mg/L. However, about 10% of myeloma patients with Bence Jones proteinuria excrete less than 60 mg/L.

Immunoglobulin D Myeloma

Immunoglobulin D myeloma has some unusual features that are worth mentioning. This entity is rare, seen in about 1% of myeloma patients. In IgD myeloma, the light chain of the abnormal IgD molecule is lambda type in about 90% of cases, whereas in other types of myeloma about 66% are kappa and about 33% are lambda. Also, Bence Jones proteinuria occurs in more than 90% of IgD cases, compared with an incidence of about 75% in IgG and IgA myeloma (literature range, 60%–80%). It is claimed that IgD myeloma is more likely to be associated with extraosseus myeloma spread, although about 50%–75% of myeloma patients display microscopic extramedullary (nonbone) foci (predominantly in liver, spleen, and lymph nodes), which usually are not evident clinically.

Amyloidosis

A word should be said about amyloidosis. There are several categories of amyloidosis, including primary, secondary, familial, localized, and senile. The amyloid of primary amyloidosis is derived from the variable region of immunoglobulin light chains (most often lambda), and myeloma is associated with 20%–30% of these patients. Standard electrophoresis is said to detect a monoclonal peak in serum and urine in about 50% of cases, whereas immunoelectrophoresis of serum and urine is abnormal in 90% of cases. Diagnosis is made through tissue biopsy and special stains with or without polarized light. Biopsy can be obtained from clinically affected tissue (e.g., the carpal ligament in those patients with carpal tunnel syndrome) or from certain other tissues such as subcutaneous fat aspirates (in two reports, positive in 75% or more cases). However, the yield from subcutaneous fat aspiration is only about 17% if the patient has amyloid-induced carpal tunnel syndrome without any other clinical evidence of amyloidosis, and is only 0%–40% if the patient has amyloidosis but is on renal dialysis.

Solitary Plasmacytoma

About 3% (literature range, 2%–5%) of patients with plasma cell dyscrasias present with a single plasma cell localized tumor. There is considerable confusion in the literature as to the nomenclature of these lesions. In general, those within bone tend to be regarded as solitary myeloma, whereas those in soft tissue are usually called "extramedullary plasmacytomas." The most common location for extramedullary plasmacytoma is the upper respiratory tract, whereas solitary bone lesions are found most often in the spine. About 60% of patients with solitary (bone) myeloma lesions when first seen develop disseminated myeloma by 10 years after diagnosis. Extramedullary plasmacytomas are usually regarded as having a better prognosis than myeloma, with some being cured by therapy, some recurring, and some metastasizing or developing into myeloma in spite of treatment. In one review of the literature, only about 20% of patients with localized plasma cell tumors in bone were found to have monoclonal proteins in serum on standard electrophoresis and about 25% on immunoelectrophoresis.

Heavy Chain Disease

Whereas light chain myeloma involves selective production of the light chain fragment of immunoglobulin molecules, there is a rare condition known as "Franklin's disease" (heavy chain disease) that is characterized by selective production of the heavy chain fragment. The clinical picture most often resembles that of malignant lymphoma. Bone marrow aspiration findings are variable, and lymph node biopsy may suggest lymphoma or contain a mixed cell infiltrate.

OTHER MONOCLONAL GAMMOPATHIES (TABLE 21–1)

Waldenström's (Primary) Macroglobulinemia

Waldenström's macroglobulinemia is a lymphoproliferative disorder characterized by monoclonal IgM (molecular weight 1,000,000 daltons or 19S) production, with classic clinical features of lymphadenopathy, hepatosplenomegaly, anemia, hyperglobulinemia with rouleaux formation, and the hyperviscosity syndrome. From 10%–30% of patients with

TABLE 21–1.
Distribution of Monoclonal Gammopathy Etiologies*

Disease	% of Total Monoclonal Gammopathy
Multiple myeloma	65 (52–66)
IgG, 60% (50%–71%)	
IgA, 25% (22%–28%)	
Bence Jones (light chain) only, 20% (10%–26%)	
Waldenström's	5–10 (3–20)
Franklin's disease (heavy chain disease)	0.5 (0–1)
Lymphomas and leukemias	6 (0.5–20)
Cancer	8 (5–15)
Not associated with neoplasia	15 (8–64)

*Numbers represent average figures. Numbers in parentheses represent literature range.

Waldenström's macroglobulinemia (literature range 0%–60%) excrete Bence Jones protein in the urine. Although typical biopsy findings are a mixture of mature lymphocytes and plasmacytoid lymphocytes, in some cases the histologic picture is suggestive of a diffuse type of lymphocytic lymphoma. Bone marrow aspiration may yield either normal findings, nonspecific lymphoid infiltration, or lymphoma-like infiltrate. On skeletal x-ray film, punched-out osteolytic lesions of the type seen in myeloma are usually absent. The hyperviscosity syndrome consists of shortness of breath, various neurologic abnormalities, and visual difficulty with sausage-shaped segmentation of retinal veins. Serum viscosity (as measured by the Ostwald viscosimeter or other method) is increased. In some patients the disease could be interpreted as malignant lymphoma or lymphocytic leukemia with IgM production. In a few instances, plasma cells predominate, and osteolytic bone lesions compatible with an IgM myeloma are present. Since plasma cells are derived from lymphocytes, many are inclined to view these disorders as a spectrum. However, since clinicians usually insist on a specific diagnosis, the "intermediate" forms create a problem.

Idiopathic Monoclonal Gammopathy

Idiopathic monoclonal gammopathy is defined as monoclonal protein in the absence of disease known to be associated with monoclonal proteins. True incidence is hard to define, since in many reports in the literature patients with nonneoplastic "secondary" paraproteinemia frequently are not segregated from patients with paraproteinemia but without other disease. The incidence of nonneoplastic monoclonal gammopathy apparently is increased with advanced age. Some investigators found an incidence of 0.3%–3.0% in populations tested, with the higher rates in the elderly. There is disagreement about whether overt myeloma will develop if patients are followed long enough, although it is reported in some cases.

SECONDARY MONOCLONAL GAMMOPATHY

Secondary monoclonal gammopathy may be further subdivided into diseases associated with neoplasia and those associated with nonneoplastic disorders. In the neoplasm group, monoclonal proteins are most often found with malignant lymphoma and chronic lymphocytic leukemia. Among carcinomas, those of the rectosigmoid are most frequent, followed by carcinomas of the prostate, breast, and lung. The incidence in one large cancer hospital ranged from 0.2% in the fourth decade of life to 5.7% in the ninth. In three large series of patients with monoclonal gammopathy, 6%–8% of cases were associated with lymphoma or lymphocytic leukemia and 4%–8% with other types of neoplasms. Nonneoplastic diseases that have been associated with monoclonal proteins are many and varied, but the greatest number appear in the rheumatoid-collagen-autoimmune group, cirrhosis, chronic infection (particularly tuberculosis and chronic infection of the biliary tract, urinary tract, and lung), Gaucher's disease, osteitis deformans (Paget's disease of bone), and sarcoidosis. One study detected monoclonal or oligoclonal serum proteins in 9% of patients who had human immunodeficiency virus I infection without the criteria for acquired immunodeficiency syndrome (AIDS). There is also increased incidence in AIDS. Most of these nonneoplastic conditions are ordinarily associated with polyclonal hyperglobulinemia rather than monoclonal gammopathy. The incidence of nonneoplastic monoclonal protein in the three series mentioned varied from 4%–10%. Monoclonal protein type in the secondary paraproteinemias may be IgG, IgA, or IgM. Occasional patients in either the neoplastic or nonneoplastic group excrete Bence Jones protein in the urine, usually in small amounts. In some cases the heat test gives false positive results due to an increase in normal light chains associated with polyclonal gammopathy.

Diagnostic Techniques

In many instances the diagnosis of myeloma or Waldenström's macroglobulinemia can be made by serum protein electrophoresis, followed by bone marrow aspiration. In patients without a monoclonal-type serum peak, urine electrophoresis on a concentrated specimen is essential to detect cases in which the only protein abnormality is urinary excretion of Bence Jones protein. In problem cases, it is necessary to resort to serum and urine immunoelectrophoresis. Many authorities advocate immunoelectrophoresis in all patients since this is the only way to classify monoclonal immunoglobulin disorders with certainty (even subgrouping of IgG and IgA is now possible.) Although subclassification of myeloma into immunoglobulin categories at present has more academic than practical application from the standpoint of therapy, such classification may become important in the future, and in any event, it provides additional confirmation of the diagnosis. About 1%–2% of myeloma patients fail to secrete abnormal proteins that are detectable in either serum or urine by immunoelectrophoresis ("nonsecretory" myeloma).

Immunoelectrophoresis consists of three steps. First, the unknown (patient's) serum is subjected to ordinary electrophoresis in a substance such as agar gel; this separates the immunoglobulins from one another to some extent. Second, antiserum against a specific type of human globulin (or a polyvalent antiserum against several types) is added to a trench cut nearby and parallel to the electrophoretic separation bands. Then the immunoglobulins and anti-immunoglobulin antibodies diffuse toward each other. Finally, the reaction between the patient's immunoglobulin fractions and any specific antibodies against one or more of those immunoglobulin fractions forms visual precipitin lines (Fig 21–4). The combination of electrophoresis and agar diffusion antigen-antibody reaction produces better separation of the immunoglobulin components and demonstrates abnormal quantities of any type present. Immunofixation is a modification of the immunoelectrophoresis technique that takes a little longer to perform but is easier to interpret and may be a little more sensitive. Immunoelectrophoresis or immunofixation are currently most useful in differentiating macroglobulinemia from other types of monoclonal gammopathy. If the monoclonal peak is shown to be IgM, this is evidence against myeloma, since only a few cases of IgM myeloma have been reported. On the other hand, if the peak is not IgM, this rules out Waldenström's macroglobulinemia. The idiopathic or secondary paraproteinemias can be of the IgG, IgA, or IgM class.

There are two types of immunoglobulin light chains: kappa and lambda. Normally about twice as much kappa is produced as lambda. Immunoelectrophoresis can detect these light chains, differentiate kappa from lambda, demonstrate whether one is increased or decreased in relation to the other, and afford a rough visual estimate whether either one is increased or

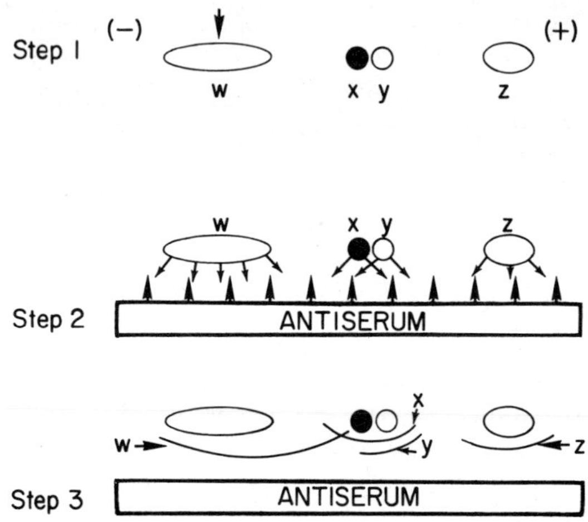

FIG 21–4.
Procedure for immunoelectrophoresis (modified from Terry and Fahey). *Step 1*, electrophoretic separation of human serum globulins on agar gel (*arrow* indicates area where the sample is applied). *Step 2*, addition of anti–human globulin antibody mixture to a nearby trough and diffusion of the separated globulin fractions and the antibody mixture components toward each other. *Step 3*, formation of precipitin lines at interaction of globulin fractions and specific antibodies to these fractions from the antiglobulin mixture. The globulin fractions have different rates of diffusion and thus produce precipitin lines in different areas.

decreased in quantity. Malignant monoclonal gammopathies, such as myeloma or Waldenström's macroglobulinemia, usually have an abnormal predominance of either kappa or lambda, with the other markedly decreased or absent. Unfortunately, commercial companies have had problems in producing consistently good antisera to kappa and lambda light chains. Controls must be run with every lot of antiserum to guard against false results.

Differentiation of Benign and Malignant Monoclonal Gammopathies

Patients with monoclonal gammopathies are usually detected in one of two ways. Either clinical symptoms suggest myeloma and electrophoretic studies are performed, or the studies are ordered for some other reason and monoclonal abnormality is discovered by accident. In 80%–90% of patients with myeloma, bone marrow aspiration findings make the correct diagnosis relatively easy. In those patients with monoclonal gammopathy but normal or equivocal results of bone marrow aspirate, diagnosis becomes a problem. As listed in Table 21–1, nonmyelomatous monoclonal gammopathies include Waldenström's macroglobulinemia, leukemia and lymphoma (usually the lymphocytic B-cell types), secondary monoclonal gammopathies (carcinomas and inflammatory disease), and idiopathic cases without known associated disease. Some investigators divide the monoclonal gammopathies into two categories, malignant (myeloma, Waldenström's macroglobulinemia, and lymphoproliferative disorders) and benign (secondary and idiopathic types). The majority of diagnostic problems involve the secondary and idiopathic monoclonal gammopathies, and the usual difficulty consists of excluding a plasma cell or lymphocytic malignancy when bone marrow results are normal and other studies are negative.

In general, if the monoclonal serum protein is greater in quantity than 3.0 gm/100 ml (30 g/L), if the bone marrow contains more than 20% plasma cells, or if the patient excretes more than 60 mg/L of Bence Jones protein, the disorder is probably malignant. On the other hand, if serum monoclonal protein does not exceed 2.0 gm/100 ml, marrow plasma cells do not exceed 5%, and Bence Jones protein does not exceed 60 mg/L, the condition is more likely to be benign. However, up to 5% of those with benign monoclonal gammopathies are reported to exceed at least one of the three criteria for malignancy, although usually not more than one criterion. About 15% of myeloma patients are reported to have less than 10% plasma cells in their initial bone marrow aspirate, with about 5% of myeloma patients having less than 5%. About 30% of myeloma patients have monoclonal protein in serum less than 3.0 gm/100 ml, and about 20% (literature range, 17%–22%) have less than 2.0 gm/100 ml. About 20%–30% have no Bence Jones protein in the urine, and of those who do, about 10% excrete less than 60 mg/L. Thus, the criteria for malignancy are more reliable than those for benign monoclonal etiology. In addition, in one study about 10% of patients thought to have benign monoclonal gammopathy developed myeloma or macroglobulinemia within 5 years.

Some patients require quantitation of one or more immunoglobulin groups. The most frequent reasons include serial quantitation of monoclonal protein to monitor the effects of therapy and immunoglobulin quantitation to detect deficiency of one or more specific immunoglobulin groups. The current standard method to quantitate immunoglobulins is some type of immunologic technique (radial immunodiffusion, immunonephelometry, immunoassay, and others). It must be emphasized that immunoelectrophoresis is not suitable for immunoglobulin quantitation. Immunoelectrophoresis detects and classifies immunoglobulins, but the quantity of any detectable immunoglobulin can only be very roughly estimated as normal, increased, or decreased rather than measured. Serum protein electrophoresis is sometimes used to monitor myeloma protein response to therapy. However, protein electrophoresis is not ideal for this purpose, since standard methods depend on measuring total protein, finding the percentage that each protein fraction contributes to total protein, and then multiplying the total protein numerical value by the percentage representing each protein fraction to derive the numerical quantity of each protein fraction. This means that abnormality in one fraction (e.g., albumin) can change total protein and secondarily change the percentage of all the protein fractions relative to total protein. This can produce some degree of artifactual change in quantity of protein fractions calculated from percent of total protein. Finally, if serial determinations of a specific protein fraction are necessary, the same laboratory should perform the assays, since different techniques can yield somewhat different results on the same specimen.

Cryoglobulins

Occasionally there may be other types of abnormal serum proteins in myeloma, Waldenström's macroglobulinemia, malignancy, and some of the other diseases, such as lupus. Among these are cryoglobulins. These are abnormal globulins that have the interesting property of coagulating when cooled to certain temperatures. They are not generally demonstrable as distinct peaks on paper electrophoresis but are incorporated into areas occupied by other globulins.

There are screening tests for both cryoglobulins and macroglobulins. The cryocrit is essentially a cold precipitation test for cryoglobulins adapted to yield a rough quantitative result. Serum of the patient is refrigerated overnight, then centrifuged in a Wintrobe hematocrit tube. Normally, less than 2% of precipitate is found. To test for cryofibrinogen, heparinized plasma is used for the same procedure. Macroglobulins are screened by the Sia test, which is actually a test for euglobulin. The procedure entails adding a drop of the patient's serum to distilled water. Most of the macroglobulins are insoluble in water, so the formation of a precipitate suggests the presence of macroglobulins. The test is not very reliable.

SERUM COMPLEMENT

Serum complement is an important immunologic enzyme system that comprises about 10% of the serum globulins. Complement has many activities, some of which are undoubtedly still unknown. Most attention has been focused on its role in the immunologic system, where effects have been demonstrated on vascular permeability, chemotaxis, phagocytosis, immune adherence, and immune cell lysis. The best-known laboratory procedure directly involving complement is the complement fixation (CF) test method. There are nine major components of complement, ranging from alpha to gamma in electrophoretic mobility. There are also inhibitors of some of these components. Nomenclature for this system has been confusing because numbers assigned to the components do not correspond to the sequence in which the components are activated and also because subcomponents exist in some of the components. Total complement is abbreviated C (some use the symbol C′ instead of C). Total complement is sometimes referred to as total hemolytic complement, or CH_{50}. The major complement components are numbered C1 through C9. Component C1 has three subcomponents: C1q, C1r, and C1s. Component C3 has also been called beta-1C.

The actual order of complement component activation in the classic complement pathway is C1, C4, C2, C3, C5, C6, C7, C8, and C9. There is an alternate pathway involving properdin, which activates C3 directly and bypasses C1, C4, and C2.

Complement has been assayed in two ways: methods that test complement overall functional activity and methods that depend on immunologic quantitative measurement of individual components of the complement system. Functional assessment is usually done through a hemolytic system using antibody-coated sheep RBCs in which complement is necessary for RBC lysis. The assay is dependent on proper function of the entire complement pathway. The end point is lysis of 50% of a standard antibody-coated RBC suspension with the results being reported in complement hemolytic (CH_{50}) units per milliliter of test specimen (this refers to the dilution of patient serum required to produce the end point). The total hemolytic complement (CH_{50}) test assesses overall function of the entire complement pathway. Immunologic measurement involves use of antibodies against single components of the complement system. This permits direct quantitation of the component being measured. The amount of the component is assumed to be directly related to its functional activity. A decreased C4 level suggests some defect in the classic pathway. A decreased C3 level with normal C4 level suggests abnormality in the alternate pathway.

The most common congenital disease associated with complement is hereditary angioedema. This is due to absence of C1 inhibitor, and the diagnosis is established by assay of C1 (C1 esterase) inhibitor. In 10%–20% of cases C1 inhibitor is present but nonfunctional. If immunologic methods are used for assay, this would lead to apparent normal results. Since C1, when activated, will split C2 and C4, lack of C1 inhibitor leads to decrease of CH_{50}, C2, and C4 levels during an acute attack. During remission the C4 level usually remains decreased, but CH_{50} and C2 levels may return to their reference ranges. These assays permit the diagnosis of functional decrease in the C1 esterase inhibitor level even if immunologic C1 esterase inhibitor values are within reference range.

Acquired complement abnormalities are much more common than congenital ones. Total complement is temporarily elevated following onset of various acute or chronic inflammatory diseases or acute tissue damage, although hepatitis virus type B infection is associated with decreased complement. Most of the clinical conditions in which complement measurement is useful are associated with decreased levels, either because of decreased production secondary to severe liver disease or to increased consumption secondary to glomerulonephritis or because of activation by circulating immune complexes. Total complement

(C or CH_{50}), C3, and C4 levels are all usually reduced in active systemic lupus erythematosis (SLE) nephritis. They may also be decreased in serum sickness, infectious endocarditis (subacute bacterial endocarditis), immune complex disease, and renal transplant rejection. They are normal in most patients with rheumatoid arthritis but may be reduced in a subgroup with severe disease accompanied by vasculitis. Total complement and C3 levels are usually reduced (but the C4 level is often normal) in poststreptococcal acute glomerulonephritis and in membranoproliferative nephritis.

Complement C3 function is unstable and may decrease significantly in blood or serum left standing at room temperature for more than 1–2 hours. This results in low CH_{50} levels with normal C3 and C4 levels. Serum or plasma that must be preserved should be frozen immediately.

Complement assays are not available in most laboratories and must be done by university hospitals or large reference laboratories. Problems with maintaining complement levels in specimens and the length of time before results are available have limited the popularity of complement assay. The assays currently are used mainly to diagnose angioedema, evaluate some patients with poststreptococcal or SLE nephritis, and to monitor therapy in some patients with SLE nephritis or membranoproliferative nephritis.

LIPOPROTEINS

Lipoproteins are molecules composed of lipids and proteins in varying proportions. Lipids, in general, are insoluble in water and most biologic fluids and are dependent for transport on protein incorporated into the molecule or on binding to plasma protein. The major lipoproteins are outlined in Table 21–2. The protein fraction of lipoproteins is composed predominantly of several polypeptides called "apoproteins." The major lipoprotein subgroups have specific apoprotein patterns (see Table 21–7). Some of the apoproteins have a functional role in lipoprotein metabolism. A short summary of lipoprotein metabolism will help to introduce the laboratory tests useful in lipid assay or in diagnosis of lipid disorders.

TABLE 21–2.
Major Lipoprotein Subgroups

Lipid-Protein Fractions	Ultracentrifuge S_f	Ultracentrifuge Specific Gravity	Electrophoresis	Approximate Composition
Chylomicrons	400–40,000	...	Neutral fat zone (point of application)	85% triglyceride 5% cholesterol 5% phospholipid 2% protein
Very low-density (beta) lipoproteins (VLDLs)	20–400	< 1.006	Prebeta	60% triglyceride 15% cholesterol 15% phospholipid 10% protein
Low-density (beta) lipoproteins (LDLs)	10–20 0–10	1.006–1.019 1.019–1.063	Beta Beta	45% cholesterol 10% triglyceride 20% phospholipid 25% protein
High-density (alpha) lipoproteins (HDLs)	—	> 1.063	Alpha	50% protein 15% cholesterol 5% triglyceride 30% phospholipid
Albumin-unesterified fatty acids (or free fatty acids, FFAs)	—	—	—	—

Lipoprotein Metabolism

Triglycerides enter the blood from exogenous (food) and endogenous (liver) sources. Food provides neutral fat, which is primarily triglyceride and which is hydrolyzed by pancreatic lipase into free fatty acids (FFA) and monoglycerides. These are taken into small intestine mucosal cells. The lipid fractions are recombined within the intestinal mucosa and are formed into chylomicrons. Chylomicrons have a thin outer shell of phospholipid and unesterified cholesterol with protein in the form of apoprotein B (and small quantities of other apoproteins). There is a central core of triglyceride and some cholesterol esters. When chylomicrons are released into plasma, they acquire some apoprotein C. Chylomicrons give postprandial plasma its characteristic milky appearance.

Chylomicrons enter the capillary network of adipose tissue, heart muscle, and skeletal muscle, where an enzyme called "lipoprotein lipase" splits off much of the triglyceride and hydrolyzes it to FFAs and glycerol. Some FFA is taken to the liver coupled to albumin, and some enters tissue cells. Free fatty acid is used for energy in heart and skeletal muscle or stored for future use in fat. Some glycerol likewise travels to the liver, and some is taken up by adipose tissue, where it is combined with FFA for storage as triglyceride. Some of the surface components of chylomicrons (phospholipids, unesterified cholesterol, and apoprotein C) are transferred to HDL molecules. The chylomicrons with reduced triglyceride and surface molecule content are called "chylomicron remnants." High-density lipoprotein molecules have an enzyme called "lecithin-cholesterol acyltransferase" (LCAT), produced by the liver, which esterifies the transferred cholesterol material; the cholesterol esters are then transferred back to the remaining chylomicron remnants to form LDL molecules.

The liver synthesizes triglyceride from FFA and glucose. Triglyceride is coupled to protein (apoprotein B) and released VLDL molecules. Very low-density lipoproteins are subjected to the action of lipoprotein lipase and metabolized in a manner similar to chylomicrons, with a considerable amount of VLDL being converted to LDL.

Body cholesterol is derived from exogenous dietary sources and from endogenous synthesis by the liver from acetate. The majority is produced by the liver. The liver excretes some cholesterol as a component of bile.

Low-density lipoprotein differs from VLDL in that LDL has lower triglyceride content, higher cholesterol content, and no C or E apoproteins. Low-density lipoprotein molecules are taken into tissue cells from specific receptor sites in the cell membrane. Inside the cell, the LDL molecules are metabolized into their component parts. Some of the cholesterol is utilized by the cell, and some can leave the cell under proper conditions. Thus, LDLs are thought to have a major role in providing body cells with cholesterol and thereby are an important part of the atherogenic process.

High-density lipoproteins have two contrasting roles in lipid metabolism. On one hand, they help create LDL from VLDL and thus enhance the possibility of atherogenesis. On the other hand, they are thought to help transport cholesterol out of peripheral tissues to the liver (although the mechanism for this is still not completely understood) and thus help "protect" against atherosclerosis.

Laboratory Tests Used to Assess Risk of Coronary Heart Disease

There has been much interest in the significance of the lipoproteins in atherosclerosis. Large numbers of studies have been carried out, different populations have been examined, various diets have been tried, and endless pages of statistics have been published. Several laboratory assays that have general, but sometimes not unanimous, acceptance as predictors of atherosclerotic risk have emerged from these data. Descriptions of these follow.

Serum (Total) Cholesterol.—Total serum cholesterol comprises all of the cholesterol found in various lipoproteins. Cholesterol is the major component of LDLs and a minority component of VLDLs and HDLs. Since LDL has consistently been associated with risk of atherosclerosis, and since LDL is difficult to measure, serum total cholesterol has been used for many years as a substitute. There is general agreement that a strong correlation exists between considerably elevated serum cholesterol levels and an increased tendency for atherosclerosis. Disadvantages include the following:

1. There is considerable overlap between

TABLE 21–3.

Upper Normal Limits for Fasting Serum Total Cholesterol and Triglyceride Derived in the Usual Statistical Way from Clinically Normal U.S. Population

	Age (yr)				
	10–19	20–29	30–39	40–49	50–59
Cholesterol (mg/100 ml)					
Frederickson et al.	230	240	270	310	330
Heiss et al.					
Male	200	234	267	275	276
Female	200	222	251	267	296
Triglyceride (mg/100 ml)					
Frederickson et al.	140	140	150	160	190
Heiss et al.					
Male	150	204	316	279	262
Female	130	128	174	192	280

cholesterol values found in populations and individuals at normal risk for atherosclerosis and those at higher risk. This leads to controversy over what values should be established as "normal" for the serum cholesterol reference range. A related problem is a significant difference between the reference range values for cholesterol based on "ideal" populations (i.e., derived from populations with a low incidence of atherosclerosis) compared with reference ranges from populations with a higher incidence of atherosclerosis (e.g., unselected clinically asymptomatic persons in the United States). This has led to objections that data from many persons with significant but subclinical disease are being used to help derive the reference values for populations with higher risk of coronary heart disease (CHD). Some evidence of this is seen when population cholesterol reference values in Table 21–3 are compared with the cholesterol values found to be correlated with increased risk of CHD in the Framingham coronary disease study (Table 21–4).

Whereas the upper limit of statistically derived U.S. values is about 275–300 mg/100 ml, some investigators favor 225 mg/100 ml as the acceptable upper limit since that is the value representing average risk for CHD in the Framingham study (see Table 21-4). However, the average risk for CHD in the U.S. population of the Framingham study is higher than the average risk for a low-risk population. The National Institutes of Health (NIH) Consensus Conference on cholesterol in heart disease in 1984 proposed age-related limits based on degree of CHD risk (Table 21–5). The NIH Conference guidelines were widely adopted. In some studies, serum cholesterol (as well as triglyceride) reference values are sex related as well as age related.

To make matters more confusing, many investigators believe that 200 mg/100 ml (5.15 mmol/L) should be considered the acceptable upper limit because that is the approximate upper limit for low-risk populations. The Expert Panel of the National Cholesterol Education Program (NCEP, 1987) chose 200 mg/100 ml without regard to age or sex (Table 21–6). Although the NCEP advocated use of total cholesterol as the basic screening test for CHD risk, they recommended that therapy should be based on LDL cholesterol values.

The NCEP Guidelines seem to be replacing the NIH Consensus Guidelines. One possible drawback is lack of consideration of HDL cholesterol effects (discussed later), which may be important since HDL is an independent risk factor.

2. Serum cholesterol can have a within-

TABLE 21–4.

Relative Risk of Coronary Heart Disease at Various Total Cholesterol Levels

Relative CHD Risk*	Total Serum Cholesterol (mg/100 ml)	(mmol/L)
1/2 average risk	150	3.90
Average risk	225	5.85
2× average risk	260	6.70
3× average risk	300	7.75

*Based predominantly on Framingham coronary disease study.

TABLE 21–5.

Risk of Coronary Heart Disease at Different Total Cholesterol Levels (NIH Consensus Conference)*

	Total Cholesterol (mg/100 ml)		
Age (yr)	Low Risk	Moderate Risk	High Risk
2–19	≤ 170	170–185	> 185
20–29	≤ 200	200–220	> 220
30–39	≤ 220	220–240	> 240
> 40	≤ 240	240–260	> 260

*Data based predominantly on Framingham coronary disease study.

TABLE 21–6.

National Cholesterol Education Program Total Cholesterol Criteria to Screen for Coronary Heart Disease Risk and Low-Density Lipoprotein Criteria Used to Plan Therapy

	Total Cholesterol (mg/100 ml)		LDL Cholesterol (mg/100 ml)
Desirable total cholesterol	< 200 (5.15)*	Desirable LDL	< 130 (3.36)*
Borderline high-risk total cholesterol	200–239 (5.15–6.18)*	Borderline high-risk LDL	130–159 (3.36–4.11)*
High total cholesterol	≥ 240 (6.20)*	High-risk LDL	≥ 160 (4.14)*

*mmol/L.

day variation that averages about 8% (range, 4%–17%) above or below mean values during any 24-hour period (±8% variation represents about ±20 mg/100 ml if the mean value is 250 mg/100 ml).

3. Day-to-day cholesterol values in the same individual can fluctuate by 10%–15% (literature range, 3%–44%).

4. Serum cholesterol values may decrease as much as 10% (literature range 7%–15%) when a patient changes from the erect to the recumbent position, as would occur if blood were drawn from an outpatient and again from the same person as a hospital inpatient. Two studies have shown less than 5% average difference between serum cholesterol obtained from venipuncture and from fingerstick capillary specimens in the same patient.

5. Various lipid fractions are considerably altered during major illnesses. For example, total cholesterol values often begin to decrease 24–48 hours after an acute myocardial infarction (MI). Values most often reach their nadir in 7–10 days with results as much as 30%–50% below previous levels. The effect may persist to some extent as long as 6–8 weeks. In one study not all patients experienced postinfarct cholesterol decrease. Although theoretically one could obtain valid cholesterol results within 24 hours after onset of acute MI, the true time of onset is often not known. Surgery has been shown to induce similar changes in total cholesterol to those following acute MI. High-density lipoprotein cholesterol also temporarily fell in some studies but not in others. Triglyceride levels were relatively unchanged in some studies and increased in others. In bacterial sepsis and in viral infections, total cholesterol levels tend to fall and triglyceride levels tend to increase. Besides effects of illness there are also effects of posture and diet change, stress, medications, and other factors that make hospital conditions different from outpatient basal condition. For example, thiazide diuretic therapy is reported to increase total cholesterol levels about 5%–8% (range, 0%–12%) and decrease HDL cholesterol to a similar degree. However, several studies reported return to baseline levels by 1 year. Certain medications can interfere with cholesterol assay. For example, high serum levels of ascorbic acid (vitamin C) can reduce cholesterol levels considerably using certain assay methods.

6. Certain diseases are well-known causes of hypercholesterolemia; these include biliary cirrhosis, hypothyroidism, and the nephrotic syndrome. A high-cholesterol diet is another important factor that must be considered.

All of the major lipoprotein fractions, including chylomicrons, contain some cholesterol. Therefore, an increase in any of these fractions rather than in LDL alone potentially can elevate serum total cholesterol values. Of course, for lipoproteins with low cholesterol content the degree of elevation must be relatively great before the total cholesterol value becomes elevated above reference range.

In summary, according to the NCEP, 200 mg/100 ml (5.15 mmol/L) is the upper acceptable limit for any age (see Table 21–6). Lipid values obtained during hospitalization may be misleading, and borderline or mildly elevated values obtained on a reasonably healthy outpatient may have to be repeated over a period of time to obtain a more accurate baseline. Changes between one specimen and the next up to 20–30 mg/100 ml (or even more) may be due to physiologic variation rather than alterations from disease or therapy.

Although one would expect cholesterol in food to raise postprandial serum cholesterol values, actually serum cholesterol levels are very little affected by food intake from any single meal. Cholesterol specimens are traditionally collected fasting in the early morning because serial cholesterol specimens should all be drawn at the same time of day after the patient has been in the same body position (upright or recumbent) and because triglyceride (which is greatly affected by food intake) or HDL cholesterol assay are frequently performed on the same specimen.

Low-Density Lipoprotein Cholesterol.—The LDL (beta electrophoretic) fraction has been shown in various studies to have a better correlation with risk of atherosclerosis than total serum cholesterol alone, although the degree of improvement is not marked. As noted previously, the NCEP bases its therapy recommendations on LDL values (see Table 21–6). The major disadvantage of this approach is difficulty in isolating and measuring LDL. The most reliable method is ultracentrifugation. Since ultracentrifugation is available only in a relatively few laboratories and is expensive, it has been standard procedure to estimate LDLs as LDL cholesterol by means of the Friedewald formula. This formula estimates LDL cholesterol from results of triglyceride, total cholesterol, and HDL cholesterol, as follows: LDL cholesterol = total cholesterol − (HDL cholesterol − triglycerides/5). One report suggests that modifying the formula by dividing triglyceride by 6 rather than 5 produces a more accurate estimate of LDL levels. A disadvantage of the Friedewald formula is dependence on results of three different tests. Inaccuracy in one or more of the test results can significantly affect the formula calculations. In addition, the formula cannot be used if the triglyceride level is greater than 400 mg/100 ml.

High-Density Lipoprotein Cholesterol.— Several large-scale studies have suggested that HDL levels (measured as HDL cholesterol) have a strong inverse correlation with risk of atherosclerotic CHD (the higher the HDL level, the less the risk). High-density lipoprotein seems to be a risk factor that is independent of LDL or total cholesterol. Some believe that HDL cholesterol assay has as good or better correlation with risk of CHD than total or LDL cholesterol. In general, the Framingham study suggested that every 20 mg/100 ml reduction of HDL cholesterol corresponds to approximately a doubling of CHD risk (Table 21–7). Disadvantages include certain technical problems that affect HDL assay, although methodology is becoming more simple and reliable. These problems include different methods that produce different results and need for two procedure steps (separation or extraction of HDL from other lipoproteins and then measurement of the cholesterol component), all of which produce rather poor correlation of results among laboratories. Ascorbic acid (vitamin C) may interfere (5%–15% decrease) with some test methods but not others. Reliability of risk pre-

TABLE 21–7.

Relative Risk of Coronary Heart Disease as Suggested by HDL Cholesterol and the Total Cholesterol/High-Density Lipoprotein*

Relative CHD Risk†	HDL Cholesterol (mg/100 ml)		Total Cholesterol/HDL Cholesterol Ratio	
	Male	Female	Male	Female
1/2 average	60	70	3.4	3.3
Average	45	55	5.0	4.4
2× average	25	35	10.0	7.0
3× average	—	—	24.0	11.0

*Based predominantly on Framingham coronary disease study.

†Average = average risk level of unselected U.S. population (a risk level higher than the average risk level of selected low-risk populations).

diction is heavily dependent on accurate HDL assay, since a relatively small change in assay values produces a relatively large change in predicted risk. High-density lipoprotein values are age and sex dependent. High-density lipoprotein values tend to decrease temporarily after acute MI, as do total serum cholesterol values. Hypothyroidism elevates HDL values and hyperthyroidism decreases them; therefore, in thyroid disease HDL values are not reliable in estimating risk of CHD. The possible effects of other illnesses are not as well known. Certain antihypertensive medications (thiazides, beta-blockers without intrinsic sympathomimetic activity, sympathicolytic agents) decrease HDL by a small but significant degree.

Since serum total cholesterol and HDL are independent risk factors, some patients may have values for one that suggest abnormality but values for the other that remain within reference limits. As independent risk factors, a favorable value for one does not entirely cancel the unfavorable effect of the other.

Serum Cholesterol/High-Density Lipoprotein Cholesterol Ratio.—Some investigators use this ratio as a convenient way to visualize the joint contribution of risk from these important risk factors. The ratio for normal risk is 5, for double risk is 10, and for triple risk is 20. Some believe that the ratio is the best single currently available predictor of CHD risk. Others believe that the ratio does not adequately demonstrate the independent contributions of the two factors and may be misleading in cases in which one or both factors may be abnormal, but the ratio does not suggest the actual degree of abnormality.

Apoprotein Assay.—Apoprotein A is uniquely associated with HDL (Table 21–8), and measurement of apoprotein A-1 has been proposed as a better index of atherogenic risk than assay of HDL cholesterol. Apoprotein B is the predominant protein of LDL but is also present in significant quantity in VLDL. The subgroup known as B-48 is a major structural protein in chylomicrons, whereas the subgroup called B-100 is the major B apoprotein in VLDL. Some research suggests that apoprotein B may have a role of its own in cholesterol synthesis and that apoprotein B measurement may provide a better indication of atherosclerotic risk than LDL cholesterol measurement (Table 21–9). The apoprotein A-1/apoprotein B ratio has been reported by some to be the best single predictor of CHD. However, there is some controversy over the role of apoprotein assay in current management of CHD. The apoproteins have been quantitated mostly by immunoassay, using radioimmunoassay, radial immunodiffusion, and immunonephelometry. Apoprotein assay is still not widely available or widely used, and quality control surveys have shown problems in accuracy between laboratories with one international survey finding within-lab CVs of 5%–10% and between-lab CVs of 15%–30%.

Triglyceride Measurement.—Triglyceride is found in chylomicrons and in VLDLs. In fasting plasma, chylomicrons are usually absent, so triglyceride provides a reasonably good estimate of VLDL. The usefulness of VLDL or triglyceride as an indicator of atherosclerotic risk has been very controversial. The current majority opinion is that triglyceride levels do not of themselves have a strong predictive value for atherosclerosis. There is a roughly inverse relationship between triglyceride and HDL levels, so that elevated triglyceride levels tend to be associated with low HDL levels. Elevated triglyceride levels therefore tend to be associated with increased risk for CHD. However, other factors that influence triglyceride levels are frequently present. Nonfasting specimens are a frequent source of elevated triglyceride levels. Postprandial triglyceride levels increase about 2 hours (range, 2–10 hours) after food intake with average maximal effect at 4–6 hours. Therefore, a 12- to 16-hour fast is recom-

TABLE 21–8.

Apoprotein Patterns of Major Lipoprotein Classes

Approximate Apoprotein Composition		
VDL	LDL	HDL
B = 40%	B = 98%	AI = 66%
C = 50%		AII = 22%
E = 10%		C + D = 12%

TABLE 21–9.

Relative Risk of CHD as Suggested by Apo-1/Apo-2 Ratio

Relative Risk	Males	Females
Average	1.4	1.6
2× average	1.1	1.1
3× average	1.0	1.0

mended before obtaining a specimen. Within-day variation for triglyceride averages about ± 40% (range, 26%–64%), with between-day average variation about ± 25%–50% (range, 18%–100%). Obesity, severe acute stress (trauma, sepsis, burns, acute MI), estrogen therapy, alcohol intake, high-fat diet, and a considerable number of diseases (e.g., diabetes, acute pancreatitis, nephrotic syndrome, and uremia) increase triglyceride levels. Levels more than 1,000 mg/100 ml (11.29 mmol/L) interfere with many laboratory tests (see Table 36–2, IX), and levels more than 1,500 mg/100 ml predispose to or often accompany acute pancreatitis. Currently, the major use of triglyceride measurement is not in estimating risk of atherogenesis but in screening for hyperlipidemia and establishing lipoprotein phenotypes (discussed later).

Triglyceride fasting values of 250 mg/100 ml (2.82 mmol/L) were considered to be upper limit of normal in adults by an NIH Consensus Conference on hypertriglyceridemia in 1984. Fasting values more than 500 mg/100 ml (5.65 mmol/L) were considered definitely abnormal. Some investigators consider 200 mg/100 ml (2.25 mmol/L) as the upper limit of the reference range; this value is derived from the 90th percentile of the 1980 NIH Lipid Research Clinics (NIH-LRC) Prevalence Study. The NIH-LRC values are derived from plasma; plasma values are about 2%–4% less than results obtained from serum.

Other Risk Factors for Coronary Heart Disease.—Besides lipoprotein abnormality, epidemiologic studies suggest that cigarette smoking, diabetes, obesity, male sex, hypertension, and increasing age are all factors that increase the risk for CHD.

Summary.—The most widely used current procedure to estimate risk of coronary heart disease is to obtain serum or plasma total cholesterol levels (as a substitute for LDL assay) and HDL cholesterol levels. If desired, the total cholesterol/HDL ratio can be calculated, and LDL cholesterol levels can be derived from the same data plus triglyceride assay by means of the Friedewald formula. These studies are best performed when the patient is in a basal state. It is important to note that many investigators caution that such studies may be misleading when performed on hospitalized patients, due to the effects of disease and hospital environment. Accuracy of the values is increased if more than one specimen is obtained several weeks apart (e.g., one each month for 3 months, each obtained fasting at the same time of the day) to establish an average value to compensate for physiologic and laboratory-induced fluctuations in lipoprotein measurements.

Lipoprotein Phenotyping

In 1965, Frederickson, Levy, and Lees published an article that caught the attention of the medical world. They divided lipoprotein disorders into five basic "phenotypes," based primarily on electrophoresis of serum obtained after 10 hours of overnight fasting. The sixth phenotype was added later when type II was split into IIa and IIb (Fig 21–5). Lipoprotein phenotyping was originally proposed as a means of classifying congenital disorders of lipid metabolism according to the lipoprotein abnormality involved to provide more specific therapy. In this way abnormal serum levels of specific lipids such as cholesterol could be traced to abnormalities in specific lipoprotein groups, which, in turn, could suggest certain congenital or acquired etiologies. In time, however, the original intent and limitations of the system were sometimes forgotten, and treatment was sometimes begun—based on the phenotype suggested by the patient's lipid profile or lipoprotein electrophoretic pattern—as though the patient had a congenital lipoprotein disease. Congenital disease cannot be treated directly, so therapy is directed against the abnormal lipids. Since congenital disease is present in only a small percentage of persons with abnormal serum lipid values, and since lipid disorders due to acquired conditions are best treated by therapy directed at the condition responsible for the lipid abnormality, some of these persons were not being managed appropriately. In other words, the symptoms (abnormal levels of lipids or lipoproteins) were being treated rather than the underlying etiology.

Laboratory Tests in Lipoprotein Disorders

Screening tests for lipoprotein abnormality include determination of serum cholesterol and triglyceride levels plus visual inspection of serum (or plasma) for presence of chylomi-

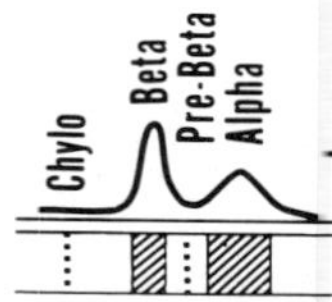

← NORMAL →

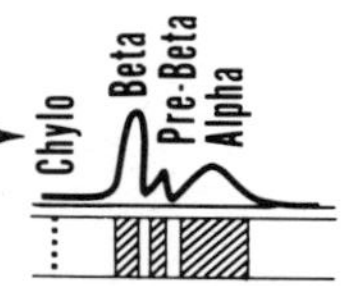

TYPE	CHOLESTEROL	TRIGLYCERIDES	LIPOPROTEINS	COMMENTS ON PATTERNS	SECONDARY CAUSES
I Rare	MILD INCR. (20% NORMAL)	MARK. INCR.	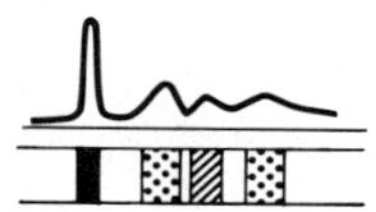	CHYLOMICRONS INCREASED PRE-BETA NORMAL OR SLIGHT INCR. BETA AND ALPHA DECR. Notes 1. "Thick cream" layer when plasma stands at 4° C 2. Plasma below "thick cream" layer is clear	Dysglobulinemia Diabetes Mellitus Pancreatitis
IIa Common	MARK. INCR.	NORMAL	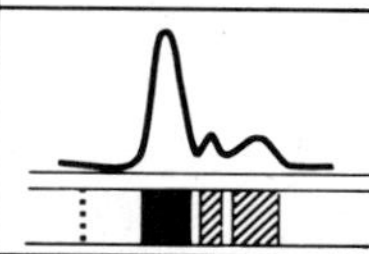	BETA MARKED INCR. PRE-BETA NORMAL OR DECR. ALPHA NORMAL CHYLOMICRONS NORMAL	Hypothyroid; Nephrotic Syndrome; Biliary Obstruction; Dysglobulinemia High Cholesterol diet
IIb Probably Common	INCR. (usually)	INCR.	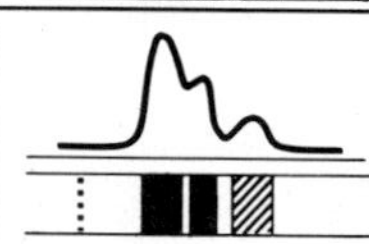	BETA INCR. PRE-BETA INCR. ALPHA NORMAL CHYLOMICRONS NORMAL	Same as type IIa Gout

<table>
<tr><td>III
Uncommon</td><td>INCR.
(20% NORMAL)</td><td>INCR.
(10% NORMAL)</td><td>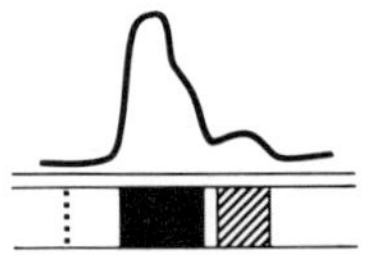</td><td>BETA INCR. ("BROAD BETA" IN 2/3 CASES)
PRE-BETA NORMAL OR MILD INCR.
ALPHA NORMAL
CHYLOMICRONS NORMAL
Notes
Need ultracentrifugation for diagnosis (Demonstration of "floating beta")</td><td>Diabetes Mellitus
Hepatic Disease
Hypothyroid</td><td></td></tr>
<tr><td>IV
Most
Common</td><td>NORMAL
(20% INCR.)</td><td>INCR.</td><td>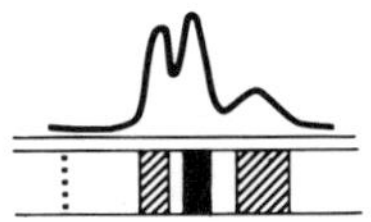</td><td>PRE-BETA MOD. OR MARK. INCR.
BETA AND ALPHA NORMAL OR MILD DECR.
CHYLOMICRONS NORMAL
Notes
Sometimes called "Carbohydrate-induced hyperlipemia"</td><td>Hypothyroid
Nephrotic Syndrome
Pregnancy; Estrogen
Diabetes Mellitus
Pancreatitis
Dysglobulinemia</td><td>Alcohol
Uremia
"Lp beta"
Gout</td></tr>
<tr><td>V
Uncommon</td><td>INCR.
(40% NORMAL)</td><td>INCR.</td><td>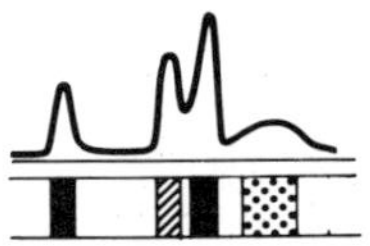</td><td>CHYLOMICRONS INCR.
PRE-BETA INCR.
BETA AND ALPHA DECR.
Notes
1. "Thick cream" layer when plasma stands at 4° C
2. Plasma below "thick cream" layer is cloudy or turbid</td><td>Pancreatitis
Alcohol
Diabetes Mellitus
Dysglobulinemia</td><td></td></tr>
</table>

FIG 21–5.
Classification of lipoproteinemias.

TABLE 21–10.
Probability of Detecting Hyperlipoproteinemia by Lipid Analysis Alone*

Type	Percentage Detectable by Lipid Assay Values		
	Abnormal Cholesterol	Abnormal Triglyceride	Abnormal Cholesterol or Triglyceride
I	80	100	100
II	89	24	92
III	82	91	91
IV	22	100	100
V	61	100	100

*From Frederickson DS, et al: The typing of hyperlipoproteinemia: A progress report (1968), in Holmes WL, et al (ed): *Drugs Affecting Lipid Metabolism.* New York, Plenum Press, 1969. Used by permission.

crons after the specimen has been kept overnight at refrigerator temperature. The specimen should be obtained after a 10- to 12-hour fast. This triad of tests serves not only as a screening procedure but in the majority of cases is sufficient to establish the phenotype. Normal results on all three tests are reasonable evidence against serious lipoprotein disease (Table 21–10. However, occasional patients with disease can be missed, due sometimes to laboratory variation, borderline abnormality, or the overlap of normal and abnormal persons in statistically established reference ranges referred to earlier. Lipoprotein electrophoresis and ultracentrifugation are useful in a minority of cases as confirmatory or diagnostic tests. Electrophoresis is helpful in differentiating Frederickson type I from type V disease, some cases of type IIa from IIb, and some cases of type II from type IV. Ultracentrifugation is useful mainly in diagnosis of type III disease. Electrophoresis is not needed in the majority of patients. Lipoprotein phenotyping is done preferably on outpatients rather than hospitalized patients due to the short-term effects of serious illness on lipid metabolism as well as the other factors mentioned in the previous discussion of serum cholesterol measurement. However, screening of hospital inpatients can detect possible abnormality that can be verified later under more basal conditions.

A short summary of lipoprotein phenotype patterns shows that the presence of a creamlike layer of chylomicrons after overnight incubation of fasting serum in the refrigerator indicates type I or type V. If the serum below the chylomicron layer is clear, this suggests type I; if the serum below the chylomicron layer is cloudy or turbid, this suggests type V. Fasting serum obtained from patients with the other phenotypes does not contain chylomicrons. If fasting serum does not contain chylomicrons, elevation of serum cholesterol levels with normal triglyceride levels suggests type II disease, whereas the reverse suggests type IV disease. If both cholesterol and triglyceride levels are significantly abnormal, the disease may be type II or type III. Type II disease has recently been subdivided into IIa and IIb. Type IIa has increased cholesterol but normal triglyceride. Type IIb has elevated cholesterol and triglyceride. Type III is uncommon. It is similar to IIb in that both cholesterol and triglyceride levels are elevated, but it frequently has a slightly different electrophoretic pattern (broad beta) and always has a peculiar "floating beta" component (a beta-mobility protein that floats at 1.006 density instead of 1.013), which can be demonstrated only by ultracentrifugation. Type IV phenotype has elevated triglyceride and normal cholesterol levels.

Although the majority of patients can be phenotyped using the triad of biochemical tests, some overlap occurs among the phenotypes because cholesterol is present to some extent in all of the major lipoprotein fractions and because triglyceride is found in both chylomicrons and the VLDL fractions. Also, the laboratory reference range may inadvertently influence a phenotype decision in some cases, depending on whether the upper limit of the reference range was derived from a sample of the local population, obtained from data published in the literature, or structured according to findings in populations with low risk of atherosclerosis.

Phenotypes I, III, and V are uncommon. Phenotypes II and IV constitute the majority of hyperlipoproteinemias. Type IV is probably more common than type II. Most type IV patients have the acquired form. The majority of type II patients also have the acquired form (the most common etiology being a high-cholesterol diet), but type II is more frequently congenital than type IV.

Some serum specimens from patients with types IIb, III, or IV disease may have a somewhat cloudy or faintly milky appearance. This must be differentiated from the thicker, creamlike precipitate characteristic of increased chylomicrons.

Certain considerations affect interpretation of these laboratory results. Patients should be on a normal diet for several days previous to testing and must be fasting for at least 10 hours before a specimen is drawn. If a test cannot be done the same day, the serum must be refrigerated but not frozen; freezing alters prebeta and chylomicron fractions, although cholesterol and triglyceride determinations can be done. Various diseases may produce certain phenotype patterns or may falsely change one pattern into another. Changes in diet, medications, activity levels, stress, and other factors may alter a mild or borderline abnormality or produce mild abnormality. In addition, the laboratory results have ± 5%–10% built-in variability for technical reasons.

On electrophoresis, occasional persons display increased prebeta but normal triglyceride levels. If laboratory error is ruled out, these patients may have a congenital variant called "Lp system" or "sinking prebeta." This is found in up to 10% of the U.S. population and is currently not thought to have any clinical significance. However, one group of investigators has raised the question whether Lp(a) may constitute some degree of independent risk factor for coronary atherosclerosis, with high Lp(a) levels having some association with increased incidence of MI. Plasma or serum may be used for lipoprotein analysis. Plasma collected with ethylenediamine tetraacetic acid (EDTA) is preferred if the specimen cannot be tested the same day. Plasma values for triglyceride are about 2%–4% lower than for serum.

Two rare diseases display characteristic lipoprotein patterns on electrophoresis. Tangier disease has no alpha peak. Bassen-Kornzweig syndrome (associated with "pincushion" RBCs called acanthocytes, and neurologic abnormalities) lacks a beta peak.

BIBLIOGRAPHY

Lardinosi CK, Neuman SL: The effects of antihypertensive agents on serum lipids and lipoproteins. *Arch Intern Med* 1988; 148:1280.

Gertz MA, et al: Utility of subcutaneous fat aspiration for the diagnosis of systemic amyloidosis (immunoglobulin light chain). *Arch Intern Med* 1988; 148:929.

Cohen HJ: Monoclonal gammopathies and aging. *Hosp Pract* 1988; 23(3A):75.

Peddicord CH, Barnes WA: Ascorbic acid interferogram for cholesterol in the Demand and TDX. *Clin Chem* 1988; 34:773.

Lavie CJ, et al: Management of lipids in primary and secondary prevention of cardiovascular diseases. *Mayo Clin Proc* 1988; 63:605.

Painter PC, Copas PR: Cholesterol testing and drug interactions. *Lab Mgmt* 1988; 26(5):37.

Grinstead GF, Ellefson RD: Heterogeneity and lipoprotein Lp(a) and apolipoprotein (a). *Clin Chem* 1988; 34:1063.

National Heart, Lung, and Blood Institute: Report of the National Cholesterol Education Program: Expert panel on detection, evaluation, and treatment of high blood cholesterol levels in adults. *Arch Intern Med* 1988; 148:36.

Palumbo PJ: National Cholesterol Education Program: Does the emperor have any clothes? *Mayo Clin Proc* 1988; 63:88.

Laboratory Standardization Panel, National Cholesterol Education Program: Current status of blood cholesterol measurement in clinical laboratories in the United States. *Clin Chem* 1988; 34:193.

Naito HK: Apolipoproteins as biochemical markers of cardiac risk. *Am Clin Prod Rev* 1988; 7(1):27.

Meis JM, et al: Solitary plasmacytomas of bone and extramedullary plasmacytomas. *Cancer* 1987; 59:1475.

Ruff ME: Phenytoin-induced IgA depression. *Am J Dis Child* 1987; 141:858.

Theil KS, et al: Diagnosing plasma cell leukemia. *Lab Med* 1987; 18:684.

Bartl R, et al: Histologic classification and staging of multiple myeloma. *Am J Clin Pathol* 1987; 87:342.

Weingerg RB: Lipoprotein metabolism: hormonal regulation. *Hosp Pract* 1987; 22(6):223.

Maciejko JJ: Apolipoprotein A-1 and B and their relationship to coronary heart disease. Beckman Co monograph APO-1, 1987.

Crapper RM: Paraproteinemias in homosexual men with HIV infection. *Am J Clin Pathol* 1987; 88:348.

Weinsier RL: Hyperlipoproteinemias and heart disease. *Ala J Med Sci* 1987; 24:420.

Rubio-Felix D, et al: Nonsecretory multiple myeloma. *Cancer* 1987; 59:1847.

Crawford J, et al: Evaluation of monoclonal gammopathies in the "well" elderly. *Am J Med* 1987; 82:39.

Kyle RA, Garton JP: The spectrum of IgM

monoclonal gammopathy in 430 cases. *Mayo Clin Proc* 1987; 62:719.

Fassett RT, Kagnoff MF: Clinical significance of selective IgA deficiency. *Intern Med Specialist* 1987; 8:93.

Papadea C, Check IJ: Immunoglobulin G subclasses. *Clin Chem Newslett* 1987; 13(6):10.

Naito HK: Triglycerides: Part II. *Clin Chem Newslett* 1987; 13(9):8.

Gerbaut L, Macart M: Is standardization more important than methodology for assay of total protein in cerebrospinal fluid? *Clin Chem* 1986; 32:353.

Buss DH: Initial bone marrow findings in multiple myeloma. *Arch Pathol Lab Med* 1986; 110:30.

Wolf BC, et al: Bone marrow morphology and immunology in systemic amyloidosis. *Am J Clin Pathol* 1986; 86:84.

DeLong DM, et al: A comparison of methods for the estimation of plasma low- and very low-density lipoprotein cholesterol. *JAMA* 1986; 256:2372.

Naito HK: The clinical significance of apolipoprotein measurements. *J Clin Immunoassay* 1986; 9:11.

Superko HR, et al: High-density lipoprotein cholesterol measurements. *JAMA* 1986; 256:2714.

Blank DW, et al: The method of determination must be considered in interpreting blood cholesterol levels. *JAMA* 1986; 256:2867.

Rifai N: Lipoproteins and apolipoproteins. *Arch Pathol Lab Med* 1986; 110:694.

Castelli WP, et al: Incidence of coronary heart disease and lipoprotein cholesterol levels. *JAMA* 1986; 256:2835.

McManus BM: Reference ranges and ideal patient values for blood cholesterol. *Arch Pathol Lab Med* 1986; 110:469.

Nishi HH, Elin RJ: Three turbimetric methods for determining total protein compared. *Clin Chem* 1985; 31:1377.

Friedlander Y, et al: Variability of plasma lipids and lipoproteins. *Clin Chem* 1985; 31:1121.

NIH Consensus Conference: Lowering blood cholesterol to prevent heart disease. *JAMA* 1985; 253:2080.

Nusinow SR, et al: The hereditary and acquired deficiencies of complement. *Med Clin North Am* 1985; 69:487.

Crawford J, et al: Evaluation of hyperviscosity in monoclonal gammopathies. *Am J Med* 1985; 79:13.

Keshgegian AA, Van Tran N: Mixed cryoglobulinemia causing pseudoleukocytosis. *Clin Chem* 1985; 31:769.

Goldman JN, Goldman MB: The genetics of antibody production. *JAMA* 1984; 251:774.

NIH Consensus Conference: Treatment of hypertriglyceridemia. *JAMA* 1984; 251:1196.

Oken MM: Multiple myeloma. *Med Clin North Am* 1984; 68:757.

Kyle RA: "Benign" monoclonal gammopathy. *JAMA* 1984; 251:1849.

Kyle RA, Greipp PR: Amyloidosis (AL). *Mayo Clin Proc* 1983; 58:665.

Rifkind BM, Segal P: Lipid research clinics program reference values for hyperlipidemia and hypolipidemia. *JAMA* 1983; 250:1869.

Warnick GR, et al: Interlaboratory proficiency survey of high-density lipoprotein cholesterol measurement. *Clin Chem* 1983; 29:516.

Deuel TF, Davis P: Waldenstrom's Macroglobulinemia. *Arch Intern Med* 1983; 143:986.

Schenck J, et al: Laboratory evaluation of complement. *Clin Lab Prod* 1983; 12(9):19.

Duggan J, Duggan PF: Albumin by Broncresol Green: A case of laboratory conservatism. *Clin Chem* 1982; 28:1407.

Wester SM, et al: The histopathology of gamma heavy chain disease. *Am J Clin Pathol* 1982; 78:427.

Gibson JC, Brown WV: HDL assays: Methods and their rationale. *Lab Mgmt* 1981;19(9):25.

Penn GM: The monoclonal gammopathies: Laboratory detection. *Lab Mgmt* 1981; 19:30.

Uhl GS, et al: Relation between high density lipoprotein cholesterol and coronary artery disease in asymptomatic men. *Am J Cardiol* 1981; 48:903.

Tarnoky AL: Albumin. *Ann Clin Biochem* 1981; 18:61.

Ritzmann SE, et al: Bence-Jones protein. *Lab Mgmt* 1981; 19(9):17.

Heiss G, et al: Lipoprotein-cholesterol distributions in selected North American populations: The lipid research clinics prevalence study. *Circulation* 1980; 61:302.

Hulley SB: Epidemiology as a guide to clinical decisions: The association between triglyceride and coronary heart disease. *New Engl J Med* 1980; 302:1383.

Ritzmann SE: Radial immunodiffusion revisited. *Lab Med* 1978; 9:23, 27.

22 Bone and Joint Disorders

RHEUMATOID DISEASES

The relationship between the rheumatoid diseases and diseases of the so-called collagen-vascular group is both close and uncertain. Many of the clinical symptoms found classically in one disease or syndrome may be found in another; the difference is on emphasis of certain aspects over others. This similarity extends to laboratory tests and makes it even more difficult to place borderline or problem cases into one group or the other. Until the exact etiology of each disease is known, overlap in laboratory test results is likely to continue. Fortunately, most patients can be assigned to satisfactory diagnostic categories using available clinical and laboratory data.

Rheumatoid Arthritis

Rheumatoid arthritis (RA) is a chronic systemic disease whose most prominent symptom is inflammation of joints. The small joints of the hands and feet, especially the proximal interphalangeal joints, are most frequently affected; involvement of larger joints of the extremities is somewhat less frequent, and occasionally nonextremity joints may be affected. Polyarticular involvement is much more common than monoarticular disease. Articular disease activity may or may not be preceded or accompanied by systemic symptoms, such as low-grade fever, myalgias, malaise, and fatigue. Rheumatoid arthritis tends to be a slow, intermittently active, migratory process that is frequently symmetric. Onset is gradual in 75%–80% of affected adults and more severe and abrupt in 20%–25%. Subcutaneous nodules with distinctive microscopic appearance occur in 15%–20% of patients, most frequently distal to (but not far from) the elbows. Inflammatory involvement of nonarticular organs or tissues such as the heart or lungs may sometimes occur. Patients with RA have increased frequency of the antigen HLA-DR4.

Laboratory Findings.—In active adult-onset RA, anemia is present in about 40% of men and 60% of women. The anemia usually appears within 2 months after onset of clinical disease, usually does not become more severe, and is usually of mild or moderate degree, with a hemoglobin value less than 10 gm/100 ml (100 g/L) in fewer than 10% of cases. There is said to be some correlation between the degree of anemia and the initial severity of illness. The anemia of RA is usually included with the anemia of chronic disease, which typically is normocytic and normochromic. However, anemia in RA is more likely to be hypochromic (reported in 50%–100% of cases), although microcytosis is found in less than 10% of cases.

White blood cell (WBC) counts are most often normal or only minimally elevated. About 25% of RA patients are said to have leukocytosis, usually not exceeding 15,000/cu mm (15×10^9/L), which is more apt to be present when onset of disease is severe and abrupt. Leukopenia is found in about 3% of cases, usually as part of Felty's syndrome (RA plus splenomegaly and leukopenia).

Anemia and leukocytosis are more common in juvenile-onset RA than adult-onset RA.

In active RA, nonspecific indicators of acute

inflammation, such as the erythrocyte sedimentation rate (ESR) and C-reactive protein level, are elevated in most (but not all) patients. The serum uric acid level is normal in most patients. The serum iron level is generally low-normal or decreased, and iron-binding capacity is also low-normal or decreased.

Rheumatoid Factor.—Rheumatoid arthritis and related diseases are associated with production of a group of immunoglobulins called rheumatoid factors that include IgG, IgM, and IgA varieties. These immunoglobulins (antibodies) have specificity for IgG that has been altered in certain ways. It is still not certain whether the altered IgG is the cause of the inflammatory abnormalities in RA or is a body response against the inflammatory process. From the laboratory standpoint, the most important of the rheumatoid factors is the one that is an IgM macroglobulin. Rheumatoid factor combines with its altered IgG antigen in vivo, accompanied by complement fixation. Immunoglobulin M rheumatoid factor, like other antibodies, is produced by lymphocytes and plasma cells of B-cell origin. In some persons, especially in infants, IgM antibody production against some infectious organism not associated with rheumatoid disease may result in concurrent production of varying amounts of IgM rheumatoid factor. Outside the body, IgM rheumatoid factor can combine with normal gamma globulin without complement fixation (in fact, some patient serum contains excess C1q component of complement, which may cause a nonspecific rheumatoid factor test reaction that can be avoided by heat inactivation of complement prior to the test).

Serologic Tests.—Serologic tests are the usual method of laboratory diagnosis in adult-onset RA. Various types of serologic tests may be set up utilizing reaction of IgM rheumatoid factor with IgG gamma globulin, differing mainly in the type of indicator system used to visually demonstrate results (see Table 36–17). The original method was known as the "Rose-Waaler test," or "sheep cell agglutination test." Anti-sheep red blood cell (RBC) antibodies were reacted with tannic acid–treated sheep RBCs, then the rheumatoid factor in the patient's serum was allowed to combine with the antibody gamma globulin coating the sheep cells. Clumping of RBCs indicated a positive test result. It was found subsequently that synthetic particles such as latex could be coated with gamma globulin and the coated particles could be clumped by rheumatoid factor, thus giving a flocculation test. Just as happened with the serologic test for syphilis (chapter 31), many combinations of ingredients have been tried, with resulting variations in sensitivity and specificity. These tests are too numerous to discuss individually, but a distinction must be made between tube tests and rapid slide tests. The slide tests in general have a slightly greater sensitivity than tube tests but also produce more false positive results. Therefore, slide tests should be used mainly for screening purposes. As noted previously, some patient serum contains a nonspecific C1q agglutinator that can be eliminated by inactivating patient serum by heating at 56°C for 30 minutes.

The latex fixation tube test for RA, known also as the "Plotz-Singer latex test," currently is considered the standard diagnostic method. The average sensitivity in well-established clinical cases of adult RA is about 76% (range, 50%–95%). Clinically normal controls have about 1%–2% positive results (range, 0.2%–4%). Latex slide tests offer an average sensitivity of approximately 85% (literature range, 78%–98%), with positive results seen in approximately 5%–8% of normal control persons (range, 0.2%–15%). It may take several weeks or months after onset of clinical symptoms, even as long as 6 months, before RA serologic test results become abnormal.

False Positive Results.—Certain diseases, especially those associated with increased gamma globulin ("hyperglobulinemia"), produce a significantly high number of positive reactions in a manner analogous to the "biologic false positive" reactions of syphilis serology. These include collagen diseases, sarcoidosis, syphilis, chronic hepatitis and cirrhosis, bacterial infections (especially subacute bacterial endocarditis [SBE]), and even old age. The incidence of reactive RA tests is higher with the slide than the tube tests. The percentage of positive reactions in the diseases listed ranges from 5%–40%. Sjögren's syndrome (75%–96%) and SBE (50%) are the most likely to produce false positive results.

Differential Diagnosis.—Rheumatoid arthritis is usually part of the differential diagnosis of joint pain. However, other causes must be considered, especially if symptoms, location of joint involvement, laboratory test results, or other features are atypical. Even a positive rheumatoid factor test result is not conclusive evidence for RA. Other diseases that frequently enter the differential diagnosis are the so-called seronegative spondyloarthropathies, septic (infectious) arthritis, systemic lupus erythematosus (SLE) and other collagen-vascular diseases, crystal-deposition arthritis, and acute rheumatic fever (ARF). These conditions will be discussed later in this chapter.

Juvenile Rheumatoid Arthritis

Juvenile rheumatoid arthritis (JRA), also known as "juvenile chronic polyarthritis," or "Still's disease," is the most common disorder of childhood involving chronic joint inflammation (synovitis). Since there is a spectrum of signs and symptoms, diagnosis partially depends on exclusion of other recognized arthritis syndromes (some of which are discussed later). There are three subdivisions of JRA. Polyarticular JRA accounts for 40%–50% of all JRA cases and produces inflammation of multiple joints (more than four), typically in a symmetric distribution. There is no eye involvement, and those affected are predominantly girls. There are two subgroups. In one subgroup, accounting for about 10% of JRA cases, the RA test result is positive, and there is a high incidence of positive antinuclear antibody (ANA) test results. This form occurs more often in late childhood and frequently is associated with severe arthritis; it more closely resembles standard adult RA. The other subgroup accounts for about 30% of JRA cases. Rheumatoid arthritis test results are negative, there is a low incidence of positive ANA test results, and severe arthritis is rare. This form of JRA resembles minimal severity adult RA. Polyarticular JRA frequently is associated with a mild normocytic-normochromic anemia. White blood cell counts are normal or mildly elevated, usually not more than 20,000/cu mm (20×10^9/L).

Pauciarticular JRA accounts for 30%–40% of all JRA cases and affects only a few joints (less than four) in asymmetric distribution. There are also two subgroups (although this is disputed). The early-onset type occurs before age 5 years and accounts for about 30% of JRA cases. There is no hip or spine involvement, but about one half of affected patients develop iridocyclitis. Rheumatoid arthritis test results are negative, but ANA test results are positive in about 50% of patients. The late-onset subgroup overlaps with ankylosing spondylitis and is not included in JRA by some investigators. This form affects predominantly boys. Hip and sacroiliac involvement is frequent but not iridocyclitis. There is a high incidence of the HLA-B27 antigen, and RA or ANA test results are usually negative.

Systemic-onset JRA accounts for approximately 20% of JRA cases. Slightly more boys are affected than girls, and onset can occur at any age. There are one or two high fever spikes each day, especially in the evening, for several weeks, with the temperature rapidly dropping after each spike to normal or even low values. There may be chills at the same time as the fever spikes. Some 90% or more of patients develop a macular skin rash that often appears and disappears with the fever spikes. There is splenomegaly or lymphadenopathy in 80%–85% of cases, pleuritis or pericarditis in 30%–60%, and abdominal pain in 30%. Anemia is frequent and may sometimes be severe. Leukocytosis is found in 95%, and WBC counts are often in the range of 20,000–30,000/cu mm. Eventually a polyarthritis develops. Rheumatoid arthritis and ANA test results are negative.

Seronegative Spondyloarthropathies

In these conditions arthritis is associated with inflammation that affects the spine and lumbosacral joints (ankylosing spondylitis), the urethra (Reiter's syndrome), the skin (psoriasis), or the intestinal tract. These conditions were (and are) frequently referred to as "rheumatoid arthritis variants." This name has been discarded by most rheumatologists because the diseases have relatively little in common with classic RA except for involvement of joints and are considered separate entities. As a group they have certain similarities. There frequently is a component of inflammation at the attachment of ligaments to bone (enthesiopathy) rather than only synovial involvement. Except for ankylosing spondylitis, they are found in association with other well-known diseases, and there is a tendency for spine and large joint involvement in a minority of cases. Spondylitis develops in about 5%–10% of patients with inflammatory bowel arthritis, in about 20% of patients with psoriatic arthritis, and in more than 50% of those with the chronic form of Reiter's syndrome. Iritis is common in patients with spondylitis, and conjunctivitis is a typical feature of Reiter's syndrome. The RA test results are usually negative. There is a hereditary component and an increased incidence of HLA-B27.

Ankylosing Spondylitis.—Ankylosing spondylitis (Marie-Strumpell disease) involves primarily the spine and sacroiliac joints, with peripheral joint arthritis present in about 30% of cases. Iritis may develop in 30%–40% of cases. In the United States, the incidence in blacks is much less than in whites. Males are predominantly affected. Mild anemia is found in about 25%. The ESR is elevated in 80%–90% of those with active disease. HLA-B27 is present in more than 90% of affected persons. Since HLA-B27 is normally found in 6%–7% of white and 3%–4% of black Americans, and the incidence of ankylosing spondylitis is about 1 in 1,000 of the general population, most persons who have positive HLA-B27 results do not have ankylosing spondylitis. Since HLA-B27 is found in about 92% of patients (literature range 83%–98%), absence of HLA-B27 in whites is some evidence against the diagnosis in clinically borderline cases.

Reiter's Syndrome.—Reiter's syndrome typically consists of joint, urethral, mucocutaneous, and eye lesions. These are manifested by a (usually) self-limited nongonococcal urethritis found predominantly in males that may be accompanied by conjunctivitis or iritis and by mucocutaneous ulcers or other lesions. The disease may appear spontaneously, may follow a gonococcal infection (possibly due to concurrent *Chlamydia* or *Mycoplasma* infection) or may be precipitated by genitourinary or colon infection. *Shigella* infection is followed by Reiter's syndrome in 1%–2% of cases. About 85% (literature range, 63%–100%) of whites with Reiter's syndrome have HLA-B27 antigen. The arthritic component primarily involves the lower extremities and may be accompanied by tendinitis. Behçet's syndrome (oral and genital ulceration, iritis, and arthritis) may mimic some components of Reiter's syndrome. Reiter's syndrome may occur in females, in which case the urethritis component may not be recognized.

Psoriatic Arthritis.—Psoriatic arthritis most commonly involves the distal interphalangeal joints of the hands and feet, although the spine or pelvis is affected in about 20% of cases. HLA-B27 is found in about 35% of cases (literature range, 20%–90%, the higher percentages being found when spondylitis was present). About 10% (range, 5%–20%) of patients with psoriasis develop psoriatic arthritis.

Arthritis Associated With Inflammatory Bowel Disease.—Inflammatory bowel disease may be accompanied by peripheral arthritis and by spondylitis. The two types of arthritis behave independently of each other, although either type may be present or the two may coexist. Twelve percent to 20% of patients with ulcerative colitis or regional enteritis (Crohn's disease) and up to 30% of patients with infection by *Yersinia enterocolitica* are affected. Arthritis may develop in 1%–2% of patients with *Shigella* infection and in occasional patients with *Salmonella* or *Campylobacter jejuni* infection. Whipple's disease may also be associated with arthritis. Spondylitis is said to occur in about 5% of patients with chronic inflammatory bowel disease, and sacroiliitis in about 15%. HLA-B27 is reported in about 60% of those with spondylitis (literature range, 37%–75%). Iritis is also more common in these patients. Therefore, the arthritis of inflammatory bowel disease in some patients has similarities in several respects to Reiter's syndrome except for lack of urethritis.

COLLAGEN-VASCULAR DISEASES

Collagen-vascular diseases are an ill-defined collection of syndromes that have certain points of similarity, among which the most striking are fibrinoid necrosis of collagenous tissue and involvement of various subdivisions of arteries by an inflammatory process. Some diseases emphasize one aspect and some the other. Because blood vessel inflammation and other abnormalities found in the collagen diseases may also be found to a certain extent in some patients with RA, some investigators prefer the term "rheumatoid-collagen diseases." Others do not wish to use the designation collagen disease at all. Some justification to group together these often quite dissimilar syndromes is the overlap in signs, symptoms, and labo-

TABLE 22–1.
Serologic Tests in Rheumatoid-Collagen Diseases*

Test	% Abnormal Results							
	SLE	RA	Scleroderma	Polyarteritis	Dermatomyositis	Mixed CT Disease	Normal Controls	Persons > 60 yr
LE prep	70–80† (40–100)	15 (0–24)	15 (0–25)	10 (8–15)	12–15	20	0	—
ANA test	97 (91–100)	30–40 (10–60)	70 (25–100)	20–25 (5–95)	25–30 (10–95)	100	3–4 (0–7)	20 (0–49)
Anti-DNA (ds DNA)	70–80 (35–100)	15 (0–40)	30 (0–55)	—	15 (0–25)	25 (11–50)	1–2 (0–4)	—
RA tests	20–30 (20–40)	75 (50–98)	30 (25–33)	15 (5–25)	15 (10–50)	—	2–3 (0.2–8)	15 (10–24)

*Data are in percent. Numbers in parentheses refer to range in the literature. CT = connective tissue; LE prep = lupus erythematosus preparation.
†At some time during the illness; 60–70% when first seen.

ratory abnormalities between the different conditions as well as the probability that their basic etiology is a disorder involving immunologic hypersensitivity. Those conditions usually included in the connective tissue ("collagen") disease group will be discussed first; then other diseases involving joints; and finally, certain conditions primarily due to vasculitis.

Systemic Lupus Erythematosus (SLE)

Systemic lupus erythematosus features various combinations of facial skin rash, arthritis, nephritis, systemic symptoms such as fever and malaise, and inflammation of serous membranes such as the pericardium. The disease is by far more frequent in women, predominantly young or middle-aged adults. In one large series the mean age at diagnosis was 30 years, with a skewed distribution: the majority between ages 14 and 40 years, a lesser but significant number between ages 40 and 55 years, and a few scattered from infancy to age 14 years and over age 55 years. Hepatomegaly is found in about 30% of patients (literature range, 23%–44%), splenomegaly in nearly 20% (range, 9%–41%), and adenopathy in nearly 50% (range, 37%–68%).

Laboratory Findings.—Anemia is present in 60%–75% of SLE patients, most often mild or moderate and of the normocytic-normochromic type. About 30% (literature range, 18%–65%) of patients have a positive direct Coombs' test result, although only 10% or less develop autoimmune hemolytic anemia. Leukopenia is found in about 50% of patients (literature range, 43%–65%) and thrombocytopenia in about 15% (literature range, 5%–26%). There are often one or more manifestations of abnormal plasma proteins; these may include cold-precipitable cryoglobulins, circulating anticoagulants, autoantibodies, elevated gamma-globulin levels, circulating immune complexes, false positive RA and syphilis serologic reactions, and certain even rarer phenomena.

In SLE with active nephritis, total serum complement (C, C′, or CH_{50}, chapter 21), C3, and C4 levels are usually all decreased. This complement pattern is not absolutely specific for lupus nephritis and may be found in serum sickness, SBE, and immune complex disease.

Autoantibodies and Autoantibody Tests in System Lupus Erythematosus.—Almost all patients with SLE develop autoantibodies of some type. Several of the laboratory tests that are most useful for detecting and diagnosing SLE are based on the presence of certain autoantibodies. These include the lupus erythematosus (LE) cell phenomenon, screening tests for antinuclear antibodies (ANAs), and more specific assays of individual antibodies such as that against double-stranded DNA (dsDNA). Table 22–1 provides data on the sensitivity and specificity of the most commonly used tests (see also Table 36–18). Interpretation of these data requires discussion of the individual procedures.

Lupus Erythematosus Cell Preparation.—The first reasonably good test for lupus, and one that is still useful, is the LE prep. This test detects antibody against nuclear deoxyribonucleoprotein (DNP, soluble nucleoprotein [sNP], DNA-histone complex; see Table 22–3) that is produced in SLE. The LE prep technique first provides a source of nuclei from laboratory-damaged cells, either tissue cells or WBCs. The nuclei are then incubated with patient serum, during which time the nuclear material is converted by the ANA against sNP into a homogeneous amorphous mass that stains basophilic with Wright's stain. This mass is then phagocytized by nondamaged polymorphonuclear neutrophils; these neutrophils containing the hematoxylin (blue-staining) bodies in their cytoplasm are the so-called LE cells. These LE cells are considered by many to be strongly suggestive of SLE. However, certain drugs may induce an SLE-like syndrome, and some patients with RA, other collagen diseases, or a subgroup of chronic active hepatitis or cirrhosis called "lupoid hepatitis" may have a positive LE prep result. The number of LE cells in LE preps from patients with SLE tends to be greater than in the other conditions; but a sufficient number of patients with SLE have only small numbers of LE cells so that LE cell quantitation is not very helpful unless the slide contains many LE cells. There is also the possibility that at least some of the patients who appear to have conditions other than SLE, in fact, might have subclinical or underlying SLE. In some patients, such as those with RA, it becomes almost a matter of philosophy whether the diagnosis is RA with LE cells or SLE with predominantly rheumatoid-type symptoms. Finally, artifacts may be confused with true LE cells. To be definitive, the basophilic hematoxylin body must be completely amorphous, without any remaining nuclear structure whatever. In many LE preps one finds neutrophils or monocytes with phagocytized nuclear material that still retains some identity as a nucleus, such as a residual chromatin pattern. These are not true LE cells; they are called "Tart cells." Increased numbers of these may be seen in SLE, but they do not have any diagnostic significance. Neutrophils with ingested RBCs can also be misdiagnosed as LE cells by inexperienced persons.

Different methods may be used for LE prep. Their common denominator is some way to traumatize a number of the WBCs. After this, there is an incubation period during which the nuclei of the damaged cells are converted to hematoxylin bodies and then ingested by some of the living neutrophils. The preparation is centrifuged, and smears of the neutrophil layer are made. After staining with Wright's stain, the smears are searched for LE cells. When hematoxylin bodies are formed, groups of neutrophils sometimes are found surrounding one of the bodies preparatory to one neutrophil phagocytizing it. These groupings are called "rosettes" and are considered by some investigators as equal in importance to true LE cells; others insist on finding classic LE cells for definite diagnosis. It must be emphasized that the LE phenomenon is often intermittent, sometimes present for varying periods and sometimes absent. There is some correlation with the activity of the disease, in that patients with active SLE are more likely to have a positive LE prep result than those with inactive disease. In patients who have only small numbers of LE cells on smears, it is possible (although not usual) for LE preps to give positive results one day and not the next. This may be referable in some way to the disease itself or may result from technical factors such as the method of preparing the LE cell slide and the expertise of the person reading it. Adrenocorticosteroid therapy often suppresses LE cell production.

In SLE, positive LE prep results are reported in 70%–80% of cases, with a range in the literature of 40%–100%. The great differences in the literature are due to several factors. First, many of the studies report data based on LE preps obtained at various times during the entire illness rather than the result obtained on the first test at the first admission. Cumulative or repeated studies would result in a higher percentage of patients with positive results. Various modifications of the basic LE prep technique are widely used, and the modifications differ in sensitivity. Finally, patients with active disease are more likely to have a positive LE prep than those with inactive disease. A realistic figure for likelihood of a positive LE prep result in a person with SLE on initial workup is probably 60%–70%.

Antinuclear Antibody Test.—The antinuclear factor responsible for the LE cell phenomenon is not the only autoantibody or "factor" demonstrable in SLE. A wide variety of such factors has been demonstrated, reactive against either nuclear or cytoplasmic constituents with varying degrees of tissue and cellular constituent specificity. An ANA test usually involves incubating patient serum with nucleated cells. Afterward, a tagged antibody against gamma globulin is added to detect patient ANA coating the cell nuclei. The antibody tag can be fluorescent (FANA test) or can be an enzyme (EANA test). Various types of tissue cells have been used as sources of cell nuclei. Most of these tests yield initial-visit positive results in 95% or more of patients with SLE, compared with positive results on the LE prep of 60%–70%. However, the ANA test is more frequently abnormal than the LE prep in conditions other than SLE. Therefore, current practice is to employ the ANA procedure as a screening test. If the ANA test result is negative, chances that the patient has SLE are very low. If the ANA test result is positive, other studies must be done to obtain a definitive diagnosis.

Like all laboratory tests, the ANA test is not perfect. Both tissue culture cells (tumor-derived Helen Lake [HeLa] cells, human epithelial cell–derived cells [HEp-2 cells, originally obtained from a laryngeal tumor], and human amniotic cells) and thin tissue sections derived from various sources (most commonly rat liver) have been used to provide cell nuclei for the procedure; and the different nuclear sources do not all have equal sensitivity. Most of the early work on ANA tests was done with rat liver tissue sections. Tissue culture cells generally are reported to be more sensitive than rat liver. On the other hand, the more sensitive tissue culture cells detect more low-titer ANA reactions, of which some are produced by disorders other than SLE (if screening for SLE is the only consideration, these would be considered false positive reactions. However, they may be a clue to the other diseases). Also, tissue culture cells demonstrate chromosome centromere staining in patients with scleroderma (progressive systemic sclerosis, or PSS), whereas discrete centromere structures are very difficult to see on rat liver sections and instead tend to have a nonspecific speckled appearance. Similarly, rat liver sections will usually not detect ANA against the Sjögren's syndrome A, or SS-A (Ro), antigen (found most frequently in SLE and in Sjögren's syndrome but also in some patients with other connective tissue disorders). The anti-human globulin used to detect ANAs can be either a polyclonal type or specific for IgG. Specific anti-IgG eliminates a certain number of false positive reactions due to rheumatoid factor or other IgM antibodies. This is said to reduce positive test results due to RA, drug-induced problems, and old age. On the other hand, about 4% of SLE patients are reported to produce IgM-type ANA. Results of procedures that use acetone-fixed cell substrates are more likely to be positive with ANA against saline-extractable antigens (extractable nuclear antigens, or ENAs) such as Smith (Sm) and ribonucleoprotein (RNP) than those that omit substrate fixation. There have been scattered reports of patients with symptoms suggestive of SLE and positive LE prep results but negative ANA test results. In some cases the investigators decided that the LE prep results were reported incorrectly and, in others that the ANA test result was falsely negative. In addition, there appears to be a small subset of SLE patients with anticytoplasmic antibodies rather than ANAs. To date, these anticytoplasmic antibodies have been identified mostly as Ro type, the same ones that are considered strongly associated with Sjögren's syndrome (discussed later). When they are associated with SLE, the predominant clinical symptom seems to be a photosensitive skin rash.

Antinuclear Antibody Test Patterns.—The method of reporting ANA results deserves some comment. Both the titer of positive results and the pattern (distribution) of nuclear fluorescence are important. In general, the higher the titer of certain ANA patterns known to be associated with SLE, the more likelihood that the patient has SLE. In addition, the ANA staining pattern can sometimes provide useful information. There are several recognized patterns that appear to be produced by ANAs against certain nuclear proteins (Fig 22–1). It must be emphasized that none of the fluorescent patterns is specific for only one autoantibody or exclusive for the diseases with which it is traditionally associated. Also, some investigators disagree with the findings of others regarding which pattern is found more often in various diseases.

Rim (Peripheral) Pattern.—Fluorescence is much more intense on the nuclear border. This was originally thought to be specific for antibody against dsDNA (see Table 22–3). However, it is now known to be produced by ANA against several additional nucleoproteins, including sNP, single-stranded DNA (ssDNA), and histones. However, a high ANA titer (1:160 or greater) with a rim pattern strongly suggests SLE. Drug-induced SLE usually does not have a rim pattern, nor is a rim pattern common in other rheumatoid-collagen diseases (present in < 10% of those patients). However, when the ANA titer is borderline or only mildly elevated, the rim pattern is less helpful because of overlap with the other diseases.

Solid (Homogeneous) Pattern.—Fluorescence is uniform throughout the nucleus. This is the second most common ANA pattern and, like the rim pattern, can be produced by ANA against dsDNA, ssDNA, sNP, and histones. This is the most frequently seen pattern in SLE, but it is less suggestive of SLE, since it is found more frequently than the rim pattern in other rheumatoid-collagen diseases and is also seen in some patients with drug-induced ANA. The ANA titer is usually less than 1:160 in diseases other than SLE, so that the possibility of SLE is increased in patients with higher titers.

Speckled Pattern.—There are many small fluorescent dots throughout the nucleus that do not involve the nucleoli. This is the most commonly encountered ANA pattern. Antinuclear antibodies responsible include those against acidic nuclear proteins, such as ENA (Sm and RNP), SS-A (Ro), Sjögren's syndrome B (SS-B), and scleroderma 70 (Scl-70). This pattern is the one most frequently associated with the mixed connective tissue (MCT) diseases (discussed later), although the MCT disease does not produce the majority of speckled ANA reactions. It has also been reported in about 25% of patients with SLE (due to anti-Sm) and in some patients with RA, progressive systemic sclerosis, Sjögren's syndrome, drug-induced ANAs, and some aged persons. However, if the ANA titer is very high with a speckled pattern, this suggests MCT disease. At least one report indicates that many fluorescence patterns reported as speckled actually consist of small rods or filaments with dots, which is not a true speckled configuration. This pseudospeckled pattern is said to represent most of the conditions other than MCT disease that others include in the speckled category. If the speckled pattern is present in moderately elevated or high titer, specific antibody testing is useful since specific ANA against Sm is strongly suggestive of SLE, ANA against RNP suggests MCT disease, ANA against SS-B suggests Sjögren's syndrome, and ANA against Scl-70 suggests scleroderma (progressive systemic sclerosis; PSS).

Nucleolar Pattern.—Fluorescence only in the nucleolar areas of the nucleus is seen as several small areas of irregular shape and different sizes. This is due to ANA against nucleolar RNA (4–6s RNA). It suggests PSS (55%–90% of PSS patients), especially if the titer is high. Lower titers may be found in SLE and occasionally in other collagen diseases.

Centromere Pattern.—The centromere pattern is made up of moderate-sized speckles that vary in size and are fewer in number than expected with a speckled pattern. Chromosomes of mitotic cells show the same speckles

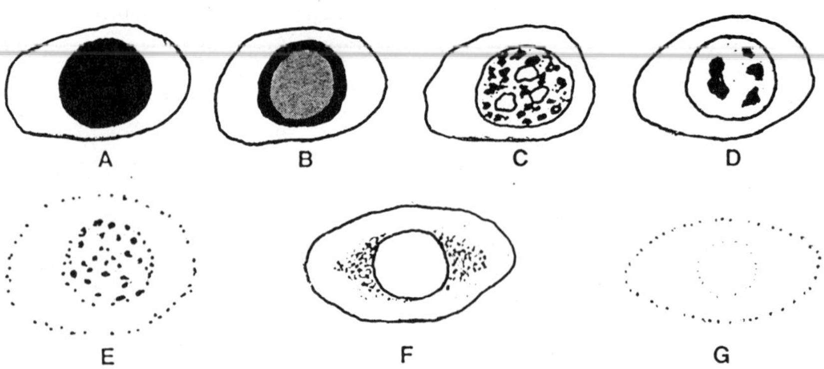

FIG 22–1.
Fluorescent ANA test patterns (HEp-2 cells). *A*, solid (homogeneous). *B*, peripheral (rim). *C*, speckled. *D*, nucleolar. *E*, anticentromere. *F*, antimitochondrial. *G*, normal (nonreactive).

along the chromosomal spindles. This pattern is due to ANA against centromere antigen and is highly suggestive of the CREST (calcinosis, Raynaud's phenomenon, esophageal motility dysfunction, sclerodactyly, and telangiectasia) variant of PSS.

Assays for Specific Antinuclear Antibodies.—At present, with the possible exception of the anti-DNA assay using the *Crithidia* method, the various assays for specific ANAs can be obtained only in large reference laboratories or laboratories specializing in autoimmune disease. It should be emphasized that correlation of specific autoantibodies with specific diseases usually depends on the presence of substantial titer elevations of the antibody; low titers are more likely to be less specific.

Anti-DNA Assay.—Assays for various specific autoantibodies have been developed (Table 22–2). Currently the most popular of these assays detects antibody against dsDNA. This is usually referred to as anti-DNA, although there is a different antibody against ssDNA. There are currently three well-recognized techniques for measurement of anti-DNA antibody. The Farr method is the oldest; it is a radioimmunoassay (RIA) technique using radioactive tritium (^3H) or carbon 14 which depends on ammonium sulfate precipitation or Millipore filter filtration to separate the antigen-antibody complex from nonbound antigen. At least two commercial companies have marketed kits using more traditional radioactive iodine reagents. Assays have also been developed that use a protozoan organism named *Crithidia luciliae;* this has a large intracytoplasmic structure called a "kinetoplast" composed mostly of dsDNA. Various commercial companies have kits with the dead organisms on prepared slides. Patient serum is added, and the anti-DNA antibodies attach to the kinetoplasts of the organisms. A fluorescent anti–human globulin antibody is added that demonstrates fluorescence of the kinetoplast if anti-DNA antibody is attached (the technique is basically similar to that used for the ANA test). In general, reports indicate that the Farr technique is a small but significant percent more sensitive than commercial RIA kits. There is some disagreement in the literature as to whether the sensitivity of the *Crithidia* procedure is equal to or less than the RIA procedures. Some of the disagreement is attributable to comparison of the *Crithidia* kits to the Farr technique vs. comparison to a commercial RIA method.

TABLE 22–2.

Some Autoantibodies Found in Systemic Lupus Erythematosus and Other Autoimmune Disorders

I. Anti-DNA
  A. Double-stranded ("native") DNA (dsDNA)
  B. Single-stranded DNA (ssDNA)
II. Antinucleoprotein (soluble nucleoprotein [sNP]; DNA-histone)
III. Antibasic nuclear proteins (histones)
IV. Antiacidic nuclear proteins (extractable nuclear antigens [ENAs]: includes Sm and RNP)
  A. Nuclear glycoprotein (Sm)
  B. Ribonucleoprotein (RNP)
  C. Sjögren's syndrome A and B (SS-A [Ro] and SS-B)
V. Antinucleolar (nuclear RNA)
VI. Anticytoplasmic (ribosomal RNA and others)

There have been claims in the literature that the anti-DNA test is highly sensitive and specific for SLE. However, review of the published evaluations discloses that overall sensitivity and specificity (as a composite of all anti-DNA methods) is about the same as those of the LE prep (Table 22–2). Data from the *Crithidia* assay, which is now the most widely used procedure, suggest that overall sensitivity of *Crithidia* is about the same as the LE prep, but that specificity for SLE is better than the LE prep, with somewhat fewer positive results in diseases other than SLE. However, positive results do occur in diseases other than SLE. Some data suggest that anti-DNA assay results by any method are more likely (by 20%–40% of cases) to be positive in patients with active SLE than in patients with inactive SLE. Also, SLE is more likely than other conditions to produce a high antibody titer. Test results of drug-induced ANA are usually negative, and if positive are usually not greatly elevated.

Anti-sNP antibody reacts against a deoxyribonucleoprotein complex with histone. Antibody to the sNP complex is reported in about 50% of SLE patients, fewer than 10% of patients with RA, Sjögren's syndrome, or MCT disease, and uncommonly in patients with scleroderma, dermatomyositis, polyarteritis nodosa, or discoid lupus. When anti-sNP antibody is present, the ANA test shows a solid (homogeneous) ANA pattern. Anti-sNP antibody is thought to produce the LE cell phenomenon. Since anti-sNP antibody is not the only autoantibody to evoke a solid ANA pattern, data on the incidence of sNP in various diseases and on the incidence of the solid ANA pattern in the same diseases may not correlate exactly.

Anti-ENA is not really a specific antibody but includes a small group of antibodies to certain antigens consisting of RNA and protein, of which the most important are Sm and RNP (discussed separately in the next paragraphs). The ENA antigen is extracted from thymus using phosphate-buffered saline and therefore, as previously mentioned, is sometimes referred to as saline-extractable antigen. An order for anti-ENA antibodies would generate assays for anti-Sm and anti-RNP. These two ANAs both produce a speckled ANA pattern.

Anti-nuclear glycoprotein (Sm) antibody is present in about 30% of patients with SLE and 8% of patients with MCT disease but not in patients with most of the other rheumatoid-collagen diseases. Therefore, anti-Sm antibody is fairly specific for SLE, but the sensitivity of the test is poor. Anti-Sm antibody is associated with the speckled ANA pattern.

Anti-RNP antibody is reported in nearly 100% of patients with the mixed connective tissue syndrome and about 25% of patients with SLE, discoid lupus, and progressive systemic sclerosis (scleroderma). Anti-RNP antibody (like anti-Sm antibody) is associated with a speckled ANA pattern. In high titer, anti-RNP antibody is suggestive of MCT disease.

Antinucleolar antibody is reported in about 55% of patients with PSS, 25% of patients with SLE, and 10% of patients with RA. In high titer it is very suggestive of PSS.

Anticentromere antibody is directed against the centromere area of chromosomes and is reported to be suggestive of the CREST syndrome.

Anti-SS-A and *Anti-SS-B* antibodies are against nuclear antigens extracted from human B lymphocytes (Wil$_2$ cell line) grown in tissue culture. The SS-A is found in about 70% of patients with Sjögren's syndrome without RA symptoms, 10% of Sjögren's patients with RA, and 25% of patients with SLE but usually not in patients with RA. The SS-B is found in about 50% of patients with Sjögren's syndrome without RA, less than 5% of patients with Sjögren's syndrome with RA, but not in patients with SLE or RA. Therefore, high titers of the SS-A or SS-B anti-Sjögren antibodies are fairly good markers for Sjögren's syndrome, although sensitivity is not good.

Rheumatoid arthritis precipitin (RAP) is an autoantibody against RA nuclear antigen (RANA) derived from reaction of Epstein-Barr virus with human lymphocytes in tissue culture. Rheumatoid arthritis precipitin is present in about 65% of patients with RA, 70% of patients with Sjögren's syndrome and RA, but in less than 10% of patients with SLE or other rheumatoid-collagen diseases. High titers of the RAP antibody are useful markers for RA when RA symptoms are present in other collagen diseases. The SS and RAP antibodies may be present in patients who have a negative ANA test result.

Skin Biopsy With Immunofluorescence Staining.—It is possible to obtain a full-thickness biopsy specimen from an uninvolved area of epidermis next to a skin lesion, prepare frozen section from the biopsy tissue, and apply immunofluorescent techniques using antisera against IgG, IgM, and IgA. Several characteristic immunofluorescent patterns have been described in certain diseases. In SLE, there is either a solid or stippled band involving the epidermis basement membrane area using IgG antiserum. This pattern is said to be present in up to 90% of patients with SLE or discoid LE if the disease is active. The incidence is considerably less if the disease is not active. Other diseases associated with characteristic skin immunofluorescent patterns are pemphigus vulgaris (intraepidermal fluorescence of spaces between squamous epithelial cells using IgG), bullous pemphigoid ("tubular" or linear solid staining of the basement membrane using IgG), and dermatitis herpetiformis (short irregular speckled band at the basement membrane confined to the tips of the dermal papillae, using IgA antiserum).

Slide Latex Tests for Systemic Lupus Erythematosus.—Commercial companies have marketed 2-minute slide latex agglutination tests for SLE based on latex particles coated with DNA (most often, thymus-derived DNA). The tests available so far have substantial differences in sensitivity but in general yield fewer positive results in SLE than the LE preparation or anti-DNA assay by the *Crithidia* method. Some of the tests do not have adequate clinical evaluations; in some cases, I was not able to obtain any published evaluations.

Serum Complement in Systemic Lupus Erythematosus.—Total serum complement (C, C′, CH_{50}; chapter 21), as well as the complement fractions C3 and C4, is often reduced in SLE patients with lupus nephritis. In one study, 38% of SLE patients had decreased C3 levels on initial workup and 66% had decreased C3 levels at some time during that illness. One report suggests that the combination of increased anti-dsDNA levels plus decreased C3 levels is highly specific for SLE; this combination was found in 32% of SLE patients on initial workup and 61% at some time during their illness.

Drug-Induced Systemic Lupus Erythematosus.—A syndrome very similar to SLE can be produced by certain medications (drug-induced SLE). The three drugs considered proven SLE-inducing agents are procainamide, hydralazine (Apresoline), and isoniazid. Patients on procainamide therapy develop clinical SLE in about 20% of cases. About 50% of patients taking more than 1.5 gm of procainamide/day develop positive LE prep results, and 75% have detectable ANAs. About 8%–13% of patients taking hydralazine develop SLE, and about 24%–50% have positive ANA test results. A small number (< 1%) of patients taking isoniazid develop the SLE syndrome, and about 20% have detectable ANAs. Certain other drugs (e.g., methyldopa, phenytoin, quinidine, and chlorpromazine) have, on occasion, been reported to induce positive LE prep results or ANA test results, but are usually not associated with the SLE syndrome. Drug-induced SLE produces ANAs that are most often directed against histones, whereas spontaneous SLE produces ANAs most often directed against dsDNA. Although both spontaneous SLE and drug-induced SLE may produce a solid (homogeneous) ANA test pattern, spontaneous SLE often produces a rim (peripheral) pattern not seen with the drug-induced syndrome, whereas drug-induced ANA results frequently show a speckled pattern, which is uncommon in spontaneous SLE. Assay for anti-dsDNA (usually ordered as "anti-DNA") is helpful to differentiate SLE and drug-induced ANA or SLE symptoms. High titers of anti-DNA are suggestive of SLE, whereas drug-induced ANA results are either negative or only minimally elevated.

Progressive Systemic Sclerosis (Scleroderma)

Progressive systemic sclerosis leads to progressive dense connective tissue replacement in certain areas that normally contain only small amounts of loose collagen. These include the dermis of the skin, the submucosa of the esophagus or other parts of the gastrointestinal (GI) tract, and the heart. The lungs frequently develop a slowly progressive type of diffuse fibrosis, radiologically most prominent in the lung bases. In addition, the kidneys are often affected by a somewhat different histologic process, similar to malignant hypertension. The disease is most common in middle-aged women. Clinically, the skin changes produce tautness and lack of elasticity; these changes most often occur in the hand and are often accompanied by Raynaud's phenomenon. Esophageal involvement leads to dysphagia, and small bowel changes may produce localized dilation. Laboratory tests usually show normal hemoglobin levels. There may be an increased ESR, and there may be associated hypergammaglobulinemia of a diffuse type, although this is not a consistent feature.

Laboratory Aspects.—Progressive system sclerosis gives a positive ANA test result in about 70% of cases, and the LE prep result may be positive in about 15% of cases. Various autoantibodies have been reported in a minority of cases. Antinucleolar antibodies in high titer are very suggestive of PSS. Rheumatoid factor test results are positive in about 15% of cases, and there may be a biologic false positive agglutination test result for syphilis.

Diagnosis usually can be made clinically but may be suggested by barium swallow esophageal x-ray studies in patients who have esophageal symptoms. Biopsy of an affected skin area is the procedure of choice if the diagnosis cannot be made clinically.

Mixed Connective Tissue Disease

As the name implies, MCT disease contains elements of several rheumatoid-collagen entities, including SLE, PSS, and dermatomyositis. Clinically, there is arthralgia or arthritis in 90%–95% of patients, Raynaud's phenomenon in about 80%–90%, abnormal esophageal motility in about 70%, muscle pain in about 70%, and fever in about 30%. There is a low incidence of renal disease. Various autoantibodies have been found, and there is a positive ANA test result in more than 95% (usually with a speckled pattern), a positive LE prep result in about 20%, and elevated anti-dsDNA antibody in about 25%. The characteristic serologic feature of MCT disease is a high titer of autoantibody against RNP. Lesser degrees of RNP elevation are found in some patients with SLE and PSS.

Sjögren's Syndrome

The parotid gland disease formerly known as "Mikulicz's syndrome" now is usually included with Sjögren's syndrome. Some reports indicate that Sjögren's syndrome affects 2%–5% of adults over age 55 and is second only to RA in frequency among the rheumatoid-collagen diseases. Sjögren's syndrome occurs in primary and secondary forms. Primary Sjögren's syndrome, sometimes called the "sicca syndrome," involves both the major and minor salivary glands, the lacrimal glands, and the labial glands. There is destruction of the salivary gland parenchymal cells with dense lymphoid reaction. Loss of lacrimal gland function makes the patient unable to produce tears and leads to injury of the cornea and conjunctiva (keratoconjunctivitis sicca). There are many other abnormalities that appear in a minority of patients; such as renal tubular acidosis, pericarditis, chronic hepatobiliary disease with antimitochondrial antibodies present, pancreatitis, disturbances of esophageal motility, and an increased tendency for lung infections. About 20% of patients with primary Sjögren's syndrome develop multifocal brain and spinal cord dysfunction closely resembling multiple sclerosis, both from clinical and laboratory aspects (chapter 18). Some of these patients develop cerebrospinal fluid oligoclonal bands and elevated IgG production indices.

Secondary Sjögren's syndrome is the coexistence of substantial components of primary Sjögren's syndrome with some other disease. The disorders that overlap with Sjögren's syndrome include most conditions that have a strong autoimmune component. The diseases most frequently reported to be associated with Sjögren's syndrome are RA (10%–25% of RA patients) and SLE (up to 30% of SLE patients). Some investigators report elements of Sjögren's syndrome in many patients with PSS and primary biliary cirrhosis.

Laboratory Aspects.—Patients with Sjögren's syndrome have various detectable autoantibodies. About 50%–80% have a positive ANA test result, about 15%–20% have positive LE prep test results, and about 75%–90% have detectable rheumatoid factor. About 25% have anti-dsDNA antibodies. The most characteristic autoantibodies are SS-A (Ro) and SS-B. The SS-A antibody is reported in about 75% (13%–88%) of patients with primary Sjögren's syndrome, about 10% of Sjögren's syndrome with RA, and about 50% of patients with SLE. The SS-B antibody is found in about 60% (literature range 48%–73%) of patients with primary Sjögren's syndrome, 75%–85% of SLE Sjögren's syndrome, and 2%–8% of SLE without Sjögren's syndrome. Rheumatoid arthritis precipitin (RAP) autoantibodies are reported in 60%–80% of Sjögren's syndrome with RA and 5%–30% of Sjögren's syndrome without RA. Therefore, elevated SS-A or SS-B antibody levels, especially in high titer, suggest primary Sjögren's syndrome or Sjögren's syndrome with SLE, with SS-B less sensitive but more specific for primary Sjögren's syndrome. Rheumatoid arthritis precipitin autoantibodies are useful markers for the RA-associated secondary form of Sjögren's syndrome. The data on autoantibodies in primary and secondary Sjögren's syndrome are rather contradictory except for larger trends, probably due to differences in antigens used in the research laboratories and differences in diagnostic criteria in the populations tested. Standardized test reagents and diagnostic criteria are needed for final evaluation of these tests.

Diagnosis of Sjögren's syndrome can be made from clinical symptoms, biopsy of salivary or labial glands, or presence of SS-A or SS-B autoantibodies in high titer. The SS-B is more specific for Sjögren's syndrome than SS-A but is less sensitive. High titers of SS-B suggest primary Sjögren's syndrome or SLE with Sjögren's syndrome.

SYNDROMES DUE PRIMARILY TO VASCULITIS

Polyarteritis Nodosa

Polyarteritis nodosa features inflammation of small and medium-sized arteries. Single organs or multiple systems may be involved, although usually the lungs are spared. The kidney is the organ that most frequently shows abnormalities, with hematuria the main sign. Hypertension is fairly common. Laboratory studies usually show moderate leukocytosis with neutrophilic increase and immaturity of the ordinary type seen with infections. Mild anemia is also common. There often is an increase in serum gamma-globulin levels. The main diagnostic procedure is biopsy. The most common specimen is muscle, and the usual region is the gastrocnemius because it is easy to reach. However, if biopsy is done, it should be from some muscle with a painful area if any is present; random samples give poor detection rates. The biopsy specimen should be generous, since the lesions of polyarteritis occur in small arteries. The incidence of positive single muscle biopsy specimens in fairly definite cases of polyarteritis ranges from 20%–40%; obviously, it is on the lower side in mild or questionable cases. Another difficulty is that occasionally patients with classic RA may have arteritis nearly identical to polyarteritis. Systemic lupus erythematosus patients also may have arteritis, but the lesions tend to be in arterioles. Other more rare syndromes of the collagen-vascular group may create histologic difficulty. Therefore, the clinical picture has as much importance as the biopsy report.

Patients with polyarteritis may have various autoantibodies. The ANA test result is positive in about 20%–25% of cases. There may be a positive LE prep result in about 10% of cases (usually with only a few LE cells) and a positive RA latex test result in about 15% of cases.

Allergic Vasculitis

The most common and well-known entity in this category is Henoch-Schönlein purpura. The primary abnormality is necrotizing inflammation of small venules, characterized by infiltration of the vessel wall by segmented neutrophils accompanied by destruction of some neutrophils with release of nuclear fragments ("leukocytoclastic vasculitis"). Immunohistologic methods can demonstrate IgA deposition in the vessel wall due to presence of IgA immune complexes. Schönlein's purpura features flat or nodular purpuric skin lesions, usually small but of varying size, most often on the lower extremities but which may occur elsewhere. There is no GI involvement. Henoch's purpura features involvement of and bleeding into the GI tract without emphasis on skin manifestations. Renal involvement with hematuria may occur in either entity. The syndrome may follow an upper respiratory tract infection or may be due to a drug hypersensitivity reaction and may include systemic symptoms such as malaise, myalgia, and arthralgias. Platelet counts and other coagulation tests usually are normal, except for the tourniquet test, results which are frequently abnormal. Diagnosis is usually made through biopsy of an abnormal area in association with the clinical symptoms.

Granulomatous Vasculitis

Wegener's granulomatosis, characterized by granulomatous inflammation containing foci of vasculitis involving the nasopharynx and kidneys, is the most important entity in this group. Biopsy is necessary for diagnosis in association with the clinical picture. Laboratory test abnormalities reflect a culture-negative ongoing inflammatory process. The WBC count and ESR are usually elevated when the disease is active.

Temporal Arteritis (Giant Cell Arteritis)

Actually, temporal arteritis is a subdivision of giant cell arteritis. The disorder involves medium-sized and large arteries, including the aorta. There is a granulomatous inflammation with varying numbers of multinucleated giant cells that involves the vessel wall in a discontinuous, or "skip," fashion and disrupts the artery's internal elastic membrane. Most (but not all) patients are whites over age 50 years. More than one half of the patients experience headache and have physical abnormality in one or both temporal arteries (tender or nodular to palpation). Important symptoms occurring in less than one half of the patients include visual disturbances and often systemic symptoms such as fever, weight loss, jaw claudication, and myalgias or arthralgias. However, the number of symptoms varies greatly. Occasional patients present as fever of unknown origin.

Laboratory abnormalities include anemia in more than 50% of patients, with the characteristics of the anemia of chronic disease, and sometimes a leukocytosis. Liver function tests are mildly abnormal in about 30% of patients, with the alkaline phosphatase level being most frequently elevated. Liver biopsy findings are most often normal. The most characteristic laboratory abnormality is ESR elevation, most often more than 50 mm/hour (Westergren method). This test has been used both for screening, as a part of diagnostic criteria, and to follow therapy effects. However, sometimes the ESR is within reference range when the patient first presents and becomes elevated later; and a small number of patients (exact number unknown but estimated at 2%–9%) never develop an elevated ESR. Definitive diagnosis requires temporal artery biopsy. The detection rate of biopsy is said to be about 90% (range, 65%–97%). About one third of patients have temporal arteries that are not painful and feel normal. It has been emphasized that a 3- to 5-cm temporal artery segment should be obtained, since the lesions are scattered. If this biopsy result is normal on serial section, biopsy of the other artery increases detection rate about 5%–10%.

Polymyalgia Rheumatica

This condition overlaps with temporal arteritis in many respects. Both occur in the same age group and both have the same general systemic symptoms and laboratory abnormalities, including elevated ESR, in about the same frequency. The major difference is that the principal symptom of polymyalgia is aching and stiffness in proximal joints such as the shoulders or hips; more noticeable after a period of inactivity, especially after sleep. Besides overlap in systemic symptoms and laboratory results with temporal arteritis, about 50% of patients with giant cell arteritis have symptoms compatible with polymyalgia rheumatica, and about 15% of patients (range, 10%–40%) with typical symptoms of polymyalgia (and normal-appearing temporal arteries on physical examination) have temporal artery biopsy findings of giant cell arteritis.

Circulating Immune Complexes

Immune complexes involve the binding of antigen to specific antibody and form part of the normal host response to foreign antigens. In some cases, immune complexes apparently can be deposited in tissues or organs and produce tissue injury. Blood vessels are most frequently involved. Although immune complexes quently involved. Although immune complexes may involve IgG, IgA, or IgM antibody, immunoglobulin G is the most common type. Immune complexes bind C1q and C3 components of complement. Cryoglobulins are immune complexes consisting either of monoclonal immunoglobulin complexes or, much more commonly, rheumatoid factor complexed with immunoglobulins ("mixed cryoglobulins"). Immune complexes may be fixed to tissue, circulating in the blood, or both. Diseases associated with circulating immune complexes include certain parasitic (schistosomiasis), protozoal (malaria), viral (hepatitis virus and cytomegalovirus), and bacterial (SBE and meningococcemia) infections; various malignancies; and various inflammatory diseases with an autoimmune component, such as the rheumatoid-collagen diseases and the vasculitides. However, circulating immune complexes have been detected in some way by some investigators in a great number of diseases.

Immune complexes can be detected in various ways. Immunofluorescent stains can be applied to tissue sections and visually demonstrate immunoglobulin binding to specific tissue locations. Circulating immune complexes (CICs) can be detected and assayed. The two most common methods include assays that detect C1q binding and methods that detect C3 activation such as the Raji cell assay. The C1q methods detect only CIC that activate complement by the classic pathway. The Raji cell assay uses tissue cultured cells derived from Burkitt's lymphoma that have high-affinity binding capability for the C3b component of complement. This detects complement activation by either the classic or the alternate pathways. Currently, the Raji cell assay method seems to be used most frequently. An EIA method has also become available. Unfortunately, assay of CIC has not achieved clinical usefulness in any way comparable to their immunologic and basic science interest. Most diseases associated with CIC average at least 10% or more false negative results with current assay methods, so that a negative result does not exclude the disease or presence of the complexes. The frequent presence of detectable CIC in many conditions hinders interpretation of a positive result. Also, use of CIC levels as a parameter of therapeutic response has yielded contradictory and inconstant results in the literature. Circulating immune complexes assay seems to have been most useful in diagnosis and therapy of SBE, especially when related to prosthetic valves. In a patient with a prosthetic valve, absence of detectable CICs is some evidence against SBE. Serial measurement of CICs in SBE apparently has been more helpful in assessing effectiveness of therapy than in most other diseases.

ACUTE RHEUMATIC FEVER

Acute rheumatic fever is a disease that has a specific etiologic agent yet has some similarities to the rheumatoid-collagen-vascular group. The etiologic agent is the beta-hemolytic Lancefield group A *Streptococcus.* Apparent hypersensitivity or other effect of this organism causes connective tissue changes manifested by focal necrosis of collagen and the development of peculiar aggregates of histiocytes called "Aschoff bodies." Symptoms of ARF include fever, a migratory type of polyarthritis, and frequently cardiac damage manifested by symptoms or only by ECG changes. Diagnosis or confirmation of diagnosis often rests on appropriate laboratory tests.

Culture.—Throat culture should be attempted; the finding of beta-hemolytic streptococci, Lancefield group A, is a strong point in favor of the diagnosis if the clinical picture is highly suggestive. However, throat cultures often show negative results by the time ARF symptoms develop, and a positive throat culture is not diagnostic of ARF (since group A streptococci may be present in 15%–20% of clinically normal children). Blood culture findings are almost always negative.

Streptolysin-O Tests.—Beta streptococci produce an enzyme known as streptolysin-O. About 7–10 days after infection, antibodies to this material begin to appear. The highest incidence of positive results is during the third week after onset of ARF. At this time, 80%–85% (range, 45%–95%) abnormal results are obtained; thereafter the antibody titer drops steadily. At the end of 2 months only 70%–75% of test results are positive; at 6 months, 35%; and at 12 months, 20%. Therefore, since the *Streptococcus* most often cannot be isolated, antistreptolysin-O (ASO) titers of more than 200 Todd units may be helpful evidence of a recent infection. However, this does not actually prove that the disease in question is ARF. Group A streptococcal infections are fairly frequent, so that occasionally a group A infection or the serologic effects of such an infection may coexist with some other arthritic disease. Another problem with ASO elevation is that the elevation persists for varying periods of time, raising the question whether the streptococcal infection that produced the antibodies was recent enough to cause the present symptoms. Commercial tests vary somewhat in reliability, and variations of 1 or 2 dilutions in titer on the same specimen tested by different laboratories are not uncommon.

Antibodies Against Other Streptococcal Enzymes.—Commercial slide latex agglutination tests that simultaneously detect ASO plus several other streptococcal antibodies, such as antideoxyribonuclease-B (ADN-B) are available. The best known of these multiantibody tests is called Streptozyme. Theoretically, these tests ought to be more sensitive for detection of group A beta-hemolytic streptococcal infections than the streptolysin-O test alone, since patients who develop acute glomerulonephritis are more apt to produce antibodies against ADN-B than streptolysin-O, and the antibodies against streptococcal enzymes may be stimulated unequally in individual patients. However, there is considerable debate in the literature on the merits of the combination-antibody tests vs. the single-antibody tests. With some dissenters, the consensus seems to be that the combination tests are either as sensitive as any single test alone or are more sensitive. If both the streptolysin-O test plus the ADN-B test are performed, the combined results are better than either test alone and even a little better than the single combination-antibody slide test. However, relatively few laboratories perform the ADN-B test, and even fewer routinely set up both the ASO test plus the ADN-B test in response to the usual order for an ASO titer.

Diagnosis.—When a patient presents with acute-onset sore throat and the question involves etiology (group A *Streptococcus* vs. some other infectious agent), throat culture is the procedure of choice, because it takes 7–10 days before ASO antibody elevation begins to occur. On the other hand, ARF and acute glomerulonephritis develop some time after the onset of the initiating streptococcal infection. The average latent period for ARF is 19 days, with a reported range of 1–35 days. Therefore, the ASO (or Streptozyme and its equivalents) is more useful than throat culture to demonstrate recent group A streptococcal infection in possible ARF or acute glomerulonephritis.

Other Tests.—The ESR is usually elevated during the clinical course of ARF and is a useful indication of current activity of the disease. However, the ESR is very nonspecific and indicates only that there is an active inflammatory process somewhere in the body. In a minority of ARF patients, peculiar subcutaneous nodules develop, most often near the elbows. These consist of focal collagen necrosis surrounded by palisading of histiocytes. In some cases, therefore, biopsy of these nodules may help confirm the diagnosis of ARF. However, biopsy is not usually done if other methods make the diagnosis reasonably certain. Also, the nodules are histologically similar to those of RA. During the acute phase of the disease there usually is moderate leukocytosis, and most often there is mild to moderate anemia.

ARTHRITIS DUE TO CRYSTAL DEPOSITION (CRYSTALLINE ARTHROPATHIES)

Gout

Gout usually involves single specific joints, usually including some of the small joints of the extremities. The most typical location is the metatarsal-phalangeal joint of the great toe, which is affected in about 75% of patients. The knee and ankle are involved in about 50% of patients. One third or more of patients have more than one joint involved during their first attack. The disease is seven times more common in males than females. Acute attacks are frequently accompanied by fever and leukocytosis. Attacks of gout typically respond to colchicine as specific therapy.

Laboratory Tests Useful in Diagnosis of Gout

Serum Uric Acid.—Patents with gout usually have elevated serum uric acid levels. However, 7%–8% have uric acid levels within reference limits at the time of the first attack. Some studies have shown elevated serum uric acid levels in about 10% of patients with RA, 15% of patients with pseudogout, and about 15% of patients with septic arthritis. Therefore, elevated serum uric acid levels are not diagnostic for gout, and normal serum uric acid levels do not conclusively rule out gout. On the other hand, positive latex test results for rheumatoid factor have been reported in 7%–11% of patients with primary gout. Serum uric acid reference values are sex related, with values in males about 1 mg/100 ml higher than values in females. One report indicates considerable week-to-week variation (about 30%–40%) in serum uric acid values in the same individual. Stress has been reported to raise uric acid levels. One investigator found that serum uric acid levels increased after exposure to sunlight.

Although elevation of serum uric acid is traditionally associated with gout, the majority of serum uric acid elevations are not due to gout. By far the most frequent cause of hyperuricemia, especially in hospitalized patients, is renal disease with azotemia.

Disorders of hyperuricemia can be divided into those due to increased intake, those due to decreased excretion, and those due to increased production.

Increased Intake.—Increased intake of purine-rich food usually does not produce hyperuricemia by itself, although it may affect the clinical symptoms of gout or add to the effect of other hyperuricemic agents.

Decreased Excretion.—Uric acid is excreted predominantly through the kidneys, with about 25% excreted by the GI tract. There is good correlation between severely decreased renal function, as indicated by elevated blood urea nitrogen (BUN) or serum creatinine levels (chapter 13) and increase in the serum level of uric acid, although the correlation is not linear. According to the literature, more than 90% of patients with elevated BUN and serum creatinine levels also have elevated serum uric acid values. However, when I examined the laboratory work of 156 newly admitted patients with elevated BUN levels, serum creatinine levels, or both, 31% of the patients had uric acid values within the reference range (even in those patients with BUN and creatinine levels both elevated, 31% still had normal uric acid levels). On the other hand, of a total of 222 patients, 30% had normal BUN and creatinine levels but elevated uric acid levels. Besides chronic renal disease, acute renal failure, and severely decreased renal blood flow, other conditions associated with hyperuricemia due to decreased renal excretion include treatment with certain drugs (including most diuretics, but especially the thiazides), ketoacidosis of diabetes or starvation, lactic acidosis, toxemia of pregnancy, lead poisoning, alcoholism, and hypothyroidism. In some of these conditions increased renal tubular reabsorption of urate is a major factor, with or without decreased renal function.

Increased Production.—Increased uric acid production can be demonstrated by increased uric acid excretion, if renal function is adequate. The standard method of evaluation is a 24-hour urine collection. Most investigators place the patient on a severely restricted (or "purine-free") purine diet before collecting the urine specimen (e.g., 4 days of diet, with the specimen collected on the fourth day and collection completed before the diet is terminated). The test is more accurate when the patient is asymptomatic, since acute inflammation may increase urine excretion of urate. Under these controlled conditions, the most commonly accepted upper limit of the reference range is 600 mg/24 hours (3,570 mmol/d). About 15%–25% of patients with primary gout have increased excretion of uric acid. The other 75%–85% have normal production and urine excretion levels. Conditions in which a substantial number of patients have increased uric acid production, increased excretion of uric acid, and hyperuricemia, include myeloproliferative syndromes (chronic myelocytic leukemia, polycythemia vera, etc.); chronic lymphocytic leukemia; myeloma; various malignancies (including the aforementioned leukemias and lymphomas); tumor or tissue cell destruction from chemotherapy or radiation therapy (including the tumor lysis syndrome); sickle cell anemia and severe hemolytic anemias; extensive psoriasis (30%–50% cases); sarcoidosis (30%–50% cases); and a congenital enzymatic defect in uric acid metabolism known as the "Lesch-Nyhan syndrome."

There is also an association of hyperuricemia with hypertension (22%–27% without renal disease), diabetes mellitus, obesity, and atherosclerotic heart disease. In some of these associated conditions there is a demonstrable etiology for hyperuricemia and in some there is not. One report indicates that up to 20% of males on long-term coumarin therapy develop elevated serum uric acid.

Measurement of urine uric acid to creatinine clearance ratio on a midmorning urine specimen has been proposed as a means to circumvent the problems involved with 24-hour urine collection. However, there is rather poor correlation between results obtained by the two methods in the same patients. One reason may be a reported diurnal variation in uric acid excretion, with about 40%–45% of daily quantity found in the 8 hours between 8 A.M. and 4 P.M.

The two most common laboratory assay methods for uric acid assay are colorimetric (based on uric acid reduction of phosphotungstic acid reagent) and enzymatic (using the specific enzyme uricase). Various reducing substances, such as levodopa and large quantities of glucose, ascorbic acid, acetaminophen, caffeine, and theophylline, can falsely elevate the colorimetric method.

Joint Fluid Aspiration.—The most accurate readily available laboratory test for gout is demonstration of uric acid crystals in synovial fluid aspirated from an acutely inflammed joint. The needle-like crystals of sodium monophosphate may be seen within neutrophils or lying free. These may be seen with the ordinary microscope but are best visualized using compensated polarized light. With the color compensator, urate crystals exhibit negative birefringence (yellow against a red background, with the axis of the crystal parallel to the axis of the compensator). When injected into a joint, some steroids form needle-like crystals that may mimic nonpolarized uric acid crystals. It has been reported that uric acid crystals cannot be demonstrated in joint aspirates from about 15% of patients with acute gout.

Pseudogout

Pseudogout is caused by calcium pyrophosphate crystal deposition. It clinically resembles gout to some degree but tends to affect large joints such as the knee rather than small peripheral joints. Joint x-ray films indicate some differences from classic gout but are frequently not a sufficient basis for diagnosis. Synovial fluid examination discloses calcium pyrophosphate crystals, either within neutrophil cytoplasm or extracellularly. These appear as short small rectangular structures or short rods, but sometimes color-compensated polarized light (imparting a positive birefringence, blue on red background) is necessary for reliable differentiation from uric acid.

Septic Arthritis

Septic arthritis is most often monoarticular but may affect more than one joint. Bacteria responsible for joint infection vary with age group, similar to the organisms producing meningitis. *Haemophilus influenzae, Staphylococcus aureus*, and gram-negative bacteria predominate in early childhood; *S. aureus*, pneumococci, and streptococci in later childhood; and *S. aureus*, pneumococci, streptococci, and gonococci in adults. Conditions that predispose to gram-negative bacilli include neoplasia, immunosuppression or decreased immunologic defenses, intravenous drug addicts, and urinary tract infections. Septic arthritis is diagnosed by direct aspiration and culture of the synovial fluid. Gram stain is reported to be positive in 40%–75% (range, 30%–95%) of infected joint aspirates, with detection of gram-positive aerobic organisms accomplished more readily than gram-negative organisms.

OTHER CONDITIONS ASSOCIATED WITH ARTHRITIS

Arthritis and arthralgia may be present in 4%–23% of patients with primary biliary cirrhosis. One report indicates that many more have radiologic abnormalities of erosive arthritis but have no symptoms. About 50% of patients with hemochromatosis and about 25% of patients with chronic active hepatitis develop arthritis or arthralgias; up to 40% of patients with hepatitis virus hepatitis have arthralgia (usually not true arthritis); and arthritis may occasionally be found in patients with viral infections of various type (e.g., rubella). Patients with cancer may develop joint symptoms due to direct extension from or a reaction to a nearby primary site or from joint area metastasis. Joint metastasis usually involves one of the knees and is most often due to carcinoma of the lung or breast. Metastasis to the hand is most often due to lung carcinoma. Childhood acute leukemia rather frequently appears to produce joint pain for a variety of reasons. Neoplasia have been associated with gout, vasculitis, and occasionally, syndromes resembling some of the collagen diseases.

Synovial Fluid Analysis

When synovial fluid is aspirated, 1 ml or more should be placed into a sterile tube for possible culture and a similar quantity into a heparinized tube for cell count. The remainder can be used for other procedures. A cell count is performed on anticoagulated fluid using 0.9% saline as the WBC pipette diluent (the usual diluent, Turk's solution, contains acetic acid, which coagulates synovial fluid mucin and produces clots that interfere with accuracy of the WBC count).

Synovial Fluid Tests

Mucin Clot.—The Ropes test for mucin clot is performed by adding a few drops of aspirate to 10–20 ml of 5% acetic acid in a small beaker. After 1 minute, the beaker is shaken. A well-formed clot remains compact; a poor clot is friable and shreds apart easily. In general, noninflammatory arthritides form a good clot. In noninfectious inflammation, the clot may be good to poor, whereas the clot of acute bacterial infection is poor.

Viscosity (String Sign).—Aspirate is allowed to drip slowly from the end of a needle. The length of the strand formed by each drop before it separates is the end point. In normal fluid and in noninflammatory arthritides the strands string out more than 3 cm. In acute inflammatory conditions fluids drip with little, if any, stringing.

Synovial Fluid Glucose.—Synovial fluid glucose value is usually within 10 mg/100 ml (0.5 mmol/L) of the serum glucose value and is always within 20 mg/100 ml. A blood specimen for glucose should be obtained as close as possible to the time of joint aspiration. The patient should have fasted at least 6–8 hours to achieve baseline values and to compensate for delay in glucose level equilibration between blood and synovial fluid. In degenerative arthritis, synovial fluid glucose levels are usually normal. In acute inflammatory noninfectious arthritis (SLE, RA, gout, etc.) there may be a mild or even a moderate decrease (up to 40 mg/100 ml below serum levels). In acute bacterial (septic) arthritis there typically is a marked decrease of more than 40 mg/100 ml (2.22 mmol/L) below serum glucose levels, but a decrease of this extent is said to occur in only about 50% of cases.

Microbiologic Studies of Synovial Fluid.—Gram stain is reported to demonstrate organisms in 40%–75% of patients with septic arthritis (literature range, 30%–95%), more often with gram-positive than with gram-negative bacterial infection. However, Gram stain is not always easy to interpret, especially when only a small number of organisms are present, due to debris from the joint which may take up some of the stain. Culture of synovial fluid is the mainstay of diagnosis in septic arthritis. Since gonococci are a major cause of joint infection, provision should be made for the special conditions necessary to culture these organisms. It has been reported that blood cultures may be positive and synovial fluid cultures negative in 15% of patients with septic arthritis. Previous antibiotic therapy considerably decreases the chance of diagnosis by culture.

Synovial Fluid White Blood Cell Count.—There is considerable overlap between WBC counts of noninflammatory conditions and noninfectious inflammatory diseases in the area of 500–2,000 WBCs/cu mm (0.5–2.0 × 10^9/L) and between infectious disease and noninfectious inflammatory conditions in the area of 10,000–100,000 WBCs/cu mm (10–100 × 10^9/L) (Table 22–3). Thus, only very high or very low WBC counts are of great help without other information. A very high percentage of neutrophils (> 75%, usually > 90%) is said to occur in most cases of untreated acute bacterial infectious arthritis. A neutrophil percentage of more than 90% may therefore be a more reliable indicator of bacterial infection than cell count, synovial glucose level, or Gram stain (unless the cell count is > 100,000, the synovial glucose level is > 40 mg/100 ml below the fasting, simultaneously drawn serum glucose level, or the Gram stain discloses unequivocal organisms).

Typical synovial fluid findings are summarized in Table 22–3.

Other Examinations.—Other examinations include a serologic test for RA. The RA tests on synovial fluid occasionally show positive results before serum tests. In SLE, LE cells sometimes form in synovial fluid and can be demonstrated on the same Wright's-stained smear used for differential cell count. Synovial fluid total complement (CH_{50}, chapter 21), is said to be decreased in SLE and active RA (more often if the patient with RA has a positive latex tube agglutination test result). Total complement is reported to be increased in Reiter's syndrome. Most other noninflammatory and inflammatory arthritic diseases are associated with normal synovial fluid complement levels. However, there are sufficient exceptions to these general observations that synovial fluid complement assay has not become popular. For example, in one study, 15% of SLE patients had normal synovial fluid total complement values and only about 40% of patients with Reiter's syndrome had elevated levels.

Synovial Fluid Specimen Collection

An anticoagulated tube is necessary for cell count, WBC differential, and examination for crystals. Heparin is preferred, but liquid ethylenediamine tetraacetic acid can be used. Without anticoagulation, spontaneous small or large clots may form that trap WBCs and alter the cell count. A sterile tube should be used for fluid that is to be cultured; heparin anticoagulant is preferred. This must be sent to the laboratory immediately. A tube without anticoagulant is needed for the mucin test, complement assay, and glucose assay. Some prefer a tube with fluoride anticoagulant for glucose to help preserve the specimen. Fluid for complement assay should be frozen immediately if the assay is not performed within 1–2 hours.

RADIONUCLIDE JOINT SCANNING

Besides synovial fluid examination, radionuclide joint scanning is a procedure that may offer useful information. For screening purposes, the scan could be performed with one of the isotope-labeled phosphate compounds used for bone scanning. These scans reveal abnormality in most joints that have a significant degree of inflammation, even when subclinical. Joint scanning permits a reasonably accurate assessment of the number, location, and degree of activity of involved joints and offers an objective (although only semiquantitative)

TABLE 22–3.
Synovial Fluid Findings*

Condition	Viscosity	Cell Count (per cu mm)	% PMN	Glucose Level	Mucin Clot	Other Tests or Findings
Normal	Normal (high)	0–200 (0–600)	0–25	Normal	Good	—
Trauma with hemorrhage/ coagulation abnormalities	Normal	> 5,000	50 (25–50)	Normal	Good	Many RBCs
Osteoarthritis/ osteochondritis dissecans/ trauma without hemorrhage	Normal	500 (200–2,000)	25	Normal	Good	Cartilage fragments
Acute rheumatic fever	Low	2,000–15,000 (0–60,000)	50 (50–60)	Occasional small decrease	Good to poor	—
SLE	Normal or low	2,000–5,000 (0–10,000)	25 (10–30)	Normal to 20 mg below blood glucose level	Good to fair	LE prep
RA RA variants	Low	2,000–50,000† (200–100,000)	70–85 (25–85)	Normal to 30 mg below blood glucose level	Fair, 50% Poor, 45%	RA latex test
Gout (acute attack)	Low	2,000–50,000‡ (100–100,000)	75 (40–90)	Normal to 30 mg below blood glucose level	Fair, 50% Poor, 40%	Urate crystals
Pseudogout	Low	2,000–50,000‡ (100–100,000)	75 (35–85)	Normal	Fair, 40% Poor, 35%	Calcium pyrophosphate crystals
Acute bacterial arthritis	Low	> 50,000§ (2,500–300,000)	90 (75–95)	More than 40 mg below blood glucose level‖	Poor (85% of cases)	Culture Gram stain¶

*Parentheses indicate ranges from the literature. PMN = polymorphonuclear leukocytes.
†More than 50,000/cu mm in 4% of cases; 2,500 in 6% of cases.
‡More than 50,000/cu mm in 12% of cases; 1,000 in 15% of cases.
§Less than 50,000/cu mm in 30% of cases; 20,000 in 11% of cases.
‖More than 40 mg/100 ml below blood glucose level in 40%–50% of cases.
¶Gram stain reported positive in 55%–95% of gram-positive and 30%–55% of gram-negative infections.

method for evaluating results of therapy. Although fairly sensitive, the phosphate agents are not ideal for joint scanning, since increased concentration denotes increased activity of bone osteoblasts in response to adjacent synovial abnormality rather than a primary synovial reaction. Other etiologies for osteoblastic stimulation, such as osteochondritis dissecans, traumatic joint disease, active osteoarthritis, healing fractures, and the later stages of aseptic necrosis, may all produce abnormal bone scan images, which sometimes are hard to differentiate from arthritis. In such cases other compounds may be employed, including technetium pertechnetate or labeled albumin. These tend to remain in blood vessels, thereby indicating regions of increased vascularity or hyperemia such as the synovial membrane when involved by active arthritis. These compounds are a little less sensitive than the phosphates but are more specific for synovial disease.

RADIONUCLIDE BONE SCANNING

Certain disorders affecting bone are discussed elsewhere (hyperparathyroidism, metastatic tumor in bone). The commonest diagnostic problems involve fractures, osteomyelitis, and metastatic tumor. The nonradiologic procedures most frequently used in bone disease are serum alkaline phosphatase and bone scanning.

Strontium 85 was the first agent to be widely used in bone scanning. Its relatively high patient radiation dose and problems with excretion by the colon led to replacement by fluorine 18, which, in turn, has been superseded by the technetium-labeled phosphates. Bone scan abnormality is due to increased osteoblastic activity, whether neoplastic, reactive, reparative, or metabolic. Local hyperemia is also a factor.

Bone scan provides important information in the evaluation of trauma and unexplained pain in areas where an occult fracture is a possibility. Whereas some fractures are immediately evident on x-ray film, in many cases the fracture line cannot be seen, especially in the spine, ribs, face, and smaller bones of the extremities. The radiologist is then forced to look for secondary changes produced by healing, which will not become evident before 10–14 days and in some cases may never be detectable. On bone scan, many fracture sites become abnormal by 3 days after trauma, and the great majority in 5 days. Once evident, the abnormality persists for a variable length of time, the average being approximately 2 years. A fracture site revealed on x-ray film but not on scan at least 7 days after trauma usually represents an old healed injury. Severe osteoporosis or severe malnutrition retards osseous reaction and may result in an equivocal or false negative scan. As noted previously, various types of joint disease can be visualized on the bone scan and may on occasion present problems in differentiation of the disease from possible fracture in the neighborhood of the joint.

Osteomyelitis is another disease in which bone scan may be invaluable. X-ray changes do not usually appear before 10–14 days after onset and may be delayed further or be difficult to interpret. Bone scan shows abnormalities days or weeks before x-ray films. Although the exact time after onset necessary for most patients to display abnormality is not as clearly defined in osteomyelitis as in fracture, the literature seems to suggest 5–7 days. If the bone scan is normal and osteomyelitis is strongly suspected, a gallium scan may be helpful, or the bone scan may be repeated after several days. Certain conditions resemble osteomyelitis clinically and to some degree on scan. These include cellulitis, arthritis, and focal bone necrosis or infarct. Patients already receiving steroid or antibiotic therapy before onset of osteomyelitis may display changes in normal bone response. These changes can affect the bone scan latent period or the image characteristics.

Metastatic tumor detection is the reason for most bone scan requests. All malignancies capable of metastasis may reach bone. Some of these, including prostate, breast, lung, kidney, urinary bladder, thyroid follicular carcinoma and possibly malignant lymphoma, are more likely to do so than other tumors (see chapter 36). Formerly, bone scanning was widely used to establish operability of these neoplasms by excluding bone metastases after a primary tumor was discovered. Most reports on breast carcinoma patients in early (potentially operable) stage disclosed a very small incidence of abnormal bone scans (usually $< 10\%$) unless there was some other evidence of bone metastases such as bone pain or elevated alkaline phosphatase levels. For example, in stage I and II breast carcinoma, there is an average reported incidence of 6% bone scan abnormality (literature range, 1%–40%). False positive abnormality due to conditions other than metastasis is also a problem (3%–57% of cases, average about 10%). Therefore, bone (and also liver or brain) scans are not being recommended in most institutions as routine preoperative tests in breast carcinoma. Fewer data are available for lung carcinoma, but there may be a better case for preoperative bone scans in potentially resectable patients based on higher rates of detectable occult metastases and the greater magnitude of the operation, which becomes unnecessary if metastases are found.

Tumor-related bone scanning is indicated in several situations: (1) to investigate bone pain when x-ray films do not show a lesion; (2) to document extent of tumor in nonresectable malignancies known to have a high rate of bone metastasis to follow results of therapy; and (3) in some cases, to help investigate unexplained symptoms that may be due to occult tumor. Until bone scanning became available, skeletal x-ray survey was the mainstay of diagnosis. Numerous comparisons have shown that bone scanning detects 15%–40% more bone metastases (literature range, 7%–57%) than x-ray. This difference is related to osteoblastic reaction induced by the tumor, which may occur even when the lesion is osteolytic on x-ray film. On the other hand, about 5% of metastases are seen on x-ray film but not on scan (literature range, 3%–8%); these are usually pure osteolytic lesions. The implication of these figures is that bone scan is sufficient for routine detection of metastases in the major bone-seeking tumors and that x-ray should be reserved for specific anatomical areas in which the scan is equivocal or the etiology of scan abnormality is in doubt. X-ray is also useful when there is strong suspicion of bone malignancy yet the scan is normal, when the scan is normal in areas of bone pain, and to help differentiate metastasis from focal severe osteoarthritis.

Bone scanning does have disadvantages, chief of which is nonspecificity. The variety of conditions that may produce abnormal bone scans include fractures (even those of long duration), osteomyelitis, active osteoarthritis, joint synovial inflammation, areas of bone necrosis or infarct, myositis ossificans, renal osteodystrophy, Paget's disease of bone, certain benign bone tumors such as fibrous dysplasia and osteoid osteoma, and various artifacts such as ossification centers in the sternum or costochondral junction calcification. On the other hand, when tumor produces widespread bone marrow invasion, the spine or other bones may sometimes have a homogeneous appearance on scan that may be misinterpreted as normal unless certain other findings are taken into account. As a general rule, the greater the number of focal asymmetric lesions on bone scan, the more metastatic tumor should be suspected. Healing fractures (which actually may have occurred at different times) and Paget's disease create the most interpretative difficulty. Some institutions routinely scan only the spine, pelvis, and ribs instead of the total body. A question may arise about the probability of metastases elsewhere. One large study encompassing a wide variety of tumors indicates that the incidence of solitary uptake (other skeletal areas negative) in the skull is about 4%; in the extremities as a unit, about 9%; in the humerus, about 1%; in the femur, 5%; in the tibia or fibula, 2%; and elsewhere in the extremities, quite rare.

BIBLIOGRAPHY

Larsson A, Sjoquist J: False-positive results in latex agglutination tests caused by rheumatoid factor. *Clin Chem* 1988; 34:767.

Molden DP, Raskin R: Deciphering systemic rheumatic disease. *Lab Mgmt* 1988; 26(1):43.

Slemenda CW, Johnston CC: Bone mass measurement: Which site to measure? *Am J Med* 1988; 84:643.

Riggs BL, Wahnwe HW: Bone densitometry and clinical decision-making in osteoporosis. *Ann Intern Med* 1988; 108:293.

Olson NY, Lindsley CB: Neonatal lupus syndrome. *Am J Dis Child* 1987; 141:908.

McKenna F, Wright V: Inflammatory bowel disease and arthritis. *Intern Med Specialist* 1987; 8:163.

Ditzian-Kadanoff R, et al: The enthesopathies. *Intern Med Specialist* 1987; 8:95.

Zwas ST, et al: Interpretation and classification of bone scintigraphic findings in stress fractures. *J Nucl Med* 1987; 28:452.

Hutton C, Maddison PJ: Systemic lupus erythematosus in the elderly. *Intern Med Specialist* 1987; 8:119.

Jansen EM, et al: Comparison of commercial kits for the detection of anti-nDNA antibodies using *Crithidia luciliae*. *Am J Clin Pathol* 1987; 87:461.

Feldkamp CS: Immune complexes. *Clin Chem Newslett* 1987; 13(4):5.

Kunnamo I, et al: Clinical signs and laboratory tests in the differential diagnosis of arthritis in children. *Am J Dis Child* 1987; 141:34.

Chestnut CH: Noninvasive technique for measuring bone mass: A comparative review. *Clin Obstet Gynecol* 1987; 30:812.

McCarty GA: Autoantibodies and their relation to rheumatic diseases. *Med Clin North Am* 1986; 70:237.

Rice JR: "Fibrositis" syndrome. *Med Clin North Am* 1986; 70:455.

Wong RL, Korn JH: Temporal arteritis without an elevated erythrocyte sedimentation rate. *Am J Med* 1986; 80:959.

Allen NB, Studenski SA: Polymyalgia rheumatica and temporal arteritis. *Med Clin North Am* 1986; 70:369.

Hunder GG: Polymyalgia rheumatica and giant cell arteritis. *Drug Ther* 1986; 16(7):73.

Haynes BF, et al: Diagnostic and therapeutic approach to the patient with vasculitis. *Med Clin North Am* 1986; 70:355.

Caldwell DS, McCallum RM: Rheumatologic manifestations of cancer. *Med Clin North Am* 1986; 70:385.

German DC, Holmes EW: Hyperuricemia and gout. *Med Clin North Am* 1986; 70:419.

Gaylis NB: Initial evaluation of the arthritic patient. *Postgrad Med* 1986; 80(5):65.

Krane SM, Simon LS: Rheumatoid arthritis: clinical features and pathogenetic mechanisms. *Med Clin North Am* 1986; 70:263.

Kredich DW: Chronic arthritis in childhood. *Med Clin North Am* 1986; 70:305.

Eichenfeld AH, et al: Limited diagnostic value of rheumatoid factor in juvenile rheumatoid arthritis. *Pediatrics* 1986; 78:480.

Sonnett RW: Serodiagnosis of systemic lupus erythematosus. *J Med Technol* 1986; 3:280.

Calin A: Seronegative spondyloarthritides. *Med Clin North Am* 1986; 70:323.

Hench PK, Mitler MM: Fibromyalgia. *Postgrad Med* 1986; 80:47.

Pisetsky DS: Systemic lupus erythematosus. *Med Clin North Am* 1986; 70:337.

Molina R, et al: Primary Sjögren's syndrome in men. *Am J Med* 1986; 80:23.

Endo L, et al: Clinical utility of assays for circulating immune complexes. *Med Clin North Am* 1985; 69:623.

Cush JJ, Goldings EA: Drug-induced lupus. *Am J Med Sci* 1985; 290:36.

Handmaker H: The role of nuclear medicine in suspected osteomyelitis. *Curr Concepts in Diagn Nucl Med* 1985; 2(2):9.

Harmon CE: Antinuclear antibodies in autoimmune disease. *Med Clin North Am* 1985; 69:547.

Molden DP: ANA profiles in systemic rheumatic disease. *Diagn Med* 1985; 8(6):12.

Kale SA: Drug-induced systemic lupus erythematosus. *Postgrad Med* 1985; 77:231.

Nakamura RM, et al: Advances in laboratory tests for autoantibodies to nuclear antigens in systemic rheumatic diseases. *Lab Med* 1984; 15:190.

Nichols WS, Nakamura RM: Antibody patterns in autoimmune disease. *Lab Mgmt* 1984; 22(5):39.

Sontheimer RD, et al: Antinuclear and anticytoplasmic antibodies. *J Am Acad Dermatol* 1983; 9:335.

Gruber HE, Seegmiller JE: The clinical and laboratory significance of uric acid assay. *Lab Mgmt* 1983; 21(10):21.

Resnik CS, Resnick D: Crystal deposition disease. *Semin Arthritis Rheum* 1983; 12:390.

Masi AT, et al: Seronegative rheumatoid arthritis; fact or fiction? *Arch Intern Med* 1983; 143:2167.

Fox AL: Anti-dsDNA in SLE: A specificity myth. *Am J Clin Pathol* 1982; 77:776.

McKendry RJR, et al: A comparison of the clinical usefulness of eight tests for IgM rheumatoid factor. *Am J Clin Pathol* 1982; 78:517.

Calebro JJ: Three patient profiles point to JRA. *Diagnosis* 1981; 3:52.

Sams WM: Allergic vasculitis. *Postgrad Med* 1981; 70:193.

Kaplan EL, Huwe BB: The sensitivity and specificity of an agglutination test for antibodies to streptococcal extracellular antigens: A quantitative analysis and comparison of the Streptozyme test with the anti-streptolysin-O and the anti-deoxyribonuclease B tests. *J Pediatr* 1980; 96:367.

Strand V, Talal N: Advances in the diagnosis and concept of Sjögren's syndrome. *Bull Rheum Dis* 1980; 30:1046.

Citrin DL, Fogelman I: A review of bone scanning in the evaluation of the cancer patient. *Appl Radiol* 1980; 9:102.

Silberstein EB: Nuclear orthopedics. *J Nucl Med* 1980; 21:997.

Khan MA: Clinical application of the HLA-B27 test in rheumatic diseases. *Arch Intern Med* 1980; 140:177.

Bayer AS: Nongonococcal bacterial septic arthritis. *Postgrad Med* 1980; 67:157.

Treves S: Skeletal scintigraphy in the diagnosis of acute osteomyelitis. *Hosp Pract* 1979; 14:66.

Fauci AS, et al: The spectrum of vasculitis. *Ann Intern Med* 1978; 89:660.

23 Acid-Base and pH Measurements

Fluid and electrolyte problems are common in hospitalized patients. Most of these problems are secondary to other diseases or are undesirable side effects of therapy. There are a few diseases regularly associated with certain pH or electrolyte alterations, which can help suggest the diagnosis and which can be used to monitor therapy.

Fluid and electrolytes in one form or another make up nearly all of the human body. It is useful to think of these constituents as though they were contained in three separate compartments between which are variable degrees of communication: individual cells, containing intracellular fluid; vascular channels, containing blood or lymph; and the extracellular nonvascular tissue containing the interstitial fluid. Shifts of fluid and electrolytes between and within these compartments take place continually as the various activities concerned with homeostasis, cell metabolism, and organ function go on. To some degree, these changes can be monitored clinically by their effects on certain measurable parameters, including the pH and concentration of certain ions (electrolytes) in a fairly accessible substance, the blood. This chapter covers blood pH and its disturbances; the next chapter discusses certain electrolyte and fluid disorders.

BLOOD pH: THE BICARBONATE–CARBONIC ACID SYSTEM

The term pH comes from the French puissance hydrogen, meaning the strength or power of hydrogen. The hydrogen ion concentration of blood expressed in gram molecular weights of hydrogen per liter (moles/L) is so much less than 1 (e.g., 0.0000001) that it is easier to communicate this information in terms of logarithms; thus, 0.0000001 becomes 1×10^{-7}. The symbol pH represents an even greater simplification, because pH is defined as the negative logarithm of the hydrogen ion concentration (in the preceding example, 1×10^{-7} becomes 10^{-7}, which then becomes 7.0). In this way, a relatively simple scale is substituted for very cumbersome tiny numbers. In the pH scale, therefore, a change of 1.0 pH unit means a tenfold change in hydrogen ion concentration (a change of pH from 7.0 to 6.0 represents a change from 10^{-7} to 10^{-6} moles/L).

The normal pH of arterial blood is 7.4, with a normal range between 7.36 and 7.44. Blood pH must be maintained within relatively narrow limits, because a pH outside the range 6.8–7.8 is incompatible with life. Therefore, the hydrogen ion content is regulated by a series of buffers. A buffer is a substance that can bind hydrogen ions to a certain extent without inducing a marked change in pH. Among substances that act as buffers are hemoglobin, plasma protein, phosphates, and the bicarbonate–carbonic acid system. Bicarbonate is by far the body's most important buffer substance; it is present in large quantities and can be controlled by the lungs and kidneys.

A brief review of the bicarbonate–carbonic acid system recalls that carbon dioxide (CO_2) in aqueous solutions exists in potential equilibrium with carbonic acid ($CO_2 + H_2O = H_2CO_3$). The enzyme carbonic anhydrase catalyzes this reaction toward attainment of equilibrium; otherwise the rate of reaction would be minimal. Carbon dioxide is produced by cellular metabolism and is released into the bloodstream. There, most of it diffuses into the red blood cells (RBCs), where carbonic anhydrase catalyzes its hydration to H_2CO_3. Carbonic acid readily dissociates into hydrogen ions (H^+) and bicarbonate ions (HCO_3^-). Eventually only a small amount of dissolved CO_2 and a much smaller amount of undissociated H_2CO_3 remain in the plasma. Therefore, the great bulk of the original CO_2 (amounting to 75%) is carried in the blood as bicarbonate, with only about 5% still in solution (as dissolved CO_2 or undissociated H_2CO_3) and about 20% coupled with hemoglobin as a carbamino compound or, to a much lesser extent, coupled with other buffers, such as plasma proteins.

This situation can best be visualized by means of the Henderson-Hasselbalch equation. This equation states that

$$\text{pH} = \text{pK} + \log \frac{\text{base}}{\text{acid}}$$

where pK is the dissociation constant (ability to release hydrogen ions) of the particular acid chosen, such as H_2CO_3. The derivation of this equation will be disregarded to concentrate on the clinically useful parts, the relationship of pH, base, and acid. If the bicarbonate-acid system is to be interpreted by means of the Henderson-Hasselbalch equation, then

$$\frac{\text{base}}{\text{acid}} = \frac{HCO_3^-}{H_2CO_3}$$

since bicarbonate is the base and carbonic acid is the acid. Actually, most of the carbonic acid represented in the equation is dissolved CO_2, which is present in plasma in an amount greater than 100 times the quantity of undissociated H_2CO_3. Therefore the formula should really be

$$\frac{HCO_3^-}{H_2CO_3 + CO_2}$$

but it is customary to let H_2CO_3 stand for the entire denominator. The next step is to note from the Henderson-Hasselbalch equation that pH is proportional to base/acid. This means that in the bicarbonate–carbonic acid system, pH is proportional to

$$\frac{HCO_3^-}{H_2CO_3}$$

The kidney is the main regulator of HCO_3^- production (the numerator of the equation) and the lungs primarily control CO_2 excretion (the denominator).

The kidney has several means of excreting hydrogen ions. One is the conversion of monohydrogen phosphate to dihydrogen phosphate (HPO_4^{2-} to $H_2PO_4^-$). Another is the formation of ammonia (NH_3) in renal tubule cells by deamination of certain amino acids, such as glutamine. Ammonia then diffuses into the urine, where it combines with H^+ to form ammonium ion (NH_4^+). A third mechanism is the one of most concern now, the production of HCO_3^- in the renal tubule cells. These cells contain carbonic anhydrase, which catalyzes the formation of H_2CO_3 from CO_2. The H_2CO_3 dissociates, leaving HCO_3^- and H^+. The H^+ is excreted in the urine by the phosphate or ammonium pathways or combined with some other anion. The HCO_3^- goes into the bloodstream where it forms part of the pH buffer system. Not only does HCO_3^- assist in buffering H^+ within body fluids, but HCO_3^- filtered at the glomerulus into the urine can itself combine with urinary H^+ (produced by the renal tubule cells from the H_2CO_3 cycle and excreted into the urine).

The lungs, on the other hand, convert H_2CO_3, into CO_2 and water with the aid of carbonic anhydrase and blow off the CO_2. In this process, a mechanism for excreting H^+ exists, because the HCO_3^- in the plasma can combine with free H^+ to form H_2CO_3, which can then be eliminated from the lungs in the form of CO_2, as was just described. This process can probably handle excretion of most normal and mildly abnormal H^+ quantities. However, when large excesses of free H^+ are present in body fluids, the kidney plays a major role, because not only is H^+ excreted directly in the urine, but HCO_3^- is formed, which helps buffer additional amounts of H^+ in the plasma.

Going back to the Henderson-Hasselbalch equation, which is now modified to indicate that pH is proportional to HCO_3^-/H_2CO_3, it is easy to see that variations in either the numerator or denominator will change pH. If HCO_3^- is increased without a corresponding increase in H_2CO_3, the ratio will be increased and the pH will rise. Conversely, if something happens to increase H_2CO_3 or dissolve CO_2, the denominator will be increased, the ratio will be decreased, the pH will fall, and so on. Clinically, an increase in normal plasma pH is called "alkalosis" and a decrease is called "acidosis." The normal ratio of HCO_3^- to H_2CO_3 is 20:1.

LABORATORY DETERMINATION OF pH AND CARBON DIOXIDE

This section describes the laboratory tests used in pH abnormalities, which, incidentally, are often called "acid-base problems" because of the importance of the bicarbonate and carbonic acid changes involved.

Carbon Dioxide Combining Power.—Venous blood is drawn aerobically with an ordinary syringe and the serum is then equilibrated to normal alveolar levels of 40 mm Hg by the technician blowing his or her own alveolar air into the specimen through a tube arrangement. This maneuver adjusts the amount of dissolved CO_2 to the normal amounts found in normal arterial blood. Bicarbonate of the serum is then converted to CO_2 by acid hydrolysis in a vacuum, and the released gas is measured. The released CO_2 thus consists of the dissolved CO_2 of the specimen already present plus the converted HCO_3^- (and thus the denominator plus the numerator of the Henderson-Hasselbalch equation). Subtraction of the known amount of dissolved CO_2 and H_2CO_3 in normal blood from this measurement gives what is essentially a value for serum HCO_3^- alone (called the "combining power," since HCO_3^- combines with H^+). The inaccuracy that may be caused by these manipulations should be obvious.

Carbon Dioxide Content.—Total CO_2 content is determined from heparinized arterial or venous blood drawn anaerobically. This may be done in a vacuum tube or a syringe that is quickly capped. (Mineral oil is not satisfactory for sealing.) The blood is centrifuged and the plasma removed. At this point, all the CO_2 present is still at the same CO_2 tension or partial pressure of dissolved gas that the patient possessed. Next, the plasma is analyzed for CO_2 by a method that converts HCO_3^- and H_2CO_3 to the gas form. Thus, CO_2 content measures the sum of HCO_3^-, H_2CO_3, and dissolved CO_2. Since the amount of dissolved CO_2 and H_2CO_3 in blood is very small, normal values for CO_2 content are quite close to those of the CO_2 combining power (which measures only HCO_3^-). Since the specimen has been drawn and processed with little or no contact with outside air, the result is obviously more accurate than that obtained from the CO_2 combining power.

Serum Bicarbonate.—An order for serum CO_2, serum HCO_3^-, or venous CO_2 will usually result in serum being obtained from venous blood drawn aerobically and assayed for HCO_3^- without equilibration. This technique is used in most automated equipment that assays "CO_2" (really, bicarbonate) in addition to performing other tests, and is also popular in many laboratories using manual methods since the patients usually have other test orders that require serum. It is somewhat less accurate than CO_2 combining power. The serum is frequently exposed to air for relatively long periods of time. Only relatively large changes in CO_2 or HCO_3^- will be detected.

Partial Pressure of Carbon Dioxide.—Direct measurement of the partial pressure of CO_2 (PCO_2) using a PCO_2 electrode was popularized by Astrup and is based on the fact that most of the denominator of the Henderson-Hasselbalch equation represents dissolved CO_2. Since the partial pressure of CO_2 (the PCO_2) of the specimen is proportional to the amount of dissolved CO_2, the PCO_2 is therefore proportional to the denominator of the Henderson-Hasselbalch equation and may be used as a substitute for the denominator. In practice, a small amount of whole blood (plasma can be used), collected anaerobically, is analyzed for PCO_2, using a CO_2 electrode. The HCO_3^- may then be calculated (from the Henderson-Hasselbalch equation), or the PCO_2 value itself may be used in conjunction with pH to differentiate acid-base abnormalities. PCO_2 determined by electrode is without question the method of choice for acid-base problems. The pH is usually measured at the same time on the same specimen.

pH Measurement.—pH determination originally involved measuring the difference in electric charge between two electrodes placed in a solution (e.g., plasma or whole blood). Present-day equipment uses a single direct-reading pH electrode, which makes pH determination very simple and reliable and enables pH determination to be a routine part of blood gas measurement. On the technical side, it should be noted that at room temperature, plasma pH decreases at the rate of about 0.015 pH unit every 30 minutes. Unless measurement is done within 30 minutes after drawing, the blood should be refrigerated immediately; it can then be kept up to 4 hours.

ACID-BASE TEST SPECIMENS

In the early days, acid-base studies were performed on venous blood. Venous specimens are nearly as accurate as arterial blood for pH and HCO_3 (or PCO_2) measurements if blood is obtained anaerobically from a motionless hand or arm before the tourniquet is released. Nevertheless, arterial specimens have mostly replaced venous ones because venous blood provides less accurate data in some conditions such as decreased tissue perfusion due to shock. Even more important, one can also obtain blood oxygen measurements (PO_2) with arterial samples. Arterial blood is most often drawn from the radial artery in the wrist. Arterial puncture is a little more difficult than venipuncture, and there is a small but definite risk of extravasation and hematoma formation that could compress the artery. In general, glass syringes are preferred to plastic syringes or vacuum blood collection devices for technical reasons and to diminish the chance of room air contamination. The specimen tube or syringe should be placed in ice immediately for transport to the laboratory, both to prevent artifact from blood cell metabolism and to diminish gas exchange between the syringe and room air. The blood must be rewarmed just before analysis.

Heparin is the preferred anticoagulant for blood gas specimens. The usual method is to wash the syringe with a heparin solution and then expell the heparin (which leaves about 0.2 ml of heparin in the dead space of the syringe and needle). If too much heparin remains or the blood sample size is too small (usually when the sample is < 3 ml), there is a disproportionate amount of heparin for the amount of blood. PCO_2 (and bicarbonate) and hemoglobin values are often significantly decreased, with a much smaller (often negligible) decrease in pH. These artifactual decreases in PCO_2 are especially apt to occur when the sample is obtained from indwelling catheters flushed with heparin.

CLINICAL DISTURBANCES OF pH

With this background, one may proceed to the various clinical disturbances of pH. These have been clinically termed "acidosis," when the pH is decreased toward the acid side of normal and alkalosis, when the pH is elevated toward the alkaline side of normal. Acidosis, in turn, is usually subdivided into metabolic and respiratory etiology, and the same for alkalosis.

Metabolic Acidosis

This type of acidosis has at least three main causes.

Acid-Gaining Acidosis.—Hydrogen ions not included in the CO_2 system are added to the blood. The common situations are:

1. Direct administration, such as treatment with ammonium chloride, or the late effects of salicylate poisoning. Ammonium chloride (NH_4Cl) releases H^+ ions and Cl^- ions as the liver utilizes this compound for NH_3 to synthesize urea. Aspirin is acetylsalicylic acid, which in large quantities will eventually add enough H^+ ions to cause acidosis, even though in the early stages there is respiratory alkalosis (to be discussed later).
2. Excess metabolic acid formation is found in diabetic ketoacidosis, starvation, or severe dehydration. These conditions cause utilization of body protein and fat for energy instead of carbohydrate, with production of ketone bodies and various metabolic acids.

The results of acid-gaining acidosis are a decrease in free HCO_3^-, which is used up trying to buffer the excess H^+. Thus, the numerator of the Henderson-Hasselbalch equation is decreased, the normal 20:1 ratio is decreased, and the pH is, therefore, decreased. The CO_2 content (or CO_2 combining power) is also decreased because the bicarbonate, which it measures, has been decreased as a primary response to the addition of excess acid.

Base-Losing Acidosis.—Base-losing acidosis is caused by severe intestinal diarrhea, especially if prolonged or in children. Diseases such as cholera or possibly ulcerative colitis or severe dysentery might cause this. The mechanism is direct loss of HCO_3^- from the lumen of the small intestine. Normally, HCO_3^- is secreted into the small intestine, so that the contents of the small intestine are alkaline in contrast to the acidity of the stomach. Most of the HCO_3^- is reabsorbed; however, prolonged diarrhea or similar conditions could mechanically prevent intestinal reabsorption enough to cause significant HCO_3^- loss in the feces. In addition, the H^+ ions that were released from H_2CO_3 in the formation of HCO_3^- by carbonic anhydrase are still present in the bloodstream and help decrease pH. However, the primary cause is the direct loss of HCO_3^-; the numerator of the Henderson-Hasselbalch equation is decreased, the 20:1 ratio is decreased, and the pH is decreased. Naturally, the CO_2 content is also decreased.

Renal Acidosis.—Renal acidosis occurs in kidney failure that produces the clinical syndrome of uremia. As mentioned previously, the kidney has the major responsibility for excreting large excesses of H^+. In uremia, H^+ from metabolic acids that normally would be excreted this way is retained in the bloodstream due to loss of renal tubular function. As in acid-gaining acidosis, the excess H^+ must be buffered; therefore, part of the available body fluid HCO_3^- is used up. This decreases the numerator of the Henderson-Hasselbalch equation, decreases the normal 20:1 ratio, and therefore decreases pH. Again, the CO_2 content is decreased.

Respiratory Acidosis

The second major category of acidosis is that called respiratory acidosis. This may be due to any condition that causes pulmonary CO_2 retention. These conditions include the respiratory muscle paralysis of poliomyelitis, the respiratory brain center depression sometimes seen in encephalitis or with large doses of such drugs as morphine, primary lung disease (e.g., pulmonary fibrosis or severe emphysema) that destroys oxygen exchange ability, and sometimes heart diseases (e.g., chronic congestive heart failure). The basic problem is H_2CO_3 excess produced by CO_2 retention. Thus, the denominator of the Henderson-Hasselbalch equation is increased, the normal 20:1 ratio is decreased, and the pH is decreased. The CO_2 content is sometimes normal but is usually increased, because of kidney attempts to handle the excess CO_2 by forming more HCO_3^- and excreting more H^+ ions.

Metabolic Alkalosis

Alkalosis may also be divided into metabolic and respiratory types. In metabolic alkalosis, three relatively common situations should be discussed.

Alkali Administration.—Alkali administration most commonly occurs when sodium bicarbonate is taken in large quantities for the treatment of peptic ulcer symptoms. If this happens, excess HCO_3^- is absorbed above the amount needed to neutralize stomach hydrochloric acid (HCl). The numerator of the Henderson-Hasselbalch equation is increased, the normal 20:1 ratio is increased, and the pH therefore rises. The CO_2 content also rises because of the additional HCO_3^-. Lactate, citrate, or acetate in sufficient quantities may also produce alkalosis, since they are metabolized to HCO_3^-.

Acid-Losing Alkalosis.—Acid-losing alkalosis most frequently results from severe or protracted vomiting, as may occur with pyloric stenosis. Gastric HCl is lost in vomiting. Gastric HCl was originally produced by conversion of H_2CO_3 to HCO_3^- and H^+, mediated by carbonic anhydrase of the gastric mucosa. The HCO_3^- is kept in the bloodstream, but the H^+ is secreted into the gastric lumen as HCl. When HCl is lost through vomiting, the H^+ component of HCl is also continually being lost. The CO_2 content becomes increased, because the HCO_3^- that is released when HCl is produced remains in the bloodstream and increases when additional HCl is formed to replace that which is being lost. Therefore, the 20:1 ratio is increased and the pH is increased. Since H_2CO_3 is decreased, as it is being continually used to produce more HCl, the lungs tend to retain CO_2 to compensate. Therefore, PCO_2 may actually increase, although not enough to prevent increase of the 20:1 ratio.

Hypokalemic Alkalosis.—Hypokalemic alkalosis is most commonly due to excess potassium ion (K^+) loss by the kidney, as might happen with overuse of certain diuretics that cause K^+ as well as sodium ion (Na^+) loss. Normally, most body K^+ is intracellular, whereas most Na^+ and H^+ is extracellular. When excess K^+ is lost in the urine, intracellular K^+ diffuses out of the cells to replace some of that being lost from plasma; Na^+ and H^+ move into the cells to replace the K^+ that has moved out. Thus, H^+ is lost from extracellular fluid and plasma. A second mechanism depends on the fact that sodium is reabsorbed from the urine into the renal distal tubule cells by an active transport mechanism. This transport mechanism involves excretion of H^+ and K^+ into the urine to replace the reabsorbed Na^+. In this exchange (or transport) system, H^+ and K^+ compete with each other. Therefore, if an intracellular deficit of K^+ exists (in the tubule cells), more H^+ is excreted into the urine to allow the reabsorption of the same quantity of sodium without losing as much K^+. The result of renal H^+ loss and extracellular H^+ loss is an acid-losing type of alkalosis. Therefore, more H^+ is manufactured by the kidney from H_2CO_3 to replace lost extracellular fluid H^+: more HCO_3^- ions are thereby formed, and the numerator of the Henderson-Hasselbalch equation is increased. The denominator is eventually increased if the lungs attempt to compensate by increasing CO_2 retention by slower breathing. However, respiratory compensation is frequently minimal or insignificant in hypokalemic alkalosis, so that the PCO_2 frequently remains normal. Also, the urine pH is decreased because of the excess H^+ being excreted in the urine. This is the opposite of what one would ordinarily expect, because in acidosis, the kidney usually attempts to compensate by excreting more H^+ (acid urine), whereas in alkalosis it normally tries to conserve H^+ and thus produces a urine of higher pH (alkaline urine).

Respiratory Alkalosis

The other major subdivision of alkalosis is respiratory alkalosis, which occurs when the respiratory mechanism blows off more CO_2 than it normally would due to respiratory center stimulation from some cause. The main conditions in which this happens are the hyperventilation syndrome caused by hysteria or anxiety, high fever, and direct stimulation of the respiratory center by drugs. Overdose of aspirin can cause respiratory alkalosis in the early stages, although later, after more of the aspirin is absorbed, a metabolic acidosis develops. In hyperventilation of whatever cause, respirations are increased and deeper, blowing off more CO_2. This creates an H_2CO_3 deficit since it is being used up to replenish CO_2 by the lung carbonic anhydrase enzymes. Therefore the denominator of the Henderson-Hasselbalch equation is decreased, the 20:1 ratio is increased, and plasma pH increased. The CO_2 content will decrease, because when H_2CO_3 is lost due to formation of CO_2 in the lungs, HCO_3^- is converted to H_2CO_3 in the kidney to compensate secondarily for or to replace the decreasing plasma carbonic acid.

SUMMARY OF ACID-BASE CHANGES

To summarize plasma pH problems, in metabolic acidosis there is eventual HCO_3^- deficit, leading to decreased plasma pH and decreased CO_2 content (or CO_2 combining power). In respiratory acidosis there is primary H_2CO_3 excess, which causes decreased plasma pH, but the CO_2 content is increased due to renal attempts at compensation. In metabolic alkalosis there is eventual bicarbonate excess leading to increased plasma pH and increased CO_2 content. In respiratory alkalosis there is primary carbonic acid deficit, which causes increased plasma pH, but the CO_2 content is decreased due to renal attempts at compensation. The urine pH usually reflects the status of the plasma pH except in hypokalemic alkalosis, where there is acid urine pH despite plasma alkalosis.

As noted, CO_2 content or combining capacity essentially constitutes the numerator of the Henderson-Hasselbalch equation. PCO_2 is essentially a measurement of the equation denominator and can be used in conjunction with pH to indicate acid-base changes. This is the system popularized by Astrup and Siggaard-Andersen. PCO_2 follows the same direction as the CO_2 content in classic acid-base syndromes. In metabolic acidosis, PCO_2 is decreased, because acids other than H_2CO_3 accumulate, and CO_2 is blown off by the lungs in attempts to decrease body fluid acidity. In metabolic alkalosis, PCO_2 is increased if the lungs compensate by hypoventilation; in mild or acute cases, PCO_2 may remain normal. In respiratory alkalosis, PCO_2 is decreased because increased ventilation blows off more CO_2. In respiratory acidosis, PCO_2 is increased because of CO_2 retention due to decreased ventilation.

PARTIAL PRESSURE OF CARBON DIOXIDE (PCO_2) AS A MEASURE OF RESPIRATORY FUNCTION

In addition to its use in the Henderson-Hasselbalch equation, PCO_2 provides information on pulmonary alveolar gas exchange (ventilation). If PCO_2 is high, there is not a sufficient degree of alveolar ventilation. This may be due to primary lung disease (inability of the lungs to ventilate properly) or to some other reason. If PCO_2 is low, there is alveolar hyperventilation, again either from primary or secondary etiology.

ACID-BASE COMPENSATION

Compensation refers to the degree of PCO_2 change when there is, or has been, an abnormality in pH.

An uncompensated disorder is a primary metabolic or respiratory condition that has not been altered by any significant degree of correction. In the case of a primary metabolic condition the respiratory counterbalance (change in ventilation which is reflected by a change in arterial PCO_2) is not evident; pH is abnormal but PCO_2 remains normal. In the case of a primary respiratory condition, both PCO_2 and pH are abnormal, and the degree of abnormality on both tests is relatively severe. In that case the renal counterbalance (increased bicarbonate formation to bring pH back toward normal) is not evident.

A partially compensated disorder is present when both pH and PCO_2 are outside their reference ranges. In primary respiratory disorders, the degree of pH abnormality is not as severe as in uncompensated cases.

A fully compensated (sometimes referred to only as compensated) condition is a primary metabolic or respiratory disorder in which PCO_2 is outside its reference range but pH has returned to its reference range.

BUFFER BASE AND BASE EXCESS

The concepts of buffer base and base excess form part of the Astrup acid-base system. The term buffer base refers to all substances in the buffering system of whole blood that are able to bind excess H^+. Bicarbonate forms slightly more than one half of the total buffer base; hemoglobin makes up about one third of the total buffer base, consisting of three fourths of the nonbicarbonate buffer system. Normal buffer base values for any patient are therefore calculated on the basis of the actual hemoglobin concentration as well as normal values for pH and HCO_3^-. The term base excess refers to any difference in the measured total quantity of blood buffer base from the patient's calculated normal value. Thus, an increase in total buffer base (e.g., an increase in HCO_3^-) is considered a positive base excess; a decrease in total buffer base from calculated normal (e.g., a decrease in HCO_3^-) is considered a negative base excess (some prefer to use the terms "base excess" and "base deficit" rather than positive or negative base excess). Venous blood has a base excess value about 2.0–2.5 mEq/L higher than arterial blood.

INTERPRETATION OF ACID-BASE DATA

Acid-base data interpretation has always been one of the more difficult areas of laboratory medicine. In most uncomplicated untreated cases the diagnosis can be achieved with reasonable ease. There are several ways of approaching an acid-base problem. One way is to examine first the arterial PCO_2 value. Since primary respiratory disorders result from hypoventilation or hyperventilation, which, in turn, are reflected by a change in arterial PCO_2, normal PCO_2 with abnormal pH is strong evidence against a primary respiratory disorder and should be an uncompensated metabolic disorder.

If PCO_2 is decreased, there are two major possibilities:

1. The primary disorder could be respiratory alkalosis (hyperventilation). If so, pH should be increased in acute (uncompensated) cases or partially compensated cases. In fully compensated cases pH is within reference range,

but frequently it is more than 7.40 even within the reference range.

2. The primary disorder could be metabolic acidosis. If so, pH should be decreased in partially compensated cases. In fully compensated cases pH is within its reference range (similar to fully compensated respiratory alkalosis), but frequently it is less than 7.40 even within the reference range.

If PCO_2 is increased, there are also two major possibilities:

1. The primary disorder could be respiratory acidosis (hypoventilation). If so, pH should be decreased in acute (uncompensated) cases or partially compensated cases. In fully compensated cases pH is within reference range, but frequently it is less than 7.40 even within reference range.

2. The primary disorder could be metabolic alkalosis. If so, pH should be increased in partially compensated cases. In fully compensated cases pH is within its reference range (similar to fully compensated respiratory acidosis), but pH frequently is more than 7.40 even within the reference range.

There is another way to interpret the data. If one first inspects pH, decreased pH means acidosis and increased pH means alkalosis. One then inspects the PCO_2 value. If the PCO_2 has changed in the same direction as the pH, the primary disorder is metabolic. If the PCO_2 has changed in the opposite direction from that of the pH, the primary disorder is respiratory.

Base excess analysis is not a vital part of this type of algorithm. However, base excess can sometimes be helpful, both as additional evidence for certain types of acid-base disorders or to help detect the presence of active acid-base disorder in fully compensated cases. A negative base excess is found in metabolic acidosis and, to a lesser extent, in respiratory alkalosis. A positive base excess is found in metabolic alkalosis and, to a lesser extent, in respiratory acidosis.

Some of the preceding data are summarized in Tables 23–1 and 23–2.

TABLE 23–1.

PCO_2 Values in Metabolic and Respiratory Acid-Base Disorders

PCO_2 normal

An abnormality in pH means an uncompensated metabolic process.

PCO_2 abnormal

PCO_2 decreased

Could be respiratory (hyperventilation) in origin (respiratory alkalosis). If so, pH should be *increased* (acute onset), or *normal, but more than 7.40* (chronic-compensated).

Could be metabolic acidosis. If so, pH should be *decreased* (partial compensation), or *normal but more than 7.4* (fully compensated).

PCO_2 increased:

Could be respiratory (hypoventilation) in origin (respiratory acidosis). If so, pH should be *decreased* (acute onset), or *normal but less than 7.40* (chronic-compensated)

Could be metabolic alkalosis. If so, pH should be *increased* (partial compensation), or *normal but more than 7.40* (fully compensated).

OTHER COMMENTS ON ACID-BASE PROBLEMS

The preceding discussion applies to an acid-base problem involving a single primary metabolic or primary respiratory abnormality, with or without body attempts at compensation. Unfortunately, in some cases the laboratory picture is more complicated; for example, when there are superimposed attempts at therapy or when two different acid-base processes coexist (referred to as "mixed acid-base disorders"). An example is diabetic acidosis (metabolic acidosis) in a patient with chronic lung disease (compensated respiratory acidosis). In this circumstance it is very important to decide what serious clinical condition the patient has (e.g., renal failure, diabetic acidosis, chronic lung disease) that might affect the acid-base status and then what other condition may be superimposed (such as vomiting, diuretic therapy, or shock) that could alter the acid-base picture in a certain direction.

In some cases of acid-base disturbance, such as classic diabetic acidosis, the diagnosis may be obvious. In other cases the diagnosis is made from the first set of arterial blood gas measurements. In these two situations, continued acid-base studies are needed only to gauge the severity of the disorder and response to therapy. If the PO_2 does not indicate respiratory impairment, it may be sufficient to obtain PCO_2 or HCO_3 values, with or without pH determi-

TABLE 23–2.
Summary of Laboratory Findings in Primary Uncomplicated Respiratory and Metabolic Acid-Base Disorders*

Disorder	PCO_2	pH	Base Excess
Acute primary respiratory hypoactivity (respiratory acidosis)	Increase	Decrease	Normal/ positive
Acute primary respiratory hyperactivity (respiratory alkalosis)	Decrease	Increase	Normal/ negative
Uncompensated metabolic acidosis	Normal	Decrease	Negative
Uncompensated metabolic alkalosis	Normal	Increase	Positive
Partially compensated metabolic acidosis	Decrease	Decrease	Negative
Partially compensated metabolic alkalosis	Increase	Increase	Positive
Chronic primary respiratory hypoactivity (compensated respiratory acidosis)	Increase	Normal	Positive
Fully compensated metabolic alkalosis	Increase	Normal	Positive
Chronic primary respiratory hyperactivity (compensated respiratory alkalosis)	Decrease	Normal	Negative
Fully compensated metabolic acidosis	Decrease	Normal	Negative

*Base excess results refer to negative (−) values more than −2 and positive (+) values more than +2.

nation, on venous specimens rather than make repeated arterial punctures.

ANION GAP

Once metabolic acidosis is apparent, the problem becomes one of identifying the cause. Calculation of the anion gap may be helpful. The anion gap is the difference between the major cations (sodium, or sodium plus potassium) and the major anions (chloride and bicarbonate). The anion gap formula is: AG = Na − (Cl + HCO_3). If the anion gap is increased, and especially when it is more than 10 mEq/L above the upper limit of the reference range, excess organic acids or acidic foreign substances should be suspected. Conditions in which these may appear include diabetic ketoacidosis, ethyl alcohol–induced ketoacidosis, renal failure, lactic acidosis, salicylate overdose, and methanol or ethylene glycol poisoning. The normal anion gap is 8–16 mEq/L (mmol/L). However, there is some disagreement in the literature whether to use a range of 8–12 or 8–16 mEq/L for a normal anion gap. Some investigators use the sum of sodium plus potassium in the equation rather than sodium alone. Although one would expect this to decrease the normal anion gap, the reference values reported in the literature are the same or even greater than those for the formula using sodium alone, with some listing a range of 8–16 mEq/L and others 8–20 (values in the literature can be found extending from 7–25 mEq/L). Anion gap reference ranges established on hospitalized patients tend to be higher than those established on outpatients.

A decreased anion gap has been associated with multiple myeloma. However, one report indicates that most calculated anion gaps that are decreased result from laboratory error in test results included in the equation, with hypoalbuminemia and hyponatremia the next most common associated findings.

BLOOD OXYGEN STUDIES

The greatest stimulus for arterial as opposed to venous specimens for blood gas studies is to obtain measurement of blood oxygen. The usual information reported is PO_2, obtained with a direct-reading PO_2 electrode. PO_2 represents the dissolved oxygen content of plasma, analogous to the relationship of PCO_2 to carbon dioxide. Reference ranges for PO_2 are age related. In persons under age 60 (breathing room air), 80–95 mm Hg is considered normal. Over age 60, 1 mm Hg per year, but no more than 20 mm Hg, is subtracted from the lower limit of the reference range. A PO_2 of 60–80 mm Hg is classified as mild hypoxemia, a PO_2 of 40–60 mm Hg represents moderate hypoxemia, and a PO_2 less than 40 mm Hg represents severe hypoxemia.

Blood oxygen studies are done for three reasons. First, they help indicate the current status of alveolar gas exchange with inspired air. PO_2 provides this information. A normal PO_2 while breathing room air indicates adequate pulmonary ventilation.

The second reason is to determine the amount of oxygen available to body cells. PO_2 is less adequate for this purpose, because most of the oxygen in the blood is not dissolved oxygen but oxygen bound to RBC hemoglobin. The measurement one really needs is oxygen saturation, which is the actual amount of oxygen bound to hemoglobin compared with the theoretical maximum amount that could be bound. Then, the quantity of hemoglobin times percent saturation times the factor 1.34 gives the total quantity of oxygen in the blood (except for the very small amount of dissolved oxygen). When the hemoglobin level is normal and PO_2 is normal, the percent saturation and total oxygen content are usually adequate. In fact, many blood gas machines provide a calculated oxygen saturation value derived from PO_2, normal hemoglobin levels, and data from the normal oxygen-hemoglobin dissociation curve. Although there is adequate correlation between calculated oxygen saturation and oxygen saturation measured in a special instrument (e.g., one known as a CO-Oximeter) at normal hemoglobin and PO_2 values, there is poor correlation between the two measurements at subnormal PO_2 values, due to the sigmoid (S) shape of the oxygen-hemoglobin dissociation curve. In the steep midportion of the S curve, a relatively small decrease in PO_2 leads to a relatively large decrease in oxygen saturation. In addition, there are a considerable number of conditions that shift the curve to greater or lesser degree and affect oxygen saturation. Nevertheless, a decreased PO_2 suggests the possibility of tissue hypoxia, and the degree of PO_2 decrease provides a rough estimate of the probability and severity of tissue hypoxia. Certain conditions decrease blood oxygen content or tissue oxygen independently of PO_2. These include anemia (decreased hemoglobin level), carbon monoxide poisoning (CO replaces O_2 on the hemoglobin molecule), acidosis (which increases oxygen dissociation from hemoglobin), and congestive heart failure (which slows blood flow and decreases tissue perfusion rate).

The third reason for PO_2 measurement is to monitor effects of oxygen therapy. The usual goal is to raise PO_2 above the lower limit of the reference range. However, in some patients, oxygen therapy may be adequate but unable to provide a normal PO_2.

EFFECT OF PHYSIOLOGIC PATIENT VARIATION ON BLOOD GAS INTERPRETATION

There is a surprising degree of fluctuation in blood gas values in normal persons and in stabilized sick persons. In one study of normal persons using arterialized capillary blood, changes of at least 10% in bicarbonate or total CO_2, 15% in PCO_2, and 170% in base excess were required to exceed normal day-to-day variation. In another study, this time using arterial samples from stabilized intensive care unit (ICU) patients, average fluctuations within patients without known cause were found of 3.0 mm Hg (range 1–8 mm Hg) for PCO_2, 0.03 pH units (range 0.01–0.08 units) for pH, and 16 mm Hg (range 1–45 mm Hg) for PO_2. There were sufficient variation in repeat samples drawn at 10 minutes and at about 1 hour that a change of about 10% at 10 minutes and of about 20% at 1 hour was necessary to be considered significant. This suggests caution in making decisions based on small changes in acid-base or PO_2 values.

NONINVASIVE MEASUREMENT OF PCO_2, PO_2, AND OXYGEN SATURATION

There are now several ways to measure carbon dioxide and oxygen in blood without drawing a blood sample. The two most popular methods at present are *transcutaneous electrode systems* and *pulse oximetry*. Both systems can provide continuous readings.

The transcutaneous systems use PCO_2 and PO_2 electrodes similar to those of standard arterial blood gas analysis applied directly to the skin over a gel sealant. Skin has capillaries close to the surface, and the tissues are permeable to some extent for carbon dioxide and oxygen. The apparatus heats the skin to 44°C to produce arterialized blood, thereby dilating the capillaries and increasing oxygen loss. The electrode sensors detect the carbon dioxide and oxygen diffusing from the capillaries. The apparatus must be moved at least every 4–6 hours in adults and 2–4 hours in infants to avoid thermal burns. The apparatus must be calibrated with a standard arterial blood gas sample obtained by arterial puncture each time the apparatus is positioned due to variability from differences in fat content (which interferes with gas diffusion) and skin thickness. Patient edema, hypothermia, or poor tissue perfusion (shock or vasoconstriction) interfere to varying degrees with accurate measurements.

Pulse oximetry measures functional oxygen saturation (percentage of available oxygen saturated with oxygen) rather than oxygen tension (PO_2). The method uses two light beams, one red and the other infrared, which are passed through tissue that contains arterial blood. Opposite to the light emitters are light detectors. The light detectors perform two tasks. First, they recognize and analyze arterial blood exclusively by differentiating those areas that have pulsation, and therefore changes in light transmission, from nonvascular tissue and nonarterial vascular components. Then oxygen saturation is measured in the pulsating vessels using the fact that changes in oxygen content have a significant effect on absorption of red light. The amount of red light absorption (transmission) is compared to that of the infrared light, which is affected much less. This system does not have to be calibrated by arterial puncture blood and does not have to be moved frequently. The instrument is accurate between saturation levels of about 70%–100%. When PO_2 is above 100 mm Hg, hemoglobin is usually 100% saturated, reaching the upper limit of the oximeter. Below 70% saturation, accuracy becomes less, but trends in saturation change can be recognized. Carboxyhemoglobin can interfere with measurement. Since the instrument measures only oxygenation, acid-base abnormalities must be detected or investigated by some other method.

Abnormal results from either transcutaneous monitors or pulse oximeters must be confirmed by arterial puncture blood gas measurement. The pulse oximeter is usually attached to a toe in infants, to a finger in adults, and to the nose in obese adults.

Noninvasive continuous oxygen monitors are especially useful during anesthesia since most serious problems involve episodes of hypoxia; in premature or sick neonates and infants; in patients on ventilators; and in ICU or other unstable seriously ill adults.

BIBLIOGRAPHY

Sarnquist FH: Clinical pulse oximetry. *Lab Med* 1988; 19:417.

Harding PJ, Fraser CG: Biological variation of blood acid-base status: consequences for analytical goal-setting and interpretation of results. *Clin Chem* 1987: 33:1416.

Rooth G, et al: Transcutaneous oxygen monitors are reliable indicators of arterial oxygen tension (if used correctly). *Pediatrics* 1987; 79:283.

Miller WW, et al: Performance of an in-vivo, continuous blood-gas monitor with disposable probe. *Clin Chem* 1987; 33:1538.

Raffin TA: Indications for arterial blood gas analysis. *Ann Intern Med* 1986; 105:390.

Smoker JM, et al: A protocol to assess oxygen therapy. *Respir Care* 1986; 31:35.

Swedlow DB: Capnometry and capnography: The anesthesia disaster early warning system. *Semin Anesth* 1986; 5:194.

Townsend-Collymore LA, Buffone CT: Transcutaneous PO_2 and PCO_2 monitoring in the newborn. *Lab Mgmt* 1985; 23(4):41.

Rothstein F, Fisher JE: pH measurement. *Am Clin Prod Rev* 1985; 4(8):26.

Walmsley RN, White GH: Mixed acid-base disorders. *Clin Chem* 1985; 31:321.

Bloom SA, et al: Spurious assessment of acid-base status due to dilutional effect of heparin. *Am J Med* 1985; 79:528.

Deckardt R, Steward DJ: Noninvasive arterial hemoglobin oxygen saturation versus transcutaneous oxygen tension monitoring in the preterm infant. *Crit Care Med* 1984; 12:935.

Goodkin DA: Acid-base disturbances in the geriatric patient. *Geriatr Med Today* 1984; 3(8):85.

Narins RG: Laboratory parameters in metabolic acidosis. *Lab Mgmt* 1984; 22(9):46.

Thorson SH, et al: Variability of arterial blood gas values in stable patients in the ICU. *Chest* 1983; 84:14.

Lolekha PH: Value of the anion gap in clinical diagnosis and laboratory evaluation. *Clin Chem* 1983; 29:279.

Garg AK, Nanji AA: The anion gap and other critical calculations. *Diagn Med* 1982; 5(2):38.

Narins RG, Gardner LB: Simple acid-base disturbances. *Med Clin North Am* 1981; 65:321.

Bandi ZL: Estimation, prevention, and quality control of carbon dioxide loss during aerobic sample processing. *Clin Chem* 1981; 27:1676.

Lott JA, Bibby D: Determination of pH, PCO_2, and PO_2 on whole blood: Steps to maximize accuracy. *Lab Med* 1980; 11:455.

Quintanilla AP: Abnormalities of acid-base balance. *Cont Ed Fam Phys* 1980; 12:67.

24 Serum Electrolytes and Protein-Calorie Malnutrition

Chapter 23 discussed pH and its clinical variations. The present chapter will attempt to cover the most frequent conditions associated with abnormalities of the major body electrolytes sodium, potassium, and chloride, as well as certain cations such as calcium, magnesium, and aluminum. A clear distinction must be made between total body electrolyte concentration and serum concentration. The total body concentration of any electrolyte such as sodium includes an intravascular component (comprising the concentration of the electrolyte within serum and within red blood cells [RBCs]), an interstitial fluid component, and an intracellular component. Since most ions are diffusible to variable degrees among the three compartments, the serum concentration often does reflect the concentration in other fluid compartments. However, since the concentration of various electrolytes (e.g., sodium and potassium) differs in cells and extracellular fluid, in many situations the serum concentration does not accurately reflect intracellular electrolyte conditions. Furthermore, the serum electrolyte concentration depends on the amount of water present (plasma volume). A normal quantity of a particular electrolyte such as sodium may appear to have a low serum value if it is diluted by an excess of water. Likewise, an actual electrolyte deficit may be masked by normal serum values if the plasma volume is decreased by excess water loss. Therefore, the serum levels of any electrolyte may or may not reflect the total body concentration, depending on the situation. Unfortunately, serum levels are the only electrolyte measurement that is readily available. A knowledge of what happens to total body levels as well as serum levels is essential to understanding problems in certain situations.

SERUM SODIUM ABNORMALITIES

The most frequent electrolyte abnormalities, both clinically and as reflected in abnormal laboratory values, involve sodium. This is true because sodium is the most important cation of the body, both from a quantitative standpoint and because of its influence in maintaining electric neutrality. The most common causes of low or high serum sodium values are enumerated in Table 24–1. Some of these conditions and the mechanisms involved require further explanation.

Technical problems in sodium measurement may affect results. For many years the primary assay technique for sodium and potassium was flame photometry. Since 1980, instrumentation has been changing to ion-selective electrodes (ISEs). Ion-selective electrodes generate sodium results that are about 2% higher than those obtained by flame photometry (in patient blood specimens this difference is equivalent to 2–3 mEq/L [2–3 mmol/L]). Potassium values are about the same with both techniques. Many, but not all, laboratories automatically adjust their ISE sodium results to make them correspond to flame photometer values. Sodium concentration can be decreased in blood by large amounts of glucose (which attracts intracellular fluid, creating a dilutional

TABLE 24–1.

Clinical Situations Frequently Associated With Serum Sodium Abnormalities

- I. Hyponatremia
  - A. Sodium and water depletion (deficit hyponatremia)
    - 1. Loss of gastrointestinal (GI) secretions with replacement of fluid but not electrolytes
      - a. Vomiting
      - b. Diarrhea
      - c. Tube drainage
    - 2. Loss from skin with replacement of fluids but not electrolytes
      - a. Excessive sweating
      - b. Extensive burns
    - 3. Loss from kidney
      - a. Diuretics
      - b. Chronic renal insufficiency (uremia) with acidosis
    - 4. Metabolic loss
      - a. Starvation with acidosis
      - b. Diabetic acidosis
    - 5. Endocrine loss
      - a. Addison's disease
      - b. Sudden withdrawal of long-term steroid therapy
    - 6. Iatrogenic loss from serous cavities
      - a. Paracentesis or thoracentesis
  - B. Excessive water (dilution hyponatremia)
    - 1. Excessive water administration
    - 2. Congestive heart failure
    - 3. Cirrhosis
    - 4. Nephrotic syndrome
    - 5. Hypoalbuminemia (severe)
    - 6. Acute renal failure with oliguria
  - C. Inappropriate antidiuretic hormone (IADH) syndrome
  - D. Intracellular loss (reset osmostat syndrome)
  - E. False hyponatremia (actually a dilutional effect)
    - 1. Marked hypertriglyceridemia
    - 2. Marked hyperproteinemia
    - 3. Severe hyperglycemia
- II. Hypernatremia

  Dehydration is the most frequent overall clinical finding in hypernatremia.
    - 1. Deficient water intake (either orally or intravenously)
    - 2. Excess water output (excessive sweating, diabetes insipidus, osmotic diuresis)
    - 3. Cases of severe protracted vomiting or diarrhea without fluid therapy
    - 4. Accidental sodium overdose
    - 5. High protein tube feedings

effect). Each 62 mg of glucose/100 ml (3.4 mmol/L) above the serum glucose upper reference limit results in a decrease in serum sodium concentration of 1.0 mEq/L. Large amounts of serum protein (usually in patients with myeloma) or lipids (triglyceride concentration > 1,500 mg/100 ml [17 mmol/L]) can artifactually decrease the serum sodium level when sodium is measured by flame photometry (values obtained by the ISE method are not affected). One report suggests a formula whose result can be added to flame photometry values to correct for severe hyperlipidemia (triglyceride > 1,500 mg/100 ml): % increase = 2.1 × [triglyceride (gm/100 ml) − 0.6]. There is an interesting and somewhat inexplicable variance in reference range values for sodium in the literature, especially for the upper end of the range. This makes it highly desirable for each laboratory to determine its own reference range. Another problem is a specimen drawn from the same arm that already has an intravenous (IV) line; this usually happens when the phlebotomist cannot find a vein in the opposite arm. However, this may lead to interference by the contents of the IV system.

Hyponatremia

Iatrogenic Sources of Hyponatremia

Diuretic therapy and administration of IV hypotonic fluids (dextrose in water or half-normal saline) form a very important and frequent etiology for hyponatremia, either as the sole agent or superimposed on some condition predisposing to hyponatremia. In several studies of patients with hyponatremia, diuretic use was considered to be the major contributing factor or sole etiology in about 30% of cases (range, 7.6%–46%). In two series of patients with severe hyponatremia (serum sodium < 120 mEq/L), diuretics were implicated in 30%–73% of cases. Hyponatremia due to diuretics without any predisposing or contributing factors is limited mostly to patients over the age of 55 years. Intravenous fluid administration is less often the sole etiology for hyponatremia (although it occurs) but is a frequent contributing factor. In one study of postoperative hyponatremia, 94% of the patients were receiving hypotonic fluids. If renal water excretion is impaired, normal maintenance fluid quantities may lead to dilution, whereas excessive infusions may produce actual water intoxication or pulmonary edema. There may also be problems when excessive losses of fluid or various electrolytes occur for any reason and replacement therapy is attempted but either is not adequate or is excessive. The net result of any of the situations mentioned is a fluid disorder with or without an electrolyte problem that must be carefully and logically reasoned out, beginning from the primary deficit (the cause of which may still be active) and proceeding through subsequent events. Adequate records of fluid and electrolyte administration are valuable in solving the problem. In nonhospitalized persons a similar picture may be produced by dehydration with conscious or unconscious attempts at therapy by the patient or relatives. For example, marked sweating leads to thirst, but ingestion of large quantities of water alone dilutes body fluid sodium, already depleted, even further. A baby with diarrhea may be treated at home with water or sugar water; this replaces water but does not adequately replace electrolytes and so has the same dilutional effect as in the preceding example. On the other hand, the infant may be given boiled skimmed milk or soup, which are high-sodium preparations; the result may be hypernatremia if fluid intake is not adequate.

Hyponatremic Depletional Syndromes

In protracted and severe vomiting, as occurs with pyloric obstruction or stenosis, gastric fluid is lost in large amounts and a hypochloremic (acid-losing) alkalosis develops, as described in chapter 23. Gastric contents have a relatively low sodium content and water loss relatively exceeds electrolyte loss. Despite relatively low electrolyte content, significant quantities of electrolytes are lost with the fluid, leading to some depletion of total body sodium. The dehydration from fluid loss is partially counteracted by increased secretion of antidiuretic hormone (ADH) in response to decreased fluid volume. Antidiuretic hormone promotes fluid retention. Whether hyponatremia, normal-range serum sodium values, or hypernatremia will develop depends on how much fluid and sodium are lost and the relative composition and quantity of replacement water and sodium, if any. Oral or parenteral therapy with sodium-free fluid tends to encourage hyponatremia. On the other hand, failure to supply fluid replacement may produce severe dehydration and even hypernatremia. Serum potassium values are most often low due to direct loss and to alkalosis that develops when so much hydrochloric acid is lost. Similar findings are produced by continuous gastric tube suction if continued over 24 hours.

In severe or long-standing diarrhea, the most common acid-base abnormality is a base-losing acidosis. Fluid loss predominates quantitatively over loss of sodium, chloride, and potassium despite considerable depletion of total body stores of these electrolytes, especially of potassium. Similar to what occurs with vomiting, decrease in fluid volume by fluid loss is partially counteracted by increased secretion of ADH. Again, whether serum sodium becomes decreased, normal, or increased depends on degree of fluid and electrolyte loss and the amount and composition of replacement fluid (if any). Sufficient electrolyte-free fluids may cause hyponatremia. Little or no fluid replacement would tend toward dehydration, which, if severe, could even produce hypernatremia. The diarrhea seen in sprue differs somewhat from the electrolyte pattern of diarrhea from other causes in that hypokalemia is a somewhat more frequent finding.

In extensive sweating, especially in a patient with fever, large amounts of water are lost. Although sweat consists mostly of water, there is a small but significant sodium chloride content. Enough sodium and chloride loss occurs to produce total body deficits, sometimes of surprising degree. The same comments previously made regarding GI content loss apply here also.

In extensive burns, plasma and extracellular fluid (ECF) leak into the damaged area in large quantities. If the affected area is extensive, hemoconcentration becomes noticeable and enough plasma may be withdrawn from the circulating blood volume to bring the patient close to or into shock. Plasma electrolytes accompany this fluid loss from the circulation. The fluid loss stimulates ADH secretion. The serum sodium level may be normal or decreased, as discussed earlier. If the patient is supported over the initial reaction period, fluid will begin to return to the circulation after about 48 hours. Therefore, after this time, fluid and electrolyte replacement should be decreased, so as not to overload the circulation. Silver nitrate treatment for extensive burns may itself cause clinically significant hyponatremia (due to electrolyte diffusion into the hypotonic silver nitrate solution).

Diabetic acidosis and its treatment provide very interesting electrolyte problems. Lack of insulin causes metabolism of protein and fat to provide energy that normally is available from carbohydrates. Ketone bodies and other metabolic acids accumulate; the blood glucose level is also elevated, and both glucose and ketones are excreted in the urine. Glucosuria produces an osmotic diuresis; a certain amount of serum sodium is lost with the glucose and water, and other sodium ions accompany the strongly acid ketone anions. The effects of osmotic diuresis, as well as of the accompanying electrolyte loss, are manifested by severe dehydration. Nevertheless, the serum sodium and chloride levels are often low in untreated diabetic acidosis, although (because of water loss) less often they may be within normal range. In contrast, the serum potassium level is usually normal. Even with normal serum levels, considerable total body deficits exist for all of these electrolytes. The treatment for severe diabetic acidosis is insulin and large amounts of IV fluids. Hyponatremia may develop if sufficient sodium and chloride are not given with the fluid to replace the electrolyte deficits. After insulin administration, potassium ions tend to move into body cells as they are no longer needed to combine with ketone acid anions. Also, potassium is apparently taken into liver cells when glycogen is formed from plasma glucose under the influence of insulin. In most patients, the serum potassium level falls to nearly one-half the admission value after 3–4 hours of fluid and insulin therapy (if urine output is adequate) due to continued urinary potassium loss, shifts into body cells, and rehydration. After this time, potassium supplements should be added to the other treatment.

Role of the Kidney in Electrolyte Physiology

In many common or well-recognized syndromes involving electrolytes, abnormality is closely tied to the role of the kidney in water and electrolyte physiology. A brief discussion of this subject may be helpful in understanding the clinical conditions discussed later.

Urine formation begins with the glomerular filtrate, which is similar to plasma except that plasma proteins are too large to pass the glomerular capillary membrane. In the proximal convoluted tubules, about 85% of filtered sodium is actively reabsorbed by the tubule cells. The exchange mechanism is thought to be located at the tubule cell border along the side opposite the tubule lumen; thus, sodium is actively pumped out of the tubule cell into the renal interstitial fluid. Sodium from the urine passively diffuses into the tubule cell to replace that which is pumped out. Chloride and water passively accompany sodium from the urine into the cell and thence into the interstitial fluid. Most of the filtered potassium is also reabsorbed, probably by passive diffusion. At this time, some hydrogen ions are actively secreted by tubule cells into the urine but not to the extent that occurs farther down the nephron (electrolyte pathways and mechanisms are substantially less well known for the proximal tubules than for the distal tubules).

In the ascending (thick) loop of Henle, sodium is still actively reabsorbed, except that the tubule cells are now impermeable to water. Therefore, since water cannot accompany reabsorbed sodium and remains behind in the urine, the urine at this point becomes relatively hypotonic (the excess of water over what would have been present had water reabsorption continued is sometimes called "free water" and from a purely theoretical point of view is sometimes spoken of as though it were a separate entity, almost free from sodium and other ions).

In the distal convoluted tubules, three processes go on. First, sodium ions continue to be actively reabsorbed. (In addition to the sodium pump located at the interstitial side of the cell, which is pushing sodium out into the interstitial fluid, another transport mechanism on the tubule lumen border now begins actively to extract sodium from the urine into the tubule cells.) Intracellular hydrogen and potassium ions are actively excreted by the tubule cells into the urine in exchange for urinary sodium. There is competition between hydrogen and potassium for the same exchange pathway. However, since hydrogen ions are normally present in much greater quantities than potassium, most of the ions excreted into the urine are hydrogen. Second, the urinary acidification mechanisms other than bicarbonate reabsorption ($NaHPO_4$ and NH_4) operate here. Third, distal tubule cells are able to reabsorb water in a selective fashion. Permeability of the distal tubule cell to water is altered by a mechanism under the influence of ADH. There is a limit to the possible quantity of water reabsorbed, because reabsorption is passive; ADH simply acts on cell membrane permeability, controlling the ease of diffusion. Therefore, only free water is actually reabsorbed.

In the collecting tubules, the tubular membrane is likewise under the control of ADH. Therefore, any free water not reabsorbed in the distal convoluted tubules plus water that constitutes actual urine theoretically could be passively reabsorbed here. However, three factors control the actual quantity reabsorbed: (1) the state of hydration of the tubule cells and renal medulla in general, which determines the osmotic gradient toward which any reabsorbed water must travel; (2) the total water reabsorption capacity of the collecting tubules, which is limited to about 5% of the normal glomerular filtrate; and (3) the amount of free water reabsorbed in the distal convoluted tubules, which helps determine the total amount of water reaching the collecting tubules.

Whether collecting tubule reabsorption capacity will be exceeded, and if so, to what degree, is naturally dependent on the total amount of water available. The amount of water reabsorbed compared to the degree of dilution (hypotonicity) of urine reaching the collecting tubules determines the degree of final urine concentration.

Effects of Adrenal Cortex Dysfunction

Certain adrenal cortex hormones control sodium retention and potassium excretion. Aldosterone is the most powerful of these hormones, but cortisone and hydrocortisone also have some effect. In primary Addison's disease there are variable degrees of adrenal cortex destruction. This results in deficiency of both aldosterone and cortisol, thereby severely decreasing normal salt-retaining hormone influence on the kidney. Sometimes there is just enough hormone to maintain sodium balance at a low normal level. However, when placed under sufficient stress of any type, the remaining adrenal cortex cells cannot provide a normal hormone response and therefore cannot prevent a critical degree of sodium deficiency from developing. The crisis of Addison's disease is the result of overwhelming fluid and salt loss from the kidneys and responds to adequate replacement. Serum sodium and chloride levels are low, the serum potassium level is usually high normal or elevated, and the patient is markedly dehydrated. The carbon dioxide (CO_2) content (or serum bicarbonate; chapter 23) may be normal or may be slightly decreased due to the mild acidosis that accompanies severe dehydration. In secondary Addison's disease, due to pituitary insufficiency, glucocorticoid hormone production is decreased or absent but aldosterone production is maintained. However, hyponatremia sometimes develops due to an increase in ADH production by the hypothalamus. In primary aldosteronism (chapter 29) there is oversecretion of aldosterone, which leads to sodium retention and potassium loss. However, sodium retention is usually not sufficient to produce edema, and the serum sodium value remains within the reference range in more than 95% of cases. The serum potassium value is decreased in about 80% of cases (literature range, 34%–92%). In Cushing's syndrome (chapter 29) there is overproduction of hydrocortisone (cortisol), which leads to spontaneous mild hypokalemia and hypochloremic alkalosis in 10%–20% of patients (usually those with more severe degrees of cortisol excess). Use of diuretics will induce hypokalemia in other patients. The serum sodium level usually remains within reference range.

Dilutional Syndromes

Cirrhosis is frequently associated with hyponatremia and hypokalemia, either separately or concurrently. There are a variety of etiologies: ascitic fluid sequestration; attempts at diuresis, often superimposed on poor diet or sodium restriction; paracentesis therapy; and hemodilution. Electrolyte abnormalities are more likely to appear when ascites is present and are more severe if azotemia complicates liver disease. Hemodilution is a frequent finding in cirrhosis, especially with ascites; this may be due to increased activity of aldosterone, which is normally deactivated in the liver, or sometimes is attributable to inappropriate secretion of ADH.

Congestive heart failure is frequently associated with hyponatremia and much less frequently with hypokalemia. The most frequent cause of hyponatremia is overtreatment with diuretic therapy, usually in the context of dietary sodium restriction. However, sometimes the hyponatremia may be dilutional, due to retention of water as the glomerular filtration rate is decreased by heart failure or by inappropriate secretion of ADH. If hypokalemia is present, it usually is a side effect of diuretics.

Disorders of Antidiuretic Hormone Secretion

Antidiuretic hormone has been mentioned as one regulator of plasma volume via its action on renal distal tubule water reabsorption. It is produced by the posterior pituitary under the control of the hypothalamus. Several factors influence ADH production: blood osmotic changes (concentration and dilution, acting on osmoreceptors in the hypothalamus), blood volume changes, certain neural influences such as pain, and certain drugs such as morphine and alcohol.

Diabetes insipidus is a syndrome caused by lack of or insufficient production of ADH. In diabetes insipidus the kidney is not able to retain water normally. A continual diuresis of dilute urine is produced, and marked dehydration results, producing increased serum sodium values. Pitressin (a synthetic compound with some ADH-like activity) given parenterally corrects the defect.

Inappropriate ADH syndrome (IADH syndrome) is another syndrome involving ADH that is now well recognized. It results from water retention due to secretion of ADH when ADH would not ordinarily be secreted. The criteria for IADH syndrome include (1) hyponatremia, (2) continued renal excretion of sodium despite hyponatremia, (3) serum hypo-osmolality, (4) urine osmolality that shows a significant degree of concentration (instead of the maximally dilute urine one would expect), (5) no evidence of blood volume depletion, and (6) normal renal and adrenal function (this criterion is necessary to rule out continuous sodium loss due to renal disease or Addison's disease. Diuretic-induced urine sodium loss should also be excluded). These criteria attempt to demonstrate that ADH is secreted despite hemodilution, decreased serum osmolality, or both. The reason for increased sodium excretion is not definitely known; it is thought that increase of interstitial fluid volume by water retention may lead to suppression of sodium reabsorption (in order not to reabsorb even more water). Most patients with IADH syndrome do not have edema, since interstitial fluid expansion is usually only moderate in degree.

In the diagnosis of IADH syndrome a problem may arise concerning what urine osmolality values qualify as a significant degree of concentration. If the serum and urine specimens are obtained at about the same time and the serum demonstrates significant hyponatremia and hypo-osmolality, a urine osmolality greater than the serum osmolality is considered more concentrated than usual. However, in some cases of IADH syndrome the urine need not be higher than the serum osmolality for the diagnosis to be made, if it can be demonstrated that water retention is taking place despite a hypotonic plasma. With significant serum hypo-osmolality, urine osmolality should be maximally dilute. This value is about 60–80 milliosmoles (mOsm)/L. A urine osmolality greater than 100 mOsm/L (literature range, 80–120 mOsm/L) can be considered a higher osmolality than expected under these circumstances. The urine sodium level is usually more than 20 mEq/L in patients with IADH syndrome, but can be decreased if the patient is on sodium restriction or has volume depletion. In patients with borderline normal or decreased urine sodium levels, the diagnosis of IADH may be assisted by administering a test dose of sodium. In IADH syndrome, infusion of 1,000 ml of normal saline will greatly increase urine sodium excretion but will not correct the hyponatremia as long as the patient does not restrict fluids (fluid restriction will cause sodium retention in IADH syndrome). Water restriction is the treatment of choice and may provide some confirmatory evidence. However, water restriction is not diagnostic, since it may also benefit patients with extracellular fluid (ECF) excess and edema. Uric acid renal clearance is increased in IADH syndrome, resulting in decreased serum uric acid levels in most, but not all, patients. Decreased serum uric acid levels in a patient with hyponatremia is another finding that is nondiagnostic but that raises the question of IADH syndrome.

In some patients, assay of serum ADH levels may be helpful to confirm the diagnosis. The ADH levels should be elevated in IADH syndrome. However, ADH assay is expensive, technically very difficult, and is available only in a few reference laboratories. The specimen should be placed immediately into a precooled anticoagulant tube, centrifuged at low temperature, frozen immediately, and sent to the laboratory packed in dry ice.

Inappropriate ADH syndrome may be induced by a variety of conditions, such as: (1) central nervous system neoplasms, infections, and trauma; (2) various malignancies, most often in bronchogenic carcinoma of the undifferentiated small cell type; (3) various types of pulmonary infections; (4) several endocrinopathies, including myxedema and Addison's disease; (5) certain medications, such as antineoplastics (vincristine, cyclophosphamide), oral antidiabetics (chlorpropamide, tolbutamide), hypnotics (opiates, barbiturates), and certain others such as carbamazepine; and (6) severe stress, such as pain, trauma, and surgery.

Normal physiologic response to surgery is a temporary moderate degree of fluid and electrolyte retention, occurring at least in part from increased secretion of ADH. In the first 24 hours after surgery there tends to be decreased urine output, with fluid and electrolytes remaining in the body that would normally be excreted. Because of this, care should be taken not to overload the circulation with too much IV fluid on the first postoperative day. Thereafter, adequate replacement of normal or abnormal electrolyte daily losses is important, and excessive hypotonic fluids should be avoided. In certain patients, such as those undergoing extensive surgical procedures and those admitted originally for medical problems, it is often useful to obtain serum electrolyte values preoperatively so that subsequent electrolyte problems can be better evaluated.

Disorders Simulating Inappropriate Antidiuretic Hormone

Refractory dilutional syndrome is a moderately frequent condition in which many features of IADH are seen but the classic syndrome is not present. The dilutional hyponatremia of cirrhosis and congestive heart failure may sometimes be of this type, although usually other mechanisms can better account for hyponatremia, such as overuse of diuretics. However, in some cases, IADH syndrome seems to be contributory. These patients differ from those with the classic IADH syndrome in that edema is often present and the urine contains very little sodium. In other words, the main feature is water retention with dilutional hyponatremia. Treatment with sodium can be dangerous, and therapy consists of water restriction.

Reset osmostat syndrome is another syndrome involving hyponatremia without any really good explanation, although, again, IADH syndrome may contribute in part. These persons have a chronic wasting illness such as carcinomatosis or chronic malnutrition or may simply be elderly and without known disease. Serum sodium levels are mildly or moderately decreased. As a rule, affected persons do not exhibit symptoms of hyponatremia and seem to have adjusted physiologically to the lower serum level. Treatment with salt does not raise the serum values. Apparently the only cure is to improve the patient's state of nutrition, especially the body protein, which takes considerable time and effort. This condition has also been called the "tired cell syndrome."

Laboratory Investigation of Hyponatremia

When the serum sodium level is unexpectedly low, one must determine whether it is due to false (artifactual) hyponatremia, sodium depletion, hemodilution, the IADH syndrome, or the reset osmostat syndrome. The first step is to rule out artifactual causes. The serum sodium tests should be repeated and blood redrawn if necessary, avoiding areas receiving IV infusions. Then, other causes for artifact, such as hyperlipemia or myeloma protein (if a flame photometer is being used), should be excluded. Next, iatrogenic causes should be considered, including sodium-poor IV fluids (producing dilution) and diuretics (producing sodium depletion). If none of these possibilities is the cause, measurement of urine sodium excretion and serum or urine osmolality may be useful.

Urine Sodium.—In hyponatremia, the kidney normally attempts to conserve sodium, so that the urine sodium level is low (< 20 mEq/L, usually < 10 mEq/L). If the patient has hyponatremia and is not receiving IV fluids containing sodium, and if the urine sodium concentration is normal or high (e.g., early morning random urine sodium > 20 mEq/L), this suggests inappropriate sodium loss through the kidneys. Possible etiologies are: (1) acute or chronic renal failure, such as diffuse, bilateral, renal tissue injury (blood urea nitrogen [BUN] and serum creatinine levels confirm or eliminate this possibility); (2) effect of diuretics or osmotic diuresis; (3) Addison's disease; (4) IADH syndrome; and (5) some patients with the reset osmostat syndrome.

A low urine sodium concentration is a normal response to a low serum sodium level and suggests (1) nonrenal sodium loss (sweating or GI tract loss); (2) some patients with the reset osmostat syndrome; and (3) ECF dilution. Presence of edema favors ECF dilutional etiology (e.g., cirrhosis, congestive heart failure, nephrotic syndrome). Measurement of certain relatively stable constituents of blood, such as hemoglobin and total protein, may provide useful information. However, one must have previous baseline values to assist interpretation. A significant decrease in hemoglobin and total protein levels—possibly in other substances such as serum creatinine and uric acid—suggests hemodilution. Similar changes in several blood constituents are more helpful than a change in only one, since any constituent could change due to disease that is independent of vascular fluid shifts. A significant increase in hemoglobin level and other blood constituents suggests nonrenal sodium loss with accompanying dehydration.

The best way to determine hemodilution or hemoconcentration is by plasma volume measurement, most often by using albumin tagged with radioactive iodine. However, the diagnosis usually can be made in other ways.

Serum and Urine Osmolality.—Osmolality (chapter 13) is the measurement of the number of osmotically active particles in a solution. It is determined by either the degree of induced freezing point change or measurement of vapor pressure in special equipment. Units are milliosmoles per liter of water. Therefore, osmolality depends not only on the quantity of solute particles but also on the amount of water in which they are dissolved. Sodium is by far the major constituent of serum osmolality. Plasma proteins have little osmotic activity and normally are essentially noncontributory to serum osmolality. Serum (or plasma) osmolality may be calculated from various formulas, such as:

$$\text{mOsm/L} = 2\text{Na} + \frac{\text{BG}}{20} + \frac{\text{BUN}}{3}$$

where blood glucose (BG) and BUN are in mg/100 ml and Na (sodium) is in mEq/L. The adult reference range is 275–300 mOsm/L. The ratio of serum sodium concentration to serum osmolality (Na/Osm) is normally 0.43–0.50.

Increased Serum Osmolality.—Increased serum osmolality may be caused by loss of hypotonic (sodium-poor) water, producing dehydration. Some etiologies include diabetes insipidus; fluid deprivation without replacing the daily insensible water loss of 0.5–1.0 L; and hypotonic fluid loss from skin, GI tract, or osmotic diuresis. It may also be caused by sodium overload; hyperglycemia (100 mg of glucose/100 ml increases osmolality about 5.5 mOsm/L); uremia (10 mg of urea/100 ml increases osmolality about 3.5 mOsm/L); unknown metabolic products; or various drugs or chemicals, especially ethyl alcohol. Ethanol is one of the more common etiologies for increased serum osmolality. Each 100 mg of ethanol/100 ml (equivalent to a serum concentration of 0.1%) raises serum osmolality about 22 mOsm/L. An "osmolal gap" (the difference between the calculated and the measured osmolality) of more than 10 mOsm/L provides a clue to the presence of unusual solutes. Osmolality is one of the criteria for diagnosis of hyperosmolar nonketotic acidosis (chapter 27) and of the IADH syndrome (discussed previously). Renal dialysis units sometimes determine the osmolality of the dialysis bath solution to help verify that its electrolyte composition is within acceptable limits.

Decreased Serum Osmolality.—Serum osmolality is usually decreased (or borderline low) in true noncomplicated hyponatremia. Hyponatremia with definitely normal or elevated serum osmolality can be due to: (1) artifactual hyponatremia, due to interference by hyperlipidemia or elevated protein with flame photometer methods; (2) the presence of abnormal quantities of normal hyperosmolar substances, such as glucose or urea; or (3) the presence of abnormal hyperosmolar substances, such as ethanol, methanol, lactic acid or other organic acids, or unknown metabolic products. In categories 2 and 3, measured osmolality is more than 10 mOs/L above calculated osmolality (alcohol does not produce this osmolal gap when the vapor pressure technique is used). Most of the hyperosmolar substances listed here, with the exception of ethanol, are associated with metabolic acidosis and will usually produce an elevated anion gap (chapter 23).

An appreciable minority of patients with hyponatremia (especially of mild degree) have serum osmolality results in the low-normal range, although theoretically the osmolality value should be decreased. Some of these patients may be dehydrated; others may have cardiac, renal, or hepatic disease. These diseases characteristically reduce the Na/Osm ratio, this being partially attributed to the effects of increased blood glucose, urea, or unknown metabolic substances. Especially in uremia, osmolality changes cannot always be accounted for by the effects of BUN alone. Patients in shock may have disproportionately elevated measured osmolality compared with calculated osmolality; again, this points toward circulating metabolic products. Besides elevating osmolality, these substances displace a certain amount of sodium from serum, thus lowering sodium levels.

Urine Osmolality.—In patients with hyponatremia, urine osmolality is most helpful in diagnosis of the IADH syndrome (discussed previously). Otherwise, urine osmolality values parallel the amount of sodium excreted, except that osmolality values may be disproportionately increased when large quantities of hyperosmotic substances (glucose, urea, ethanol, etc.) are also being excreted, causing an increased urine osmolality gap.

Summary of Laboratory Findings in Hyponatremia

1. When hyponatremia is secondary to exogenous hemodilution from excess sodium-deficient fluid (e.g., excess IV fluids or polydipsia), serum osmolality is low, urine osmolality is low, and the urine sodium level is low. There may be other laboratory evidence of hemodilution.

2. When hyponatremia is secondary to endogenous hemodilution in cirrhosis, nephrotic syndrome, or congestive heart failure, serum osmolality is decreased and the urine sodium concentration is low. There may be other laboratory evidence to suggest hemodilution. The patient may have visible edema. The underlying condition (e.g., cirrhosis) may be evident.

3. When hyponatremia is due to sodium loss not involving the kidney (skin or GI tract), serum osmolality is usually decreased (or low normal due to dehydration if there is water intake that is inadequate). The degree of dehydration would influence the serum osmolality value. The urine sodium concentration is low. There may be other laboratory and clinical evidence of dehydration.

4. When hyponatremia is due to sodium loss through the kidneys (diuretics, renal failure, Addison's disease), there is low serum osmolality and the urine sodium concentration is increased. Both BUN and serum creatinine levels are elevated in chronic renal disease (although they can be elevated from prerenal azotemia with normal kidneys).

5. In IADH syndrome, serum osmolality is low, urine osmolality is normal or increased, and urine sodium concentration is normal or high. Serum ADH level is elevated.

6. In false hyponatremia due to marked serum protein or triglyceride elevation, serum sodium concentration is mildly decreased, serum osmolality is normal, and urine sodium concentration is normal.

7. In hyponatremia secondary to marked hyperglycemia, serum osmolality is increased; this suggests the presence of hyperosmotic substances, of which glucose can be confirmed by a blood glucose measurement.

The laboratory findings described earlier and summarized above apply to untreated classic cases. Diuretic or fluid therapy, or therapy with various other medications, may alter fluid and electrolyte dynamics and change the typical laboratory picture, or may even convert one type of hyponatremia into another. There is also a problem when two conditions coexist, for example, depletional hyponatremia from GI tract loss (which should produce dehydration and low urine sodium concentration) in a patient with poor renal function (whose kidneys cannot conserve sodium and who thus continues to excrete normal amounts of sodium into the urine despite dehydration).

Certain other test results or clinical findings suggest certain diseases. Hyperkalemia with hyponatremia raises the possibility of renal failure or Addison's disease. If the patient's hyponatremia is at least moderate in degree and is asymptomatic, it may reflect chronic hyponatremia rather than acute. If the patient has the reset osmostat syndrome, water restriction does not correct the hyponatremia, whereas water restriction would correct the hyponatremia of the IADH syndrome. If the serum osmolality is well within reference range in a patient with hyponatremia, and the sodium assay was done using flame photometry, serum total protein measurement and examination of the serum for the creamy appearance of hypertriglyceridemia can point toward pseudohyponatremia. If ion selective electrodes were used to assay sodium, and serum osmolality is normal or elevated in hyponatremia, calculation of the osmolal gap can point toward the presence of unexpected hyperosmolal substances.

Hypernatremia

Hypernatremia is much less common than hyponatremia. It is usually produced by a severe water deficit that is considerably greater than the sodium deficit and is most often accompanied by dehydration (see Table 24–1). The water deficit can be due to severe water deprivation, severe hypotonic fluid loss (renal or nonrenal) without replacement, or a combination of the two. The serum sodium concentration and serum osmolality are increased. Urine volume is low and urine specific gravity or osmolality are high in water deprivation or in dehydration due to nonrenal water loss. Urine volume is high and urine specific gravity or osmolality is low in dehydration due to water loss through the kidneys. Other laboratory test values may suggest dehydration, and clinical signs of dehydration may be present. Although serum sodium level is increased, total body sodium level may be normal or even decreased, the sodium deficit being overshadowed by the water deficit. Occasionally, hypernatremia is caused by excess intake of sodium, which is usually not intentional.

SERUM POTASSIUM ABNORMALITIES

The potassium level in serum is about 0.4–0.5 mEq/L higher than the potassium level in whole blood or plasma (literature range 0.1–1.2 mEq/L). This is attributed at least in part to potassium released from platelets during clotting. Serum specimens may have artifactual potassium level increase additional to that of normal clotting in patients with very high white blood cell (WBC) counts or platelet counts. The sodium concentration is about the same in serum, plasma, and whole blood. Potassium values increase 10%–20% if the patient follows the common practice of opening and closing his or her hand after a tourniquet is applied to the arm before venipuncture. Potassium can be increased in patient specimens by RBC hemolysis, sometimes considerably increased, which, unfortunately, is most often a laboratory artifact produced during venipuncture or when processing the specimen after venipuncture. Therefore, a pink or red color of plasma or serum usually means very inaccurate potassium values. There may be some artifactual increase during the clotting process in specimens with very high WBC counts or platelet counts.

Hypokalemia

Hypokalemia has been reported in about 5% of hospitalized patients. Abnormalities in potassium have many similarities to those of sodium (Table 24–2). Some conditions with potassium abnormalities are also associated with sodium abnormalities and were discussed earlier. Several different mechanisms may be involved.

Inadequate Intake.—Ordinarily, 90% of ingested potassium is absorbed, so that most diets are more than adequate. Inadequate intake is most often due to anorexia nervosa or to severe illness with anorexia, especially when combined with administration of potassium-free therapeutic fluids. Alcoholism is often associated with inadequate intake, and various malabsorption syndromes may prevent adequate absorption.

Gastrointestinal Tract Loss.—Severe prolonged diarrhea, including diarrhea due to lax-

TABLE 24–2.
Clinical Conditions Commonly Associated With Serum Potassium Abnormalities

Hypokalemia
Inadequate intake (cachexia or severe illness of any type)
Intravenous infusion of potassium-free fluids
Renal loss (diuretics; primary aldosteronism)
Protracted vomiting; severe prolonged diarrhea
Treatment of diabetic acidosis without potassium supplements
Treatment with large doses of adrenocorticotropic hormone; Cushing's syndrome
Cirrhosis; some cases of secondary aldosteronism
Hyperkalemia
Renal failure
Dehydration
Excessive parenteral administration of potassium
Artifactual hemolysis of blood specimen
Tumor lysis syndrome
Hyporeninemic hypoaldosteronism
Spironolactone therapy
Addison's disease and salt-losing congenital adrenal hyperplasia

ative abuse, can eliminate substantial amounts of potassium. One uncommon but famous cause is large villous adenomas of the colon. Protracted vomiting is another uncommon cause. Patients with ileal loop ureteral implant operations after total cystectomy frequently develop hypokalemia if not closely watched.

Renal Loss.—Twenty percent to 30% (range, 10%–40%) of hypertensive patients receiving diuretic therapy, particularly with the chlorothiazides, are reported to be hypokalemic. Combined with other conditions requiring diuretics, this makes diuretic therapy the most frequent overall cause of hypokalemia. Renal tubular acidosis syndromes might also be mentioned. Finally, there is a component of renal loss associated with several primarily nonrenal hypokalemic disorders. These include the various endocrinopathies (discussed next), diabetic ketoacidosis, and administration of potassium-poor fluids. The kidney is apparently best able to conserve sodium and to excrete potassium (since one way to conserve sodium is to excrete potassium ions in exchange), so that when normal intake of potassium stops, it takes time for the kidney to adjust and to stop losing normal amounts of potassium ions. In the meantime, a deficit may be created. In addition, renal conservation mechanisms cannot completely eliminate potassium excretion, so that 5–10 mEq/day is lost regardless of total body deficit.

Endocrinopathies.—These conditions are discussed in detail elsewhere. Patients with primary aldosteronism (Conn's syndrome) are hypokalemic in about 80% of cases. Patients with secondary aldosteronism (cirrhosis, malignant hypertension, renal artery stenosis, increased estrogen states, hyponatremia) are predisposed toward hypokalemia. Cirrhosis may have other predisposing causes, such as poor diet or attempts at diuretic therapy. About 20%–25% of patients with Cushing's syndrome have a mild hypokalemic alkalosis. Congenital adrenal hyperplasia (of the most common 11-β-hydroxylase type) is associated with hypokalemia. Hypokalemia may occur in Bartter's syndrome or the very similar condition resulting from licorice abuse. Most of the conditions listed in this section, except for cirrhosis, are also associated with hypertension.

Diabetic Ketoacidosis.—Extracellular fluid may lose potassium both from osmotic diuresis due to hyperglycemia and from shift of extracellular to intracellular potassium due to insulin therapy. Nevertheless, these changes are masked by dehydration, so that 90% of patients have normal or elevated serum potassium values when first seen in spite of substantial total body potassium deficits. These deficits produce overt hypokalemia if fluid therapy of diabetic acidosis does not contain sufficient potassium.

Hypokalemic Alkalosis.—Hypokalemia has a close relationship to alkalosis. Increased plasma pH (alkalosis) results from decreased ECF hydrogen ion concentrations; the ECF deficit draws hydrogen from body cells, leading to decreased intracellular concentration and therefore less H^+ available in renal tubule cells for exchange with urinary sodium. This means increased potassium excretion in exchange for urinary sodium and eventual hypokalemia. Besides being produced by alkalosis, hypokalemia can itself lead to alkalosis, or at least a tendency toward alkalosis. Hypokalemia results from depletion of intracellular potassium (the largest body store of potassium). Hydrogen ions diffuse into body cells to partially replace the intracellular cation deficit caused by potassium deficiency; this tends to deplete ECF hydrogen levels. In addition, more hydrogen is excreted into the urine in exchange for sodium since the potassium that normally would participate in this exchange is no longer available. Both mechanisms tend eventually to deplete extracellular fluid hydrogen. As noted in chapter 23, in alkalosis due to hypokalemia an acid urine is produced, contrary to the usual situation in alkalosis. This incongruity is due to the intracellular acidosis that results from hypokalemia.

Medication-Induced Hypokalemia.—Certain nondiuretic medications may sometimes produce hypokalemia. Ticarcillin, carbenicillin, and amphotericin B may increase renal potassium loss. Theophylline, especially in toxic concentration, may decrease serum potassium to hypokalemic levels.

In one group of hospitalized patients with serum potassium levels less than 2.0 mEq/L, apparent etiology was potassium-insufficient

IV fluids in 17%, diuretic therapy in 16%, GI loss in 14%, acute leukemia receiving chemotherapy in 13%, dietary potassium deficiency in 6%, renal disease with urinary potassium loss in 6%, diabetic acidosis in 5%, and all other single causes less than 5% each.

Urine Potassium Assay in Hypokalemia

Measurement of urine potassium may sometimes be useful in differentiating etiologies of hypokalemia. Those conditions associated with decreased urine potassium include:

1. Loss from the GI tract (diarrhea, villous adenoma, ileal conduit). Vomiting, however, is associated with alkalosis, which may increase renal potassium excretion.
2. Shift of extracellular potassium to intracellular location (insulin therapy). However, hyperglycemic osmotic diuresis may confuse the picture.
3. Inadequate potassium intake, in the absence of conditions that increase urine potassium excretion.
4. Potassium deficiency associated with renal excretion of potassium (e.g., diuretic induced) after the stimulus for potassium loss is removed and renal loss ceases.

Besides the first three categories, the other etiologies for hypokalemia usually demonstrate normal or increased urine potassium levels while active potassium loss is occurring.

Hyperkalemia

High potassium values are not uncommon in hospitalized patients, especially in the elderly. One study reported serum potassium levels more than 5 mEq/L in 15% of patients over age 70. However, hyperkalemia is found in relatively few diseases.

Decreased Renal Potassium Excretion.—Renal failure is the most common etiology of hyperkalemia, both in this category and including all causes of hyperkalemia.

Pseudohyperkalemia.—Dehydration can produce apparently high-normal or mildly elevated electrolyte values. Artifactual hemolysis of blood specimens may occur, which results in release of potassium from damaged RBCs, and the laboratory may not always mention that visible hemolysis was present. In one series of patients with hyperkalemia, 20% were found to be due to a hemolyzed specimen, and an additional 9% were eventually thought to be due to some technical error. Rarely, mild hyperkalemia may appear with very marked elevation of platelets.

Exogenous Potassium Intake.—Examples include excessive oral potassium supplements or parenteral therapy that either is intended to supplement potassium (e.g., potassium chloride) or contains medications (e.g., some forms of penicillin) that are supplied as a potassium salt or in a potassium-rich vehicle. Some over-the-counter salt substitutes contain a considerable amount of potassium.

Endogenous Potassium Sources.—Potassium can be liberated from tissue cells in muscle crush injuries, burns, and therapy of various malignancies, or released from RBCs in severe hemolytic anemias. In some cases where liberated potassium reaches hyperkalemic levels, there may be a superimposed element of decreased renal function.

Endocrinologic Syndromes.—As noted previously, hyperkalemia may be produced by dehydration in diabetic ketoacidosis. Hyperkalemia is found in about 50% of patients with Addison's disease. In one series, hyporeninemic hypoaldosteronism (chapter 29) was found in 10% of patients with hyperkalemia. Decreased renal excretion of potassium is present in most endocrinologic syndromes associated with hyperkalemia, with the exception of diabetic acidosis.

Drug-Induced Hyperkalemia.—Some medications supply exogenous potassium, as noted previously. A few, including beta-adrenergic blockers such as propranolol and pindolol; digoxin overdose; certain anesthetic agents at risk for the malignant hyperthermia syndrome such as succinylcholine; therapy with or diagnostic infusion of the amino acid arginine; hyperosmotic glucose solution; or insulin, affect potassium shifts between intracellular and extracellular location. In the case of insulin, deficiency rather than excess would predispose toward hyperkalemia. Most other medications that are associated with increase in serum potassium produce decreased renal excretion of potassium. These include certain potassium-sparing diuretics such as spironolactone and triamterene; several nonsteroidal anti-inflammatory agents such as indomethacin and ibuprofen; angiotensin-converting enzyme inhibitors such as captopril; heparin therapy, including low-dose protocols; and cyclosporine immunosuppressant therapy.

CLINICAL SYMPTOMS OF ELECTROLYTE IMBALANCE

Before I conclude the discussion of sodium and potassium, it might be useful to describe some of the clinical symptoms of electrolyte imbalance. Interestingly enough, they are very similar for low-sodium, low-potassium, and high-potassium states. They include muscle weakness, nausea, anorexia, and mental changes, which usually tend toward drowsiness and lethargy. The ECG in hypokalemia is very characteristic, and with serum values less than 3.0 mEq/L usually shows depression of the ST segment and flattening or actual inversion of the T wave. In hyperkalemia the opposite happens: the T wave becomes high and peaked; this usually begins with serum potassium values more than 7.0 mEq/L (reference values being 4.0–5.5 mEq/L). Hypokalemia may be associated with digitalis toxicity with digitalis doses that ordinarily are nontoxic because potassium antagonizes the action of digitalis. Conversely, very high concentrations of potassium are toxic to the heart, so IV infusions should never administer more than 20.0 mEq/hour even with good renal function.

There is disagreement in the medical literature regarding preoperative detection and treatment of hypokalemia. On one hand, various reports and textbooks state that clinically significant hypokalemia (variously defined as less than 2.8, 3.0, or 3.2 mEq/L) produces a substantial number of dangerous arrhythmias. On the other hand, several investigators did not find any significant difference in intraoperative arrhythmias, morbidity, or mortality between those patients with untreated hypokalemia and those who were normokalemic.

SERUM CHLORIDE

Chloride is the most abundant extracellular anion. In general, chloride is affected by the same conditions that affect sodium (the most abundant extracellular cation) and in roughly the same degree. Thus, in the great majority of cases, serum chloride values change in the same direction as serum sodium values (except in a few conditions such as the hyperchloremic alkalosis of prolonged vomiting). For example, if the serum sodium concentration is low, one can usually predict that the chloride concentration will also be low (or at the lower edge of the reference range). To confirm this I did a study comparing sodium and chloride values in 649 consecutive patients. There were 37 discrepancies (5.7%) in the expected relationship between the sodium and chloride values. On repeat testing of the discrepant specimens, 21 of the 37 discrepancies were resolved, leaving only 16 (2.5%). Of these, 6 (1%) could be classified as minor in degree and 10 (1.5%) as significant. Thus, in 649 patients only 1.5% had a significant divergence between serum sodium and chloride values.

SERUM ELECTROLYTE PANELS

Many physicians order serum "electrolyte panels" or "profiles" that include sodium potassium, chloride, and bicarbonate ("CO_2"; when "CO_2" is included in a multitest electrolyte panel using serum, bicarbonate comprises most of what is being measured). In my experience, chloride and "CO_2" are not cost effective as routine assays on electrolyte panels. If there is some necessity for serum chloride assay, as for calculation of the anion gap, it can be ordered when the need arises. Assay of serum bicarbonate is likewise questionable as a routine test. In most patients with abnormal serum bicarbonate values, there is acidosis or alkalosis that is evident or suspected from other clinical or laboratory findings (e.g., as severe emphysema or renal failure). In patients with acid-base problems, blood gas measurement or PCO_2 measurement is more sensitive and informative than serum bicarbonate assay.

TESTS IN CALCIUM DISORDERS

Hypercalcemia

Symptoms referable to hypercalcemia itself are very nonspecific; they include vomiting, constipation, polydipsia and polyuria, and mental confusion. Coma may develop in severe cases. There may be renal stones or soft tissue calcification. Hypercalcemia is most often detected on routine multitest biochemical screening panels, either in asymptomatic persons or incidental to symptoms from some disease associated with hypercalcemia (Table 24–3). By far the commonest of these is malignancy. The next most common is primary hyperparathyroidism.

TABLE 24–3.
Selected Etiologies of Hypercalcemia

Relatively common
- Neoplasia (noncutaneous)
  - Bone primary
    - Myeloma
    - Acute leukemia
  - Bone metastatic
    - Breast
    - Lung
    - Kidney
  - Neoplasm secretion of PTH ("ectopic PTH")
- Primary hyperparathyroidism (PHPT)
- Thiazide diuretics
- Tertiary (renal) hyperparathyroidism
- Idiopathic
- Spurious (artifactual) hypercalcemia
  - Dehydration
  - Serum protein elevation
  - Lab technical problem

Relatively uncommon
- Neoplasia (less common tumors)
- Sarcoidosis
- Hyperthyroidism
- Immobilization (especially in children and young adults)
- Diuretic phase of acute renal tubular necrosis
- Vitamin D intoxication
- Milk-alkali syndrome
- Addison's disease
- Lithium therapy
- Idiopathic hypercalcemia of infancy
- Acromegaly
- Theophylline toxicity

Regulation of Serum Calcium Levels

Regulation of serum calcium levels is somewhat complex. The major control mechanism is parathyroid hormone (PTH). Normally, parathyroid secretion of PTH is regulated by a feedback mechanism involving the blood calcium level. A decreased serum calcium level induces increased secretion of PTH, whereas an acute increase of the serum calcium level decreases secretion of PTH. Parathyroid hormone has a direct action on bone, increasing bone resorption and release of bone calcium and phosphorus. In addition, PTH increases the activity of the activating enzyme cyclic adenosine monophosphate (AMP) in the proximal tubules of the kidney, which increases conversion of calcidiol (25-hydroxyvitamin D) to calcitriol (1,25-dihydroxyvitamin D). Calcitriol has metabolic effects that help to increase serum calcium levels, such as increased renal reabsorption of calcium, increased GI tract absorption of calcium, and the drawing out of some calcium from bone. On the other hand, an increased calcitriol level also initiates a compensatory series of events that prevents the calcium-elevating system from overreacting. An increased calcitriol level inhibits renal tubule phosphate reabsorption, which results in loss of phosphorus into the urine. This leads to a decreased serum phosphate level, which, in turn, inhibits production of calcitriol. The actions of PTH, phosphate, and calcitriol produce a roughly reciprocal relationship between serum calcium and phosphate levels, with elevation of one corresponding to a decrease of the other. Both PTH (through cyclic AMP) and phosphate act on the same enzyme (25-OH-D 1α-hydroxylase), which converts calcidiol to calcitriol.

Besides PTH, a hormone called "calcitonin" has important, although subsidiary, effects on calcium metabolism. Calcitonin is produced in the thyroid gland, and secretion is at least partially regulated by serum calcium levels. Acute elevation of serum calcium leads to increased calcitonin secretion. Calcitonin inhibits bone resorption, which decreases withdrawal of calcium and phosphorus and produces a hypocalcemic and hypophosphatemic effect that opposes calcium-elevating mechanisms.

Primary Hyperparathyroidism

Primary hyperparathyroidism is caused by overproduction or inappropriate production of PTH by the parathyroid gland. The most common cause is a single adenoma. The incidence of parathyroid carcinoma is listed in reviews as 2%–3%, although the actual percentage is probably less. About 15% (possibly more) of cases are due to parathyroid hyperplasia, which involves more than one parathyroid gland. The most frequent clinical manifestation is renal stones (Table 24–4). The reported incidence of clinical manifestations varies widely, most likely depending on whether the patient group analyzed was gathered because of the symptoms, whether the group was detected because of routine serum calcium screening, or whether the group was mixed in relation to the method of detection. About 5% (literature range, 2%–10%) of patients with renal stones have PHPT.

Laboratory Tests.—Among nonbiochemical tests, the hemoglobin level is decreased in less than 10% of cases (2%–21%) without renal failure or bleeding peptic ulcer. A large number of biochemical tests have been advocated for diagnosis of PHPT. The classic findings on biochemical testing are elevated serum calcium, PTH, and alkaline phosphatase levels and a decreased serum phosphate level.

Serum Calcium (Total Serum Calcium).—Most investigators consider an elevated serum calcium level the most common and reliable standard biochemical test abnormality in PHPT. Even when the serum calcium level falls within the population reference range, it can usually be shown to be inappropriately elevated compared with other biochemical indices. However, PHPT may exist with serum calcium values remaining within the reference range; reported incidence is about 10% of PHPT patients (literature range, 0%–50%). Normocalcemic PHPT has been defined by some as PHPT with at least one normal serum calcium determination and by others as PHPT in which no calcium value exceeds the upper reference limit. Some of the confusion and many of the problems originate from the various factors that can alter serum calcium values in normal persons, as listed here.

TABLE 24–4.

Symptoms or Clinical Syndromes Associated With Primary Hyperparathyroidism, With Estimated Incidence*

Urologic: nephrolithiasis, 30%–40% (21%–81%); renal failure
Skeletal: 15%–30% (6%–55%); Osteoporosis, fracture, osteitis fibrosa cystica
Gastrointestinal: peptic ulcer, 15% (9%–16%); pancreatitis, 3% (2%–4%)
Neurologic: weakness, 25% (7%–42%); mental changes 25% (20%–33%)
Hypertension: 30%–40% (18%–53%)
Multiple endocrine neoplasia syndrome: 2% (1%–7%)
Asymptomatic hypercalcemia: 45% (2%–47%)

*Numbers in parentheses refer to literature range.

1. Reference range limits used. Reference range values may be derived from the literature or from the reagent manufacturer or may be established by the laboratory on the local population. These values may differ significantly. For example, the values supplied by the manufacturer of our calcium method are 8.7–10.8 mg/100 ml (2.17–2.69 mmol/L), whereas our values derived from local blood donors (corrected for effects of posture) are 8.7–10.2 mg/100 ml (2.17–2.54 mmol/L).

2. The patient's normal serum calcium value before developing PHPT compared with population reference values. If the predisease value was in the lower part of the population reference range, the value could substantially increase and still be in the upper part of the range.

3. Diet. A high-calcium diet can increase serum calcium levels up to 0.5 mg/100 ml. A high-phosphate diet lowers serum calcium levels, reportedly even to the extent of producing a normal calcium value in PHPT.

4. Posture. Changing from an upright to a recumbent posture decreases the serum calcium concentration by an average of 4% (literature range, 2%–7%). A decrease of 4% at the 10.5 mg/100 ml level is a decrease of 0.4 mg/100 ml. Therefore, reference ranges derived from outpatients are higher than those established in blood donors or others who are recumbent. This means that high-normal results for outpatients would appear elevated by inpatient standards.

5. Tourniquet stasis. Prolonged stasis is reported to produce a small increase in serum calcium and total protein values.

6. Changes in serum albumin concentration (discussed under ionized calcium).

7. Laboratory error or, in borderline cases, usual laboratory test degree of variation.

Hypercalcemia in Malignancy

Primary hyperparathyroidism is not the

TABLE 24–5.
Hypercalcemia in Neoplasia*

	Avg (%)	Literature Range (%)
Breast	15	7–23
Renal	11	10.5–13
Lung	10	7–13
Myeloma	30	20–50
Leukemia	3	2–11.5
Non-Hodgkin's lymphoma	5	3–13
Cervix	7	
Colon	5	

*Overall incidence about 10% (8.5%–20%) of noncutaneous malignancies.

only or even the most frequent cause of hypercalcemia. A list of selected etiologies was given in Table 24–3. The most common cause is malignancy, either metastatic tumor to bone or multiple myeloma. Table 24–5 gives data on the common neoplasias associated with hypercalcemia. Malignancy may produce hypercalcemia in three ways. The first is primary bone tumor; the only common primary bone tumor associated with hypercalcemia is myeloma (chapter 21), which begins in the bone marrow rather than in bone itself. Hypercalcemia is found in about 30% of myeloma patients (literature range, 20%–50%). The alkaline phosphatase level is usually normal (literature range, 0%–48%) unless a pathologic fracture develops. About 5% of acute lymphocytic leukemia patients develop hypercalcemia. The most common cause of hypercalcemia in malignancy is metastatic carcinoma to bone. The breast is the most frequent primary site, followed by lung and kidney. Although prostate carcinoma is frequent in males, prostatic bone lesions are usually osteoblastic rather than osteolytic, and serum calcium is usually not elevated. A third condition associated with malignancy is tumor production of a hormone resembling PTH. This is known as the"ectopic PTH syndrome," sometimes called "pseudohyperparathyroidism" because ectopic PTH produces a condition very similar to PHPT. The most frequent source is lung carcinoma, followed by renal cell carcinoma. The tumor need not directly involve bone.

Selected Nonneoplastic Causes of Hypercalcemia

Among the conditions traditionally associated with hypercalcemia is sarcoidosis. There seems to be a much lower incidence of hypercalcemia in these patients today than in the past. Estimated frequency of hypercalcemia in sarcoidosis is about 5%–10% (literature range, 1%–62%). Serum phosphate levels are usually normal. Many of these patients have increased urine calcium excretion; the exact percentage is difficult to determine from the literature. Bone lesions are reported in 5%–16% of cases. Another etiology of hypercalcemia is tertiary hyperparathyroidism. In chronic renal failure, secondary hyperparathyroidism develops, consisting of decreased serum calcium, elevated PTH, elevated serum phosphate, and elevated alkaline phosphatase levels and development of renal osteodystrophy. If renal failure persists for a long time, secondary hyperparathyroidism may become tertiary hyperparathyroidism, which displays elevated serum calcium, elevated PTH, decreased serum phosphate, and elevated alkaline phosphatase levels and bone lesions (i.e., most of the biochemical changes usually associated with PHPT, but with diffuse hyperplasia of the parathyroid glands rather than a single adenoma). Hypercalcemia is reported in about 15% of patients with hyperthyroidism, and alkaline phosphatase elevation in about 40%. Lithium therapy frequently increases serum total calcium levels. Although most calcium values remain within population reference range, about 12% of patients on long-term lithium therapy become hypercalcemic and about 16% are reported to develop elevated PTH assay results. Thus, discovery of hypercalcemia becomes a problem of differential diagnosis, with the major categories being artifact, neoplasia, PHPT, and "other conditions." The incidence of asymptomatic hypercalcemia in unselected populations subjected to biochemical test screening ranges from 0.1%–6%. Many of the diagnostic procedures for PHPT have been developed to separate PHPT from other possible causes of hypercalcemia.

Tests Useful in Differential Diagnosis of Hypercalcemia

Ionized Calcium.—Routine serum calcium assay measures the total serum calcium value. Total serum calcium contains about 50% bound calcium (literature range, 35%–55%) and about 50% nonbound calcium (literature range, 35%–65%). (Traditionally, nonbound calcium was called "ionized" calcium and is also known as "free" or "dialyzable" calcium.) Bound calcium is subdivided into calcium bound to protein and calcium complexed to nonprotein compounds. About 45% of total calcium (30%–50%) is protein-bound, of which 70%–80% is bound to albumin. The remaining 5% (5%–15%) of total calcium is complexed to ions such as citrate, phosphate, sulfate, and bicarbonate, which are not part of the serum proteins. Ionized calcium levels can be measured directly by ion-selective electrode techniques or can be estimated from total serum calcium and albumin or total protein values using certain formulas. Ionized calcium values are affected by serum pH (a decrease of 0.1 pH unit increases ionization by 1.5–2.5%). If serum is exposed to air and stands too long, the pH slowly increases.

Ionized calcium is not affected by changes in serum albumin concentration, which is a significant advantage over total calcium assay. A decrease in the serum albumin level by 1 gm/100 ml produces an approximate decrease in the (total) serum calcium level of approximately 0.8 mg/100 ml from previous levels (this is an average value, and could be more or less in any individual patient). Since a decrease in the serum albumin level is frequent in patients with severe acute or chronic illness, an artifactual decrease of the serum calcium level is likewise frequent in hospitalized patients. The ionized calcium value is regarded by many investigators as more sensitive and reliable than the total calcium value in detection of PHPT. A certain number of their PHPT patients had elevated ionized calcium levels but normal total calcium levels. However, some investigators do not find that ionized calcium materially assists detection or diagnosis of PHPT. Also, certain conditions that produce hypercalcemia, such as myeloma, sarcoidosis, hypervitaminosis D, and metastatic carcinoma to bone, may in some cases be associated with increased ionized calcium levels. Most laboratories do not have the equipment necessary to perform ionized calcium assay, and although there are formulas that estimate ionized calcium from total calcium plus serum protein levels, there is disagreement in the literature concerning which formula is best. There is also disagreement whether such estimates are reliable enough to be used in the diagnosis of PHPT. The consensus in the literature seems to be that ionized calcium may be helpful in the diagnosis of PHPT in a relatively few patients, such as those with borderline total calcium values or those with hypoalbuminemia, and is best determined using ion-selective electrode methodology.

Serum Phosphate.—Decreased serum phosphate is one of the classic biochemical findings in PHPT. Phosphate usually is measured as the phosphorus ion. Only about 10%–15% is protein bound. There is a diurnal rhythm, with higher values in the afternoon and evening, which may be as much as double those in the morning. Serum phosphate (phosphorus) has not proved as useful as the earliest studies suggested, since phosphate levels in PHPT that are below the population reference range tend to be limited to patients with more severe disease. In fact, the serum phosphate level is decreased in only about 40%–50% of PHPT cases (literature range, 22%–80%). The reference range is fairly wide, which can mask small decreases. A high-phosphate diet or low-calcium diet increases serum phosphate levels. Renal dysfunction severe enough to produce an increased BUN level raises the serum phosphate level. Various conditions decrease serum phosphate levels (discussed later in this chapter). Among those associated with hypercalcemia and hypophosphatemia, besides PHPT, are some patients with malignancy and occasional patients with sarcoidosis, myeloma, hyperthyroidism, and vitamin D intoxication.

Serum Alkaline Phosphatase.—Alkaline phosphatase in nonneoplastic calcium disorders is an index of bone involvement. X-ray bone abnormalities in PHPT are reported in 23%–36% of patients, with most of the relatively few reports being in the older literature. X-ray studies of the fingers demonstrate the most typical changes. The current incidence of x-ray abnormality in PHPT is probably about 15%. It is estimated that alkaline phosphatase elevation occurs in about 95% of patients with PHPT who have bone x-ray changes but in only about 10%–15% of those who do not. Metastatic malignancy can produce elevated alkaline phosphatase levels due to either bone or liver involvement.

Urine Calcium Excretion.—Excretion of calcium in urine is increased in about 75% of patients with PHPT (literature range, 50%–91%). In addition to PHPT, a considerable number of other conditions may produce hypercalciuria (e.g., idiopathic hypercalciuria, said to be present in nearly 5% of the population; bone immobilization syndrome; Cushing's syndrome; milk-alkali syndrome; hypervitaminosis D; renal tubular acidosis; and sarcoidosis). Assay is performed on 24-hour urine specimens. There is disagreement in the literature on whether to collect the specimens with the patient on a normal diet, a normal diet minus milk, cheese, and other milk products, or a standard 200-mg low calcium diet. Most investigators and urologists seem to prefer a normal diet, at least for screening purposes. Reference ranges differ according to type of diet. The Sulkowitch test is a semiquantitative chemical procedure for urine calcium measurement that was widely used before 1960 but is rarely performed today.

Urine Phosphate Excretion.—The older literature states that phosphate excretion is increased in most patients with PHPT. There are surprisingly little data on this subject in recent literature. However, hyperphosphaturia probably is not as frequent today, just as decreased serum phosphate levels are seen much less frequently. Increased urine phosphate excretion in PHPT is expected in 70%–75% of cases. Phosphate depletion (due to prolonged vomiting, nasogastric suction, or ingestion of aluminum-type antacids) and chronic renal disease can reduce or eliminate phosphate hyperexcretion. Conditions that can produce increased urine phosphate excretion besides PHPT include renal triple phosphate lithiasis, osteomalacia, and, in some patients, hyperthyroidism, sarcoidosis, Cushing's syndrome, and malignancy. Reference values depend on diet.

Table 24–6 summarizes classic expected results for the tests that have been discussed thus far in various disorders of calcium metabolism.

Parathyroid Hormone Measurement.—Serum PTH can now be measured directly by radioimmunoassay (RIA). The parathyroids synthesize intact hormone, consisting of 84 amino acid residues (1–84 complete amino acid sequence), which is metabolized to several fragments. Breakdown of intact PTH outside the parathyroid takes place in the liver and, to a much lesser extent, in the kidney. Some of the RIA antisera that are available to measure PTH react with a small PTH fragment consisting of the 1–34 amino acid sequence of intact PTH that contains a terminal amino group ("N terminal"). Other antisera react with a larger PTH fragment consisting of the 53–84 amino acid sequence of intact PTH that contains a terminal carboxy group ("C terminal"). Still other antisera react with a PTH fragment containing the amino acid sequence 44–68 from the interior of the molecule ("midregion" or "midmolecule"). Currently it is thought that the intact PTH molecule and the N-terminal

TABLE 24–6.

Classic Laboratory Findings in Selected Conditions Affecting Serum Calcium and Phosphorus*

	Serum Calcium	Serum Phosphorus	Alkaline Phosphorus	Acidosis	Urine Calcium
PHPT	H	N/L†	N/H†		H
Ectopic PTH syndrome	H	L	H		H
Vitamin D excess	H	N/L	N/H		H
Sarcoidosis	N/H	N	H		N/H
Secondary hyperparathyroidism	L/N	H	H	+	H
Renal acidosis	L/N	N/L	H	+	H
Sprue	L/N	N/L	H		L
Osteomalacia	L/N	L/N	H		L
Paget's disease	N	N	H		N/H
Metastatic neoplasm to bone‡	N/H	N	N/H		N/H
Hypoparathyroidism	L	H	N		L
Osteoporosis	N	N	N		N/H
Hyperthyroidism	N/H	N/H	N/H		N/H

*Incidence of these findings varies in individual patients. H, N, and L = high, normal, and low; second letter, if present, indicates less common finding.

†Alkaline phosphatase level is high and serum phosphate level is low in "textbook cases" of PHPT.

‡Depends on primary tumor and type of bone lesion produced. Metastatic carcinoma to bone is one of the most common etiologies of hypercalcemia, perhaps the most common.

fragment have metabolic activity, whereas the C-terminal fragment and midregion fragment are metabolically inactive. The C-terminal fragment is eliminated through the kidneys by glomerular filtration. Although the antisera react with a specific portion of the PTH molecule, there may be fragments of different size that contain the same detectable PTH location. For example, anti-N reacts both with intact PTH and its N-terminal fragment. Anti-C reacts with intact PTH, the C-terminal fragment, and a very large fragment consisting of the combined midregion and C-terminal areas. Antimidregion reacts with intact PTH, the midregion fragment, and the combined midregion and C-terminal fragment. Therefore, the anti-C and antimidregion antibodies detect several of the same fragments. The measurable half-life of intact PTH in serum is only about 20 minutes and that of the N-terminal fragment is even shorter, so that turnover of material measured by N-terminal assay is very fast. Therefore, anti-N measures short-duration hormone, which is indicative of acute changes in PTH secretion. Anti-C reacts with intact PTH plus its C-terminal fragment; the C-terminal fragment is measurable for a relatively long time (hours or days). Therefore, since intact PTH is present in low concentration due to its fast turnover, C-terminal assay primarily measures the large long-duration fragments of PTH, which are more influenced by long-term or chronic PTH changes. N-terminal assay is considered more useful than C-terminal assay in measuring hormone from neck vein catheterization when attempting to localize a parathyroid adenoma. C-terminal assay is generally considered more useful for peripheral vein blood (although there is disagreement on this subject, based on antisera produced in different institutions). Both antisera may show PTH elevation in patients with renal failure, although more patients demonstrate elevation on C-terminal than on N-terminal assay since severe renal disease markedly reduces glomerular filtration and thus interferes with elimination of the C-terminal fragment. Generally speaking, the comments regarding C-terminal assay also hold true for midregion assay.

Problems in Parathyroid Hormone Assay and Current Solutions. Theoretically, PTH assay should differentiate parathyroid tumor from various other etiologies of hypercalcemia, since PHPT should have increased PTH serum levels and hypercalcemia of all other etiologies should show decreased PTH secretion. Unfortunately, when tested with presently available antisera, some patients with PHPT may have PTH values within laboratory reference range (5%–73% in reports from different laboratories). In addition, some patients with hypercalcemia not due to PHPT may have values that are within the reference range rather than decreased. In most publications, results in hypercalcemia of malignancy fall within the reference range or below, but a few antisera permit some elevated values. In most reports there is substantial overlap between patients with PHPT and patients with hypercalcemia of malignancy when their values fall within the reference range, averaging about 10%–20% (literature range, 0%–73%). Diagnosis of parathyroid adenoma can be assisted by correlating PTH assay with serum calcium levels, based on the fact that the PTH level normally decreases as the serum calcium level increases. A parathyroid adenoma may produce a PTH level that is within population normal range but is higher than expected in relation to the degree of calcium elevation. A nomogram should be constructed for each PTH antiserum, correlating PTH values with serum calcium values obtained from patients with surgically proved PHPT. This nomogram also should provide data on PTH and calcium findings in other calcium-phosphorus disorders, such as metastatic carcinoma to bone, ectopic PTH syndrome, myeloma, and renal disease. The nomogram may permit separation of these conditions when it would be impossible with the numerical values alone. For example, in one report 45% of PHPT patients had PTH values within the PTH reference range; but with the use of the nomogram, 87% of the PHPT patients could be separated from normal persons. Therefore, with the majority of antisera, such a nomogram is almost essential when PTH values are interpreted, especially since results from different reference laboratories on the same patient specimens have shown considerable difference in behavior among different antisera when tested on patients with calcium disorders. These differences in results exist not only between C-terminal, midregion, and N-terminal categories of antisera but also between individual antisera within the same category. Use of a nomogram can reduce overlap between PHPT and malignancy to 5%–10% (literature

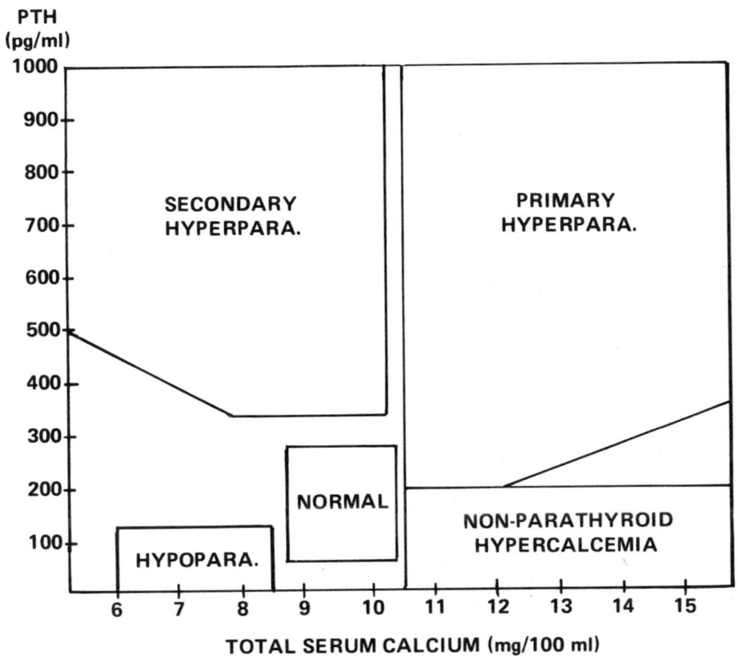

FIG 24–1.
Representative (but hypothetical) nomogram for differentiation of calcium disorders using serum calcium and PTH levels.

range, 0%–15%). A sample nomogram is shown in Figure 24–1.

Although nomograms in the form of a block diagram, as depicted in Figure 24–1, are useful, they may not be competely truthful. The diagram block areas appear to clearly separate different categories of calcium disease, but, in fact, there may be overlap between patient values in certain disorders, and the amount of overlap is different with each individual antiserum. To choose the best laboratory for PTH assay, I strongly suggest that each laboratory under consideration be required to supply a nomogram for each type of PTH assay they perform showing actual values from patients with proven calcium diseases, including hypercalcemia of malignancy, plotted on the diagram in the form of individual symbols, the symbols (dots, circles, triangles) representing the different diseases. It is necessary to have a substantial number of patient results in each disease category, especially in both PHPT and malignancy, to obtain an accurate picture. This way, it is possible to obtain a more meaningful comparison of actual PTH test results in different laboratories. The best PTH assay is one that not only clearly separates different diseases from the reference range but also has the least overlap between disease categories, especially in the area between PHPT and hypercalcemia of malignancy.

Ectopic Parathyroid Hormone Syndrome.—Nonparathyroid tumors that secrete PTH or PTH-like hormones (ectopic PTH syndrome) can produce considerable diagnostic problems. In one study, 19% of patients with tumor-associated hypercalcemia had no evidence of bone metastases. On the average, PTH assay values in ectopic PTH syndrome are lower than PTH values in PHPT. Although there is some overlap, the degree of overlap depends on the individual antiserum. There is disagreement regarding the nature of the ectopically produced hormone, that is, whether it is true PTH or a nonidentical molecule with a similar structure and PTH-like action that cross-reacts with most present-day PTH antisera. To further confuse matters, it is estimated that 5%–10% of patients with malignancy and hypercalcemia also will have a coexisting parathyroid adenoma with PHPT. It has also been stated that 15% of patients with PHPT have some coexisting disorder that could produce hypercalcemia.

Parathyroid Hormone Assay Interpretation.—Among diseases associated with hypercalcemia, PTH values are elevated in PHPT, in most cases of ectopic PTH syndrome, and in most cases of tertiary hyperparathyroidism. The actual percentage of elevated results in each category varies with the particular antiserum used (e.g., 8%–73% of PHPT patient values have been reported to be within the reference range with different antisera). In metastatic carcinoma to bone, the PTH value is normal with the majority of antisera, but there is overlap with PHPT in a significant minority of patients with nearly all antisera (the exact percentage varying with the particular antiserum). Parathyroid hormone values are usually normal or decreased in other conditions producing hypercalcemia.

Parathyroid hormone values are elevated in many (but not all) conditions associated with true hypocalcemia (false hypocalcemia from hypoalbuminemia must be excluded). These include osteomalacia, vitamin D deficiency of dietary origin and in some patients with malabsorption, renal failure, and pseudohypoparathyroidism (congenital nonresponse of kidney to PTH). In PHPT, serum PTH and serum calcium levels are both increased.

There are additional factors in PTH assay interpretation. Parathyroid hormone has a diurnal variation, with the lowest values (trough, nadir) about noon (10 A.M.–2 P.M.) and the peak about 2 A.M. (midnight–4 A.M.). Specimens should be drawn when patients are fasting at about 7-8 A.M. without using specimen anticoagulants. Specimens should be processed at cold temperatures, frozen immediately, and transported in dry ice. Assay of PTH at present is difficult. Reliable antisera are not yet readily available from commercial sources, and, as noted previously, homemade antisera in reference laboratories differ in reactivity.

Tubular Reabsorption of Phosphate (Phosphate Reabsorption Index).—This procedure indirectly measures PTH by estimating PTH action on renal phosphate reabsorption. The patient should be on a normal phosphate diet; a low-phosphate diet ($<$ 500 mg/day) raises tubular reabsorption of phosphate (TRP) normal values, whereas a high-phosphorus diet (3,000 mg/day) lowers normal limits.

The patient drinks several glasses of water and then voids completely. One hour after voiding, a blood sample is obtained for phosphorus and creatinine measurement. Exactly 2 hours after beginning the test, the patient again voids completely, and the urine volume and urine concentration of creatinine and phosphate are determined. It is then possible to calculate the creatinine clearance rate and find the amount of phosphorus filtered per minute by the glomeruli. Comparing this with the actual amount of phosphate excreted per minute gives the amount reabsorbed by the tubules per minute, or the TRP value. A rough approximation is afforded by the formula:

$$\%\text{TRP} = \left[1 - \frac{\text{Urine PO}_4 \times \text{serum creatinine}}{\text{Urine creatinine} \times \text{serum PO}_4}\right] \times 100$$

An index value of less than 80% means diminished TRP value and suggests PHPT. This test becomes increasingly unreliable in the presence of renal insufficiency. About 5% of patients with renal stones but without parathyroid tumor have TRP values of 70%–80%, whereas about 20% of patients with parathyroid tumors have normal TRP values. Therefore, a TRP reduction is more significant than a normal result. Hypercalcemia due to malignancy is usually associated with a decreased TRP value. In addition, some patients with other conditions such as sarcoidosis and myeloma have been reported to have reduced TRP values.

X-Ray Findings.—Bone changes highly suggestive of hyperparathyroidism may be found radiologically in about 15% of PHPT patients (literature range, 9%–36%), although the older literature reports some type of change in up to 46% of cases with skeletal surveys. The incidence of bone change has considerably decreased because of earlier diagnosis. The most typical findings are subperiosteal cortical bone resorption in the phalanges. Patients with chronic renal disease (secondary or tertiary hyperparathyroidism) may also demonstrate these abnormalities but do not have elevated serum calcium levels (except in tertiary hyperparathyroidism, in which case there should be obvious long-term renal failure). Serum alkaline phosphatase elevation in PHPT is highly correlated with the presence of bone changes. It would be unlikely to find skeletal changes in hand x-ray films if the serum alkaline phosphatase level is not elevated. Of course, the serum alkaline phosphatase level could be elevated for a variety of reasons in any individual patient with hypercalcemia.

Serum Chloride.—Primary hyperparathyroidism tends to develop a hyperchloremic acidosis. Serum chloride is often elevated in PHPT (40%–50% of cases, if one excludes patients with conditions that lower serum chloride levels such as vomiting, diarrhea, or diuretic use). Less than 10% of patients with non-PHPT etiologies of hypercalcemia have elevated serum chloride levels. In one series, these were all patients with thyrotoxicosis or the ectopic PTH syndrome. A chloride/phosphorus ratio has also been proposed. This was found to be greater than 33 in about 94% of PHPT patients (without renal failure). However, results in other hypercalcemias have been variable, with the percentage of patients with a ratio greater than 33 ranging from 4%–39%.

Serum Calcitonin Assay.—Calcitonin (thyrocalcitonin, TCT) is secreted by nonfollicular C cells of the thyroid. An increased serum calcium level induces thyroid C cells to produce more calcitonin as part of hypercalcemia compensatory mechanisms. A major exception if PHPT, where the TCT level is usually normal or low, for poorly understood reasons (one report indicates an elevation in 10% of cases). The TCT level may be elevated in a considerable percentage of certain tumors known to metastasize to bone, such as lung carcinoma (about 30%–50% of cases, literature range 21%–62%) and breast carcinoma (about 50%, range 38%–75%). Medullary thyroid carcinoma (MTC) produces elevated basal TCT in about 75% of cases (range, 33%–100%). Total serum calcium in MTC is usually normal. MTC or C-cell hyperplasia is found in > 95% of patients with multiple endocrine neoplasia (MEN) syndromes type 2A and 2B (Chapter 32). Type 2A also includes pheochromocytoma (about 50% cases) and PHPT (10%–25% cases). PHPT also is part of MEN type 1, which does not include MTC. The TCT level may be increased in the Zollinger-Ellison syndrome, as well as in certain nonneoplastic conditions such as chronic renal failure or pernicious anemia, and values may overlap with MCT. In summary, and elevated TCT level in a patient with possible PHPT raises the question of medullary carcinoma of the thyroid or some other malignancy, if the patient is not in renal failure.

Hypercalcemia and Malignancy.—In patients with confirmed hypercalcemia, the differential diagnosis is usually among PHPT, malignancy (metastatic to bone or the ectopic PTH syndrome), and all other etiologies. In most cases the differential eventually resolves into PHPT vs. malignancy. There is no single laboratory test that can distinguish between PHPT and malignancy with certainty, with the possible exception of hand x-rays if typical changes of PHPT are found (but this occurs in only a small percentage of cases). Renal stones are common in PHPT and uncommon in tumor. The quickest and easiest screening test for myeloma is serum protein electrophoresis, although serum and urine immunoelectrophoresis is more sensitive. A serum chloride value at the upper limit of the reference range or above is evidence against metastatic tumor. A bone scan and x-ray skeletal survey are useful to detect metastatic tumor. Parathyroid hormone assay may be able to differentiate PHPT from other conditions if the result falls into a nomogram area clearly distinct from any other disease group. Some investigators advocate the assay of calcitonin, which is elevated with varying frequency in tumors associated with hypercalcemia and is usually not elevated in PHPT (some investigators report mild elevation in some patients). Unfortunately, regardless of the test results, one still might have a patient with concurrent PHPT and nonparathyroid malignancy.

Hypocalcemia

Hypocalcemia may be subdivided into laboratory hypocalcemia (decrease in serum total calcium value) and true hypocalcemia (decrease in ionized calcium value). Symptoms of decreased ionized calcium include neuromuscular irritability (Chvostek's or Trousseau's sign), which may progress to tetany in severe cases, mental changes (irritability, psychotic symptoms), and sometimes convulsions. The most common cause of laboratory hypocalcemia is a decrease in the serum albumin level, which lowers the total serum calcium value by decreasing the metabolically inactive bound fraction without changing the nonbound "ionized" metabolically active fraction. Therefore, this type of hypocalcemia is artifactual as far as the patient is concerned, since the metabolically active fraction is not affected. Sometimes laboratory hypocalcemia occurs with serum albumin values within the lower part of the population reference range, presumably because the previous albumin level was in the upper portion of the reference range. Although laboratory hypocalcemia is fairly common in hospitalized patients, true hypocalcemia is considerably less common than hypercalcemia. In one study, only 18% of patients with a decreased total serum calcium level had true hypocalcemia. Some causes of hypocalcemia are listed in Table 24–7.

Laboratory Tests

Laboratory tests helpful in differential diagnosis are serum albumin, BUN, calcium, phosphorus, pH, and PCO_2. These help to exclude hypoalbuminemia, chronic renal disease (BUN and phosphorus levels are elevated, pH is decreased), and alkalosis (respiratory or metabolic). Medication effect can be detected by a good patient history. Serum magnesium assay can exclude magnesium deficiency. If malabsorption is possible, serum carotene is a good screening test (chapter 25). Parathyroid hormone assay is needed to diagnose hypoparathyroidism (PTH deficiency with decreased PTH levels) or pseudohypoparathyroidism (renal or skeletal nonresponse to PTH with increased PTH levels). N-terminal PTH assay is better for this purpose than midregion or C-terminal assay if the patient has renal failure, since midregion and C-terminal fragments have a long half-life and thus accumulate in renal failure more than N-terminal fragments. If the BUN level is normal, there should be no difference between the various PTH assays.

TABLE 24–7.
Selected Etiologies of Hypocalcemia

Primary hypoparathyroidism
Pseudohypoparathyroidism
Malabsorption
Renal failure
Sepsis
Alkalosis (respiratory or metabolic)
Magnesium deficiency
Vitamin D deficiency
Tumor lysis syndrome
Rhabdomyolysis
Acute pancreatitis
Drug-induced hypocalcemia
Large doses of magnesium sulfate
Anticonvulsants
Mithramycin
Gentamicin
Cimetidine
Artifactual
Hypoalbuminemia
Hemodilution

Neonatal Hypocalcemia.—Neonatal serum calcium levels are lower than adult levels, with adult levels being attained at about 2 weeks of life for full-term infants and at about 4 weeks for premature infants. Neonates may develop hypocalcemia early (within the first 48 hours of life) or later (between age 4–30 days). Late-onset hypocalcemia can be due to a high-phosphate diet (cow's milk), malabsorption, dietary vitamin D deficiency, alkalosis, and congenital disorders. The etiology of early-onset hypocalcemia is poorly understood. Symptoms include muscular twitching, tremor, and sometimes convulsions. Since one or more episodes of tremor or twitching are not uncommon in neonates, hypocalcemia is a rather frequent consideration in the newborn nursery. Conditions that predispose to early-onset neonatal hypocalcemia include maternal insulin-dependent diabetes, birth hypoxia, acidosis, respiratory distress, and low birth weight (usually associated with prematurity). There is a general inverse relationship between serum calcium level and birth weight or infant gestational age. Infants who are severely premature or have very low birth weight tend to develop hypocalcemia very early; in one study of such patients, one-third became hypocalcemic by 15 hours after birth. In adult hypocalcemia, the diagnosis can be easily made with a serum total calcium assay if the patient has typical symptoms and if hypoalbuminemia is excluded. Ionized calcium assay may be necessary in equivocal cases. Although several formulas exist to predict ionized calcium using total calcium and serum albumin data, there is considerable disagreement in the literature whether these formulas are sufficiently accurate to be clinically useful. In one study on seriously ill adult patients, only about 20% of those who had formula-predicted ionized calcium deficit had measured ionized calcium abnormality. In newborns, serum calcium assay is much more difficult to interpret. First, neonatal calcium reference values increase with increasing gestational age, so that the reference range for prematures is different from the range for term infants. Second, there are surprisingly few data on neonatal reference ranges for calcium in the literature, and the data available are contradictory. For example, in laboratories with adult calcium reference range values of 9–11 mg/100 ml, the lower limit for premature infants varies in the literature from 6.0 to 8.0 mg/100 ml; and for full-term infants, from 7.3 to 9.4 mg/100 ml. If some other laboratory's adult reference range were lower than 9–11 mg/100 ml, presumably the neonatal reference lower limit could be even lower than those quoted. High levels of bilirubin or hemoglobin (hemolysis) can affect (falsely decrease) several methodologies for serum calcium. Thus, laboratory results in possible early-onset neonatal hypocalcemia may be difficult to interpret.

Vitamin D Compound Assay.—Vitamin D is a fat-soluble steroid-related molecule that is absorbed in the small intestine. After absorption it is carried in chylomicrons or bound to an alpha-1 globulin called "transcalciferin." Normally, about one-third is metabolized to calcidiol in the liver, and the remainder is stored in adipose tissue. Estrogen increases calcidiol formation. Calcidiol is altered to calcitriol in kidney proximal tubules by a 1α-hydroxylase enzyme. About 10% is metabolized to 24,25-dihydroxyvitamin D by a different enzyme. As noted previously, calcitriol has actions affecting calcium availability in bone, kidney, and intestine. Parathyroid hormone and blood phosphate levels can influence the hydroxylase enzyme, with the effects of PTH being produced through its action on cyclic AMP.

Laboratory assays for both calcidiol and calcitriol are available in some of the larger reference laboratories. These assays are useful mainly in patients with possible vitamin D overdose (hypervitaminosis D), in children with rickets, and in some adults with osteomalacia (the adult equivalent of rickets). Both osteomalacia and rickets are characterized by defective calcification of bone osteoid, and both involve some element of vitamin D deficiency.

Vitamin D excess can produce hypercalcemia, hyperphosphatemia, soft tissue calcification, and renal failure. Calcidiol assay is the test of choice; the calcidiol level should be considerably elevated. In some patients with PHPT, the serum calcium level may be normal or borderline, and PTH assay may be equivocal. In these few patients, calcitriol assay may be useful, since it should be elevated in PHPT.

The major usefulness of vitamin D compound assays is in persons with hypocalcemia, especially those with rickets or osteomalacia. Laboratory findings in some disorders involving vitamin D are listed in Table 24–8.

SERUM MAGNESIUM ABNORMALITIES

Magnesium is the fourth most common body cation (after sodium, potassium, and calcium) and the second most common intracellular cation (after potassium). About half is located in soft tissue and muscle cells and about half is in bone. Only 1%–5% is extracellular. Most body magnesium is derived from food intake. About one third of dietary magnesium is absorbed, with the absorption site being the small intestine. Body magnesium is excreted by the kidney, primarily through glomerular filtration. Some tubular reabsorption also takes place. About 33% of serum magnesium (literature range, 15%–45%) is bound to serum proteins, 15% is complexed, and about 50% is free in the ionized form. Of the protein-bound fraction, about 75% is attached to albumin and most of the remainder to alpha-1 and alpha-2 globulin. Albumin thus carries about 30% (range, 25%–33%) of total serum magnesium. Parathyroid hormone is a very important regulator of magnesium blood levels through regulation of renal tubule reabsorption.

Magnesium is important in protein synthesis, enzyme activation, and oxidative phosphorylation. It influences renal exchange of potassium and hydrogen ions and affects calcium levels. It also has an important role in nervous system control of muscle at the neuromuscular junction, where it slows neuromuscular impulse transmission by inhibiting acetylcholine. The major clinical symptoms of magnesium disorders are neuromuscular. Magnesium deficiency enhances muscle fiber excitability due to increased activity of acetylcholine; this is manifested by muscle tremor, which can progress to seizures and tetany. Mental abnormalities include confusion, anxiety, and hallucination. Magnesium excess conversely displays antagonism of nerve impulse transmission and results in muscle weakness. Magnesium also exerts some effect on heart muscle. Decreased magnesium levels may produce or aggravate cardiac arrythmias, whereas toxic levels of magnesium may be associated with heart block. Hypomagnesemia also potentiates the toxic effects of digitalis.

TABLE 24–8.
Laboratory Findings in Some Disorders Involving Vitamin D

	Calcium	Phosphorus	PTH	Calcidiol	Calcitriol
Primary hypoparathyroidism (PTH deficiency)	L	H	L	N	L
Pseudohypoparathyroidism (nonresponse of kidney and bone to PTH)	L	H	H	N	L
Failure of calcitriol formation (severe renal disease = secondary hyperparathyroidism)	L	H	H	N	L
Vitamin D deficiency (dietary, malabsorption)	L	L	H	L	L/LN
Decreased calcidiol formation (severe liver disease)	L	L	H	L	L/LN
Type I (autosomal recessive) vitamin D–dependent rickets (pseudo–vitamin D deficiency; due to decreased renal 1α-hydroxylase enzyme)†	L	N/L	H	N/H	L
Type II vitamin D–dependent rickets with alopecia (bone nonresponsiveness to calcitriol)†	L	N/L	H	N	H
X-linked familial hypophosphatemic rickets (defect in renal phosphate reabsorption and intestinal phosphate absorption; may also occur with magnesium deficiency)	N	L	N/H	N	N/L

*L = low; N = normal; H = high; LN = low normal. The results listed are those most frequently reported in the literature. Some investigators had different findings for one or more assay, especially for PTH (probably due to differences in PTH antibody characteristics).
†Also known as vitamin D–resistant rickets.

Magnesium Deficiency.—Magnesium deficiency has been reported in about 10% (range, 7%–11%) of hospitalized patients. Some of the etiologies of hypomagnesemia are listed in Table 24–9. In addition, it has been reported that hypomagnesemia frequently accompanies hyponatremia (22%–27% of hyponatremic patients); hypocalcemia (22%–32% of patients); and hypophosphatemia (25%–29% of patients). Several studies also found that hypomagnesemia is frequent in patients with hypokalemia (38%–42%), but one study reported only 7%. Postoperative patients on IV feeding are reported to have a short-term, temporary 20% decrease in serum magnesium levels. Similar findings have been reported 12–24 hours after acute myocardial infarction, returning to previous levels by 48 hours, but not all studies agree.

Excess Magnesium.—Increased serum magnesium levels are most often due to oliguric renal failure, which prevents excretion of magnesium. Overuse of magnesium compounds is an occasional etiology.

Laboratory Tests.—Red blood cells contain two–three times the concentration of magnesium found in serum. Artifactual hemolysis thus may produce a significant increase in assay values. Skeletal muscle contains about 10 times the serum concentration. Since about 30% of serum magnesium is bound to albumin, and assays measure total magnesium levels, hypoalbuminemia will artifactually decrease serum magnesium levels.

Various reports emphasize that serum magnesium values may not always truly reflect total body magnesium levels, since serum values may be falsely elevated in dehydration and falsely decreased in hemodilution with or without clinical edema or hypoalbuminemia. However, this problem is not unique to magnesium.

TABLE 24–9.
Magnesium Disorders

Magnesium deficiency
Alcoholism
Malabsorption
Malnutrition
IV fluids without magnesium
Severe diarrhea
Diabetic ketoacidosis
Hemodialysis
Hypercalcemia
Congestive heart failure
Artifact (hypoalbuminemia)
Certain medications
Loop and thiazide diuretics
Cyclosporine
Cisplatin
Gentamicin
Magnesium excess
Oliguric renal failure
Overuse of magnesium-containing compounds
Artifactual (specimen hemolysis)

PHOSPHORUS AND PHOSPHATE ABNORMALITIES

Phosphorus and phosphate are often spoken of interchangeably, although phosphorus is only one component of phosphate. The semantic problem is even more confusing because an order for "phosphate" assay usually results in laboratory measurement of inorganic phosphorus. However, much of the body phosphorus is a part of phosphate compounds. About 80%–85% of body phosphorus is found in bone and about 10% in skeletal muscle. Most body phosphorus is intracellular, where it represents the most abundant intracellular anion. Phosphorus is a part of phospholipid compounds in all cell membranes, adenosine triphosphate energy-transfer compounds, nucleic acids, the compound 2,3-diphosphoglyceric acid (which regulates oxygen affinity for hemoglobin), various enzymes, and the principal urinary acid-base buffer system. Phosphorus is acquired through food and absorbed through the small intestine. About 90% is extracted from serum by the kidney with about 85%–90% being normally reabsorbed by the renal proximal tubules. Serum phosphorus values change considerably during the day (variation of 2 mg/100 ml within a reference range of 2.5–4.5 mg/100 ml; 0.81–1.45 mmol/L), with values generally higher in the afternoon and evening than in the morning. Some of these changes are due to dietary factors and some to shifts between intracellular and extracellular localization. Administration of glucose leads to a temporary shift of phosphorus from an extracellular to an intracellular location. If a glucose load is given orally, trough serum phosphorus values are found about 2 hours postprandially, and preingestion values are regained about 5 hours postprandially.

Hypophosphatemia

Most clinical abnormalities involving phosphorus are associated with hypophosphatemia. Symptoms include confusion, disorientation, delerium, and sometimes seizures, thus resembling the symptoms of hyponatremia and other metabolic encephalopathies. In addition, there is skeletal muscle weakness that may progress to actual myopathy. In chronic severe hypophosphatemia there may be bone abnormalities such as osteomalacia and pseudofractures, as well as hematologic abnormalities such as decrease in oxygen delivery by RBCs and a tendency toward hemolysis. White blood cell function may be disturbed, with an increased incidence of fungal and bacterial infection. Mild hypophosphatemia, on the other hand, is usually asymptomatic clinically and biochemically.

The overall incidence of hypophospha-

TABLE 24–10.
Selected Disorders Associated With Serum Phosphate Abnormality

Phosphate decrease
Severe decrease
Parenteral hyperalimentation
Diabetic acidosis
Alcohol withdrawal
Severe metabolic or respiratory alkalosis
Antacids that bind phosphorus
Malnutrition with refeeding using low-phosphorus nutrients
Moderate decrease
Glucose administration
Nasogastric suction
Malabsorption
Gram-negative sepsis
PHPT
Phosphate excess
Renal failure
Severe muscle injury
Phosphate-containing antacids
Hypoparathyroidism

temia ranges from 2%–22% in hospitalized patients. The great majority of patients demonstrate only a mild degree of abnormality and no clinical effects. Table 24–10 lists conditions more likely to be associated with severe hypophosphatemia. For example, severe hypophosphatemia may appear in chronically malnourished persons who undergo rapid refeeding with low-phosphate nutrients (nutritional recovery syndrome). In many of the conditions listed under severe phosphate deficiency, onset of hypophosphatemia may not appear until 1 or more days after onset of illness. The other conditions on the list frequently produce hypophosphatemia but usually only of moderate degree. Even more conditions may produce mild disorder. There is an association of hypophosphatemia with hypomagnesemia, especially in alcoholics.

Hyperphosphatemia

The most common cause of hyperphosphatemia is renal failure. Other causes are listed in Table 24–10. Hyperphosphatemia may lead to hypocalcemia.

TRACE ELEMENTS

A considerable number of elements are found in the body in tiny amounts. Only a few will be mentioned. Lead is discussed in chapter 34, copper in chapter 33, and iodine in chapter 28.

Zinc

Zinc is a component of certain important enzymes, such as carbonic anhydrase, lactic dehydrogenase, alkaline phosphatase, DNA and RNA polymerases, and δ-aminolevulinic acid dehydratase. Zinc is obtained primarily through food. About 30% of that ingested is absorbed in the small intestine. About 80% of zinc in blood is found in RBCs, mostly as part of the enzyme carbonic anhydrase. Of that portion not in RBCs, about 50% is bound to albumin, about 30% is bound to alpha-2 macroglobulin or transferrin, and about 5% is bound to histidine and certain other amino acids, leaving about 15% free in plasma. Excretion occurs predominantly in the stool, with a much smaller amount excreted in urine and sweat.

Zinc deficiency is usually not clinically evident until it becomes severe. Severe deficiency may produce growth retardation, delayed sexual development, acrodermatitis enterohepatica (dermatitis, diarrhea, and alopecia), decreased taste acuity, and poor wound healing. Acrodermatitis enterohepatica can either be congenital (autosomal recessive trait) or can appear in severe acquired zinc deficiency.

Conditions producing zinc deficiency include inadequate diet intake (most often in hospitalized patients on IV feeding, including hyperalimentation patients), conditions that interfere with intestinal absorption (high-fiber or phytate diet, prolonged severe diarrhea, steatorrhea), excess zinc loss (sickle cell anemia), increased zinc requirement (pregnancy, lactation, wound healing), and certain diseases such as alcoholism and cirrhosis.

Assay of plasma zinc is usually done by atomic absorption spectrophotometry. Contamination is a major problem. Rubber stoppers or gaskets are well known for this. Glassware must be specially prepared. Another major problem is considerable variation in reference range between laboratories for both adults and infants. Serum is reported to have slightly higher levels than plasma. Since a substantial amount of plasma zinc is bound to albumin, changes in albumin can change (total) plasma zinc levels without reflecting patient body zinc levels. Hemolysis invalidates zinc measurement due to the high levels in RBCs. There is a circadian rhythm, with values somewhat higher in the morning.

Aluminum

Normally, small amounts of aluminum are ingested with food. Other sources include aluminum leached from aluminum cooking utensils by acidic juices, and alum-containing baking soda, processed cheese, and beer. Aluminum in serum is predominantly bound to transferrin, with a small amount bound to citrate in extracellular fluid. The only source of excretion is the kidney. Most interest in aluminum is focused on aluminum toxicity in patients with renal failure. These patients develop microcytic anemia, osteodystrophy (osteomalacia) resistant to Vitamin D, and encephalopathy. The osteodystrophy is caused by deposition in bone of excessive aluminum, where it interferes with bone mineralization. Initially, aluminum toxicity was thought to be due to aluminum contamination of water used for renal dialysis. More recently, the source of aluminum has been traced to aluminum-containing preparations used to bind phosphates in the GI tract to prevent phosphate absorption, with subsequent phosphate accumulation and development of secondary hyperparathyroidism. The gold standard test for aluminum osteodystrophy is bone biopsy with either (or both) chemical analysis or histochemical staining for aluminum content. However, other procedures have been used to estimate likelihood of aluminum bone toxicity. The serum aluminum level has been most commonly used for this purpose. Values greater than 50 ng/ml are generally considered abnormal, and values greater than 100 ng/ml are generally considered suggestive of possible aluminum bone toxicity. However, in one series about 30% of patients with serum aluminum values greater than 100 ng/ml failed to show definite evidence of aluminum toxicity on bone biopsy (70% specificity), and about 20% with serum values less than 100 μg/ml had biopsy evidence of aluminum toxicity (80% sensitivity). Many patients with aluminum toxicity develop a microcytic anemia (although it must be emphasized that microcytic anemia is not specific for aluminum toxicity). In one series, about 20% of renal hemodialysis patients with a microcytic mean cell volume (MCV) had a serum aluminum level less than 50 ng/ml; about 40% had a level between 50 and 100 ng/ml; and about 40% had a level more than 100 ng/ml. About 25% of patients with serum aluminum values greater than 100 ng/ml had a normal MCV. However, no patient with a value more than 140 ng/ml had a normal MCV. Another test involves infusion of a chelating drug desferrioxamine, which extracts some aluminum from tissues and increases serum aluminum levels by a certain amount over baseline if the tissues contain excess aluminum. Serum aluminum assay is difficult and is available only at large reference laboratories and some medical centers. The major problem is contamination by aluminum in laboratory apparatus and in the environment. Some sources of contamination include aluminum needles used for specimen collection, rubber stoppers on blood tubes, contaminated pipets or other glassware, and aluminum contamination of environmental dust.

EVALUATION OF PROTEIN-CALORIE NUTRITIONAL STATUS

Various studies have shown that a significant degree of malnutrition is frequent in hospitalized persons, ranging from 25%–50% of patients (depending on whether the population screened was a general or specialty group). In one report, 97% of surgical patients had at least one abnormal result on tests for nutritional status.

Classification of Protein-Calorie Malnutrition

Although protein or caloric deficiency exists in grades of severity, a classification of patients according to pathophysiology and laboratory abnormalities requires analysis of late-stage deprivation. At a late stage, three basic patient types have been described: kwashiorkor, marasmus, and a mixed picture.

Kwashiorkor results from protein deficiency without total calorie deficiency. This condition is produced by a diet with adequate calories that are obtained almost exclusively from carbohydrate. This may result from a nonhospital diet that is low in protein or may be seen in hospitalized patients who are maintained primarily on IV dextrose. Severe stress, major illness, or surgery results in greatly increased utilization of body protein and may rapidly lead to protein depletion if there is not adequate replacement. These patients externally seem to be of normal weight or even overweight and may have edema. Kwashiorkor involves depletion of primarily visceral (nonmuscle) protein.

Marasmus is produced by prolonged deficiency of both protein and carbohydrates. Examples are starvation due to inability to eat and anorexia nervosa. These patients lose both fat and muscle mass and appear emaciated. Marasmus involves loss of primarily somatic (fat and muscle) protein rather than visceral protein.

The *mixed category* combines various degrees of protein deprivation with various degrees of carbohydrate and total calorie deficiency. It may also result from end-state marasmus (when both somatic and visceral protein are consumed) or may occur in a patient with moderate marasmus who undergoes severe stress, thus accelerating visceral protein loss.

Besides classic end-state cases there are far

greater numbers of patients with malnutrition of lesser severity. In general, the greater the degree of deficiency, the greater the chance of unwanted consequences. These include increased postoperative morbidity and mortality and certain defined complications such as increased tendency toward infection, poor wound healing, and extended hospitalization.

Tests Useful in Patients With Malnutrition

Functional categories of tests (i.e., information that tests can supply) in protein-calorie malnutrition include:

1. Tests that screen patients for protein-calorie deficiency
2. Tests that assess degree of deficiency
3. Tests that differentiate the various types of deficiency
4. Tests used to guide therapy

Procedures or Tests Available

1. Anthropometric measurements: triceps skinfold thickness; midarm circumference
2. Calculation of undernourishment based on body height and weight (percent of ideal weight or percent of preillness weight)
3. Biochemical tests reflecting visceral (nonmuscle) protein status: serum albumin and serum transferrin (also, serum iron-binding capacity, retinol-binding protein, serum prealbumin)
4. Metabolic indices: creatinine-height index (somatic protein or muscle mass) and urinary nitrogen excretion (protein catabolism)
5. Tests of immune status: skin tests with various antigens, total lymphocyte count

Anthropometric Measurements

These procedures are designed to estimate fat and muscle wasting, which reflects somatic protein depletion. Triceps skin fold measurement is performed with special calipers and measures fat reserves. Midarm circumference is used to estimate lean body mass. Patient measurements are compared with values in standard tables.

Weight Deficiency (Weight Loss)

Weight deficiency may be calculated either as a percentage of preillness weight (current weight/preillness weight) or as a percentage of ideal weight (current weight/ideal weight). Ideal weight requires measurement of height and use of ideal weight tables. Percent weight loss after hospitalization is also useful. In all the various measurements, a 10% weight loss is considered suspicious for protein-calorie deficiency. If this occurred before admission, it probably developed over a relatively extended period of time (there is no standard time period, but at least 4 weeks has been suggested and seems reasonable) rather than over a short period of time, which is more likely to be a fluid problem. After hospitalization, there is no time limit if the weight loss is not due to diuretics, fluid removal, or some other obvious cause. Edema and obesity may produce error in nutritional assessment by these methods.

Tests for Visceral Protein Status

Serum Albumin.—Albumin is the major force maintaining plasma oncotic pressure. It is synthesized by the liver from amino acids. Decreased serum albumin levels result from decreased production, either from defective synthesis because of liver cell damage, deficient intake of amino acids (absolute protein intake deficit); or from disease- or stress-induced catabolism of body protein, which increases the need for dietary protein without a corresponding increase in dietary protein intake (relative protein intake deficit). The serum albumin level is thus considered an indicator of visceral (nonmuscle) protein status. Other serum proteins that have been used for the same purpose include transferrin, prealbumin, and retinol-binding protein.

Serum albumin has a serum half-life of about 20 days and begins to decrease about 2 weeks after onset of protein depletion. Mild protein deficiency is said to correlate with albumin levels of 3.0–3.5 gm/100 ml (30–35 g/L); moderate deficiency, 2.1–3.0 gm/100 ml (21–30 g/L); and severe deficiency, less than 2.1 gm/100 ml (21 g/L). Other etiologies for albumin decrease besides deficient protein intake include disorders of liver synthesis (cirrhosis, severe acute liver disease); extravascular protein loss (nephrotic syndrome, acute or chronic protein-losing enteropathy, extensive burns); and hemodilution (congestive heart failure). Albumin decrease, whether within or below reference limits, is seen in many severe acute and chronic illnesses. The exact mechanism is frequently uncertain or is sometimes due to more than one cause. Overhydration and dehydration also may change apparent albumin levels.

Serum Transferrin.—Transferrin has a serum half-life of about 9 days and begins to decrease about 1 week after onset of protein depletion. However, chronic iron deficiency, therapy with estrogen or estrogen-containing contraceptives, and the same severe acute and chronic illnesses that decrease albumin levels tend to elevate serum transferrin levels and could mask early change due to nutritional depletion. Transferrin can be measured directly in a variety of ways, usually by immunologic (antitransferrin antibody) techniques, or can be estimated using serum total iron-binding capacity (TIBC). Total iron-binding capacity is easier and less expensive for most laboratories. The formula most commonly used is: transferrin = (0.8 × TIBC) − 43. Mild protein deficiency correlates with transferrin levels of 150–175 mg/100 ml (1.5–1.7 g/L); moderate deficiency, 100–150 mg/100 ml (1.0–1.5 g/L); and severe deficiency, less than 100 mg/100 ml (1.0 g/L).

Serum Prealbumin.—Prealbumin is a carrier protein for retinol-binding protein and for a small part of serum thyroxine. Its serum half-life is about 2 days. Its serum concentration decreases in many severe illnesses. It is measured by immunologic techniques, most commonly by radial immunodiffusion or immunonephelometry. Prealbumin levels begin to decrease within 48–72 hours in response to protein malnutrition. However, like albumin, it is decreased by severe liver disease or as a temporary short- or long-term result of many severe acute or chronic illnesses.

Retinol-Binding Protein.—Retinol-binding protein is the specific binding protein for vitamin A. Its serum half-life is only about 10 hours. It begins to decrease within 48–72 hours after onset of protein malnutrition and otherwise behaves like prealbumin. However, in addition, retinol-binding protein may decrease when renal function decreases (as frequently occurs in severely ill persons).

Most investigators have accepted serum albumin as the most practical marker for visceral protein depletion. When serial measurements of visceral protein indices are necessary, transferrin may be substituted because it responds faster than albumin to change in nutrition status. Transferrin can also be used if albumin measurement is invalidated by therapeutic administration of albumin. Comparisons of serum albumin with other parameters of malnutrition have generally shown that serum albumin levels have the best single-test correlation with patient outcome.

Metabolic Indices

Creatinine Height Index (CHI).—This calculated value is thought to provide an estimate of lean body mass, based on the theory that urinary creatinine (UC) output is related to body muscle mass. Height is used to relate patient data to data of normal ("ideal") persons. The formula used is:

$$\text{CHI (in \% of ideal)} = \frac{\text{Measured UC (mg/24 h)}}{\text{Ideal UC (mg/24 h)}} \times 100$$

The creatinine height index (CHI) has the advantage that it relates to skeletal muscle mass (somatic protein) rather than to liver production of serum protein (visceral protein). In classic marasmus, the CHI is markedly decreased, whereas the serum albumin concentration may be either within reference range or close to it. Another advantage is that edema does not greatly affect the CHI, whereas it might affect arm circumference measurement. The major disadvantage is need for accurate 24-hour urine collection. Also, urine ketone bodies can interfere with creatinine assay. Data for ideal urine creatinine excretion are presented in Table 36–19.

Nitrogen Balance Estimates.—Nitrogen balance (NB), as measured by urine urea nitrogen (UUN), may be helpful in assessing the quantitative and compositional adequacy of nutritional therapy. The formula most often used is:

$$\text{NB} = \frac{\text{Protein intake}}{6.25} - (\text{UUN} + 4)$$

when nitrogen balance is in terms of net gain (+) or loss (−) in grams of nitrogen per day and both protein intake and urine urea output are in grams per day. Reference limits are +4 to −20 gm of nitrogen/day. Protein intake (in grams/day) is usually estimated but can be measured if feeding is entirely through nasogastric tube or hyperalimentation. If the patient has oral food intake, only the food actually eaten rather than food provided should be used in the calculation. The 4-gm correction factor is supposed to compensate for urine non–urea nitrogen loss additional to the urea nitrogen. If additional loss occurs from the GI tract, fistulas, and so forth, such loss must be estimated and incorporated into the correction factor. The 24-hour urine collection must be complete, because incomplete collection results in a falsely higher value.

Tests of Immune Status

Moderate or severe protein-calorie malnutrition of any type often results in depression of the body immune system. This is reflected in decreased immune response (especially, delayed hypersensitivity response) to various stimuli.

Total Lymphocyte Count.—There is a rough correlation of total lymphocyte count with degree of malnutrition. The correlation is closest in kwashiorkor (visceral protein depletion). Total lymphocyte counts of 1,200–2,000/cu mm ($1.2–2.0 \times 10^9$/L) are said to be associated with mild protein depletion; counts of 800–1,200/cu mm with moderate depletion, and counts of less than 800/cu mm with severe depletion. However, there is considerable overlap between immunologic impairment and nonimpairment with counts higher than 1,000/cu mm. Values less than 1,000/cu mm (1.0×10^9/L) are generally considered evidence of definite significant immunologic impairment. Total lymphocyte count is easy to obtain (WBC count × percent lymphocytes in the peripheral smear WBC differential result). Most investigators have found less correlation with eventual patient outcome than with serum albumin levels. One reason is that various other conditions may cause a decrease in total lymphocytes. Best correlation of total lymphocyte count to patient well-being seems to be associated with infection and with cancer therapy. When both albumin and total lymphocyte counts are significantly decreased, there is some reinforcement of significance compared with abnormality in either test alone.

Skin Tests.—Skin test response to various intradermally injected delayed hypersensitivity antigens such as *Candida*, mumps, and streptokinase-streptodornase provides an in vivo method to evaluate immune response. Reactions are measured at 24 and 48 hours. Various studies have shown a substantial correlation between lack of skin test reactivity to multiple antigens and an increased incidence of sepsis or postoperative complications and mortality. There is some disagreement in the literature on the predictive value of skin tests vs. serum albumin levels, with the majority opinion favoring albumin. The major drawbacks to skin testing are the time interval required and the necessity for good injection technique.

TABLE 24–11.

Nutritional Deficiency Syndromes and Screening Tests

Overall nutritional status
1. Percent weight loss (at least 10% nondiuretic loss)

Marasmus (somatic protein and fat deficit due to total calorie deficiency; somatic protein = skeletal muscle lean body mass)
1. Somatic protein
   Creatinine-height index
   Midarm circumference
2. Fat
   Triceps skin fold thickness

Kwashiorkor (visceral protein deficit due to protein intake deficiency; visceral protein = liver-produced protein, including plasma proteins)
1. Serum albumin (transferrin, prealbumin, retinol-binding protein)
2. Total lymphocyte count
3. Cell-mediated immunity

Mixed kwashiorkor and marasmus (deficit in both protein intake and total calories)
1. Tests abnormal in both deficiency groups

Current Status of Tests for Protein-Calorie Malnutrition (Table 24–11)

Patient Screening for Protein-Calorie Malnutrition.—Although various institutions have different protocols, the most common practice that is emerging is to determine the percent of weight loss and the serum albumin level, either one alone or in combination, and to take into consideration the type of illness or therapy involved. Total lymphocyte count also seems to be widely used as an adjunctive test. The CHI is helpful if marasmus is suspected; serum albumin levels could be misleading if albumin were the sole criterion for possible malnutrition.

Tests to Assess Degree of Deficiency.—Serum albumin level is the most widely used single test. The CHI is also widely employed if marasmus is present. Anthropometric measurements, serum transferrin determination, and tests of immune function are available but seem to be ordered more in university or research centers.

Tests to Differentiate Categories of Malnutrition.—In classic kwashiorkor, anthropometric measurements and CHI values are relatively normal, whereas serum albumin levels and other tests of visceral protein status are decreased. In classic marasmus, anthropometric measurements and the CHI are decreased, whereas results of visceral protein adequacy tests may be normal. Although immune status test results are depressed in severe marasmus, over the broad spectrum of marasmus severity they are not as severely affected as in kwashiorkor. It must be emphasized that patients may have some combination of overall protein-calorie deficiency and of severe protein loss and therefore may not have clear-cut differential test patterns.

Tests to Guide Nutritional Therapy.—Serum albumin levels and total lymphocyte count are still the most commonly used parameters of therapeutic response. Because serum albumin has a relatively long half-life and changes relatively slowly in response to renourishment, and also because fluid shifts influence albumin levels, an increasing number of investigators use serum transferrin or prealbumin levels rather than albumin levels to monitor therapy. Some find that urinary nitrogen excretion data are very helpful in determining when a positive nitrogen balance has been achieved, but others do not believe that it is necessary.

Additional tests relevant to this chapter are discussed in chapter 35, and additional data are listed in Table 36–20.

BIBLIOGRAPHY

Stein HJ: Hypokalemia: Common and uncommon causes. *Hosp Pract* 1988; 23(3A):55.

Halery J, Bulvik S: Severe hypophosphatemia in hospitalized patients. *Arch Intern Med* 1988; 148:153.

Arieff AI: Osmotic failure: Physiology and strategies for treatment. *Hosp Pract* 1988; 23(5):173.

Hirsch IA, et al: The overstated risk of preoperative hypokalemia. *Anesth Analg* 1988; 67:131.

Elin RJ: Assessment of magnesium status. *Clin Chem* 1987; 33:1965.

Avioli LV: Primary hyperparathyroidism: Recognition and management. *Hosp Pract* 1987; 22(9A):69.

Knochel JP: Etiologies and management of potassium deficiency. *Hosp Pract* 1987; 22(1):153.

Lufkin EG, et al: Parathyroid hormone radioimmunoassays in the differential diagnosis of hypercalcemia due to primary hyperparathyroidism or malignancy. *Ann Intern Med* 1987; 106:559.

Whitlock EP: Selenium, vitamin E and vitamin A: Nutritional and physiologic findings. *Lab Mgmt* 1987; 25(5):49.

AMA Council on Scientific Affairs: Vitamin preparations as dietary supplements and as therapeutic agents. *JAMA* 1987; 257:1929.

Durham JR, et al: Hypocalcemia following total thyroidectomy. *Ill Med J* 1987; 171:135.

Flink EB: Magnesium deficiency: Causes and effects. *Hosp Pract* 1987; 22:116A.

Vargas SJ, et al: Comparison of commercially available parathyroid hormone immunoassays in the differentiated diagnosis of hypercalcemia. *Am J Med Sci* 1987; 294:415.

Cannon-Babb ML, Schwartz AB: Drug-induced hyperkalemia. *Hosp Pract* 1986; 21(9A):99.

Buckalew VM: Hyponatremia: Pathogenesis and management. *Hosp Pract* 1986; 21:49.

Zantvoort FA, et al: Theophylline and serum electrolytes. *Ann Intern Med* 1986; 104:134.

Chung H-M, et al: Postoperative hyponatremia. *Arch Intern Med* 1986; 146:333.

Zaloga GP, Chernow B: Hypocalcemia in critical illness. *JAMA* 1986; 256:1924.

Venkataraman PS, et al: Early neonatal hypocalcemia in extremely preterm infants. *Am J Dis Child* 1986; 140:1004.

Rasmussen HS, et al: Magnesium and acute myocardial infarction. *Arch Intern Med* 1986; 146:872.

Bowers GN, et al: Measurement of ionized calcium in serum with ion-selective electrodes: A mature technology that can meet the daily service needs. *Clin Chem* 1986; 32:1437.

Schoeff L: Antidiuretic hormone and water regulation. *J Med Technol* 1986; 3:342.

Armitage EK: Parathyrin (parathyroid hormone): Metabolism and methods for assay. *Clin Chem* 1986; 32:418.

Julian BA: Aluminum-associated renal osteodystrophy. *Ala J Med Sci* 1986; 23:414.

McCarthy JT, et al: Interpretation of serum aluminum values in dialysis patients. *Am J Clin Pathol* 1986; 86:629.

Rettmer RL, Labbe RF: Monitoring total parenteral nutrition. *Lab Med* 1985; 16:476.

Puri S, Chandra RK: Nutritional regulation of host resistance and predictive value of immunologic tests in assessment of outcome. Pediatr Clin North Am 1985; 32:499.

Fields M: Newer understanding of copper metabolism. *Intern Med Specialist* 1985; 6:91.

Gundberg CM: Osteocalcin and gamma-carboxyglutamic acid. *Clin Chem News* 1985; 11:22.

Kopyt N, Narins RG: Should hypokalemia be treated? *Drug Therapy* 1985; 15:156.

Edes TE, Sunderrajan EV: Heparin-induced hyperkalemia. *Arch Intern Med* 1985; 145:1070.

Maas AHJ: Ion-selective electrodes for sodium and potassium. *Clin Chem* 1985; 31:482.

Robinson AG: Disorders of antidiuretic hormone secretion. *Clin Endocrinol Metab* 1985; 14:55.

Zaloga GP: Assessment of calcium homeostasis in the critically ill surgical patient. *Ann Surg* 1985; 202:587.

Audrian M, Kumar R: The physiology and pathophysiology of vitamin D. *Mayo Clin Proc* 1985; 60:851.

Katz SA: Collection and preparation of biological tissues and fluids for trace element analysis. *Am Clin Prod Rev* 1985; 4(4):8.

Levine MA: Laboratory investigation of disorders of the parathyroid glands. *Clin Endocrinol Metab* 1985; 14:257.

Klein G, Rivera D: Adverse metabolic consequences of total parenteral nutrition. *Cancer* 1985; 55:305.

Campbell JA: Nutritional evaluation of hospital patients. *Lab Med* 1984; 15:666.

Walmsley RN: Hyperkalemia in the elderly. *Clin Chem* 1984; 30:1409.

Walmsley RN, White GH: Occult causes of hypokalemia. *Clin Chem* 1984; 30:1406.

Williams DM: Copper deficiency in humans. *Sem in Hematol* 1983; 20:118.

Narins RG, et al.: Diagnostic strategies in disorders of fluid, electrolyte, and acid-base homeostasis. *Am J Med* 1982; 72:496.

Tiber AM, Mukherjee MD: Clinical manifestations of zinc deficiency. *Am Fam Phys* 1982; 26:167.

Agus ZS, et al: Disorders of calcium and magnesium homeostasis. *Am J Med* 1982; 72:473.

Stoff JS: Phosphate homeostasis and hypophosphatemia. *Am J Med* 1982; 72:489.

Dourville P, et al: Potential usefulness of serum prealbumin in total parenteral nutrition. *Clin Chem* 1982; 28:1706.

Anderson CF, Wochos DN: The utility of serum albumin values in the nutritional assessment of hospitalized patients. *Mayo Clin Proc* 1982; 57:181.

Feig PU: Hypernatremia and hypertonic syndromes. *Med Clin North Am* 1981; 65:271.

Tan SY, Burton M: Hyporeninemic hypoaldosteronism: An overlooked cause of hyperkalemia. *Arch Intern Med* 1981; 141:30.

25 Gastrointestinal Function

MALABSORPTION

The function of the gastrointestinal (GI) tract is to perform certain mechanical and enzymatic procedures on food to prepare food for absorption, to absorb necessary dietary constituents into the bloodstream, and to excrete whatever is not absorbed. When the usual dietary constituents are not absorbed normally, symptoms may develop that form part of the syndrome known as malabsorption (Table 25–1). There are three basic types of malabsorption. The first type involves the interruption of one of the stages in fat absorption (indicated in Table 25–1 by categories I, II, and III); this concerns primarily fat absorption and also those substances dependent on the presence of lipid. The second type is related to intrinsic defect of the small bowel mucosa (category IV, A–D). In this kind of malabsorption there is interference not only with fat and fat-soluble substances but also with absorption of carbohydrates and many other materials. The third type of malabsorption is associated with altered bacterial flora (category IV, E) and also with the deficiency disease called "pernicious anemia." In malabsorption of this kind, lack of a single specific substance normally produced by the GI tract leads to malabsorption of other substances dependent on that substance for absorption. Some of these conditions and their laboratory diagnosis are discussed in detail elsewhere (e.g., lactase deficiency in chapter 33, *Giardia lamblia* in chapter 17, Zollinger-Ellison syndrome in chapter 32).

Clinical Findings.—Steatorrhea, or the appearance of excess quantities of fat in the stool, is a frequent manifestation of most malabsorption syndromes. Many patients with steatorrhea also have diarrhea, but the two are not synonymous; a patient can have steatorrhea without diarrhea. In children, the principal diseases associated with steatorrhea and malabsorption are celiac disease and cystic fibrosis of the pancreas. In adults, the most common causes are tropical sprue, nontropical sprue (the adult form of celiac disease), and pancreatic insufficiency. The clinical picture of all these diseases is roughly similar but varies according to etiology, severity, and duration. The most common chief complaints of severe malabsorption are diarrhea and weakness, weight loss, and mild functional GI complaints (anorexia, nausea, mild abdominal pain). Physical findings and laboratory test results tend to differ with the various etiologies. In severe cases of sprue, tetany, bone pain, tongue surface atrophy, and even bleeding may be found. Physical examination may show abdominal distention and also peripheral edema in nearly half the patients. In pancreatic insufficiency, physical examination may be normal or show malnutrition. Neurologic symptoms are found with moderate frequency in pernicious anemia but may be present in malabsorption of other causes as well.

Laboratory Findings.—Laboratory test findings vary according to severity and etiology of the malabsorption, but in sprue they most often include one or more of the following: anemia, steatorrhea, hypoproteinemia, hypocalcemia, and hypoprothrombinemia. In pancreatic insufficiency, the main laboratory test abnormalities are steatorrhea and decreased car-

TABLE 25–1.

Classification of Malabsorptive Disorders (With Comments on Occurrence and Associated Abnormalities)

I. Inadequate mixing of food with bile salts and lipase. Mild chemical steatorrhea common, but clinical steatorrhea uncommon. Actual diarrhea uncommon. Anemia in approximately 15%–35%; most often iron deficiency, rarely megaloblastic.
    A. Pyloroplasty
    B. Subtotal and total gastrectomy (occasional megaloblastic anemias reported)
    C. Gastrojejunostomy

II. Inadequate lipolysis—lack of lipase or normal stimulation of pancreatic secretion. Steatorrhea only in far-advanced pancreatic destruction, and diarrhea even less often.
    A. Cystic fibrosis of the pancreas
    B. Chronic pancreatitis
    C. Cancer of the pancreas or ampulla of Vater
    D. Pancreatic fistula
    E. Severe protein deficiency
    F. Vagus nerve section

III. Inadequate emulsification of fat—lack of bile salts. Clinical steatorrhea uncommon, sometimes occurs in very severe cases. Usually no diarrhea.
    A. Obstructive jaundice
    B. Severe liver disease

IV. Primary absorptive defect—small bowel
    A. Inadequate length of normal absorptive surface. Unusual complication of surgery.
        1. Surgical resection
        2. Internal fistula
        3. Gastroileostomy
    B. Obstruction of mesenteric lymphatics (rare)
        1. Lymphoma
        2. Hodgkin's disease
        3. Carcinoma
        4. Whipple's disease
        5. Intestinal tuberculosis
    C. Inadequate absorptive surface due to extensive mucosal disease. Except for *Giardia* infection and regional enteritis, most of these diseases are uncommon. Steatorrhea only if there is extensive bowel involvement.
        1. Inflammatory
            a. Tuberculosis
            b. Regional enteritis or enterocolitis (diarrhea very common)
            c. *Giardia lamblia* infection (diarrhea common; malabsorption rare)
        2. Neoplastic
        3. Amyloid disease
        4. Scleroderma
        5. Pseudomembranous enterocolitis (diarrhea frequent)
        6. Radiation injury
        7. Pneumatosis cystoides intestinalis
    D. Biochemical dysfunction of mucosal cells
        1. "Gluten-induced" (steatorrhea and diarrhea very common)
            a. Celiac disease (childhood)
            b. Nontropical sprue (adult)
        2. Enzymatic defect
            a. Disaccharide malabsorption (diarrhea frequent symptom)
            b. Pernicious anemia (deficiency of "gastric" intrinsic factor)
        3. Cause unknown. Uncommon except for tropical sprue (which is common only in the tropics).
            a. Tropical sprue (diarrhea and steatorrhea common)
            b. Severe starvation
            c. Diabetic visceral neuropathy
            d. Endocrine and metabolic disorder (e.g., hypothyroidism)
            e. Zollinger-Ellison syndrome (diarrhea common; steatorrhea may be present)
            f. Miscellaneous

TABLE 25–1 (cont.).

E. Malabsorption associated with altered bacterial flora (diarrhea fairly common)
   1. Small intestinal blind loops, diverticula, anastomoses (rare)
   2. Drug (oral antibiotic) administration (infrequent but not rare)

bohydrate tolerance (sometimes overt diabetes). In pernicious anemia the patient has only anemia without diarrhea, steatorrhea, or the other test abnormalities previously listed. Most stomach operations do not cause diarrhea or abnormalities of fat absorption.

Steatorrhea is caused by excess excretion of fat in the stools due to inability to absorb lipids. Anemia is most often macrocytic but sometimes is caused by iron deficiency or is a mixed type due to various degrees of deficiency of folic acid, vitamin B12, and iron. Calcium may be decreased both from hypoalbuminemia and GI loss from diarrhea. Prothrombin formation by the liver is often impaired to some degree because of lack of vitamin K. Vitamin K is a fat-soluble vitamin that is obtained from food and also is produced by bacteria in the small bowel. Long-term oral antibiotic use may reduce the bacterial flora by killing these bacteria and thus may interfere with vitamin K formation. Inability to absorb fat secondarily prevents vitamin K and vitamin A, which are dependent on fat solubility for intestinal absorption, from entering the bloodstream. Malnutrition resulting from lack of fat and carbohydrate absorption leads to hypoalbuminemia because of decreased production of albumin by the liver. This also contributes to the peripheral edema that many patients develop.

The majority of patients with malabsorption usually present in one of two ways. In the first group the major finding on admission is anemia, and once malabsorption is suspected, either by the finding of megaloblastic bone marrow changes or by other symptoms or signs suggestive of malabsorption, the problem becomes one of differentiating pernicious anemia from other types of malabsorption. In the second group, the patients present with one or more clinical symptoms of malabsorption, either mild or marked in severity. The diagnosis must be firmly established and the etiology investigated. There are several basic tests for malabsorption which, if used appropriately, usually can lead to the diagnosis and in some cases reveal the cause.

Useful Individual Laboratory Tests

Qualitative Fecal Fat.—Fat in the feces can be stained with Sudan III dye. Neutral fat can be seen as bright orange droplets, but the fatty acids normally do not stain. Both these fatty acids and the original neutral fat can be converted to stainable fatty acids by heat and acid hydrolysis. The preparation is then stained and examined a second time to determine if the number of droplets has increased from the first examination. The reliability of this procedure is debated in the literature, but it seems reasonably accurate if the technician is experienced. Naturally, there will be difficulty in distinguishing normal results from low-grade steatorrhea. It is possible to get some idea of etiology by estimating the amount of neutral fat vs. fatty acid: lack of fatty acid suggests pancreatic disease.

Quantitative Fecal Fat.—The basic diagnostic test for steatorrhea is quantitative fecal fat. Stool collections are taken over a minimum of 3 full days. The patient should be on a diet containing approximately 50–150 gm/day of fat (average 100 gm/day) beginning 2 days before the test collection. It is necessary to make sure that the patient is actually eating enough of this diet to take in at least 50 gm of fat/day; it is also obviously important to make sure that all the stools are collected and the patient is not incontinent of feces. Patient noncompliance with complete stool collection is probably the most common cause of false negative results. If the patient is constipated (and some are), it may be necessary to use a bedtime laxative. Normal diet results in an average excretion of less than 7 gm of fat/24 hours. Excretion of 5–7 gm/24 hours is equivocal, since many patients with minimal steatorrhea and a small but significant percentage of normal persons have excretion in this range. Finally, some patients with partial or complete malabsorption syndromes may have normal fecal fat excretion. This is most common in tropical sprue.

Plasma Carotene.—Carotene is the fat-soluble precursor of vitamin A and is adequately present in most normal diets that contain green or yellow vegetables. Normal values are considered 70–300 μg/100 ml (1.3–5.6 μmol/L). Values of 30–70 μg/100 ml are usually considered moderately decreased, and levels less than 30 μg/100 ml (0.56 μmol/L) indicate severe depletion. Other causes of low plasma carotene, besides malabsorption, are poor diet, severe liver disease, and high fever. There is considerable overlap between the carotene values of malabsorption and the carotene values in normal control patients, but such overlap usually is over the 30-μg level. However, this test is valuable mostly as a screening procedure. The patient must be eating a sufficient quantity of carotene-rich food to draw valid conclusions from a low test result.

X-ray Examination.—A small bowel series is done by letting barium pass into the small intestine. There are several changes in the normal radiologic appearance of the small bowel that are suggestive of malabsorption. These changes appear in 70%–90% of patients, depending on the etiology and severity of the disease and the interpretative skill of the investigator. The radiologic literature agrees that many chronic diseases, especially when associated with fever and cachexia, may interfere with digestion so severely as to produce a pattern that may be confused with sprue. Secondary malabsorption cannot be distinguished from primary malabsorption except in certain rare cases such as tumor. The so-called diagnostic patterns of sprue are thus characteristic of, but not specific for, primary small intestine absorption and are not present in about 20% of patients.

Radioisotope Techniques.—To test for fat malabsorption, a neutral fat called "triolein," which combines glycerol and fatty acid, has been tagged with iodine 131. It is also possible to tag a simple fatty acid such as oleic acid with ^{131}I. The radioactive fat can be administered in several ways, usually as a capsule or as part of a fatty meal. After a certain period, a specimen of blood is drawn and measured for radioactivity. The stool also can be measured for radioactivity. Either procedure gives an idea of how much fat was either absorbed or rejected by the intestinal mucosa. In malabsorption due to pancreatic disease, radioactive fatty acid (oleic acid) is absorbed normally but not radioactive neutral fat (triolein). In primary small bowel malabsorption, both types of fat are not absorbed normally. There have been many reports on this subject. The main problem with the test is a technical one and concerns the way the radioactive fat is administered. Apparently results differ quite markedly according to whether the radiosotope is given as a capsule or as an integral part of a fatty meal, and even the type of fatty vehicle has some influence on absorption. Radioisotope labeling is a promising technique but is not yet standardized. For the present, it is probably better to avoid using this technique, since the same information usually can be obtained in other ways and the accuracy of radioisotope fat labeling is open to considerable question.

Schilling Test.—Pernicious anemia is an interesting disease in which a combination of specific (anatomical) lesions and factor deficiency leads to a characteristic clinical picture (see chapter 3). Briefly, patients with pernicious anemia have atrophic gastritis, a complete lack of gastric hydrochloric acid (anacidity), and a partial or complete deficiency of intrinsic factor. Intrinsic factor is a substance produced by the stomach that is necessary for the absorption of vitamin B12 in the ileum. Laboratory findings vary according to the duration and severity of the disease but classically consist of a macrocytic anemia and megaloblastic changes in the bone marrow. The bone marrow changes are often accompanied by peripheral blood leukopenia and thrombocytopenia, with hypersegmentation of some mature neutrophil nuclei. In true pernicious anemia, oral administration of usual dietary amounts of vitamin B12 (1–2 μg/day) has no measurable effect on the clinical course or the hematologic picture. A few patients respond to a dose of as little as 5 μg, and nearly all respond to a dose of 100 μg, presumably because of the effect of mass action on the small intestine mucosa despite intrinsic factor deficiency.

Test Protocol.—The Schilling test entails oral administration of vitamin B12 that has been tagged with radioactive cobalt. The usual dose is 0.5 μg, although a 1981 publication of the International Committee for Standardization in Hematology (ICSH) recommends 1.0 μg. Next,

1,000 μg of nonisotopic vitamin B12 is given subcutaneously or intramuscularly to saturate tissue-binding sites to allow a portion of any labeled B12 absorbed from the intestine to be excreted or flushed out into the urine. This "flushing dose" of nonradioactive B12 is usually administered 2 hours after the radioactive B12 (investigators have reported administration times of 2–6 hours, with extremes ranging from simultaneous injection with the radioactive dose to as much as 12 hours later). In a normal person, more than 8% (literature range, 5%–16%) of the oral radioactive B12 dose appears in the urine. In classic pernicious anemia, the Schilling test result is positive; that is, there is less than 8% urinary excretion of the radioisotope if no intrinsic factor has been given with the test dose. The test is then completely repeated after at least 24 hours, administering adequate amounts of oral intrinsic factor with the radioactive B12 dose. Urinary B12 excretion should then become normal, since the added intrinsic factor permits normal vitamin B12 absorption.

Urine collection.—Although the ICSH recommends a single 24-hour urine collection and the majority of laboratories follow this protocol, some reports indicate that certain patients without B12 malabsorption may take up to 72 hours to excrete normal amounts of the radioactive B12. One report indicated that 14% of patients with normal B12 excretion took 48 hours and 7% took 72 hours. Some of those with delayed excretion had an elevated blood urea nitrogen (BUN) level, but some did not. Poor renal function is known to delay Schilling test B12 excretion and frequently produces low 24-hour results. Reports indicate that cumulative results over a 48-hour time period, and sometimes even a 72-hour period, may be required to reach a normal recovery level. Normal values for a 48- or 72-hour excretion period are the same as those for a 24-hour collection. Therefore, at least a 48-hour collection should be considered if the BUN level is elevated. If extended urine collection periods are used, it is recommended that one additional nonradioactive B12 parenteral dose be administered each 24 hours, since this has been reported to increase the B12 excretion. Because renal function can be significantly decreased with the BUN level remaining within reference range, and because of uncertainty reported for individual patient response, some laboratories routinely collect two consecutive 24-hour urine specimens. If the first 24-hour specimen contains a normal amount of radioactive B12, the second collection can be discontinued. If the total 48-hour specimen radioactivity is low but relatively close to the lower limit of normal, a third 24-hour specimen might be desirable. One relatively frequent 24-hour Schilling test problem is inadvertent loss of a portion of the urine collection. If this occurs, in my experience it is useful to order completion of the 48-hour collection period. In the meantime, if the urine actually collected before the accident is counted, it may contain a normal amount of radioactivity, in which case the additional collection can be terminated. If not, the radioactivity in the initial specimen can be added to that in the remainder of the collection.

One precaution to be observed when performing a Schilling test is having the patient fast overnight since food may contain B12 and also to prevent food interference with gastric emptying or protein in food from binding any radioactive B12. Two hours after the radioactive dose is administered, the patient is permitted a light meal that does not contain any B12 (the ICSH recommends toast and jelly as an example). A 12- to 24-hour urine specimen should be obtained just prior to starting the test to demonstrate that no previously administered radioactivity (e.g., from a nuclear medicine scan) is present.

Repeat Schilling Tests.—If the Schilling test result without intrinsic factor is abnormal (low result), the test is repeated with intrinsic factor. In some cases it may have to be repeated without intrinsic factor to correct a test problem or to verify results. There is some debate over what time interval should elapse between the end of the first test and beginning of the second (with or without intrinsic factor). Various investigators have recommended intervals ranging from 1–7 days. The ICSH states that it is not necessary to wait more than 24 hours. However, there are some reports that nonradioactive B12 from the flushing dose might be excreted in bile sufficient to compete with radiolabeled B12 for absorption in the ileum. Also, if only a 24-hour collection is used for the first Schilling test, a few persons with considerably delayed excretion might contribute a significant, although small, amount of radioactivity to the next test. Therefore, a 48-hour wait might be a reasonable compromise.

False positive results (falsely low values) may be produced by bladder retention of urine (incomplete voiding) and by spilled or lost urine already voided; in either case the problem is incomplete urine collection (normal output is > 600 ml/24 hours and usually is > 800 ml). Measurement of urine creatinine excretion is also helpful as a check on complete collection. Delayed B12 excretion could produce falsely decreased values in a 24-hour collection. As noted previously, some laboratories routinely collect two consecutive 24-hour urine specimens, since the initial 24-hour collection may be incomplete, and vitamin B12 excretion during the second 24 hours may be sufficient to bring total 48-hour excretion to normal range. False negative results (falsely normal values) are much less of a problem than false positive results but may be caused by fecal contamination of the urine or by presence of radioactivity from a previous nuclear medicine procedure. One report indicates that folic acid deficiency (manifested by low blood folate level) significantly increases urine B12 excretion with or without intrinsic factor, which potentially might produce a borderline or low normal Schilling test result when the result ordinarily would be decreased.

Interpretation.—The Schilling test, with and without intrinsic factor, is extremely helpful in distinguishing pernicious anemia from various other malabsorption syndromes, which may show part or all of the classic pernicious anemia clinical and laboratory findings. The typical pattern of malabsorption without intrinsic factor deficiency is abnormal Schilling test results, both with and without intrinsic factor. A considerable number of patients with sprue, up to 40% of patients with severe chronic pancreatitis, a few patients with some of the other malabsorption diseases, and possibly some persons with severe gastric acid secretion deficiency may have positive Schilling test results without intrinsic factor, but B12 malabsorption will not be corrected by the addition of intrinsic factor. This differential procedure is especially helpful because other laboratory test results may be confusing. For example, some patients with primary malabsorption do not have steatorrhea, and some may have anacidity, especially in the older age groups. In fact, about 30% of normal patients over age 70 apparently do not produce hydrochloric acid (HCl). Finally, occasional patients with classic pernicious anemia also show impaired results in some of the other absorptive function tests that one would expect in other malabsorption syndromes. The Schilling test can thus be very helpful and, incidentally, can be performed even if the patient already has been started on treatment as long as intrinsic factor is not being given.

One Additional Caution.—Some patients with pernicious anemia may have abnormal Schilling test results with added intrinsic factor, thus simulating sprue or similar malabsorption diseases, but then revert to the typical pernicious anemia test pattern of normal absorption response with added intrinsic factor after treatment for several weeks with parenteral vitamin B12.

If a bone marrow aspiration to document megaloblastic change is contemplated, it should be performed before the Schilling test. The nonisotopic B12 parenteral flushing dose will quickly convert the megaloblastic changes to normal. In fact, the flushing dose is actually a treatment dose. The nonradioactive B12 is not completely eliminated for 6 months or more and therefore can interfere with serum B12 assay. It also can produce a reticulocyte response in persons with folate deficiency; and, likewise, folic acid therapy can produce a reticulocyte response in persons with B12 deficiency. Folic acid therapy can also increase serum B12 levels in patients with B12 deficiency.

D-Xylose Test.—Besides quantitative (fecal) fat studies, the most important test for malabsorption is the D-xylose test. Rather than a screening test for malabsorption per se, it is a test that identifies the sprue-type diseases and differentiates them from other malabsorption etiologies. Originally, an oral glucose tolerance test (OGTT) was used in malabsorption, since it was found that most patients with sprue showed a flat curve. A "flat" OGTT is usually defined as an OGTT peak with a value no greater than 25 mg/100 ml (1.4 mmol/L) above the baseline fasting level, although there is some disagreement about this criterion. However, some patients with obvious malabsorption have a normal curve, and it was also found in several large series that up to 20% of apparently normal persons had a flat curve, so this test was abandoned.

Test Protocol.—D-Xylose is a pentose isomer that is absorbed in much the same manner as glucose from the jejunum. The standard test dose is 25 gm of D-xylose in 250 ml of water, followed by another 250 ml of water. The patient is fasted overnight, since xylose absorption is delayed by other food. After the test dose, the patient is kept in bed for 5 hours without food. The normal person's peak D-xylose blood levels are reached in approximately 2 hours and fall to fasting levels in approximately 5 hours. D-Xylose is excreted mostly in the urine with approximately 80%–95% of the excretion in the first 5 hours and the remainder in 24 hours. Side effects of oral D-xylose administration are mild diarrhea and abdominal discomfort in a small number of patients.

Interpretation.—Normal values for (2-hour) blood D-xylose levels are more than 25 mg/100 ml (1.66 mmol/L); values of 20–25 mg/100 ml are equivocal, and values less than 20 mg/100 ml (1.33 mmol/L) are strongly suggestive of malabsorption. The 5-hour urinary D-xylose normal values are more than 5 gm/5 hours. It is obviously very important to make sure that urine collection is complete and that there is no fecal contamination of the urine. A catheter may have to be used if the patient is incontinent of urine or if there is a question of fecal contamination, but catheterization should be avoided if at all possible. Two main physiologic circumstances may affect the 5-hour urinary excretion—renal insufficiency and advanced age. There may be abnormally low 5-hour urinary excretion of D-xylose in persons over age 65. However, one study claims that the 24-hour urine collection is normal (also > 5 gm) unless actual malabsorption is present. If the serum creatinine level is borderline or elevated, the 5-hour urinary D-xylose excretion is also likely to be abnormally low, and again the 24-hour excretion may be useful. In these cases, however, the 2-hour blood levels may help, because they should be normal and are not affected by age or renal insufficiency. Otherwise, the 5-hour urinary excretion is more reliable than the blood levels, which tend to fluctuate.

Clinical Correlation.—The D-xylose test may be helpful in determining if the patient has malabsorption and also provides some clues as to etiology. Most patients with cystic fibrosis and pancreatic insufficiency are said to have normal urinary D-xylose values. This is also true of most patients with liver disease. Patients with classic pernicious anemia have normal D-xylose test results, although it must be remembered that many of these patients are aged and for that reason may have low 5-hour urine results. Some patients with megaloblastic anemia of pregnancy have abnormal D-xylose test results, although probably the majority have normal values. A small percentage of patients with partial gastrectomy reportedly have abnormal urine values. Patients with functional diarrhea and duodenal ulcer have normal results.

In malabsorption diseases, there is excellent correlation of D-xylose excretion with proved sprue and celiac disease. The urine results are more often clear-cut than the blood levels. There is no correlation with the degree of steatorrhea. Patients with regional enteritis involving extensive areas of the jejunum may have abnormal results, whereas normal results are associated with this disease when it is localized to the ileum. Patients with Whipple's disease, "blind loop" syndrome (isolated small intestine area of bacterial overgrowth), post-gastrectomy, small intestine lymphoma, multiple jejunal diverticula, and some infants with cow's milk allergy may also have abnormal results. Certain patients with diseases other than classic malabsorption may have an abnormal D-xylose test result. These diseases include myxedema, diabetic neuropathic diarrhea, rheumatoid arthritis, acute or chronic alcoholism, and occasionally severe congestive heart failure. Ascites is reported to produce abnormal urine excretion with normal plasma levels. Although D-xylose excretion is frequently depressed in myxedema, abnormal test results occur in only a small number of patients with the other conditions listed. Some of these conditions can produce decreased absorption of substances other than D-xylose, although such problems are usually mild or moderate in degree and may be due to multiple factors.

D-Xylose tests thus may be abnormal in diseases other than sprue. In nontropical sprue, about 10% of untreated patients have normal D-xylose 5-hour urine test results (literature range, 0%–40%). There is also sufficient overlap in the urine excretion range of 4–5 gm/5 hours from persons without primary small intestine malabsorption to warrant routine collection of a 19-hour urine specimen immediately following the 5-hour specimen (to have a total of 24 hours, if necessary).

Hydrogen Breath Test.—An oral test dose of a specific carbohydrate is administered. If the carbohydrate is not absorbed normally in the small intestine, it reaches the colon, where bacteria metabolize the carbohydrate and release various metabolic products, among which is hydrogen gas. About 15%–20% of the hydrogen is absorbed and then released from the lungs in expired air. Expired air is collected in a single-breath collection bag or other apparatus and analyzed for hydrogen content by some variant of gas chromatography. This technique has been used to test for various types of malabsorption. It has proved most useful in diagnosis of deficiency involving the enzyme lactase (disaccharide malabsorption, discussed in chapter 33), small intestine "blind loop" syndrome, and some cases of rapid intestine transit ("intestinal hurry syndrome"). In the case of the blind loop syndrome or rapid transit, the test dose consists of a carbohydrate that normally is not absorbed. The hydrogen breath test has not proved reliable in diagnosis of sprue or glutin-associated malabsorption.

There are various conditions that interfere with the test. Recent use of antibiotics can affect the bacterial flora, sometimes when discontinued as long as 2 weeks before the test. Use of colon enemas can partially wash out some of the flora. Delayed or unusually swift gastric emptying can change the quantity of the carbohydrate or the time that it reaches the colon. Breath collected during sleep contains two–three times the amount of hydrogen obtained when the patient is awake. Cigarette smoking produces large amounts of hydrogen. Finally, the collection apparatus and the analysis equipment are relatively expensive, and the test is usually available only in larger institutions or medical centers.

Small Intestine Biopsy.—In classic sprue, both tropical and nontropical, the mucosa of the small intestine shows characteristic histologic abnormalities. Instead of the normal monotonous finger-like villous pattern, the villi are thickened and blunted, with flattening of the cuboidal epithelium, and the villi may eventually fuse or disappear altogether. Depending on the degree of change in the villi, biopsy results may show moderate or severe changes. These same changes may be found to a much lesser degree in many of the other conditions causing malabsorption, including even subtotal gastrectomy. However, these usually are not of the severity seen in sprue and generally can be differentiated by the clinical history or other findings. Other causes of malabsorption, such as Whipple's disease (which characteristically shows many periodic acid–Schiff-positive macrophages in the mucosa) may be detected on biopsy. In infants less than 1 year of age, transient small intestinal mucosal abnormalities similar to those of sprue have been reported in some patients with acute gastroenteritis and in some with cow's milk allergy. Eosinophilic gastroenteritis is another cause in older children.

Workup for Possible Malabsorption

This section has considered certain tests for intestinal malabsorption. In the opinion of many gastroenterologists, the most useful tests in initial screening for malabsorption syndromes are the D-xylose, plasma carotene, and qualitative fecal fat. If the results of all these tests are normal, the chances of demonstrating significant degrees of steatorrhea by other means are low. If one or more results are abnormal and confirmation is desirable, it may be necessary to perform a 72-hour fecal fat study.

Once steatorrhea is strongly suspected or established, many investigators proceed to a D-xylose test. If the test is abnormal, many will attempt a small intestine mucosal biopsy, both to confirm a diagnosis of sprue and to rule out certain other conditions such as Whipple's disease. Some prefer a trial period of oral antibiotics to eliminate the possibility of bacterial overgrowth syndrome and then repeat the D-xylose test before proceeding to biopsy. In some centers a biopsy is done without a D-xylose test. If results of the small intestine biopsy are normal, possibilities other than sprue are investigated, such as pancreatic enzyme deficiency and bile salt abnormalities. A trial of pancreatic extract or an endoscopic retrograde cholangiopancreatography examination (chapter 26) to investigate pancreatic or common bile duct status might be considered in these patients. Small intestine x-ray series may demonstrate some of the secondary causes of steatorrhea, such as lymphoma, diverticula, blind loops, and regional enteritis. However, barium may interfere with certain tests, such as stool collection for *Giardia*.

If small intestine biopsy is not available, a therapeutic trial of a gluten-free diet could be attempted. However, this requires considerable time and patient cooperation, and adults with nontropical sprue may respond slowly.

If pernicious anemia is suspected, a Schilling test is the best diagnostic procedure. Bone marrow aspiration could be performed prior to the Schilling test to demonstrate megaloblastic changes, which, in turn, would be useful mainly to suggest folate deficiency if the Schilling test result is normal. It may also reveal coexistent iron deficiency. More widely used than bone marrow aspiration are serum B12 and folic acid (folate) assay.

GASTRIC ANALYSIS

Gastric analysis has two main uses: to determine gastric acidity and to obtain material for exfoliative cytology. I shall discuss only the first here.

When gastric aspiration is performed to determine gastric acidity, the usual purpose is either (1) to determine the degree of acid production in persons with ulcer or ulcer symptoms or (2) to determine if the stomach is capable of producing acid as part of a workup for pernicious anemia. Since passing the necessary large-caliber tube is not met with enthusiasm by the patient, it is important that the physician understand what information can be obtained and be certain that this information is really necessary.

Outdated Gastric Acidity Method.—One problem in evaluating gastric acid secretion data from the literature is the term "achlorhydria," which is often used as a synonym for "anacidity." The classic method of gastric analysis involved titration with 0.1N sodium hydroxide to the end point of Topfer's reagent (pH, 2.9–4.0); this represented "free HCl." Next the specimen was titrated to the end point of phenolphthalein (pH, 8.3–10.0); this represented "total acid." The difference was said to represent "combined acid," thought to consist of protein-bound and weak organic acids but probably including small amounts of HCl. Achlorhydria technically is defined as absence of free acid (pH will not drop below 3.5 on stimulation) but not necessarily complete lack of all acid. True anacidity is absence of all acid, now defined as a pH that does not fall below 6.0 or decrease more than 1 pH unit after maximum stimulation. Therefore, achlorhydria is not the same as anacidity. Nevertheless, the two terms are often used interchangeably. Gastric acidity by the old method was reported in degrees or units; this was the same as milliequivalents per liter. Reference values for total 12-hour gastric secretion were 20–100 ml and for 12-hour total acid content were 10–50 mEq/L (literature range, 2–100 mEq/L).

Currently Recommended Gastric Acidity Procedure.—All authorities today recommend that the old gastric acidity procedure be replaced by a timed collection protocol with results reported in milliequivalents per hour, that is, secretion rate instead of concentration. A 1-hour basal specimen is collected (basal acid output; BAO). Reference values are not uniform but seem most often to be quoted as 1–6 mEq/hour. An acid production stimulant is then injected. Either pentagastrin, betazole (Histolog), or histamine can be used; pentagastrin has the fewest side effects and histamine the most. After injection of the acid stimulant, four 15-minute consecutive specimens are collected (using continuous suction if possible). Maximum acid output (MAO) is the sum of all four 15-minute poststimulation acid collections. Acidity can be measured by titration with the chemical indicator methyl red, but many laboratories now use a pH electrode.

Proper placement of the gastric tube is critical; many recommend assistance by fluoroscopy. Reference values for MAO are less than 40 mEq/hour. The BAO/MAO ratio should be less than 0.3.

Conditions in Which Gastric Analysis is Useful

Diagnosis of Pernicious Anemia.—Presence of acid secretion rules out pernicious anemia. Complete lack of acid secretion after maximum stimulation is consistent with pernicious anemia but may occur in up to 30% of persons over age 70 and occasionally in presumably normal younger persons. If basal secretion fails to demonstrate acid, stimulation is necessary. Alcohol or caffeine stimulation has been used, but since these agents do not produce maximal stimulation of acid production, it would be necessary to repeat the test using pentagastrin, betazole, or histamine if no acid production were found. Therefore, a stronger stimulant, such as pentagastrin, is preferred as the original stimulation agent. Anacidity rather than achlorhydria is the classic gastric analysis finding in pernicious anemia, but, as noted previously, the older term achlorhydria is still being used with the same meaning as anacidity.

Many hematologists perform the Schilling test without preliminary gastric analysis if they suspect pernicious anemia. If the Schilling test produces clear-cut evidence either for or against pernicious anemia, gastric aspiration usually is not necessary. This is especially true if test results are definitely normal, since the greatest technical problem of the Schilling test is incomplete urine collection leading to a falsely low result. If the Schilling test result is equivocal, or if there is some doubt regarding an excretion value suggesting pernicious anemia, gastric aspiration can still be carried out since it is not affected by the Schilling test.

Diagnosis of Gastric Cancer.—Given a known gastric lesion, anacidity after maximum stimulation is strong evidence against peptic ulcer. However, only about 20% of gastric carcinomas are associated with complete anacidity, so gastric analysis in most cases has been replaced by fiberoptic gastroscopy with direct visualization and biopsy of the lesion.

Diagnosis of Zollinger-Ellison Syndrome.—These patients have a gastrin-producing tumor, usually in the pancreas (chapter 32), and typically demonstrate a high basal acid secretion with minimal change after stimulation. Specifically, gastric analysis is strongly suggestive when the BAO is 15 mEq/hour or the BAO/MAO ratio is 0.6 or greater (i.e., BAO is 60% or more of the MAO after maximum stimulation). Some consider a BAO of 10 mEq/hour and a BAO/MAO ratio greater than 0.4 as evidence suggesting a need for further workup so as not to miss a gastrin-producing tumor. About 70% of Zollinger-Ellison patients have a BAO more than 15 mEq/hour (literature range, 50%–82%) as opposed to about 8% of duodenal ulcer patients (literature range, 2%–10%). About 55% of patients with Zollinger-Ellison syndrome (literature range, 35%–75%) have a BAO/MAO ratio higher than 0.6 as opposed to about 2% (literature range, 1%–5%) of duodenal ulcer patients. The definitive diagnostic procedure for gastrinoma is serum gastrin assay. If Zollinger-Ellison syndrome is a possibility, many physicians proceed directly to serum gastrin assay without gastric acid studies.

Diagnosis of Marginal Ulcer.—After partial gastric resection with gastrojejunostomy (Billroth II procedure or one of its variants), abdominal pain or GI bleeding may raise the question of ulcer in the jejunum near the anastomosis. An MAO value above 25 mEq/hour is strongly suggestive of marginal ulcer; one less than 15 mEq/hour is evidence against this diagnosis.

Differentiation of Gastric From Duodenal Ulcer.—Duodenal ulcer patients as a group tend to have gastric acid hypersecretion, whereas gastric ulcer patients most often have normal or even low rates. Patients with gastric ulcer usually have MAO values less than 40 mEq/hour. About 25%–50% of duodenal ulcer patients have MAOs greater than 40 mEq/hour. Conversely, very low acid secretion rates are evidence against duodenal ulcer. Basal secretion greater than 10 mEq/hour is evidence against gastric ulcer.

Determining Type and Extent of Gastric Resection.—Knowing the amount of acid is sometimes helpful in the surgical treatment of duodenal ulcer. Some surgeons prefer to do a hemigastrectomy (removal of one half of the stomach) rather than a subtotal gastrectomy (two-thirds resection) because postoperative complications are fewer with a hemigastrectomy. If the patient is a hypersecretor, the surgeon may add vagotomy to a hemigastrectomy or may perform a subtotal resection to reduce HCl-producing cells or lessen stimulation of those that remain.

Evaluation of Vagotomy Status.—Patients undergoing a surgical procedure that includes bilateral vagotomy may later experience symptoms that might be due to recurrent ulcer or manifest a proved recurrent ulcer. The question then arises whether vagotomy is complete. The

Hollander test employs insulin hypoglycemia (20 units of regular insulin, or 0.1 unit/kg) to stimulate gastric acid secretion through intact vagal nerve fibers. Although disagreement exists on what values are considered normal, most physicians use (1) a BAO less than 2 mEq/hour; and (2) for postinsulin values, either total acid output less than 2 mEq/hour in any 1-hour period or an increase in acid concentration of less than 20 mEq/hour in 2 hours. Most agree that a "positive" response means incomplete vagal section. Interpretation of the "negative" response (failure to secrete sufficient acid under stimulus of hypoglycemia) is more controversial. Antrectomy or partial gastrectomy removes HCl-secreting cells, and a negative response thus could be due either to vagal section or to intact vagus but insufficient total gastric HCl secretory activity.

DIARRHEA

Differential Tests

There are many conditions that produce a chronic diarrhea, which must be differentiated from the relatively common types that last only a few days and usually respond to ordinary treatment (Table 25–2). Diarrhea in infants will not be specifically discussed, since this is a special problem peculiar to that age group.

In patients of all ages with long-term or chronic diarrhea, a stool should be obtained for culture to rule out the presence of *Salmonella* or *Shigella* bacteria. In some areas, *Campylobacter* or *Yersinia* infection might be the etiology. A stool should also be obtained for ova and parasites, with special emphasis on the possibility of amebae or *Giardia* being present. As discussed in chapter 25, chronic diarrhea is one of the two major presenting symptoms of the various malabsorption diseases (anemia being the other). In children, malabsorption is caused either by cystic fibrosis of the pancreas or celiac disease. In adults, the various forms of sprue and, more rarely, some of the secondary malabsorption causes might be considered. In children and young and middle-aged adults, ulcerative colitis is a possibility, especially if there is blood in the stools. This calls for a sigmoidoscopic or colonoscopic examination. In adults over age 40 years, carcinoma of the colon is the cause of diarrhea in a significant number of cases. A barium enema and colonoscopic examination are necessary. In the aged, in addition to carcinoma, fecal impaction is a frequent cause of diarrhea, and this usually can be determined easily by ordinary rectal examination. One study reports that diarrhea is more frequent in patients with serum albumin levels less than 2.5 g/100 ml (25 g/L). In many cases no organic etiology for persistent diarrhea can be found. This situation is often called "functional diarrhea" and is attributed to psychiatric causes. The organic diseases listed here must be ruled out before deciding that a patient has a psychosomatic disorder.

Persons infected by the human immunodeficiency virus I (HIV-I) often develop diarrhea, especially if they progress to the stages of disease known as acquired immunodeficiency syndrome (AIDS) or AIDS-related complex (chapter 16). Common infecting organisms in these patients are *Mycobacterium avium-intracellulare, Salmonella, Cryptosporidium,* cytomegalovirus, *Giardia, Strongyloides stercoralis, and Isospora belli*. However, numerous other organisms have been reported.

TABLE 25–2.
Differential Diagnosis of Diarrhea

Infection—bacterial
- *Salmonella, Shigella, Campylobacter, Yersinia enterocolitica,* enteropathic *Escherichia coli, Clostridium difficile* enterocolitis.

Infection—virus
- Rotovirus

Infection—parasites
- *Giardia lamblia, Entamoeba histolytica*

Ulcerative colitis—regional enteritis

Partial obstruction of colon
- Colon carcinoma
- Fecal impaction

Malabsorption—steatorrhea
- Celiac disease: nontropical sprue, tropical sprue, disaccharide enzyme deficiency

Other
- Diabetic neuropathy
- Zollinger-Ellison syndrome
- Hypoalbuminemia-associated

GASTROINTESTINAL TRACT CANCER

Detection

The most frequent major diseases affecting the GI tract may be divided into benign or malignant and localized to the upper GI tract (stomach and duodenum) or lower GI tract (colon). The major benign disease of the upper GI tract area is peptic ulcer; those of the lower GI tract are diverticulosis and mucosal polyp. The malignant disease usually affecting either area is the same—adenocarcinoma. As a general rule, GI carcinoma is not common in persons under age 40 years (although it can occur) and increases steadily in probability after that age, as do many other types of cancer. The major clinical symptom of peptic ulcer is epigastric pain that occurs between meals and is relieved by food or antacids. Patients with gastric carcinoma may have similar pain, nonspecific pain, or simple gastric discomfort. The major symptom of colon carcinoma is change in bowel habits, either toward chronic diarrhea or constipation. However, either upper or lower GI tract carcinoma may be relatively asymptomatic until very late.

Detection methods for these GI lesions are of three kinds: tests for occult blood in the stool, x-ray examination, and direct visualization.

Stool Occult Blood.—The most useful laboratory screening test is examination of the feces for blood. Usually this blood is occult (not grossly visible), although sometimes it is grossly visible. If it is from the upper GI tract the stool is often black ("tarry"), whereas lower GI bleeding may still show unchanged blood and color the stool red. Anemia of the chronic iron deficiency type is often present, although not always, and sometimes may be severe. Occult blood in the feces can be demonstrated by simple chemical tests for hemoglobin. All are based on peroxidase activity of hemoglobin, which is detected when it catalyzes the oxidation of a color reagent by a peroxide reagent. The most popular test agents are benzidine, guaiac (as powder, tablet, or impregnated filter paper), and orthotolidine. Many studies have been done evaluating one or more of these methods. Results have often been conflicting and, at times, completely contradictory. Nevertheless, some consensus emerges. Benzidine is the most sensitive of the reagents but yields a great number of false positive results. It is currently not available in the United States. Orthotolidine (most commonly in the form of a tablet called Hematest) has intermediate sensitivity, consistently detecting 10–15 ml of blood placed in the stomach experimentally. False positive results (in patients on an unrestricted diet) are most often reported as 20%–30%. Guaiac in powder form provides surprisingly divergent results for different investigators, but the majority report a lesser degree of sensitivity than with Hematest. Guaiac-impregnated filter paper slides have been available since 1966 under various trade names, of which the earliest and best known is Hemoccult. The guaiac-impregnated filter papers are said to be approximately 25% as sensitive as guaiac powder or orthotolidine. Limits of consistent detection (> 90% sensitivity) are variously reported as 6–20 mg of hemoglobin/gm of stool. Some of the discrepancies in the literature may reflect an increase in sensitivity of the newer guaiac-impregnated filter paper tests compared to the older versions. In patients on an unrestricted diet, false positive results are reported in 1%–12% of cases, most being trace or weak reactions. In vitro tests on specimens with added blood in amounts considered to be normal (usually 2 mg of hemoglobin/gm of feces) similarly yields about 10% false positive results.

Interfering Substances.—False positive results may be caused by ingestion of meat that has not been cooked sufficiently to inactivate its peroxidase. Plant material also may contain peroxidase. False negative results may be caused by large doses of ascorbic acid (vitamin C). This is more likely to occur with oral doses more than 500 mg/day. False negative results are frequently caused by bleeding that is intermittent rather than continuous and by blood that is not uniformly distributed within a stool specimen.

Useful Precautions.—Certain precautions must be taken to minimize false positive or false negative reactions and increase detection of true lesions:

1. The patient should be on a meat-free high-residue diet beginning at least 24 hours prior to collections of the stool. Eliminating meat decreases weak false positive reactions. In addition, some investigators advocate preparation and boiling of a fecal suspension to destroy plant peroxidases, although few laboratories do this routinely. Some protocols eliminate any vitamin C intake for at least 48 hours before the test. The diet high-residue component increases detection of significant lesions. If patients must be screened on an unrestricted diet, someone who manifests a weakly

positive result could be restudied on a restricted diet.

2. At least three stool specimens should be collected, each specimen obtained at least 1 day apart but with the collection days as close together as possible. Testing should be performed on two well-separated areas from each specimen, since the blood may not be evenly distributed. A single stool specimen yields about 40%–50% positive results in colon carcinoma, whereas increasing the number of stool specimens to three or more increases sensitivity to approximately 60%–70%.

3. Stool specimens should be tested within 48 hours after collection. Conversion of positive to negative results or vice versa has been reported after storage, although data are conflicting.

Other Guaiac Tests.—Collecting or working with stool specimens has never appealed to most persons. Compliance rates have been low in various stool guaiac programs. It is not unusual for less than 50% of specimen kits distributed to be returned to the laboratory. Several variations of the guaiac method have been devised to improve rates of patient specimen collection. One variant is a guaiac-impregnated paper that is placed in the toilet bowl water with the stool specimen. Water leaching hemoglobin from the outside portions of the stool react with the guaiac reagent in the paper to produce a blue color. Another variant obtains the specimen by wiping the anal area with a special guaiac-impregnated paper system, from which the grossly contaminated portion is discarded and the remaining area tested. Whether these techniques will substantially improve cancer detection awaits adequately controlled clinical trials.

Nonguaiac Stool Tests.—Immunologic tests specific for hemoglobin have been reported but to date have not been widely used due to their relatively high cost and relatively long time needed for assay. An assay method specific for heme called HemoQuant has been developed based on extraction and measurement of porpyrins from hemoglobin in the patient sample. This method also has not yet been widely used, since a measured amount of specimen must first be heated in an acid reagent to extract the porphyrins, purified by extraction with another acid reagent, and then quantitated with a fluorometer.

Other Considerations.—Besides ulcer, polyp, or malignancy, many other conditions affecting the nasopharynx (nasal bleeding) to the anus (hemorrhoids) may produce a guaiac-positive stool. Some of the more common serious conditions include ulcerative colitis, regional enteritis, and diverticulitis.

X-rays.—Radiologic procedures include an upper GI series for stomach and duodenum and a barium enema for the colon. In the upper GI series, the patient swallows a barium mixture, and a series of x-ray films shows this radiopaque material filling the stomach and duodenum. In a barium enema study the barium is washed into the colon through a tube after all feces have been eliminated by laxatives and regular enemas. The major cause of poor barium enema studies is inadequate colon preparation. If feces remain in the colon after cleansing, obviously the barium cannot fill these areas, and small lesions may be missed. Barium enema may be performed by two techniques: regular and air contrast. Air contrast is more sensitive for colon lesions than standard barium enema, especially for polyps, but is somewhat more difficult to perform well and is even more dependent on good preparatory cleansing of the colon.

Direct Visualization Techniques.—Direct visualization techniques include gastroscopy for stomach lesions and proctoscopy, sigmoidoscopy, and fiberoptic colonoscopy for rectal and colon lesions. Proctoscopy examines the anus and rectum. Sigmoidoscopes have two variants: the rigid type permits vision only to 25 cm, whereas the flexible type can reach as high as 40–50 cm. The fiberoptic colonoscope in experienced hands can be used to view almost the entire colon. Biopsy specimens can be obtained at the same time. Simple digital rectal examination detects many rectal and prostate cancers. For this reason, rectal examination is always included as a part of any good physical examination.

Carcinoembryonic Antigen.—Carcinoembryonic antigen is an antigen found in embryonic GI tract epithelium. After serologic tests

TABLE 25–3.
Sensitivity of Tests for Colon Carcinoma*

Procedure	Sensitivity (%)	
Digital rectal examination	15–40	(12–56)
Proctoscopy/sigmoidoscopy	55–65	(47–78)
Barium enema	75–85	(64–94)
Colonoscopy	⩾ 95	
Stool blood (Hemoccult test)	50–65	(33–100)
Single stool specimen	40–50	
Three or more specimens	60–70	
CEA		
All colon carcinomas	65–75	(59–93)
Dukes' A tumors†	20–25	(18–50)

*Numbers in parentheses refer to ranges found in the literature.
†Dukes' A = tumor not penetrating completely through the muscle wall of the colon (corresponds roughly to T2N0 in the TNM tumor stage classification).

were devised using antibodies against extracted CEA, elevated CEA levels were found in many patients with colon cancer, and the test was publicized as a specific and sensitive means of detecting colon adenocarcinoma. Since then, elevated CEA levels have been found in a considerable number of patients with other tumors and various nonneoplastic conditions. A more complete discussion is located in chapter 32. In brief, the test has not proved as useful as was originally hoped. It is much more likely to be positive (elevated level) in larger and more advanced colon carcinomas than in smaller and earlier lesions. Overall sensitivity is recorded in Table 25–3. A positive result does not differentiate colon tumors from those of other primary sites. There is considerable overlap between malignancy and various benign conditions in the area up to four times the upper reference limit (2.5–10 mg/ml, normal being 0–2.5 ng/ml), especially in the area up to twice the upper reference limit (2.5–5 ng/ml). At present, CEA use in colon cancer is limited mostly to follow-up of patients after therapy. A significant and sustained increase in titer suggests recurrence or metastasis. Since the test requires technical expertise and considerable attention to technical details, repeat assay is suggested if one individual value deviates significantly from previous values and major decisions would be based on that value.

Sensitivity of Tests for Colon Cancer

It is important to have some idea of the sensitivity of the various tests available to detect colon cancer, since one must make decisions on the basis of these test results. This information was presented in Table 25–3. In some cases it is difficult to compile accurate data, since a technique (e.g., barium enema) may be carried out by different methods that are not specified in the report. In the case of stool guaiac (as noted previously) there is significant improvement in detection rate when more than one specimen is obtained; this is not adequately reflected in the overall statistics provided by the studies summarized in Table 25–3. Nevertheless, most reports indicate that 20%–30% of colon cancers will be missed with Hemoccult using multiple stool specimens. In fact, at least one investigator concluded that a careful history, emphasizing symptoms commonly associated with colon carcinoma (change in bowel habits toward diarrhea, constipation, or narrowing of the stool; vague abdominal pain; increased flatus or mucous discharge) was at least as sensitive as, if not more than, stool testing for occult blood in raising suspicion of colon cancer.

In summary, rectal examination and stool tests for occult blood are the best simple screening procedures for GI tumor. If these are positive or arouse strong clinical suspicion, one can proceed to x-ray studies of the area indicated. When possible, direct visualization techniques are extremely helpful. Fiberoptic colonoscopy can detect lesions throughout the colon.

Predisposition to Colon Cancer

Certain conditions either predispose to colon cancer or are frequently associated with it. These include age over 40 years; family history of cancer; the syndromes of multiple polyposis, Gardner's syndrome, and Peutz-Jegher's syndrome; and ulcerative colitis present for more than 8 years. The chance of having a second colon cancer simultaneously with one newly discovered is quoted as 1.5%–5%, and the chance of developing a second carcinoma at some time after resection of the first is about 5%–10%.

TESTS FOR GASTRIC BLOOD

Until the middle of the 1980s, there was no commonly accepted method to test for blood in gastric contents. Methods I have personally seen used in different laboratories include urine dipsticks, orthotolidine tablets, and guaiac-impregnated filter paper. Studies have indicated that small numbers of red blood cells (RBCs) are present in most gastric aspirates without clinical evidence of bleeding. These RBCs are often sufficient to produce a reaction with orthotolidine or the urine dipsticks. The guaiac-impregnated filter paper tests used for stool occult blood are less sensitive and also appear to detect clinically significant amounts of blood but were shown to lose sensitivity at pH levels below 3.0 (literature range, 2.5–4.0). In addition, cimetadine, a medication frequently used to decrease gastric acid production, can produce false negative guaiac tests. A new guaiac test introduced in 1985 called Gastroccult is buffered so as to maintain sensitivity down to pH 1.0. In addition, the reagent contains a substance that inhibits plant peroxidase and thereby decreases chances of a false positive result from that source. Also, Gastroccult is not affected by cimetadine. Gastroccult has a sensitivity of approximately 5 mg of hemoglobin/100 ml of gastric contents (equivalent to about 50 μl of whole blood/100 ml of gastric contents), with a detection range in the literature of 30–200 μl of blood/100 ml of diluent. Although there is no consensus regarding the exact amount of gastric blood considered significant, 50 μl/100 ml seems to be acceptable. Ascorbic acid (vitamin C) inhibits both the standard guaiac test and Gastroccult. Large amounts of antacids may also inhibit the test reaction; the manufacturer states that this possibility must be taken into consideration if testing is done within 1 hour after administering the antacid.

BIBLIOGRAPHY

Trier JS: Intestinal malabsorption: Differentiation of cause. *Hosp Pract* 1988; 23(5):195.

Fleming JL, et al: Whipple's disease: Clinical, biochemical, and histopathological features and assessment of treatment in 29 patients. *Mayo Clin Proc* 1988; 63:539.

Levine JJ, et al: Screening tests for enteropathy in children. *Am J Dis Child* 1987; 141:435.

Barry MJ, et al: Effect of workup strategy on the cost-effectiveness of fecal occult blood screening for colorectal cancer. *Gastroenterology* 1987; 93:301.

Gryska PV, et al: The need for total colonoscopy in screening of high risk patients. *Dis Colon Rectum* 1987; 30:18.

Antony MA, et al: Infectious causes of diarrhea in patients with AIDS. *Gastroenterology* 1987; 92:1297.

Brinson RR, Kolts BE: Hypoalbuminemia as an indicator of diarrheal incidence in critically ill patients. *Crit Care Med* 1987; 15:506.

Mastropaolo G, et al: Evaluation of the hydrogen breath test in man: Definition and elimination of the early hydrogen peak. *Gut* 9187; 28:721.

Nilsson-Ehle H, et al: Cyanocobalamin absorption in the elderly. *Clin Chem* 1986; 32:1368.

Hardcastle JD, et al: Fecal occult blood screening for colorectal cancer in the general population. *Cancer* 1986; 58:397.

Feczko PJ, Halpert RD: Reassessing the role of radiology in Hemoccult screening. *AJR* 1986; 146:697.

Aldridge MC, et al: Colonoscopy findings in symptomatic patients without X-ray evidence of colonic neoplasms. *Lancet* 1986; 2:833.

Gelfand DW: Correlative studies reveal efficacy of GI radiology. *Diagn Imag Clin Med* 1986; 8(5):114.

Cacciari E, et al: Can antigliadin antibody detect symptomless coeliac disease in children with short stature? *Lancet* 1985; 1:1469.

Rodney WM, Ruggiero C: The coloscreen self-test for detection of fecal occult blood. *J Fam Pract* 1985; 21:200.

Wardlaw SC, et al: A new sample collecting and testing system for the detection of occult blood in feces. *Conn Med* 1985; 49:151.

Ahlquist DA, et al: Fecal blood levels in health and disease. *N Engl J Med* 1985; 312:1422.

Colebunders R, Van Royen E: The Schilling test. *Mayo Clin Proc* 1984; 59:53.

Rosenthal P, et al: Detection of occult blood in gastric juice. *J Clin Gastroenterol* 1984; 6:119.

Solomans NW: The use of H2 breath-analysis tests in gastrointestinal diagnosis. *Curr Concepts Gastroenterol* 1983; 8:30.

Salom IL: Results of the Schilling test. *Mayo Clin Proc* 1983; 58:839.

Winower SJ: Detection and diagnosis of colorectal cancer. *Cancer* 1983; 51:2519.

Layne EA, et al: Insensitivity of guaiac slide tests for detection of blood in gastric juice. *Ann Intern Med* 1981; 94:774.
Bliss CM: Fat absorption and malabsorption. *Arch Intern Med* 1981; 141:1213.
Simko V: Fecal fat microscopy. *Am J Gastroenterol* 1981; 75:204.
Pettit JE, et al: International Committee for Standardization in Hematology: Recommended methods for the measurement of vitamin B_{12} absorption. *J Nucl Med* 1981; 22:1091.
Toskes PP: Current concepts of cobalamin (vitamin B_{12}) absorption and malabsorption. *J Clin Gastroenterol* 1980; 2:287.
Herbert V: The nutritional anemias. *Hosp Pract* 1980; 15:65.
Bayless TM: Malabsorption in the elderly. *Hosp Pract* 1979; 14:57.

26 Pancreatic Function

The pancreas is an important gastrointestinal (GI) accessory organ and may be involved in disease from both its exocrine and endocrine aspects. Pancreatic enzymes consist mainly of starch-digesting amylase, fat-digesting lipase, and protein-digesting trypsin, as well as bicarbonate and certain other substances. These are secreted through the pancreatic duct, which enters the duodenum close by the common bile duct. Intrinsic diseases of the pancreatic parenchyma or obstruction of the pancreatic duct by tumor and by disease in surrounding areas such as the ampulla of Vater may cause diminution or complete absence of pancreatic secretions and secondarily lead to symptoms from lack of these important digestive enzymes. The diseases of the endocrine system that involve the islands of Langerhans in the pancreas will be discussed in the next chapter.

The most important parenchymal diseases are acute and chronic pancreatitis and carcinoma of the pancreas.

ACUTE PANCREATITIS

Classic acute pancreatitis is manifested by sudden onset of severe epigastric pain (90%–100% of patients) that may radiate elsewhere, often to the back. There may be vomiting (30%–96%), fever (60%–95%), abdominal distention (70%–80%), and paralytic ileus (50%–80%). Jaundice occasionally is present (8%–30%). Hypotension or shock develops in 30%–40% of cases. In severe and classic disease, the diagnosis is frequently obvious; unfortunately, various symptoms found in acute pancreatitis regardless of severity may occur in other diseases as well. In disease of mild or moderate degree or in patients with chronic low-grade or intermittent pancreatitis, symptoms may be vague or atypical. The most common diseases that clinically are confused with acute (or sometimes chronic) pancreatitis are perforated peptic ulcer, biliary tract inflammation or stones, intestinal infarction, and intra-abdominal hemorrhage. Myocardial infarct may sometimes enter the differential diagnosis since the pain occasionally radiates to the upper abdomen; in addition, the aspartate aminotransferase (formerly serum glutamate oxaloacetate transaminase) level may be elevated in more than one half of patients with acute pancreatitis.

Acute pancreatitis is associated with alcohol abuse or biliary tract stones in 60%–90% of cases. A substantial number of patients with acute pancreatitis also have cirrhosis or alcoholic liver disease. Drug hypersensitivity is another factor. Alcohol is thought to be the most common cause of chronic relapsing pancreatitis.

Nonspecific Laboratory Tests

In acute pancreatitis there is some variation in laboratory findings according to the severity of the disease. Mild or moderate leukocytosis with a neutrophil shift to the left is reported in about 80% of patients, more frequently in the more severe cases. Moderate postprandial hyperglycemia or even mild fasting hyperglycemia may be present in about one third of patients (literature range, 10%–66%). There is hyperbilirubinemia (usually mild) in 10%–20% (literature range, 10%–50%), which could be due to biliary tract stones, liver disease, or edema around the ampulla of Vater.

Decreased serum calcium levels may be found in 10%–30% of cases (literature range, 10%–60%). However, since total calcium measurements include both protein-bound and nonprotein-bound (ionized) calcium, since about one half of total calcium is protein-bound, since the protein-bound fraction is predominantly bound to albumin, and since hypoalbuminemia occurs in at least 10% of acute pancreatitis cases, the serum calcium level must be correlated with the serum albumin level. Of course, there could be a coexisting artifactual and actual calcium decrease. When a calcium decrease that is not artifactually caused by hypoalbuminemia occurs, the decrease often appears 3–14 days after onset of symptoms, most frequently on the fourth or fifth day. It is attributed to the liberation of pancreatic lipase into the peritoneal cavity, with resulting digestion of fat and the combination of fatty acids with calcium, which we see grossly as fat necrosis. Again, in very severe disease there may be hemorrhagic phenomena due either to release of proteolytic enzymes such as trypsin into the blood or to release of blood into the abdominal cavity from a hemorrhagic pancreas.

Serum Amylase

In acute pancreatitis, the most commonly used laboratory test is measurement of alpha amylase. Alpha amylase actually has several components (isoenzymes), some derived from the pancreas and some from salivary glands. Clearance from serum takes about 2 hours. A significant portion is cleared via the kidney by glomerular filtration and the remainder (some data indicate > 50%) by other pathways. Serum levels become abnormal 2–12 hours after onset of acute pancreatitis in many patients and within 24 hours in about 85%-90% of cases (literature range, 17%–100%). Those studies reporting less than 75% sensitivity were in a minority and were mostly published before 1975. In most patients the serum amylase level reaches a peak by 24 hours and returns to normal in 48–72 hours. If there is continuing pancreatic cell destruction, the serum amylase level will remain elevated longer in some patients but will return to reference range in others.

Falsely Normal Results.—In certain situations there may be falsely low or normal serum amylase levels. The administration of glucose causes a decrease in the serum amylase level, so that values obtained during intravenous fluid therapy containing glucose may be unreliable, and one should wait at least 1 hour and preferably 2 after the patient has eaten before measuring the serum amylase value. In massive hemorrhagic pancreatic necrosis there may be no serum amylase elevation at all because no functioning cells are left to produce it. Pancreatic destruction of this degree is uncommon, however. Serum lipemia produces artifactual decrease in serum amylase values using most current methodologies. Since hypertriglyceridemia occurs in about 10%–15% of patients with acute pancreatitis (literature range, 5%–38%) and since many laboratories cannot be depended on to recognize the problem or to report the appearance of the serum, the possibility of lipemia should be considered if serum amylase results do not agree with the clinical impression.

Important Causes of Elevated Serum Amylase Levels.—Following is a list of important causes of elevated serum amylase levels.

1. Primary acute pancreatitis or chronic relapsing pancreatitis: idiopathic; traumatic; and pancreatitis associated with alcohol, drug sensitivity (thiazides, furosemide, oral contraceptives, tetracyclines), viral hepatitis, and hyperparathyroidism.
2. Hyperamylasemia associated with biliary tract disease: cholecystitis, biliary tract lithiasis, tumor, spasm of the sphincter of Oddi produced by morphine and meperidine (Demerol) or following biliary tract cannulation.
3. Hyperamylasemia associated with nonbiliary acute intra-abdominal disease: perforated or nonperforated peptic ulcer, peritonitis, intra-abdominal hemorrhage, intestinal obstruction or infarct, and recent abdominal surgery.
4. Nonpancreatic or nonalpha amylase: acute salivary gland disease, and macroamylase.
5. Miscellaneous: renal failure; diabetic ketoacidosis in the recovery phase (41%–80% of cases), pregnancy, cerebral trauma, extensive burns, and cholecystography using radiopaque contrast medium (the contrast medium effect may last up to 72 hours in some cases).

In some instances of biliary tract disease

there is probably a retrograde secondary pancreatitis, in other cases there is release of amylase into the circulation when pancreatic duct obstruction takes place, and in still others there is no convincing anatomical explanation. Likewise, in some cases of acute nonbiliary tract intra-abdominal disease there is a surface chemical pancreatitis; when intestinal obstruction or infarction occurs, there may be escape of intraluminal enzyme, but in other instances no definite cause is found.

Serum amylase levels are elevated in about 10%–15% of patients following abdominal surgery (literature range, 9%–32%). About one half of the cases have been traced to elevation of salivary amylase levels and about one half to elevation of pancreatic amylase levels.

Several studies have reported that serum amylase levels more than five times the upper reference limit are much more likely to be secondary pancreatitis caused by biliary tract disease (cholecystitis or stones in the gallbladder or common bile duct) than by idiopathic or alcoholic acute pancreatitis. However, this is not sufficiently reliable by itself to differentiate primary and secondary pancreatic disease. The serum amylase level is said to be normal in most patients with pancreatic carcinoma, but occasionally some degree of acute pancreatitis may coexist with the tumor.

Patients with poor renal function may have false elevation of serum amylase, pancreatic amylase isoenzyme, lipase, immunoreactive trypsin, and amylase/creatinine clearance ratio. In one study it was reported that a creatinine clearance value of 40 ml/min represented the degree of renal function beyond which false enzyme elevation began to occur. However, regardless of severity of renal failure, some patients had enzyme values that remained within the normal range (60% [literature range, 40%–81%] had elevated amylase and 60% had elevated lipase). One study found that the highest false amylase elevation was 5 times normal (4 times normal in chronic renal failure); for lipase, 6 times normal; and for trypsin, 5.5 times normal. Patients with acute renal failure have higher values than those with chronic renal failure.

Sensitivity and specificity of alpha amylase as a test for acute pancreatitis has varied considerably in reports using different manufacturer's kits and even between investigators using the same kit. As noted previously, the average sensitivity in acute pancreatitis seems to be about 85%–90% (range, 17%–100%), with specificity about 45%–50% (range, 0%–89%). In nonpancreatic diseases with elevated amylase levels, the frequency of elevated values above three times the upper reference limit was about 15% (range, 0%–36%).

Urine Amylase

Urine amylase determination may also be helpful, especially when the serum amylase level is normal or equivocally elevated. Urine amylase usually rises within 24 hours after serum amylase and as a rule remains abnormal for 7–10 days after the serum concentration returns to normal. Various investigators have used 1-, 2-, and 24-hour collection periods with roughly equal success. The shorter collections must be very accurately timed, whereas the 24-hour specimen may involve problems in complete collection. It is important to have the results reported in units per hour. Frequently the values are reported in units/100 ml, which is inaccurate because it is influenced by fluctuating urine volumes. One drawback to both serum and urine amylase determination is their relation to renal function. When renal function is sufficiently diminished to produce serum blood urea nitrogen elevation, amylase excretion also diminishes, leading to mild or moderate elevation in serum amylase levels and a decrease in urine amylase levels.

Amylase/Creatinine Clearance Ratio

Because renal excretion of amylase depends on adequate renal function, amylase urinary excretion correlates with creatinine clearance. In acute pancreatitis, however, there seems to be increased clearance of amylase compared with creatinine. The amylase/creatinine clearance ratio (A/CCR) is based on this observation. Determination of A/CCR involves "simultaneous" collection of one serum and one urine specimen and does not require a timed or complete urine collection. The A/CCR becomes abnormal 1–2 days after elevation of serum amylase levels but is said to remain abnormal about as long as urine amylase. The A/CRR has been the subject of widely discrepant reports. Early investigators found more than 90% sensitivity for acute pancreatitis. Later reports indicated a sensitivity varying from 33%–75%. One great problem in evaluating reports of sensitivity for any biochemical pancreatic function test is the fact that there is no noninvasive perfect way to detect all cases of acute pancreatitis (while at the same time not producing false abnormality due to nonpancreatic disease) against which the various tests may be compared, and even the invasive diagnostic procedures may fail to detect relatively mild disease.

The A/CCR is more specific for pancreatitis than changes in the serum amylase level. Many of the etiologies for hyperamylasemia that do not evoke a secondary pancreatitis are associated with normal A/CCR values. The exact degree of specificity is not yet established; reports have appeared that A/CCR may be elevated in some cases of diabetic ketoacidosis and burns. Behavior in renal failure is variable. In mild azotemia, the A/CCR may be normal, but in more severe azotemia or in uremia sufficient to require dialysis, it may be elevated. In addition, different investigators have adapted different ratio numbers as upper limits of normal, and there have been suggestions that the particular amylase method used can influence results. More data are needed before final conclusions about A/CCR can be made.

Notwithstanding the limitations of the A/CCR previously noted and the ongoing debate in the literature regarding its usefulness, the sensitivity and specificity results for other tests suggest that the A/CCR is probably the most reliable of the readily available tests for acute pancreatitis. However, since there are serious questions about its sensitivity, serum and urine amylase measurements would be helpful if the A/CCR result is within reference limits. The A/CCR formula includes both serum and urine amylase, as follows:

$$\text{A/CCR (in \%)} = \left[\frac{\text{Urine amylase}}{\text{Serum amylase}} \times \frac{\text{Serum creatinine}}{\text{Urine creatinine}}\right] \times 100$$

(All values are in units/100 ml.) Therefore, if the urine amylase specimen is collected as a timed specimen, the urine amylase test result as well as the serum amylase would be available as a single test result. Urine amylase is especially useful since it remains elevated longer than serum amylase and is not affected by macroamylasemia. Poor renal function can be a disruptive factor in all of these tests.

Macroamylase is a macromolecular complex that contains alpha amylase bound to other molecules. Although macroamylase is thought to be uncommon, two studies detected it in 1.1%–2.7% of patients with elevated serum amylase levels. Macroamylase does not pass the glomerular filter but accumulates in serum; if a serum amylase test is performed, the macroamylase will be included in the amylase measurement and may produce an elevated test result. This could simulate pancreatic disease. Since macroamylase does not reach the urine, the urine amylase level is normal or low. The combination of an elevated serum amylase level and a normal or low urine amylase level produces a low A/CCR, and the elevated serum amylase level plus reduced A/CCR has been used to diagnose macroamylasemia. However, in early acute pancreatitis the serum amylase level may be elevated before the urine amylase level becomes elevated. Also, since occasional patients with elevated serum amylase levels due to salivary (rather than pancreatic) amylase may have a reduced A/CCR, macroamylase should be confirmed by special techniques such as selective chromatography. Renal failure introduces an additional source of confusion, since both serum amylase and lipase levels are frequently elevated and the A/CCR may not be reliable. Other hints that an elevated serum amylase level might be due to macroamylase would include a normal serum lipase level and failure of the elevated serum amylase level to decrease significantly over several additional days.

Amylase Isoenzyme Fractionation

Alpha amylase consists of two groups of isoenzymes: pancreatic and salivary. Each group consists of more than one isoenzyme. Separation of serum amylase into its component isoenzymes is possible by selective enzymatic or chemical inhibition or by electrophoresis. In clinical acute pancreatitis, reports indicate that the expected increase in pancreatic-type isoenzymes is observed. In hyperamylasemia without clinical pancreatitis (e.g., may occur during diabetic ketoacidosis or after abdominal surgery), some patients exhibit increased salivary type isoenzymes and others, increased pancreatic type. Pancreatic isoenzyme kits have only recently become commercially available. The majority use an enzyme derived from wheat germ that inhibits salivary isoenzyme. Most evaluations to date found that isoenzyme fractionation was very helpful, especially since the finding of elevated salivary-type isoamylase without the pancreatic type would suggest a nonpancreatic amylase source. Although theoretically the pancreatic-type isoenzyme should be specific for pancreatic origin, a minority of investigators reported relatively frequent elevation of pancreatic-type isoenzyme in several nonpancreatic conditions.

Serum Lipase

The serum lipase level is considered more specific for pancreatic damage than the amylase level. Lipase levels rise slightly later than the serum amylase levels, although usually within 24 hours, and tend to remain abnormal longer, in most instances returning to normal in 7–10 days. Urine lipase assay is not currently used. Evaluation of serum lipase sensitivity and specificity for acute pancreatitis have been subject to the same wide variation as those of serum amylase, with sensitivity averaging about 75%–80% (range, 18%–100%) and with specificity averaging about 70% (range, 40%–99%). In general, the consensus in the literature is that lipase is probably about 10% less sensitive than serum amylase but is about 20%–30% more specific. In those reports that indicated less specificity, lipase elevations were found in many of the same conditions associated with elevated serum amylase. Renal failure is the nonpancreatic condition most frequently associated with elevated serum lipase levels. Lipemia produces falsely decreased serum lipase levels as well as serum amylase levels.

Serum Immunoreactive Trypsin

Several investigators in recent years have developed radioimmunoassay (RIA) procedures for serum trypsin, and at least one manufacturer has a commercial kit available. Trypsin is produced exclusively by the pancreas. In serum a considerable proportion is bound to alpha-1 antitrypsin, and some is also complexed to alpha-2 macroglobulin. Normally the trypsin activity in serum (as measured by current RIA techniques) actually is not trypsin but the trypsin precursor trypsinogen. In acute pancreatic disease there is activation of trypsinogen to form trypsin. Some of the RIA techniques described in the literature measure trypsin bound to alpha-1 antitrypsin as well as trypsinogen, and some do not. None measure trypsin complexed to alpha-2 macroglobulin.

Serum immunoreactive trypsin (SIT) levels are reported to be elevated in 95%–100% of patients with acute pancreatitis or acute exacerbation of chronic pancreatitis. They are also elevated in 80%–100% of patients with renal failure. There are insufficient and conflicting data on SIT behavior in nonpancreatic disorders, with some investigators reporting normal results in patients with cirrhosis and biliary tract disease and others reporting elevation in more than one half of patients with common duct stones and 6%–16% of patients with cirrhosis (the larger incidence being alcoholic cirrhosis). One investigator found elevated values in patients with viral infections such as mumps. In one report 50% of patients with pancreatic carcinoma had elevated values, whereas 19% had subnormal values.

Because only large medical centers or reference laboratories currently offer the test, the time delay necessary for results makes SIT less useful for diagnosing acute pancreatitis.

Endoscopic Retrograde Cholangiopancreatography

As the term implies, endoscopic retrograde cholangiopancreatography (ERCP) entails placing a special side-viewing fiberoptic duodenoscope into the duodenum under fluoroscopic control, finding the ampulla of Vater, cannulating the ampulla, and injecting x-ray contrast media into either the common bile duct or the pancreatic duct, or both. In the case of the pancreas, alterations in pancreatic duct x-ray morphology can suggest acute pancreatitis, chronic pancreatitis, pancreatic carcinoma, and pancreatic cyst. Clear separation of all of these entities from each other is not always possible in every patient. Current consensus is that ERCP is the most sensitive and reliable single procedure to detect clinically significant degrees of pancreatic dysfunction and to establish normal function (this does not take into account minimal or minor degrees of pancreatic disease, since the test depends on alteration of duct structure from abnormality in surrounding parenchyma). It is said to be especially useful when pancreatic ductal surgery or drainage procedures are being considered, in patients with possible traumatic injury to the pancreas, in cases where other diagnostic modalities fail to yield a clear-cut diagnosis, and in cases where strong clinical suspicion of pancreatic disease exists but other modalities are normal.

Disadvantages of ERCP are insensitivity to mild or minimal pancreatic disease as noted previously, the invasiveness of the procedure, the need for very experienced endoscopists and radiologists, and the considerable cost involved. About 10%–20% of attempts fail for various technical reasons. Complications of ERCP are uncommon (< 2%), with sepsis and self-limited episodes of acute pancreatitis being the most frequent problems. There is a transient increase in serum amylase levels after ERCP in about 40% of patients. If there is barium in the GI tract that could obscure x-ray visualization of the pancreatic duct system, ERCP of the pancreas cannot be performed.

Computerized Tomography and Ultrasound

Both computerized tomography (CT) and ultrasound can visualize the pancreas, and both have their enthusiasts. Ultrasound is a little better in very thin persons, and CT is better in obese persons. Both can detect abnormality of the pancreas in about 80%–85% of patients. Neither ultrasound nor CT can always delineate the normal pancreas, although failure is less frequent with newer CT models. In general, in the average hospital CT of the pancreas is easier to perform and interpret than ultrasound. However, ultrasound is generally considered the best procedure for the diagnosis of pancreatic pseudocyst. Both CT and ultrasound depend on focal or generalized gland enlargement, so that small tumors or mild generalized disease are likely to be missed.

CHRONIC PANCREATITIS

Chronic pancreatic insufficiency may occur as a result of pancreatitis or hemochromatosis in adults and in the disease known as cystic fibrosis of the pancreas in children. The diagnosis may be quite difficult, since the disease either represents an end-stage phenomenon with an acute process going on or else may take place slowly and subclinically over a long period. The classic case of chronic pancreatitis consists of diabetes, pancreatic calcification on x-ray study, and steatorrhea. The diagnosis of diabetes will be discussed in the next chapter. Steatorrhea may be demonstrated by quantitative fecal fat studies, as described in chapter 25. Either of these parameters may be normal or borderline in many patients. The sensitivity of this test, and that of other pancreatic function tests, depends on the amount and degree of pancreatic tissue destruction and whether it occurs acutely or in a low-grade fashion.

Tests Useful in Diagnosis of Chronic Pancreatitis

Serum Amylase.—The serum amylase level in chronic pancreatitis is important, although it is much less reliable than in acute disease. In about one half of the patients it is within normal range. Repeated determinations are necessary at intervals of perhaps 3 days. Moreover, the values may be borderline or only slightly elevated, leading to confusion with other causes of elevated amylase levels mentioned previously. In this situation, the urine amylase level or the A/CCR is the most helpful test.

Serum Immunoreactive Trypsin.—Serum immunoreactive trypsin was discussed earlier as a test for acute pancreatitis. In chronic pancreatitis with pancreatic insufficiency there is variation in SIT data, depending on the severity of deficiency. In severely deficient cases 75% or more patients are reported to have decreased SIT values. In mild or moderate cases the values are more often within reference limits. One report indicated decreased values in nearly 40% of childhood diabetics on insulin therapy.

Bentiromide Test.—Bentiromide is a synthetic peptide linked to a *p*-aminobenzoic acid (PABA) molecule. The patient must fast overnight and remain fasting until the test is begun. A control urine specimen is collected just prior to starting the test. A 500-mg test dose of bentiromide is given orally with sufficient food to stimulate the pancreas. After the bentiromide passes into the duodenum, the pancreatic enzyme chymotrypsin splits off the PABA molecule. The PABA is then absorbed into the bloodstream, conjugated in the liver, and excreted by the kidneys as arylamines. The arylamines are assayed in a 6-hour urine collection beginning with the oral dose. Decreased excretion (< 50% of the test dose) suggests decreased absorption from the duodenum, which, in turn, suggests deficient activity of pancreatic chymotrypsin due to decreased pancreatic function. Sensitivity of the test for chronic pancreatitis depends to some extent on the severity of the disease, with greater sensitivity correlating with greater severity. Overall sensitivity appears to be 75%–80% (range, 39%–100%), with specificity about 90% (range, 72%–100%).

Various conditions such as severe liver disease (interfering with conjugation), poor renal function (impaired excretion), malabsorption, incomplete urine collection, diabetes mellitus, previous gastrectomy, and inflammatory bowel disease may produce falsely decreased excretion (false positive test result). Certain medications (acetaminophen, phenacetin, lidocaine, procainamide, sulfas, thiazide diuretics, sunscreens containing PABA, and pancreatic enzyme supplements) may produce false normal results. The baseline (pretest) urine specimen can be tested to exclude presence of exogenous PABA metabolites. If there is a question of diffentiating pancreatic from primary small intestine malabsorption, a D-xylose test can be done.

Endoscopic Retrograde Cholangiopancreatography.—Duodenal intubation using the ERCP technique with injection of x-ray contrast medium into the common bile duct and pancreatic ducts provides useful information about biliary tract stones or pancreatic disease in 61%–81% of cases and may be the only method that can obtain a diagnosis. However, as noted previously, ERCP requires considerable expertise and does not always succeed.

Pancreatic Stimulation Tests.—A tube can be passed into the duodenum with direct assay of pancreatic fluid constituents collected by duodenal tube drainage before and after injection of secretin, the pancreatic stimulating hormone. This procedure used to be considered the best diagnostic test for chronic pancreatitis and still can be useful. However, with the advent of ERCP this test has lost much of its importance. The stimulation tests do not become abnormal until 75% of pancreatic exocrine function is lost.

Other Tests.—As noted previously, the D-xylose test may be useful if the patient has demonstrable steatorrhea. A normal D-xylose result is usually found in pancreatic insufficiency or in cystic fibrosis. Stool examination can be performed in a patient with steatorrhea, with differentiation of neutral fat and fatty acid. Theoretically, in pancreatic insufficiency there should be a large amount of neutral fat but very little fatty acid. Unfortunately, some of the colon bacteria apparently are able to convert neutral fat to fatty acid, so some fatty acids might be present in spite of pancreatic insufficiency in some patients. Presence of undigested meat fibers also suggests abnormal pancreatic function.

CYSTIC FIBROSIS OF THE PANCREAS

A few words should be said about the diagnosis of cystic fibrosis, a hereditary disease carried by a recessive gene. Symptoms usually begin in childhood but may not be manifested until adolescence or occasionally not until adulthood. The disease affects the mucous glands of the body but for some reason seems to affect those of the pancreas more than other organs. The pancreatic secretions become thick and eventually block pancreatic acinar ducts, leading to secondary atrophy of the pancreatic cells. The same process may be found elsewhere, as in the lungs, where inspissated secretions may lead to recurrent bronchopneumonia, and in the liver, where thickened bile may lead to plugging of the small ducts and to a secondary cirrhosis in very severe disease. These patients usually do not have a watery diarrhea, but this is not always easy to ascertain by the history. The diagnosis is made because the sweat glands of the body are also involved in the disease. Although these patients excrete normal volumes of sweat, the sodium and chloride concentration of the sweat is much higher than in normal persons. Cystic fibrosis and its diagnosis are discussed in chapter 33.

Cystic fibrosis in children should be differentiated from celiac disease. Celiac disease is basically the childhood form of the nontropical sprue seen in adults, both of which in many cases seem due to hypersensitivity to gluten. Gluten is found in wheat, oats, and barley and causes both histologic changes and clinical symptoms that are indistinguishable from those of tropical sprue, which is not influenced by gluten. These patients have normal sweat electrolytes, often respond to a gluten-free diet, and behave as ordinary malabsorption syndrome patients.

BIBLIOGRAPHY

Moreau JA, et al: Gallstone pancreatitis and the effect of cholecystectomy. *Mayo Clin Proc* 1988; 63:466.

Royse VL, et al: Pancreatic enzymes in chronic renal failure. *Arch Intern Med* 1987; 147:537.

Ansher AF, et al: Amylase, lipase, isoamylase, and trypsin in patients with renal insufficiency and renal failure. *Gastroenterology* 1987; 92:1296.

Scharpe S, Iliano L: Two indirect tests of exocrine pancreatic function evaluated. *Clin Chem* 1987; 33:5.

Busch M: An oral test of pancreatic function: NBT-PABA. *Pathologist* 1986; 40(6):33.

Lott JL: Assays of serum lipase. *Clin Chem* 1986; 32:1290.

Tietz NW, et al: Laboratory tests in the differential diagnosis of hyperamylasemia. *Clin Chem* 1986; 32:301.

Kleinman DS, O'Brien JF: Macroamylase. *Mayo Clin Proc* 1986; 61:669.

Geokas MC, et al: Acute pancreatitis. *Ann Intern Med* 1985; 103:86.

Steinberg WM, et al: Diagnostic assays in acute pancreatitis. *Ann Intern Med* 1985; 102:576.

Lott JA, et al: Is serum amylase an obsolete test in the diagnosis of acute pancreatitis? *Arch Pathol Lab Med* 1985; 109:314.

Moossa AR: Diagnostic tests and procedures in acute pancreatitis. *N Engl J Med* 1984; 311:639.

Jacobson DG, et al: Trypsin-like immunoreactivity as a test for pancreatic insufficiency. *N Engl J Med* 1984; 310:1307.

Freeny PC, et al: Impact of high resolution computed tomography of the pancreas on utilization of endoscopic retrograde cholangiopancreatography and angiography. *Radiology* 1982; 142:35.

Frey CF, et al: Endoscopic retrograde cholangiopancreatography. *Am J Surg* 1982; 144:109.

Thomas FB: Drug-induced pancreatitis: Facts vs fiction. *Drug Ther* 1982; 12(11):229.

Fahrenkrug J, et al: Immunoreactive trypsin and pancreatic isoamylase activity in serum of patients with chronic renal failure or hepatic cirrhosis. *Clin Chem* 1981; 27:1655.

Silverstein W, et al: Diagnostic imaging of acute pancreatitis. *AJR* 1981; 137:497.

27 Tests for Diabetes and Hypoglycemia

DIABETES

Besides secreting exocrine digestive enzymes into the duodenum, the pancreas has endocrine functions centered in the islands of Langerhans. These structures are found primarily in the tail and body of the pancreas, the hormones involved are glucagon and insulin, and secretion is directly into the bloodstream (Table 27–1). Diabetes mellitus results from abnormality in the production or the utilization of insulin. Production abnormality involves the islet beta cells and can be of two types: deficient beta-cell insulin production, or relatively normal synthesis but abnormal release. Besides production abnormality, diabetes may result from extrapancreatic factors such as peripheral tissue cell receptor dysfunction, producing resistance to the cellular action of insulin, or abnormalities of nonpancreatic hormones that affect insulin secretion or blood glucose metabolism.

Categories

The two types of idiopathic islet cell insulin abnormalities are associated with two of the most important clinical categories of diabetics. The first is the type I, or insulin-dependent, category of the National Diabetes Data Group (NDDG). Type I diabetes usually (but not always) begins relatively early in life and is more severe. Patients require insulin for management and show severe insulin deficiency on blood insulin assay. The second type of diabetes mellitus is the NDDG type II, or noninsulin-dependent diabetes, affecting about 80% of diabetics. Type II diabetes usually (but not always) begins in middle age or afterward, is frequently associated with overweight body status, is associated with less severe blood glucose abnormality, and can be treated by diet alone, oral medication, or small doses of insulin. Some type II persons show significantly elevated or normal insulin production on insulin blood level assay but a decrease in liver and peripheral tissue insulin utilization (insulin resistance). Others have varying degrees of decreased insulin production, although usually not as severe as the insulin deficiency of textbook type I diabetics.

There is a small subgroup of teen-aged diabetics who have disease resembling type II adult diabetes. There are also a few adult diabetics with type II disease who are not overweight, and a small subgroup of adult diabetics who have disease resembling type I.

The NDDG has two other categories of diabetics. The first group is associated with various nonidiopathic conditions and syndromes ("secondary diabetes") that either destroy pancreatic tissue (pancreatitis, pancreatic carcinoma, hemochromatosis) or produce abnormal glucose tolerance due to various extrapancreatic influences such as hormones, drugs, and insulin receptor abnormalities. The second category is gestational diabetes, diabetes that begins in pregnancy.

Laboratory Tests

Most laboratory tests for diabetes attempt to demonstrate pancreatic islet cell malfunction, either deficient insulin production or ab-

TABLE 27–1.
Cell Types in Pancreatic Islets of Langerhans

Cell Type	Hormone
A	Glucagon
B	Insulin
D	Somatostatin
F	Vasoactive intestinal polypeptide
G	Gastrin

normal insulin release, using either direct or indirect blood insulin measurement. For many years direct blood insulin measurement was technically too difficult for any but a few research laboratories. Therefore, emphasis in clinical medicine was placed on indirect methods, whose end point usually demonstrated the action of insulin on a relatively accessible and easily measurable substance, blood glucose. Radioimmunoassay (RIA) methods for insulin measurement are now commercially available. However, in most cases direct insulin assay has not proved more helpful than blood glucose measurement in the diagnosis of diabetes, since in general the quantitative result and the pattern of blood glucose values permit one to separate diabetics into the two basic type I and type II groups with a reasonable degree of accuracy. In addition, blood glucose measurement is far less expensive, more readily available, and less technically demanding than current RIA methods.

For reasons already noted, blood glucose measurement is still the mainstay for diagnosis of diabetes. Unfortunately, certain flaws are inherent in all systems using blood glucose for this purpose. These problems derive from any technique that attempts to assay one substance by monitoring its action on another. Ideally, one should measure a substrate that is specific for the reaction or enzyme in question under test conditions that eliminate the effects on utilization by any other factors. The blood glucose level does not meet any of these criteria.

Blood Glucose Regulation

The blood glucose level depends primarily on the liver, which exerts its effect on blood glucose homeostasis via its reversible conversion of glucose to glycogen, as well as via gluconeogenesis from fat and protein. Next most important is tissue utilization of glucose, which is mediated by pancreatic insulin but is affected by many factors in addition to insulin.

The actual mechanisms involved in the regulation of blood glucose levels are complex and in many cases only partially understood. Insulin is thought to increase glucose transport into cells of most tissues (except red blood cells (RBCs) and possibly brain and intestinal mucosa) and to stimulate glucose oxidation and synthesis of fat, glycogen, and protein. In addition, insulin has a direct effect on the liver by suppressing glucose formation from glycogen (glycogenolysis).

The liver is affected by at least three important hormones: epinephrine, glucagon, and hydrocortisone (cortisol). Epinephrine from the adrenal medulla stimulates breakdown of glycogen to glucose by converting inactive hepatic cell phosphorylase to active phosphorylase, which mediates the conversion of glycogen to glucose-1-phosphate. In addition, there is evidence that gluconeogenesis from lactate is enhanced by the action of the enzyme adenosine 3,5-monophosphate. Glucagon is a hormone produced by the pancreatic alpha cells and released by the stimulus of hypoglycemia. It is thought to act on the liver in a manner similar to that of epinephrine. Cortisol, cortisone, and similar 11-oxygenated adrenocroticosteroids also influence the liver but in a different manner. One fairly well-documented pathway is enhancement of glycogen synthesis from amino acids. This increases the carbohydrate reserve available to augment blood glucose levels; thus, steroids like cortisol essentially stimulate gluconeogenesis. In addition, cortisol deficiency leads to anorexia and also causes impairment of carbohydrate absorption from the small intestine.

Methods of Blood Glucose Assay

The technique of blood glucose determination must be considered because different methods vary in specificity and sensitivity to glucose. The blood specimen itself is important; according to several reports (and my own experience), during each hour of standing at room temperature, whole blood glucose values decrease about 10 mg/100 ml unless a preservative is added. Fluoride is considered the best preservative at present. Plasma and serum are more stable than whole blood. If serum can be removed from the cells before 2 hours, serum glucose values remain stable for up to 24 hours at room temperature (although some authors report occasional decreases). Refrigeration assists this preservation. Serum or plasma values are 10%–15% higher than those of whole blood. Most present-day automated equipment uses serum. Venous blood is customarily used for glucose measurement. Capillary (arterial) blood values are about the same as those for venous blood when the patient is fasting. Nonfasting capillary values, however, average about 30 mg/100 ml (1.6 mmol/L) higher than venous blood, and this difference may sometimes be as great as 100 mg/100 ml (5.55 mmol/L).

Biochemical Methods.—There are a considerable number of methods for blood glucose determination. These may be conveniently categorized as nonspecific reducing substance methods, which yield values significantly above true glucose values (Folin-Wu manual method and neocuproine SMA 12/60 automated method); methods that are not entirely specific for glucose but that yield results fairly close to true glucose values (Somogyi-Nelson, orthotoluidine, ferricyanide); and methods using enzymes that are specific for true glucose (glucose oxidase and hexokinase). There are certain technical differences and interference by certain medications or metabolic substances that account for nonuniformity of laboratory methodology and that in some instances may affect interpretation (see Table 36–22). Reference values mentioned in this chapter are for serum and for true glucose unless otherwise specified.

Paper Strip Methods.—Another test for glucose consists of rapid quantitative paper strip methods (Dextrostix, Visidex, Chemstrip-BG, and others) available from several manufacturers. A portion of the paper strip is impregnated with glucose oxidase, an enzyme specific for glucose, plus a color reagent. One drop of whole blood, plasma, or serum is placed on the reagent area, and the color that develops is compared with a reference color chart. Visidex has two reagent areas that correspond to low- and high-glucose value areas. Small electronic readout meters are available for several of the manufacturer's paper strips. The meters have generally been reported to make a substantial improvement in accuracy. Evaluations of the various paper strip methods provide a consensus that, with experience and with the use of a readout meter, experiments using quality control material or glucose solutions generally agree with standard laboratory methods within about ± 5%. Using actual patient fingerstick capillary blood specimens, values between 40 and 130 mg/100 ml (2.2–7.2 mmol/L) usually agree within about ± 15% (range, 8%–40%) with values obtained by standard laboratory methods. Persons without much familiarity with the technique may obtain more erratic results. These paper strip methods have been used with venous whole blood or finger puncture blood as a fast way to diagnose hypoglycemia and hyperglycemia in comatose or seriously ill persons and to provide guidance for patient self-adjustment of insulin dosage at home.

Some cautions include possible differences between capillary (finger puncture) blood and venous blood values, alluded to previously, and effects of hematocrit on results, since blood with a low hematocrit (< 35%) produces a higher result, whereas blood with a high hematocrit (> 55%) produces a lower result. This creates a special problem with newborns, who normally have a high hematocrit compared to adults. Also, evaluation of methods by using glucose solutions may not accurately predict results using patient blood specimens. Very high serum levels of ascorbic acid (vitamin C) or gross lipemia may interfere. Patients with hyperosmolar hyperglycemia, with or without ketosis, may show test strip results that are lower than true values.

Glucose Tolerance Test

The diagnosis of diabetes is made by demonstrating abnormally increased blood glucose values under certain controlled conditions. If insulin deficiency is small, abnormality is noted only when an unusually heavy carbohydrate load is placed on the system. In uncompensated insulin deficiency, fasting glucose is abnormal; in compensated insulin deficiency, a variety of carbohydrate tolerance test procedures are available to unmask the defect. To use and interpret these procedures, one must thoroughly understand the various factors involved.

Glucose tolerance tests (GTTs) are provocative tests in which a relatively large dose of glucose challenges the body homeostatic mechanisms. If all other variables are normal, it is assumed that the subsequent rise and fall of the blood glucose is due mainly to production of insulin in response to hyperglycemia and that the degree of insulin response is mirrored in the behavior of the blood glucose. Failure to realize that this assumption is predicated on all other variables being normal explains a good deal of the confusion that exists in the literature and in clinical practice.

Test Standardization

The most important factor in the GTT is the need for careful standardization of the test procedure. Without these precautions any type of GTT yields such varied results that an abnormal response cannot be interpreted. Previous carbohydrate intake is very important. If diet has been low in both calories and carbohydrates for as little as 3 days preceding the test, glucose tolerance may be diminished temporarily and the GTT may shift more or less toward diabetic levels. This has been especially true in starvation, but the situation does not have to be this extreme. Even a normal caloric diet that is low in carbohydrates may influence the GTT response. A preparatory diet has been recommended that includes approximately 300 gm of carbohydrates/day for 3 days preceding the test, although others believe that 100 gm for each of the 3 days is sufficient. The average American diet contains approximately 100–150 gm of carbohydrates; it is obviously necessary in any case to be certain that the patient actually eats at least 100 gm/day for 3 days.

Factors That Affect the Glucose Tolerance Test

Inactivity has been reported to have a significant influence on the GTT toward the diabetic side. One study found almost 50% more diabetic GTT responses in bedridden patients compared with ambulatory patients identical in most other respects. The effect of **obesity** is somewhat controversial. Some believe that obesity per se has little influence on the GTT. Others believe that obesity decreases carbohydrate tolerance; they have found significant differences after weight reduction, at least in obese mild diabetics. **Fever** tends to produce a diabetic-type GTT response; this is true regardless of the etiology but more so with infections. **Diurnal variation** in glucose tolerance has been reported, with significantly decreased carbohydrate tolerance during the afternoon in many persons whose GTT curves were normal in the morning. This suggests that tests for diabetes should be done in the morning. **Stress,** when severe, results in release of various hormones (e.g., epinephrine and possibly cortisol and glucagon), which results in decreased glucose tolerance. **Acute myocardial infarction, trauma, burns, and similar conditions** frequently are associated with transient postprandial hyperglycemia and occasionally with mild fasting hyperglycemia. This effect may persist for some time. It has been recommended that definitive laboratory testing for diagnosis of diabetes be postponed for at least 6 weeks. However, if the fasting blood glucose (FBG) level is considerably elevated and there is substantial clinical evidence of diabetes, the diagnosis can be made without additional delay.

There is a well-recognized trend toward a decreasing carbohydrate tolerance with **advanced age.** Although the degree of abnormality is not enough to affect the FBG normal range, glucose tolerance curve upper limits in clinically normal persons increase about 1 mg/100 ml/year beyond age 50. There are three schools of thought as to the interpretation of this fact. One group believes that effects of aging either unmask latent diabetes or represent true diabetes due to impairment of islet cell function in a manner analogous to subclinical renal function decrease through arteriosclerosis. Another group applies arbitrary correction formulas to decrease the number of abnormalities to a predetermined figure based on estimates of diabetes incidence in the given population. A third group, representing the most widely accepted viewpoint, regards these changes as physiologic rather than pathologic. In fact, to avoid labeling many elderly persons diabetic who have no other evidence of diabetes, some experts used to deliberately extend the upper limits of the oral GTT (OGTT) reference range by adding 1 mg/100 ml for each year over age 50 to the acceptable reference limit for each point on the OGTT curve (not including the fasting value). The NDDG diabetes criteria (discussed later) incorporate some of this shift of the reference range.

The question arises occasionally as to what serum glucose values are normal when a patient is receiving intravenous 5% dextrose. In 20 patients at our hospital who had no evidence of disease known to affect serum glucose, values ranged from 86–232 mg/100 ml (4.74–12.78 mmol/L), with a mean value of 144 mg/100 ml.

Oral Glucose Tolerance Test

The OGTT is more reliable when the patient is ambulatory and does not have other severe acute or chronic illnesses. The test should be preceded by at least 3 days of adequate carbohydrate diet and should be performed in the morning after the patient has fasted at least 10 hours (but no longer than 16 hours). The test dose has been standardized by the NDDG at 75 gm of glucose or dextrose for nonpregnant persons and 100 gm for pregnant women. The dose may be calculated from body weight. Various ready-made commercial preparations can be used, or the dose can be given in up to 300 ml of water, usually flavored with a substance such as lemon juice. The dose should be consumed by the patient within 5 minutes. The test officially begins when the patient begins to drink. The NDDG recommends that the patient should remain seated during the test and should not smoke. One should also beware of medication that could affect test results, such as oral contraceptives, steroids, diuretics, and anticonvulsants.

Test Protocol.—Blood specimens are taken fasting, then 0.5, 1, 2, and 3 hours after dextrose ingestion. After ingestion of the test dose, a lag period occurs, after which the blood glucose curve rises sharply to a peak, usually in 15–60 minutes. In one study, 76% had maximal values at 30 minutes and 17% at 1 hour. The curve then falls steadily but more slowly, reaching normal levels at 2 hours. These may be fasting values or simply within normal blood glucose ranges.

Occasionally, after the fasting level is reached, there may follow a transient dip below the fasting level, usually not great, then a return to fasting values. This relative hypoglycemic phase of the curve (when present) is thought to be due to a lag in the ability of the liver to change from converting glucose to glycogen (in response to previous hyperglycemia) to its other activity of supplying glucose from glycogen. In some cases, residual insulin may also be a factor. This "hypoglycemic phase," if present, is generally between the second and fourth hours. Several reports indicate that so-called terminal hypoglycemia, which is a somewhat exaggerated form of this phenomenon, occurs in a fairly large number of patients with a GTT response indicative of mild diabetes. They believe that an abnormally marked hypoglycemic dip often appears in mild diabetics 3–5 hours after meals or a test dose of carbohydrates and may be one of the earliest clinical manifestations of the disease.

Flat OGTT.—This is an OGTT the peak of which has been defined variously as less than 40 mg, 25 mg, or 20 mg/100 ml above the FBG value. The most commonly used definition is 25 mg/100 ml (1.38 mmol/L). The condition most frequently associated with a flat OGTT is small intestinal carbohydrate malabsorption due to sprue or celiac disease, with a lesser number of cases seen in myxedema and some cases reported in pituitary insufficiency. Flat OGTT results may also occur in clinically normal persons. When the 40 mg definition was used, one study reported a flat OGTT in 90% of patients with sprue, but also in up to 40% of clinically normal persons. When the 25 mg definition was used, another study reported a flat OGTT in about 60% of patients with sprue. Using the 20 or 25 mg definition, several investigators found a flat OGTT result in about 20% of clinically normal persons (range, 7%–25%).

Oral Glucose Tolerance Test Interpretation.—In the past, criteria for interpretation of the OGTT have varied widely. This situation is brought about because of the absence of a sharp division between diabetics and nondiabetics, variations in methodology, and variations in adjustment for the many conditions that may affect the GTT quite apart from idiopathic diabetes mellitus; some of these factors have been mentioned previously, and others will be discussed later. The NDDG criteria are rapidly replacing previous criteria as world-recognized standards (other previously widely used criteria are listed in Table 36–23) . The NDDG criteria are listed in Table 27–2. All values are for venous serum or plasma in milligrams per 100 ml using true glucose methods unless otherwise stated.

The NDDG has permitted a diagnosis of diabetes mellitus to be made in any one of three different ways:

1. Sufficient classical symptoms of diabetes mellitus (e.g., polydipsia, polyuria, ketonuria, and weight loss) plus either an unequivocal elevation of the FBG level or an elevation of the non-FBG level greater than 200 mg/100 ml (11.1 mmol/L).

2. Elevation of the FBG level (venous serum or plasma) greater than 140 mg/100 ml (7.8 mmol/L) on more than one occasion (assuming no condition is present that falsely increases blood glucose values).

3. A normal FBG level but OGTT peak and 2-hour values both greater than 200 mg/100 ml on more than one occasion.

Three points should be noted. First, the diagnosis of diabetes can be made in nonpregnant adults if typical clinical symptoms are present plus a nonfasting serum specimen more than 200 mg/100 ml. Second, the diagnosis can be made without requiring a GTT if the FBG level is sufficiently elevated. Third, when the diagnosis is based predominantly on blood glucose measurement, either the FBG level or the OGTT, diagnosis requires sufficient abnormality on 2 different days rather than only one occasion.

Oral Glucose Tolerance Test Criteria for Children.—In children, criteria for diagnosis of diabetes mellitus are rather similar to those of nonpregnant adults, but there are a few significant differences. First, the upper limit of the FBG reference range is set at 130 mg/100 ml (7.2 mmol/L) instead of the nonpregnant adult upper limit of 115 mg/100 ml (6.4 mmol/L). However, FBG values necessary for diagnosis of diabetes are the same for children and adults (140 mg/100 ml; 7.8 mmol/L). Second, the glucose dose for children is calculated on the basis of patient weight (1.75 gm/kg of ideal weight to a maximum of 75 gm). Third, elevation of the FBG level alone is not sufficient in children. The FBG level must be more than 140 mg/100 ml (7.8 mmol/L) and either the peak or the 1-hour value must be more than 200 mg/100 ml (11.1 mmol/L) (if the FBG level is normal, both the peak and the 2-hour value must be more than 200 mg/100 ml, which is the same requirement listed for adults).

Impaired Glucose Tolerance.—The NDDG recognizes a category of OGTT curve that it calls impaired glucose tolerance, which is abnormal but not sufficiently abnormal to make a diagnosis of diabetes Table 27–3). This involves an FBG level less than 140 mg/100 ml and a single point on the OGTT curve above 200 mg/100 ml (either the peak or the 2-hour value greater than 200 mg/100 ml but not both).

Gestational Diabetes

The NDDG definition of gestational diabetes is abnormal glucose tolerance with onset or recognition during pregnancy. After the end of pregnancy, the patient should be retested using the standard nonpregnant OGTT with standard nonpregnant NDDG criteria and reclassified into previous abnormal glucose tolerance (if the postpartem standard nonpregnant OGTT result is normal); impaired glucose tolerance (if the standard nonpregnant OGTT result is abnormal but not sufficiently abnormal to fit the NDDG criteria for diabetes); or diabetes mellitus. The American Diabetes Association (1986) recommends that pregnant women who are not known to have abnormal

TABLE 27–2.

National Diabetes Data Group Criteria for Diagnosis of Diabetes Mellitus in Nonpregnant and Pregnant Adults*

OGTT	Serum (mg/100 ml) Normal	Serum NGDM†	Serum GDM‡	Whole Blood (mg/100 ml) Normal	Whole Blood NGDM†	Whole Blood GDM‡
Fasting	70–115	(≥ 140)	≥ 105	60–100	≥ 120	≥ 90
Peak (0.5–1.5 hr)	< 200	≥ 200	≥ 190	< 180	≥ 180	≥ 170
2 hr	< 140	≥ 200	≥ 165	< 120	≥ 180	≥ 145
3 hr	70–115	—	≥ 145	60–100	—	≥ 125

*NGDM = nongestational diabetes mellitus; GDM = gestational diabetes mellitus.
†The serum FBG level is ≥ 140 mg/100 ml. If the serum FBG level is < 140 mg/100 ml, both the peak and the 2-hr value must be ≥ 200 mg/100 ml (75-gm glucose dose).
‡Two GTT curve values must be diabetic (100-gm glucose dose).

TABLE 27–3.

National Diabetes Data Group Classification of Glucose Tolerance Abnormalities

New (NIH-NDDG) Classification		Old Classification	
Diabetes mellitus (DM)	Unequivocal clinical signs or symptoms and/or FBG test or OGTT result diagnostic of DM	Overt diabetes	FBG level usually abnormal; clinical symptoms present
Impaired GTT	FBG level normal; *either* OGTT peak *or* 2-hr value (but not both) > 200.	Latent (chemical) diabetes	OGTT result abnormal; FBG level normal or abnormal; no clinical symptoms
Previous abnormality of glucose tolerance	Normal OGTT result, but previous abnormal GTT level or hyperglycemia, known or unknown cause	Subclinical diabetes	Cortisone GTT result abnormal; OGTT result normal
Potential abnormality of glucose tolerance	All laboratory test results normal; genetic predisposition to DM	Prediabetes	All laboratory test results normal; genetic predisposition to DM
Gestational DM*	Onset of unequivocal DM and/or OGTT results exceeding special pregnancy criteria	Diabetes of pregnancy	Onset of diabetes during pregnancy; clinical signs or symptoms of DM and/or abnormal OGTT result

*Should be retested and possibly reclassified after end of pregnancy.

glucose tolerance should be screened between the 24th and 28th week with a test dose of 50 gm of oral glucose (fasting or nonfasting) and a single postdose 1-hour venous plasma specimen. A 1-hour value of 140 mg/100 ml (7.8 mmol/L) or more suggests the need for the full NDDG gestational OGTT.

Screening Tests for Diabetes

Screening tests for diabetes attempt to circumvent the multiple blood glucose determinations required for the GTT. The FBG level and the 2-hour postprandial (2 hours after a meal) or blood glucose level have been widely used. Since these essentially are isolated segments of the GTT curve, interpretation of their results must take several problems into consideration in addition to those inherent in the GTT.

An abnormality in the FBG level for example, raises the question of whether a full GTT is needed for confirmation of diabetes. Most authorities, including the NDDG panel, believe that if the FBG level is sufficiently elevated, there is no need to do the full GTT. Whatever the etiology of the abnormal FBG level, the GTT result will also be abnormal. Since it is known in advance that the GTT result will be abnormal, no further information is gained from performing the GTT. Most also agree that a normal FBG value is not reliable in ruling out possible diabetes. In one study, 63% of those with diabetic GTT results had normal FBG values. Others have had similar experiences, although perhaps with less striking figures.

Most investigators believe that of all the postprandial GTT values, the 2-hour level is the most crucial. The 2-hour value alone has therefore been proposed as a screening test. This recommendation is based on the fact that with a normal FBG level, the diagnosis of diabetes mellitus cannot be made with confidence on the basis of an abnormal peak blood glucose level if it is accompanied by a normal 2-hour blood glucose level in the OGTT. The main reason for this lies in the effect of gastric emptying on glucose absorption. It has been fairly well proved that normal gastric emptying does not deliver a saturation dose to the duodenum. Therefore, slow gastric emptying tends to produce a low, or "flat," GTT curve. On the other hand, either unusually swift gastric transit or delivery of a normal total quantity of glucose to the small intestine within a markedly shortened time span results in abnormally large amounts of glucose absorbed during the initial phases of the tolerance test. Since homeostatic mechanisms are not instantaneous, the peak values of the tolerance curve reach abnormally high figures before the hyperglycemia is brought under control. An extreme example of this situation occurs in the "dumping syndrome" produced by gastrojejunostomy.

If previous time interval specimens are considered unreliable, the question then is justified as to whether the 2-hour value alone is sufficient for diagnosis of diabetes. According to the NDDG criteria, both the peak level and the 2-hour level must be greater than 200 mg/100 ml (11.1 mmol/L), so that a full GTT is necessary, even though it is uncommon to find a 2-hour value more than 200 mg/100 ml and a peak value less than 200 mg/100 ml. The NDDG recommendation may be based on reports that one variant of the normal OGTT drops relatively swiftly to normal at approximately 1.5 hours and then rebounds above 140 mg/100 ml (7.8 mmol/L) by 2 hours. In one report this phenomenon occurred in as many as 5%–10% of patients.

Glucose Tolerance in Other Diseases

Besides the intrinsic and extrinsic factors that modify response to the OGTT, other diseases besides diabetes mellitus regularly produce diabetic-type GTT patterns or curves. Among these are adrenal, thyroid, and pituitary hormone abnormalities that influence liver or tissue response to blood glucose levels. **Cushing's syndrome** results from hypersecretion of hydrocortisone. Since this hormone stimulates gluconeogenesis among its other actions, 70%–80% of patients with Cushing's syndrome exhibit decreased carbohydrate tolerance, including 25% who exhibit overt diabetes. One report suggests that patients with gestational diabetes who are in the third trimester have fasting plasma cortisol levels higher than those of nonpregnant women. **Pheochromocytomas** of the adrenal medulla (or elsewhere) have been reported to produce hyperglycemia in nearly 60% of affected patients and glucosuria in a lesser number. These tumors produce norephinephrine or epinephrine, either continually or intermittently. The diabetogenic effects of epinephrine were mentioned earlier, and it has been noted that pheochromocytomas that secrete norepinephrine rather than epinephrine are not associated with abnormalities of carbohydrate metabolism. **Primary aldosteronism** leads to the overproduction of aldosterone, the chief electrolyte-regulating adrenocortical hormone. This increases renal tubular excretion of potassium and retention of sodium. Patients with primary aldosteronism frequently develop decreased carbohydrate tolerance. According to Conn, this is most likely due to potassium depletion, which in some manner adversely affects the ability of pancreatic beta cells to respond normally to a hyperglycemic stimulus. Parenthetically, there may be some analogy in reports that **chlorothiazide diuretics** may cause added decrease in carbohydrate tolerance in diabetics, thus acting as diabetogenic agents. Some say that no such effect exists without some degree of preexisting glucose tolerance abnormality, but others maintain that it may occur in a few clinically normal persons. Chlorothiazide often leads to potassium depletion as a side effect; indeed, one report indicates that potassium supplements will reverse the diabetogenic effect. However, other mechanisms have been postulated.

Thyroid hormone has several effects on carbohydrate metabolism. First, thyroxine acts in some way on small intestine mucosal cells to increase hexose sugar absorption. In the liver, thyroxine causes increased gluconeogenesis from protein and increased breakdown of glycogen to glucose. The metabolic rate of peripheral tissues is increased, resulting in an increased rate of glucose utilization. Peripheral tissue glycogen is depleted. Nevertheless, the effect of **hyperthyroidism** on the GTT is variable. Apparently the characteristic hyperthyroid curve is one that peaks at an unusually high value, sometimes with glucosuria, but that returns to normal ranges by 2 hours. However, in one extensive survey, as many as 7% of hyperthyroid patients were reported to have diabetic curves, and another 2% had actual diabetes mellitus. Surprisingly, the type of curve found in any individual patient was not related to the severity of the hyperthyroidism. In **myxedema,** a flat OGTT curve (defined as a peak rise of < 25 mg/100 ml [1.4 mmol/L] above the FBG value) is common. However, since absorption defects vary in degree and are counterposed against decreased tissue metabolism, one investigator reported that 50% of hypothyroid patients tested had a diabetic type of OGTT curve with the FBG value usually normal.

Acromegaly is reported to produce an elevated FBG level in 25% of cases and a diabetic OGTT curve in 50% of cases. Growth hormone (somatotropin) is thought to be able to stimulate gluconeogenesis independently. Actually, the influence of the pituitary on carbohydrate metabolism has been mainly studied in conditions of pituitary hypofunction; in hypopituitarism, a defect in gluconeogenesis was found that was due to a combination of thyroid and adrenocorticosteroid deficiency rather than to deficiency of either agent alone.

In **acute pancreatitis,** perhaps 25%–50% of patients may have transient hyperglycemia. In chronic pancreatitis, abnormal glucose tolerance or outright diabetes mellitus is extremely common.

A variety of nonendrocrine disorders may produce diabetogenic effects on carbohydrate tolerance. **Chronic renal disease with azotemia** frequently yields a diabetic curve of varying degree, sometimes even to the point of fasting hyperglycemia. The reason is not definitely known. Hyperglycemia with or without glucosuria occurs from time to time in patients with **cerebral lesions,** including tumors, skull fracture, cerebral infarction, intracerebral hemorrhage, and encephalitis. The mechanism is not known, but experimental evidence suggests some type of center with regulatory influence on glucose metabolism located in the medulla and the hypothalamus, and perhaps elsewhere. Similar reasoning applies to the transient hyperglycemia, sometimes accompanied by glucosuria, seen in severe **carbon monoxide poisoning.** This is said to appear in 50% of these patients and seems to be due to a direct toxic effect on the cerebral centers responsible for carbohydrate metabolism. **Type IV lipoproteinemia** (chapter 21) is frequently associated with some degree of decreased carbohydrate tolerance, which sometimes may include fasting hyperglycemia.

Malignancies of varying types are reported to produce decreased carbohydrate tolerance in varying numbers of patients, but the true incidence and the mechanism involved are difficult to ascertain due to the presence of other diabetogenic factors such as fever, cachexia, liver dysfunction, and inactivity.

Liver disease often affects the OGTT response. This is not surprising in view of the importance of the liver in carbohydrate homeostasis. Abnormality is most often seen in cirrhosis; the degree of abnormality has a general (although not exact) correlation with degree of liver damage. In well-established cirrhosis, the 2-hour postprandial blood glucose level is usually abnormal. The FBG level is variable but is most often normal. Fatty liver may produce GTT abnormality similar to that of cirrhosis. In hepatitis virus infection there is less abnormality than in cirrhosis; results become normal during convalescence and may be normal at all times in mild disease.

Acute myocardial infarction has been shown to precipitate temporary hyperglycemia, glucosuria, or decreased carbohydrate tolerance. In one representative study, 75% of patients had abnormal GTT responses during the acute phase of infarction, with 50% of these being frankly diabetic curves; follow-up showed that about one third of the abnormal curves persisted. Besides the well-known increased incidence of atherosclerosis (predisposing to infarction) in overt or latent diabetics, emotional factors in a stress situation and hypotension or hepatic passive congestion with liver damage may be contributory.

Emotional hyperglycemia is considered a well-established entity presumably related to epinephrine effect.

Oral glucose tolerance test responses in **pregnancy** are the subject of dispute. Some investigators believe that the OGTT curve in gravid women does not differ from that in nulliparas, and thus any abnormalities in the curve are indicative of latent diabetes. Others believe that pregnancy itself, especially in the last trimester, tends to exert a definite diabetogenic influence. This view is reinforced by observations that the original synthetic estrogen-progesterone combinations used for contraception (with higher estrogen content than most current types) often mimicked the diabetogenic effects of pregnancy. This occurred in 18%–46% of patients, and, as in pregnancy, the FBG level was most often normal. The exact mechanism is not clear; some suggest altered intestinal absorption.

Salicylate overdose in children frequently produces a clinical situation that closely resembles diabetic acidosis. Salicylate in large quantities has a toxic effect on the liver, leading to decreased glycogen formation and to increased breakdown of glycogen to glucose. Therefore, there may develop a mild to moderate elevation in blood glucose level, accompanied by ketonuria. Plasma ketone test results may even be positive, although usually only to mild degree. Salicylic acid metabolites give positive results on tests for reducing substances such as Clinitest (chapter 12), so that results of such tests falsely suggest glucosuria. In addition, salicylate stimulates the central nervous system (CNS) respiratory center in the early phases of overdose, so that increased respiration may suggest the Kussmaul breathing of diabetic acidosis. The carbon dioxide (CO_2) content (or partial pressure of CO_2, PCO_2) is decreased. Later on, a metabolic acidosis develops.

Differentiation from diabetic acidosis can be accomplished by simple tests for salicylate in plasma or urine. A dipstick test called Phenistix is very useful for screening purposes. A positive plasma Phenistix reaction for salicylate is good evidence of salicylate poisoning. A positive result in urine is not conclusive, since in urine the procedure will detect nontoxic levels of salicylate, but a negative urine result is strong evidence against the diagnosis. Definitive chemical quantitative or semiquantitative tests for blood salicylate levels are available. It is important to ask about a history of medication given to the patient or the possibility of accidental ingestion in children with suspicious clinical symptoms.

Salicylate intoxication is not frequent in adults. When it occurs, there is much less tendency toward development of a pseudodiabetic acidosis syndrome. In fact, in adults, salicylate in nontoxic doses occasionally produces hypoglycemia, which tends to occur 2–4 hours postprandially.

Phenytoin (Dilantin) is reported to decrease glucose tolerance, and overdose occasionally produces a type of nonketotic hyperglycemic coma.

Posthypoglycemic hyperglycemia (Somogyi phenomenon) refers to fasting hyperglycemia produced by hormonal (epinephrine, catecholamines, growth hormone) response to previous hypoglycemia induced by too much administered insulin. This can produce the false appearance of treatment failure due to insufficient insulin.

Dawn phenomenon refers to circadian increase in plasma insulin levels between 3 A.M. and 7 A.M. This occurs in response to increased plasma glucose level produced by circadian increase in pituitary growth hormone secretion. In nondiabetic persons the plasma glucose level remains normal in response to the insulin. In diabetics, including those who are insulin dependent and some who are noninsulin dependent, impaired glucose tolerance permits plasma glucose levels to become elevated to some degree over baseline values during this time. In some patients the 6 A.M. or 7 A.M. fasting glucose level becomes sufficiently elevated to simulate necessity for higher doses of daily insulin, whereas more insulin is needed only during this limited time period.

Controversy on Clinical Relevance of the Oral Glucose Tolerance Test

Complete discussion of the OGTT must include reference to various studies that attack the clinical usefulness of the procedure. These consist of reports of large series of normal persons showing up to 20% flat GTT results, studies that showed different curves in repeat determinations after time lapse, and others in which various types of curves were obtained on repeated tests in the same individual. Based on the criteria in use before the NDDG recommendations, some investigators believed there is inadequate evidence that GTT abnormality actually indicates true diabetes mellitus, since many persons with abnormal GTT responses failed to progress to clinical diabetes, and the population incidence of diabetes was far short of that predicted by GTT screening. Since the NDDG criteria require somewhat more abnormality than previous criteria to make a diagnosis of diabetes mellitus, these problems have been partially corrected. Even so, not all drawbacks of the OGTT have been solved regarding problems of sensitivity, specificity, reproducibility, and clinical relevance even when the test is performed under optimal conditions. Nevertheless, at present the OGTT is still the standard test of carbohydrate tolerance and the laboratory basis for the diagnosis of diabetes mellitus.

Intravenous Glucose Tolerance Test

The intravenous glucose tolerance test (IVGTT) was devised to eliminate some of the objections to the OGTT. Standard procedure for the IVGTT is as follows: The patient has a 3-day high-carbohydrate preparatory diet. After the FBG level is measured, a standard solution of 50% glucose is injected intravenously over a 3- to 4-minute period (see Table 36–21). Blood samples are obtained at 0.5, 1, 2, and 3 hours, although it would seem more informative to omit the 30-minute specimen and substitute a 1.5-hour sample. The curve reaches a peak immediately after injection (300–400 mg/100 ml [16.7–22.2 mmol/L], accompanied by glucosuria), then falls steadily but not linearly toward fasting levels. Criteria for interpretation are not uniform. However, most believe that a normal response is indicated by return to fasting levels by 1–1.25 hours. The height of the curve has no significance. Most agree that the IVGTT response is adequately reproducible. In diabetes, fasting levels are not reached in 2 hours and often not even by 3 hours. The curve in liver disease most characteristically returns to normal in 1.25–2 hours; however, some patients with cirrhosis have a diabetic-type curve. Many of the same factors that produce a diabetogenic effect on the OGTT do likewise to the IVGTT; these include carbohydrate deprivation, inactivity, old age, fever, uremia, stress, neoplasms, and the various steroid-producing endocrine diseases. There are, however, several differences from the OGTT. Alimentary problems are eliminated. The IVGTT is said to be normal in pregnancy and also in hyperthyroidism, although one report found occasional abnormality in thyrotoxicosis. The IVGTT is conceded to be somewhat less sensitive than the OGTT, although, as just noted, a little more specific.

Plasma (or Serum) Insulin Assay

Insulin was the first hormone measured successfully by radioisotope immunoassay, and insulin assay is now available in most sizable reference laboratories. In general, juvenile diabetics have low fasting insulin levels, and an OGTT using insulin determinations will usually produce a flat curve. Mild diabetics have normal fasting insulin levels and display an insulin GTT curve that has a delayed rise, either to normal height or to a point moderately above normal; in either case the curve thereafter falls in a normal fashion. Decreased tolerance due to many other causes produces similar curves; an insulin OGTT has not been more efficient in uncovering subclinical diabetes than blood glucose OGTT. Some maintain that the ratio of insulin values to glucose values obtained on the same specimen during the OGTT is more reliable than insulin values alone. At any rate, most investigators believe that, at present, plasma insulin levels should not be used for diagnosis of diabetes mellitus.

Plasma anticoagulated with ethylenediamine tetraacetic acid (EDTA) is reported to produce plasma insulin values equal to serum, but heparin is said to be associated with plasma insulin values greater than serum.

Patients being treated with insulin frequently develop anti-insulin antibodies after approximately 6 weeks. These antibodies interfere with insulin RIA measurement by competing with insulin antibodies used in the test. Whether values will be falsely increased or decreased depends on the method used. Endogenous antibodies do not interfere with tolerance tests, since the quantity of endogenous antibody remains unchanged throughout the test; only the baseline value is affected.

Glycosylated Hemoglobin Assay

In adults, hemoglobin A (Hb A) constitutes about 97%–98% of normal hemoglobin; the remainder includes about 2.5% hemoglobin A_2 and about 0.5% hemoglobin F (Hb F). About 6%–7% of Hb A consists of Hb A molecules that have been partially modified by attachment of a glucose molecule to the terminal valine amino acid of the beta chain. This process is called "glycosylation," and the glycosylated hemoglobin is called "hemoglobin A_1" (Hb A_1). Glycosylated hemoglobin (Hb A_1) is formed by exposure of RBCs to plasma glucose; hemoglobin and glucose can form a bond that initially is labile but then becomes stable. Once stable bonding occurs, it is very slowly and poorly reversible. The labile bonding fraction normally constitutes about 10% of total glucose bonding. Formation of Hb A_1 occurs very slowly during the entire 120 day life span of the RBC, and the number of Hb A molecules affected by glycosylation depends on the degree and duration of RBC exposure to glucose. Hemoglobin A_1 is actually composed of three hemoglobins: A_{1a}, A_{1b}, and A_{1c}. Of these, Hb A_{1c} is about 70% glycosylated, whereas the other two are less than 20% glycosylated. In addition, Hb A_{1c} constitutes about 60%–70% of total Hb A_1, so that Hb A_{1c} represents the majority of glycosylated hemoglobin. The term glycosylated hemoglobin has been used for both Hb A_1 and its major component Hb A_{1c}, which sometimes is confusing.

An increase in glycosylated hemoglobin quantity can be produced by recent very high short-term increases in blood glucose (in which case labile bonding is primarily affected), but is most often caused either by relatively continual elevation of blood glucose or by intermittent elevations that are frequent enough to produce abnormally high average glucose levels (in both of these cases stable glycosylation is primarily affected). A measurable increase in glycosylated (stable) hemoglobin begins about 2–3 weeks (literature range, 1–4 weeks) after a sustained increase in the average blood glucose level and takes at least 4 weeks to begin decreasing after a sustained decrease in the average blood glucose level. Hemoglobin A_1 assay represents the averaged blood glucose levels during the preceding 2–3 months (literature range, 1–4 months). In contrast, blood glucose increases or decreases of "moderate" (100 mg/100 ml; 5.55 mmol/L) degree that occur within the 3 days just before Hb A_1 measurement add sufficient labile component so as to constitute as much as 15% (range, 12%–19%) of the glycosylated hemoglobin result. Spontaneous sudden decreases in blood glucose of this magnitude are not common, so that under most circumstances a normal glycosylated hemoglobin level is good evidence of relatively normal average blood glucose during at least the preceding 4 weeks. Most of the clinical problems with labile bonding component occur with false increases in glycosylated hemoglobin levels. In summary, an elevated glycosylated hemoglobin level is most often due to long-term average blood glucose elevation over the preceding 2–3 months, but the possibility exists for elevation due to marked short-term blood glucose increase if an assay method is used that is not specific for stable bonding.

Glycosylated hemoglobin measurement has been used to monitor effectiveness of (long-term) diabetic therapy, to monitor patient compliance with therapy, and to differentiate between stress-related glucose tolerance abnormality (e.g., acute myocardial infarction) and diabetes. Of these, the most widely accepted indications are monitoring of diabetic therapy effectiveness and monitoring of patient compliance. Glycosylated hemoglobin assay has also been used to diagnose diabetes mellitus, but this is controversial.

Laboratory Methods

Glycosylated hemoglobin can be measured as either Hb A_1 or Hb A_{1c} (since most of Hb A_1 is Hb A_{1c}). Most commercially available kits measure Hb A_1 and report the result as a percentage of total hemoglobin. There are a variety of assay methods. Currently, most commercial kits use some method involving ion exchange resin. Most resin-based kits do not differentiate between labile and stable glucose bonding to hemoglobin. Certain techniques available can eliminate the labile fraction before testing the patient serum. The method known as "affinity chromatography," using a boronic acid resin, measures only the stable fraction without needing pretreatment. To date there are surprisingly few evaluations of different glycosylated hemoglobin kits. In several kits evaluated in my laboratory there was significant variation in reproducibility and accuracy.

Sources of Error.—Hemoglobins S and C form glycosylated hemoglobin in the same manner as Hb A. However, with ion exchange resin methods, Hb S and Hb C remain on the resin with nonglycosylated Hb A. Therefore, Hb S and Hb C produce glycosylated hemoglobin assay values that are less than true levels because these abnormal hemoglobins have a glycosylated component that is not measured along with Hb A_1. On the other hand, Hb F and Hb H elute from the resin in the same fraction as Hb A_1. Therefore, an increased Hb F value or the presence of Hb H will falsely increase glycosylated hemoglobin values since they are included with Hb A_1 assay. Hemoglobin F may be increased in young infants, in up to 17% of pregnant women, and in some of the hemoglobinopathies. Chronic renal failure has been reported to produce falsely high results with resin methods. Single reports have described false increase with aspirin, alcoholism, and lead poisoning. Affinity (boronic acid) chromatography is not affected by abnormal hemoglobin levels or by renal failure. Hemolytic and megaloblastic anemia produce falsely low glycosylated hemoglobin values with any method because RBCs have a shortened life span and therefore are not exposed to blood glucose as long as normal RBCs. Finally, there is some difficulty in calibration of assay kits because primary standards (i.e., material with substance values that are known with absolute certainty) are not available.

In summary, glycosylated hemoglobin assay provides information of great value in the treatment of diabetes and in certain cases may help in the diagnosis. However, the sensitivity and reliability of some commercial kits still need improvement.

Serum Fructosamine Assay

Besides Hb A, albumin and various globulins may undergo nonenzymatic glycosylation. In contrast to hemoglobin, which has a serum half-life of about 60 days, albumin has a half-life of about 17–20 days, and total protein (roughly one half albumin and one half globulins) has a half-life of about 30 days. Either glycosylated albumin or glycosylated total protein can be assayed, but most laboratories assay total protein using the fructosamine procedure. This is based on biochemical reaction with glucose bound to protein with a ketoamine linkage. Serum fructosamine assay results indicate average glycosylation within the preceding 2-week time period (range, 1–3 weeks). This time period is considerably shorter than that of glycosylated hemoglobin but substantially longer than that for labile hemoglobin glycosylation. Drawbacks of fructosamine assay include changes in serum level due to changes in albumin rather than blood glucose. According to one report, changes in albumin affect fructosamine levels significantly only if decreased albumin levels are due to increased catabolism (decreased half-life) or increased albumin loss, but not when there is decreased metabolism of protein. Reducing substances in serum may interfere with the assay in some methods.

Glucosuria

Besides measurement of blood glucose or carbohydrate tolerance, certain other procedures are widely used or proposed for the detection of diabetes mellitus. The appearance of glucose in the urine has long been utilized both for detection and as a parameter of treatment. As a clue to diagnosis, urine glucose depends on hyperglycemia that exceeds the renal tubular threshold for glucose. This threshold is most often considered to be a venous plasma true glucose value of 180 mg/100 ml (1.0 mmol/L) (however, there is a range in the literature of 150–200 mg/100 ml). Of some interest regarding the threshold concept in diabetics is evidence that some diabetics (especially in the elderly) possess unusually high thresholds (up to 300 mg/100 ml; 16.6 mmol/L). It has also been shown that arterial blood glucose levels are much better correlated with glucosuria than venous ones. Nevertheless, routine urine testing provides one method for practical continuous outpatient monitoring of therapy and for the prevention of ketoacidosis. This aspect provides another argument for more routine use of the full GTT, since glucosuria can be correlated with degree of hyperglycemia. Incidentally, many diabetic patients and many of those involved in mass surveys have a urine glucose test before breakfast, which is the least likely time to produce glucosuria.

The problem of causes of hyperglycemia not due to diabetes mellitus was discussed earlier. Renal threshold assumes importance in another way because of the condition known as "renal glucosuria." This may be congenital or acquired; the acquired type may be idiopathic or secondary to certain diseases such as Fanconi's syndrome, acute tubular necrosis, or renal rickets. In all these conditions there is glucosuria at lower blood glucose levels than normal renal threshold values. Some report that a significant number of patients with the nonfamilial idopathic variety of renal glucosuria eventually develop overt diabetes mellitus, although others do not agree.

Glucosuria of pregnancy occurs in the last trimester. Reported incidence depends on the sensitivity of the testing methods used, ranging from 5%–35% or even 70%. The etiology seems to be a combination of increased glomerular filtration rate and temporarily decreased renal threshold. Lactosuria is even more common. Glucosuria without hyperglycemia occurs in 20% of patients with lead poisoning. This is due to a direct toxic effect on the renal tubule cells. Glucosuria of a transient nature has been reported in 24% of normal newborn infants. A study utilizing paper chromatography found galactosuria, usually in amounts too small for detection by routine techniques, to be even more common.

Mentioned here only for the sake of completeness are the two main types of urine glucose tests: the copper sulfate tests for reducing substances and the glucose oxidase enzyme papers. The merits, drawbacks, and technical aspects of these tests, as well as a general discussion of glucosuria, are presented in chapter 12.

Diagnosis of Diabetic Coma

Diabetic coma may occur without a history of diabetes or in circumstances where history is not available. Other major etiologies of coma must be considered, including insulin hypoglycemia, meningitis or cerebrovascular accident, shock, uremia and barbiturate overdose. A clear-cut, fast diagnosis of diabetic coma can be made with a test for plasma ketones (frequently called "acetone," although acetone is not the only ketone substance). Anticoagulated blood is obtained, a portion is centrifuged for 2–3 minutes, and the plasma is tested for ketones. Diabetic acidosis severe enough to produce coma will be definitely positive (except for the rare cases of lactic acidosis or hyperosmolar coma). The other etiologies for coma will be negative, since they rarely produce the degree of acidosis found in diabetic coma. The presence of urinary glucose and ketones strongly suggests diabetes but may occur in other conditions. Such findings would not entirely rule out insulin overdose (always a consideration in a known diabetic), since the urine could have been produced before the overdose. An elevated blood glucose level also is strong evidence of diabetic coma, especially if the degree of elevation is marked. Other conditions that might combine coma with hyperglycemia (cerebrovascular accident, acute myocardial infarction) have only mild or moderate hyperglycemia in those instances where hyperglycemia is produced. Besides blood glucose determination, a simple empirical test to rule out hypoglycemia is to inject some glucose solution intravenously. Cerebral damage is investigated by cerebrospinal fluid examination or computerized tomography scan. Uremia is determined by means of the blood urea nitrogen (BUN) level, although other etiologies of coma besides primary renal disease may be associated with an elevated BUN level. Drug ingestion is established by careful history, analysis of stomach contents, and identification of the drug in blood samples (one anticoagulated and one clotted specimen are preferred) or urine samples. Shock is diagnosed on the basis of blood pressure; further laboratory investigation depends on the probable etiology.

Hyperosmolar Nonketotic Coma.—Hyperosmolar nonketotic coma is uncommon but is being reported with increased frequency. The criterion for diagnosis is very high blood glucose level (usually well above 500 mg/100 ml; 28.0 mmol/L) without ketones in either plasma or urine. The patients usually become severely dehydrated. Plasma osmolality is high due to dehydration and hyperglycemia. Most patients are maturity-onset mild diabetics, but nondiabetics may be affected. Associated precipitating factors include infections, severe burns, high-dose corticosteroid therapy, and renal dialysis. Occasional cases have been reported due to phenytoin and to glucose administration during hypothermia.

Lactic Acidosis Syndrome.—Lactic acidosis syndrome is rare and may have several etiologies. It used to be most frequently reported with phenformin therapy of diabetes but now is encountered as a nonketotic form of diabetic acidosis. The most common cause of elevated blood lactate levels is tissue hypoxia from shock. Arterial blood is said to be more reliable than venous for lactic acid determination. Tourniquet blood stagnation must be avoided, and the specimen must be kept in ice until analyzed.

Hypoglycemia

Hypoglycemia is a topic that has generated a great deal of confusion. Although the word means "low blood glucose," the diagnosis of hypoglycemia is controversial, because it is sometimes defined strictly on the basis of an arbitrary blood glucose level (chemical hypoglycemia), sometimes in terms of symptoms (clinical hypoglycemia), and sometimes as a combination of glucose level and symptoms. The most readily accepted aspect of hypoglycemia is division into two clinical categories: one in which symptoms occur after fasting (fasting hypoglycemia) and one in which symptoms occur after eating (postprandial hypoglycemia). If the blood glucose level drops rapidly, symptoms tend to be similar to those associated with release of epinephrine (adrenergic) and include anxiety, sweating, palpitation, tremor, and hunger. If hypoglycemia persists, CNS glucose deprivation occurs (neuroglycopenia) and symptoms resemble those of cerebral hypoxia, such as lethargy, headache, confusion, bizarre behavior, visual disturbances, syncope, convulsions, and coma. Symptoms associated with fasting hypoglycemia tend to be one or more of those associated with CNS neuroglycopenia, and those associated with postprandial hypoglycemia tend to be adrenergic. However, there is some overlap in symptoms between the two groups. In general, symptoms due to fasting hypoglycemia have a much higher incidence of visual disturbances, bizarre behavior or personality changes, convulsions, and loss of consciousness, especially prolonged loss of consciousness. Postprandial hypoglycemia tends to be more abrupt in onset and is usually self-limited.

Fasting Hypoglycemia

Of the two clinical categories, fasting hypoglycemia is by far the more straightforward. The two chief mechanisms are insulin excess (either absolute or relative) and effects of carbohydrate deprivation. Conditions acting through these mechanisms are:

1. The most well-known etiology of insulin excess is the beta-cell insulin-producing pancreatic islet cell tumor (insulinoma). About 80% of these tumors are single adenomas, about 10% are multiple adenomas, and about 10% are carcinomas. Although insulinomas typically are associated with fasting hypoglycemia, one study reported that nearly 50% of their insulinoma patients developed symptoms less than 6 hours postprandially, which would clinically suggest a postprandial (reactive) etiology.

2. Overdose of insulin in a diabetic person. Since the patient may be found in coma without any history available, insulin overdose must be a major consideration in any emergency room comatose patient.

3. Hypoglycemia may be associated with deficiency of hormones that normally counteract the hypoglycemic effect of insulin. This group includes pituitary insufficiency (deficiency of growth hormone and cortisol) and adrenal insufficiency (cortisol). Glucagon and thyroxine also have a hyperglycemic effect, but hypoglycemia due to a deficiency of these hormones is rare.

4. Prolonged carbohydrate deprivation, even when total calories are relatively adequate, has been reported to predispose to hypoglycemia. Occasional patients with severe liver disease develop hypoglycemia, but this is uncommon.

5. Certain nonpancreatic tumors have occasionally been reported to cause hypoglycemia, presumably either by glucose utilization or by production of an insulin-like substance. The great majority have been neoplasms of large size described as fibrosarcomas or spindle cell sarcomas, usually located in the abdomen (in one study, about two-thirds occurred in the abdomen and one-third occurred in the thorax). Hepatoma is next most frequent.

6. Alcoholic hypoglycemia may occur in either chronic alcoholics or occasional drinkers. Malnutrition, chronic or temporary, is an important predisposing factor. In those persons who develop hypoglycemia, fasting for 12–24 hours precedes alcohol intake. Symptoms may occur immediately but most often follow 6–34 hours later. Therefore, alcohol-related hypoglycemia is most often a fasting type but occasionally may appear to be reactive.

Laboratory Tests

The major consideration in these patients is to discover a pancreatic islet cell tumor or eliminate its possibility. Diagnosis of islet cell tumor is important since the condition is surgically correctable, but accurate diagnosis is a necessity to avoid unnecessary operation.

Whipple's Triad.—Whipple's triad remains the basic screening procedure for insulinoma:

1. Symptoms compatible with hypoglycemia while fasting.
2. A fasting blood glucose (FBG) level of 10 mg/100 ml (0.55 mmol/L) or more below FBG normal lower limits at some time. This is most reliable when the specimen is obtained while the patient is having symptoms.
3. Relief of symptoms by glucose.

Plasma (or Serum) Insulin/Glucose Ratio.—In functioning insulinomas, one would expect serum insulin levels to be elevated. In some cases the insulin level remains within population reference limits but is disproportionately high in relationship to the glucose level. Therefore, the ratio of immunoreactive insulin to glucose (IRI/G ratio) is considered more sensitive and reliable than blood levels alone of either glucose or insulin. Normally the IRI/G ratio should be less than 0.3 (the immunoreactive insulin is measured in microunits per milliliter, the glucose in milligrams per 100 ml). The ratio is abnormal if it is greater than 0.3 in nonobese persons and greater than 0.3 in obese persons with serum glucose values less than 60 mg/100 ml. Hyperinsulinism due to insulinoma results in serum insulin levels inappropriately high in relation to the low serum glucose values. In some institutions a G/IRI ratio is used instead of an IRI/G ratio.

Prolonged Fasting.—A considerable number of patients do not display symptoms or laboratory evidence of insulinoma after overnight fasting. When this occurs, the most useful procedure is prolonged fasting for a time period up to 72 hours long, with periodic insulin plus glucose measurements, or such measurements if symptoms develop. After an overnight fast, approximately 50% of insulinomas are revealed by the FBG level alone and about 66% by the IRI/G ratio. After a 48-hour fast, the blood glucose value uncovers about 66% of tumors and the IRI/G ratio about 85%. In 72 hours, the blood glucose level alone detects about 70% of patients and the IRI/G ratio is abnormal in more than 95%. Serum insulin assay alone reveals about the same percentage of patients with elevated values as the blood glucose level does with low values.

Tolbutamide Tolerance Test.—Tolbutamide (Orinase) is a sulfonylurea drug that has the ability to stimulate insulin production from pancreatic islet cells. The drug has been used to treat diabetics who produce insulin but not in sufficient quantity. In the tolbutamide test, a special water-soluble form of tolbutamide (not the therapeutic oral form) is given intravenously. In normal persons there is a prompt fall in blood glucose levels to a minimum at 30–45 minutes, followed by a return to normal values between 1.5 and 3 hours. In patients with insulinoma the fall in the blood glucose level is greater than that of most normal persons, declining to 40%–65% of baseline, whereas normal persons usually do not fall as low as 50% of baseline.

Since there is occasional overlap between normal persons and those with insulinoma, of greater significance is the fact that hypoglycemia from insulinoma persists for more than 3 hours, whereas in most normal individuals the blood glucose level has returned to fasting values by 3 hours. In a few normal individuals and in those with functional hypoglycemia, values return to at least 80% of FBG levels by 3 hours. Adrenal insufficiency also returns to at least 80% of FBG levels by 3 hours, although the initial decrease may be as great as that for insulinoma. Some patients with severe liver disease have curves similar to those of insulin-producing tumor. However, this is not frequent and usually is not a real diagnostic problem. The tolbutamide test is definitely more sensitive than the OGTT for the diagnosis of islet cell tumor but has the disadvantage that the characteristic responses of diabetic or alimentary hypoglycemia to the OGTT cannot be demonstrated.

The major drawback to the tolbutamide test is the necessity in some patients to stop the test prematurely because of severe hypoglycemic symptoms. Patients must be closely watched during the test. Sensitivity of the test for insulinoma seems to be approximately 80%–85% using the extended 3-hour time period (literature range, 75%–97%). A major advantage of the test is the short time required to obtain an answer. The tolbutamide test is usually not performed if the FBG value is already in the hypoglycemic range.

Proinsulin.—Insulin is derived from a precursor called proinsulin, which is synthesized in the pancreas, is metabolically inactive, and is larger in size ("big insulin"). Proinsulin consists of an alpha and a beta chain connected by an area called "connecting peptide" (C-peptide). Proinsulin is enzymatically cleaved within beta cells into equal quantities of insulin and C-peptide. Radioimmunoassay measurement of insulin includes both proinsulin and regular insulin. Normally, about 5%–15% of so-called immunoreactive insulin (that which is measured by RIA) is proinsulin. In many (but not all) patients with insulinomas, the amount of circulating proinsulin is increased relative to total insulin. In diabetics with insulin deficiency who are being treated with insulin, the proinsulin fraction of the individual's own immunoreactive insulin values may be increased. Measurement of proinsulin necessitates special procedures such as Sephadex column chromatography and is not widely available. Sensitivity of proinsulin assay for detection of insulinoma is reported to be about 80%.

Serum Connecting Peptide Measurement.—As noted previously, C-peptide is a byproduct of insulin production. Although it is released in quantities equal to insulin, serum C-peptide levels do not exactly parallel those of insulin, due to differences in serum half-life and catabolic rate. Nevertheless, C-peptide values correlate well with insulin values in terms of the position of each in relation to its own normal range (i.e., if one is decreased, the other likewise is decreased). Therefore, C-peptide can be used as an indicator of insulin secretion.

Present-day insulin is derived from animal pancreas (synthetic human insulin is available but not yet widely used). Use of this foreign substance may lead to anti-insulin antibody production. Pork insulin is less antigenic than beef insulin. Insulin antibodies falsely increase insulin assay values in most commercial kits (although in a few systems the values are decreased instead). Connecting peptide assay kits do not react with animal-origin insulin and therefore reflect only actual patient insulin production without being affected by the presence of insulin antibodies.

Connecting peptide assay has been used in several ways: (1) most commonly, to detect or prove factitious (self-medication) insulin hypoglycemia; (2) to detect insulinoma in diabetic patients requiring insulin therapy; (3) to evaluate pancreatectomy status; and (4) to evaluate insulin reserve or production in diabetics who have taken or are taking insulin.

Occasional patients become hypoglycemic by self-administration of insulin. Since insulin assay cannot differentiate between exogenous insulin and that produced by insulinoma, C-peptide assay should be performed on the same specimen that showed elevated insulin levels. In hyperinsulinism from islet cell tumor, C-peptide levels are elevated; in that due to exogenous (self-administered) insulin, C-peptide levels are low. Another cause of low C-peptide levels is a type I diabetic who cannot produce insulin, but the insulin assay value would be low. An elevation of the C-peptide level classically suggests insulinoma but may also be seen after taking oral hypoglycemic agents (since these agents stimulate the production of insulin).

Connecting peptide assay has been used after pancreatectomy to evaluate the possibility of residual pancreatic islet tissue.

Some investigators have used C-peptide assay in diabetics previously treated with insulin to see how much insulin production is possible. Those who have substantial capability for insulin production are treated differently from those who do not. This method can help diagnose the syndrome of peripheral insulin resistance. Also, if the diabetic patient has significant capability for insulin production, frequent and severe episodes of diabetic ketoacidosis may suggest some factor other than insulin deficiency. There is still controversy over criteria dividing type I and type II diabetics based on insulin or C-peptide assay and what therapeutic changes, if any, should be made based on the amount of insulin production using insulin or C-peptide information.

Other Tests.—The 5-hour OGTT after overnight fasting was widely used in the past for detection of insulinoma. Patients characteristically had a low or low-normal FBG level and a normal sharp rise after glucose administration (the peak remaining within normal OGTT limits), then a slower fall to hypoglycemic levels that did not rapidly return to the reference range. However, the OGTT has been virtually abandoned for diagnosis of insulinoma because a considerable minority of insulinomas are reported to demonstrate a flat curve or sometimes even a diabetic-type curve, or the curve may be normal. The 5-hour OGTT, however, is sometimes used in patients with the postprandial type of hypoglycemia. Leucine and glucagon provocative tests for insulinoma have been reported. However, these are rarely used since they are somewhat less sensitive than tolbutamide and substantially less sensitive than the IRI/G ratio after prolonged fasting.

Tumor Localization.—Once the diagnosis of insulinoma has been made, it is important to localize the tumor within the pancreas if surgery is contemplated. Most tumors are located in the body and tail of the pancreas. Pancreatic artery selective angiography may be able to pinpoint the exact location of the tumor, but the detection rate is only about 50%.

Current Status of Tests for Insulinoma

At present, most investigators use Whipple's triad and prolonged fasting (with the IRI/G ratio) as the primary screening tests for insulinoma, with the tolbutamide test available in equivocal or problem cases.

Postprandial Hypoglycemia

Some of the most common etiologies of postprandial hypoglycemia (which is also known as "reactive hypoglycemia") include the following etiologies.

Alimentary.—Postprandial hypoglycemia of gastrointestinal tract origin (sometimes called the "dumping syndrome") most often occurs after gastric surgery and results from unusually swift or complete gastric emptying of ingested carbohydrate into the duodenum, resulting in abnormally high blood glucose levels and temporary hypoglycemia after hastily produced insulin has overcome the initial hyperglycemia. Initial blood glucose elevation is definitely greater than that of a normal person.

Diabetic.—Some persons with subclinical or early diabetes mellitus of the NDDG type II (noninsulin-dependent) category may develop mild and transitory hypoglycemia 3–5 hours after eating. This seems to be an early manifestation of their disease, which often disappears as the disease progresses. The exact incidence in diabetics is unclear but is probably low. However, because of the large number of diabetic persons, it may be a relatively frequent cause of postprandial hypoglycemia. Initial elevation of blood glucose values may or may not be higher than in normal persons, but the 2-hour postprandial value is elevated. The rise in plasma insulin after eating tends to be delayed, and the insulin peak (when finally achieved) may be somewhat elevated, resulting in the hypoglycemic episode.

Functional.—Some patients develop symptoms of hypoglycemia after eating without known cause. This most often occurs 3–4 hours postprandially (range, 1–5 hours). In some cases symptoms can be correlated with acceptably low blood glucose values, in which case many physicians make a diagnosis of functional hypoglycemia (although there is controversy on this point, to be discussed later with the 5-hour OGTT). In other cases, probably the majority, symptoms cannot be adequately correlated with acceptably low blood glucose values. Either the OGTT serum glucose value is low but no symptoms occur or (less commonly) symptoms occur at a relatively normal glucose level. In these cases some have used the diagnosis of "idiopathic postprandial syndrome." Perhaps a better term would be "pseudohypoglycemia." The peak blood glucose elevation after eating is not higher than in a normal person, and the 2-hour value is also normal.

Other.—A few patients with insulinoma or alcoholism may develop postprandial hypoglycemia, although fasting hypoglycemia is much more common.

Laboratory Tests

The first consideration is to rule out a fasting hypoglycemia, especially when hypoglycemic symptoms occur several hours after food intake. Self-administered hypoglycemic agents are also possible, although for some reason this is not often mentioned when associated with postprandial symptoms. The best test would be a blood glucose measurement drawn at the same time that symptoms were present. Because symptoms in daily life usually occur at times when blood specimens cannot be obtained, the traditional laboratory procedure in postprandial hypoglycemia has been the 5-hour OGTT. In alimentary hypoglycemia the classic OGTT pattern is a peak value within 1 hour that is above OGTT reference limits, followed by a swift fall to hypoglycemic levels (usually between 1 and 3 hours after glucose). In diabetic hypoglycemia, there is an elevated 2-hour postprandial value, followed by hypoglycemia during the 3–5 hours postglucose time interval. In functional hypoglycemia, there is a normal OGTT peak and 2-hour level, followed by hypoglycemia during the 2- to 4-hour postglucose time interval (Fig 27–1).

Unfortunately, diagnosis has not been as simple as the classic OGTT findings just mentioned would imply. Many investigators have found disturbing variability in OGTT curves, which often change when testing is repeated over a period of time and may change when testing is repeated on a day-to-day basis. In some cases this is related to factors known to influence the OGTT, such as inadequate carbohydrate preparation, but in other cases there is no obvious cause for OGTT discrepancies. Another major problem is disagreement regarding what postprandial blood glucose value to accept as indicative of hypoglycemia. Most investigators use 50 mg/100 ml (2.76 mmol/L) of plasma glucose as the dividing line. However, there is considerable controversy in the literature on this point. In some cases it is not clear whether serum or whole blood was assayed (reference values for whole blood are 15% less than those for serum or plasma). An additional problem involves the concept of chemical hypoglycemia vs. clinical hypoglycemia. A number of studies have shown that a certain percentage of clinically normal persons may have OGTT curves compatible with functional hypoglycemia without developing any symptoms. In some instances asymptomatic OGTT serum levels as low as 30 mg/100 ml (1.65 mmol/L) were observed. Moreover, in some studies continuous blood glucose monitoring systems disclosed hypoglycemic dips not evident in standard OGTT specimens. On the other hand, some persons with symptoms compatible with hypoglycemia do not develop OGTT values below reference limits. To make matters more

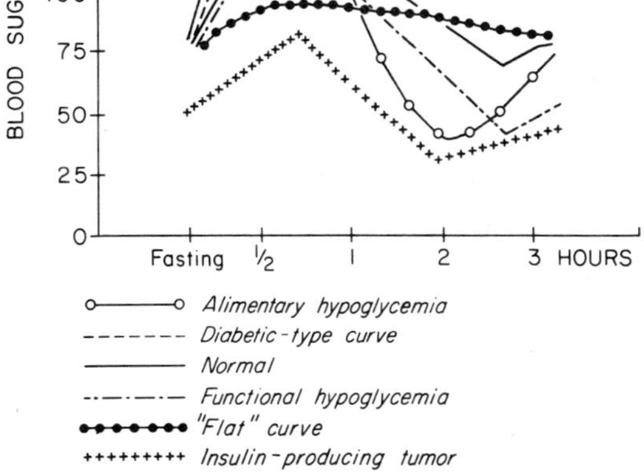

FIG 27–1.
Representative oral glucose tolerance curves.

confusing, some studies have found that when the 5-hour OGTT was repeated after it had initially displayed a hypoglycemic dip, a substantial number of the repeat OGTT results became normal (about 65% of cases in one report). Finally, several studies have indicated that hypoglycemic values found during an OGTT usually disappear when an ordinary meal is substituted for the carbohydrate dose. Since actual patients do not usually ingest pure carbohydrate meals, this casts doubt on the reliability and usefulness of the OGTT in the diagnosis of functional hypoglycemia. One study found that patients with symptoms of functional hypoglycemia had an increase in the plasma epinephrine level of at least 250 pg/ml over baseline at the time of the OGTT lowest ("nadir") serum glucose level, regardless of the actual value, whereas those who did not develop symptoms had an epinephrine increase at the time of the glucose nadir that was less than 250 pg/ml.

In summary, the diagnosis of postprandial hypoglycemia is clouded by controversy, especially the category of functional hypoglycemia. Probably the least debatable diagnosis would be one established by a serum glucose level less than 50 mg/100 ml obtained less than 5 hours after a regular meal while the patient is having hypoglycemic symptoms. A 5-hour OGTT could be done with a regular meal instead of the pure glucose dose. This would also help to exclude alimentary or diabetic etiologies.

Neonatal and Childhood Hypoglycemia

Neonatal and childhood hypoglycemia will be considered together, although some are of the fasting type and some are postprandial.

Idiopathic Hypoglycemia of Infancy.—It has been reported that as many as 10% of all neonates have at least one low blood glucose value. Neonatal reference values are lower than the adult reference range, and there is disagreement as to what level should be considered hypoglycemic. Values considered hypoglycemic in the literature range from 20–40 mg/100 ml (1.10–2.20 mmol/L). The most widely quoted reference value lower limits are 20 mg/100 ml for premature or low birth weight newborns and 30 mg/100 ml for term normal weight newborns during the first day of life. These values were originally derived from whole blood assay. Conversion to serum or plasma glucose assay values (15% higher than whole blood) would bring the premature lower limit on serum specimens to about 25 mg/100 ml (1.38 mmol/L) and the mature infant lower limit on serum to about 35 mg/100 ml (1.93 mmol/L). The other frequently used reference range consists of premature infant serum lower limit of 30 mg/100 ml (1.65 mmol/L) and mature infant serum lower limit of 40 mg/100 ml (2.20 mmol/L) during the first day of life. Use of these reference values results in at least 10% more diagnoses of hypoglycemia than use of the lower reference limits. Since a substantial number of these infants are asymptomatic, the lower values are more commonly used. In both systems, the serum glucose lower limit after the first day of life is 40 mg/100 ml. Idiopathic neonatal hypoglycemia is more common in male infants with low birth weight for age and in premature infants. In some cases the condition is aggravated by delay in beginning milk feeding. Clinical symptoms occur within 72 hours of birth and include some combination of tremors, twitching, cyanosis, respiratory difficulties, high-pitched or weak cry, refusal to eat, limpness, apnea, and convulsions. These symptoms are nonspecific and could be due to a wide variety of serious or life-threatening neonatal illnesses.

Neonatal hypoglycemia is thought to be caused at least in part by low hepatic glycogen levels. The condition is usually transient and is treated by oral milk and glucose (if mild) or by parenteral glucose (if severe). If the infant does not develop a clinical problem until after milk feeding is begun and the problem continues, the possibility of leucine sensitivity should be considered.

Leucine Sensitivity.—Symptoms of leucine sensitivity usually begin within the first 2 years of life and spontaneously disappear by age 5–6 years. Intake of foods that are rich in the amino acid leucine (e.g., cow's milk) apparently stimulate the pancreatic beta cells to overproduce insulin, rather similar to the effect of tolbutamide. The patients typically have a low FBG level and demonstrate marked hypoglycemia after leucine administration. Diagnosis is made by a leucine tolerance test, similar to the OGTT but using oral leucine. Since leucine also stimulates 50%–70% of insulinomas, the possibility of insulin-producing tumor or nesidioblastosis must also be considered.

Nesidioblastosis.—Occasional children with hypoglycemia have diffuse pancreatic islet cell hyperplasia known as nesidioblastosis. Insulinomas also occur but are rare. Diagnosis is the same as for insulinomas and is based on demonstrating inappropriate elevation of insulin when blood glucose levels are low.

Galactosemia.—Galactosemia is an inborn error of metabolism produced by deficiency of an enzyme necessary to metabolize galactose to glucose. Galactose is produced by metabolism of lactose, which is present in milk. Some of these patients develop hypoglycemic episodes, presumably due to abnormality of liver production of glucose from glycogen. A more complete summary of this condition, including laboratory diagnosis, is found in chapter 33.

Ketosis.—Ketosis is said to be the most common etiology of hypoglycemia in childhood. Onset is usually between age 1.5 and 5 years, and the condition usually disappears by age 10 years. It is more common in males of lower than normal birth weight. Episodes of hypoglycemia tend to be precipitated by prolonged lack of food intake or by a low-calorie, low-carbohydrate diet. The cause is thought to be at least partially due to depletion of hepatic glycogen. The child is normal between episodes. Hypoglycemic attacks are usually associated with readily detectable plasma ketone bodies and frequently with urine ketonuria. Blood glucose levels and plasma insulin values are both low.

Other.—Hypoglycemia may be associated with maternal toxemia of pregnancy or poorly controlled diabetes mellitus or with neonatal severe hypoxia or neonatal sepsis. Diagnosis would be based on recognition that these conditions are present.

Additional tests relevant to this chapter are discussed in chapter 35.

BIBLIOGRAPHY

Nelson RL: Oral glucose tolerance test: Indications and limitations. *Mayo Clin Proc* 1988; 63:263.

Grunberger G, et al: Factitious hypoglycemia due to surreptitious administration of insulin. *Ann Intern Med* 1988; 108:252.

Becket NM, Belsey R: Reagent strip testing: Blood glucose error in a teaching hospital. *Lab Med* 1988; 19:26.

Armbruster DA: Fructosamine: Structure, analysis, and clinical usefulness. *Clin Chem* 1987; 33:2153.

Sacks DA: Screening for gestational diabetes with the one-hour 50-g glucose test. *Obstet Gynecol* 1987; 70:89.

Mosca A, et al: Plasma protein glycation as measured by fructosamine assay. *Clin Chem* 1987; 33:1141.

Heck LJ, Erenberg A: Serum glucose levels in term neonates during the first 48 hours of life. *J Pediatr* 1987; 110:119.

Gerich JE: Pathogenesis and differentiation of the Dawn and Somogyi phenomena in patients with diabetes mellitus. *Pract Cardiol* 1987; 13:81.

NIH Consensus Conference: Consensus statement on self-monitoring of blood glucose. *Diabetes Care* 1987; 10:95.

Gerich JE: Insulin-dependent diabetes mellitus: Pathophysiology. *Mayo Clin Proc* 1986; 61:787.

Weiner CP, et al: The relationship between capillary and venous glucose concentration during pregnancy. *Am J Obstet Gynecol* 1986; 155:61.

Threatte GA, et al: Accuracy of instruments for bedside monitoring of whole blood glucose. *Clin Chem* 1986; 32:1184.

American Diabetes Association: Gestational diabetes mellitus. *Ann Intern Med* 1986; 105:461.

Coustan DR, et al: Should the fifty-gram, one-hour plasma glucose screening test for gestational diabetes be administered in the fasting or fed state? *Am J Obstet Gynecol* 1986; 154:1031.

Van Dieijen-Visser MP, et al: Influence of variations in albumin or total-protein concentration on serum fructosamine concentration. *Clin Chem* 1986; 32:1640.

Chalew SA, et al: Diagnosis of reactive hypoglycemia: Pitfalls in the use of the oral glucose tolerance test. *South Med J* 1986; 79:285.

Licinio-Paixao J, et al: Ingestion of a mixed meal does not affect the metabolic clearance rate of biosynthetic human C-peptide. *J Clin Endocrinol Metab* 1986; 63:401.

Srinivasan G, et al: Plasma glucose values in normal neonates: A new look. *J Pediatr* 1986; 109:114.

Rasaiah B: Self-monitoring of the blood glucose level: Potential sources of inaccuracy. *Can Med Assoc J* 1985; 132:1357.

Kilzer P: Glycated hemoglobin and diabetes. *Clin Chem* 1985; 31:1060.

Nelson RL: Hypoglycemia: Fact or fiction? *Mayo Clin Proc* 1985; 60:844.

Bakerman S, Bakerman P: Hypoglycemia in pediatric patients: Sources and diagnosis. *Lab Mgmt* 1985; 23(12):15.

Mazze RS, et al: Reliability of blood glucose monitoring by patients with diabetes mellitus. *Am J Med* 1984; 77:211.

Yatscoff RW, et al: Quantification of nonenzymically glycated albumin and total serum protein by affinity chromatography. *Clin Chem* 1984; 30:446.

Chalew SA, et al: The use of the plasma epinephrine response in the diagnosis of idiopathic postprandial syndrome. *JAMA* 1984; 251:612.

Sexon WR: Incidence of neonatal hypoglycemia: A matter of definition. *J Pediatr* 1984; 105:149.

Yatscoff RW, et al: Interference of fetal hemoglobin and labile glycosylated hemoglobin with measurements of glycosylated hemoglobin. *Clin Chem* 1983; 29:543.

Goldman JM: Fasting hypoglycemia. *Arch Intern Med* 1983; 143:1496.

Hogan MJ, et al: Oral glucose tolerance test compared with a mixed meal in the diagnosis of reactive hypoglycemia. *Mayo Clin Proc* 1983; 58:491.

Nanji AA: Hypoglycemia: When it's the real thing. *Diagn Med* 1983; 6(7):60.

Lev-Ran A: Nadirs of oral glucose tolerance tests are independent of age and sex. *Diabetes Care* 1983; 6:405.

Nathan DM, et al: Rapid method for eliminating labile glycosylated hemoglobin from the assay for hemoglobin A1. *Clin Chem* 1982; 28:512.

Hammond GT: Glycosylated hemoglobin and diabetes mellitus. *Lab Med* 1981; 12:213.

Barden TP, Knowles HC: Diagnosis of diabetes in pregnancy. *Clin Obstet Gynecol* 1981; 24:3.

National Diabetes Data Group: Classification and diagnosis of diabetes mellitus and other categories of glucose intolerance. *Diabetes* 1979; 28:1039.

Randall M, et al: C-peptide as a clinical assay. *Ligand Q* 1979; 2:20.

Anderson N, Lokich JJ: Mesenchymal tumors associated with hypoglycemia. *Cancer* 1979; 44:785.

28 Thyroid Function Tests

THYROID HORMONE PRODUCTION

Thyroid hormone production and utilization involve several steps (Fig 28–1). Thyroid gland activity is under the control of thyroid-stimulating hormone (TSH, or thyrotropin), produced by the anterior pituitary. Pituitary TSH secretion is regulated by thyrotropin-releasing hormone (TRH, thyroliberin, protirelin) from the hypothalamus. The main raw material of thyroid hormone is inorganic iodide provided by food. Thyroid hormone synthesis begins when inorganic iodide is extracted from the blood by the thyroid. Within the thyroid, inorganic iodide is converted to organic iodine, and one iodine atom is incorporated into a tyrosine nucleus to form monoiodotyrosine. An additional iodine atom is then attached to form diiodotyrosine. Two diiodotyrosine molecules are combined to form tetraiodothyronine (thyroxine, T_4), or one monoiodotyrosine molecule can be combined with one diiodotyrosine molecule to form triiodothyronine (T_3). Thyroid hormone is stored in the thyroid acini as thyroglobulin, to be reconstituted and released when needed. Under normal conditions the greater part of thyroid hormone secretion is T_4, with only about 7% being T_3. In the blood, more than 99% of both T_4 and T_3 is bound to serum proteins. About 80%–85% of T_4 attaches to T_4-binding globulin (TBG), an alpha-1 globulin; about 10%–15% to prealbumin; and about 5% to albumin. Parenthetically, although only a small percentage binds to albumin, there is a large quantity of albumin, so that large changes in serum albumin (usually a decrease) may significantly affect the amount of T_4 bound to protein. About 70% of T_3 is bound to TBG and most of the remainder to albumin. Protein-bound hormone is metabolically inactive, as though it were in a warehouse for storage. The unbound ("free") T_4 and T_3 are metabolically active in body cells. Within body cells, particularly the liver, about 80% of daily T_3 production takes place by conversion of free T_4 to T_3. Thyroxine is also converted into a compound known as "reverse T_3," which is not biologically active. Finally, there is a feedback system of control over thyroid hormone production and release. Decreased serum levels of free T_4 and T_3 stimulate TRH production, whereas increased levels of free T_4 and T_3 directly inhibit pituitary secretion of TSH as well as inhibit TRH production.

Certain drugs affect aspects of thyroid hormone production. Perchlorate and cyanate inhibit iodide trapping by the thyroid. The thionamide compounds propylthiouracil (PTU) and methimazole (Tapazole) inhibit thyroid hormone synthesis within the gland from iodine and tyrosine. In addition, PTU inhibits liver conversion of T_4 to T_3. Iodine in large amounts tends to decrease thyroid vascularity and acinar hyperplasia and to have some inhibitory effect on thyroid hormone release in Graves' disease. Cortisol has some inhibitory effect on pituitary TSH secretion.

SIGNS AND SYMPTOMS OF THYROID DISEASE

Many persons have at least one sign or symptom that could suggest thyroid disease.

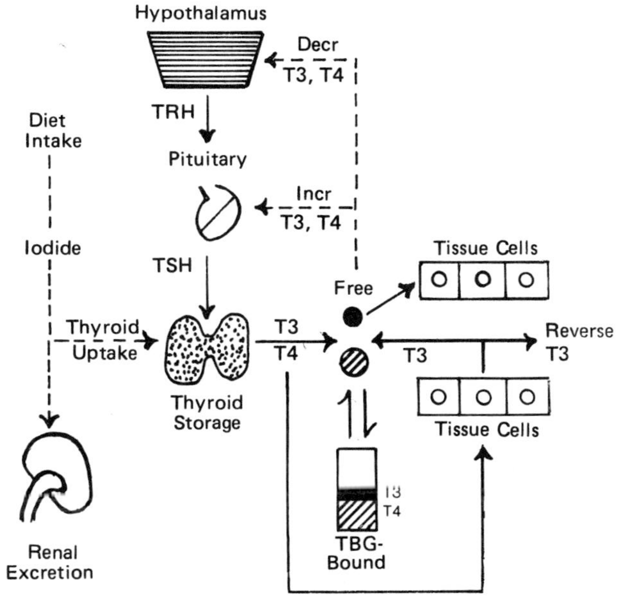

FIG 28–1.
Iodine and thyroid hormone metabolism.

Unfortunately, most of these signs and symptoms are not specific for thyroid dysfunction. Enumeration of the classic signs and symptoms of thyroid disease is the best way to emphasize these facts.

Hyperthyroidism

Thyrotoxicosis from excess secretion of thyroid hormone is usually caused by a diffusely hyperactive thyroid (Graves' disease, about 75% of hyperthyroid cases) or by a hyperfunctioning thyroid nodule (Plummer's disease, about 15% of hyperthyroid cases). A much less common cause is iodine-induced hyperthyroidism (Jod-Basedow disease), and rare causes include pituitary overproduction of TSH, ectopic production of thyroid hormone by the ovary (struma ovarii), high levels of chorionic gonadotropin (with some thyroid-stimulating activity) from trophoblastic tumors, and functioning metastic thyroid carcinoma. Thyroiditis (discussed later) may produce symptoms of thyrotoxicosis (producing about 10% of hyperthyroid cases), but the symptoms are caused by leakage of thyroid hormones from damaged thyroid tissue rather than oversecretion from intact tissue. Many hyperthyroid patients have eye signs such as exophthalmos, lid lag, or stare. Other symptoms include tachycardia; warm, moist skin; heat intolerance; nervous hyperactive appearance; loss of weight; and tremor of fingers. Less frequent symptoms are diarrhea, atrial fibrillation, and congestive heart failure. The hemoglobin level is usually normal; the white blood cell count (WBC) is normal or slightly decreased. There is sometimes an increase in the lymphocyte level. The serum alkaline phosphatase level is elevated in 42%-89% of patients. In elderly patients the clinical picture is said to be more frequently atypical, with a higher incidence of gastrointestinal symptoms, atrial fibrillation, and apathetic appearance.

Hypothyroidism

Myxedema develops from thyroid hormone deficiency. Most common signs and symptoms include nonpitting edema of eyelids, face, and extremities; loss of hair in the outer third of the eyebrows; large tongue; cold, dry skin; cold intolerance; mood depression; lethargic appearance; and slow mental activity. Cardiac shadow enlargement on chest x-ray film is common, with normal or slow heart rate. Anorexia and constipation are frequent. Laboratory tests show anemia in 50% or more of myxedema patients, with a macrocytic but nonmegaloblastic type in approximately 25%.

The WBC count is usually normal. The cerebrospinal fluid (CSF) usually has an elevated protein level with normal cell counts, for unknown reasons. Total serum CPK level is elevated in about 80% (range, 20%–100%) of patients, and the aspartate aminotransferase (AST; formerly SGOT) level is elevated in about 40%–50%.

Hypothyroidism in the infant is known as "cretinism." Conditions that superficially resemble or simulate cretinism include mongolism and Hurler's disease (because of mental defect, facial appearance, and short stature); various types of dwarfism, including achondroplasia (because of short stature and retarded bone age); and nephrosis (because of edema, high cholesterol levels, and low T_4 levels). Myxedema in older children and adults may be simulated by the nephrotic syndrome, mental deficiency (because of mental slowness), simple obesity, and psychiatric depression.

THYROID FUNCTION TESTS

The classic picture of hyperthyroidism or hypothyroidism is frequently not complete and may be totally absent. There may be only one noticeable symptom or sign, and even that may be vague or misleading or suggestive of some other disease. The physician must turn to the laboratory to confirm or exclude the diagnosis.

There is a comparatively large group of laboratory procedures that measure one or more aspects of thyroid function (Table 28–1). The multiplicity of these tests implies that none is infallible or invariably helpful. To get best results, one must have a thorough knowledge of each procedure, including what aspect of thyroid function is measured, sensitivity of the test in the detection of thyroid conditions, and the rate of false results caused by nonthyroid conditions. In certain cases, a brief outline of the technique involved when the test is actually performed helps clarify some of these points.

Radioactive Iodine Uptake

Radioactive iodine uptake is an indirect estimate of thyroid hormone production based on the need of the thyroid for iodine to make thyroid hormone, which, in turn, depends on the rate of thyroid hormone synthesis. A small dose of radioactive iodine is given, and a radiation detector measures the amount present in the gland at some standard time (usually 24 hours after the dose). The RAIU measurement is one of the oldest currently used thyroid function tests, but it has several drawbacks, as listed:

1. The RAIU result is falsely normal in 50%–70% (literature range, 20%–80%) of patients with hyperthyroidism due to toxic nodules.
2. The RAIU results are affected by a considerable number of medications (see Table 36–24) and may be elevated during the last trimester of pregnancy.
3. Any condition that alters thyroid requirements for iodine will affect the RAIU response. Iodine deficiency goiter elevates RAIU results, and some reports indicate that elevation for similar reasons occur in 25%–50% of patients with cirrhosis. Excess iodine in the blood contained in certain medicines (inorganic iodide) or in x-ray contrast media (organic iodine) competes with radioactive iodine for thyroid uptake, thereby preventing uptake of some radioactive iodine and falsely decreasing test results.
4. The standard 24-hour uptake requires two patient visits and 2 days.
5. Normal values are uncertain due to increasing environmental and foodstuff iodine

TABLE 28–1.
Thyroid Function Tests*

- I. Thyroid uptake of iodine
  - A. RAIU
- II. Thyroxine tests
  - A. "Direct" measurement
    - 1. T_4 by RIA or EIA
    - 2. Free T_4 assay
  - B. "Indirect" measurement
    - 1. THBR (T_3 uptake, or T_3U)
    - 2. Free T_4 index
- III. Triiodothyronine tests
  - A. T_3-RIA
- IV. Pituitary and hypothalamic function tests
  - A. TSH assay
  - B. TRH assay
- V. Other
  - A. Stimulation and suppression tests
  - B. Thyroid scan
  - C. Thyroid autoantibody assay

*RAIU = radioactive iodine uptake; RIA = radioimmunoassay; EIA = enzyme immunoassay; THBR = thyroid hormone–binding ratio; TRH = thyrotropin-releasing hormone.

content. Before 1960 the average 24-hour RAIU reference range was 15%–40%. Reports from 1960–1970 suggest a decrease of the range to 8%–30%. There have been little recent data on this subject, and most nuclear medicine departments are unable to obtain reference values for their own locality.

6. Occasional patients with hyperthyroidism have unusually fast synthesis and release (turnover) of T_4 and T_3. The RAIU measurement depends not only on uptake of radioactive iodine but also on retention of the radioactive iodine (incorporated into hormone) within the gland until the amount of radioactivity within the gland is measured. By 24 hours a significant amount of newly formed hormone may already be released, providing falsely lower thyroid radioactivity values compared with earlier (2–6 hours) uptake measurements.

7. The RAIU provides relatively poor separation of normal from hypothyroid persons. Prior to 1960, approximate sensitivity of the RAIU was 90% for hyperthyroidism and 85% for hypothyroidism. Current RAIU sensitivity in thyroid disease is difficult to determine because of reference range problems. However, sensitivity is probably about 80% for hyperthyroidism and about 50%–60% for hypothyroidism.

8. The patient receives a certain small amount of radiation (especially if a scan is done), whereas thyroid hormone assays, even those using radioisotopes, are performed outside the patient's body and therefore do not deliver any radiation to the patient.

These difficulties have precluded use of the RAIU measurement for screening purposes. However, RAIU in conjunction with the thyroid scan has definite value in patients when there is laboratory evidence of hyperthyroidism. As will be discussed later, the RAIU can help differentiate between primary hyperthyroidism and hyperthyroidism secondary to thyroiditis or self-administration of thyroid hormone; and the thyroid scan can differentiate Graves' disease from Plummer's disease.

Thyroid Hormone–Binding Ratio (THBR; T_3 Uptake)

The THBR is a variant of what is commonly known as the T_3 uptake, or T_3U. T_3U does not measure T_3, as its name might imply, but instead estimates the amount of nonoccupied (unsaturated) thyroid hormone–binding sites on serum protein. Therefore, the American Thyroid Association has recommended that the name thyroid hormone–binding ratio replace the name T_3 uptake. The T_3U was originally used as a substitute for direct T_4 measurement. Radioactive T_3 placed into patient serum competes for binding sites both with patient serum proteins and with a special hormone-binding resin (or other added binding material). The number of T_3 binding sites available on serum proteins depends primarily on the amount of T_4 occupying the protein binding sites, since T_4 molecules greatly outnumber T_3 molecules. Radioactive T_3 not able to bind to protein is forced onto the resin. Therefore, the greater the amount of T_4 bound to protein, the fewer protein binding sites are available for radioactive T_3, and the greater is the radioactive T_3 uptake by the resin.

Several modifications of the basic resin uptake procedure are sold by commercial companies. Although the various kits in general give similar results, in my experience there have been definite and significant differences between some of the kits. In particular, some may produce occasional and inexplicable mildly decreased results. There also is some confusion in the way that resin uptake results are reported. Most T_3 uptake kits use a reference range expressed in percent of resin uptake. A few count radioactivity in the serum proteins, which produces opposite values to those derived from resin uptake. Some kits (including the THBR) report results as a ratio between resin uptake and a "normal" control.

Results in Thyroid Disease.—As a thyroid function test, THBR becomes an indirect estimate of T_4 when the quantity of thyroxine-binding protein is normal, since the number of T_3 binding sites is determined primarily by the amount of T_4 and the amount of binding protein. There are rather widely variant opinions on diagnostic accuracy of THBR in thyroid disease. Some reports were highly favorable, although recent ones tend to be less so. There is reasonably good sensitivity for hyperthyroidism (approximately 80%, with a literature range of 46%–96%). The test is not affected by iodine. However, there is relatively poor separation of normal from hypothyroid conditions (sensitivity for hypothyroidism is approximately 50%–

60%, with a literature range of 27%–92%).

Drawbacks.—Problems in diagnosis of hypothyroidism were mentioned previously. Also, since the test depends on the number of binding sites, changes in the amount of thyroxine-binding protein will affect results. These alterations may be congenital, drug induced, or produced by nonthyroid illness (Table 28–2). There is interference by a considerable number of medications, the majority of which also affect serum T_4 assay (see Table 36–24). In addition, atrial fibrillation and severe acidosis have been reported to sometimes falsely increase the THBR. Current use of the THBR is mainly as an adjunct to a T_4 assay to provide a warning of alterations in thyroxine-binding protein. The THBR can also be of some help in ruling out laboratory error as a cause for T_4 elevation; if both the T_4 and resin uptake levels are increased, the T_4 elevation is probably genuine.

TABLE 28–2.

Causes for Increased or Decreased Thyroxine-Binding Globulin

- I. Increased TBG
  - A. Increased estrogens
    1. Pregnancy
    2. Oral contraceptives
    3. Estrogen therapy
  - B. Other medications
    1. Perphenazine (Trilafon) occasionally
    2. Heroin and methadone (variable degree)
  - C. Severe liver disease
    1. Severe acute hepatitis
    2. Severe cirrhosis (occasionally)
  - D. Congenital
  - E. Acute intermittent porphyria
- II. Decreased TBG
  - A. Certain medications
    1. Androgens
    2. Drugs (e.g., phenytoin and salicylate) that compete with T_4 and T_3 for binding sites on TBG or albumin
  - B. Severe nonthyroidal illness
  - C. Congenital decrease
  - D. Nephrotic syndrome or conditions leading to severe hypoproteinemia

Total Serum Thyroxine

Thyroxine can be measured directly by radioassay (or, more recently, by enzyme-linked assay). Radioassay involves competition of patient hormone and radioactive hormone for a hormone binder. In T_4 by radioimmunoassay (T_4-RIA) the binder is anti-T_4 antibody; in T_4 competitive binding (T_4-CPB) or T_4 displacement methods (T_4-D) the binder is T_4-binding serum protein. After patient T_4 and radioactive T_4 have reacted with the T_4 binder, the bound complex is separated from the free (unbound) hormone and the radioactivity in either the bound or free fraction is counted. The amount of patient T_4 determines the amount of radioactive T_4 allowed to attach to the binder.

Results in Thyroid Disease.—The sensitivity of T_4 assay is approximately 95% (literature range, 90%–100%) for hyperthyroidism, and approximately 92% (literature range, 54%–100%) for hypothyroidism. There is some difficulty in evaluating T_4 data for hypothyroidism from the literature since patients with a temporary T_4 decrease from thyroiditis or severe nonthyroid illness may be included with patients having true primary hypothyroidism in some reports.

Drawbacks.—As noted previously, more than 99% of total serum T_4 is protein bound, so that the contribution of free T_4 to the test results is negligible. Therefore, serum T_4 by any present-day method essentially measures protein-bound T_4 and will be affected by alterations in T_4-binding proteins. These alterations may be congenital, drug induced, or secondary to severe nonthyroid illness. As a rule of thumb, estrogens from pregnancy or birth control medication increase T_4 levels by increasing TBG levels, and amphetamine abuse is reported to increase T_4 levels in some patients by increasing pituitary secretion of TSH. Most other drugs that affect T_4 produce decreased T_4 levels by decreasing TBG levels or T_4 binding to TBG (or albumin). Medications that may affect T_4 assay are listed in Table 36–24. The most commonly encountered medication problems, in my experience, are associated with administration of levothyroxine (Synthroid), estrogens, or phenytoin (Dilantin). Like phenytoin, furosemide and some of the nonsteroidal anti-inflammatory drugs can decrease T_4 levels by displacing T_4 from it's binding proteins. However, these medications, especially furosemide, are often administered to patients who already have severe nonthyroid illness, so that it may be difficult to separate the effect of the drug from the effect of the illness.

With the possible exception of TBG alterations, the most frequent false abnormalities in T_4 are produced by severe nonthyroidal illness. Severe nonthyroid illnesses or malnutrition of various etiologies may decrease T_4 below the lower limits of the T_4 reference range. The incidence of decreased T_4 is roughly proportional to the severity of illness. Therefore, the overall incidence of decreased T_4 in nonthyroid illness is low but in severe illness reports indicate decreased T_4 levels in approximately 20%–30% of cases (literature range, 9%–59%); and in a lesser number of cases even free T_4 assay is reduced below reference limits. As discussed later, serum TSH levels often decrease in nonthyroid illness somewhat parallel to T_4 but to a lesser extent, usually (but not always) remaining within reference range. In the recovery phase, TSH levels increase before or with T_4 and could temporarily even become elevated. Table 28–3 lists various causes of T_4 decrease.

Cushing's syndrome produces a mild or moderate T_4 decrease below lower limit of reference range in two thirds or more of patients. Free T_4 levels are usually normal.

Conditions producing an increase in T_4 levels without hyperthyroidism are listed in Table 28–5, Table 28–8, and portions of Table 28–10. One group of conditions involves certain iodine-containing substances. For many years it was thought that neither organic iodine nor inorganic iodide would interfere with the T_4-RIA method. However, it was subsequently found that a few x-ray contrast media such as ipodate (Oragrafin) and iopanoic acid (Telepaque) and also the iodinated antiarrhythmic drug amiodarone can increase T_4 values somewhat. These compounds do not affect the T_4 assay directly but can increase T_4 values by certain metabolic actions (e.g., blocking of T_4 deiodination) that are still being investigated. Effects of iodine on the thyroid will be discussed in detail later.

TABLE 28–3.

Decrease in Thyroxine Without Primary Hypothyroidism*

Laboratory error
Severe nonthyroid illness†
Decreased TBG levels (congenital, disease or drug induced)
Thyroiditis (some patients)‡
Certain drugs (e.g., lithium,‡ phenytoin)
Large doses of inorganic iodide (SSKI)‡§
Pituitary failure
Cushing's syndrome
Severe iodine deficiency‡

*Not all patients with any of these conditions have decreased T_4 levels.
†Some patients may have elevated TSH levels.
‡Those patients who have decreased T_4 levels usually have elevated TSH levels.
§SSKI = saturated solution of potassium iodide.

Free Thyroxine Index

The American Thyroid Association has recommended that the entity most commonly known as the free thyroxine index (FTI, or T-7, T-12, Clark and Horn index) be renamed the free T_4 index (FT_4I). The FT_4I was developed to correct the T_4 assay for effects of thyroxine-binding protein alterations. It consists basically of the serum T_4 result multiplied by the THBR result. This manipulation takes advantage of the fact that THBR (T_3U) and T_4 values travel in opposite directions when TBG alterations are present, but they proceed in the same direction when the TBG value is normal and the only variable is the amount of T_4. For example, in hyperthyroidism both the T_4 and THBR values are increased, and the two high values, when multiplied together, produce an elevated FTI. On the other hand, estrogen in birth control medication or pregnancy elevates TBG levels. Normally, TBG is about one third saturated with T_4. If the TBG level is increased, the additional TBG also becomes one third saturated. Thus, the total T_4 value is increased due to the normal amount of T_4 plus the extra T_4 on the extra TBG. Thyroxine-binding globulin binding sites are similarly increased by the additional TBG, leading to a decreased THBR, because additional radioactive T_3 is bound to the additional TBG, with less T_3 attracted to the resin. Therefore, if estrogens increase the TBG value, the T_4 level is increased and the THBR is decreased; the high number multiplied by the low number produces a middle-range normal index number. Actually, if one knows the reference values for the T_4 assay and the THBR, one simply decides whether assay values for the two tests have equivalent positions in their separate reference ranges (i.e., both increased or both near the middle of the reference range) or whether the values are divergent (i.e., one near the upper limit and the other near the lower limit). If the values are considerably divergent, there is a question of possible thyroxine-binding protein abnormality. Therefore, it is more helpful to have the T_4 and THBR values than the index number alone, because these values are sometimes necessary to interpret the index or provide a clue to technical error.

Results in Thyroid Disease.—In general, the FT_4I does an adequate job in canceling the effects of thyroxine-binding protein alterations without affecting results in thyroid dysfunction. Reported sensitivity in hyperthyroidism is approximately 95% (literature range 90%–100%). Reported sensitivity in hypothyroidism is approximately 90%–95% (literature range, 78%–100%). Therefore, as with T_4, there seems to be more overlap in the hypothyroid than the hyperthyroid area.

Drawbacks.—Although there is general agreement in the literature that the FT_4I is more reliable than T_4 in the diagnosis of hypothyroidism when the T_4 value is decreased, and also more accurate in the diagnosis of thyroid dysfunction when TBG alteration is present, the FT_4I itself gives misleading results in a significant minority of cases. In TBG alteration due to estrogen in oral contraceptives or in pregnancy, the reported incidence of T_4 elevation is approximately 40% of cases, whereas the reported incidence of FT_4I elevation is approximately 10%–15% (literature range, 0%–29%). The FT_4I is usually normal in nonthyroid illness, but in severe illness it may be decreased in approximately 10%–15% of cases (literature range, 4%–43%). There is some correlation with the severity of illness.

"Corrected" Thyroxine Assays

Several manufacturers have devised techniques for internally "correcting" T_4 results for effects of TBG alterations. Depending on the manufacturers these have been called ETR, Normalized T_4, and other brand names. The ETR is the only test from this group for which there are evaluations from a substantial number of laboratories. In general, results were not as favorable as those obtained with the FT_4I.

Free T_4 Assay

Another approach to the problem of thyroxine-binding protein alteration is to measure free T_4 rather than total T_4. The amount of protein-bound inactive T_4 by itself has no direct influence on the serum level of metabolically active free hormone. The original Sterling technique involved separation of free from protein-bound T_4 by a dialysis membrane. The procedure was complicated and was available only in a few reference laboratories. Since then, at least four FT_4 nondialysis methods have been introduced that are based on different principles but that are simple enough to be within the technical ability of most ordinary laboratories. At present, most kit manufacturers use the "analogue" method, because it is the easiest and least expensive. A synthetic molecule similar to T_4 (T_4 analogue) is created that will not bind to TBG but will compete with nonbound (free) T_4 for anti-T_4 antibody. This analogue is labeled with an isotope or enzyme system, so that the amount of analogue bound to the antibody is proportional to the amount of free T_4 available. The analogue kits appear to function as well or slightly better than the FT_4I in differentiating euthyroid persons from hyperthyroid and hypothyroid patients.

Drawbacks.—Unfortunately, in patients with severe nonthyroid illness most of the first-generation analogue kits were falsely decreased as often as the ordinary T_4 methods and more often than the FT_4I. Although the reasons for this have been disputed, the consensus indicates that the analogues bind to albumin to some degree and also are affected by nonesterified fatty acids. Albumin is often decreased in severe nonthyroid illness. The manufacturers now attempt to "correct" their analogue kits in various ways, most often by adding a blocking agent that is supposed to prevent analogue binding to albumin. At present, most analogue kits are less affected by nonthyroid illness than previously, but they still are affected, with a rate of false decrease about the same as the FT_4I. However, not all FT_4 kits perform equally well.

Total Serum Triiodothyronine (T_3-RIA)

Serum T_3 may be assayed by the same technique as T_4-RIA. Total serum T_3 (T_3-RIA) is a specific, direct measurement of T_3 using anti-T_3 antibody and should not be confused with the test formerly called the T_3U. As previously mentioned, the T_3U (THBR) is primarily an estimate of serum protein unsaturated binding sites, which secondarily provides an indirect estimate of T_4 but not of T_3. It is unfortunate that many used to speak of the T_3U as "the T_3 test," making it difficult to be certain whether T_3U or T_3-RIA was meant. Analogous to T_4 assay, serum T_3 consists mostly of protein-bound T_3. Therefore, serum T_3 measurement is affected by alterations in thyroxine-binding proteins in the same direction as serum T_4, although to a slightly lesser degree than serum T_4. One may obtain a free T_3 index using T_3-RIA and THBR (T_3U) values.

Results in Thyroid Disease.—Under usual circumstances, T_3-RIA has at least as good sensitivity as T_4 in detecting thyrotoxicosis. In fact, some investigators have stated that T_3-RIA is the most sensitive test for standard hyperthyroidism associated with increase of both T_4 and T_3, occasionally demonstrating elevation at an early stage before T_4 values have risen above reference range upper limits. In addition, T_3-RIA helps to detect that form of hyperthyroidism known as "T_3 toxicosis" in which the T_3 level is elevated but not the T_4 level. Triiodothyronine toxicosis has been estimated to comprise about 3%–4% of hyperthyroid patients.

Drawbacks.—Unfortunately, T_3-RIA has several substantial drawbacks. First, although T_3-RIA test kits are as easy to use as T_4-RIA kits, there seems to be more variation in results among T_3 kits from different manufacturers than among T_4 kits. Second, as noted previously, T_3-RIA is affected by thyroxine-binding protein alterations similarly to T4. Third, perhaps the most serious drawback is the strong tendency of many severe acute or chronic nonthyroid illnesses to decrease T_3-RIA values even though the patient remains clinically euthyroid. In many of these cases T_4 conversion to T_3 in peripheral tissues is temporarily decreased and instead is shunted toward reverse T_3 production. The effects of nonthyroid illness considerably decrease the usefulness of the T_3-RIA in hospitalized patients. Fourth, T_3-RIA is not reliable in hypothyroidism, because there is considerable overlap between values from hypothyroid patients and the low-normal reference range. A few reports suggest that occasional persons have mildly hypothyroid T_4 levels but enough T_3 secretion by the thyroid to maintain a clinically euthyroid state. Fifth, T_3-RIA is increased in iodine deficiency.

A sixth problem affecting T_3-RIA is difficulty in defining the reference range. Persons over age 60 may have reference limits that are significantly lower than those for persons under age 60. Most studies have found a 10%–30% decrease in mean values after age 60, although reports have varied from 0%–52%, possibly because of differences in response by different manufacturer's kits or differences in the populations tested. If the kit used by any individual laboratory is affected, this implies that a result in an elderly person within the reference range but near the upper limit of the range may, in fact, be elevated for that patient if the reference range is not age corrected. A few studies report a lifelong decrease of 5–10 ng/ml/10 years. This implies that T_3-RIA values in childhood are higher than those for adults.

Serum Thyrotropin Assay (TSH)

Thyrotropin previously was known as thyroid stimulating hormone (TSH), and the abbreviation TSH is still used. Direct assay of TSH is now possible with commercially available kits that are as easy to use as those for T_4 assay. Thyrotropin has a diurnal variation of two to three times baseline (literature range, 33%–600%), with highest levels occurring at about 10–11 P.M. (range, 6 P.M.–2 A.M.) and lowest levels at about 10 A.M. (range, 8 A.M.–4 P.M.).

Results in Thyroid Disease.—Serum TSH levels are elevated in about 95% of patients with myxedema due to primary thyroid disease, which comprises 95%–96% of hypothyroid patients. Serum TSH levels are low in most cases of secondary (pituitary or hypothalamic) myxedema (about 4% of hypothyroid patients). Some patients with secondary hypothyroidism have normal TSH values when one would expect low TSH levels. The pituitary of these patients is able to secrete a small amount of TSH, not enough to maintain normal T_4 levels but enough to leave TSH values within reference range. The T_3-RIA values in these patients may be decreased, but in some instances may be low normal; either because of preferential secretion of T_3 rather than T_4 by subnormal TSH stimulation or because of problems with kit sensitivity in low ranges. In primary hyperthyroidism, serum TSH is decreased, the percentage of patients with decreased values depends on the sensitivity of the particular kit used. Prior to 1985, most commercially available kits were poorly sensitive in the lower part of their range, and could not easily differentiate low values from zero or from low normal values. About 1985, manufacturers began modifying their TSH kits so as to increase sensitivity at the lower end of the TSH range in order to detect the decreased TSH levels found in primary hyperthyroidism. These "ultrasensitive" TSH kits are sensitive enough in the low range that the decreased values in hyperthyroid patients can be reliably separated from low-normal euthyroid patient values. Since efficiency in detecting the elevated values of hypothyroidism are still excellent, some endocrinologists have advocated use of these ultrasensitive TSH assays as the only test necessary to screen for and diagnose thyroid disease.

Drawbacks.—Evaluations in the literature and my own experience have shown that not all TSH kits (either "standard" or "ultrasensitive") perform equally well. Laboratory error may produce false normal or abnormal results. In addition, there are conditions other than hypothyroidism or hyperthyroidism that can produce abnormal TSH results (see Tables 28–4 and 28–10).

Some causes of increased TSH results are listed in Table 28–4. There is some controversy whether or not elevated TSH levels in some of these conditions (except adrenal insufficiency and heterophil or anti-TSH antibodies) represent a mild hypothyroid state with the pituitary forced to secrete more TSH to maintain clinical euthyroidism. The serum TSH level in primary hypothyroidism is usually elevated to values more than twice normal and frequently to more than three times normal; whereas TSH levels in the other conditions frequently are less than twice normal and in most cases are less than three times normal.

Some cases of elevated free T_4 levels accompanied by TSH values that were inappropriately elevated (above the lower third of the TSH reference range) rather than depressed have been reported. These cases have been due to TSH-producing pituitary tumors, defective pituitary response to thyroid hormone levels, or peripheral tissue resistance to the effects of thyroid hormone (laboratory error in T_4 or TSH assay also must be excluded). Some (a minority) of the current TSH kits (predominantly the solid-phase double-antibody technique) may cross-react with hCG if hCG is present in very large amounts. These TSH kits will indicate varying degrees of (false) TSH increase during pregnancy and in the rare syndrome of hyperthyroidism due to massive hCG production by a hydatidiform mole or choriocarcinoma. Likewise, some (a minority) of the double antibody kits using the "sandwich" technique, when one of the antibodies has been produced in mice, may become falsely elevated due to interference by a heterophil-type antibody in the patient serum that reacts with the mouse-derived antibody. These antimouse antibodies usually occur without known cause and in one study were found in 9% of blood donors. Some manufacturers have attempted to counteract or neutralize the effect of these antibodies, with a variable degree of success. Another antibody problem of a different type concerns artifactual interference in TSH assay procedure by anti-TSH antibodies in patients who had previous TSH injections and who developed antibodies against the injected material.

In severe nonthyroid illness, it was soon noticed that a considerable number of the "ultrasensitive" TSH kits were producing abnormal results in clinically euthyroid patients. Previous "standard" TSH kits, although less sensitive in the lower range, generally produced normal TSH values in severe nonthyroid illness. The percentage of abnormal results in

TABLE 28–4.
Elevation of Thyrotropin Without Primary Hypothyroidism

- Laboratory error
- Pituitary TSH–secreting tumor
- Euthyroid goiter with enzyme defect
- Some patients with
  - Severe nonthyroid illness
  - Thyroiditis
  - Large doses of inorganic iodide (e.g., SSKI)
  - Primary Addison's disease
  - Iodine deficiency goiter
  - Postsubtotal thyroidectomy
  - After iodine 131 thyroid radiotherapy
  - Hypothermia
- TSH diurnal variation peak 6 P.M.–2 A.M.
- Presence of anti-TSH antibodies
- Cross-reaction in some TSH methods with alpha subunit of hCG*
- Interference in some TSH methods by patient antimouse antibodies

*hCG = human chorionic gonadotropin.

the "ultrasensitive" kits varies between different kits and also depends on the severity of illness. Most abnormality is reported in severe nonthyroid illness, and is manifested by decreased TSH in about 15% of cases (range, 0%–72%) and elevated TSH in about 7% of cases (range, 0%–17%). Of those elevated, most (but not all) were less than twice the upper limit of the reference range. The decreased values return toward normal as the patient recovers; in some reports, most of the elevated values occurred in the recovery phase. This has been interpreted as pituitary inhibition during the acute phase of the illness and release of inhibition in the recovery phase. As mentioned, some kits are less likely to produce abnormal TSH results than other kits in severe nonthyroid illness.

The antiarrhythmic drug amiodarone contains a considerable amount of inorganic iodide. In some patients it may cause iodine-induced thyrotoxicosis (Jod-Basedow disease; more common in patients with preexisting iodine deficiency). In others, it may lead to iodine suppression of the thyroid (similar to SSKI therapy), producing decreased T_4 and elevated TSH values. A third effect is inhibition of peripheral tissue conversion of T_4 to T_3; the patients remain euthyroid, but there is elevation of T_4 and TSH in some patients, while T_3-RIA is relatively normal. In patients with amiodarone-induced T_4 elevation, T_3-RIA is said to be normal in euthyroid patients with T_4 artifact due to peripheral T_4 conversion abnormality but elevated in those with Jod-Basedow hyperthyroidism.

Thyroid Stimulation and Suppression Tests

Thyrotropin Stimulation Test.—In some patients with myxedema, the question arises as to whether the etiology is primary thyroid disease or a malfunction secondary to pituitary deficiency. Normally, administration of TSH more than doubles a baseline RAIU or T_4 value. Failure of the thyroid to respond to TSH stimulation strongly suggests primary thyroid failure, whereas normal gland response implies either a pituitary or hypothalamic problem or else some artifactual abnormality in the original screening tests. The same procedure can be used to confirm the diagnosis of primary hypothyroidism, since the thyroid should not be able to respond to TSH. The test may be helpful in patients who have been on long-term thyroid hormone treatment and who must be reevaluated as to whether the original diagnosis of hypothyroidism was correct. The TSH stimulation test can be done while thyroid hormone is still being administered, whereas it would take several weeks after cessation of long-term therapy for the pituitary-thyroid relationship to reach pretherapy equilibrium.

Drawbacks.—The TSH stimulation test is performed using bovine TSH. Some persons form antibodies against this material that may interfere with future TSH assay or produce allergic reaction if TSH is used again. Therefore, the test is infrequently used today. To avoid this potential problem, some investigators use a T_3 withdrawal test rather than TSH stimulation.

Triiodothyronine Withdrawal Test.—The patient is placed on T_3 therapy for 1 month (instead of other therapy). The T_3 is then discontinued for 10 days, after which a serum TSH assay is performed. With medication containing T_4 it is necessary to wait at least 4 weeks after withdrawal before routine thyroid function tests (T_4, T_3, TSH), are performed to allow the thyroid-pituitary-hypothalamic feedback system to regain normal equilibrium. After T_3 withdrawal, it takes only 10 days to achieve the same effect. If the patient has primary hypothyroidism, the serum TSH level will be elevated after 10 days without T_3. In euthyroid persons or those with secondary and tertiary hypothyroidism, the TSH level will be normal or decreased. The major drawbacks to this procedure are the long time intervals necessary and the fact that not enough experience with this test has been reported to ascertain how many exceptions or false results may be expected. This test also is rarely used today.

Thyroid Suppression Test.—This is frequently called "T_3 suppression," although T_4 could be used instead of T_3, and the pituitary rather than the thyroid is the actual organ directly suppressed by T_3 administration (the thyroid is affected secondarily). A standard dose of T_3 is given daily for 1 week. In normal persons, exogenous T_3 (added to the patient's own T_4) suppresses pituitary secretion of TSH, leading to a decrease in patient thyroid hormone manufacture. Values of RAIU or T_4 after T_3

administration drop to less than 50% of baseline. In hyperthyroidism, the thyroid is autonomous and continues to manufacture hormone (with little change in RAIU or T_4 level), although the pituitary is no longer stimulating the thyroid. The suppression test is thought to be very reliable in confirming borderline hyperthyroidism, although there are reports that 25% or more of patients with nontoxic nodular goiter may fail to show suppression. The same basic technique may be used in conjunction with the thyroid scan to demonstrate that a nodule seen on original scan is autonomous. This may be helpful, since reports indicate that 50%–80% of toxic nodular goiter patients have normal RAIU values and many have normal T_4 test results. The procedure must be used with caution in elderly persons or patients with cardiac disease. The T_3 suppression test has been largely replaced by the TRH test.

Thyrotropin-Releasing Hormone (TRH) Test

Synthetic TRH (Thypinone) is now available. Intravenous bolus administration of TRH normally results in a marked rise in serum TSH levels by 30 minutes after the dose. Serum prolactin levels also increase. There is some disagreement as to how much TRH to administer, with doses reported in the literature ranging from 100–500 μg. Early studies reported that at least 400 μg was needed to obtain full TRH effect. Interpretation depends on whether the patient has evidence of hyperthyroidism or hypothyroidism (see Table 36–25).

Thyrotropin-Releasing Hormone Results in Hyperthyroidism.—In hyperthyroidism, pituitary TSH production is suppressed by direct effect of excess circulating T_4/T_3 on the pituitary, and TSH assay after TRH fails to demonstrate a significant degree of TSH increase from pretest baseline values (positive test result). Unfortunately, about 5% false positive results (failure to elevate serum TSH levels after TRH) have been reported in persons without demonstrable hyperthyroidism. A flat or blunted TSH response to TRH has also been reported in patients with autonomous thyroid nodules but no clinical evidence of hyperthyroidism; in a considerable number of patients after adequate treatment of Graves' disease; and in some patients with multinodular goiter. Certain other conditions (discussed later) may also affect results. A flat TRH test result is therefore considered very suggestive but not conclusive evidence of thyrotoxicosis. A normal result (normal degree of TSH elevation after TRH) is considered very reliable in excluding thyrotoxicosis. For this reason the TRH test is currently considered the most reliable confirmatory procedure for hyperthyroidism and is the standard against which all other tests are compared for accuracy.

Thyrotropin-Releasing Hormone Results in Hypothyroidism.—In primary hypothyroidism the TRH test usually demonstrates an exaggerated TSH response. This may render the test useful in the occasional patient with both equivocal symptoms and equivocal serum TSH values. One problem, however, is disagreement in the literature concerning how much TSH increase over baseline is considered exaggerated. The normal limit of increase over baseline varies in the literature from 20–35 μU/ml, so that 25 μU/ml seems to be a reasonable compromise. Theoretically, the TRH test should be able to differentiate between hypothyroidism from inability of the pituitary to secrete TSH due to pituitary disease (secondary hypothyroidism) and inability of the hypothalamus to secrete TRH (tertiary hypothyroidism). In pituitary disease, the serum TSH level should not rise significantly after TRH adminstration, whereas in hypothalamic disease there characteristically is a TSH response that is normal in degree but that is delayed for approximately 30 minutes. Unfortunately, a substantial number of patients with pituitary lesions demonstrate relatively normal or delayed TRH test reponse. Therefore, absent or markedly blunted response is strongly suggestive of primary pituitary disease, but response to TRH is not diagnostic of hypothalamic disease.

Thyrotropin-Releasing Hormone Results in Psychiatric Patients.—There have been reports that the TRH test is useful in differentiating unipolar (primary depression only) from bipolar (manic-depressive) psychiatric illness and from secondary types of depression. In unipolar depression, TRH-induced TSH response is said to be blunted in up to two thirds of patients, whereas most patients with other categories of depression have normal TSH response. Occasional patients with symptoms of depression may actually have thyrotoxicosis ("apathetic hyperthyroidism") and some may have hypothyroidism.

Drawbacks.—There is conflicting evidence in the literature regarding the effects of severe nonthyroidal illness on TRH test results. At least one report indicates that a blunted response may occur in some apparently euthyroid patients with depressed T_4 levels associated with severe nonthyroidal illness and also in some patients with hypothyroidism under the same conditions. This would complicate the diagnosis of hypothyroidism in some cases as well as the differential diagnosis of primary vs. secondary etiology. In addition, certain conditions such as psychiatric unipolar depression, fasting more than 48 hours' duration, and therapy with aspirin, levodopa, or adrenocorticosteroids depress TSH response to TRH. Patients should discontinue dessicated thyroid or T_4 therapy for 3–4 weeks (literature range, 2–5 weeks) before a TRH test. Another (although not major) drawback is the $30–$40 cost for TRH and the need for two or three TSH assay specimens.

Thyroid Scan

Thyroid uptake of radioactive isotopes of iodine or technetium may be counted by a special radiation detector that produces a visual overall pattern of gland radioactivity. This permits visual localization of areas that may be hyperactive or hypoactive. Thyroid scan has two major applications:

1. In patients with hyperthyroidism, the scan can differentiate between diffuse hyperplasia and a hyperfunctioning nodule ("toxic nodule"), entities that require different treatment. In addition, occasional patients with symptoms of hyperthyroidism have chronic lymphocytic thyroiditis. Serum T_4 and T_3 levels are frequently elevated. Both elevated and low 24-hour RAIU values have been reported. Early (2–6 hours) RAIU values may be elevated more frequently than the 24-hour uptake. Thyroid scan frequently has a rather characteristic nonuniform appearance that can be helpful in suggesting the diagnosis. Factitious (self-medication) hyperthyroidism and subacute thyroiditis usually are associated with a low RAIU value in conjunction with an elevated T_4 level (falsely low RAIU due to excess iodine or previous antithyroid therapy must be ex

2. In patients with a palpable thyro ule, the scan may demonstrate lack of ra activity in that area ("cold" nodule), suggestin a lack of functional activity that would increase suspicion of carcinoma. Most reports agree that a hyperfunctioning nodule is rarely malignant. Single nonfunctioning nodules have a 10%–20% incidence of malignancy. Truly nonfunctioning nodules are much more likely to be malignant than nodules that retain some function. At times, however, normal thyroid tissue above or below a nodule may contribute some degree of apparent function to a nonfunctioning area. However, there is some controversy over the usefulness of thyroid scanning in the evaluation of thyroid nodules for possible malignancy (see chapter 32).

EFFECTS OF IODINE ON THYROID TESTS

Iodine Deficiency

Iodine deficiency goiter is rare in the United States but still might be encountered by a physician. Iodine deficiency leads to an increase in RAIU. In mild or moderate iodine deficiency there is said to be a decrease in T_4 and THBR values, but values usually remain within their reference range. Often T_3-RIA is increased. Assay levels of TSH are usually normal. In severe iodine deficiency, T_4 and THBR values often decrease and T_3-RIA increases. The TSH level may be elevated but only to a mild or moderate degree. Thus, iodine deficiency may simulate thyrotoxicosis (goiter and RAIU increases), T_3 toxicosis (goiter with normal or decreased T_4 levels and elevated T_3-RIA) or even hypothyroidism (decreased T_4 level).

Iodine Excess

As noted previously, excess iodine usually results from inorganic iodide, most commonly found in respiratory tract medications such as SSKI, or from organic iodine present in x-ray contrast media and in certain medications such as the antiarrhythmic drug amiodarone. **With long-term SSKI therapy,** when the medication is initially administered, there is a decrease in T_4 values of varying degree, accompanied by an increase in TSH values, followed by a return of the T_4 and TSH values toward baseline levels in days or weeks. However, some of those whose

T_4 level stabilizes within reference range have persisting mildly elevated TSH level. A minority of patients have persistently decreased T_4 and increased TSH values, which tend to be more frequent in patients with preexisting thyroid diseases such as Hashimoto's thyroiditis, therapy with lithium carbonate, previous iodine deficiency, and patients with treated Graves' disease or toxic nodules. On the other hand, inorganic iodide can occasionally induce thyrotoxicosis (Jod-Basedow's disease), most commonly when administered to persons who are iodine deficient. As noted previously, **certain x-ray contrast media** (ipodate and iopanoic acid) may temporarily increase T_4 levels (due to inhibition of T_4 to T_3 conversion) but usually only to a mild degree (20%–40% over baseline). This may or may not be accompanied by a mild increase in TSH values. Marked T_4 elevation suggests Jod-Basedow's disease. If this occurs, it is usually associated with a decreased RAIU value. **Amiodarone** produces more frequent and substantial abnormalities than does x-ray contrast media. The T_4 level is elevated over reference range upper limit in 20%–30% (range, 10%–40%) of patients; there are no clinical signs of hyperthyroidism, and the elevated T_4 level is accompanied by increased reverse T_3 and normal T_3-RIA, THBR, and TSH values. The RAIU value can be decreased or normal. A few patients develop thyrotoxicosis that is thought to represent Jod-Basedow's disease. This is said to be more frequent in iodine-deficient persons. The T_4, FT_4, FT_4I, THBR, and T_3-RIA values are elevated, whereas the TSH value is low. On the other hand, decreased T_4 and elevated TSH values with clinical hypothyroidism occurs in 15%–20% of patients. In those patients with thyroid test abnormalities, the test results usually return to normal in 3–7 months after the end of amiodarone therapy.

THYROID TESTS IN PHENYTOIN THERAPY

There are conflicting statements in the literature on the effect of phenytoin (diphenylhydantoin; Dilantin) on certain thyroid tests. Dilantin is known to compete for binding sites on TBG, but it may also affect thyroid tests due to activation ("induction") of liver microsomal enzymes, resulting in accelerated metabolic alteration of T_4. The majority of reports indicate that T_4, free T_4, and T_3-RIA values are somewhat decreased from pretreatment levels. The T_4 level is said to decrease about 25%–33% from pretreatment level, whereas the T_3-RIA value decreases about 15%. In one study, the T_4 level decreased below reference range in 40% of patients, whereas the T_3-RIA value remained within reference range in all patients. The THBR, TSH and TRH tests are not significantly affected.

LABORATORY TEST PATTERNS IN HYPERTHYROIDISM

The diagnosis of thyroid disease now depends as much on laboratory results as it does on clinical findings. One might therefore use the term "laboratory hyperthyroidism" when considering the spectrum of test results in thyrotoxicosis in the same manner that one employs the term "clinical hyperthyroidism" when evaluating patient signs and symptoms. Laboratory diagnosis is usually based on elevated values of serum T_4 and T_3, the two active thyroid hormones. Laboratory hyperthyroidism can be subdivided into three categories, depending on T_4 and T_3-RIA results:

1. Standard T_4/T_3 toxicosis (both T_4 and T_3-RIA elevated).
2. Triiodothyronine toxicosis (T_3-RIA elevated, T_4 not elevated).
3. Thyroxine toxicosis (T_4 elevated, T_3-RIA not elevated).

Standard T_4/T_3 toxicosis includes nearly 95% of cases of hyperthyroidism.

Triiodothyronine toxicosis is estimated to occur in 3%–5% of hyperthyroidism patients (literature range, 2.4%–30%). Although T_3-RIA values are increased in T_3 toxicosis, the T_4, THBR, and RAIU values are usually all normal. There is some evidence that T_3 toxicosis is more common in patients with atrial fibrillation, and it may be associated more often with Plummer's disease than with Graves' disease (although not all investigators agree). One report indicates that T_3 toxicosis is more common in iodine-deficiency areas (although some of these cases might have been pseudo-T_3 toxicosis with T_4 levels decreased because of the iodine deficiency). TSH is decreased in T_3 toxicosis.

Thyroxine toxicosis has not received much attention, and it was assumed to be less frequent than T_3 toxicosis. In the more recent articles on this subject in the literature, incidence ranged from 0%–21% of hyperthyroid patients, although the true incidence is probably less than that of T_3 toxicosis. Several investigators report that T_4 toxicosis is more commonly found with iodine-induced hyperthyroidism (Jod-Basedow's disease). Thyroxine toxicosis is also found more commonly in elderly persons, but in some reports it is difficult to be certain that some cases were not actually T_4/T_3 toxicosis with depressed T_3-RIA values due to concurrent severe illness.

Deceptive (Misleading) Test Patterns of Laboratory Hyperthyroidism

Each of the three categories of true laboratory thyrotoxicosis has a counterpart in which the apparent pattern does not reflect true thyroid hormone status. I would like to call the resulting test patterns "deceptive laboratory hyperthyroidism." These patterns are misleading because of nonthyroidal alteration of one or both thyroid hormone levels. Deceptive laboratory hyperthyroidism represents a significant (although relatively small) percentage of hyperthyroid patients. Therefore it is important to recognize these patients and to anticipate a potential problem when situations associated with deceptive test results arise.

1. Pseudo-T_4/T_3 hyperthyroidism (both T_4 and T_3-RIA test results are elevated in a euthyroid patient).
2. Pseudo-T_3 hyperthyroidism (T_3-RIA value elevated; T_4 test result not elevated).
3. Pseudo-T_4 hyperthyroidism (T_4 test result elevated; T_3-RIA value not elevated).

Laboratory error may produce apparent abnormality in a euthyroid person or may reduce one or both of the hormone levels in true thyrotoxicosis. Therefore, unexpected test patterns or results may require repetition of one or more of the tests before a definitive diagnosis is made. Abnormality of the same type on two tests (i.e., both test results elevated) is more helpful for diagnosis than abnormality of only one.

Pseudo–T_4/T_3 Hyperthyroidism (T_4 a. RIA Both Elevated)

Causes of pseudo-T_4/T_3 hyperthyroidism in euthyroid patients are listed in Table 28–5. Pseudo-hyperthyroidism is most commonly produced by increase of thyroid binding proteins, principally TBG. The most common etiology is increased estrogens, either in pregnancy or through use of birth control pills. Both T_4 and T_3-RIA values are elevated in many of these patients. However, in some, the T_3-RIA value may remain in upper reference range while only the T_4 value is elevated.

Effects of TBG alterations on T_4 levels can be counteracted in most instances by using the FT_4I or by measuring FT_4 rather than total T_4 values. The FT_4I or FT_4 value will usually be normal in TBG abnormalities. If the T3-RIA value is measured, it will appear to be elevated since TBG alterations affect T_3-RIA as well as T_4, and the combination of elevated T_3-RIA plus normal FT_4I values or FT_4 value would suggest T_3 toxicosis. Therefore, correction of only T_4 may avoid pseudo-T_4/T_3 toxicosis but produce pseudo-T_3 toxicosis. This hazard can be prevented by either applying the same basic FT_4I formula to T_3-RIA (thus generating an FT_3I) or simply inspecting the two separate components of the FT_4I, the T_4 and THBR (T_3 uptake). If T_4 and TBHR are at the opposite ends of their respective reference ranges, this suggests artifact due to TBG alteration. Unfortunately, many laboratories that generate FT_4I report only the single FT_4I result without separate T_4 and THBR values. The FT_4I value has no feature that could lead anyone to suspect TBG abnormality.

There are other causes of pseudo-T_4/T_3 toxicosis listed in Table 28–5. Occasional patients have been discovered with the syndrome of peripheral tissue resistance to thyroid hormone. These patients are euthyroid but have elevated T_4 and T_3-RIA values. TSH is normal or elevated.

TABLE 28–5.
Pseudo-T_4/T_3 Hyperthyroidism

Increased TBG values
Thyroiditis
Subacute
Painless (silent) thyroiditis
Some patients with Hashimoto's thyroiditis
Peripheral resistance to thyroid hormones
Factitious (self-medication with thyroid hormone)

TABLE 28–6.

Etiologies of Decreased Radioactive Iodine Uptake Values

Hypothyroidism, primary or secondary
Technical error
Excess organic iodine or inorganic iodide with euthyroidism
Subacute thyroiditis
Painless (silent) thyroiditis
Postpartum transient toxicosis
Some patients with chronic (Hashimoto's) thyroiditis
Amiodarone-induced hyperthyroidism
Self-administered (factitious) thyroid hormone intake
Iodide-induced (Jod-Basedow) hyperthyroidism
Struma ovarii

Factitious ingestion of T_4 compounds by a patient may be deliberate, may be due to prior therapy that is not mentioned by the patient, or may represent T_4 included in diet-control pills unknown to the patient. In both factitious T_4 ingestion and subacute thyroiditis the RAIU value is typically low. Spurious causes for a low RAIU value must be excluded, such as iodine ingestion (e.g., SSKI or amiodarone) or x-ray contrast medium administration within the past 3–4 weeks (Table 28–6).

Thyrotoxicosis in thyroiditis is usually temporary and is produced by release of thyroid hormone from damaged thyroid tissue rather than by hypersecretion. Subacute thyroiditis typically has pain in the thyroid area and is accompanied by a low RAIU value. The erythrocyte sedimentation rate (ESR) is usually elevated (> 50 mm/hour, Westergren method). Occasional cases of thyroiditis ("painless thyroiditis") may present with the clinical picture of subacute thyroiditis, including hyperthyroidism, but without a painful thyroid gland and with a normal ESR. Chronic lymphocytic thyroiditis (Hashimoto's thyroiditis) typically is associated with normal thyroid hormone blood levels, normal or decreased 24-hour RAIU value, normal ESR, and increased thyroid autoantibody levels. However, in occasional patients, chronic lymphocytic thyroiditis presents with hyperthyroidism that is clinically similar to nonpainful thyroiditis. The 24-hour RAIU value is typically decreased (although a few patients are reported to have normal values, and one study included a few patients with elevated values). Thyroid hormone levels are elevated, and the ESR is normal. Therefore, an elevated ESR favors subacute thyroiditis rather than factitious hyperthyroidism, painless thyroiditis, or thyrotoxic chronic lymphocytic thyroiditis.

Other entities with elevated T_4 or elevated T_3-RIA values associated with low RAIU values include T_4/T_3 toxicosis with artifactual RAIU suppression by exogenous iodine, iodine-induced hyperthyroidism (Jod-Basedow disease), radiation-induced active thyroid disease (caused by RAI therapy or external radiotherapy), and ectopic T_4 production (struma ovarii).

Pseudo-T_3 Hyperthyroidism (T_3-RIA Elevated; T_4 Not Elevated)

Pseudo-T_3 toxicosis may be of two types: (1) true hyperthyroid type, T_4/T_3 hyperthyroidism with normal-range T_4 test result; and (2) false hyperthyroid type, elevated T_3-RIA test result without hyperthyroidism (Table 28–7).

True Hyperthyroid Type.—Such cases are uncommon. It is said that T_3 values may rise before T_4 values in early thyrotoxicosis, and T_3-RIA values are usually elevated to a greater degree than T_4 values. Examples of isolated T_3 elevation that eventually was joined by T_4 elevation have been reported. An early or mild T_4 abnormality may be masked in the upper area of population reference range (if a person's normal T_4 value were in the lower part of population reference range, the T_4 value could double and still remain within reference range).

False Hyperthyroid Type.—This type of pseudo-T_3 toxicosis may be produced by measurement of T_3-RIA plus either the FT_4I or the FT_4 in patients with increased TBG values. Since FT_4I and FT_4 values usually remain normal when TBG values are altered, an increased TBG value would be associated with normal

TABLE 28–7.

Pseudo-T_3 Hyperthyroidism

True hyperthyroidism
Rise of T_3 level before T_4 level in early T_4/T_3 hyperthyroidism
False hyperthyroidism
Increased TBG with FTI (or FT_4) and T_3-RIA results
1–2 hr after dose of T_3 (liothyronine [Cytomel])
For several hours after dose of dessicated thyroid
Severe iodine deficiency

TABLE 28–8.
Pseudo-T_4 Hyperthyroidism

True hyperthyroidism (patient is hyperthyroid)
- Factitious ingestion of levothyroxine
- T_4/T_3 hyperthyroidism plus decrease in T_3-RIA result due to:
  - Severe nonthyroid illness
  - Advanced age
  - Certain medications (e.g., dexamethasone, propranolol)

False hyperthyroidism (patient is euthyroid)
- Increased TBG value plus decrease in T_3-RIA result
- Severe nonthyroid illness occasionally producing falsely elevated T_4 levels
- Increased TBG value with disproportionate T_4 increase relative to T_3-RIA
- Acute psychiatric illness (some patients)
- Amphetamine abuse
- Certain x-ray contrast media
- Certain medications (e.g., propranolol, amiodarone)
- Specimen obtained 1–4 hr after levothyroxine dose rather than just before the dose
- Patient taking therapeutic levothyroxine

FT_4I or FT_4 values plus artifactual increase in T_3-RIA value. The T_3-RIA value may be increased alone for 1–2 hours after T_3 (liothyronine) administration. It may also be temporarily increased for several hours after dessicated thyroid intake. Iodine deficiency of moderate degree usually is associated with normal T_3-RIA and T_4 levels, although mean T_3-RIA values are higher than in normal persons. In severe iodine deficiency, T_3-RIA values are sometimes increased, T_4 values may be decreased, and TSH values may be increased. The RAIU value is increased in iodine deficiency, providing additional potential for misdiagnosis. As noted previously, one report indicates that occasional free T_3 index elevations can be found in amphetamine abusers.

Pseudo-T_4 Hyperthyroidism (T_4 Elevated; T_3-RIA Not Elevated)

Pseudo-T4 toxicosis may be of two types: (1) true hyperthyroidism, T_4/T_3 toxicosis with (temporarily) reduced T_3-RIA test result; and (2) false hyperthyroidism, elevated T_4 test result in euthyroid patient (Table 28–8).

True Hyperthyroidism.—Ordinarily, both T_4 and T_3-RIA values are elevated in T_4/T_3 toxicosis or when the TBG value is incre Pseudo-T_4 toxicosis may be produced in p tients who have T_4/T_3 toxicosis if the T_3-RIA level becomes decreased for some reason while the T_4 level remains elevated. The most common causes for T_3-RIA decrease in T_4/T_3 toxicosis are severe nonthyroid illness and effect on T_3-RIA of old age. Many severe nonthyroid illnesses, particularly when chronic (see Table 28–3), depress T_3-RIA levels, often to very low levels. The free T_3 index also decreases but to a lesser extent. The effect of severe illness persists for variable periods of time and usually involves a shift from production of T_3 toward reverse T_3. Another factor that depresses T_3-RIA levels but not T_4 levels is the effect of advanced age. After age 60 years, most T_3-RIA kits have demonstrated a progressive decrease with time of approximately 10%–30% (literature range, 0%–52%). The degree of effect differs with individual manufacturers' kits. Unfortunately, very few laboratories determine age-related values for the particular kit that they use. There is general but not unanimous agreement that T_4 values are not greatly changed in old age. Certain medications (propranolol, dexamethasone) have been reported to decrease T_3-RIA levels, although not severely.

False Hyperthyroidism.—Artifactual T_4 elevation may result when TBG levels are increased, artifactually elevating both T_4 and T_3-RIA results, but some condition is superimposed that decreases T_3-RIA results, leaving only the T_4 value elevated. As noted previously, the most common reason for artifactual T_3-RIA decrease is severe nonthyroid illness. Another possibility is the effect of advanced age. In patients with normal TBG levels, severe nonthyroidal illness may be associated with T_4 values that are increased, decreased, or that remain within normal population range. Thyroxine levels most commonly display slight or mild decreases but still remain within normal limits. In a significant minority of patients (depending on the severity of illness), the T_4 level is decreased below its reference range to varying degrees, producing pseudohypothyroidism (clinical euthyroidism with laboratory test results falsely suggesting hypothyroidism). A small minority of patients exhibit an increase in T_4 results for poorly understood reasons. In these patients, pseudo-T_4 toxicosis would be produced without clinical hyperthyroidism or increased TBG levels (designated "T_4 euthyroidism" by some investigators). The TSH value in severe nonthyroidal illness is most often normal but may be mildly increased. The THBR level may be normal but is sometimes mildly increased, reflecting decreased TBG levels. Occasionally the THBR level is decreased, mainly in acute hepatitis.

Certain conditions produce artifactual elevation of T_4 values but not T_3-RIA values. In some patients with increased TBG values without severe nonthyroid illness, T_3-RIA values remain within upper reference range while the T_4 levels are elevated. One explanation is that increase in binding proteins affects T_4 levels somewhat more than T_3-RIA values. However, an increased TBG level frequently produces an elevated T_3-RIA value as well as a T_4 value. Elevated T_4 values with normal T_3-RIA values have been reported in some patients with acute psychiatric illness who were clinically euthyroid and where T_4 values returned to the reference range after treatment of the psychiatric problem. However, the possibility of true thyrotoxicosis should not be ignored.

Amphetamine abuse has been reported to increase serum T_4 values without affecting T_3-RIA values. Both the FTI and FT_3I are elevated in some of these patients. Some of these patients had mildly elevated serum TSH values and some did not. Increased FT_3I was also found in some cases without increase of FT_4 index.

Certain x-ray contrast media such as ipodate and iopanoic acid gallbladder visualization agents decrease T_3-RIA values and may increase T_4 values somewhat. Dexamethasone and propranolol are reported to decrease T_3-RIA values, as noted previously. Propranolol has been reported to increase T_4 values, but there is some disagreement as to whether this occurs.

If a patient is taking therapeutic levothyroxine (Synthroid, Levothroid), and a blood specimen happens to be drawn 1–4 hours after a dose has been administered, a result above steady-state level will often be obtained that might be above the reference range. Peak values after an oral dose are reached in 2–4 hours and average 1–3 μg above steady-state level. Even at steady-state levels and drawn just before the scheduled dose, patients who are clinically normal and whose TSH and T_3-RIA values are within reference range may have a steady state T_4 level as much as 2 μg above the upper limit of the T_4 reference range (discussed later). This is a problem because the dose is not always given at the scheduled time, the laboratory usually does not know what medications the patient is receiving to schedule the time of venipuncture, and sometimes the physician is unaware that a new patient is taking levothyroxine.

It has been reported that some hyperthyroid patients with elevated T_4 levels but normal-range T_3-RIA values have an elevated FT_3I.

Hyperthyroidism With False Laboratory Euthyroidism

One final category of deceptive hyperthyroidism may be added, clinical hyperthyroidism with falsely normal T_4 and T_3-RIA values (Table 28–9). Patients with decreased TBG levels may have falsely decreased T_4 and T_3-RIA levels that could convert elevated values to normal-range assay results. Severe nonthyroidal illness decreases T_3-RIA values and may decrease T_4 values. This could mask expected thyroid test results in T_3 toxicosis and in some cases of T_4/T_3 or T_4 toxicosis.

Isolated Graves' Ophthalmopathy

Besides the two classic types of clinical hyperthyroidism, there is one additional form known as isolated Graves' ophthalmopathy, or "euthyroid Graves' disease." This consists of eye signs associated with hyperthyroidism but without other clinical evidence of thyrotoxicosis and with normal RAIU, T_4, and T_3-RIA values. Evidence of true hyperthyroidism consists of reports that about 50%–70% of these patients fail to demonstrate thyroid suppression on the T_3 suppression test (literature range, 50%–100% in several small series of patients). About two thirds have a flat or blunted TSH response on the TRH test, suggestive of thyroid autonomy. A considerable number of these patients have detectable thyroid-stimulating immunoglobulins (TSI test, chapter 35). However, published reports of the latest versions of this test show considerable differences in

TABLE 28–9.

Hyperthyroidism With False Laboratory Euthyroidism
Hyperthyroidism plus decreased TBG value (see Table 28–1)
Hyperthyroidism plus severe nonthyroid illness (see Table 28–2)

sensitivity between laboratories. Similar differences were reported in detection rates for Graves' disease.

Confirmatory Tests for Hyperthyroidism

The existence of deceptive laboratory hyperthyroidism with the various forms of pseudotoxicosis accentuates the need for reliable confirmatory tests. This is especially true when the patient has severe nonthyroidal illness and symptoms such as atrial fibrillation that may be due to thyrotoxicosis. At present, the two most useful confirmatory procedures for hyperthyroidism are the T_3 suppression test and the TRH test. Of these, the main advantage of T_3 suppression over TRH is lower cost. Major disadvantages include potential danger in persons with cardiac disease and the prolonged time period necessary for the test. The TRH test has emerged as the gold standard for diagnosis of hyperthyroidism. The procedure appears to be safe, with relatively minor side effects. It can be completed in less than 1 day and can be used in most (but not all) patients with nonthyroidal illness. The major disadvantage is that a small minority of persons without clinical or biochemical evidence of thyrotoxicosis are reported to demonstrate TRH test results compatible with hyperthyroidism. A relative disadvantage is the high cost of the test, although the cost is not prohibitive and is comparable to the cost of nuclear medicine scans or radiologic procedures such as laminograms or skeletal surveys.

From the preceding discussion, several conclusions seem warranted:

1. The basic screening test for hyperthyroidism is serum T_4. Some are using the newer ultrasensitive TSH assay instead.
2. The THBR when ordered with the T_4 may be useful for two reasons: (1) the assurance it provides for hyperthyroidism when the THBR value is elevated in association with an elevated T_4 value and (2) as an indicator of TBG alterations when the results are compared with those of T_4 assay.
3. Free thyroxine index or FT_4 assay provide T_4 values corrected for effects of TBG alterations; but if the TBG value is elevated and thereby produces falsely elevated T_3-RIA values, a normal FT_4I or FT_4 assay result may lead to misdiagnosis of T_3 toxicosis.
4. Decreased or mildly elevated T_4 results must be interpreted with caution when a patient has severe nonthyroid illness.
5. The T_3-RIA results are not reliable when a patient has moderate or severe nonthyroid illness. A normal or reduced T_3-RIA result must be interpreted with caution if the patient is over age 60 or has any significant degree of nonthyroid illness.
6. An RAIU test is not recommended as a screening test but is helpful as a follow-up procedure to detect factitious hyperthyroidism and thyroiditis.
7. Thyroid scan is useful to differentiate between Graves' disease and Plummer's disease and to help reveal thyroiditis.
8. The TRH test may be necessary to confirm or exclude the diagnosis of hyperthyroidism when the patient has nonthyroidal illness (not severe enough to decrease T_4 below reference range), when thyroid function tests disagree, when test results are equivocal, and when test results do not fit the clinical picture. A normal test result is reasonably conclusive in ruling out hyperthyroidism, whereas an abnormal test result (abnormally low TSH response) is suggestive evidence of hyperthyroidism but is not completely reliable in confirming the diagnosis.

LABORATORY TEST PATTERNS IN HYPOTHYROIDISM

The physiology of thyroid hormone production in hypothyroidism is similar to that described in hyperthyroidism. Hypothyroidism may be divided into three types, depending on functional defect. Each of these categories may have various etiologies: (1) primary (primary thyroid T_4/T_3 secretion defect), (2) secondary (pituitary TSH secretion defect), and (3) tertiary (hypothalamus TRH secretion defect).

From the laboratory standpoint there are three basic laboratory test patterns:

1. Decreased T_4 value and markedly elevated TSH value (usually more than three times reference range upper limit). This pattern is diagnostic of primary hypothyroidism (with the possible exception of very severe iodine deficiency) and is found in the great majority of primary hypothyroid patients.
2. Thyroxine level in the lower half of the reference range with markedly elevated TSH

level. This pattern may be seen in patients with early or mild primary hypothyroidism.

3. Decreased T_4 level with decreased TSH values. This pattern suggests secondary or tertiary hypothyroidism.

THYROID TESTS IN HYPOTHYROIDISM

Serum Thyroxine.—Thyroxine is frequently used as the major screening test for hypothyroidism, since the T_4 level is low in most cases. There is some overlap between hypothyroid patients and normal persons in the lower part of the T_4 reference range, since persons with mild, early, or subclinical disease may be inadvertently included in groups of clinically normal persons used to establish the reference range. There is some evidence that nearly all hypothyroid patients within euthyroid population reference limits have T_4 values in the lower 50% of the reference range, so that T_4 values in the upper half of the reference range are generally reliable in excluding hypothyroidism. Laboratory error, of course, must be considered if the laboratory result does not conform to the clinical picture. If the patient specimens are kept at room temperature for more than 48–72 hours, as might happen when they are sent by mail, increase in fatty acids during transit may falsely increase T_4 values when competitive binding (displacement) T_4 methods rather than RIA methods are used. Conditions that alter T_4 results, such as TBG changes, nonthyroidal illness, and certain medications (see Table 36–24) must be remembered. Some endocrinologists are using TSH assay as a screening test instead of T_4.

Triiodothyronine-Radioimmunoassay.—T_3-RIA has not proved very useful in the diagnosis of hypothyroidism. The majority of reports indicate that one fourth to one third of hypothyroid patients have T_3-RIA values within normal range. In some cases, typically in Hashimoto's thyroiditis or after treatment of hyperthyroidism with radioactive iodine, it is thought that normal-range T_3-RIA values are due to preferential secretion of T_3 in what has been called the "failing gland syndrome." Test alterations due to nonthyroidal illness, age-related decrease, and TBG alterations further complicate interpretation.

Thyroid Hormone–Binding Ratio.—The THBR (T_3U) test is another test that has not been very helpful in screening for myxedema because of substantial overlap with the euthyroid reference range. The major benefit from its use in possible hypothyroidism is for detection of TBG abnormality.

Serum Thyrotropin (TSH) Assay.—Serum TSH levels are increased in the great majority of patients with primary hypothyroidism, and serum TSH assay is currently the most useful first-line confirmatory test. Since secondary hypothyroidism (pituitary failure) is uncommon and dysfunction due to hypothalamic etiology is rare, TSH assay has also been advocated as a screening test. Until recently TSH assay had not found wider use in screening for thyroid disease in general because of considerable overlap in the low range between hyperthyroid and euthyroid persons. This occurred because in most TSH assay kits the lower limit of the euthyroid reference range is relatively close to zero. In addition, these kits had relatively poor sensitivity in the low range, so that it was difficult to separate hyperthyroid values, which typically are subnormal, from zero on one hand and lower limit of normal on the other. Some euthyroid lower-normal specimens demonstrated the same problem. Therefore, TSH assay was restricted mostly to diagnosis of hypothyroidism. As mentioned earlier, several ultrasensitive TSH kits have recently become available that have adequate sensitivity in the low range to reliably separate decreased TSH values from low normal values. The ultrasensitive TSH is now being advocated by some investigators as the best single screening test for thyroid disease in general. But as I mentioned earlier, in my experience, at present all ultrasensitive TSH kits are not equally reliable. The TSH levels may be increased, usually (but not always) to mild degree, in some clinically euthyroid patients with a variety of conditions (see Table 28–4). When the TSH level is elevated in conditions other than primary hypothyroidism, TSH values are usually less than twice the upper reference range limit. However, sometimes they may be as high as three times the upper limit and occasionally even higher.

Primary hypothyroidism constitutes 95% or more of hypothyroid cases. The TSH assay in conjunction with the serum T_4 assay is sufficient for diagnosis in the great majority of these patients (decreased T_4 level with TSH level elevated more than twice and preferably more than three times the upper reference limit). In equivocal cases, a TRH test may be useful either to confirm primary hypothyroidism or to differentiate primary from secondary or tertiary etiology. As noted in the section on the TRH test, usefulness of the TRH test may be limited in severe nonthyroidal illness. In those circumstances, a TSH stimulation test might be useful.

It has been reported that there are several subgroups of patients with primary hypothyroidism, ranging from those with classic symptoms and markedly elevated TSH values to those with milder symptoms and only mildly elevated TSH values to those with equivocal or single symptoms and T_4 and TSH values remaining within population reference range and only the TRH test result abnormal.

About 5%–10% of patients referred to psychiatrists with symptoms of mood depression ("melancholia") have been reported to have laboratory evidence of hypothyroidism. This evidence ranges from decreased T_4 and elevated TSH levels to an exaggerated TRH test response as the only abnormality.

Thyrotropin-Releasing Hormone (TRH) Test.—A more complete discussion of the TRH test is located in the early part of this chapter. The TRH test has been mentioned as a confirmatory test for hypothyroidism. The TRH test has also been used to differentiate secondary from tertiary hypothyroidism. A significant increase in TSH after administration of TRH should theoretically suggest a hypothalamic rather than pituitary etiology for nonprimary hypothyroidism. Unfortunately, 40% of TSH hyposecretors of pituitary origin demonstrate adequate response to TRH stimulation. Therefore, only proof of pituitary hyposecretion by a poor response is considered sufficiently reliable for definite diagnosis. Even a poor response may not be reliable in the presence of severe nonthyroidal illness.

Pseudohypothyroidism

Pseudohypothyroidism may be defined as a decreased T_4 level in a euthyroid person. This may occur with (1) decreased TBG or TBG binding (congenital or drug induced), (2) certain medications (e.g., phenytoin, lithium, dopamine, corticosteroids), (3) some patients with severe nonthyroidal illness, (4) some clinically euthyroid patients with Hashimoto's thyroiditis, (5) after recent therapy of hyperthyroidism or thyroid cancer with radioactive iodine (some patients eventually develop true hypothyroidism), (6) Cushing's syndrome, (7) in some patients with SSKI therapy, and (8) severe iodine deficiency.

Most of these conditions have been discussed previously (see Table 28–3). The TSH levels are normal when the TBG level is decreased and in most of the drug-induced causes of nonhypothyroid T_4 decrease. Cushing's syndrome is associated with decreased T_4, T_3-RIA, TSH, and TBG levels in most patients. The TRH test results usually show a blunted TSH response. The TSH level becomes elevated in some (usually a minority) of patients with the remainder of the conditions listed above (also see Table 28–4); TSH values are usually (but not always) less than three times the upper limit of the reference range and most frequently are less than twice that limit. Decreased T_4 levels with elevated TSH levels in thyroiditis and following radioiodine therapy might be considered true hypothyroidism, even if it is only temporary, especially since some of these patients go on to develop clinical as well as laboratory hypothyroidism. Lithium carbonate therapy might be included in pseudohypothyroidism since the abnormalities it produces are reversible. About 8%–10% of patients have decreased T_4 levels, and about 15% (range, 2.3%–30%) of patients develop some degree of elevated serum TSH levels. In about 5% of patients the clinical as well as laboratory indices are compatible with true myxedema.

False Laboratory Euthyroidism in Hypothyroid Patients

Normal T_4 values in a hypothyroid patient may occur:

1. In early or very mild hypothyroidism. Serum TSH values are usually elevated. Some investigators have reported patients in whom the T_4 and TSH values were both within reference range, but the TRH test result exhibited an exaggerated response suggestive of hypothyroidism.

2. When the T_4 level in a hypothyroid person is artifactually increased into the normal population reference range. This may be due to elevated TBG levels or because the reference range overlaps with values for some patients with mild hypothyroidism. The TSH level should be elevated in most cases, unless the reason for the patient's hypothyroidism is pituitary insufficiency.

Summary of Laboratory Tests in Hypothyroidism

From the preceding discussion, several conclusions seem warranted:

1. Serum T_4 is the most widely used screening test for hypothyroidism, but some physicians use FT_4 or serum TSH assay instead. Values in the upper half of the T_4 and FT_4 reference range are strong evidence against hypothyroidism unless the TBG level is increased (congenital, pregnancy, or estrogen induced).
2. The THBR test is useful to detect TBG-induced alterations in T_4.
3. The new FT_4 methods circumvent the majority of TBG-induced problems and significantly reduce the number of pseudohypothyroid cases due to severe nonthyroidal illness. However, even the FT_4 may give falsely decreased results in seriously ill patients.
4. The TSH assay is the most useful single test to confirm primary hypothyroidism. In occasional patients a TRH test may be necessary.
5. Certain conditions may produce decreased T_4 levels, increased TSH levels, or both in occasional patients without primary hypothyroidism.

COMMENTS REGARDING USE OF THYROID TESTS

As previously noted, some thyroidologists and laboratorians advocate screening for thyroid disease with a single test, often citing need for cost containment. The ultrasensitive TSH appears to be advantageous for this purpose. The T_4 test result is more frequently normal in mild disease and more frequently abnormal in the absence of thyroid disease than is the ultrasensitive TSH. The FT_4 test has many of the same problems as the T_4 test, although the FT_4 is less frequently affected by nonthyroid conditions. The major problem with the one-test approach is that the clinician becomes very dependent on the laboratory to select a reliable method or commercial kit. I can verify that not all commercially available kits are equally reliable and that it takes search for published evaluations of the exact manufacturer's kit under consideration in addition to extensive evaluation of the kit in the potential user's own laboratory to establish proof of reliability. In addition, each laboratory should establish its own reference range using a statistically satisfactory number (at least 20) of blood donors or other clinically normal persons.

Finally, one has to consider the possibility of laboratory error, even though it may not be frequent on a statistical basis. For these and other reasons, some order two tests rather than one for screening purposes, such as the FT_4 plus the ultrasensitive TSH. If both test results are normal, this is very reassuring. If one or both are abnormal, either or both can be repeated to verify abnormality. The diagnosis sometimes can be made with this evidence plus clinical findings, or additional tests may be needed.

Since the T_4 (or its variants) and the ultrasensitive TSH are being used extensively to screen for and diagnose thyroid disease, it might be useful to catalog the patterns encountered using these two tests and some of the conditions that produce these patterns (Table 28–10).

MONITORING OF REPLACEMENT THERAPY

Desiccated thyroid and presumably other T_4 and T_3 combinations result in T_3-RIA values that may become elevated for several hours after administration and then decrease into the reference range. Thyroxine values remain within the reference range if replacement is adequate. In the few instances when clinical evidence and T_4 results disagree, TSH assay is helpful. Elevated TSH values suggest insufficient therapy. Unfortunately, low TSH values using standard TSH kits is not a reliable indicator of overtreatment since most of these kits produce considerable overlap between normal persons and those with decreased values in the low reference range area. Ultrasensitive TSH kits should solve this problem if the kit is reliable.

TABLE 28–10.

Interpretation of Abnormal T_4 and TSH Patterns (FT_4 and FTI Findings Can Be Substituted for T_4; Not Every Possible Etiology is Included)

T_4 low; TSH low
- Lab error (T_4 or TSH)
- Pituitary insufficiency
- Some patients with severe nonthyroid illness*
- Cushing's syndrome

T_4 low; TSH normal
- Lab error (T_4 or TSH)
- Severe nonthyroid illness
- Severe TBG or albumin deficiency
- Moderate iodine deficiency
- Dilantin therapy

T_4 low; TSH elevated
- Lab error (T_4 or TSH)
- Primary hypothyroidism
- Few patients with severe nonthyroid illness*
- Large doses of inorganic iodide (e.g., SSKI)
- Severe iodine deficiency
- Some patients on amiodarone therapy
- Some patients on lithium therapy

T_4 normal; TSH low
- Lab error (T_4 or TSH)
- T_3 toxicosis
- Pituitary insufficiency plus increased TBG
- Mild hyperthyroidism with decreased TBG and/or severe nonthyroidal illness
- Synthroid therapy with slightly high dose
- Few patients with severe nonthyroid illness*

T_4 normal; TSH elevated
- Lab error (T_4 or TSH)
- Mild hypothyroidism
- Hypothyroidism plus increased TBG
- Hypothyroidism with inadequate dose of replacement therapy
- Few patients with iodine deficiency (T_4 is usually decreased)
- Addison's disease (some patients)
- TSH specimen drawn in the evening (peak of diurnal variation)
- Few patients with severe nonthyroid illness*

T_4 elevated; TSH low
- Lab error (T_4 or TSH)
- Primary hyperthyroidism
- Jod-Basedow's disease
- Some patients with thyroiditis (subacute, "painless," early active chronic)
- Postpartum transient toxicosis

T_4 elevated; TSH normal
- Lab error (T_4 or TSH)
- TBG increase
- T_4 sample drawn 2–4 hr after T_4 dose
- Peripheral resistance to T_4
- Some patients with pituitary TSH-secreting tumor
- Some patients with Synthroid therapy, inadequate dosage
- Some patients with amiodarone therapy
- Occasional patients on propranolol therapy
- Certain x-ray contrast media

T_4 elevated; TSH elevated
- Lab error (T_4 or TSH)
- Pituitary TSH-secreting tumor
- TBG increase (T_4 elevation) plus TSH drawn at peak of diurnal variation
- Some patients with certain x-ray contrast media

*Depends on individual TSH kit (see text).

L-Thyroxine (Synthroid, Levothroid) results in T_3-RIA values that, in athyrotic persons, are approximately two thirds of those expected at a comparable T_4 level when thyroid function is normal. This is due to peripheral tissue conversion of T_4 to T_3. The T_3-RIA values are more labile than T_4 values and are more affected by residual thyroid function. The standard test to monitor L-thyroxine therapy is the T_4 assay. There is disagreement whether T_4 values must be in the upper half of the T_4 reference range or whether they can be mildly elevated. In general, when the TSH value returns to its reference range, the T_4 level stabilizes somewhere between 2 μg above and below the upper limit of the T_4 range. Thyroxine elevation more than 2 μg above reference range probably suggests too much dosage. A minority believe that T_4 values should not be above the reference range at all. On the other hand, T_4 values in the lower half of the reference range are usually associated with elevated TSH levels and probably represent insufficient replacement dose. Some investigators favor T_3-RIA to monitor therapy rather than T_4 or TSH. The THBR value is most often within reference range with adequate replacement dose but has not been advocated for monitoring therapeutic effect.

One report indicates that dosage requirement decreases after age 65 years.

THYROIDITIS

The usual classification of thyroiditis includes acute thyroiditis, subacute thyroiditis, chronic thyroiditis, and Riedel's struma.

Acute thyroiditis is generally defined as acute bacterial infection of the thyroid. Signs, symptoms, and laboratory data are those of acute localized infection.

Riedel's struma consists of thyroid parenchymal replacement by dense connective tissue. In some cases at least this presumably represents scar tissue from previous thyroiditis. Thyroid function tests are either normal (if sufficient normal thyroid remains) or indicate primary hypothyroidism.

Subacute thyroiditis (granulomatous thyroiditis or de Quervain's disease) features destruction of thyroid acini with a granulomatous reaction consisting of multinucleated giant cells of the foreign body reaction type and large histiocytes. The etiology is unknown but possibly is viral or autoimmune. The classic syndrome of subacute thyroiditis includes thyroid enlargement (usually less than twice normal size) with pain and tenderness, symptoms of thyrotoxicosis, substantially increased ESR, increased T_4, T_3-RIA, and THBR (T_3U) values, and decreased RAIU values. Thyroid scans demonstrate patchy isotope concentration throughout the thyroid gland (occasionally, only in focal areas) or else very little uptake. Classic cases have been reported to progress through four sequential stages: hyperthyroidism, followed by transient euthyroidism, then hypothyroidism, and then full recovery. Recovery in most cases takes place in 3–5 months. The classic syndrome is estimated to occur in approximately 50%–60% of patients with subacute thyroiditis. Milder or nonclassic cases lack the symptoms and laboratory findings of thyrotoxicosis. However, the ESR is usually elevated, and the RAIU value is usually decreased.

Painless thyroiditis (also called "silent thyroiditis") describes a group of patients with a syndrome combining some elements of subacute thyroiditis with some aspects of chronic thyroiditis (Hashimoto's disease). These patients have nonpainful thyroid swelling with or without clinical symptoms of thyrotoxicosis. Laboratory data include increased T_4, T_3-RIA, and THBR values, decreased RAIU value, patchy thyroid scan, and normal or minimally elevated ESR. Painless thyroiditis thus differs from subacute thyroiditis by lack of pain in the thyroid area and by normal ESR. Although some consider this syndrome to be a painless variant of subacute thyroiditis, biopsies of most cases have disclosed histologic findings of chronic lymphocytic thyroiditis rather than subacute thyroiditis. The reported incidence of this condition has varied from 5%–30% of all cases of hyperthyroidism. However, one report suggests that the incidence varies with geographic location, with the highest rates being in the Great Lakes region of the United States and in Japan.

Postpartum transient toxicosis is a syndrome that is said to occur in as many as 5%–6% (literature range, 5%–11%) of previously euthyroid postpartum women. There is transient symptomatic or asymptomatic thyrotoxicosis with elevated T_4 and low RAIU values, similar to the findings in thyrotoxic silent thyroiditis. This episode in some cases is followed by transient hypothyroidism. Thyroid autoantibody titers are elevated, suggesting lymphocytic thyroiditis.

Chronic thyroiditis is characterized histologically by dense lymphocytic infiltration of the thyroid with destruction of varying amounts of thyroid parenchyma. Chronic thyroiditis is frequently divided into two subdivisions: lymphocytic thyroiditis, most frequent in children and young adults; and Hashimoto's disease, found most often in adults aged 30–50 years. In both cases females are affected much more often than males. In approximately one half of chronic thyroiditis patients, serum T_4 levels are normal and the patients are clinically euthyroid. In 20%–40% the T_4 level is decreased, and there may be variable degrees of hypothyroidism. In some patients with decreased T_4 levels the T_3-RIA may be normal and presumably is responsible for maintaining clinical euthyroidism. The RAIU value is normal in 30%–50% of cases. In 10%–30% the RAIU value is increased, especially in the early stages of the disease. In fact, an elevated RAIU value with a normal T_4 value definitely raises the possibility of active (early) chronic thyroiditis. The

ESR is usually normal. Thyroid scan discloses generalized patchy isotope distribution in approximately 50% of cases and focal patchy or reduced uptake in 5%–10% more. In approximately one third of cases various precursors of T_4 or abnormal thyroglobulin derivatives are released from damaged thyroid acini. In about 5% of patients with chronic thyroiditis, release of thyroid hormone derivatives produces hyperthyroidism with increased serum T_4 levels. The RAIU value may be elevated or decreased. If the RAIU value is decreased, these patients might be considered part of the "thyrotoxic silent thyroiditis" group. On the other hand, some patients with chronic thyroiditis eventually develop sufficient damage to the thyroid to produce permanent hypothyroidism.

Lymphocytic thyroiditis and Hashimoto's disease are very similar, and some do not differentiate between them. However, in lymphocytic thyroiditis the goiter tends to enlarge more slowly, abnormal iodoproteins tend to appear more often, and the RAIU value tends to be elevated more frequently. Hashimoto's disease tends to have more histologic evidence of a peculiar eosinophilic change of thyroid acinar epithelial cells called "Askenazi cell transformation." Exact diagnosis of chronic thyroiditis is important for several reasons: to differentiate the condition from thyroid carcinoma; because a diffusely enlarged thyroid raises the question of possible thyrotoxicosis; and because treatment with thyroid hormone gives excellent results, especially in childhood lymphocytic thyroiditis.

Thyroid Autoantibodies.—Both subgroups of chronic thyroiditis are now considered to be either due to or associated with an autoimmune disorder directed against thyroid tissue. Autoantibodies against one or another element of thyroid tissue have been detected in most cases. In addition, there is an increased incidence of serologically detectable thyroid autoantibodies in rheumatoid-collagen disease patients, conditions themselves associated with disturbances in the body autoimmune mechanisms. There are two major subgroups of thyroid autoantibodies, those active against thyroglobulin and those directed against the microsome component of thyroid cells. There are several different techniques available to detect these antibodies, including, in order of increasing sensitivity: latex agglutination (antithyroglobulin antibodies only), immunofluorescence, hemagglutination (also known as the tanned [tannic acid–treated] red blood cell [or TRC] test), and radioassay. At present RIA and immunofluorescence are not widely available, and most reference laboratories use some modification of the hemagglutination test.

In general, antimicrosomal antibodies are found more often in chronic thyroiditis than antithyroglobulin antibodies. Antithyroglobulin antibodies are found less often in diseases other than chronic thyroiditis; but this increase in specificity is only moderate, and neither test has adequate selectivity for chronic thyroiditis (Table 28–11). High titers are much more likely to be associated with chronic thyroiditis than with nontoxic nodular goiter or thyroid carcinoma. High titers of antimicrosomal antibodies (or both antimicrosomal and antithyroglobulin antibodies) are not specific for chronic thyroiditis, because patients with Graves' disease or primary hypothyroidism may have either high or low titers. Normal or only slightly elevated titers, however, constitute some evidence against the diagnosis of chronic thyroiditis.

NEONATAL HYPOTHYROID SCREENING

Congenital hypothyroidism occurs in approximately 1 in 6,000 infants (literature range, 1–3/10,000), which makes it about three times as common as phenylketonuria (PKU). Approximately 85% of cases are due to thyroid agenesis and 10% are defects of enzymes in thyroid hormone synthesis, so that about 95% of all cases are primary hypothyroidism and

TABLE 28–11.

Thyroid Autoantibody Test Results in Thyroid Diseases (Hemagglutination Method)*

	% Abnormal	
Disease	Thyroglobulin	Microsomal
Hashimoto's disease	70 (50–86)	97 (92–100)
Graves' disease	55 (29–65)	75 (71–86)
Primary myxedema	55 (50–64)	75 (67–86)
Nontoxic nodular goiter	(5–50)	(27)
Thyroid carcinoma	(20)	(20†)
Normal male	(0–2)	(0–3)
Normal female	(2–20)	(15†)

*Numbers in parentheses are ranges from the literature.
†Immunofluorescence method.

3%–5% are secondary to pituitary or hypothalamic malfunction. Screening tests that have received the most attention include T_4, TSH, and reverse T_3.

There is minimal T_4 and T_3 placental transfer from mother to fetus in utero. At birth, cord blood T_4 values range from the upper half of normal to mildly elevated, compared with nonpregnant adult reference values (e.g., cord blood average levels of 11–12 μg/100 ml [142–154 nmol/L] compared with nonpregnant adult average values of about 9 μg/100 ml [116 nmol/L]). The T_3-RIA level is about one-third to one-half adult levels, the reverse T_3 level is about five times the adult levels, and the TSH has a mean value about twice that of adults but ranges from near zero to nearly three times adult upper limits. There is a strong correlation between birth weight and neonatal T_4 and TSH values. At birth, premature infants have T_4 values averaging one third lower than those of normal birth weight infants (although individual measurements are variable), with the subsequent changes in T_4 levels between premature and full-term infants remaining roughly parallel for several days. The TSH value at birth is also about one third lower in premature than in full-term infants but becomes fairly close to full-term infant levels at 24 hours of age.

After birth, the TSH value surges about five–seven times birth values to a peak at 30 minutes, then falls swiftly to levels about double birth values at 24 hours. The fall continues much more slowly to values about equal to those at birth by 48 hours and values about one half of birth levels at 4–5 days. After birth, the T_4 level increases about 30%–40%, with a plateau at 24–48 hours, and returns to birth levels by about 5 days. The TBG value does not change appreciably.

There is some disagreement in the literature regarding the best specimen to use for neonatal screening (heel puncture blood spot on filter paper versus cord blood) and the best test to use (T_4 vs. TSH assay). Most screening programs use filter paper methods because cord blood is more difficult to obtain and transport. Most programs use T_4 assay as the primary screening test because T_4 assay in general is less expensive than TSH assay, because TSH is more likely to become falsely negative when the specimen is subjected to adverse conditions during storage and transport, and because TSH assay values will not be elevated in the 10% of cases that are due to pituitary or hypothalamic dysfunction. Disadvantages of T_4 assay include occasional mildly hypothyroid infants with T_4 levels in the lower portion of the reference range but with clearly elevated TSH values. In one series this pattern occurred in 2 of 15 hypothyroid infants (13%). Some institutions therefore retest all infants whose T_4 values fall in the lower 10% of the reference range. Another problem concerns approximately 20% of neonatal T_4 results in the hypothyroid range that prove to be false positive (not hypothyroid), most of which are due to prematurity or decreased TBG.

Some additional thyroid function tests not discussed in this chapter are described in chapter 35.

BIBLIOGRAPHY

Desai RK, et al: Autoantibodies to thyroxine and triiodothyronine. *Clin Chem* 1988; 34:944.

Nordyke RA, et al: Graves' disease: Influence of age on clinical findings. *Arch Intern Med* 1988; 148:626.

Hardy MJ, et al: Pituitary-thyroid function in chronic renal failure assessed by a highly sensitive thyrotropin assay. *J Clin Endocrinol Metab* 1988; 66:233.

Larsen PR, et al: Revised nomenclature for tests of thyroid hormones and thyroid-related proteins in serum. *Arch Pathol Lab Med* 1987; 111:1141.

Bayer MF, et al: Diagnostic performance of sensitive measurements of serum thyrotropin during severe nonthyroidal illness: Their role in the diagnosis of hyperthyroidism. *Clin Chem* 1987; 33:2178.

Brennan MD: Heterophilic serum antibodies: A cause for falsely elevated serum thyrotropin levels. *Mayo Clin Proc* 1987; 62:894.

Bambini G, et al: Serum sex hormone-binding globulin in amiodarone-treated patients. *Arch Intern Med* 1987; 147:1781.

Spencer C, et al: Specificity of sensitive assays of thyrotropin (TSH) used to screen for thyroid disease in hospitalized patients. *Clin Chem* 1987; 33:1391.

Midgley JEM, et al: Validity of analog free thyroxin immunoassays. Part II. *Clin Chem* 1987; 33:2145.

Thornes HM, et al: Economy and efficiency in routine thyroid-function testing: Use of a sensitive immunoradiometric assay for

thyrotropin in a general hospital laboratory. *Clin Chem* 1987; 33:1635.
Ratnaike S, et al: Anomalous thyrotropin values. *Clin Chem* 1987; 33:1213.
Jackson JA, et al: Euthyroid hyperthyroxinemia and inappropriate secretion of thyrotropin. *Arch Intern Med* 1987; 147:1311.
Smallridge RC: Thyrotropin-secreting pituitary tumors. *Endocrinol Metab Clin* 1987; 16:765.
Blank MS, Tucci JR: A case of thyroxine thyrotoxicosis. *Arch Intern Med* 1987; 147:863.
Mechlis S, et al: Amiodarone-induced thyroid gland dysfunction. *Am J Cardiol* 1987; 59:833.
Gruhn JG: The development of tests of thyroid function. *Arch Pathol Lab Med* 1987; 111:84.
Goldman JM: Postpartem thyroid dysfunction. *Arch Intern Med* 1986; 146:1296.
Levin RM: Sick euthyroid syndrome. *Hosp Pract* 1986; 21:110C.
Hamburger JI: The various presentations of thyroiditis. *Ann Intern Med* 1986; 104:219.
Alexander NM: Free thyroxin in serum: Labeled thyroxin-analog methods fall short of their mark. *Clin Chem* 1986; 32:417.
Tibaldi JM, et al: Thyrotoxicosis in the very old. *Am J Med* 1986; 81:619.
Stockigt JR, et al: Interaction of furosemide with serum thyroxine-binding sites. *J Clin Endocrinol Metab* 1985; 60:1025.
Sawin CT: Hypothyroidism. *Med Clin North Am* 1985; 69:989.
Emerson CH: Central hypothyroidism and hyperthyroidism. *Med Clin North Am* 1985; 69:1019.
Liewendahl K, et al: Free thyroxine and free triiodothyronine as measured by equilibrium dialysis and analog radioimmunoassay in serum of patients taking phenytoin and carbamazepine. *Clin Chem* 1985; 31:1993.
Vitug A, Goldman JM: Silent (painless) thyroiditis. *Arch Intern Med* 1985; 145:473.
Kaplan MM: Clinical and laboratory assessment of thyroid abnormalities. *Med Clin North Am* 1985; 69:863.
Tibaldi JM, Surks MI: Effects of nonthyroidal illness on thyroid function. *Med Clin North Am* 1985; 69:899.
Woolf PD: Thyroiditis. *Med Clin North Am* 1985; 69:1035.
Tibaldi J, Barzel US: Thyroxine supplementation. *Am J Med* 1985; 79:241.
Silva JE: Effects of iodine and iodine-containing compounds on thyroid function. *Med Clin North Am* 1985; 69:881.
Spaulding SW, Lippes H: Hyperthyroidism. *Med Clin North Am* 1985; 69:937.
Jacobson DH, Gorman CA: Diagnosis and management of endocrine ophthalmopathy. *Med Clin North Am* 1985; 69:973.
Walfish PG, Chan JYC: Post-partum hyperthyroidism. *Clin Endocrinol Metab* 1985; 14:417.
Studer H, et al: Toxic nodular goiter. *Clin Endocrinol Metab* 1985; 14:351.
Nicoloff JT: Thyroid storm and myxedema coma. *Med Clin North Am* 1985; 69:1005.
Jurney TH, Wartofsky L: Thyrotropin-releasing hormone tests in an outpatient clinic. *South Med J* 1985; 78:774.
Kolesnick RN, Gershengorn MC: Thyrotropin-releasing hormone and the pituitary. *Am J Med* 1985; 79:729.
Martino E, et al: Twenty-four hour radioactive iodine uptake in 35 patients with amiodarone associated thyrotoxicosis. *J Nucl Med* 1985; 26:1402.
Himsworth RL: Hyperthyroidism with a low iodine uptake. *Clin Endocrinol Metab* 1985; 14:397.
Walfish PG: The best way to screen for neonatal hypothyroidism. *Diagn Med* 1984; 7(2):67.
Wilke TJ: Free thyroid hormone index, thyroid hormone/thyroxine-binding globulin ratio, triiodothyronine uptake, and thyroxine-binding globulin compared for diagnostic value regarding thyroid function. *Clin Chem* 1983; 29:74.
Szpunar WE, et al: Screening for minimal hypothyroidism. *Postgrad Med* 1983; 74:259.
Chan DW, et al: Meaning of serum free-thyroxin values in nonthyroidal illnesses: Seven methods compared. *Clin Chem* 1983; 29:1091.
Deam DR, et al: Effect of oral intake of thyroxine on results of thyroid function tests in patients receiving thyroid replacement therapy. *Med J Aust* 1983; 2:374.
Melmed S, et al: A comparison of methods for assessing thyroid function in nonthyroidal illness. *J Clin Endocrinol* 1982; 54:300.
Stoffer SS: Menstrual disorders and mild thyroid insufficiency. *Postgrad Med* 1982; 72:75.
Chervu S, et al: Thyroid uptake measurements with I-123: Problems and pitfalls. *J Nucl Med* 1982; 23:667.
Fisher DA, Klein AH: Thyroid development and disorders of thyroid function in the newborn. *N Engl J Med* 1981; 304:702.
Gold MS, et al: Hypothyroidism and depression. *JAMA* 1981; 245:1919.

Witherspoon LR: The triiodothyronine uptake test: An assessment of methods. *Clin Chem* 1981; 27:1272.

Wenzel KW: Pharmacological interference with in vitro tests of thyroid function. *Metabolism* 1981; 30:717.

Wong MM, Volpe R: What is the best test for monitoring levothyroxine therapy? *Can Med Assoc J* 1981; 124:1181.

Cohen KL, Swigar ME: Thyroid function screening in psychiatric patients. *JAMA* 1979; 242:254.

29 Adrenal Function Tests

ADRENAL CORTEX HORMONES

This chapter will begin with adrenal cortex hormones and conclude with adrenal medulla hormones. The adrenal medulla produces epinephrine and norepinephrine. The relationships of the principal adrenal cortex hormones, their actions, and their metabolites are shown in Figure 29–1. The adrenal cortex is divided into three areas. A narrow outer (subcapsular) region is known as the "zona glomerulosa." It is thought to produce aldosterone. The cortex middle zone, called the "zona fasciculata," mainly secretes 17-hydroxycortisone, also known as "hydrocortisone" or "cortisol." This is the principal agent of the cortisone group. A thin inner zone, called the "zona reticularis," manufactures compounds with androgenic or estrogenic effects. Pathways of synthesis for adrenal cortex hormones are outlined in Figure 29–2. Production of cortisol is controlled by pituitary secretion of adrenal cortex–stimulating hormone, or adrenocorticotropic hormone (ACTH). The pituitary, in turn, is regulated by a feedback mechanism involving blood levels of cortisol. If the plasma cortisol level is too high, pituitary action is inhibited and ACTH production is decreased. If more cortisol is needed, the pituitary increases ACTH production.

Excess or deficiency of any one of adrenal cortex hormones leads to several well-recognized diseases, which are diagnosed by assay of the hormone or its metabolites. In diseases of cortisol production, three assay techniques form the backbone of laboratory diagnosis: 17-hydroxycorticosteroids (17-OHCS), 17-ketosteroids (17-KS), and direct measurement of cortisol. Before the use of these steroid tests in various syndromes is discussed, it is helpful to consider what actually is being measured.

17-Hydroxycorticosteroids

These are C21 compounds that possess a dihydroxyacetone group on carbon number 17 of the steroid nucleus (Fig 29–3). In the blood, the principal 17-OHCSs is hydrocortisone. In urine, the predominating 17-OHCS are tetrahydro metabolites (breakdown products) of hydrocortisone and cortisone. Therefore, measurement of 17-OHCS levels can be used to estimate the level of cortisone and hydrocortisone production. Estrogen therapy (including oral contraceptives) will elevate plasma 17-OHCS values, although degradation of these compounds is delayed and urine 17-OHCS levels are decreased.

17-Ketosteroids

These are C19 compounds with a ketone group on carbon number 17 of the steroid nucleus (see Fig 29–3). They are measured in urine only. In males, about 25% of 17-KS are composed of metabolites of testosterone. The remainder of 17-KS in males and nearly all 17-KS in females is derived from androgens other than testosterone, although lesser amounts come from early steroid precursors and a small percentage from hydrocortisone breakdown products. Testosterone itself is not a 17-KS. The principal urinary 17-KS is a compound known as dehydroisoandrosterone (dehydroepian-

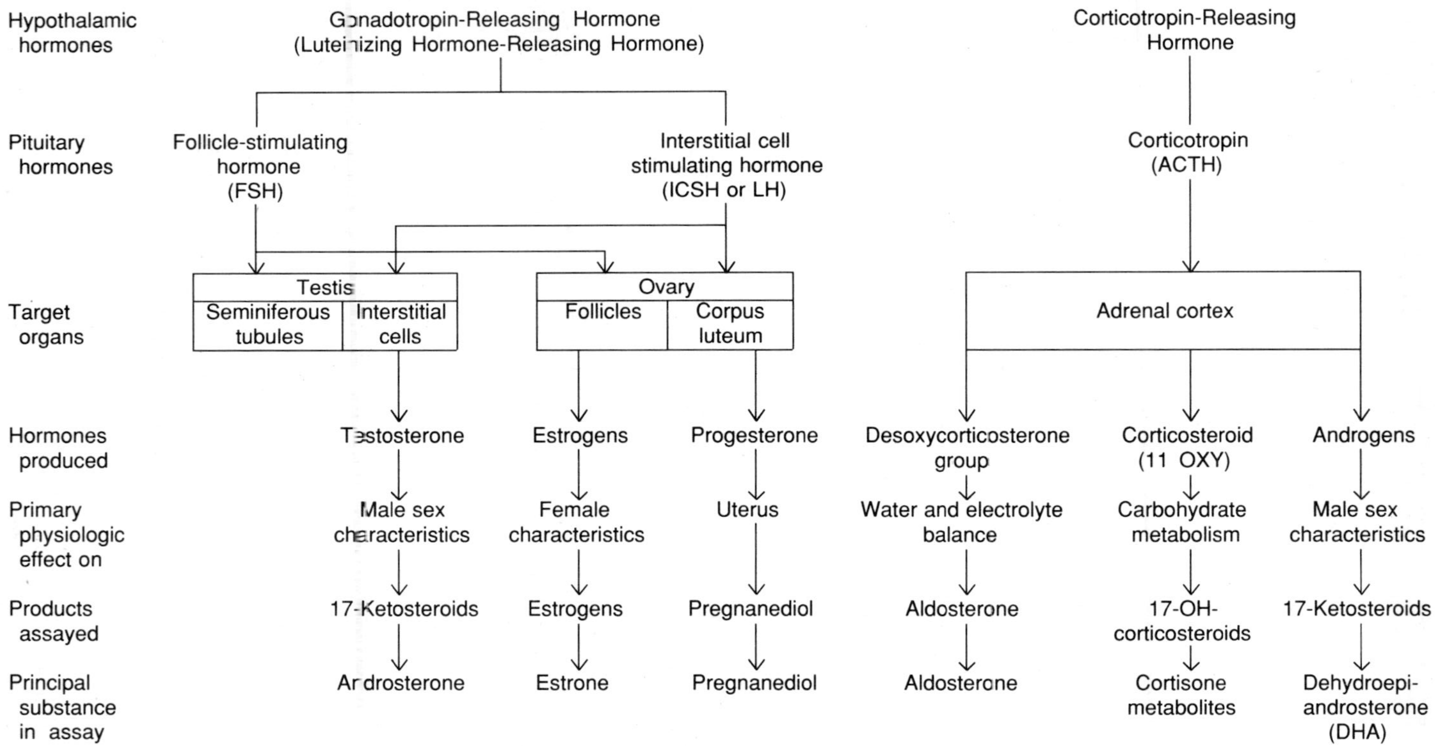

FIG 29–1.
Derivation of principal urinary steroids. (Modified from *Handbook of Specialized Diagnostic Laboratory Tests*, ed 7. Van Nuys, Calif, Bioscience Laboratories, 1966, p 5.)

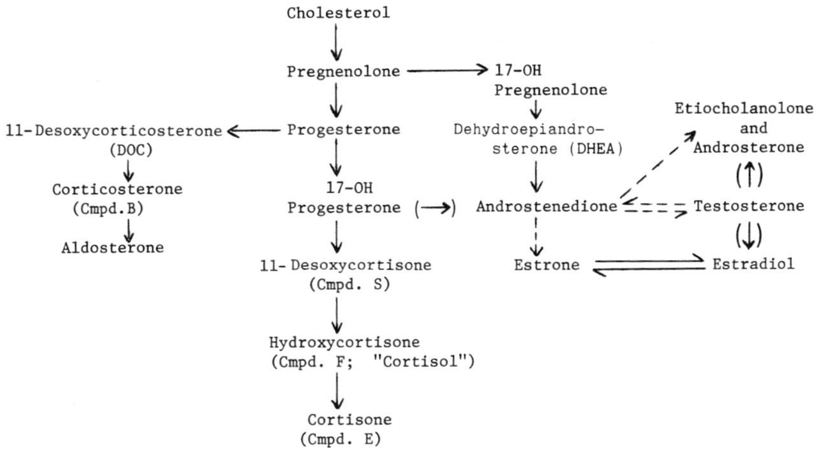

FIG 29–2.
Adrenal cortex steroid synthesis. Important classic alternate pathways are depicted in parentheses, and certain alternate pathways are omitted. *Dotted lines* indicate pathway that normally continues in another organ, although adrenal capability exists.

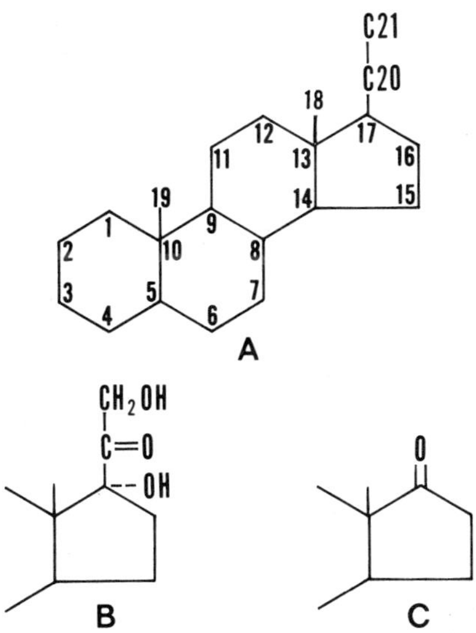

FIG 29–3.
Adrenal cortex steroid nomenclature. **A**, basic 17-OHCS nucleus with standard numerical nomenclature of the carbon atoms. **B**, configuration of hydrocortisone at the C-17 carbon atom. **C**, configuration of the 17-KS at the C-17 carbon atom.

drosterone; DHEA). This compound is formed in the adrenal gland and has a weak androgenic effect. It is not a metabolite of cortisone or hydrocortisone, and therefore 17-KS cannot be expected to mirror or predict levels of hydrocortisone production.

In adrenogenital or virilization syndromes, high levels of 17-KS usually mean congenital adrenal hyperplasia in infants and adrenal tumor in older children and adults. In both conditions, steroid synthesis is abnormally shifted away from cortisone formation toward androgen production. High 17-KS levels are occasionally found in testicular tumors if the tumor produces androgens greatly in excess of normal testicular output. In Cushing's syndrome, 17-KS production is variable, but adrenal hyperplasia is often associated with mild to moderate elevation, whereas adrenal carcinoma frequently produces moderate or marked elevation in urinary values. In adrenal tumor, most of the increase is due to DHEA.

Low levels of 17-KS are not very important because of normal fluctuation and the degree of inaccuracy in assay. Low levels are usually due to a decrease in DHEA. This may be caused by many factors, but the most important is stress of any type (e.g., trauma, burns, or chronic disease). Therefore, normal 17-KS levels are indirectly a sign of health.

Plasma Cortisol

Plasma cortisol, like thyroxine, exists in two forms, bound and unbound. About 75% is bound to an alpha-1 globulin called "transcortin," about 15% is bound to albumin, and about 10% is unbound ("free"). The bound cortisol is not physiologically active. Increased estrogens or hyperthyroidism elevates transcortin (raising total serum cortisol values without affecting free cortisol), whereas increased androgens or hypothyroidism decreases transcortin. A marked decrease in serum albumin level can also lower total serum cortisol levels. There is a diurnal variation in cortisol secretion, with values in the evening being about one half those in the morning. Lowest values are found about 11 P.M.

Cortisol Test Methods.—All current widely used assays for serum cortisol measure total cortisol (bound plus free). There are three basic assay techniques: (1) Porter-Silber colorimetric, (2) Mattingly fluorescent, and (3) radioassay. The Porter-Silber technique is the most widely used of the older chemical methods. It measures cortisol, cortisone, and compound S (see Fig 29–2), plus their metabolites. Ketosis and various drugs (see chapter 36) may interfere. The Mattingly fluorescent procedure is based on fluorescence of certain compounds in acid media at ultraviolet wavelengths. It is more sensitive than the Porter-Silber technique, faster, requires less blood, and measures cortisol and compound B but not compound S. Certain drugs that fluoresce may interfere. Radioassay has two subgroups, competitive protein binding (CPB) and radioimmunoassay (RIA). The CPB technique is the older of the two. It is based on competition of patient cortisol-like compounds with isotope-labeled cortisol for space on cortisol-binding protein. Competitive protein binding measures cortisol, cortisone, compound S, and compound B. Advantages are small specimen requirement and less interference by drugs. Radioimmunoassay is based on competition of patient cortisol with isotope-labeled cortisol for anticortisol antibody. The method is nearly specific for cortisol, with less than 20% cross-reaction with compound S. In certain clinical situations, such as congenital adrenal hyperplasia or the metyrapone test, it is important to know what "cortisol" procedure is being performed to interpret the results correctly.

All techniques measure total blood cortisol, so that all will give falsely increased values if increases in cortisol-binding protein levels occur due to estrogens in pregnancy or from birth control pills. Stress, obesity, and severe hepatic or renal disease may falsely increase plasma levels. Androgens and phenytoin (Dilantin) may decrease cortisol-binding protein levels. In situations where cortisol-binding protein levels are increased, urine 17-OHCS or, better, urine free cortisol assay may be helpful, since urine reflects blood levels of active rather than total hormone.

CONGENITAL ADRENAL HYPERPLASIA

Congenital adrenal hyperplasia (CAH), also known as the "adrenogenital syndrome," is an uncommon condition caused by a congenital defect in one of several enzymes that take part in the chain of reactions whereby cortisol is manufactured from its precursors. There are at least six fairly well-defined variants of CAH that result from the various enzyme defects (see Table 36–26). The most common of these are types I and II, which are due to C21-hydroxylase enzyme deficiency. All CAH variants are inherited as autosomal recessive traits. The clinical and laboratory findings depend on which metabolic pathway—and which precursor in the metabolic pathway—is affected. All variants affect the glucocorticoid (cortisol) pathway in some manner. In CAH due to 21-hydroxylase defect (types I and II) and in CAH type III, although formation of cortisone and cortisol is blocked, the precursors of these glucocorticoids are still being manufactured. Most of the early precursors of cortisone are estrogenic compounds, which also are intermediates in the production of androgens by the adrenal cortex (see Fig 29–2). Normally, the quantitative production of adrenal androgen is small; however, if the steroid precursors pile up (due to block in normal formation of cortisone), some of this excess may be used to form more androgens.

Three things result from these metabolic pathway abnormalities. First, due to abnormally high production of androgen, secondary sexual characteristics are affected. If the condition is manifest in utero, pseudohermaphroditism (masculinization of external genitalia) or ambiguous genitalia occur in girls and macrogenitosomia praecox (accentuation of male genitalia) occurs in boys. If the condition does not become clinically manifest until after birth, virilism (masculinization) develops in girls and precocious puberty in boys. In CAH variants IV, V, and VI there is some degree of interruption of the adrenal androgen pathway, so that the external appearance of the female genitalia is not significantly affected and subsequent virilization is minimal or absent. External genitalia in genotypic boys appear to be female or ambiguous.

Second, the adrenal glands themselves increase in size due to hyperplasia of the steroid-producing adrenal cortex. This results because normal pituitary production of ACTH is controlled by the amount of cortisone and hydrocortisone produced by the adrenal. In all variants of congenital adrenal hyperplasia, cortisone production is partially or completely blocked, the pituitary produces more and more ACTH in attempts to increase cortisone production, and the adrenal cortex tissue becomes hyperplastic under continually increased ACTH stimulation.

Third, when the mineralocorticoid pathway leading to aldosterone is blocked, there are salt-losing crises similar to those of Addison's disease. This occurs in CAH types II, IV, and VI. On the other hand, hypertension may develop if there is accumulation of a salt-retaining precursor (CAH type III) in the mineralocorticoid pathway or a mineralocorticoid production increase due to block in the other adrenal pathways (CAH type V).

Since 21-hydroxylase deficiency is responsible for more than 90% of the CAH variants and the others are rare, only laboratory data referable to this enzyme defect (CAH types I and II) will be discussed.

The CAH 21-hydroxylase deficiency is brought to the attention of the physician by either abnormalities in newborn external genitalia (CAH types I and II, the most common cause of female pseudohermaphroditism) or salt-losing crises (type II, constituting one third to two thirds of 21-hydroxylase deficiency cases). In later childhood, virilization is the most likely clinical problem. In patients with ambiguous genitalia, a buccal smear (chapter 33) and chromosome karyotype establish the correct (genotypic) sex of the infant. In salt-losing crises, the infant is severely dehydrated and may develop shock. The serum sodium level is low and the serum potassium level is high-normal or elevated. For a number of years, the diagnosis was made through elevated urine 17-KS levels (metabolites of androgens) and increased urinary pregnanetriol levels (metabolite of 17-OH-progesterone). However, 17-KS values may normally be four–five times as high in the first 2 weeks of life as they are after 4 weeks, and pregnanetriol values may be normal in some neonates with CAH in the first 24–48 hours of life. At present, plasma 17-OH-progesterone is considered the best screening test for neonatal 21-hydroxylase deficiency. After the first 24 hours of life, plasma 17-OH-progesterone is markedly elevated in most patients with CAH type I or II. Also, plasma specimens are easier to obtain in neonates or infants than 24-hour urine collections. However, plasma 17-OH-progesterone may be elevated to some extent in other severe illnesses. Also, because there is diurnal variation, the blood specimen should be drawn in the morning.

Late-onset CAH is one possible etiology of hirsutism (discussed in Chapter 30). Diagnosis is most commonly made with the cortrosyn stimulation test, also described in Chapter 30.

VIRILIZATION SYNDROME

This rare syndrome occurs in older children and in adults. It is manifested by virilism in females and by excessive masculinization in males. It may be due to idiopathic adrenal cortex hyperplasia, adrenal cortex adenoma, or cortex carcinoma. Tumor is more common than hyperplasia in these patients. Virilism in a female child or adult leads to hirsutism, clitoral enlargement, deepening of the voice, masculine contour, and breast atrophy. The syndrome may be simulated in females by idiopathic hirsutism, arrhenoblastoma of the ovary, and possibly by the Stein-Leventhal syndrome. Urinary 17-KS values are elevated with normal or decreased 17-OHCS values when the adrenal is involved. Ovarian arrhenoblastoma gives normal or only slightly elevated urine 17-KS values, since androgen is produced in smaller quantities but is more potent, thus giving clinical symptoms without greatly increased quantities. In prepubertal boys, the symptoms of virilism are those of precocious puberty; in men, excessive masculinization is difficult to recognize. A similar picture may be associated with certain testicular tumors.

CUSHING'S SYNDROME

Cushing's syndrome is caused by excessive body levels of adrenal glucocorticoids such as cortisol, either from (primary) adrenal cortex overproduction or from (secondary) therapeutic administration. This discussion will consider only the primary type due to excess adrenal production of cortisol. About 70% of cases (range 50%–80%) of Cushing's syndrome due to adrenal overproduction of cortisol are caused by pituitary hypersecretion of ACTH leading to bilateral adrenal cortex hyperplasia. About 10% of cases are due to adrenal cortex adenoma, about 10% to adrenal cortex carcinoma, and about 10% to "ectopic" ACTH production by tumors outside the adrenal or pituitary glands, most commonly lung small-cell carcinomas. One additional category is the uncommon syndrome of micronodular cortical hyperplasia, which biochemically behaves in a similar manner to adrenal cortex adenoma. Adrenal tumor is the most frequent etiology in patients younger than 10 years, and pituitary hyperactivity is the most common cause in patients older than 10. Cushing's syndrome must be differentiated from Cushing's disease, which is the category of Cushing's syndrome due to pituitary hypersecretion of ACTH (usually due to a basophilic cell pituitary adenoma or microadenoma). The highest incidence of Cushing's syndrome is found in adults, with women affected four times more often than men. Major symptoms and signs include puffy, obese-looking ("moon") appearance of the face, body trunk obesity, "buffalo hump" fat deposit on the back of the neck, abdominal striae, osteoporosis, and a tendency to diabetes, hirsutism, easy bruising, and hypertension.

Standard Test Abnormalities

General laboratory findings include impairment of glucose tolerance in about 85% of patients (literature range, 57%–94%) which is severe enough to be classified as diabetes mellitus in about 25%. There is lymphocytopenia (usually mild) in about 80%, but most patients have an overall mild leukocytosis. Hemoglobin tends to be in the upper half of the reference range, with polycythemia in about 10% of affected persons. About 20%–25% have a mild hypokalemic alkalosis. The serum sodium level is usually normal but is slightly increased in about 5%. Total circulating eosinophils are usually decreased.

Screening Tests

Urine 17-Ketosteroid Assay.—The urine 17-KS assay was one of the first tests used for diagnosis of Cushing's syndrome. However, urine 17-KS values are increased in only about 50%–55% of patients with Cushing's syndrome, and the test yields about 10% false positive results. Thus, 17-KS assay is no longer used to screen for Cushing's syndrome. The 17-KS values may be useful in patients who are already known to have Cushing's syndrome. About 45% of patients with adrenal adenoma and about 80%–85% (range 67%–91%) of patients with adrenal carcinoma have elevated urine 17-KS values. Patients with adrenal carcinoma tend to have higher urine 17-KS values than patients with Cushing's syndrome from other etiologies, so that very high urine 17-KS values of adrenal origin suggest adrenal carcinoma.

Single-Specimen Serum Cortisol Assay.—Laboratory diagnosis of Cushing's syndrome requires proof of cortisol hypersecretion. For some time, assay of 17-OHCS in a 24-hour urine specimen or a single-specimen plasma 17-OHCS assay by the Porter-Silber method was the mainstay of diagnosis. However, in Cushing's syndrome this technique yields about 15% false negative and 15% false positive results. The 17-OHCS values in urine are increased in some patients by obesity, acute alcoholism, or hyperthyroidism, whereas the 17-OHCS values in plasma are increased in many patients by stress, obesity, or an increase in cortisol-binding protein due to estrogen increase (oral contraceptive medication or pregnancy). Therefore, urine 17-OHCS assay and single determinations of plasma 17-OHCS are no longer considered reliable enough to screen for Cushing's syndrome. Plasma or urine 17-OHCS assay was also used to measure adrenal response in stimulation or suppression tests. However, it has been replaced for this purpose by serum cortisol assay, which is technically easier to do and avoids the many problems of 24-hour urine specimen collections.

Single determinations of plasma cortisol, either in the morning or in the afternoon or evening, have the same disadvantages as plasma 17-OHCS and are not considered reliable for screening of Cushing's syndrome. For example, single morning specimens detect about 65% of patients with Cushing's syndrome (range, 40%–83%) and produce false positive results in about 30% of cases (range, 7%–60%). One report in-

TABLE 29–1.
Some Conditions That Affect Serum Cortisol Diurnal Variation

Severe stress
Severe nonadrenal illness
Obesity
Psychiatric depression
Alcoholism (especially with recent intake)
Change in sleep habits
Encephalitis
Blindness
Certain medications (prolonged steroids, phenothiazines, reserpine, phenytoin, amphetamines

dicates that 11 P.M. or midnight specimens provide better separation of normal persons from those with Cushing's syndrome.

Plasma Cortisol Diurnal Variation.—If plasma cortisol assay is available, a better screening test for Cushing's syndrome than a single determination consists of assay of two plasma specimens, one drawn at 8 A.M. and the other at 8 P.M. Normally there is a diurnal variation in plasma levels (not urine levels), with the highest values found between 6 and 10 A.M. and the lowest near midnight. The evening specimen ordinarily is less than 50% of the morning value. In Cushing's syndrome, diurnal variation is absent in about 90% of patients (literature range 70%–100%). False positive results are obtained in about 20% of patients (range, 18%–25%). Therefore, significant alteration of the diurnal pattern is not specific for Cushing's syndrome, since it is found in occasional patients with a wide variety of conditions. Some of the conditions that may decrease or abolish the normal drop in the evening cortisol level in some persons are listed in Table 29–1. Therefore, a normal result (normal circadian rhythm) is probably more significant than an abnormal result (although, as already noted normal plasma cortisol circadian rhythm may be present in about 10% of patients with Cushing's syndrome).

Urine Free Cortisol.—About 1% of plasma cortisol is excreted by the kidney in the original free or unconjugated state; the remainder appears in urine as conjugated metabolites. Original Porter-Silber chromogenic techniques could not measure free cortisol selectively. Fluorescent methods or immunoassay can quantitate free cortisol, either alone or with compound S, depending on the method. Immunoassay is becoming the most frequently used technique. Urine free cortisol values in 24-hour collections are reported to be elevated in about 95% of patients with Cushing's syndrome (literature range, 90%–100%) and to produce false positive elevation in about 6% of patients without Cushing's syndrome (literature range, 0%–8%).

Urine free cortisol levels may be elevated in some patients by some of the factors that affect blood cortisol, including severe stress, acute alcoholism, psychiatric depression, and occasional patients with obesity. In cortisol-binding protein changes such as an increase produced by estrogens, most reports indicate that urine free cortisol secretion levels are usually normal. Renal insufficiency may elevate plasma cortisol levels and decrease urine free cortisol levels. Hepatic disease may increase plasma cortisol levels but usually does not affect urine free cortisol levels significantly. The major difficulty with the test involves accurate collection of the 24-hour specimen. Also, the test is not performed in most ordinary laboratories and would have to be sent to a medical center or reference laboratory.

Single-Dose Dexamethasone Suppression Test.—The most simple reasonably accurate screening procedure is a rapid overnight dexamethasone suppression test (DST). Oral administration of 1 mg of dexamethasone at 11 P.M. suppresses pituitary ACTH production, so that the normal 8 A.M. peak of plasma cortisol fails to develop. After 11 P.M. dexamethasone, normal persons and the majority of obese persons have 8 A.M. plasma cortisol values less than 50% of baseline (predexamethasone) levels. Many endocrinologists require suppression to 5 μg/100 ml (138 nmol/L) or less. The consensus is that about 95% of Cushing's syndrome patients exhibit abnormal test response (failure to suppress), although there is a range in the literature of 70%–98%. There is an average of less than 5% false positive results in normal control persons (range 1%–10%).

There is controversy in the literature regarding certain aspects of this test. Some investigators found substantial numbers of patients with a Cushingoid type of obesity, but without demonstrable Cushing's syndrome, who failed to suppress adequately (falsely suggesting Cushing's syndrome) after the overnight DST. This involved 10% of Cushingoid obese patients in one series and 53% in another. Unfortunately, there are not many reports in the literature that differentiate lean from obese persons in control series. Another controversial point is the degree that the 8 A.M. cortisol specimen must be suppressed from baseline value to separate normal persons from those with Cushing's syndrome. Some have found the standard of a 50% decrease from baseline values to be insufficiently sensitive, missing up to 30% of Cushing's syndrome patients. These investigators suggest a fixed 8 A.M. plasma cortisol value (after dexamethasone) of 5 or 7 μg/100 ml. However, establishment of such a fixed value is complicated by the variations in cortisol reference ranges found in different methods and kits. Another problem are conditions that may produce false results (failure to suppress normally). Some of these are listed in Table 29–2.

Phenytoin and phenobarbital affect cortisol by affecting the microsomal metabolic pathway of the liver. Estrogen increases cortisol-binding protein values, which, in turn, increases total plasma cortisol values. This may affect the DST when a fixed 5 μg/100 ml cutoff limit is used, since the already increased cortisol level must be suppressed even more than usual to reach that value. Spironolactone is a fluorescent compound and interferes with the Mattingly fluorescent assay technique. Immunoassay is not affected. Additional evidence to support abnormal screening test results may be obtained by using the standard DST.

TABLE 29–2.

Some Conditions That Interfere With the Low-Dose Overnight Dexamethasone Suppression Test

*Conditions producing false normal test results**
Drug-induced interference (phenytoin, phenobarbital, estrogens, possibly spironolactone)
Conditions producing false abnormal test results†
Acute alcoholism
Psychiatric depression
Severe stress
Severe nonadrenal illness
Malnutrition
Some patients with obesity
Renal failure

*Apparent suppression of 8 A.M. cortisol in patients with Cushing's syndrome.
†Failure to suppress 8 A.M. cortisol in patients without Cushing's syndrome.

The single-dose DST and diurnal variation test may be combined. Plasma cortisol specimens are drawn at 8 A.M. and 8 P.M. Dexamethasone is administered at 11 P.M., followed by a plasma cortisol specimen at 8 A.M. the next day.

Confirmatory Tests

Confirmation of the diagnosis depends mainly on tests that involve either stimulation or suppression of adrenal hormone production. It is often possible with the same tests to differentiate the various etiologies of primary hyperadrenalism. Normally, increased pituitary ACTH production increases adrenal corticosteroid release. Increased plasma corticosteroid levels normally inhibit pituitary release of ACTH and therefore suppress additional adrenal steroid production. Adrenal tumors, as a rule, produce their hormones without being much affected by suppression tests; on the other hand, they tend to give little response to stimulation, as though they behaved independently of the usual hormone control mechanism. Also, if urinary 17-KS values are markedly increased (more than twice normal), this strongly suggests carcinoma. However, hyperplasia, adenoma, and carcinoma values overlap, and 17-KS levels may be normal with any of the three etiologies.

48-Hour Dexamethasone Suppression Test.—The 48-hour DST is the most widely used confirmatory procedure. Dexamethasone (Decadron) is a synthetic steroid with cortisone-like actions but is approximately 30 times more potent than cortisone, so that amounts too small for laboratory measurement may be given to suppress pituitary ACTH production. The test is preceded by two consecutive 24-hour urine collections as a baseline. If low doses (2 mg/day) are used, patients with normal adrenal function will usually have at least a 50% decrease (suppression) in their 24-hour urine 17-OHCS values compared to baseline, whereas those with Cushing's syndrome from any etiology will have little if any change. This test result is usually normal in those patients whose low-dose overnight DST is abnormal (nonsuppressed) only because of obesity. If larger doses (8 mg/day) are used, about 85% (range, 42%–98%) of those with adrenal cortex hyperplasia due to pituitary oversecretion of ACTH have at least a 50% decrease (suppression) of their 24-hour urine 17-OHCS values. Adrenal cortisol-producing adenomas or carcinoma rarely decrease their urine 17-OHCS levels. Patients with the ectopic ACTH syndrome due to bronchial or thymus carcinoids have been reported to produce false positive test results (decrease in urine 17-OHCS levels) in up to 40% of patients. Patients with the ectopic ACTH syndrome from lung small-cell carcinoma or other tumors rarely change urine 17-OHCS levels. Since the test takes a total of 4 days (48 hours at baseline and 48 hours of test duration) and requires 24-hour urine collections, and since there are a significant number of exceptions to the general rules, plasma ACTH assay is supplementing or replacing the high-dose DST for differentiation of the various etiologies of Cushing's syndrome. Some investigators report that the metyrapone test (discussed later) is better than the 48-hour high-dose DST in differentiating pituitary oversecretion of ACTH from adrenal tumor.

Corticotropin-Releasing Hormone Test.—Corticotropin-releasing hormone (CRH) from the hypothalamus stimulates the pituitary to release ACTH. Ovine CRH is now becoming available, and several investigators have administered this hormone in attempts to differentiate adrenal tumor and the ectopic ACTH syndrome from pituitary overproduction of ACTH. Initial studies reported that after CRH administration, pituitary ACTH-producing tumors increased plasma cortisol levels by increasing their ACTH secretion, whereas primary adrenal tumors and the ectopic ACTH syndrome did not increase cortisol levels. However, several recent studies found that about 10% of pituitary ACTH-producing tumors failed to increase plasma ACTH or cortisol levels. This is similar to the failure rate for pituitary tumors in the high-dose 48-hour DST. Also, occasional patients with the ectopic ACTH syndrome have demonstrated some degree of suppressibility with the 48-hour DST and also some increase in ACTH or cortisol level with the CRH test. Therefore, differentiation of the etiologies of Cushing's syndrome by the CRH test alone is not as clearcut as theoretically would be expected.

Metyrapone Test.—Metyrapone (Metopirone) blocks conversion of compound S to cortisol. This normally induces the pituitary to secrete more ACTH to increase cortisol production. Although production of cortisol is decreased, the compound S level is increased as it accumulates proximal to the metyrapone block, and 17-OHCS or radioassay CPB methods for cortisol in either serum or urine demonstrate sharply increased apparent cortisol values (due to compound S) in normal persons and those with pituitary-induced adrenal cortex hyperplasia. Fluorescent assay or RIA for cortisol do not include compound S and therefore yield decreased cortisol values. Adrenal tumors are not significantly affected by metyrapone. Some authorities recommend measuring both cortisol and compound S. An increase in compound S verifies that lowering of the plasma cortisol level was accompanied by an increase in ACTH secretion. This maneuver also improves the ability of the test to indicate the status of pituitary reserve capacity, and the test is sometimes used for that purpose rather than investigation of Cushing's disease. To obtain both measurements, one must select a test method for cortisol that does not also measure compound S. Compound S can be measured by a specific RIA method. Phenytoin or estrogen administration interferes with the metyrapone test.

Adrenocorticotropic Hormone Stimulation Test.—Injection of ACTH directly stimulates the adrenal cortex. Patients with cortex hyperplasia and some adenomas display increased plasma cortisol and 17-OHCS levels. If urine collection is used, a 24-hour specimen taken the day of ACTH administration should demonstrate a considerable increase from preinfusion baseline values, which persists in a 24-hour specimen collected the day after ACTH injection. Normal persons should have increased hormone excretion the day ACTH is given but should return to normal in the next 24 hours. Carcinoma is not affected. The ACTH stimulation test at present does not seem to be used very frequently.

Serum Adrenocorticotropic Hormone.—Serum ACTH measurement by RIA is now available in many reference laboratories. At present, the assay techniques are too difficult for the average laboratory to perform in a re-

TABLE 29–3.
Plasma Adrenocorticotropic Hormone in Adrenal Diseases

	ACTH	Diurnal Variation
Pituitary Cushing's	Increase in 50%* Normal in 50%	Absent
Ectopic ACTH	Increase†	Absent
Adrenal Cushing's	Decrease	(Absent)
Primary Addison's disease	Increase	Normal
Secondary Addison's disease (pituitary hypofunction)	Decrease (some normal)	Normal

*When elevated, usually less than 200 pg/ml (44 pmol/L).
†About 65% are > 200 pg/ml.

liable fashion, and even reference laboratories still have problems with accuracy.

There is a diurnal variation in serum ACTH levels corresponding to cortisol secretion, with highest values at 8–10 A.M. and lowest values near midnight. Stress and other factors that affect cortisol diurnal variation may blunt or eliminate the ACTH diurnal variation. Serum ACTH data in adrenal disease are summarized in Table 29–3.

In Cushing's syndrome due to adrenal tumor or micronodular hyperplasia, pituitary activity is suppressed by adrenal-produced cortisol, so the serum ACTH level is very low. In ectopic ACTH syndrome, the serum ACTH level is typically very high (four–five times the upper reference limit) due to production of cross-reacting ACTH-like material by the tumor. However, some patients with the ectopic ACTH syndrome have serum levels that are not this high. In bilateral adrenal hyperplasia due to pituitary overactivity, serum ACTH levels can either be normal or mildly to moderately elevated (typically less than the degree of elevation associated with the ectopic ACTH syndrome). However, there is a substantial degree of overlap between pituitary tumor ACTH values and ectopic ACTH syndrome values. It has been suggested that ACTH specimens obtained at 10–12 P.M. provide better separation of normal from pituitary hypersecretion than do specimens drawn in the morning. Another study found that specimens drawn between 9:00 and 9:30 A.M. provided much better separation of normal from pituitary hypersecretion than specimens drawn at any other time in the morning. In summary, adrenal tumor (low ACTH levels) can usually be separated from pituitary-induced adrenal cortex hyperplasia (normal or increased ACTH levels) and from ectopic ACTH (increased ACTH levels). Pituitary-induced adrenal cortex hyperplasia has ACTH values that overlap with the upper range of normal persons and with the lower range of the ectopic ACTH syndrome. The time of day that the specimen is drawn may improve separation of normal persons from those with Cushing's disease.

Computerized Tomography

Computerized tomography (CT) can frequently differentiate between unilateral adrenal enlargement (adrenal adenoma or carcinoma) and bilateral enlargement (pituitary hyperactivity or ectopic ACTH syndrome). However, it has been reported that nonfunctioning adrenal cortex nodules may occur in 1%–8% of normal persons, and one of these nodules could be present coincidentally with pituitary Cushing's syndrome or ectopic ACTH. Computerized tomography is very useful, better than pituitary sella x-ray films, in verifying the presence of a pituitary adenoma. Even so, third- and fourth-generation CT detects only about 45% (range, 30%–60%) of pituitary adenomas. In addition, it has been reported that 10%–25% of normal persons have a pituitary microadenoma, and some of these nonfunctioning nodules may be seen on CT and lead to a misdiagnosis of Cushing's disease.

Summary of Tests in Cushing's Syndrome

Currently, the most frequently utilized tests to screen for Cushing's syndrome are the overnight low-dose DST and the test to detect abolishment of serum cortisol diurnal variation. Urine free cortisol determination would provide more accurate information than the diurnal variation test. Confirmatory tests (if necessary) and tests to differentiate adrenal from nonadrenal etiology that are most often used are the 48-hour DST or the metyrapone test, serum ACTH assay, and CT visualization of the adrenals.

Conditions that affect the screening and confirmatory tests should be kept in mind. In particular, alcoholism (especially with recent drinking) and psychiatric depression can closely mimic the test results that suggest Cushing's syndrome. Finally, there are some patients in each category of Cushing's syndrome etiology who do not produce the theoretically expected response to screening or confirmatory tests.

PRIMARY ALDOSTERONISM

Aldosterone is the major electrolyte-regulating steroid of the adrenal cortex. Production is stimulated by ACTH but is also influenced by serum sodium or potassium levels. In addition, aldosterone can be secreted under the influence of the renin-angiotensin system in quantities sufficient to maintain life even without ACTH. In plasma, some aldosterone is probably bound to alpha globulins. There is a circadian rhythm that corresponds to that of cortisol, with peak levels occurring in the early morning and low levels (50% or less of A.M. values) in the afternoon. Ninety percent of breakdown and inactivation takes place in the liver. Aldosterone acts primarily on the distal convoluted tubules of the kidney, where it promotes sodium reabsorption with compensatory excretion of potassium and hydrogen ions.

Primary aldosteronism (Conn's syndrome) results from overproduction of aldosterone, usually by an adrenal cortex adenoma (carcinoma, nodular hyperplasia, and glucocorticoid-suppressible aldosteronism are rare etiologies). Symptoms include hypertension, weakness, and polyuria, but no edema.

Secondary aldosteronism refers to overproduction of aldosterone in certain nonadrenal conditions:

1. Hyponatremia or low salt intake
2. Potassium loading
3. Generalized edema (cirrhosis, nephrotic syndrome, congestive heart failure)
4. Malignant hypertension
5. Renal ischemia of any etiology (including renal artery stenosis)
6. Pregnancy or use of estrogen-containing medications

Current explanations for the effects of these conditions on aldosterone point toward decreased effective renal blood flow (Fig 29–4). This triggers certain pressure-sensitive glomerular afferent arteriole cells called the "juxtaglomerular apparatus" into compensatory release of the enzyme renin. Renin acts on an alpha-2 globulin from the liver called "renin substrate" to produce a decapeptide, angiotensin I, which, in turn, is converted to an octapeptide, angiotensin II, by angiotensin-converting enzymes in lung and kidney. Angiotensin II has a very short half-life (< one minute), and is both a powerful vasoconstrictor and a stimulator of the adrenal cortex to release aldosterone. There are several feedback mechanisms, one of which is mediated by retention of salt (and accompanying water) by increased aldosterone, leading to increase in plasma volume, which, in turn, induces the juxtaglomerular apparatus of the kidney to decrease renin secretion directly. The autonomic nervous system also affects renin output. Normally, renin production follows a circadian rhythm that

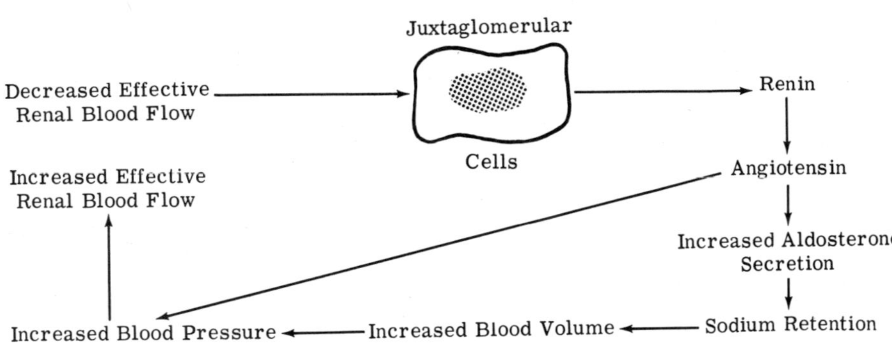

FIG 29–4.
Renal pressor system.

roughly (not exactly) parallels that of cortisol and aldosterone (highest values in early morning). There are reports that renin normal values diminish somewhat with age. Upright posture is a strong stimulus to renin secretion.

General Laboratory Findings

Hypokalemia is the most typical abnormality, and the combination of hypertension and hypokalemia in a person who is not taking diuretics suggests the possibility of primary aldosteronism. However, about 20% (range, 0%–66%) of patients with primary aldosteronism have serum potassium levels within population reference range. Most of these normokalemic patients have a serum potassium value that does not exceed 4.0 mEq/L (4 mmol/L). Also, hypokalemia in a person with hypertension who is taking diuretics does not mean that hypokalemia is invariably due only to the diuretic unless the patient had already been adequately investigated for Conn's syndrome. Some other diseases that may be associated with both hypertension and hypokalemia include Cushing's syndrome, essential hypertension combined with diuretic therapy, potassium-losing renal disease, licorice abuse, malignant hypertension, Bartter's syndrome, and the 11-β-hydroxylase variant of congenital adrenal hyperplasia.

Other frequent laboratory findings in primary aldosteronism include mild alkalosis and a low urine specific gravity. Postprandial glucose tolerance (but not the fasting glucose) is abnormal in about 50% of patients. Hypernatremia is occasionally found in classic cases, but most patients have high-normal or normal serum sodium levels. Excretion of 17-OHCS and 17-KS is normal. Hemoglobin values and white blood cell counts are also normal.

Diagnostic Tests

Serum Potassium Loading.—Diagnosis of primary aldosteronism may be suggested by failure to raise serum potassium levels on regular diet plus 100 mEq of potassium/day. (In addition, urine potassium excretion should increase during potassium loading, assuming a normal salt intake of 5–8 gm/day.)

Plasma or Urine Aldosterone.—Patients with primary aldosteronism secrete more aldosterone than normal persons, so that aldosterone levels are increased in 24-hour urine specimens and, under proper conditions, in plasma specimens. Although RIA methods are now being used, these are still too difficult for the average laboratory. Even reference laboratories are not always dependable, especially for plasma aldosterone assay. Urine assay has the advantage that short-term fluctuations are eliminated, and there appears to be less overlap between normal and abnormal values. Accurate collection of the 24-hour specimen is the major drawback. Plasma is much more convenient to obtain, but plasma levels are more likely to be affected by short-term influences and other factors. Among these are diurnal variation (lower values in the afternoon than in the morning) and upright position (which greatly increases plasma aldosterone), whereas a 24-hour urine collection dampens the effects of these changes and instead reflects integrated secretion rate. Both plasma and urine aldosterone levels are increased by low-sodium diets and by lowered body sodium content and are decreased in the presence of high sodium intake. A low serum magnesium level also stimulates production of aldosterone. Potassium has an opposite effect: high potassium levels stimulate aldosterone secretion, whereas hypokalemia inhibits it.

Since hypertensive patients are frequently treated by sodium restriction or diuretics that increase sodium excretion, and since the body may be sodium depleted while still maintaining serum sodium within a normal range, it is advisable to give patients a high-sodium diet or salt supplements for several days before collecting specimens for aldosterone (renin assay is invalidated by salt loading and would have to be done previously or at some other time). One investigator suggests adding 10–12 gm of salt/day for 5–7 days plus one additional day while a 24-hour urine for aldosterone is collected. Salt loading should not affect aldosterone values in primary aldosteronism, since the hormone is secreted autonomously and therefore production is not significantly affected by normal feedback mechanisms. As a further check, the 24-hour specimen (if urine is assayed) or a random urine specimen (if plasma is used) should be assayed for sodium. Urine sodium values less than 30 mEq/L (mmol/L) suggest decreased sodium excretion, implying a sodium deficit and therefore a falsely increased aldosterone level. Several investigators have used a saline infusion procedure (1.5–2.0 L of saline infused between 8 and 10 A.M., with plasma aldosterone samples drawn just before and after the infusion). Some data indicate that aldosterone normal values, like those of renin, decrease somewhat with age. Certain drugs may increase aldosterone secretion; most of these are agents that increase plasma renin (hydralazine [Apresoline], diazoxide [Hyperstat], nitroprusside, and various diuretics such as furosemide [Lasix]). Glucose ingestion temporarily lowers plasma aldosterone levels.

Plasma Renin.—Plasma renin characteristically is decreased in primary aldosteronism. Plasma renin assay is complicated by the fact that renin cannot be measured directly, even by RIA. Instead, angiotensin I generation is estimated. This situation is standard in laboratory measurement of enzymes: usually the action of the enzyme on a suitable substrate is measured rather than direct reaction of a chemical or antibody with the enzyme. Two related techniques are used: plasma renin activity (PRA) and plasma renin concentration (PRC). The PRA reflects the rate of angiotensin I formation per unit of time. However, renin substrate (on which renin acts) is normally not present in sufficient quantities for maximal renin effect. In PRC, excess renin substrate is added to demonstrate maximal renin effect; the result is compared with standard renin preparations to calculate the patient's renin concentration. In most cases PRA is adequate for clinical purposes and is technically a little more easy. Estrogens increase renin substrate, so PRC would be more accurate in that circumstance.

Plasma renin is a RIA technique of moderate or moderately great difficulty; accurate results are highly dependent on the manner in which a laboratory performs the test. In addition, optimum conditions under which the assay should be performed are not yet standardized. Although several kits are now commercially available, these kits demonstrate considerable variation in results when tested on the same plasma samples. In short, most laboratories cannot be depended on to produce accurate results, and even reference laboratories may at times have problems, especially with some of the kits. Renin is a very unstable enzyme, and for usable results it must be drawn into a cold tube, the tube being kept cold while it is centrifuged, and the plasma frozen immediately. Heparin cannot be used. The tourniquet should be removed before the blood sample is drawn, since stasis may lower renin levels considerably. Certain factors influence renin secretion. Sodium depletion, hypokalemia, upright posture, various diuretics, estrogens, and vasodilating antihypertensive drugs (hydralazine, diazoxide, and nitroprusside) increase plasma renin levels. Methyldopa (Aldomet), guanethidine, levodopa, and propranolol decrease renin levels. Changes in body sodium have parallel effects on renin and aldosterone (e.g., low sodium level stimulates production of both), whereas changes in potassium have opposite effects (low potassium level stimulates renin but depresses aldosterone).

Although Conn's syndrome is typically associated with low plasma renin levels, other conditions (see Table 29–4) may produce similar decreased values. In addition, nearly 25% of hypertensive patients have decreased plasma renin levels without having Conn's syndrome. In Conn's syndrome, low-salt diet plus 2 hours of upright posture may increase previously low renin values but not enough to reach the normal range. In patients who do not have Conn's syndrome, a renin level that is temporarily decreased for some reason will be stimulated enough to rise above the lower limits of normal. It has been advised not to use diuretics in addition to a low-salt diet plus upright posture, since the additional stimulation of renin production may overcome renin suppression in some patients with Conn's syndrome. Four hours of continual upright posture was originally thought to be necessary; subsequent data indicated that 2 hours is sufficient.

Several screening tests for renin abnormality have been suggested (see Table 36–27). The furosemide test seems to be the one most widely used.

Unilateral renal disease is another cause of hypertension that is potentially curable. It is estimated that 5% (or even more) of hypertensive persons have this condition, which makes it much more common than primary aldosteronism. Plasma renin is frequently elevated. Since renin assay may already be considered in a hypertensive patient to rule out Conn's syndrome, it could also serve as a screening test for unilateral renal disease. However, about one half of patients (literature range,

TABLE 29–4.
Typical Renin-Aldosterone Patterns in Various Conditions

	Plasma Renin	Aldosterone
Primary aldosteronism	Low	High
"Low-renin" essential hypertension	Low	Normal
Cushing's syndrome	Low	Low-normal
Licorice ingestion syndrome	Low	Low
High-salt diet	Low	Low
Oral contraceptives	High	Normal
Cirrhosis	High	High
Malignant hypertension	High	High
Unilateral renal disease	High	High
"High-renin" essential hypertension	High	High
Pregnancy	High	High
Diuretic overuse	High	High
Juxtaglomerular tumor (Bartter's syndrome)	High	High
Low-salt diet	High	High
Addison's disease	High	Low
Hypokalemia	High	Low

4%–80%) who have curable hypertension due to unilateral renal disease have normal peripheral vein plasma renin levels.

Summary of Tests in Primary Aldosteronism

Hypokalemia in a patient with hypertension should raise the question of possible Conn's syndrome. The typical laboratory pattern for primary aldosteronism is that of increased aldosterone and decreased renin levels. Other conditions have symptoms or laboratory findings that might suggest primary aldosteronism, but these can be differentiated by the combination of aldosterone and renin (Table 29–4). Some patients with Conn's syndrome have aldosterone values in the upper normal area rather than definitely elevated values. At times, either the renin or the aldosterone assay will have to be repeated to obtain a correct diagnosis.

Adrenal Localization Procedures in Aldosteronism

Primary aldosteronism actually comprises a group of at least four conditions. First is Conn's syndrome, produced by unilateral adrenal tumor (adenoma, rarely carcinoma). This syndrome comprises about 75% (range, 60%–90%) of primary aldosteronism cases. Second is idiopathic aldosteronism, caused by bilateral nodular adrenal hyperplasia or associated with apparently normal adrenals. This category comprises about 20%–25% (range, 10%–40%) of primary aldosterone cases. Third is intermediate hyperaldosteronism, in which elevated aldosterone levels are suppressible by infusion of deoxycorticosterone acetate. This category is uncommon. Fourth is glucocorticoid-responsive aldosteronism, in which elevated aldosterone levels are suppressible and treatable by cortisol or similar glucocorticoids. This category is also uncommon.

Of these, Conn's syndrome is responsible for about 75% of cases and is the only condition that is surgically curable. Several procedures have been advocated to help verify the diagnosis of Conn's syndrome, to help differentiate it from the other categories of primary aldosteronism, and to establish which adrenal contains the adenoma. Currently, CT visualization of the adrenals is the most widely used technique. Computerized tomography is reported to detect 60%–90% of aldosterone-producing adenomas. Radionuclide adrenal scanning using one of several new radioactive agents concentrated by the adrenal is also useful in those few institutions that do the procedure. If CT or radionuclide scans are normal, some medical centers proceed to adrenal vein catheterization for aldosterone assay from the adrenal vein on each side. A considerable difference in concentration between the two sides suggests adenoma.

ADDISON'S DISEASE

Addison's disease is primary adrenocortical insufficiency from bilateral adrenal cortex destruction. Tuberculosis used to be the most frequent etiology but now is second to idiopathic atrophy. Long-term steroid therapy causes adrenal cortex atrophy from disuse; and if steroids are abruptly withdrawn, symptoms of adrenal failure may develop rapidly. This is now the most common cause of addisonian-type crisis. Less common etiologies of Addison's disease are infection, idiopathic hemorrhage, and replacement by metastatic carcinoma. The most frequent metastatic tumor is from the lung, and it is interesting that there often can be nearly complete replacement without any symptoms.

The salt-wasting forms of congenital adrenal hyperplasia—due to congenital deficiency of certain enzymes necessary for adrenal cortex hormone synthesis—might also be included as a variant of Addison's disease.

Weakness and fatigability are early manifestations of Addison's disease, often preceded by infection or stress. Other signs and symptoms of the classic syndrome are hypotension of varying degree, weight loss, a small heart, and sometimes skin pigmentation. Anorexia, nausea, and vomiting occur frequently in adrenal crisis. The most common symptoms of adrenal crisis are hypotension and nausea.

General Laboratory Tests

Laboratory studies show low serum sodium and chloride levels. Serum potassium levels are mildly elevated in about 50% of patients. There occasionally is a mild hypoglycemia. There may be a normocytic-normochromic mild anemia and relative lymphocytosis with a decreased neutrophil count. The diagnosis may be suspected on clinical grounds and by the finding of normal or increased sodium and chloride levels in the urine despite low serum levels. Total circulating eosinophil count usually (although not always) is close to normal.

Diagnostic Tests in Addison's Disease

Screening Tests.— A single random plasma cortisol specimen has been used as a screening procedure, since theoretically the value should be very low in Addison's disease and normal in other conditions. Unfortunately, there are sufficient interfering factors so that its usefulness is very limited. Because serum cortisol normally has a circadian rhythm with its peak about 6–8 A.M., the specimen must be drawn about 6–8 A.M. in order not to misinterpret a lower value drawn later in the day. Stress increases plasma cortisol levels, although the increase is proportionately much less in Addison's disease than in normal persons. The classic patient with Addison's disease in crisis has an early morning cortisol level of less than 5 μg/100 ml (138 nmol/L), and a level of 5–10 μg/100 ml (138–276 nmol/L) is suspicious for Addison's disease, especially if the patient is under stress. Patients with milder degrees of illness or borderline deficiency of cortisol may have a morning cortisol value of more than 10 μg/100 ml. It is often difficult to determine whether mild elevation of more than 10 μg/100 ml is due to stress or is a normal level. An early morning cortisol level of more than 20 μg/100 ml is some evidence against Addison's disease. Most endocrinologists do not consider a single random cortisol level to be reliable in screening for Addison's disease. As noted previously, the serum sodium level is low in classic cases and is associated with a normal or elevated urine sodium level, but the serum sodium level may be within its reference range in up to 50% of patients.

Adrenocorticotropic Hormone Stimulation Test.— A definitive diagnosis of Addison's disease is possible using ACTH stimulation. The classic procedure is the 8-hour infusion test. If biologic rather than synthetic ACTH is used, many recommend giving 0.5 mg of dexamethasone orally before starting the test to prevent allergic reactions. A 24-hour urine specimen is taken the day before the test. Twenty-five units of ACTH in 500 ml of saline is given intravenously during an 8-hour period while another 24-hour urine specimen is obtained. In normal persons, there will be at least a twofold to fourfold increase in cortisol or 17-OHCS levels. In Addison's disease, there is practically no response. If pituitary deficiency is suspected, the test should be repeated the next day, in which case there will be a gradual, although relatively small, response. If exogenous steroids have been given over long periods, especially in large doses, the test period may have to be prolonged up to 7 days. One group has circumvented this by using a continuous 24- to 48-hour infusion. If maintenance steroids are necessary during the test period, small doses of dexamethasone should be used to avoid measuring the treatment steroid along with endogenous production.

Rapid Adrenocorticotropic Hormone Stimulation Test.— Most investigators now prefer a rapid ACTH stimulation test rather than the classic procedure, since the rapid test can serve as a screening test unless the patient is extremely ill and in some patients may provide the same information as a confirmatory test. After a baseline serum cortisol specimen is obtained, 25 units of ACTH or 0.25 mg of corsyntropin (Cortrosyn or Synacthen, a synthetic ACTH preparation) is administered by intramuscular injection. There is variation in technique among the descriptions in the literature. Some measure plasma cortisol response after administration of corsyntropin and a few assay urinary 17-OHCS. Some inject corsyntropin intramuscularly and others intravenously. Some obtain a plasma cortisol specimen 30 minutes after giving corsyntropin whereas others do so at 60 or 120 minutes. Some obtain samples at two intervals instead of one. A reasonable compromise seems to be intravenous (IV) injection of corsyntropin (after a baseline blood specimen is drawn) and measurement of plasma cortisol at 30 minutes and again at either 90 or 120 minutes after the test dose. Theoretically, patients with primary adrenal insufficiency should demonstrate little response, whereas patients with pituitary insufficiency or normal persons should have cortisol levels that increase over twice baseline values. Some patients with pituitary insufficiency demonstrate normal response to corsyntropin and some have a subnormal response. Because corsyntropin test results are not uniform in patients with pituitary insufficiency, it has been suggested that aldosterone should be measured as well as cortisol. Aldosterone levels should increase in pituitary hypofunction but should not rise significantly in primary adrenal failure. The metyrapone test is also useful to diagnose pituitary insufficiency.

Some patients may have equivocal rapid test results, and others may have been treated with substantial doses of steroids for considerable periods of time before definitive tests for etiology of Addison's disease are attempted. Under long-term steroid suppression, a normal adrenal cortex may be unable to respond immediately to stimulation. For definitive tests, the classic approach is to repeat the 8-hour ACTH infusion procedure daily for 5–7 days. Patients with primary Addison's disease should display little daily increment in cortisol values; those with secondary Addison's disease should eventually produce a stepwise increase in cortisol values. Some have used depot intramuscular synthetic ACTH preparations once daily instead of IV infusion.

Thorn Test.— If steroid measurements are not available, the Thorn test is a reasonably satisfactory substitute, although not as accurate. First, a count of total circulating eosinophils is done. Then the patient is given 25 units of ACTH, either intravenously in the same way as in the ACTH test just described or intramuscularly in the form of long-acting ACTH gel. Eight hours after ACTH administration is started, another total circulating eosinophil count is made. Normally, cortisone causes depression of eosinophil production. Therefore a normal cortisol response to ACTH stimulation would be a drop of total circulating eosinophils to less than 50% of baseline values. A drop of less than 50% is considered suspicious for adrenal insufficiency. False positive responses (less than a 50% drop) may occur in any condition that itself produces eosinophilia (e.g., acute episodes of allergy).

Plasma Adrenocorticotropic Hormone Assay.— Plasma ACTH measurement has been used to help confirm the diagnosis of Addison's disease and to differentiate primary from secondary adrenal failure. In primary adrenal failure, the ACTH value should be high and cortisol levels should be low. In hypothalamic or pituitary insufficiency, both ACTH and cortisol values theoretically should be low. Unfortunately, a considerable number of patients have cortisol or ACTH values within reference range. A specimen for plasma ACTH determination can be drawn at the same time as the specimen for baseline cortisol prior to stimulation tests and can be frozen for availability if needed.

SECONDARY ADRENAL INSUFFICIENCY

Secondary adrenal insufficiency is due to deficient production of ACTH by the pituitary. This usually results from pituitary disease but is occasionally due to hypothalamic disorders. In general, primary adrenocortical insufficiency (Addison's disease) is associated with inability of the adrenal to produce either cortisol or aldosterone. In addition, there may be cutaneous hyperpigmentation due to pituitary hypersecretion of melanocytic-stimulating hormone (MSH). In secondary adrenal insufficiency, aldosterone secretion is usually sufficient to prevent hyperkalemia, and hyponatremia tends to be less severe. Cutaneous pigmentation does not occur because the pituitary does not produce excess MSH. The major abnormality is lack of cortisol due to deficiency of ACTH. The laboratory picture may simulate inappropriate ADH syndrome.

HYPORENINEMIC HYPOALDOSTERONISM

Another adrenal cortex deficiency disease is hyporeninemic hypoaldosteronism. Since this condition is usually due to a deficiency of renin, the disorder is a secondary rather than a primary defect in aldosterone secretion. The characteristic laboratory feature is hyperkalemia, and the condition is usually discovered when a patient is found to have hyperkalemia not due to any other cause. The serum sodium level is normal or mildly decreased. There may be a mild metabolic acidosis. If dietary sodium is restricted, renal salt wasting develops, since deficiency of aldosterone makes it difficult to conserve sodium. Hyperkalemia is not diagnostic of hyporeninemic hypoaldosteronism since it may be found in Addison's disease, salt-wasting congenital adrenal hyperplasia, renal failure, and other conditions listed in the chapter on serum electrolytes and Table 24–2.

ADRENAL MEDULLA DYSFUNCTION

The only syndrome in this category is produced by pheochromocytomas. Pheochromocytoma is a tumor of the adrenal medulla that frequently secretes epinephrine or norepinephrine. This causes hypertension, which may be continuous or intermittent. Although rare, pheochromocytoma is one of the few curable causes of hypertension and so should be considered as a possible etiology in any patient with hypertension of either sudden or recent onset. This is especially true for young or middle-aged persons.

Approximately 90% of pheochromocytomas in adults arise in the adrenal. Of the 10% that are extra-adrenal, the great majority are located in the abdomen, with 1%–2% in the thorax and neck. Extra-adrenal abdominal tumors are usually found in the para-aortic sympathetic nerve chain (below the level of the renal artery), but perhaps one third are located in the remnants of the organ of Zuckerkandl (which is situated in the para-aortic region between the origin of the inferior mesenteric artery and the bifurcation of the aorta). About 20% of pheochromocytomas are multiple and about 10% are bilateral. Approximately 5%–10% of all pheochromocytomas are malignant, but the malignancy rate for extra-adrenal abdominal tumors is reported to be about 25%–30%. Although hypertension is the most common significant clinical finding, 10%–20% of pheochromocytomas do not produce hypertension (Table 29–5). Hyperglycemia is reported in about 50% of patients. In one autopsy series of 54 cases, only 25% were diagnosed during life.

About 5% of pheochromocytoma patients have neurofibromatosis, and in 5%–10% the pheochromocytoma is associated with the multiple endocrine neoplasia (MEN) syndrome type II (also known as "IIA," with medullary carcinoma of the thyroid) or III (also known as "IIB," with mucosal neuromas). The MEN syndrome pheochromocytomas are bilateral in 50%–95% of cases and multiple in about 70% of cases, whereas nonfamilial (sporadic) pheochromocytomas are usually unilateral and are multiple in about 20% of cases. About 5% of the familial cases are said to be malignant.

In children, extra-adrenal pheochromocytomas are more common (30% of cases), more often bilateral (25%–70% of cases), and more

TABLE 29–5.
Common Signs and Symptoms of Pheochromocytoma

Sign or Symptom	% of Cases
Hypertension	80–90
(paroxysmal hypertension)	(22–87)
Headache	55
Tachycardia	44–50
Dyspnea	19–27
Excess sweat	23–78
Weight loss	33
Organ abnormalities	
Cardiac	50
Retinal	80–100
Cerebrovascular	14–26
Systemic	
Fever	18–78
Hyperglycemia	40–78
Paroxysmal	
Nausea	90
Vomiting	33
Thoracic pain	12–27
Abdominal pain	15

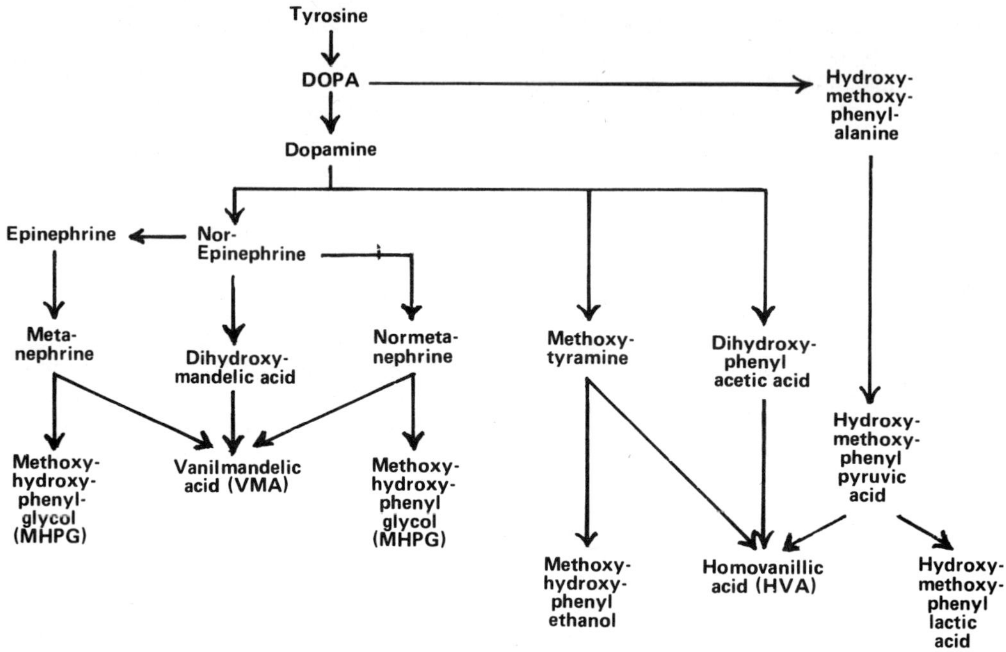

FIG 29–5.
Catecholamine metabolism.

often multiple (about 30% of cases) than in adults. About 10%–20% of adrenal or extra-adrenal childhood pheochromocytomas are reported to be malignant.

Tests for Pheochromocytoma

Regitine Test.— The first tests for pheochromocytomas were pharmacologic, based on neutralization of epinephrine effects by adrenergic-blocking drugs such as Regitine. After basal blood pressure has been established, 5 mg of Regitine is given intravenously, and the blood pressure is checked every 30 seconds. The result is positive if systolic blood pressure decreases more than 35 mm Hg or diastolic pressure decreases 25 mm Hg or more and remains decreased 3–4 minutes. Laboratory tests have proved much more reliable than the pharmacologic procedures, which yield an appreciable percentage of false positives and negatives.

Clonidine Suppression Test.— Clonidine is a centrally acting alpha-adrenergic agonist that inhibits sympathetic nervous system catecholamine release from postganglionic neurons. After a baseline blood specimen is obtained, a single 0.3-mg oral dose of clonidine is administered and a second blood specimen is drawn 3 hours later. Most patients without pheochromocytoma had postdose plasma norepinephrine values more than 25% below baseline and plasma catacholamine values less than 500 pg/ml. Most patients with pheochromocytoma showed little change in plasma norepinephrine values between the predose and postdose specimens and had a plasma catacholamine postdose level greater than 500 pg/ml. Another investigator obtained less favorable results in a small number of patients. The test has not yet been widely evaluated.

Catacholamine/Vanillylmandelic Acid/Metanephrine Assay.—The catecholamines epinephrine and norepinephrine are excreted by the kidney, about 3%–6% free (unchanged), and the remainder as various metabolites (Fig 29–5). Of these metabolic products, the major portion is vanillylmandelic (vanilmandelic) acid (VMA), and the remainder (about 20%–40%) is compounds known as metanephrines. Therefore, one can measure urinary catecholamines, metanephrines, or VMA. Of these, urine metanephrine assay is considered by many to be the most sensitive and reliable single test. There are also fewer drugs that interfere.

Most investigators report that urine metanephrine assay detects about 95% (range, 77%–100%) of patients with pheochromocytoma. Sensitivity of urine catecholamines is approximately 90%–95% (range, 67%–100%) and that of urine VMA assay is also about 90%–95% (range, 50%–100%). One report indicates that metanephrine excretion is relatively uniform and that a random specimen reported in terms of creatinine excretion can be substituted for the usual 24-hour collection in screening for pheochromocytoma. Although the metanephrine excretion test is slowly gaining preference, VMA and catecholamine assay are still widely used. All three methods have detection rates within 5%–10% of one another. A small but significant percentage of pheochromocytomas are missed by any of the three tests (fewer by metanephrine excretion), especially if the tumor secretes intermittently. The VMA test has one definite advantage in that certain screening methods are technically more simple than catecholamine or metanephrine assay and therefore are more readily available in smaller laboratories. The VMA screening methods are apt to produce more false positive results, however, so that abnormal values (or normal results in patients with strong suspicion for pheochromocytoma) should be confirmed by some other procedure.

Catecholamine production and plasma catecholamine levels may be increased after severe exercise (although mild exercise has no appreciable effect), by emotional stress, and by smoking. Uremia interferes with assay methods based on fluorescence. Other diseases or conditions that may increase plasma or urine catecholamines or urine catecholamine metabolites are hypothyroidism, diuretic therapy, heavy alcohol intake, hypoglycemia, hypoxia, severe acidosis, Cushing's syndrome, myocardial infarction, hemolytic anemia, and occasionally lymphoma or severe renal disease. In addition, bananas, coffee, and various other foods as well as certain medications may produce falsely elevated results (see Table 36–2). These foods or medications produce appreciable numbers of false-positive results in some of the standard screening techniques for VMA. An abnormal result with the "screening" VMA techniques should be confirmed by some other VMA method. Although other VMA methods or methods for metanephrine and catecholamine assay are more reliable, they too may be affected by certain foods or medications, so it is best to check with individual laboratories for details on substances that affect their particular test method. Reports differ on whether some patients with essential hypertension may have elevated serum or urine catecholamine or catecholamine metabolite results, and if so, how often it occurs and what percent are due to conditions known to elevate catecholamines, to medications, or to unknown causes.

Plasma Catecholamine Assay.— Several investigators report better sensitivity in pheochromocytoma with plasma catecholamine assay than with the particular urine metabolite assays they were using. Another advantage is the simplicity of a single blood specimen vs. 24-hour collection. However, stress and upright posture can greatly affect plasma catecholamine levels, even the stress of venipuncture, so it is best to draw the specimen in the early morning before the patient rises. Even then, some advocate placement of an indwelling venous catheter or heparinized scalp vein apparatus with an interval of 30 minutes between insertion of the catheter and withdrawal of the blood specimen. One investigator reported that plasma catecholamine values decreased rapidly if the red blood cells (RBCs) were not removed within 5 minutes after obtaining the specimen. Placing the specimen on ice was helpful but only partially retarded RBC catecholamine uptake. Plasma catecholamine assay detection rate in pheochromocytomas is about 90% (literature range, 53%–100%). Failure to detect the tumor in some instances is due to intermittent tumor secretion. Urine collection has the advantage of averaging the 24-hour excretion.

Tumor Localization Methods.—Once pheochromocytoma is strongly suspected by results of biochemical testing, certain procedures have been useful in localizing the tumor. Intravenous pyelography with nephrotomography is reported to have an accuracy of about 70% in detecting adrenal pheochromocytoma. Computerized tomography has been reported to detect 84%–93% of pheochromocytomas, including some in extra-adrenal locations. Angiographic procedures are reported to detect 60%–84% of pheochromocytomas; but angiography is somewhat controversial because it is invasive, because it yields about 10% false negative results in adrenal tumors, and because some investigators believe that the incidence of tumor bilaterality warrants exploration of both sides of the abdomen regardless of angiographic findings.

ADRENAL AND NONADRENAL CAUSES OF HYPERTENSION

Cushing's syndrome, primary aldosteronism, unilateral renal disease (rarely, bilateral renal artery stenosis), and pheochromocytoma often produce hypertension. Hypertension due to these diseases is classified as secondary hypertension, in contrast to primary idiopathic (essential) hypertension. Although patients with these particular diseases that cause secondary hypertension are a relatively small minority of hypertension patients, the diseases are important because they are surgically curable. The patient usually is protected against the bad effects of hypertension by early diagnosis and cure. Patients who must be especially investigated are those who are young (less than age 50 years), those whose symptoms develop over a short time period, or those who have a sudden worsening of their hypertension after a previous mild stable blood pressure elevation.

Additional tests relevant to this chapter are discussed in chapter 35.

BIBLIOGRAPHY

Young WF, Klee GG: Primary aldosteronism: Diagnostic evaluation. *Endocrinol Metab Clin North Am* 1988; 17:367.

Elliott WJ, Murphy MB: Reduced specificity of the clonidine suppression test in patients with normal plasma catecholamine levels. *Am J Med* 1988; 84:419.

Sheps SG, et al: Diagnostic evaluation of pheochromocytoma. *Endocrinol Metab Clin North Am* 1988; 17:397.

Knight JA, Wu JT: Catecholamines and their metabolites: Clinical and laboratory aspects. *Lab Med* 1987; 18:153.

Marks P: Endocrine hypertension. *Intern Med Specialist* 1987; 8:155.

White PC, et al: Congenital adrenal hyperplasia. *N Engl J Med* 1987; 316:1519–1580.

Hermus AR, et al: The corticotropin-releasing hormone test versus the high-dose dexamethasone test in the differential diagnosis of Cushing's syndrome. *Lancet* 1986; 2:540.

Nieman LK, et al: The ovine corticotropin-releasing hormone stimulation test and the dexamethasone suppression test in the differential diagnosis of Cushing's syndrome. *Ann Intern Med* 1986; 105:862.

Carpenter PC: Cushing's syndrome: Update of diagnosis and management. *Mayo Clin Proc* 1986; 61:49.

Findling JW, Tyrrell JB: Occult ectopic secretion of corticotropin. *Arch Intern Med* 1986; 146:929.

Tyrrell JB, et al: An overnight high-dose dexamethasone suppression test for rapid differential diagnosis of Cushing's syndrome. *Ann Intern Med* 1986; 104:180.

May ME, Carey RM: Rapid adrenocorticotropic hormone test in practice. *Am J Med* 1986; 79:679.

Bravo EL: Secondary hypertension. *Postgrad Med* 1986; 80:139.

Bravo EL: Plasma catacholamines: Their measurement and clinical utility. *Lab Med* 1986; 17:512.

Cryer PE: Phaeochromocytoma. *Clin Endocrinol Metab* 1985; 14:203.

Drury PL: Disorders of mineralocorticoid activity. *Clin Endocrinol Metab* 1985; 14:175.

Dunlap NE, et al: Cushing's syndrome. *Arch Pathol Lab Med* 1985; 109:222.

May ME: Rapid adrenocorticotropic hormone test in practice. *Am J Med* 1985; 79:679.

Wand GS, Ney RL: Disorders of the hypothalamic-pituitary-adrenal axis. *Clin Endocrinol Metab* 1985; 14:33.

Arteaga E, et al: Use of the saline infusion test to diagnose the cause of primary aldosteronism. *Am J Med* 1985; 79:722.

Gilliland PF: Endocrine emergencies. *Postgrad Med* 1983; 74:215.

Cunningham SK: Normal cortisol response to corticotropin in patients with secondary adrenal failure. *Arch Intern Med* 1983; 143:2276.

Bravo EL, et al: The changing clinical spectrum of primary aldosteronism. *Am J Med* 1983; 74:641.

Atuk NO: Pheochromocytoma: Diagnosis, localization, and treatment. *Hosp Pract* 1983; 18:187.

Zachmann M, et al: Clinical and biochemical variability of congenital adrenal hyperplasia due to 11β-hydroxylase deficiency: A study of 25 patients. *J Clin Endocrinol* 1983; 56:222.

Sindler BH, et al: The superiority of the metyrapone test versus the high-dose dexamethasone test in the differential diagnosis of Cushing's syndrome. *Am J Med* 1983; 74:657.

Nanji AA, Campbell DJ: Pheochromocytoma: Which tests are best? *Diagn Med* 1982; 5(6):52.

Horocks PM, London DR: Diagnostic value of 9 AM plasma adenocorticotrophic hormone concentrations in Cushing's disease. *Br Med J* 1982; 285:1302.

Plouin PF, et al.: Biochemical tests for diagnosis of pheochromocytoma: Urinary versus plasma determinations. *Br Med J* 1981; 282:853.

Aron DC, et al: Cushing's syndrome: Problems in diagnosis. *Medicine* (Baltimore) 1981; 60:25.

Burke MD: Adrenal dysfunction. *Postgrad Med* 1981; 69:155.

White EA: Use of computed tomography in diagnosing the cause of primary aldosteronism. *N Engl J Med* 1980; 303:1503.

Sealey JE: Renin, angiotensin, and aldosterone: Laboratory methods. *Lab Mgmt* 1980; 18(8):33.

Streeten DHP, et al: Reliability of screening methods for the diagnosis of primary aldosteronism. *Am J Med* 1979; 67:403.

Wonjg ET, et al: Urinary 17alpha-hydroxyprogesterone in diagnosis and management of congenital adrenal hyperplasia. *J Clin Endocrinol* 1979; 49:377.

Engel RH: Diagnosing and monitoring virilizing congenital adrenal hyperplasia. *Lab Mgmt* 1979; 17(10):38.

30 Pituitary and Gonadal Function Tests; Tests in Obstetrics

TESTS OF PITUITARY FUNCTION

The most common disorders resulting from pituitary dysfunction are pituitary insufficiency in adults, growth hormone (GH) deficiency of childhood, and acromegaly in adults.

Pituitary Insufficiency

Body organs affected by stimulatory hormones from the pituitary include the thyroid, adrenals, and gonads. Bone growth in childhood is dependent on pituitary GH. Pituitary failure does not produce a clear-cut syndrome analogous to syndromes produced by failure of pituitary-controlled organs ("end organs") such as the thyroid. Therefore, pituitary hormone deficiency is considered only when there is deficiency-type malfunction in one or more end-organs or metabolic processes such as growth that are dependent on pituitary hormones. Diagnosis is complicated by the fact that primary end-organ failure is much more common than pituitary hormone deficiency. Another source of confusion is that most abnormal effects that can be produced by pituitary dysfunction can also be produced or simulated by nonpituitary etiologies. In addition, the hypothalamus controls pituitary secretion of several hormones, so that hypothalamic abnormality (e.g., defects produced by a craniopharyngioma or other hypothalamic tumor) can result in pituitary dysfunction.

Pituitary insufficiency in adults most commonly results in deficiency of more than one pituitary hormone and is most frequently caused by postpartum hemorrhage (Sheehan's syndrome). Pituitary tumor is also an important etiology. Gonadal failure is ordinarily the first clinical deficiency to appear. It is followed some time later by hypothyroidism. The first laboratory abnormality is usually failure of GH to rise normally in response to stimulation.

Diagnosis

Diagnosis of pituitary insufficiency can be made by direct or indirect testing methods. Indirect methods demonstrate that a hypofunctioning organ that is pituitary dependent shows normal function after stimulation by injection of the appropriate pituitary hormone. Direct methods consist of blood level assays of pituitary hormones. Another direct method is injection of a substance that directly stimulates the pituitary. Now that pituitary hormone assays are available in most medical centers and sizable reference laboratories, indirect tests are much less frequently needed.

Assay of Pituitary Hormones.—Pituitary hormones are peptide hormones rather than steroid hormones. Currently available immunoassays are a great improvement over original bioassays and even the first-generation radioimmunoassays (RIAs). However, with the exception of thyroid-stimulating hormone (TSH), pituitary hormone assays are still ordered infrequently, so that most physician's offices and ordinary hospital laboratories do not find it economically worthwhile to perform the tests. The assays for TSH and adrenocortical-stimulating (adrenocorticotropic) hormone (ACTH) are discussed in the chapters on thyroid and adrenal function. Pituitary luteinizing hormone (LH) and follicle-stimulating hormone (FSH) assay will be discussed later. Growth hormone deficiency is probably the most frequent pituitary hormone deficiency, either in overall pituitary failure or as an isolated defect leading to growth retardation in childhood. Growth hormone assay will be discussed in detail in relation to childhood growth disorders. Growth hormone assay has been used as an overall screen for pituitary insufficiency, but not all cases of pituitary hormone secretion deficiency have associated GH secretion deficiency. Prolactin is another pituitary hormone, but prolactin secretion is one of the last pituitary functions to disappear when the pituitary is injured.

In primary end-organ failure the blood level of stimulating hormone from the pituitary is usually elevated, as the pituitary attempts to get the last possible activity from the damaged organ. Therefore, in the presence of end-organ failure, if values for the pituitary hormone that stimulates the organ are in the upper half of the reference range or are elevated, this is strong evidence against deficiency of that pituitary hormone. Theoretically, inadequate pituitary hormone secretion should result in serum assay values less than the reference range for that pituitary hormone. Unfortunately, low-normal or decreased values of some pituitary hormones may overlap with values found in normal persons, at least using many of the present-day commercial assay kits. In that situation, stimulation or suppression testing may be necessary for more definitive assessment of pituitary function.

Stimulation and Suppression Tests.—Pituitary suppression and stimulation tests available for diagnosis of pituitary hormone secretion deficiency include:

1. Metyrapone (Metopirone) test (chapter 29), based on the adrenal cortex–pituitary feedback mechanism involving ACTH and cortisol but dependent also on hypothalamic function.
2. Thyrotropin-releasing hormone (TRH) test (chapter 28), involving the ability of synthetic TRH to stimulate the pituitary by direct action to release TSH and prolactin.
3. Tests involving pituitary gonadotropins (LH and FSH) such as clomiphene stimulation (involving the hypothalamic-pituitary axis) or LH-releasing hormone (LHRH) administration (direct pituitary stimulation).
4. Tests of hypothalamic function, usually based on establishing pituitary normality by direct stimulation of the pituitary (TRH stimulation of TSH and prolactin, LHRH stimulation of LH secretion, etc.) followed by use of a test that depends on intact hypothalamic function to stimulate pituitary secretion of the same hormone. An example is the use of TRH to stimulate prolactin secretion by the pituitary, followed by chlorpromazine administration, which blocks normal hypothalamic mechanisms that inhibit hypothalamic stimulation of pituitary prolactin secretion and which leads to increased prolactin secretion if the hypothalamus is still capable of stimulating prolactin release.

Growth Hormone Deficiency

Growth hormone is a peptide that is secreted by the acidophil cells of the pituitary. Growth hormone release depends on the interplay between two opposing hormones secreted by the hypothalamus; growth hormone-releasing hormone (GHRH), which stimulates GH release, and somatostatin, which inhibits GH release. Growth hormone exerts its effect through stimulation of various tissues to produce a group of peptide growth factors called "somatomedins." The most important somatomedin is somatomedin-C, which is produced by the liver and which acts on cartilage. High levels of somatomedin participate in a GH feedback mechanism by inhibiting pituitary release of GH and also by stimulating hypothalamic secretion of somatostatin. In addition, there apparently are numerous other factors that influence GH production to varying degree, some of which act through the hypothalamus and others that apparently do not. Normal GH secretion takes place predominantly (but not entirely) during sleep in the form of short irregularly distributed secretory pulses or bursts. Growth hormone deficiency most often is suspected or questioned as part of the differential diagnosis of retarded growth or short stature. A considerable number of hormones and factors are nec-

TABLE 30–1.

Body Factors Necessary for Normal Growth

GH
Somatomedins
Insulin
Thyroxine
Sex hormones
Adequate nutritional factors

TABLE 30–2.

Partial List of Short Stature Etiologies

Familial short stature
Constitutional growth delay
Turner's syndrome
Trisomy syndromes (e.g., Down's syndrome)
GH deficiency (isolated or hypopituitarism)
Hypothyroidism
Severe malnutrition
Malabsorption
Uncontrolled type I diabetes mellitus
Severe chronic illness with organ failure (chronic renal disease, congenital heart disease, severe chronic hemolytic anemia)
Excess androgens or estrogens
Excess cortisol (Cushing's syndrome or iatrogenic)
Psychosocial retardation (abused or severely emotionally deprived children)

essary for adequate growth. Some of the most important are listed in Table 30–1. Some etiologies of short stature (whose extreme result is dwarfism) are listed in Table 30–2. Diagnosis of many of these conditions is discussed elsewhere. Deficiency of GH will be discussed in the context of pediatric or childhood growth retardation. As noted previously, GH deficiency may be part of multihormone pituitary dysfunction but may exist as an isolated defect in an otherwise apparently normal pituitary.

Tests

Growth Hormone Assay.—The most widely used screening test for GH deficiency is serum GH assay. Values are elevated by sleep, exercise of any type, and various foods. Therefore, if a single basal level is obtained, the specimen should be secured in the morning after an overnight fast, and the patient should be awake but not yet out of bed. Because basal normal range for single specimens includes some normal persons with values low enough to overlap the range of values found in patients with GH deficiency, only a result high enough to rule out GH deficiency is significant. Low results either may be due to GH deficiency or may simply be low-normal. Other conditions that increase GH levels besides those previously mentioned include severe malnutrition and chronic liver or renal disease. Patients with psychiatric depression or poorly controlled diabetes mellitus secrete more GH than normal persons during waking hours but not during sleep.

Two relatively simple screening tests for GH deficiency have been advocated. It has been found that a major part of daily GH secretion takes place in a short time period beginning approximately 1 hour after onset of deep sleep (EEG stage 3 or 4). Therefore, one method is to observe the patient until deep sleep occurs, wake the patient 60–90 minutes later, and quickly draw a blood sample for GH assay. About 70% of normal children or adults have GH values sufficiently elevated (≥7 ng/ml; 7 μg/L) to exclude GH deficiency. Strenuous exercise is a strong stimulus to GH secretion. An exercise test in which the patient exercises vigorously for 20–30 minutes and a blood sample is drawn for GH assay 20–30 minutes after the end of the exercise period has been used. About 75%–92% of normal children have sufficiently elevated levels of GH after exercise to exclude GH deficiency.

A third method involves integrated multihour time period blood specimens, which is being used in research and in some medical centers. Because of the irregular pulsatile nature of GH secretion, it was found that a more reliable estimate of GH secretion levels could be obtained by drawing blood specimens for GH assay every 20–30 minutes from an indwelling catheter over a 24-hour time period. Some investigators report that the same information can be obtained using an 8 P.M.–8 A.M. 12-hour time period while the patient is sleeping. The integration (averaging) of the GH specimen values correlate much better with clinical findings, especially in patients with partial GH deficiency (also known as "neurosecretory GH deficiency"), than does a single-specimen value. This test is being used when standard tests are equivocal or normal in spite of clinical suspicion of GH deficiency.

Somatomedin-C Assay.—Somatomedin-C assay has been proposed as a screening test for GH deficiency, pituitary insufficiency, and acromegaly. As noted previously, somatomedin serum levels depend on serum GH levels, and it has been postulated that the growth-promoting actions of GH are actually carried out by the somatomedins. Somatomedin-C is produced in the liver and circulates in serum predominantly bound to certain long-lived high molecular weight serum proteins. Normal values for females are about 10%–20% higher than those for males in both children and adults. Normal values also depend on age and developmental stage. There is a considerable increase during the pubertal adolescent growth spurt. Radioreceptor and immunoassay measurement techniques are available in large reference laboratories for somatomedin-C. Serum levels are low in most patients with isolated GH deficiency or pituitary insufficiency. The assay has some advantages in that the result does not depend on relation to food intake or time of day. Disadvantages are that only large medical centers or reference laboratories offer the assay and that various conditions besides pituitary dysfunction may produce a low result. These nonpituitary conditions include decreased caloric intake and malnutrition, malabsorption, severe chronic illness of various types, severe liver disease, hypothyroidism, and Laron dwarfism. Therefore, a clearly normal result is more diagnostic than a low result, since the low result must be confirmed by other tests. Somatomedin-C levels are elevated in acromegaly (discussed later).

Growth Hormone Stimulation Tests.—Since only a clearly normal single-specimen GH result excludes pituitary GH secretion deficiency, in patients with lower single-specimen GH values a stimulation test will be needed for detection of deficiency or confirmation of normality. The classic procedures are insulin-induced hypoglycemia and arginine infusion. Pituitary insufficiency cannot be documented on the basis of pituitary nonresponse to either test agent alone, since about 20% of normal persons may fail to respond satisfactorily to insulin alone or to arginine alone. Estrogen administration tends to increase GH secretion, and some investigators have obtained better results from arginine infusion after administration of estrogens.

Stimulation tests with other substances, including glucagon, tolbutamide, levodopa, and clonidine, have been proposed. Of these, levodopa stimulation seems to give best results; some believe that it has an accuracy equal to or better than that achieved with insulin or arginine stimulation and, in addition, is easier and safer to perform. One investigator found a greater number of unreliable results in older persons and depressed patients. Blood samples are drawn 60 and 90 minutes after oral levodopa administration. Investigators have explored various means to improve the accuracy of these tests. Sympathetic nervous system alpha-adrenergic stimulants enhance GH release while beta stimulation is inhibitory. The beta blocker propranolol, given with levodopa, enhances levodopa stimulation of GH secretion and improves identification of normal persons. For example, one investigator reported only about 5% false low GH results with the combination of levodopa and propranolol but 20% false low results with levodopa alone. Clonidine stimulation has attracted interest because it has fewer side effects and is more convenient to perform than the other tests. However, there is disagreement regarding test accuracy, partially because some investigators used lower doses that did not provide maximal effect. Overall effectiveness with higher doses is said to be similar to the other stimulation tests. The major problems with the stimulation tests are the need for more than one test to confirm a failure to stimulate GH levels and the existence of partial ("neurosecretory") GH secretion deficiency, in which GH secretion is not sufficient for normal bone growth but stimulation test results are normal. At present, the diagnosis of partial GH deficiency is made through 12-hour or 24-hour integrated GH measurements or by therapeutic trial with GH. Growth hormone–releasing hormone is now available for investigational use. Preliminary reports using GHRH as a stimulation test in GH deficiency have yielded results rather similar to those of standard stimulatory tests. Growth hormone–releasing hormone testing may be useful in differentiating hypothalamic dysfunction from pituitary GH dysfunction. However, some patients with hypothalamic dysfunction may show apparent failure to respond to initial stimulation of the pituitary by GHRH, thus simulating pituitary GH secretory dysfunction, although they respond normally after repeated stimulation.

Bone X-ray Studies.—Hand-wrist x-ray

studies for bone age (bone maturation) are strongly recommended in patients with suspected growth disorders. The actual genetic sex (which in some instances may be different from the apparent sex) must be furnished to the radiologist so that the correct reference range may be used. Bone maturation should be compared with linear growth (height) and chronologic age. Table 30–3 lists some conditions associated with retarded or accelerated bone age.

Prolactin Secretion Abnormalities

Prolactin is another peptide pituitary hormone. It stimulates lactation (galactorrhea) in females, but its function in males is less certain. The major regulatory mechanism for prolactin secretion is an inhibitory effect exerted by the hypothalamus, with one known pathway being under control of dopamine. There is also a hypothalamic stimulating effect, although a specific prolactin-stimulating hormone has not yet been isolated. Thyrotropin-releasing hormone (TRH) stimulates release of prolactin from the pituitary as well as release of TSH. Dopamine antagonists such as chlorpromazine or reserpine block the hypothalamic inhibition pathway, leading to increased prolactin secretion. Serum prolactin is measured by immunoassay. Prolactin secretion in adults has a diurnal pattern much like that of GH, with highest levels during sleep.

TABLE 30–3.

Some Conditions Associated With Generalized Retardation or Acceleration of Bone Maturation Compared to Chronologic Age (as Seen on Hand-Wrist X-ray Films

Bone age retarded
- Hypopituitarism with GH deficiency
- Constitutional growth delay
- Gonadal dysgenesis (Turner's syndrome)
- Hypothyroidism
- Cushing's syndrome
- Severe chronic disease (renal, inflammatory gastrointestinal (GI) disease, malnutrition, chronic anemia, cyanotic congenital heart disease)
- Poorly controlled severe type I diabetes mellitus

Bone age accelerated
- Excess androgens (adrenogenital syndrome; tumor; iatrogenic)
- Excess estrogens (tumor; iatrogenic)
- Albright's syndrome (polyostotic fibrous dysplasia)
- Hyperthyroidism

Prolactin Assay

Prolactin-Secreting Pituitary Tumors.— Prolactin assay has aroused interest for two reasons. First, about 65% of symptomatic pituitary adenomas (literature range, 25%–95%), including both microadenomas (<1 cm) and adenomas, produce elevated serum levels of prolactin. The pituitary cell type most often associated with hyperprolactinemia is the acidophil cell adenoma, but chromophobe adenomas (which are by far the most frequent adenoma type) are also involved. In addition, about 20%–30% of women with postpubertal (secondary) amenorrhea (literature range 15%–50%) have been found to have elevated serum prolactin levels. The incidence of pituitary tumors in such persons is 35%–45%. Many patients have been cured when pituitary adenomas were destroyed or when drug therapy directed against prolactin secretion was given. Hyperprolactinemia has also been reported to be an occasional cause of male infertility.

Some reports indicate that extension of a pituitary adenoma outside the confines of the sella turcica can be detected by assay of cerebrospinal fluid (CSF) prolactin. Prolactin in CSF rises in proportion to blood prolactin levels but is disproportionately elevated when tumor extension from the sella takes place. A CSF/plasma prolactin ratio of 0.2 or more suggests suprasellar extension of a pituitary tumor. Simultaneously obtained CSF and venous blood specimens are required.

Not all pituitary tumors secrete prolactin. Autopsy studies have demonstrated nonsymptomatic pituitary adenomas in 2.7%–27% of patients. Theoretically, nonfunctional tumors should have normal serum prolactin levels. Reports indicate, however, that some tumors that do not secrete prolactin may be associated with elevated serum prolactin levels, although the values are usually not as high as levels found with prolactin-secreting tumors.

Prolactin Assay Drawbacks.—Elevated serum prolactin levels may be associated with conditions other than pituitary tumors, idiopathic pituitary hyperprolactinemia, or hypothalamic dysfunction. Some of these conditions are listed in Table 30–4. Especially noteworthy are the empty sella syndrome, stress, and medication. The empty sella syndrome is associated with an enlarged sella turcica on x-ray film. Serum prolactin is elevated

TABLE 30–4.
Conditions Associated With Increased Serum Prolactin (% With Elevation Varies)

Sleep
Stress (including exercise, trauma, illness, etc.)
Nursing infant
Pregnancy and estrogens
Pituitary adenoma
Hypothalamic space-occupying, granulomatous, or destructive diseases
Hypothyroidism
Chronic renal failure
Hypoglycemia
Certain medications (see chapter 36)
Postpartum amenorrhea syndrome
Postpill amenorrhea-galactorrhea syndrome
Empty sella syndrome
Addison's disease (Nelson's syndrome)
Polycystic ovary (PCO) disease
Ectopic prolactin secretion (nonpituitary neoplasms)

in some of these patients, although the elevation is most often not great, and the combination of an enlarged sella plus elevated serum prolactin level could easily lead to a false diagnosis of pituitary tumor. Stress is important since many conditions place the patient under stress. In particular, the stress of venipuncture may itself induce some elevation in serum prolactin levels, so some investigators place an indwelling heparin lock venous catheter and wait as long as 2 hours with the patient resting before the sample is drawn. Estrogens and other medications may contribute to diagnostic problems. In general, very high prolactin levels are more likely to be due to pituitary adenoma than to other causes, but there is a great deal of overlap in the low- and medium-range elevations, and only a minority of pituitary adenomas display marked prolactin elevation. Statistics depend on the diagnostic cutoff level being used. The level of 100 ng/ml (100 μg/L) is most frequently quoted; the majority (45%–81%) of pituitary adenomas are above this level, but only 25%–57% of patients with prolactin levels above 100 ng/ml are reported to have a pituitary adenoma. A value of 300 ng/ml gives clear-cut separation but includes only about one third of the adenomas (literature range 12%–38%).

Prolactin Stimulation and Suppression Tests

Several stimulation and suppression tests have been used in attempts to differentiate pituitary adenoma from other causes of hyperprolactinemia. For example, several investigators have reported that pituitary adenomas display a normal response to levodopa but a blunted response to chlorpromazine. Normally there is a considerable elevation of prolactin level (at least twofold) after TRH or chlorpromazine administration and a decrease of the prolactin level after levodopa administration. In pituitary insufficiency there typically is failure to respond to TRH, chlorpromazine, or levodopa. In hypothalamic dysfunction there typically is normal response to TRH (which directly stimulates the pituitary), little, if any, response to chlorpromazine, and blunted response to levodopa. Pituitary adenomas are supposed to give a blunted response to TRH and chlorpromazine but a normal decrease with levodopa. Unfortunately, there are sufficient inconsistent results or overlap in adenoma and nonadenoma response that most investigators believe none of these tests is sufficiently reliable. There have also been some conflicting results in differentiating hypothalamic from pituitary disease. Diseases such as hypothyroidism and other factors that affect pituitary function or prolactin secretion may affect the results of these tests.

Acromegaly

Acromegaly is produced in adults by increase of GH, usually from an eosinophilic adenoma of the pituitary. About two thirds of these patients are female. Signs and symptoms include bitemporal headaches, disturbances of the visual fields, optic nerve atrophy, and physical changes in the face and hands. About 25% of patients have fasting hyperglycemia, and about 50% have decreased carbohydrate tolerance when the oral glucose tolerance test is performed. Serum prolactin is elevated in 25%–40% of patients (literature range 0%–83%). About 65%–75% of patients with acromegaly display sella turcica enlargement on skull x-ray films. Growth hormone assay usually reveals levels above the upper limit of 5 ng/ml. The standard method of confirming the diagnosis is a suppression test using glucose. Normal persons nearly always respond to a large dose of glucose with a decrease in GH levels to less than 50% of baseline, whereas acromegalic patients in theory have autonomous tumors and should show little, if any, effect of hyperglycemia. One study, however, noted relatively normal suppression in a significant percentage of acromegalics. In acromegaly (GH excess), a high somatomedin-C result is diagnostic and is found in nearly all such patients. Other causes of elevated somatomedin-C levels include the adolescent growth spurt and the last trimester of pregnancy. Some investigators believe that somatomedin-C assay is the screening test of choice for acromegaly and that a clear-cut blood level elevation of somatomedin-C might be sufficient for the diagnosis. The major problem is the surge during adolescence.

TESTS OF GONADAL FUNCTION

The most common conditions in which gonadal function tests are used are hypogonadism in males and menstrual disorders, fertility problems, and hirsutism or virilization in females. The hormones currently available for assistance include LH, FSH, testosterone, and human chorionic gonadotropin (hCG).

Luteinizing Hormone and Follicle-Stimulating Hormone

Originally FSH and LH were measured together using bioassay methods, and so-called FSH measurements included LH. Radioimmunoassay techniques are able to separate the two hormones. The LH cross-reacts with hCG in some RIA systems. Although this ordinarily does not create a problem, there is difficulty in pregnancy and in patients with certain neoplasms that secrete hCG. Several of the pituitary and placental glycopeptides (TSH, FSH, hCG, LH) are composed of at least two immunologic units, alpha and beta. All have the same immunologic response to the alpha fraction but a different response to the beta subunit. Antisera against the beta subunit of hCG eliminate interference by LH, and some investigators have reported success in producing antisera against the beta subunit of LH which does not detect hCG. There is some cross reaction between FSH and TSH, but as yet this has not seemed important enough clinically in TSH assay to necessitate substitution of TSH beta subunit antiserum for antisera already available. Assay of FSH in serum is thought to be more reliable than in urine due to characteristics of the antibody preparations available.

Serum Luteinizing Hormone

Luteinizing hormone is secreted intermittently in pulses occurring at a rate of about two–four every 6 hours, ranging from 30% to nearly 300% over lowest values. Therefore, single isolated LH blood levels may be difficult to interpret and could be misleading. It has been suggested that multiple samples be obtained (e.g., four specimens, each specimen collected at a 20-minute interval from another). The serum specimens can be pooled to obtain an average value. Follicle-stimulating hormone and testosterone have a relatively constant blood level in females.

Urine Luteinizing Hormone

In contrast to serum LH, urine LH is more difficult to obtain, since it requires a 24-hour specimen with the usual problem of complete specimen collection. It also has the disadvantage of artifact due to urine concentration or dilution. The major advantage is averaging of 24-hour secretion, which may avoid misleading results associated with serum assays due to LH pulsatile secretion. Another role for urine LH assay is detection of ovulation during infertility workups. Luteinizing hormone is rapidly excreted from plasma into urine, so that a serum LH surge of sufficient magnitude is mirrored in single urine samples. An LH surge precedes ovulation by about 24–36 hours (range, 22–44 hours). Single daily urine specimens are obtained beginning 9–10 days after onset of menstruation (so as not to miss the LH surge preceding ovulation if ovulation should occur earlier than the middle of the patient cycle). It has been reported that the best time to obtain the urine specimen is during midday (11 A.M.–3 P.M.) because the LH surge in serum usually takes place in the morning (5 A.M.–9A.M.). In one study, the LH surge was detected in 56% of morning urine specimens, 94% of midday specimens, and 88% of evening specimens. In contrast, basal body temperature, another method of predicting time of ovulation, is said to be accurate in only 40%–50% of cases. Several manufacturers have marketed simple immunologic tests for urine LH with a color change endpoint that can be used by many patients to test their own specimens. Possible problems include interference by hCG with some of the LH kits, so that early pregnancy could simulate a LH surge. Since the LH surge usually does not last more than 2 days, positive test results for more than 3 consecutive days suggest some interfering factor. Similar interference may appear in some patients with elevated serum LH levels due to ovarian failure (PCO disease, early menopause, etc.).

Finally, an estimated 10% of patients have more than one urine LH spike, although the LH surge has the greatest magnitude. It may be necessary to obtain serum progesterone or urine pregnanediol glucuronide assays to confirm that elevation of LH values is actually the preovulation LH surge.

Urine Pregnanediol

The ovarian corpus luteum formed shortly after ovulation secretes increasing amounts of progesterone. Progesterone or its metabolite pregnanediol glucuronide begin to appear in detectable quantities about 2–3 days after ovulation (3–5 days after the LH surge) and persists until about the middle of the luteal phase that ends in menstruation. Conception is followed by progesterone secretion by the placenta. A negative baseline urine pregnandiol assay before the LH surge followed by a positive pregnanediol test result on at least 1 day of early morning urine specimens obtained 7, 8, and 9 days after the LH surge confirm that the LH surge did occur and was followed by ovulation and corpus luteum formation. Urine specimens are collected in the morning rather than at the LH collection time of midday. At least one manufacturer markets a simple easy kit for urine pregnanediol assay.

Problems with interpretation of a positive urine pregnanediol glucuronide assay include the possibility that early pregnancy may be present. Also, 5%–10% of patients throughout their menstrual cycle non-ovulatory phase have slightly or mildly increased pregnanediol levels compared to the reference range. A urine sample collected before the LH surge can be tested to exclude or demonstrate this phenomenon.

Serum Androgens

The most important androgens are dehydroepiandrosterone (DHEA), a metabolite of DHEA called DHEA-sulfate (DHEA-S), androstenedione, and testosterone. Dehydroepiandrosterone is produced in the adrenal cortex, ovary, and testis (in the adrenal cortex, the precursors of DHEA are also precursors of cortisol and aldosterone, which is not the case in the ovary or testis). DHEA is the precursor of androstenedione, and androstenedione is a precursor both of testosterone and of estrogens (see Fig 29–2). About 50%–60% of testosterone in normal females is derived from androstenedione conversion in peripheral tissues, about 30% is produced directly by the adrenal, and about 20% is produced by the ovary. Dehydroepiandrosterone blood levels in females are 3 times androstenedione blood levels and about 10 times testosterone blood levels. In normal males after onset of puberty, testosterone blood levels are twice as high as all androgens combined in females. Androstenedione blood levels in males are about 60% of those in females and about 10%–15% of testosterone blood levels.

Serum Testosterone

About 60%–75% of circulating serum testosterone is bound to a beta globulin variously known as sex hormone–binding globulin (SHBG) or as testosterone-binding globulin (TBG, a misleading abbreviation because of its similarity to the more widely used abbreviation representing thyroxine-binding globulin). About 20%–40% of testosterone is bound to serum albumin and 1%–2% is unbound ("free"). The unbound fraction is the only biologically active portion. Serum assays for testosterone measure total testosterone (bound plus unbound) values. Special techniques to assay free testosterone are available in some reference laboratories and in larger medical centers. Circulating androstenedione and DHEA are bound to albumin only.

Several conditions can affect total serum testosterone levels by altering the quantity of SHBG without affecting free testosterone. Factors that elevate SHBG levels include estrogens (estrogen-producing tumor, oral contraceptives, or medication), cirrhosis, hyperthyroidism, and (in males) decreased testis function or testicular feminization syndrome. Conditions that decrease SHBG levels include androgens and hypothyroidism.

There is a relatively small diurnal variation of serum testosterone in men, with early morning levels about 20% higher than evening levels. There is little diurnal change in women. Serum levels of androstenedione in men or women are about 50% higher in the early morning than in the evening.

In males, testosterone production is regulated by a feedback mechanism with the hypothalamus and pituitary. The hypothalamus produces gonadotropin-releasing hormone (GTRH), also called LHRH, which induces the pituitary to secrete LH (and FSH). Luteinizing hormone, in turn, stimulates the Leydig cells of the testis to secrete testosterone.

Serum Estrogens

There are three major estrogens: estrone (E_1), estradiol (estradiol-17β; E_2), and estriol (E_3). All of the estrogens are ultimately derived from androgenic precursors (DHEA and androstenedione), which are synthesized by the adrenal cortex, ovaries, or testis. The adrenal is unable to convert androgens to estrogens, so estrogens are directly produced in the ovary or testis (from precursors synthesized directly in those organs) or are produced in nonendocrine peripheral tissues such as the liver, adipose tissue, or skin by conversion of androgenic precursors brought by the bloodstream from one of the organs of androgen synthesis. Peripheral tissue estrogens are derived mainly from adrenal androgens. Estradiol is the predominant ovarian estrogen. The ovary also secretes a much smaller amount of estrone. The primary pathway of estradiol synthesis is from androstenedione to estrone and then from estrone to estradiol by a reversible reaction. This takes place in the ovary and to a much lesser extent in peripheral tissues. A subsidiary pathway is peripheral conversion of testosterone to estradiol. Estrone is produced directly from androstenedione (mostly in peripheral tissues) and to a lesser extent in the ovary from already formed estradiol by the reversible reaction. Estriol in nonpregnant women is formed as a metabolite of estradiol or estrone. In pregnancy, estriol is synthesized by the placenta from DHEA (actually from DHEA-S) derived from the fetal adrenals. This is a different pathway from the one in nonpregnant women. Estriol is the major estrogen of the placenta. The placenta also produces some estradiol, derived from both fetal and maternal precursors. Nonendocrine peripheral tissues (liver, skin, fat) synthesize a small amount of estrone and estradiol in pregnancy, mainly from adrenal precursors.

In females, there is a feedback mechanism for estradiol production involving the ovaries, hypothalamus, and pituitary. As already mentioned, the hypothalamus produces GTRH. The GTRH is secreted in a pulsatile manner about every 70–90 minutes and is excreted by glomerular filtration. The GTRH stimulates FSH and LH secretion by the pituitary. Some investigators believe there may be a separate (undiscovered) factor that regulates FSH secretion. The FSH acts on the ovarian follicles to stimulate follicle growth and development of receptors to the action of LH. The LH stimulates the follicles to produce estradiol.

Estradiol values can be measured in serum, and estriol values can be measured in serum or urine by immunoassay. Total estrogen values are measured in urine by a relatively old but still useful procedure based on the Kober biochemical reaction. All of the estrogens can be assayed by gas chromatography. The DHEA and androstenedione values can also be measured by special techniques, but these are available only in large reference laboratories.

Male Infertility or Hypogonadism

About 40%–50% of infertility problems are said to be due to dysfunction of the male reproductive system. Male infertility can be due to hormonal etiology (either lack of gonadotropin or suppression of spermatogenesis), nonhormonal factors affecting spermatogenesis, primary testicular disease, obstruction to sperm passages, disorders of sperm motility or viability, or presence of antisperm antibodies (Table 30–5). About 30%–40% is reported to be associated with varicocele. Diagnosis and investigation of etiology usually begins with physical examination (with special attention to the normality of the genitalia and the presence of a varicocele), semen analysis (ejaculate quantity, number of sperm, sperm morphology, and sperm motility), and serum hormone assay (testosterone, LH, and FSH).

Testicular Function Tests.—Male testicular function is based on formation of sperm by testicular seminiferous tubules under the influence of testosterone. Follicle-stimulating hormone is necessary for testicular function because it stimulates seminiferous tubule (Sertoli cell) development. Testosterone secretion by the Leydig cells (interstitial cells) of the testis is necessary for spermatogenesis in seminiferous tubules capable of producing sperm. Luteinizing hormone (in males sometimes called "interstitial cell–stimulating hormone") stimulates the Leydig cells to produce testosterone. Testosterone is controlled by a feedback mechanism whereby testosterone levels regulate hypothalamic secretion of GTRH, which, in turn, regulates pituitary secretion of LH. The adrenals also produce androgens, but normally this is not a significant factor in males. In classic cases, serum levels of testosterone and gonadotropins (LH and FSH) can differentiate between primary testicular abnormality (failure of the testis to respond to pituitary gonadotropin stimulation, either congenital or acquired) and pituitary or hypothalamic dysfunction (either congenital or acquired). In primary gonadal (testis) insufficiency, pituitary gonadotropin levels are usually elevated. Of the various categories of primary gonadal insufficiency, Klinefelter's syndrome in its classic form shows normal FSH and LH gonadotropin levels during childhood, but after puberty both FSH and LH levels are elevated and the serum testosterone level is low. Klinefelter's syndrome exists in several variants, however, and in some cases LH levels may be within reference range (single LH samples also may be confusing because of the pulsatile nature of LH secretion). Occasional patients with Klinefelter's syndrome may have low-normal total serum testosterone levels (due to an increase in SHBG levels) but decreased free testosterone levels. Elevated pituitary gonadotropin levels should be further investigated by a buccal smear for sex chromatin to evaluate the possibility of Klinefelter's syndrome. Some investigators also perform a chromosome analysis because of possible inaccuracies in buccal smear interpretation and because some persons with Klinefelter's syndrome have cell mosaicism rather than the same chromosome pattern in all cells, or a person with findings suggestive of Klinefelter's syndrome may have a different abnormal chromosome karyotype. In the "Sertoli cell only syndrome," testicular tubules are abnormal but Leydig cells are normal. Therefore, the serum FSH level is elevated but LH and testosterone levels are usually normal. In acquired gonadal failure (due to destruction of the testicular tubules by infection, radiation, or other agents), the FSH level is often (but not always) elevated, whereas LH and testosterone levels are often normal (unless the degree of testis destruction is sufficient to destroy most of the Leydig cells, a very severe change). In secondary (pituitary or hypothalamic) deficiency, both the pituitary gonadotropin (FSH and LH) and the testosterone levels are low.

Although serum testosterone is normally an indicator of testicular Leydig cell function and, indirectly, of pituitary LH secretion, other factors can influence serum testosterone levels. The adrenal provides much of the precursor steroids for testosterone, and some types of congenital adrenal hyperplasia result in de-

TABLE 30–5.

Some Important Causes of Male Infertility, Classified According to Primary Site of the Defect

Hormonal
- Insufficient hypothalamic gonadotropin (hypogonadotropic eunuchoidism)
- Insufficient pituitary gonadotropins (isolated LH deficiency ["fertile eunuch"] or pituitary insufficiency)
- Prolactin-secreting pituitary adenoma
- Excess estrogens (cirrhosis, estrogen therapy, estrogen-producing tumor)
- Excess androgens
- Excess glucocorticosteroids
- Hypothyroidism

Nonhormonal factors affecting testis sperm production
- Varicocele
- Poor nutrition
- Diabetes mellitus
- Excess heat in area of testes
- Stress and emotion
- Drugs and chemicals
- Febrile illnesses
- Cryptochism (undescended testis, unilateral or bilateral)
- Spinal cord injuries

Primary testicular abnormality
- Maturation arrest at germ cell stage
- "Sertoli cell only" syndrome
- Klinefelter's syndrome and other congenital sex chromosome disorders
- Testicular damage (radiation, mumps orchitis, inflammation, trauma)
- Myotonic dystrophy

Posttesticular abnormality
- Obstruction of sperm passages
- Impaired sperm motility
- Antisperm antibodies

creased levels of testosterone precursors. Cirrhosis may decrease serum testosterone levels. Increase or decrease of testosterone-binding protein levels may falsely increase or decrease serum testosterone levels, since the total serum testosterone value is being measured, whereas assay of free (unbound) testosterone is not affected.

Stimulation Tests.—Stimulation tests are available to help determine which organ is malfunctioning in equivocal cases. The testis is directly stimulated by hCG, increasing testosterone secretion to at least twice baseline values. Clomiphene stimulates the hypothalamus, producing increases in both LH and testosterone levels. The medication is given for 10 days. However, clomiphene will not stimulate LH production significantly in prepubertal children. Serum testosterone and LH values must be close to normal pubertal or adult levels before the test can be performed, and the test can be used only when there is a mild degree of abnormality in the gonadal-pituitary system. Gonadotropin-releasing hormone is now available. This compound stimulates pituitary secretion of FSH and LH. Normal pituitary response is considered more significant than poor response, since deficiency of hypothalamic GTRH production may cause the pituitary to temporarily display a reduced response to exogenous (test) GTRH. In patients with hypothalamic deficiency, a normal pituitary response can be obtained after several days' pretreatment with GTRH. It has been reported that a normal pituitary response is not always a guarantee of pituitary normalcy, since pituitary tumors causing hypogonadism may exist with normal LH response to GTRH administration.

Semen Analysis.—Semen analysis is an essential part of male infertility investigation. Semen findings that are highly correlated with hypofertility or infertility include greatly increased or decreased ejaculate volume, very low sperm counts, greatly decreased sperm motility, and more than 20% of the sperm showing abnormal morphology (see Table 36–28). One particular combination of findings is known as the "stress pattern" and consists of low sperm count, decreased sperm motility, and more than 20% of the sperm being abnormal in appearance (especially with an increased number of tapering head forms instead of the normal oval head). The stress pattern is suggestive of varicocele but can be due to acute febrile illness (with effects lasting up to 60 days), some endocrine abnormalities, and antisperm agents. An abnormal semen analysis should be repeated at least once after 3 weeks and possibly even a third time, due to the large variation within the population and variation of sperm production even within the same person as well as the temporary effects of acute illness. Most investigators recommend that the specimen be obtained 2–3 days after regular intercourse to avoid artifacts that may be produced by prolonged sperm storage. The specimen should be received by the laboratory by 1 hour after it is obtained, during which time it should be kept at room temperature.

Testicular Biopsy.—Testicular biopsy may be useful in a minority of selected patients in whom no endocrinologic or other cause is found to explain infertility. Most investigators agree that complete lack of sperm in semen analysis is a major indication for biopsy but disagree on whether biopsy should be done if sperm are present in small numbers. Biopsy helps to differentiate lack of sperm production from sperm passage obstruction and can suggest certain possible etiologies of testicular dysfunction or possible areas to investigate. However, none of the histopathologic findings is specific for any one disease. The report usually indicates if spermatogenesis is seen and, if so, whether it is adequate, whether there are normal numbers of germ cells, and whether active inflammation or extensive scarring is present.

Serum Antisperm Antibody Studies.—In patients with no evidence of endocrine, semen, or other abnormality, serum antisperm antibody titers can be measured. These studies are difficult to perform and usually must be done at a center that specializes in reproductive studies or therapy. Serum antisperm antibodies are a common finding after vasectomy, being reported in about 50% of cases (literature range, 30%–70%). The incidence and significance of serum antisperm antibodies in couples with infertility problems are somewhat controversial. There is wide variance of reported incidence (3.3%–79%), probably due to different patient groups tested and different testing methods. In men, one report suggests that serum antibody titer is more significant than the mere detection of antibody. High titers of antisperm antibody in men were considered strong evidence against fertility; low titers were of uncertain significance, and mildly elevated titers indicated a poor but not hopeless prognosis. In women, serum antisperm antibodies are said to be present in 7%–17% of infertility cases but their significance is rather uncertain, since a considerable percentage of these women can become pregnant. Antisperm antibody detected in the cervical mucus of women is thought to be much more important than that detected in serum.

Precocious Puberty

Precocious puberty can be isosexual (secondary sex characteristics of the same sex) or heterosexual (masculinization in girls and feminization in boys). The syndromes have been further subdivided into those that produce true puberty with functioning gonads and those that produce pseudopuberty, in which development of secondary sex characteristics suggests puberty but the gonads do not function. The major causes of precocious puberty are idiopathic early puberty or the hypersecretion of androgens or estrogens from hypothalamic, pituitary, adrenal, gonadal, or factitious (self-medication) sources.

Hypothalamic precocious puberty is usually associated with a tumor (e.g., a pinealoma) involving the hypothalamus; or with encephalitis. The result is always an isosexual true puberty.

Pituitary precocious puberty is usually idiopathic ("constitutional"). The result is normal isosexual puberty. In girls the condition rarely may be due to Albright's syndrome (polyostotic fibrous dysplasia). Primary pituitary tumors do not cause precocious puberty.

Gonadal precocious puberty in boys results from a Leydig cell tumor of the testis that produces testosterone. This is a pseudopuberty, since FSH is not produced and no spermatogenesis occurs. In girls, various ovarian tumors may cause pseudopuberty, which may be either isosexual or heterosexual, depending on whether the tumor secretes estrogens or androgens. Granulosa-theca cell tumors are the most frequent, although their peak incidence is not until middle age. These tumors most frequently produce estrogens. Dysgerminoma and malignant teratoma are two uncommon ovarian tumors that may produce hCG rather than the usual type of estrogens.

Adrenal precocious puberty is due to either congenital adrenal hyperplasia or adrenal tumor. In early childhood, congenital adrenal hyperplasia is more likely; if onset is in late childhood or prepubertal age, tumor is more likely. In both cases a pseudopuberty results, usually isosexual in boys and heterosexual (virilization) in girls. Congenital adrenal hyperplasia may also produce pseudohermaphroditism (simulation of male genitalia) in infant girls.

Hypothyroidism has been reported to cause rare cases of true isosexual precocious puberty in both boys and girls.

Laboratory Evaluation

Laboratory evaluation depends on whether the physical examination indicates isosexual or heterosexual changes. In girls, heterosexual changes point toward congenital adrenal hyperplasia, ovarian tumor, or adrenal carcinoma. The most important test for diagnosis of congenital adrenal hyperplasia is plasma 17-hydroxyprogesterone (17-OH-P) assay (chapter 29). A 24-hour urine specimen for 17-ketosteroid (17-KS) is also very helpful, since the 17-KS values are usually elevated in adrenal carcinoma, frequently elevated in congenital adrenal hyperplasia, and sometimes elevated in ovarian carcinoma. If test results for congenital adrenal hyperplasia are negative, normal urine 17-KS levels point toward ovarian tumor. Ultrasound examination of the ovaries and adrenals and an overnight dexamethasone screening test for adrenal tumor are helpful. Computerized tomography (CT) of the adrenals is also possible, but some believe that CT is less successful in childhood than in adults. Isosexual changes suggest hypothalamic area tumor, constitutional precocious puberty, ovarian estrogen-secreting tumor, or hypothyroidism. Useful tests include serum thyroxine assay, ultrasound examination of the ovaries, and CT scan of the hypothalamus area. The possibility of exposure to estrogen-containing creams or other substances should also be investigated. Serum hCG levels may be elevated in the rare ovarian choriocarcinomas.

Female isosexual precocious puberty must be distinguished from isolated premature development of breasts (thelarche) or pubic hair (adrenarche). Female heterosexual precocious puberty must be distinguished from hirsutism, although this is a more common problem during and after puberty.

In boys, heterosexual precocious pseudopuberty suggests estrogen-producing tumor (testis choriocarcinoma or liver hepatoblastoma) or the pseudohermaphrodite forms of congenital adrenal hyperplasia. Tests for congenital adrenal hyperplasia plus serum hCG are necessary. Isosexual precocious puberty could be due to a hypothalamic area tumor, constitutional (idiopathic) cause, testis tumor (Leydig cell type), hypothyroidism, or congenital adrenal hyperplasia. Necessary tests include those for congenital adrenal hyperplasia and a serum thyroxine determination. If the results are negative, serum testosterone (to detect values elevated above normal puberty levels) and hypothalamic area CT scan are useful. Careful examination of the testes for tumor is necessary in all cases of male precocious puberty.

Female Delayed Puberty and Primary Amenorrhea

Onset of normal puberty in girls is somewhat variable, with disagreement in the literature concerning at what age to diagnose precocious puberty and at what age to suspect delayed puberty. The most generally agreed-on range of onset for female puberty is between 9 and 16 years. Signs of puberty include breast development, growth of pubic and axillary hair, and estrogen effect as seen in vaginal smears using the Papanicolaou stain. Menstruation also begins; if it does not, the possibility of primary amenorrhea arises. Primary amenorrhea may or may not be accompanied by evidence that suggests onset of puberty, depending on the etiology of the amenorrhea. Some of the causes of primary amenorrhea are listed in Table 30–6.

Physical examination is very important to detect inguinal hernia or masses that might suggest the testicular feminization type of male pseudohermaphroditism, to document the appearance of the genitalia, to see the pattern of secondary sex characteristics, and to note what evidence of puberty exists and to what extent. Pelvic examination is needed to ascertain if there are anatomical defects preventing menstruation, such as a nonpatent vagina, and to detect ovarian masses.

TABLE 30–6.

Some Etiologies of Female Delayed Puberty and Primary Amenorrhea

Müllerian dysgenesis (Mayer-Rokitansky syndrome): congenital absence of portions of the female genital tract, with absent or hypoplastic vagina. Ovarian function is usually normal. Female genotype and phenotype.

Male pseudohermaphroditism: genetic male (XY karyotype) with female appearance due to deficiency of testosterone effect.

1. Testicular feminization syndrome: lack of testosterone effect due to defect in tissue testosterone receptors.
2. Congenital adrenal hyperplasia: defect in testosterone production pathway.
3. Male gonadal dysgenesis syndromes: defect in testis function.
   a. Swyer syndrome (male pure gonadal dysgenesis): female organs present except for ovaries. Bilateral undifferentiated streak gonads. Presumably testes never functioned and did not prevent müllerian duct development.
   b. Vanishing testes syndrome (XY gonadal agenesis): phenotype varies from male pseudohermaphrodite to ambiguous genitalia. No testes present. Presumably testes functioned in very early embryologic life, sufficient to prevent müllerian duct development, and then disappeared.
   c. Congenital anorchia: male phenotype, but no testes. Presumably, testes functioned until male differentiation took place, then disappeared.

Female sex chromosome abnormalities (Turner's syndrome—female gonadal dysgenesis—and Turner variants): XO karyotype in 75%–80% of patients, mosaic in others. Female phenotype. Short stature in most, web neck in 40%. Bilateral streak gonads.

Polycystic (Stein-Leventhal) or nonpolycystic ovaries, not responsive to gonadotropins.

Deficient gonadotropins due to hypothalamic or pituitary dysfunction.

Hyperprolactinemia: pituitary overproduction of prolactin alone.

Effects of severe chronic systemic disease: chronic renal disease, severe chronic GI disease, anorexia nervosa, etc.

Constitutional (idiopathic) delayed puberty: puberty eventually takes place, so this is a retrospective diagnosis.

Other: Cushing's syndrome, hypothyroidism, and isolated GH deficiency can result in delayed puberty.

Laboratory Tests

Basic laboratory tests begin with chromosome analysis, since a substantial minority of cases have a genetic component. Male genetic sex indicates male pseudohermaphroditism and leads to tests that differentiate the various etiologies. Turner's syndrome and other sex chromosome disorders are also excluded or confirmed. If there is a normal female karyotype and no chromosome abnormalities are found, there is some divergence of opinion on how to evaluate the other important organs of puberty—the ovaries, pituitary, and hypothalamus. Some prefer to perform serum hormone assays as a group, including pituitary gonadotropins (FSH and LH), estrogen (estradiol), testosterone, prolactin, and thyroxine. Others perform these assays in a step-by-step fashion or algorithm, depending on the result of each test, which could be less expensive but could take much more time. Others begin with tests of organ function. In the algorithm approach, the first step is usually to determine if estrogen is present in adequate amount. Vaginal smears, serum estradiol level, endometrial stimulation with progesterone (for withdrawal bleeding), and possibly endometrial biopsy (for active proliferative or secretory endometrium, although biopsy is considered more often in secondary than in primary amenorrhea); all are methods to detect ovarian estrogen production. If estrogen is present in adequate amount, this could mean intact hypothalamic-pituitary-ovarian feedback or could raise the question of excess androgen (congenital adrenal hyperplasia, Cushing's syndrome, PCO disease, androgen-producing tumor) or excess estrogens (obesity, estrogen-producing tumor, iatrogenic, self-medication). If estrogen effect is absent or very low, some gynecologists then test the uterus with estrogen, followed by progesterone, to see if the uterus is capable of function. If no withdrawal bleeding occurs, this suggests testicular feminization, congenital absence or abnormality of the uterus, or the syndrome of intrauterine adhesions (Asherman's syndrome). If uterine withdrawal bleeding takes place, the uterus can function, and when this finding is coupled with evidence of low estrogen levels, the tentative diagnosis is ovarian failure.

The next step is to differentiate primary ovarian failure from secondary failure caused by pituitary or hypothalamic disease. Hypothalamic dysfunction may be due to space-occupying lesions (tumor or granulomatous disease), infection, or (through uncertain mechanism) effects of severe systemic illness, severe malnutrition, and severe psychogenic disorder. X-ray films of the pituitary are often ordered to detect enlargement of the sella turcica from pituitary tumor or suprasellar calcifications due to craniopharyngioma. Polytomography is more sensitive for sellar abnormality than ordinary plain films. Computerized tomography also has its advocates. Serum prolactin, thyroxine, FSH, and LH assays are done. It is necessary to wait 4–6 weeks after a progesterone or estrogen-progesterone test before the hormone assays are obtained to allow patient hormone secretion patterns to resume their pretest status. An elevated serum prolactin value raises the question of pituitary tumor (especially if the sella is enlarged) or idiopathic isolated hyperprolactinemia. However, patients with the empty sella syndrome and some patients with hypothyroidism may present with an enlarged sella and elevated serum prolactin levels, and the other causes of elevated prolactin levels (see Table 30–4) must be considered. A decreased serum FSH or LH level confirms pituitary insufficiency or hypothalamic dysfunction. A pituitary stimulation test can be performed. If the pituitary can produce adequate amounts of LH, this suggests hypothalamic disease (either destructive lesion, effect of severe systemic illness, or malnutrition). However, failure of the pituitary to respond does not necessarily indicate primary pituitary disease, since severe long-term hypothalamic deficiency may result in temporary pituitary nonresponsiveness to a single episode of test stimulation. Hormone therapy within the preceding 4–6 weeks can also adversely affect test results.

Table 30–7 lists some conditions associated with primary amenorrhea or delayed puberty and the differential diagnosis associated with various patterns of pituitary gonadotropin values. However, several cautionary statements must be made about these patterns. Clearly elevated FSH or LH values are much more significant than normal or mildly to moderately decreased levels. Current gonadotropin immunoassays are technically more reproducible and dependable at the upper end of usual values than at the lower end. Thus, two determinations on the same specimen could produce both a mildly decreased value and a value

TABLE 30–7.

Gonadotropin Levels in Certain Conditions Associated With Primary Amenorrhea or Delayed Puberty

*FSH and LH decreased**
- Hypopituitarism
- Hypothalamic dysfunction
- Constitutional delayed puberty
- Some cases of primary hypothyroidism
- Some cases of Cushing's syndrome
- Some cases of severe chronic illness

FSH and LH increased†
- Some cases of congenital adrenal hyperplasia
- Female gonadal dysgenesis
- Male gonadal dysgenesis
- Ovarian failure due to nonovarian agents

LH increased, FSH not increased‡
- Testicular feminization
- Some cases of PCO disease

*Decreased in a variable proportion of patients with these conditions.
†Must use age-related reference ranges.
‡FSH levels normal or minimally increased.

within the lower half of the reference range. In addition, blood levels of gonadotropins, especially LH, frequently vary throughout the day. The values must be compared with age- and sex-matched reference ranges. In girls, the levels also are influenced by the menstrual cycle, if menarche has begun. Second, the conditions listed—even the genetic ones, although to a lesser extent—are not homogeneous in regard to severity, clinical manifestations, or laboratory findings. Instead, each represents a spectrum of patients. The more classic and severe the clinical manifestations, the more likely that the patient will have "expected" laboratory findings, but even this rule is not invariable. Therefore, some patients having a condition typically associated with an abnormal laboratory test result may not show the expected abnormality. Laboratory error is another consideration. Also, the spectrum of patients represented by each condition makes it difficult to evaluate reports of laboratory findings due to differences in patient population, severity of illness, differences in applying diagnostic criteria to the patients, variance in specimen collection protocols, and technical differences in the assays used in different laboratories. In many cases, adequate data concerning frequency that some laboratory tests are abnormal are not available.

Elevated FSH and LH levels or an elevated LH level alone suggests primary ovarian failure, whether from congenital absence of the ovaries or congenital inability to respond to gonadotropins, acquired abnormality such as damage to the ovaries after birth, or PCO disease.

An elevated estrogen or androgen level raises the question of hormone-secreting tumor, for which the ovary is the most common (but not the only) location. Nontumor androgen production may occur in PCO disease and Cushing's syndrome (especially adrenal carcinoma).

As noted previously, there is no universally accepted single standard method to investigate female reproductive disorders. Tests or test sequences vary among medical centers and also according to findings in the individual patients.

When specimens for pituitary hormone as-

TABLE 30–8.

Some Etiologies of Secondary Amenorrhea Classified According to Ovarian Function

I. Pregnancy
II. Decreased ovarian hormone production
   A. Primary ovarian failure
      1. Normal menopause
      2. Some cases of gonadal dysgenesis (Turner's syndrome)
      3. Acquired ovarian failure (idiopathic, postradiation, postchemotherapy, postmumps infection)
      4. PCO disease
   B. Secondary ovarian failure
      1. High pituitary prolactin value (with or without galactorrhea)
      2. Hypothalamic failure to secrete adequate GTRH levels (tumor, trauma, infection, nonintracranial illness)
      3. Pituitary failure (primary pituitary tumor, Sheehan's syndrome, empty sella syndrome)
      4. Anorexia nervosa or severe malnutrition
      5. Rigorous athletic training
      6. Psychogenic amenorrhea
      7. Severe acute or chronic illness
      8. Increased nonovarian estrogen levels (tumor, obesity, therapy)
      9. Hypothyroidism or hyperthyroidism
      10. Cushing's disease or Addison's disease
      11. Poorly controlled diabetes
III. Increased ovarian estrogen or androgen production
   A. Androgen-secreting ovarian tumor
   B. Estrogen-secreting ovarian tumor
IV. Normal ovarian hormone production
   A. Local uterine pathology

says are collected, the potential problems noted earlier in the chapter should be considered.

Secondary Amenorrhea

Secondary amenorrhea implies ending of menstruation after menstruation has already begun. A list of etiologies of secondary amenorrhea is presented in Table 30–8, grouped according to evidence of ovarian function (from tests discussed in the section on primary amenorrhea). If menstruation definitely takes place, especially if it continues for several months or years, this eliminates some of the etiologies of primary amenorrhea such as müllerian dysgenesis and most types of male pseudohermaphroditism. Otherwise, the list of possible causes and the workup are similar to that for primary amenorrhea. Even chromosome studies are still useful, in this case, to rule out Turner's syndrome or its variants. Certain conditions are much more important or frequent in secondary, as opposed to primary, amenorrhea; these include hyperprolactinemia (with or without galactorrhea), early menopause, psychogenic cause, anorexia nervosa, severe chronic illness, and hypothyroidism. Normal pregnancy should also be excluded.

Hyperprolactinemia is found in 20%–30% of patients with secondary amenorrhea. There may or may not be galactorrhea. The condition may be idiopathic, may be due to pituitary tumor, or sometimes develops when a person taking oral contraceptives stops the medication or in the postpartum period.

Some cases of periodic amenorrhea or varying time periods without menstruation are due to anovulation. Anovulation is said to cause up to 40% of all female infertility. Some of these patients have enough estrogen production to permit the endometrium to reach the secretory phase, so these women will respond to a dose of progesterone ("progesterone challenge") by menstruating. These women frequently will ovulate if treated with clomiphene, which has an antiestrogen action on the hypothalamus. Other patients will not respond to progesterone challenge and usually do not respond to clomiphene. Some of these women have hypothalamic function deficiency, pituitary failure, exercise-induced (e.g. rigorous athletic training) or stress-related amenorrhea, anorexia nervosa, or ovarian failure.

TABLE 30–9.
Some Conditions That Produce Hirsutism

Ovary
PCO disease
(Hyperthecosis)
Ovarian tumor
Adrenal
Congenital adrenal hyperplasia (CAH)
Cushing's syndrome (nontumor)
Adrenal tumor
Testis
Leydig cell tumor
Other
Idiopathic hirsutism
Hyperprolactinemia
Starvation
Acromegaly (rare)
Hypothyroidism (rare)
Porphyria (rare)
Medications
Phenytoin (Dilantin)
Diazoxide (Hyperstat)
Minoxidil (Loniten)
Androgenic steroids
Glucocorticosteroids
Streptomycin

Female Hirsutism

Female hirsutism is a relatively common problem in which the overriding concern of the physician is to rule out an ovarian or adrenal tumor. The type and distribution of hair can be used to differentiate physiologic hair growth from nonphysiologic growth (hirsutism). In females there are two types of hair: fine, thin, nonpigmented vellus hair and coarse, curly, pigmented terminal hair. Pubic and axillary terminal hair growth is induced by androgens in the physiologic range. Growth of such hair on the face (especially the chin), sternum area, and sacrum suggests male distribution and therefore excess androgens. Virilization goes one step further and is associated with definite hirsutism, acne, deepening of the voice, and hypertrophy of the clitoris.

The major etiologies of hirsutism are listed in Table 30–9. Hirsutism with or without other evidence of virilization may occur before or after puberty. When onset is prepubertal, the etiology is more often congenital adrenal hyperplasia or tumor. After puberty, PCO disease, Cushing's syndrome, late-onset congenital adrenal hyperplasia, and idiopathic causes are more frequent. Findings suspicious for tumor are relatively sudden onset; progressive hirsutism, especially if rapidly progressive; and signs of virilization.

Laboratory Tests

There is considerable disagreement among endocrinologists regarding which tests are most useful in hirsutism. The tests that most frequently appear in the literature are urine 17-KS, serum testosterone (total or free testosterone), DHEA-S, serum androstenedione, serum dihydrotestosterone, urine 3-α-androstanediol glucuronide, serum LH and FSH, serum prolactin, serum 17-OH-P, urine free cortisol, an ACTH stimulation ("Cortrosyn") test, and the low-dose overnight dexamethasone suppression test. Each of these tests is used either to screen for one or more etiologies of hirsutism or to differentiate between several possible sources of abnormality. There is considerable disagreement concerning which tests to use for initial screening purposes, with some endocrinologists ordering only two or three tests and others using a panel of five–seven tests. Therefore, it may be worth while to briefly discuss what information each test can provide.

Urine 17-KS was one of the first tests used for hirsutism or virilization. Elevated urine 17-KS levels suggest abnormality centered in the adrenal, usually CAH or adrenal tumor. Ovarian tumors, PCO disease, or Cushing's syndrome due to pituitary adenoma usually do not produce elevated urine 17-KS levels (although some exceptions occur). However, some cases of CAH fail to demonstrate elevated 17-KS levels (more often in the early pediatric age group and in late-onset CAH). Serum 17-OH-P in neonatal or early childhood CAH and 17-OH-P after ACTH stimulation in late-onset CAH are considered more reliable diagnostic tests. Also, a significant minority (16% in one series) of patients with adrenal carcinoma and about 50% of patients with adrenal adenomas fail to show elevated 17-KS levels. In addition, 17-KS values from adrenal adenoma and carcinoma overlap, although carcinoma values in general are higher than adenoma values. The overnight low-dose dexamethasone test is more reliable to screen for Cushing's syndrome of any etiology (including tumor) than are urine 17-KS levels; and the 24-hour urine free cortisol assay is a little more reliable than the overnight dexamethasone test (chapter 29). At present most endocrinologists do not routinely obtain 17-KS levels.

Serum testosterone was discussed earlier in this chapter. Testosterone levels are elevated (usually to mild degree) in more than one half of the patients with PCO disease and in patients with Leydig cell tumors or ovarian testosterone-producing tumors. Elevated serum testosterone suggests a problem of ovarian origin because the ovaries normally produce 15%–30% of circulating testosterone; and in addition, the ovary produces about one half of circulating androstenedione from adrenal DHEA and this androstenedione is converted to testosterone in peripheral tissues. On the other hand, testosterone is produced in peripheral tissues and even in the adrenal as well as in the ovary. Serum testosterone levels therefore may be elevated in some patients with nonovarian conditions such as idiopathic hirsutism. These multiple origins make serum testosterone the current best single screening test in patients with hirsutism. Several investigators have found that serum free testosterone levels are more frequently elevated than serum total testosterone levels in patients with hirsutism although a lesser number favor total testosterone. Possible false results in total testosterone values due to changes in testosterone-binding protein is another point in favor of free testosterone. Some investigators have reported that serum androstenedione and DHEA-S levels are elevated in some patients with free testosterone values within reference range and that a test panel (e.g., free testosterone, androstenedione, dihydrotestosterone, and DHEA-S) is the most sensitive means of detecting the presence of excess androgens (reportedly with a sensitivity of 80%–90%).

Dehydroepiandrosterone-sulfate (DHEA-S) is produced entirely in the adrenal from adrenal DHEA. Therefore, elevated DHEA-S levels suggest that at least some excess androgen is coming from the adrenal. The DHEA-S test is also more sensitive for adrenal androgen excess than the urine 17-KS test. A minor difficulty is that a certain number of patients with PCO disease (in which the ovary is supposed to be the source of excess androgen production) and also certain patients with idiopathic hirsutism have some DHEA-S evidence of adrenal androgen production. For example, one third of PCO disease patients in one series were found to have increased DHEA-S levels. Although this was interpreted to mean that some adrenal factor was present as well as the ovarian component, it tends to confuse the diagnosis. Another difficulty is that some infertile women without hirsutism have been reported to have elevated DHEA-S levels. **Androstenedione,** as noted previously, is a metabolite of adrenal DHEA that is produced about equally in the adrenal and in the ovaries but then reaches peripheral tissues where some is converted to testosterone. Therefore, elevated serum androstenedione levels indicate abnormality without localizing the source. **Dihydrotestosterone** (DHT) is a metabolite of testosterone and is formed mainly in peripheral tissues. Therefore, elevated DHT levels suggest origin from tissues other than the ovaries or adrenals. **Androstanediol glucuronide** is a metabolite of DHT and has the same significance. Some investigators report that it is elevated more frequently than DHT. Serum prolactin levels are usually elevated in prolactin-producing pituitary tumors (prolactinoma). These tumors are said to be associated with hirsutism in about 20% of cases. The mechanism is thought to be enhancement of ACTH effect on formation of DHEA. However, it has also been reported that up to 30% of patients with PCO disease have mildly elevated serum prolactin levels (elevated < 1.5 times upper limit of the reference range). Prolactinomas are more likely in patients with irregular menstrual periods.

Luteinizing hormone and FSH are useful in diagnosis of PCO disease, which typically (although not always) shows elevated LH levels, with or without elevated FSH levels.

Urine free cortisol or low-dose overnight dexamethasone test are both standard tests used for diagnosis of Cushing's syndrome (see chapter 29), which is another possible cause of hirsutism.

Serum 17-OH-P is used to diagnose CAH. Levels of the 17-OH-P specimens drawn between 7 A.M. and 9 A.M. are elevated in nearly all patients with CAH who have symptoms in the neonatal period or in early childhood. However, in late-onset CAH that becomes clinically evident in adolescence or adulthood, 17-OH-P levels may or may not be elevated. The most noticeable symptom of late-onset CAH is hirsutism. Reports indicate that about 5%–10% (range, 1.5%–30%) of patients with hirsutism have late-onset CAH. The most effective test for diagnosis of late-onset CAH is an ACTH (Cortrosyn) stimulation test. A baseline 17-OH-P blood specimen is followed by injection of 25 units of synthetic ACTH, and a postdose specimen is drawn 30 minutes after intravenous injection or 60 minutes after intramuscular injection. Exact criteria for interpretation are not frequently stated. However, comparison of test results in the literature suggests that an abnormal response to ACTH consists of 17-OH-P values more than 1.6 times the upper limit of the normal 17-OH-P range before ACTH. An "exaggerated" response appears to be more than three times the upper limit of the pre-ACTH normal range. In homozygous late-onset CAH there is an exaggerated 17-OH-P response to ACTH. CAH heterozygotes may have a normal response to ACTH or may have an abnormal response to ACTH that falls between a normal response and an exaggerated response.

Suppression tests, such as a modified dexamethasone suppression test with suppression extended to 7–14 days, have been advocated in the past to differentiate between androgens of adrenal and ovarian origin. Dexamethasone theoretically should suppress nontumor androgen originating in the adrenal. However, studies have shown that the extended dexamethasone suppression test may be positive (i.e., may suppress androgen levels to < 50% of baseline) in some patients with PCO disease, and the test is no longer considered sufficiently dependable to localize the origin of increased androgen to either the adrenal or the ovary alone.

Radiologic visualization of abdominal organs is helpful if PCO disease, ovarian tumor, or adrenal tumor is suspected. Ultrasound examination of the ovaries and CT of the adrenals are able to detect some degree of abnormality in most (but not all) patients.

Polycystic Ovary Disease

Polycystic ovary (PCO) disease is considered by some to be the most common cause of female postpubertal hirsutism. It is also an important cause of amenorrhea, oligomenorrhea, and female sterility. Polycystic ovary disease is defined both clinically and by histopathology. The classic findings at operation are bilaterally enlarged ovaries (about 65%–76% of cases), which on pathologic examination have a thickened capsule and numerous small cysts (representing cystic follicles) beneath the capsule. However, PCO disease is considered to have a spectrum of changes in which there is decreasing ovarian size and a decreasing number of cysts until the ovaries are normal in size (about 25%–35% of cases) with few, if any, cysts but with an increased amount of subcapsular and interstitial stroma. There is also a condition called "hyperthecosis" in which the thecal cells of the stroma are considerably increased and have a luteinized appearance. Some consider hyperthecosis a separate entity; some include it in PCO disease but consider it the opposite end of the spectrum from the polycystic ovary type; and some combine PCO disease and hyperthecosis together under a new name, "sclerocystic ovary syndrome."

Clinically, there is considerable variety in signs and symptoms. The classic findings were described by Stein and Leventhal, and the appellation Stein-Leventhal syndrome can be used to distinguish patients with classic findings from patients with other variants of PCO disease. The Stein-Leventhal subgroup consists of women who have bilaterally enlarged polycystic ovaries and who are obese, are hirsute without virilization, have amenorrhea, and have normal urine 17-KS levels. Other patients with PCO disease may lack one or more of these characteristics. For example, only about 70% of patients have evidence of hirsutism (literature range, 17%–95%). Some patients with PCO disease have hypertension, and some have abnormalities in glucose tolerance. A few have virilization, which is said to be more common in those with hyperthecosis.

Laboratory Tests.—Laboratory findings in PCO disease are variable, as are the clinical findings. In classic Stein-Leventhal cases, serum testosterone levels are mildly or moderately elevated in about 50% of patients, and other androgen levels are elevated in many patients whose serum testosterone level remains within reference range. Free testosterone levels are elevated more frequently than total testosterone levels. Higher testosterone values tend to occur in hyperthecosis. Most investigators consider the increased androgen values to be derived mainly from the ovary, although an adrenal component has been found in some patients. Although urine 17-KS levels are usually normal, they may occasionally be mildly increased. Serum LH levels are typically elevated; FSH levels are usually normal or even mildly decreased.

Summary of Tests in Hirsutism

Most endocrinologists begin the laboratory investigation of hirsutism with a serum testosterone assay. Many prefer free testosterone rather than total testosterone. The number and choice of additional tests is controversial. Additional frequently ordered screening tests include serum DHEA-S, serum DHT, and the ACTH-stimulated 17-OH-P test. If abnormality is detected in one or more of these tests, additional procedures can help to find which organ and disease is responsible.

Gynecomastia

Gynecomastia is usually defined as enlargement of the male breast. This may be palpable only or may be grossly visible. Either type may be unilateral or bilateral. A small degree of palpable nonvisible gynecomastia is said to be present in about 30%–40% of clinically normal men. Most etiologies of gynecomastia can produce either unilateral or bilateral effects.

Etiologies.—Major etiologies of gynecomastia are presented in Table 30–10. In most cases, estrogen (estradiol) is increased relative to testosterone, even if assay values do not dem-

TABLE 30–10.
Selected Etiologies of Gynecomastia (% With Gynecomastia)

Physiologic etiologies
Neonatal
Pubertal (adolescence) (40%–70%)
Old age (40%)
Increased estrogen secretion
Testicular Leydig cell tumor (25%)
hCG-secreting tumor
Hepatoma
Adrenal cortex tumor
Increased estrogen precursors
Obesity
Cirrhosis (50%)
Hyperthyroidism (10%–40%)
Recovery from severe chronic disease
Renal failure on hemodialysis (50%)
"Refeeding" gynecomastia after malnutrition (15%)
Deficiency in androgens
Testicular failure (primary or secondary)
Klinefelter's syndrome (30%–50%)
Androgen resistance syndromes
Breast carcinoma
Medication-induced etiologies
Testosterone inhibitors (spironolactone, cimetidine)
Estrogens
Androgens
Others (methyldopa, isoniazid, various psychotropic medications, cytoxins, digitalis, reserpine, ketoconazole)

TABLE 30–11.
Possible Workup for Gynecomastia

Palpation of breast for tumor and examination of testis for tumor
Medication history
Inquire about chronic disease; especially dialysis for chronic renal disease, chronic liver disease, or refeeding conditions
Initial test screen
Serum estrogen (estradiol)
Serum free testosterone
Serum hCG
Serum LH
Additional tests (only if indicated)
Serum androstenedione
Thyroxine
γ-Glutamyltransferase
Urine 17-KS

onstrate this. Considering some of the etiologies, some degree of gynecomastia is present in 60%–70% of boys during puberty but disappears in 1–2 years. Old age demonstrates increased incidence of gynecomastia, possibly due to testicular failure. Testicular failure, either primary (congenital or testicle damage) or secondary (pituitary FSH decrease) can induce increased pituitary production of LH, which, in turn, may induce increased Leydig cell secretion of estradiol. Obesity may result in enhanced conversion of estrogen precursors to estrogen in peripheral tissues. Adrenal hyperactivity, cirrhosis, and chronic renal failure on dialysis therapy may be associated with gynecomastia in some patients due to increased estrogen formation from circulating androgenic precursors. Ten percent to 40% of patients with hyperthyroidism may develop gynecomastia due to increase in testosterone-binding protein. Breast carcinoma in males is rare but is always a possibility in unilateral gynecomastia.

Laboratory Tests.—Tests most commonly ordered in patients with gynecomastia are listed in Table 30–11. These tests screen for certain possible etiologies. Elevated serum LH levels suggest testicular failure; elevated testosterone levels, Leydig cell tumor; elevated serum estradiol levels, either an estrogen-producing tumor or elevated androgen precursors that are converted to estrogens; serum hCG, testicular or certain other tumors; liver function tests, cirrhosis. There is considerable disagreement among endocrinologists regarding how many tests to order for initial screen and what tests to include in the screen. Table 30–11 contains tests and procedures frequently mentioned that might be useful to nonendocrinologists. Serum prolactin is usually normal.

TESTS IN OBSTETRICS

Pregnancy Tests

Most pregnancy tests are based on the fact that the placenta secretes human chorionic gonadotropin (hCG), a hormone that has a luteinizing action on ovarian follicles and probably has other functions that are not completely known. Serum hCG levels of about 25 milli–international units (mIU)/ml (IU/L) are reached about 8–10 days after conception. The hCG levels double approximately every 2 days (various investigators have reported doubling times ranging from 1–3 days) during approximately the first 6 weeks of gestation. Levels of about 500 mIU/ml are encountered about 14–18 days after conception (28–32 days after the beginning of the last menstrual period). Serum levels are generally higher than urine levels for about the first 2 weeks after conception and about the same as urine levels during the third week. Thereafter, urine levels are higher than serum. The serum (and urine) hCG levels peak about 55–70 days (8–10 weeks) after conception (literature range, 40–77 days). Peak serum values are about 30,000 mIU/ml (range, 20,000–57,000 mIU/ml); peak urine values are about 100,000–200,000 mIU/ml (range, 3,500–600,000 mIU/ml). Serum and urine levels then decline rather rapidly during the last part of the first trimester and the first part of the second trimester, with average urine values falling to levels between 5,000 and 20,000 mIU/ml (range, 1,000–100,000 mIU/ml). Urine levels of 2,000–4,000 mIU/ml are not uncommon. Serum levels average about 10,000 mIU/ml. These levels are maintained for the remainder of pregnancy, although some investigators describe a brief rise and fall in the third trimester. The hCG molecule is composed of two subunits, alpha and beta. The alpha subunit is also a part of the hormones LH, FSH, and TSH. The beta subunit, however, is different for each hormone.

Biologic Tests.—The first practical biologic test for pregnancy was the Ascheim-Zondek test, published in 1928. Urine was injected into immature female mice, and a positive result was indicated by corpus luteum development in the ovaries. This took 4–5 days to perform. The next major advance took place in the late 1950s when frog tests were introduced. These took about 2 hours to complete. The result was almost always positive by the 40th day after the last menses, although it could become positive earlier.

Immunologic Tests.—In the 1960s it was discovered that antibodies to hCG could be produced by injecting the hCG molecule into animals. This was the basis for developing immunologic pregnancy tests using antigen-antibody reactions. In the late 1960s and during the 1970s, both latex agglutination slide tests and hemagglutination tube tests became available. The slide tests took about 2 minutes to perform and had a sensitivity of 1,500–3,000 mIU/ml, depending on the manufacturer. The tube tests required 2 hours to complete and had a sensitivity of 600–1,500 mIU/ml. A few procedures based on chemical reaction with urine estrogens were also being marketed. Counting from the first day of the last menstrual period, the slide or tube tests became positive between the 35th and 40th days, sometimes sooner, and were almost always positive by the 41st day (equivalent to 3.5–4 weeks after conception). Proteinuria (> 25 mg/100 ml) caused false positive results in many slide test kits, and some of the kits were affected by methadone and certain psychotropic drugs such as the phenothiazines. The antibody preparations used at that time were developed against the intact hCG molecule and cross-reacted with LH and TSH. This did not permit tests to be sensitive enough to detect small amounts of hCG, because urine LH could produce false positive results. Even so, false positive results were observed with some of the tests in some postmenopausal women because these women developed increased LH levels. False negative tests were sometimes encountered in the third trimester of pregnancy and occasionally even in the second trimester due to the much lower hCG levels compared to those in the first trimester.

Beta Subunit Antibody Tests.—In the late 1970s, methods were found to develop antibodies against the beta subunit of hCG rather than against the whole molecule. Antibody specific against the beta subunit could greatly reduce or even eliminate the cross-reaction of hCG with LH. However, the degree of present-day beta subunit antibody specificity varies with different commercial companies. By 1980, sensitivity of the slide tests using beta hCG antibody had reached 500–1,500 mIU/ml, with the majority in the 500–1,000 mIU/ml range (equivalent to 2.5–3.5 weeks after conception). Sensitivity of the beta hCG tube tests was approximately 200 mIU/ml. The tube tests detected pregnancy about 2–3 weeks after conception. Both the slide and the tube tests required a urine specimen. In the 1980s, standard immunoassay methods were developed for beta hCG in serum that provide a sensitivity of 3–50 mIU/ml (see Table 36–29). This detects pregnancy 1–2 weeks after conception. Several manufacturers developed abbreviated serum pregnancy immunoassays that compared patient serum with a single standard containing a known amount of beta hCG (usually in the range of 25 mIU/ml). A result greater than the standard means that beta hCG is present in a quantity greater than the standard value, which in usual circumstances indicates pregnancy. Present-day serum immunoassay procedures take between 15 minutes and 1 hour to perform (depending on the manufacturer), whether the standard or the abbreviated ("yes-no") type. The abbreviated method is much less expensive and is usually quicker. Several urine tests are available that detect 50 mIU/ml of hCG.

Technical Problems With Human Chorionic Gonadotropin.—Some (not all) of the kits that detect less than 25 mIU/ml of hCG may have problems with false-positive results of several different etiologies. First, of course, there may be incorrect performance of the test or patient specimen mishandling. The antibodies used in the different manufacturer's tests have different specificities. The hCG molecules may exist in different forms in some patients (whole molecule, beta subunit alone, alpha subunit alone, or hCG molecule fragments). This is more often seen with tumors. Different antibodies may detect different amounts of hCG material depending on whether the antibody detects the whole molecule, the beta segment, or both. Some beta-hCG antibodies have a certain degree of cross-reaction with LH, although theoretically a beta-specific antibody should not do so. The serum of occasional patients contains heterophil-type antibodies capable of cross-reacting with test antibodies that were produced in different animals (e.g., mice). Some kits are affected in a similar way by renal failure. Finally, it has been reported in several studies that occasional normal nonpregnant women may sometimes have low-level circulating levels of an hCG-like substance, usually less than 25 mIU/ml. This was reported in about 2.5% (range, 0%–14%) of patients in these studies, although most evaluations of hCG test kits have not reported false positive results. When one kit was reactive, sometimes one or more different kits would also be reactive, but usually some kits do not react with these substances. At present, in most laboratories there is no satisfactory way to know immediately whether a positive result is due to pregnancy, is due to hCG-producing tumor, or is false positive, especially when the test is a yes-no method. Although there are ways to investigate possible discrepancies, it usually takes a considerable period of time and retesting to solve the problem, or it may necessitate consultation with a reference laboratory.

Other Uses for hCG Assay.—Pregnancy tests are useful in certain situations other than early diagnosis of normal pregnancy. These conditions include ectopic pregnancy, spontaneous abortion, and hCG-producing neoplasms. Ectopic pregnancy and neoplasms will be discussed in detail later. When the differential diagnosis includes normal intrauterine pregnancy, ectopic pregnancy, and threatened, incomplete, or complete abortion, the pattern obtained from serum quantitative beta-hCG assays performed every other day may be helpful. During the first 4 weeks of pregnancy (beginning at conception), there is roughly a doubling of hCG every 2 days (range, 1–3 days). As noted earlier, serum beta hCG by immunoassay first detects embryonic placental hCG in titers of 2–25 IU/L between 1 and 2 weeks after conception. Ectopic pregnancy and abortions may demonstrate an increase in their hCG levels at the same rate as in normal pregnancy up to a certain point. In the case of ectopic pregnancy, that point is usually less than 4 weeks (possibly as long as 6 weeks) after conception, since the ectopic location usually limits placental growth or rupture occurs. The typical pattern of ectopic pregnancy is a leveling off (plateau) at a certain point in time. The usual pattern of abortion is either a decrease in beta-hCG levels as abortion takes place or a considerable slowing in the rate of increase. However, these are only rules of thumb. About 15% of normal intrauterine pregnancies display less increase (decreased rate of increase) than expected, and thus could be mistaken for beginning abortion by this criterion alone. Also, ectopic pregnancy values may sometimes decline rather than plateau if the fetus dies.

Ectopic Pregnancy

Ectopic pregnancy is a common gynecologic problem, either by itself or in differential diagnosis. Symptoms include abdominal pain of various types in about 97% of patients (literature range 91%–100%), abnormal uterine bleeding in about 75% (54%–80%), delayed menses in about 75% (68%–84%), adnexal tenderness on palpation in about 90%–95%, unilateral adnexal mass in about 50% (30%–76%), and fever (usually lowgrade) in about 5% (3%–9%). Hypovolemic shock is reported as the presenting symptom in about 14%. It is obvious that these signs and symptoms can suggest a great number of conditions. In one study, 31% of patients with ectopic pregnancy in the differential diagnosis had a strongly suggestive triad of abdominal pain, uterine bleeding, and an adnexal mass. Only 14% of these patients were found to have ectopic pregnancy. Some conditions that frequently mimic ectopic pregnancy are pelvic inflammatory disease, threatened, incomplete, or complete abortion, corpus luteum rupture, dysfunctional uterine bleeding, and bleeding ovarian cyst. Among routine laboratory tests, a hemoglobin value less than 10 gm/100 ml is reported in about 40% of ectopic pregnancy cases (28%–55%) and leukocytosis in about 50%. Among other diagnostic procedures, culdocentesis for fresh blood is reported to produce about 10% false negative results (5%–18%). Pregnancy test results vary according to the sensitivity of the test. The older latex agglutination slide tests with a sensitivity of 1,500–3,000 mIU/ml yielded about 50%–60% false negative results. Tests with a sensitivity of 500–1,000 mIU/ml resulted in about 25% false negative results (8%–60%). Tests with a sensitivity of 50 mIU/ml yield about 5%–10% false negative results (0%–13%). Serum beta-hCG tests with a sensitivity of 25 IU/L or better have a false negative rate of about 1%–2% (range, 0%–3%). A positive pregnancy test result is not a diagnosis of ectopic pregnancy but signifies only that the patient has increased levels of hCG, for which there could be several possible causes. Also, some manufacturers' kits are subject to a certain number of false positive results. Interpretation of a negative test result depends on the sensitivity of the test. If the test is a serum beta hCG immunoassay with a sensitivity of 25 IU/L or better, a negative test result is about 98%–99% accurate in excluding pregnancy. However, there are rare cases in which the specimen might be obtained 2–4 days prior to the time patient hCG reaches detectable levels, or there could be a technical laboratory error. A repeat test 48 hours later helps to exclude these possibilities. Ultrasound has been advocated for diagnosis and may be very helpful. However, some reports indicate a significant number of false positive and false negative results. Newer equipment may alter this assessment.

Neoplasms Producing Human Chorionic Gonadotropin

Neoplasms arising from chorionic villi, the fetal part of the placenta, are known as gestational trophoblastic neoplasms and include hydatidiform mole (the counterpart in tumor classification of benign adenoma) and choriocarcinoma (chorioepithelioma, the equivalent of carcinoma). Hydatidiform mole also has a subdivision, chorioadenoma destruens, in which the neoplasm invades the placenta but there is no other evidence of malignancy. The major importance of hydatidiform mole is a very high (⩾ 10%) incidence of progression to choriocarcinoma.

Several hormone assays have been proposed as aids in diagnosis. By far the most important is hCG, which is produced by the trophoblast cell component of fetal placental tissue. As just noted, hCG forms the basis for most pregnancy tests. Luteinizing hormone has a close biochemical and immunologic similarity to hCG (through its alpha subunit), so that the original immunologic pregnancy tests could not be made more sensitive than 700–1,000 IU/L to avoid too many false positive results from cross-reaction with LH. Unfortunately, 25%–30% of trophoblastic tumors produce hCG in amounts less than 1,000 IU/L. Antibodies to the specific beta subunit of hCG are now available, and RIA procedures using these antibodies can detect levels of 25 IU/L or less without interference by LH, permitting detection of nearly all gestational tumors. Since normal placental tissue secretes hCG, the problem then is to differentiate normal pregnancy from neoplasm. Suspicion is raised by clinical signs and also by finding hCG levels that are increased more than expected by the duration of pregnancy or that persist after removal of the placenta. Twin or other multiple pregnancies can also produce hCG levels above expected values. Although serum levels of hCG greater than 50,000 mIU/ml (or urine levels > 300,000 mIU/ml) are typically associated with gestational neoplasms, especially if these levels persist, a considerable number of patients with gestational tumors have hCG values less than this level. About 25% of patients in one report had values less than 1,000 mIU/ml. In normal pregnancies, serum hCG levels become nondetectable by about 14 days (range, 3–30 days) after delivery. In one study of elective abortions, it took 23–52 days for hCG levels to become nondetectable. After removal of a hydatidiform mole, hCG levels should become nondetectable in about 2–3 months (range, 21–278 days). Once neoplasm is diagnosed and treated, hCG measurement is a guideline for success of therapy and follow-up of the patient for possible recurrence.

Other Hormones Useful in Possible Gestational Neoplasms.—Fetal and placental tissue produces other hormones that may be useful. Progesterone (or its metabolite pregnanediol) and estradiol are secreted by the placenta in slowly increasing quantity throughout most of pregnancy. It has been reported that during the first 20 weeks of gestation, hydatidiform moles are associated with serum estradiol-17β values that are increased from values expected in normal pregnancy, with good separation of normal pregnancy from molar pregnancy. Serum progesterone levels were increased in about 75% of nonaborted moles up to the 20th week. Urinary pregnanediol levels, on the other hand, are frequently decreased. Finding increased serum progesterone and estradiol-17β levels during the time that peak hCG values are expected (between the 50th and 80th days after the last menstrual period), accompanied by a decreased urine pregnanediol level, would suggest a hydatidiform mole or possibly a choriocarcinoma. Serum human placental lactogen (hPL), or somatomammotropin, is another placental hormone that rises during the first and second trimesters and then reaches a plateau during the last 2–3 months. The association of decreased levels of hPL in the first and second trimesters with increased hCG levels suggests neoplasm. There is, however, a small degree of overlap of hPL level in patients with mole and the normal range for pregnancy. One report suggests a possible inverse ratio between hPL values and degree of malignancy (the greater the degree of malignancy, the less serum hPL produced).

Production of hCG has been reported to occur in nearly two thirds of testicular embryonal cell carcinomas and in about one third of testicular seminomas. Instances of hCG secretion by adenocarcinomas from other organs and, rarely, from certain other tumors have been reported.

Fetal or Placental Function

Several hormone assays are available to help estimate whether placental function is normal or to predict impending fetal death. The tests most widely used are urine estriol, urine total estrogens, serum unconjugated estriol, and serum placental lactogen (Fig 30–1).

Urine Estriol or Total Estrogens.—Estriol is an estrogenic compound produced by the placenta from precursors derived from fetal adrenal cortex and fetal liver. Newly synthesized estriol is unconjugated; therefore, unconjugated estriol represents a product of the entire fetoplacental unit. The unconjugated estriol reaches maternal serum (where it has a half-life of about 20 minutes) and is taken to the maternal liver, where about 90% is conjugated with a glucuronide molecule. The conjugated form of estriol is excreted in maternal urine. A lesser amount of conjugated estriol is produced by the maternal liver from nonestriol estrogens synthesized by the placenta from maternal adrenal precursors. Serum estriol can be measured either as total estriol or as unconjugated estriol. It usually is measured as unconjugated estriol to exclude maternal contribution to the conjugated fraction. Urine estriol can be measured as total estriol or as total estrogens, since estriol normally constitutes 90%–95% of urine total estrogens.

Historically, urine total estrogen was the first test used, since total estrogen can be assayed by standard chemical techniques. However, urine glucose falsely increases results (which is a problem in diabetics, who form a large segment of the obstetrical high-risk group), and certain other substances such as urobilinogen also may interfere. In addition, urine total estrogen results are a little more variable than urine estriol patterns. Eventually, other biochemical procedures that were more specific for urine estriol (in some cases, however, the "estriol" being measured using biochemical methods is actually total estrogen) were devised. These procedures also have certain drawbacks, some of which are shared by the total estrogen methods. Both urine total estrogens and urine estriol have a significant degree of between-day variation in the same patient, which averages about 10%–15% but which can be as high as 50%. Both are dependent on renal

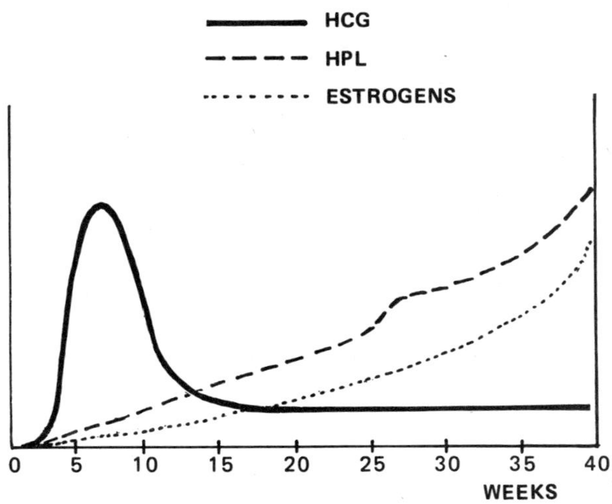

FIG 30–1.
Changes in total estrogens (or estriol), human chorionic gonadotropin (HCG), and human placental lactogen (HPL) in normal pregnancy.

excretion, and, therefore, on maternal renal function. Both have a maternal component as well as the fetal component. Urine total estrogen necessitates a 24-hour collection. The standard method for urine estriol also is a 24-hour specimen. There is substantial difficulty collecting accurate 24-hour specimens, especially in outpatients. Also, there is a 1- to 2-day time lag before results are available. Some have proposed a single voided specimen based on the estriol/creatinine ratio. However, there is controversy whether the single-voided specimen method (reported in terms of either estriol per gram creatinine or estriol/creatinine ratio) provides results as clinically accurate as the 24-hour specimen.

Estriol can be detected by immunoassay as early as the ninth week of gestation. Thereafter, estriol values slowly but steadily increase until the last trimester, when there is a more pronounced increase. Clinical use of estriol measurement is based on the fact that severe acute abnormality of the fetoplacental unit (i.e., a dead or dying placenta or fetus) is manifested either by failure of the estriol level to continue rising or by a sudden marked and sustained decrease in the estriol level. Urine specimens are usually obtained weekly in the earlier part of pregnancy, twice weekly in the last trimester, and daily for several days if a problem develops.

In general, urine estriol or estrogen excretion correlates reasonably well with fetal health. However, there are important exceptions. Only severe fetal or placental distress produces urine estrogen decrease of sufficient magnitude, sufficient duration, and sufficiently often to be reliable (i.e., mild disorder may not be detected). There is sufficient daily variation in excretion so that only a very substantial and sustained decrease in excretion, such as 40%–50% of the mean value of several previous results, is considered reliable. Some consider an estriol value less than 4 mg/24 hours (after 32 weeks of gestation) strongly suggestive of fetal distress and a value more than 12 mg/24 hours as indicative of fetal well-being. Maternal hypertension, preeclampsia, severe anemia, and impaired renal function can decrease urine estrogen or estriol excretion considerably. Decrease may also occur to variable degree in variable numbers of fetuses with severe congenital anomalies. Certain drugs such as ampicillin and cortisol may affect urine estriol or estrogen values by effects on production, and other substances such as mandelamine or glucose can alter results from biochemical interference with some test methods. Some investigators have reported a decrease shortly before delivery in a substantial minority of normal patients. Maternal Rh-immune disease may produce a false increase in urine estriol levels. Continued bed rest has been reported to increase estriol excretion values an average of 20% over levels from ambulatory persons, with this increase occurring in about 90% of patients in the third trimester.

The literature contains widely differing opinions regarding clinical usefulness of estrogen excretion assay in pregnancy. In general, investigators have found that urinary estrogen or estriol levels are decreased in about 60%–70% of cases in which fetal distress occurs (literature range 33%–80%). The more severe the fetal or placental disorder, the more likely that urine estrogen or estriol levels will be low. The percentage of falsely low values is also said to be substantial, but numerical data are not as readily available.

Serum Unconjugated Estriol.—Plasma or serum unconjugated estriol, measured by immunoassay, has been used as a replacement for urine hormone excretion. Advantages include ease of specimen collection (avoidance of 24-hour urine collection problems), increased specificity for fetoplacental dysfunction (no maternal hormone contribution), no 24-hour wait for a specimen, closer observation of fetoplacental health (due to the short unconjugated estriol half-life), little technical interference by substances such as glucose, and less dependence on maternal kidney function. Drawbacks include the majority of those drawbacks previously described for urine hormone excretion (effect of bed rest, hypertension, and other conditions, and medications affecting estrogen production). Also similar to urine excretion, there is substantial between-day variation, averaging about 15% (reported maximum variation up to 49%). However, there are also considerable within-day fluctuations, which average about 15% (with maximum variation reported as high as 51%). Thus, a single value is even more difficult to interpret than a urine value. Some believe that 24-hour urine measurements may thus have some advantage, since within-day fluctuations are averaged out. Also similar to urine values, the current trend of interpretation is to require a sustained decrease of 40%–50% from the average of several previous serum values to be considered a significant abnormality. The serum specimens should preferably be drawn at the same time of day in the same patient position and assayed by the same laboratory. Although frequency of sampling is not uniform among investigators, many obtain one or two specimens per week during the earlier part of pregnancy and one per day if there is clinical suspicion of abnormality or one serum value becomes significantly decreased. Although there is some disagreement, the majority of investigators indicate that serum unconjugated estriol has a little better correlation with clinical results than does urine hormone excretion.

Because of the problems associated with collection of urine or serum estriol specimens and interpretation of the values, as well as the disturbing number of false positive and negative test results, many clinicians depend more on other procedures (e.g., the nonstress test, which correlates the rate of fetal heartbeat to fetal movement) than on estrogen values to monitor fetal well-being.

Placental Lactogen.—Human placental lactogen is a hormone produced only by the placenta, with metabolic activity similar in some degree to that of prolactin and GH. Values correlate roughly with the weight of the placenta and rise steadily in maternal serum during the first and second trimesters before entering a relative plateau in the third. Serum levels of hPL are higher than those attained by any other peptide hormone. Serum half-life is about 30 minutes. Although hPL cross-reacts with GH in most RIA systems, the high level of hPL relative to GH at the time of pregnancy when hPL levels are measured avoids clinical problems with GH interference. Serum hPL has been evaluated by many investigators as a test of placental function in the third trimester. Its short half-life is thought to make it a more sensitive indicator of placental failure than measurements of other hormones, especially urine measurements. Since hPL levels normally can fluctuate somewhat, serial measurements are more accurate than a single determination. Estriol, which reflects combined fetal and placental function, still seems to be used more than hPL.

Fetal Maturity Tests

Tests for monitoring fetal maturity via amniocentesis are also available. Bilirubin levels in erythroblastosis are discussed in chapter 10. Amniotic creatinine assay, amniotic epithelial cell stain with Nile blue sulfate, fat droplet evaluation, osmolality, and the Clemens shake test, alone or in combination, have been tried with varying and not entirely satisfactory results. The current most widely used tests are the lecithin/sphingomyelin (L/S) ratio, assay of phosphatidylglycerol (PG), and the foam stability index (FSI).

Lecithin/Sphingomyelin Ratio.—The L/S ratio has been the most widely accepted procedure. Lecithin (phosphatidylcholine) is a phospholipid which is the major component of alveolar surfactant. Surfactant is a substance composed predominantly of phospholipids that is found in lung alveoli and that lowers the surface tension of the alveolar lining, stabilizes the alveoli in expiration, and helps prevent atelectasis. Surfactant deficiency causes neonatal respiratory distress syndrome (RDS), formerly called "hyaline membrane disease." In amniotic fluid, the phospholipid known as sphingomyelin normally exceeds lecithin before the 26th week; thereafter, lecithin concentration is slightly predominant until approximately the 35th week, when the lecithin level swiftly rises to more than twice sphingomyelin levels. After the lecithin level becomes twice that of sphingomyelin, it was originally reported that there was no longer any danger of neonatal RDS. The L/S ratio thus becomes a test for fetal maturity. Certain precautions must be taken. Presence of blood or meconium in the amniotic fluid or contamination by maternal vaginal secretions may cause a false increase in lecithin levels. The amniotic fluid specimen must be cooled immediately, centrifuged to eliminate epithelial cells and other debris, and kept frozen if not tested promptly to avoid destruction of lecithin by certain enzymes in the amniotic fluid.

Evaluations in unselected amniocentesis patients have revealed that about 55% of neonates with "immature" L/S ratios using the 2.0 ratio cutoff point do not develop RDS and about 5% (literature range 0%–17%) of neonates with a "mature" L/S ratio (ratio > 2.0) develop RDS. Some have attempted to eliminate the falsely mature cases by changing the cutoff point to a ratio of 2.5, but this correspondingly increases the number of falsely immature results. In clinically normal pregnancies, only about 3% of neonates with a mature L/S ratio, using proper technique, develop RDS. In complicated pregnancies, especially those with maternal type I insulin-dependent diabetes, hypertension, or premature rupture of the amniotic membrane, about 15% (literature range, 3%–28%) of neonates with mature L/S ratios are reported to develop RDS. The wide range in the literature reflects differences in opinion among investigators as to the effect of diabetes on neonatal L/S ratios. Also, the L/S ratio can produce falsely mature results if contaminated by blood or meconium. It takes experience and careful attention to technical details to obtain consistently accurate L/S results.

Phosphatidylglycerol.—A number of other tests have been developed in search of a procedure that is more accurate in predicting or excluding RDS and that is also technically easy to perform. Only two of these will be discussed here, but several others appear in the chapter on special category tests. Phosphatidylglycerol is a relatively minor component (about 10%) of lung surfactant phospholipids. However, PG is almost entirely synthesized by mature lung alveolar cells and therefore is a good indicator of lung maturity. In normal pregnancies PG levels begin to increase after about 30 weeks' gestation and continue to increase until birth. It normally becomes detectable about the 36th week. In conditions that produce severe fetal stress, such as maternal insulin-dependent diabetes, hypertension, and premature membrane rupture, PG levels may become detectable as early as 30 weeks' gestation. Most of the limited studies to date indicate that the presence of PG in more than trace amounts strongly suggests that RDS will not develop, whether the pregnancy is normal or complicated. Overall incidence of RDS when PG is present seems to be about 2% (range 0%–10%). It is considered to be a more reliable indicator of fetal lung maturity than the L/S ratio in complicated pregnancy. It may be absent in some patients with clearly normal L/S ratios and occasionally may be present when the L/S ratio is less than 2.0. Phosphatidylglycerol assay is not significantly affected by usual amounts of contamination by blood or meconium.

Phosphatidylglycerol can be assayed in several ways, including gas chromatography, thin-layer chromatography (TLC), enzymatically, and immunologically. The TLC technique is roughly similar to that of the L/S ratio. Some report the visual presence or absence of PG, with or without some comment as to how much appears to be present (trace or definite). Some report a PG/sphingomyelin (PG/S) ratio. A PG/S ratio of 2.0 is considered mature. The enzymatic PG method separates phospholipids from the other components of amniotic fluid (using column chromatography or other means), followed by enzymatic assay of glycerol in the phospholipid fraction. At present there is insufficient published evaluation of this technique. The immunologic methods are currently restricted to a slide agglutination kit called Amniostat. Current evaluations indicate that Amniostat detects about 85%–90% (range, 74%–100%) of patients who are positive for PG on TLC. However, the risk of RDS is only about 1%–2% if the test is reactive (positive).

Foam Stability Index (FSI).—The FSI is a surfactant function test based on the ability of surfactant to lower surface tension sufficiently to permit stabilized foaming when the amniotic fluid is shaken. This depends on the amount and functional capability of surfactant as challenged by certain amounts of the antifoaming agent ethanol. It is thought that the phospholipid dipalmitoyl lecithin is the most important stabilizing agent. The FSI is actually a modification of the Clemens shake test which used a final amniotic fluid-ethanol mixture of 47.5% ethanol. The FSI consists of a series of seven tubes containing amniotic fluid with increasing percentages of ethanol in 1% increments from 44%–50%. The endpoint is the tube with the highest percentage of ethanol that maintains foam after shaking. An endpoint of the 47% tube predicts about a 4% chance of RDS and an endpoint in the 48% tube predicts less than 1% chance. Because even tiny inaccuracies or fluctuations of ethanol concentration can influence results considerably, and also the tendency of absolute ethanol to adsorb water, some problems were encountered in laboratories making their own reagents. To solve these problems a commercial version of the FSI called Lumidex was introduced featuring sealed tubes containing the 1% increments of ethanol to which aliquots of amniotic fluid are added through the rubber caps that seal the tubes. The

FSI (or Lumidex) has been reported to be more reliable than the L/S ratio in predicting fetal lung maturity. At least two reports indicate that the FSI correctly demonstrates fetal lung maturity much more frequently than the L/S ratio in fetuses who are small for their gestational age. Drawbacks of the FSI method in general are interference (false positive) by blood, meconium, vaginal secretions, obstetrical creams, and mineral oil. A major drawback of the current Lumidex kit is a shelf-life of only 3 weeks without refrigeration. Although the shelf life is 3 months with refrigeration, it is necessary to stabilize the tubes at room temperature for at least 16 hours before the test is performed.

Amniocentesis Laboratory Problems.— Occasionally, amniotic puncture may enter the maternal bladder instead of the amniotic sac. Some advocate determining glucose and protein levels, which are high in amniotic fluid and low in normal urine. To avoid confusion in diabetics with glucosuria, it has been suggested that urea and potassium levels be measured instead; these are relatively high in urine and low in amniotic fluid. Another potential danger area is the use of spectrophotometric measurement of amniotic fluid pigment as an estimate of amniotic fluid bilirubin content. Before 25 weeks' gestation, normal pigment levels may be greater than those usually associated with abnormality.

BIOCHEMICAL TESTS FOR CONGENITAL ANOMALIES

Besides giving information on fetal well-being, amniocentesis makes it possible to test for various congenital anomalies via biochemical analysis of amniotic fluid and tissue culture chromosome studies of fetal cells (see chapter 36). In addition, certain substances of fetal origin may appear in maternal serum. In some cases it is possible to detect certain fetal malformations by screening tests in maternal serum.

Maternal Serum Alpha-Fetoprotein

One of the most widely publicized tests for congenital anomalies is the alpha-fetoprotein (AFP) test in maternal serum for detection of open neural tube defects. Although neural tube defects are much more common in infants born to families in which a previous child had such an abnormality, about 90% occur in families with no previous history of malformation. Alpha-fetoprotein is an alpha-1 glycoprotein with a molecular weight of about 70,000. It is first produced by the fetal yolk sac and then mostly by the fetal liver. It becomes the predominant fetal serum protein by the 12th or 13th week of gestation but then declines to about 1% of peak levels by delivery. It is excreted via fetal urine into amniotic fluid and from there reaches maternal blood. After the 13th week both fetal serum and amniotic fluid AFP levels decline in parallel, the fetal blood level being about 200 times the amniotic fluid level. In contrast, maternal serum levels become detectable at about the 12th to 14th week and reach a peak between the 26th and 32d week of gestation. Although maternal serum screening could be done between the 15th and 20th weeks, the majority of investigators have decided that the interval between the 16th and 18th weeks is optimal, since the amniotic fluid AFP level is still relatively high and the fetus is still relatively early in gestation. Maternal AFP normal levels differ for each week of gestation and ideally should be determined for each laboratory. Some reports suggests that maternal weight is also a factor, with heavier women tending to have lower serum AFP values. However, one group of investigators does not agree that maternal AFP values should be corrected for maternal weight.

Maternal AFP levels reportedly detect about 85%–90% (literature range, 67%–97%) of open neural tube defects; about one half are anencephaly and about one half are open or closed spina bifida. There is an incidence of about 1–2 per 1,000 live births. The test also detects a lesser (but currently unknown) percentage of certain other abnormalities, such as fetal ventral wall defects, Turner's syndrome, pilonidal sinus, hydrocephalus, duodenal atresia, multiple hypospadias, congenital nephrosis, and cystic hygroma. In addition, some cases of recent fetal death, threatened abortion, and Rh erythroblastosis produce elevated maternal AFP levels, as well as some cases of maternal chronic liver disease and some maternal serum specimens obtained soon after amniocentesis. A theoretical but unlikely consideration is AFP-producing tumors such as hepatoma. More important, twin pregnancies cause maternal values that are elevated in terms of the reference range established on single-fetus pregnancies. A large minority of elevated maternal AFP levels represent artifact due to incorrect estimation of fetal gestational age, which, in turn, would result in comparing maternal values to the wrong reference range. There is also the possibility of laboratory error. Most authorities recommend a repeat serum AFP test 1 week later to confirm an abnormal result. If results of the second specimen are abnormal, ultrasound is usually suggested to date the age of gestation more accurately, to examine the fetus for anencephaly, and to exclude twin pregnancy. However, even ultrasonic measurements may vary from true gestational age by as much as 5–7 days. Some perform ultrasonic evaluation if the first AFP test result is abnormal; if ultrasound confirms fetal abnormality, a second AFP specimen would be unnecessary. In some medical centers, about 40%–59% of elevated maternal AFP levels can be explained on the basis of technical error, incorrect fetal gestation date, and multiple pregnancy.

Some conditions produce abnormal decrease in maternal serum AFP values. The most important is Down's syndrome. It is reported that use of AFP maternal screening can increase the detection rate of Down's syndrome from about 20% using maternal age as a risk factor to about 40%. Follow-up studies that include amniocentesis with chromosome analysis of amniotic cells are necessary. Other conditions that are associated with decreased maternal serum AFP levels include overestimation of fetal age and absence of pregnancy (including missed abortion).

Amniotic Fluid Alpha-Fetoprotein

Amniocentesis is another technique that can be used to detect open neural tube defects. It is generally considered the next step after elevated maternal AFP levels are detected and confirmed and the age of gestation is accurately determined. As mentioned previously, amniocentesis for this purpose is generally considered to be optimal at 16–18 weeks of gestation. Assay of amniotic fluid AFP is said to be about 95% sensitive for open neural tube defects (literature range, 80%–98%), with a false positive rate in specialized centers less than 1%. Most false positive results are due to contamination by fetal blood, so a test for fetal red blood cells or hemoglobin is recommended when the amniotic fluid AFP level is elevated. Amniotic fluid AFP normal values are age related, similar to maternal serum values.

Amniotic Fluid Acetylcholinesterase

Acetylcholinesterase (ACE) assay in amniotic fluid has been advocated as another way to detect open neural tube defects and to help eliminate diagnostic errors caused by false positive AFP results. Acetylcholinesterase is a major enzyme in spinal fluid. Results from a limited number of studies in the late 1970s and early 1980s suggest that the test has 98%–99% sensitivity for open neural tube defects. Acetylcholinesterase assay has the further advantage that it is not as dependent as AFP on gestational age. It is not specific for open neural tube defects; amniotic fluid elevations have been reported in some patients with exomphalos (protrusion of viscera outside the body due to a ventral wall defect) and certain other serious congenital anomalies and in some patients who eventually miscarry. Not enough data are available to properly evaluate risk of abnormal ACE results in normal pregnancies, with reports in the literature ranging from 0%–6%. There is also disagreement as to how much fetal blood contamination affects ACE assay. The test is less affected than AFP assay, but substantial contamination seems capable of producing falsely elevated results.

BIBLIOGRAPHY

Hicks JM, Iosefsohn M: Home pregnancy kits: Should they be on the market? *Clin Chem* 1988; 34:1182.

New MI, Josso N: Disorders of gonadal differentiation and congenital adrenal hyperplasia. *Endocrinol Metab Clin North Am* 1988; 17:339.

Abboud CF, Laws ER: Diagnosis of pituitary tumors. *Endocrinol Metab Clin North Am* 1988; 17:241.

Swerdloff RS, et al: Evalulation of the infertile couple. *Endocrinol Metab Clin North Am* 1988; 17:301.

Reiter EO, et al: Variable estimates of serum growth hormone concentrations by different radioassay systems. *J Clin Endocrinol* 1988; 66:68.

Doran TA, et al: Maternal serum alpha-fetoprotein screening: Report of a Canadian

pilot project. *Can Med Assoc J* 1987; 137:285.
Baumann G: Acromegaly. *Endocrinol Metab Clin* 1987; 16:685.
Vance ML, Thorner MO: Prolactinomas. *Endocrinol Metab Clin* 1987; 16:731.
Jack BW, et al: Routine obstetric ultrasound. *Am Fam Phys* 1987; 35:173.
Griffin JE, Wilson JD: Syndromes of androgen resistance. *Hosp Pract* 1987; 22:159.
Kim DS, et al: Comparative review of diagnostic accuracy in tubal pregnancy. *Obstet Gynecol* 1987; 70:547.
Chalew SA, et al: Therapy in short children with subnormal integrated concentrations of growth hormone. *Am J Dis Child* 1987; 141:1195.
Richards GE, et al: Diagnostic validity of 12-hour integrated concentration of growth hormone. *Am J Dis Child* 1987; 141:553.
Brunader REA, Moore DC: Evaluation of the child with growth retardation. *Am Fam Phys* 1987; 35:165.
Bevan JS, et al: Misinterpretation of prolactin levels leading to management errors in patients with sellar enlargement. *Am J Med* 1987; 82:29.
Kubasik NP: Prolactin: Its functional effects and measurement. *Lab Mgmt* 1987; 25(8):49.
Melmed S, Rushakoff RJ: Ectopic pituitary and hypothalamic hormone syndromes. *Endocrinol Metab Clin* 1987; 16:805.
Hull ME, Kenigsberg DJ: Gonadotropin releasing hormone: Function and clinical use. *Lab Mgmt* 1987; 25(4):51.
Rittmaster RS, Loriaux DL: Hirsutism. *Ann Intern Med* 1987; 106:95.
Baskin HJ: Screening for late-onset congenital adrenal hyperplasia in hirsutism or amenorrhea. *Arch Intern Med* 1987; 147:847.
Bandi ZL, et al: Enzyme-linked immunosorbent urine pregnancy tests. *Am J Clin Pathol* 1987; 87:236.
LeMaistre A, et al: Role of qualitative choriogonadotropin assays in diagnosis of ectopic pregnancy. *Clin Chem* 1987; 33:1908.
Belyus PS, et al: An evaluation between Amniostat Ultra Sensitive and two-dimensional TLC for the determination of phosphatidylglycerol in amniotic fluid. *Am J Clin Pathol* 1987; 87:422.
Amenta JS, et al: Evaluating the clinical effectiveness of amniotic fluid assays in predicting respiratory distress syndrome in the neonate. *Clin Chem* 1987; 33:647.
Bennett B: Growth hormone: An update. *J Med Technol* 1986; 3:347.
Englehart J, et al: Clonidine and growth hormone response. *Am J Dis Child* 1986; 140:186.
Vance ML, Thorner MO: Growth-hormone-releasing hormone: A clinical update. *Ann Intern Med* 1986; 105:447.
Kao PC, et al: Somatomedin C: An index of growth hormone activity. *Mayo Clin Proc* 1986; 61:908.
Bercu BB, et al: Growth hormone (GH) provocative testing frequently does not reflect endogenous GH secretion. *J Clin Endocrinol Metab* 1986; 63:709.
Melmed S, et al: Pituitary tumors secreting growth hormone and prolactin. *Ann Intern Med* 1986; 105:238.
Moltz L, Schwartz U: Gonadal and adrenal androgen secretion in hirsute females. *Clin Endocrinol Metab* 1986; 15:229.
Elkind-Hirsch K, et al: Evaluation of the Ovustick urinary luteinizing hormone kit in normal and stimulated menstrual cycles. *Obstet Gynecol* 1986; 67:450.
Chapman JF, Herbert WNP: Current methods for evaluating fetal lung maturity. *Lab Med* 1986; 17:597.
Lockitch G, et al: Prediction of fetal lung maturity by use of the Lumadex-FSI test. *Clin Chem* 1986; 32:361.
Macri JN, et al: Maternal serum alpha-fetoprotein screening, maternal weight, and detection efficiency. *Am J Obstet Gynecol* 1986; 155:758.
Haddow JE, Knight GJ: Maternal serum alpha-fetoprotein screening: A test for the dedicated laboratory. *J Med Technol* 1986; 3:477.
Phillips JA: Genetic diagnosis: Differentiating growth disorders. *Hosp Pract* 1985; 20:85.
Hussa RO, et al: Discordant human chorionic gonadotropin results: Causes and solutions. *Obstet Gynecol* 1985; 65:211.
Hager CB: A dual radioimmunoassay for LH and FSH. *Am Clin Prod Rev* 1985; 4(10):44.
Komarmy LE: Clinical use of serum pregnancy test and human chorionic gonadotropin assays. *Pathologist* 1985; 39:46.
Morris DV, et al: The investigation of female gonadal dysfunction. *Clin Endocrinol Metab* 1985; 14:125.
Handelsman DJ, Swerdloff RS: Male gonadal dysfunction. *Clin Endocrinol Metab* 1985; 14:89.
Dunkel L, et al: GnRH and HCG tests are both necessary in differential diagnosis of male delayed puberty. *Am J Dis Child* 1985; 139:494.
Kletzky OA, et al: Help for the woman with

hirsutism. *Patient Care* 1985; 19(2):16.
Rule AH, et al: Use of beta-human chorionic gonadotropin in gestational aging. *Ann Clin Lab Sci* 1985; 15:428.
Schwartz FL, Flink EB: Hirsutism. *Postgrad Med* 1985; 77:81.
Dudley DKL, Black DM: Reliability of lecithin/sphingomyelin ratios in diabetic pregnancy. *Obstet Gynecol* 1985; 66:521.
Daughaday WH: Recognition of growth hormone secretory disorders. *JAMA* 1984; 251:2251.
Rock RC: Endocrinology of the fetoplacental unit: Role of estrogen assays. *Lab Med* 1984; 15:95.
Clemmons DR, Van Wyk JJ: Factors controlling blood concentration of somatomedin C. *Clin Endocrinol Metab* 1984; 13:113.
Wong T-W, Jones TM: Hyperprolactinemia and male infertility. *Arch Pathol Lab Med* 1984; 108:35.
Cartwright PS, DiPietro DL: Ectopic pregnancy: Changes in serum human chorionic gonadotropin concentration. *Obstet Gynecol* 1984; 63:76.
Franke HR: Plasma human chorionic gonadotropin disappearance in hydatidiform mole. *Obstet Gynecol* 1983; 62:467.
Boots LR, et al: Laboratory assessment of disappearance patterns of human chorionic gonadotropin from serum of patients with gestational trophoblastic disease. *Ala J Med Sci* 1983; 20:391.
Chihal HJ: Office gynecologic endocrinology. *Postgrad Med* 1982; 71:73.
Sampson JH, Alexander NJ: Semen analysis: A laboratory approach. *Lab Med* 1982; 13:219.
Amenta JS, Silverman SA: Amniotic fluid lecithin, phosphatidylglycerol, L/S ratio, and foam stability test in predicting respiratory distress in the newborn. *Clin Chem* 1983; 79:52.
Comerci GD: Diagnosis: Inhibited growth and delayed puberty. *Hosp Med* 1983; 14:138.
Huseman C: Endocrinologic evaluation of the short child. *Cont Ed Fam Phys* 1982; 16:55.
Frisch RE, et al.: Delayed menarche and amenorrhea of college athletes in relation to age at onset of training. *JAMA* 1981; 246:1559.
Stephenson SR, Weaver DD: Prenatal diagnosis: A compilation of diagnosed conditions. *Am J Obstet Gynecol* 1981; 141:319.
Keel BA: Cervical mucus analysis: A major component in evaluation of infertility. *Lab Med* 1981; 12:161.
Reindollar RH, McDonough PG: Etiology and evaluation of delayed sexual development. *Pediatr Clin North Am* 1981; 28:267.
Tho PT, McDonough PG: Gonadal dysgenesis and its variants. *Pediatr Clin North Am* 1981; 28:309.
Yannone ME: The problems of ambiguous external genitalia. *Cont Ed Fam Phys* 1980; 13:89.
Carlson HE: Gynecomastia. *New Engl J Med* 1980; 303:795.
Wilson JD, et al: The pathogenesis of gynecomastia. *Adv Intern Med* 1980; 25:1.
Yen SSC: Neuroendocrine regulation of the menstrual cycle. *Hosp Pract* 1979; 14(3):83.

31 Tests for Syphilis

Syphilis is caused by the spirochete *Treponema pallidum*. Clinical syphilis usually is subdivided into primary, secondary, latent, and tertiary (late) stages. The primary stage begins after an average incubation period of 3–6 weeks and is manifested by the development of a primary stage shallow ulcer, or chancre, near the site of infection. The time of appearance is variable, and the lesion often is inconspicuous and overlooked, especially in the female. The chancre usually heals. In classic cases, skin lesions and sometimes mucous membrane lesions develop about 4–6 weeks after appearance of a chancre, marking the secondary stage. After a few days or weeks, the secondary stage lesions disappear and the patient enters the latent stage. This lasts, on the average, 3–5 years. During this time, about one half of untreated patients apparently achieve spontaneous cure or at least do not develop further evidence of the infection. About 25% remain in a latent ("late latent") status, and the remaining 25% develop tertiary stage sequelae such as neurologic, cardiovascular, or ocular syphilis.

Diagnostic procedures in syphilis include dark-field examination, immunologic tests, and cerebrospinal fluid (CSF) examination, depending on the clinical situation.

DARKFIELD EXAMINATION

Darkfield is a wet-preparation method for direct visualization of living *T. pallidum* spirochetes in material from syphilitic lesions. A microscope with a special darkfield condensor is required. This condensor prevents light from passing directly through the slide being viewed into the microscope viewing lenses but instead forces the light to pass to the periphery of the slide. Objects on the slide reflect some light up into the viewing lenses, so the objects appear white on a dark background. Darkfield was the only way to make the laboratory diagnosis of syphilis before serologic tests were available. The usual indications for this test are suspected primary stage syphilitic lesions and any suitable secondary stage lesion. Darkfield examination may be the only way to make a diagnosis early in the primary stage, since immunologic test antibodies often do not appear until late in the primary stage. Obtaining the specimen without contamination by blood or surface bacteria is very important. The lesion should be cleansed thoroughly with water or 0.85% saline and a sterile gauze pad. No soap or antiseptics should be used. Care must be taken not to produce bleeding, since red blood cells (RBCs) will obscure the organisms. After the lesion is blotted dry, a clear serous exudate should accumulate in a few minutes. If it does not, the lesion may be abraded gently with gauze, but not enough to cause bleeding. The serous fluid exudate is drawn off in a pipette or capillary tube for examination with a darkfield microscope. The causative organism, *T. pallidum*, has a characteristic morphology and motility on dark-field examination, but experience is necessary for interpretation, since nonpathogenic varieties of spirochetes may be found normally in the genital areas. Darkfield examination by experienced personnel is no longer widely available in many areas because it is rarely ordered. If it is unavailable, a serologic test using the fluorescent treponemal antibody-absorbed (FTA-ABS) method could be substituted. However, the FTA-ABS test will miss 10%–20% of cases, with the possibility of error being greatest in the first week of the primary stage.

TABLE 31–1.

Types of Immunologic Syphilis Tests*

Specific	Cross-Reacting	Fortuitous
TPI	RPCF	Cardiolipin STS tests
FTA-ABS		
MHA-TP		

*TPI = *T. pallidum* immobilization; RPCF = Reiter protein complement fixation; STS = serologic test for syphilis; MHA-TP = microhemagglutination–*T. pallidum*.

IMMUNOLOGIC TESTS

Immunologic tests for syphilis depend on the fact that the diseases caused by infectious organisms are characterized by development of antibodies toward that organism. These antibodies may be specific or nonspecific (Table 31–1). Nonspecific antibodies may be either of the cross-reacting type (sharing a common antigen with another organism) or of the fortuitous type (provoked by some nonspecific portion of the organism).

CARDIOLIPIN TESTS

The first practical serologic test for syphilis (STS) was the complement fixation (CF) technique invented by Wassermann. He used extract from a syphilitic liver as the antigen that demonstrated the presence of antitreponemal antibodies. Subsequently it was found that the main ingredient of the substance he used actually had nothing to do with syphilitic infection and was present in other tissues besides liver. It is a phospholipid that is now commercially prepared from beef heart and therefore called cardiolipin. The present-day STS reagent is a mixture of purified lipoproteins that includes cardiolipin, cholesterol, and lecithin. Apparently, an antibody called "reagin" is produced in syphilis that will react with this cardiolipin-lipoprotein complex. Why reagin is produced is not entirely understood; it is not a specific antibody to *T. pallidum*. There is a lipoidal substance in spirochetes, and it is possible that this substance is similar enough to the cardiolipin-lipoprotein complex that antibodies produced against spirochetal lipoidal antigen may also fortuitously react with cardiolipin.

There are two basic types of STS procedures to detect reagin: CF and flocculation (agglutination) (Table 31–2).

Complement Fixation Reaction.—As mentioned earlier, the CF reaction was the procedure used by Wassermann. The original technique has been superseded by the Kolmer modification. There are several drawbacks when the CF test is used to detect reagin. The patient's serum may be anticomplementary (i.e., contain substances that bind and thus inactivate complement). The test takes 2 days to perform because the CF test is a two-stage procedure, and the second stage of the reaction must incubate overnight. Complement and sheep RBCs are among the reagents needed, and these readily deteriorate. Contamination of glassware may give anticomplementary results. The CF test is rarely used today.

Flocculation Reaction.—In earlier versions of the flocculation reaction the patient's serum was heated; for unknown reasons, heating seemed to enhance the reaction. Then a suspension of cardiolipin antigen particles is added to the serum and mixed. In a positive (reactive) test result, the reagin antibody in the patient serum will combine with the cardiolipin antigen particles, producing a microscopic clumping or flocculation of the antigen particles. The reaction is graded according to degree of clumping. The current standard procedure for this type of test is the Venereal Disease Research Laboratory (VDRL) test. It was found that the preliminary heating step could be eliminated if certain chemicals were added to the antigen, and this modification is called the rapid plasma reagin (RPR) test.

Drawbacks of the Cardiolipin Serologic Tests for Syphilis

Variation in Test Modifications.—Not all

TABLE 31–2.

Procedures for Serologic Tests for Syphilis

CF Tests	Flocculation Tests
Kolmer (modified Wassermann)	VDRL } Most widely used
	RPR } Most widely used
	Kahn
	Hinton
	Kline
	Mazzini

sera from known syphilitics gave positive reactions in these tests. It was discovered that the number of positives could be increased by altering the ratio of antigen ingredients. However, usually when the percentage of positive results increases significantly, more false positives are reported.

Effect of antibiotic therapy.—A peculiarity of the STS exists when antibiotic treatment is given. If the patient is treated early in the disease, the STS will revert to nonreactive state. In patients with primary syphilis, one study found that the VDRL or RPR returned to nonreactive state in 60% of patients by 4 months and 100% of patients by 12 months. In secondary syphilis, the VDRL became nonreactive in 12–24 months. Another study of patients with primary and secondary syphilis reported that successful treatment usually produced a fourfold decrease in VDRL titer by 3 months and an eightfold decrease by 6 months. The STS decline may be slower if the patient had other episodes of syphilis in the past. However, the longer the disease has been present before treatment, the longer the STS takes to become nonreactive. In many cases after the secondary stage it will never become nonreactive, even with adequate treatment (this is called "Wassermann fastness").

Spontaneous Loss of Test Reactivity.—In tertiary syphilis, there is a well-documented tendency for a previously reactive STS test result to revert spontaneously to nonreactive, even if the patient is untreated. This is reported to occur in about 20%–30% (literature range 5%–45%) of patients.

Biologic False Positive Reactions.—Some patients have definitely positive results on STS but just as definitely do not have syphilis or any exposure to it. These are called biologic false positive (BFP) reactions. The major known causes of BFP reactions can be classified under three headings:

1. Acute BFP reactions, due to many viral or bacterial infections and to many febrile reactions such as hypersensitivity or vaccination. These usually give low-grade or moderate (1 to 2+) STS reactions and return to normal within a few weeks.
2. Chronic BFP reactions, due to chronic systemic illness such as rheumatoid-collagen diseases, malaria, or chronic tuberculosis. There is also an increased incidence of BFP reactions in old age. Whereas there is less than 2% incidence of BFP reactions in men before the age of 60 years, some studies report an incidence as high as 9%–10% after age 70.
3. Nonsyphilitic treponemal diseases such as yaws or pinta.

Summary.—The cardiolipin STS is cheap, easy to do, and suitable for mass testing. Its sensitivity and specificity are adequate, and positivity develops reasonably early in the disease. Reagents are well standardized and reproducibility is good. Disadvantages are relatively poor sensitivity in primary syphilis, the tendency in late syphilis for spontaneous reversion of a reactive test result to a nonreactive result, and the problem of BPF reactions. To add further to the confusion, some patients with BFP reactions may have syphilis in addition to one of the diseases known to give BFP reactions. Because of this, everyone hoped for a way to use *T. pallidum* organisms themselves as antigen rather than depend on the nonspecific reagin system.

SPECIFIC *Treponema pallidum* TESTS

***Treponema pallidum* Immobilization (TPI) Test.**—Syphilitic spirochetes can grow in rabbits. Nelson devised a TPI test in which syphilitic spirochetes are incubated with the patient's serum. If specific antisyphilitic antibody is present, it will attack the spirochetes and immobilize them, causing them to stop moving when viewed under the microscope. This involves an antibody that is different from reagin and is specific against pathogenic *Treponema* spirochetes. Besides syphilis, other *Treponema* spirochetal diseases such as yaws may give positive reactions. The main disadvantages of this test are that it requires working with live spirochetes and use of an animal colony, is difficult to perform accurately, and is expensive. Antibiotics in serum kill the test spirochetes. Routine laboratories cannot perform the TPI using present techniques. The TPI test result can change with treatment, just as the STS procedure does. If the patient is treated early, the TPI test result will revert to negative; if the patient is treated late, it may remain permanently reactive. The TPI test is said to be positive in most patients with untreated tertiary syphilis (assuming good technique etc.), but there is a false negative rate of at least 5% and possibly as high as 10%. The TPI test has been replaced by the FTA-ABS and the MHA tests (to be discussed later), and it is now very difficult, almost impossible, to obtain a TPI study in the United States.

Reiter Protein Complement Fixation Test.—The TPI test is done using the Nichol strain of pathogenic spirochetes. It was discovered that a certain nonpathogenic *Treponema* spirochete called the "Reiter strain" could be cultured more easily and cheaply on artificial media. Antigen prepared from this organism was adapted to a CF technique, and the result was the RPCF test.

The Reiter antibody is different from the *Treponema*-immobilizing antibody of the TPI test. Apparently, the nonpathologic Reiter and the pathologic Nichol spirochete share a common protein antigen, and it is this protein that is used in the RPCF test. In addition, the Nichol organism has a specific antigen that results in the immobilizing antibody response of the TPI assay. Several investigators have found the RPCF test to be almost as sensitive and specific as the TPI test, although others are less enthusiastic about its sensitivity in late syphilis. The Reiter antibody also appears at a different time than does the TPI antibody. The disadvantages of the RPCF are those inherent in all CF tests. The RPCF test is practically never used in the United States.

Fluorescent Treponemal Antibody–Absorbed Test.—Fluorescent techniques have replaced the TPI test. Dead Nichol strain spirochetes are fixed to slides; those spirochete-containing slides can be prepared in the laboratory or obtained ready for use from commercial sources. The patient's serum is placed on the slide with the spirochetes and allowed to incubate with the organisms. Antispirochete antibody in the patient serum coats the surface of the spirochetes. The serum is then washed off and replaced by antibodies tagged with a fluorescent dye, which are produced by animals against human gamma globulin. Since human antibodies against syphilis produced after the first month of infection are gamma globulins, the antibodies against human gamma globulin, with the fluorescein dye attached, will attack and adhere to any patient antitreponemal antibody that coats the spirochetes on the slide. The spirochetes will then appear fluorescent when viewed with an ultraviolet microscope. This was known as the fluorescent treponemal antibody (FTA) test.

Unfortunately, fluorescent work is not as simple as this description or the recent literature would imply. Many technical problems remain. These tests at present are not suitable for mass screening, although they are less time-consuming than the RPCF test and easier than the TPI test. Many substances give varying degrees of natural fluorescence, and it is sometimes difficult to decide whether a preparation is actually positive or not. There may be nonspecific antigen-antibody binding of the cross-reacting type, as well as specific reaction. When the animal anti–human globulin antibody is conjugated with fluorescein, not all of the fluorescein binds to it. Any remaining free fluorescein may nonspecifically stain various proteins, including the spirochetes, when the tagged mixture is added to the patient's serum.

Because of the problem of nonspecific fluorescence, the FTA underwent modification to become the FTA test with absorption (FTA-ABS). Reiter *Treponema* antigen is used to absorb nonspecific cross-reacting antibodies out of the patient's serum. Antibody to *T. pallidum* is not absorbed out by this technique. The absorbed patient serum replaces nonabsorbed patient serum in the standard FTA procedure.

The FTA-ABS is a well-established test. It has relatively good sensitivity in primary syphilis (except in very early disease) and is reported to be even more sensitive than the TPI in tertiary syphilis. If the patient is treated adequately in the primary or secondary stage, the FTA-ABS response will usually return to nonreactive state, but after the secondary stage it usually will not become nonreactive in spite of therapy. It is said to be at least as specific as the TPI, possibly even more so.

Drawbacks.—Weak reactions may cause interpretation problems because of the way FTA-ABS results were reported. Official recommendations are that equivocal or 1+ reactive specimens should be repeated and the 1+ reclassified as borderline if the repeat test result is nonreactive. However, if a 1+ reactive serum result remains 1+ reactive when the test is repeated, for many years the rules of interpretation considered it to be reactive. Therefore, a physician who received a report that the FTA-ABS test result is reactive could not tell whether the degree of reactivity was weak (1+) or strong (2+ to 4+). This may be important, because there is some evidence that results on weakly reactive specimens sent to different laboratories may vary between nonreactive and reactive in a significant number of instances, and the physician has no way of knowing from the report which reactions are weak. For example, in one proficiency test study, 13% of participating laboratories reported borderline or reactive FTA-ABS results on specimens that the other 87% of laboratories considered nonreactive. On borderline specimens, about 30% of laboratories obtained different answers on retesting the same specimen. On specimens that most of the laboratories considered weakly reactive, about 20% reported other results (nonreactive, borderline, or more strongly reactive). Other studies have revealed a 5%–10% variance between laboratories. Thus, both false positive and false negative results may occur due to laboratory technical factors. This is much more likely to happen in weakly (1+) reactive specimens than on specimens with reactivity graded 2+ to 4+. Because of this, in 1984 the U.S. Centers for Disease Control recommended reporting a repeatable weak reaction as a 1+ reaction, rather than only as "reactive." However, some laboratories have not followed this recommendation.

No laboratory test is free from the possibility of error, and the FTA-ABS test is no exception. Occasional false positive FTA-ABS results have been reported in persons with hyperglobulinemia due to macroglobulins and in patients with antinuclear antibodies. In addition, atypical fluorescent patterns ("beaded") that could be misinterpreted as reactive have occurred in some patients with systemic lupus erythematosis. Problems of nonspecific fluorescence mentioned earlier have been reduced but not entirely eliminated. Occasional false negatives may occur even with the FTA-ABS test. One report suggests that concurrent infection by the HIV-I virus could sometimes delay or suppress the development of a positive VDRL or FTA-ABS reaction.

Microhemagglutination Test.—An MHA test is also available using formalin-treated RBCs coated with Nichol strain *T. pallidum* material. Patient serum is preabsorbed with Reiter *Treponema* reagent in the same manner as the FTA-ABS technique. Antibody to *T. pallidum* prevents normal RBC agglutination when the test is performed. About 1%–2% of sera contain nonspecific Forssman-type antibodies, so that reactive sera must be retested with nonsensitized control RBCs.

The MHA test is not as sensitive in primary syphilis as the FTA-ABS test, although it is reactive in more than 50% of patients. It seems equally as sensitive as the FTA-ABS test in secondary and possibly in late syphilis. Compared to FTA-ABS results, various studies have shown 90%–98% overall correlation. Our laboratory has performed a comparison of this type and found that nearly 85% of the disagreements represented either nonreactive or 1+ reactive MHA results and nonreactive or 1+ FTA-ABS results. Therefore, most disagreements seem to occur at low reactivity levels in which the accuracy of either test result is open to some question. This being the case, there is reason to conclude that the MHA could be substituted for the FTA-ABS, except possibly in primary syphilis (in which case an FTA-ABS test could be done if the MHA test results were nonreactive). The MHA test is much easier to perform than the FTA-ABS test and is less expensive.

SENSITIVITY AND SPECIFICITY OF SYPHILIS TESTS

The sensitivity and specificity of these tests should be discussed next. Sensitivity may be defined as the ability to detect syphilis or the percentage of positive (reactive) test results in patients with syphilis. Specificity refers to the ability of the test to be reactive only in syphilis or the percentage of positive results in persons who do not have syphilis (false positive reactions). Studies have been done in which duplicate samples from known syphilitic patients in various stages of their disease and also from normal persons were sent to various laboratories. Besides this, many reports have appeared from laboratories all over the world comparing one test with another in various clinical stages of syphilis, in nonsyphilitic diseases, and in apparently normal persons. These results are summarized in Table 31–3.

Table 31–3 demonstrates considerable variation in results. Several factors must be in-

TABLE 31–3.

Comparison of Serologic Tests for Syphilis (Approximate Percentage Reported Reactive)*

	STS	MHA	FTA-ABS
Primary	50–70 (48–96)	75–85 (50–95)	85–86 (80–91)
Secondary	98–100	99 (96–100)	99–100
Latent	75–100	–	95–96
Tertiary	60–75 (55–95)	96 (90–99)	97 (95–100)
Congenital	70 (66–95)	–	99–100
Normal	1.0 (0.5–10.0)	0.9 (0.0–3.0)	0.8 (0.0–1.0)
Nonsyphilitic disease†	5.0 (5–45)	–	1.5 (0.6–14)‡
Biologic false positive diseases§	20–45	1.5 (0–11)	1.5 (0–16)‡

*Numbers in parentheses indicate range from the literature.
†Miscellaneous nonspirochetal diseases; patients had no history or clinical evidence of syphilis.
‡FTA-ABS reactive, TPI nonreactive.
§Nonspirochetal diseases known to produce a high incidence of BFP reactions in the STS.

volved besides the inherent sensitivity and specificity of the individual tests themselves:

1. Antibiotic treatment may cause some previously reactive syphilitic patients to become nonreactive.
2. Some clinically normal persons may have unsuspected subclinical syphilis.
3. True BFP reactions, either acute or chronic, must be taken into account.
4. There is obvious variation in technique and ability between laboratories. Some laboratories introduce their own modifications into standard techniques.
5. The time of appearance differs for the various antibodies. In general, the FTA-ABS test result becomes positive in significant numbers of patients in the middle or end of the primary stage, followed by the MHA and RPCF, then the STS and finally the TPI. All of these procedures usually give positive results in the secondary stage, and also probably in the early latent stage.

SELECTION OF TESTS

The selection of tests for syphilis is dictated by the clinical situation. If the patient has possible primary syphilis, a darkfield examination would be helpful, although it is becoming difficult to find laboratories with the necessary equipment and laboratorians with sufficient expertise. If the darkfield test result is negative or cannot be performed, an FTA-ABS test should be done. If the FTA-ABS result is nonreactive and clinical suspicion is strong, the physician, for practical purposes, has the option of treating the patient without a conclusive diagnosis or of repeating the FTA-ABS test in 2–3 weeks.

If the patient has confirmed early syphilis, an STS result should nevertheless be obtained. If the STS result is reactive, the degree of reactivity should be titered, since a falling titer after treatment is evidence that treatment was effective.

If the patient has possible, equivocal, or late syphilis, an FTA-ABS (or MHA) and STS test should be done. If the FTA-ABS (or MHA) test result is reactive (2+ or more), the diagnosis is probable syphilis. If the FTA-ABS (or MHA) test result is weakly reactive (borderline or 1+ reactive), the test should be repeated in 1 month. If it is still weakly reactive, the diagnosis is possible or probable syphilis, depending on the clinical picture. The STS results are useful mainly as additional evidence in equivocal cases.

If a routine screening STS result is found to be positive in a person with no history or clinical evidence of syphilis, a confirmatory test should be done. If the confirmatory test result is negative, the patient should be screened for diseases known to cause a high incidence of BFP reactions. In this respect, a weakly positive STS result may be due only to an acute BFP etiology, and the STS result should be negative in 2–3 months. If the confirmatory test result is positive, past or present syphilis is a strong probability. Nevertheless, since even the confirmatory tests may occasionally produce a false positive (or false negative) reaction, in certain patients it may be necessary to repeat the confirmatory test.

CONGENITAL SYPHILIS

Congenital syphilis often gives a confusing serologic picture. Syphilitic infants usually have a positive STS reaction. Sometimes, however, these infants have a nonreactive STS result at birth, and the STS response may remain normal up to age 3 months before the titer begins rising. On the other hand, if the mother has a positive STS reaction, even though she was adequately treated, many infants will have a positive STS reaction due to passive transfer of maternal antibodies through the placenta. The same is true for the FTA-ABS test. To further confuse the picture, pregnancy is associated with an increased number of BFP reactions in the STS, and reportedly, on occasion, even with the FTA-ABS. If the mother was adequately treated before delivery, the infant's reactive STS will revert to nonreactive without treatment in approximately 3–4 months. Cord blood may cause problems in neonatal syphilis testing due to possible contamination with maternal blood or false negative results caused by interference from hemoglobin. A modification of the FTA-ABS test that is specific for IgM antibodies is reported to detect and diagnose most cases of congenital syphilis in the newborn. However, at least one report found as many as 10% false positive results and as many as 35% false negative results.

CENTRAL NERVOUS SYSTEM SYPHILIS

Central nervous system (CNS) syphilis can be diagnosed clinically or through tests on CSF. In two studies, cell counts were normal (< 5 cells) in 19%–62%, between 5 and 10 cells in 24%–69%, and more than 10 cells in 12%–14%. The majority of the cells were mononuclear in 60%–80% of the cases and polymorphonuclear in 20%–40% of the cases. Cerebrospinal fluid protein was normal in 14%–61% of patients, between 45 and 100 mg/dl in 34%–61%, and more than 100 mg/dl in 5%–25%. The VDRL test on CSF specimens was reactive in 54%–57% of the patients (literature range, 10%–70%). Serum VDRL test was reactive in 49%–86% of the patients. It was noted that before penicillin was discovered, CSF studies recorded much higher incidence and degree of abnormalities.

Central nervous system syphilis may also require serologic tests for diagnosis. The standard serologic tests for syphilis such as the VDRL usually, but not always, give positive results on peripheral blood specimens when they are positive on CSF. A lack of relationship is most often found in the tertiary stage, when the peripheral blood VDRL test result may revert to normal. Conversely, the CSF response is very often negative when the peripheral blood VDRL result is positive. Central nervous system syphilis usually is a tertiary form with symptoms appearing only after years of infection, and in many patients with syphilis the CNS is not clinically involved at all. Despite lack of clinical CNS symptoms, actual CNS involvement apparently is fairly common and often begins as early as the secondary stage, although the clinical symptoms, if they develop, are not seen until the tertiary stage years later. There is some evidence that concurrent infection by the HIV-I virus may increase the risk of active CNS syphilis. The best criteria of CNS disease activity are elevated CSF cell count and protein levels. A reactive CSF VDRL result indicates disease that has been present for a certain length of time, without necessarily being currently active. The CSF serology (STS) usually is normal in patients with BFP blood STS reactions. After adequate treatment CSF pleocytosis usually disappears within 3 months (range, 1.5-6 months). Cerebrospinal fluid protein elevation, however, may persist as long as several years.

The three most important forms of CNS lues are general paresis, tabes dorsalis, and vascular neurosyphilis. In general paresis, the CSF serology almost always is normal in untreated patients. In tabes dorsalis, the CSF serology is said to be abnormal in most early untreated patients, but may be normal in up to 50% of late or "burnt-out" cases. In vascular neurosyphilis, approximately 50% of results are abnormal.

The FTA-ABS response is nearly always reactive in peripheral blood when CSF shows some laboratory abnormality suggestive of neurosyphilis. The FTA-ABS response has been shown to be more frequently reactive than the VDRL when testing the CSF of patients with syphilis. Several studies reported 100% of patients with the diagnosis of CNS syphilis had a reactive CSF FTA-ABS response. However, a substantial number of patients who were asymptomatic and had normal CSF cell counts and protein also had a reactive CSF FTA-ABS response. Therefore, the U.S. Centers for Disease Control and an important segment of other investigators currently believe that a reactive CSF FTA-ABS response does not necessarily represent active CNS syphilis and that the clinical importance of a reactive FTA-ABS test on spinal fluid is uncertain when the cell count, protein, and spinal fluid VDRL results are normal. Based on their recommendations, the FTA-ABS test is usually not done on CSF, since there is no problem of BFP reactions in the spinal fluid STS (unless the CSF is contaminated with blood), and the peripheral blood FTA-ABS test is reactive in almost all cases of CNS syphilis. Unfortunately, there is currently no gold standard to determine which patients actually have CNS syphilis without reference to CNS laboratory tests.

BIBLIOGRAPHY

Fernandez-Guerrero ML, et al: The treatment of neurosyphilis in patients with HIV infection. *JAMA* 1988; 259:1495.

Hicks CB, et al: Seronegative secondary syphilis in a patient infected with the human immunodeficiency virus (HIV) with Kaposi's sarcoma. *Ann Intern Med* 1987; 107:492.

Siegel D, Washington AE: Syphilis: Updated approach to an old disease. *Postgrad Med* 1987; 81:83.

Hart G: Syphilis tests in diagnostic and therapeutic decision making. *Ann Intern Med* 1986; 104:368.

Dans PE, et al: Inappropriate use of the cerebrospinal fluid Venereal Disease Research Laboratory (VDRL) test to exclude neurosyphilis. *Ann Intern Med* 1986; 104:86.

Burke JM, Schaberg DR: Neurosyphilis in the antibiotic era. *Neurology* 1985; 35:1368.

Mascola L, et al: Congenital syphilis revisited. *Am J Dis Child* 1985; 139:575.

Brown ST, et al: Serological response to syphilis treatment. *JAMA* 1985; 253:1296.

Moyer NP, et al: Evaluation of the hemagglutination treponemal test for syphilis. *J Clin Microbiol* 1984; 19:849.

Beebe JL, Nouri NJ: Comparative evaluation of commercial fluorescent treponemal antibody-absorbed test kits. *J Clin Microbiol* 1984; 19:789.

Rathbun KC: Congenital syphilis. *Sex Trans Dis* 1983; 10(2):93.

Chang Y-W: A guideline to serologic tests for syphilis. *Diagn Med* 1983; 6(2):51.

Huber TW, et al.: Reactivity of microhemagglutination, fluorescent treponemal antibody absorption, Venereal Disease Research Laboratory, and rapid plasma reagin tests in primary syphilis. *J Clin Microbiol* 1983; 17:405.

Wormser GP: Serologic tests for syphilis: Assessment after 75 years' experience. *Lab Med* 1982; 13:20.

Goodhart GL, et al.: Blinded proficiency testing of FTA-ABS. *Arch Intern Med* 1981; 141:1045.

Dyckman JD, et al: Reactivity of microhemagglutination, fluorescent treponemal antibody absorption, and Venereal Disease Research Laboratory tests in primary syphilis. *J Clin Microbiol* 1980; 12:629.

Peter CR, et al: False positive reactions in the rapid plasma reagin-card, fluorescent treponemal antibody-absorbed, and hemagglutination treponemal syphilis serology tests. *J Clin Microbiol* 1979; 9:369.

Jaffe HW, et al: Tests for *Treponema* antibody in CSF. *Arch Intern Med* 1978; 138:252.

32 Laboratory Aspects of Cancer

Unfortunately, there is no laboratory test that will detect all cancer. There are, however, certain circumstances in which the laboratory may be of assistance. This chapter discusses laboratory tests used to detect cancer by organ or organ system. Some data on tumor metastasis to various organs are located in Table 36–31.

KIDNEY

Renal cell adenocarcinoma (hypernephroma) is about twice as frequent in males as in females. It occurs with about equal frequency in both kidneys. About 90% of cases occur after age 40, although more than 30 cases have been reported in children. About 80% of renal cell carcinomas are located in either the upper or the lower poles of the kidney.

Clinical Findings.—In renal cell adenocarcinoma, symptoms and urinary findings vary according to the location, size, and aggressiveness of the tumor. Renal carcinoma often causes hematuria (as does bladder carcinoma). Painless gross hematuria is the initial symptom in about 40% of patients and occurs with other symptoms in additional cases. These episodes are often intermittent and may be misdiagnosed as urinary tract calculus or infection. Flank pain is present in about 40% of patients, and about one third have a significant degree of weight loss. A mass is noticeable to the patient in about 10%–15% of cases and is palpable by the physician in about 50% of cases (Table 32–1). In addition, hypernephroma, on occasion, is a well-recognized cause of fever of unknown origin. It has rarely but repeatedly been associated with secondary polycythemia (about 3% of patients), although a large minority have anemia and the majority do not show hemoglobin abnormality (see Table 32–1). About 20% of patients have hypertension (range, 4%–38%). About 10% (range, 4%–28%) have no clinical symptoms suggestive of hypernephroma, and the tumor is discovered on intravenous pyelogram (IVP) performed for some other reason.

Laboratory Findings.—Hematuria, either gross or microscopic, is the most frequent abnormality, being detected at some time in about 60% of patients (range, 28%–80%). Unfortunately, most publications either do not differentiate between gross and microscopic hematuria or record gross hematuria only. In 38 patients with renal cell adenocarcinoma seen in my area, 39% had gross hematuria and an additional 27% had microscopic hematuria. Proteinuria may be present but is less frequent. About 30% of patients have a completely normal urinalysis on admission. The IVP is the most useful screening test for renal cell carcinoma and, if carefully done, will also detect many cases of carcinoma in the renal pelvis and ureters. Other procedures, such as kidney scanning or computerized tomography (CT), are also useful.

Other Procedures.—Once a space-occupying lesion is identified in the kidney, the question arises as to its nature. B-mode ultrasound, CT, and drip infusion tomography seem to be excellent methods of distinguishing a solid renal tumor from a renal cyst. However, there is coincidence of renal carcinoma and simple renal cyst in about 2%–3% (literature range, 2%–7%) of cysts explored. Selective renal an-

TABLE 32–1.
Some Clinical and Laboratory Findings in Renal Cell Adenocarcinoma (Hypernephroma)

	% Cases	% Reported Range
Clinical symptoms		
Flank pain	40–50	36–80
Weight loss	35	31–95
Fever	25	11–33
Gross hematuria	50	28–80
Laboratory findings		
Hematuria	60–80	
Anemia	25	20–50
Polycythemia	3	0.4–3.7
ESR increase	60	56–79
Alkaline phosphatase increase	15	10–21
Hypercalcemia	5	0–6

giography is also very effective and can be performed if tomography is inconclusive. No technique is infallible, however, since a few tumors may become exceptionally cystic due to internal necrosis. Urine cytology has relatively little value at present in the diagnosis of renal cell adenocarcinoma. Metastatic carcinoma or malignant lymphoma in the kidney usually does not produce significant clinical or urinary findings.

PROSTATE

Acid Phosphatase–Biochemical.—Prostatic carcinoma often may be detected chemically because normal prostatic tissue is rich in the enzyme acid phosphatase, and adenocarcinomas arising from the prostate often retain the ability to produce this enzyme. Acid phosphatase is actually a group of closely related enzymes that share certain biochemical characteristics. Members of this group are found in several tissues (e.g., kidney, bone, prostate, platelets, and spleen). For almost 30 years, standard biochemical methods were the only assay systems available for acid phosphatase. Since enzyme quantity cannot be measured directly by these systems, it is estimated indirectly by the amount of change the enzyme produces in a measured quantity of substrate (a substance that can be changed by action of the enzyme). Several different assay systems have evolved, each of which differs somewhat in sensitivity and specificity for acid phosphatase of prostate origin. This accounts for some (although not all) of the conflicting reports in the literature regarding ability of biochemical enzyme system assays for acid phosphatase to detect prostate carcinoma.

Studies have shown that about 5%–10% (literature range, 5%–15%) of patients with prostate adenocarcinoma confined to the prostate have elevated serum acid phosphatase levels. Elevation occurs in about 20%–25% (10%–56%) of patients with extension of prostate tumor outside the prostate capsule without distant metastases, and in about 75%–80% (47%–92%) of those with bone metastases.

False Positive Results.—Since acid phosphatase measurement is usually undertaken to detect prostate carcinoma, elevation in other conditions is usually considered to be a false positive result. Prostatic infarcts can temporarily elevate serum acid phosphatase levels. Acid phosphatase levels are reported to be elevated in about 5%–10% (0%–19%) of patients with benign prostatic hypertrophy without any evidence of carcinoma. Elevations have been reported in patients with several other diseases; patients with the most substantial percentage of abnormality include those with nonprostatic metastatic carcinomas to bone, certain metabolic bone diseases (Paget's disease, primary hyperparathyroidism), Gaucher's disease, and certain platelet disorders (thrombocytosis, disorders of platelet destruction). Alkaline and acid phosphatase are similar enzymes that differ predominantly in the pH at which they work best. Therefore, any condition that produces greatly increased alkaline phosphatase values may induce some elevation of acid phosphatase values because the ordinarily negligible action of the alkaline phosphatase at lower pH is magnified by a greatly increased quantity of enzyme.

There is controversy in the literature whether a rectal examination will temporarily (up to 24 hours) increase serum acid phosphatase levels. More investigators have reported no change than those who did find significant elevation, but the size of the two groups is not far apart. Therefore, the test probably should be repeated if elevated levels occur after a rectal examination. There is some evidence that elevated serum acid phosphatase values can fluctuate 25%–50% or even more during a 48-hour period.

Various methods have been used to decrease false positive results, some of which are more specific than others for prostatic acid phosphatase (see Table 36–30). However, none is completely specific. For example, it was found that various substances could inhibit either prostate or nonprostate acid phosphatase; the most widely used of these substances is L-tartrate, which inhibits prostatic acid phosphatase. Thus, acid phosphatase elevation that persists after patient serum is incubated with L-tartrate ("tartrate resistant") is likely to be of nonprostatic origin. Unfortunately, although tartrate inhibition does increase specificity, it does not produce complete specificity. Fortunately, in most situations where prostatic carcinoma is suspected, the majority of the nonprostatic conditions that produce elevated acid phosphatase levels would be unlikely (except for occult nonprostatic tumor involving bone).

False Negative Results.—Biochemical enzyme assays for acid phosphatase are heat and pH sensitive. Serum left at room temperature after exposure to air may exhibit significantly decreased activity after as little as 1 hour. The use of a preservative with prompt refrigeration is strongly recommended. Immunoassays can tolerate exposure of the sample to room temperature for 4–5 days.

Acid Phosphatase Immunoassay.—In the last half of the 1970s, methods were found to obtain antibodies against prostatic acid phosphatase. This enabled the development of immunoassays (radioimmunoassay [RIA], enzyme-linked immunosorbent assay [ELISA], and counterimmunoelectrophoresis) for determining prostatic acid phosphatase levels. In general, the immunoassays have greater specificity for prostatic acid phosphatase than biochemical enzyme procedures. The immunoassays also detect more patients with prostate carcinoma. Unfortunately, the tests uncover only about 10%–20% more patients with prostate carcinoma than the biochemical tests at comparable stages of tumor spread (Table 32–2). In addition, the immunoassays are not completely specific; for example, they become elevated in some cases of nonprostate carcinoma that is metastatic to bone. Many of the evaluations of test kits found that a certain number of patients with benign prostatic hypertrophy, without evidence of tumor, had elevated results. Moreover, there has been a very disturbing variation in sensitivity and specificity of the immunoassay kits. Another drawback is that immunoassays are three–five times more costly to perform than the biochemical enzyme methods.

Prostate-Specific Antigen (PSA).—Prostate-specific antigen is a glycoprotein enzyme that was isolated from prostate gland epithelial cells in 1979. There are claims that this enzyme is specific for prostate origin, although a few isolated instances of elevation in nonprostate tumors have been reported. Three manufacturers now have kits commercially available. Reports thus far agree that PSA detects more

TABLE 32–2.

Comparison of Biochemical and Immunologic Assays for Acid Phosphatase*

	% Abnormal		
Cancer Stage	Biochemical Enzyme Assays	RIA	PSA†
Clinical stage A (nonpalpable; no clinical symptoms)	6 (5–12)	15 (0–38)	55 (50–63)
Clinical stage B (palpable nodule; no evidence of metastasis or local spread)	15 (9–20)	30–35 (28–79)	75 (58–100)
Clinical stage C (local invasion by tumor without distant metastasis)	35 (29–52)	50 (24–79)	80–90 (68–100)
Clinical stage D (evidence of distant metastasis in bone, liver, or lymph nodes)	70–80 (60–87)	80–85 (60–92)	90 (74–100)
Benign prostatic hypertrophy (no evidence of carcinoma)	10–15 (0–19)	5–15 (0–33)	50–60 (10–83)
Nonprostatic carcinoma metastatic to bone	10–15 (0–17)	10–15 (6–80)	0–5

*Numbers represent average figures; parentheses enclose range of percentage values found in the literature. There is considerable variation in performance of different kits and methods within each of the two categories.
†PSA = prostate-specific antigen.

patients with prostate carcinoma than acid phosphatase by immunoassay or biochemical methods (see Table 32–2). Prostate carcinoma in stage A is detected in about 55% of cases. Overall prostate carcinoma detection is about 80%–90% (range, 75%–96%). Unfortunately, detection rate for patients with benign prostatic hypertrophy is about 50%–60% (range, 10%–83%). Since prostatic glandular hypertrophy is common in the same age group as prostate carcinoma, this has precluded use of present-day kits for screening and has limited the use of PSA to follow-up of prostate carcinoma after therapy. The half-life of PSA is about 2 days, and it has been calculated that there must be a delay of about 2 weeks after prostate surgery or even prostate needle biopsy before attempting to measure PSA.

Serum Alkaline Phosphatase.—Stage D prostate carcinoma metastasizes to bone in about 70% of patients (range, 33%–92%). More than 90% of these metastases have an osteoblastic component. Serum alkaline phosphatase levels are elevated in 70%–90% of cases.

GASTROINTESTINAL TRACT

Tumors of the Lower Gastrointestinal Tract.—Tumors of the lower gastrointestinal (GI) tract were discussed in chapter 25. Screening tests include rectal examination and examination of the stool for occult blood (see Table 25–3). Tumor anywhere in the GI tract, benign or malignant, frequently results in blood being present in the stool. Presence of blood may be obvious, although much more often it is detectable only with chemical tests. The most frequent malignancies arise in the colon and rectum, stomach, and the head of the pancreas. Some advocate sigmoidoscopy or even colonoscopy as a screening test for rectal and colon carcinoma in all persons over age 40.

Carcinoma of the Stomach.—Under the best conditions, x-ray examination (upper GI series) is said to be about 90% accurate in detection of gastric carcinoma. However, x-ray examination does not reveal the nature of the lesion. Gastroscopy is currently the best procedure for diagnosis, since instruments that allow visualization of most areas in the stomach and also permit biopsy are available. If gastroscopy is not available, gastric analysis for acid (after stimulation) may be helpful; achlorhydria considerably increases suspicion of carcinoma. Cytology of gastric washings is useful. However, gastric cytology is not as successful as cytology of specimens from uterine or even from pulmonary neoplasia, since small gastric tumors may not shed many neoplastic cells, and interpretation of gastric Papanicolaou smears in general is more difficult. Gastric aspiration specimens for cytology should be placed in ice immediately to preserve the cells.

Carcinoids.—Carcinoids are relatively uncommon tumors found mainly in the GI tract, although a minority are located in the lungs and a few arise in other locations. The appendix is the most frequent site of origin; these are almost always benign (Table 32–3). Carcinoids are next most frequent in the terminal ileum and colon; these are frequently malignant. Carcinoids are considered part of the amine precursor uptake and decarboxylation (APUD) system, composed of cells derived from embryonic neuroectoderm that migrate from the primitive neural crest. These cells are located in embryonic GI tract derivatives, which include the GI tract, GI tract accessory glands (pancreas, biliary system), and organs with a very early embryonic GI source (lungs, thymus, genitourinary tract). They potentially can synthesize and secrete most body hormones (amines or peptides) except for steroids. Carcinoid cells contain fluorogenic amine substances and in certain areas characteristically contain secretory granules or material that stains with silver (argentaffin or argyrophilic). Gastrointestinal carcinoid cells are considered to be derived from Kulchitsky's cells of GI epithelium.

Intestinal carcinoids may be multiple (see Table 32–3) and frequently are associated with noncarcinoid malignancies (about 30% of cases, literature range, 7%–38%).

Carcinoid Syndrome.—Carcinoids typically produce the vasoconstrictor substance serotonin, which induces several of the symptoms that are part of the carcinoid syndrome (Table 32–4). Carcinoids arising in foregut derivatives (bronchus, stomach, pancreas, duodenum, biliary tract) may produce the carcinoid syndrome and may be associated with the multiple endocrine neoplasia type I (MEN I) syn-

TABLE 32–3.
Effect of Origin Site on Carcinoid Tumors*

Carcinoids: Primary Site	% Frequency	% Malignant	% Multiple	% Carcinoid Syndrome Cases
Appendix	45 (20–60)	3 (0–25)	1	1
Ileum	28 (11–29)	35 (17–60)	28–33	60
Rectum	15 (9–25)	12 (12–41)	9	Rare
Cecum (and colon)	5 (2–11)	60 (57–100)	–	4
Stomach	3 (2–6.5)	17 (14–50)	6	6
Duodenum	5 (0.9–13)	25 (16–66)	–	4
Bronchus	10 (5–20)	10 (2–51)	–	6
Ovary	Uncommon	Uncommon	–	12
Other (thymus, biliary tract, Meckel's diverticulum)	Uncommon	20–30	–	–

*Data represent approximate percentage of cases; parentheses enclose range found in the literature.

drome (with parathyroid, pituitary, and pancreatic islet cell tumors). These carcinoids usually do not stain with silver methods. Carcinoids of midgut origin (jejunum, ileum, appendix, and right side of the colon) typically are silver positive, and the jejunum and ileum are the most frequent source of the carcinoid syndrome. Carcinoids of hindgut origin (left side of the colon, rectum, and anus) usually do not have stainable argentaffin granules and usually do not produce the carcinoid syndrome.

When carcinoid cells produce serotonin, in most cases the venous drainage of the tumor is routed through the liver, which metabolizes or alters the hormone and prevents the carcinoid syndrome. If liver metastases develop in sufficient quantity or location, serotonin from carcinoid tumor in the liver bypasses hepatic portal vein drainage into the liver and exerts its effect unaltered. The same thing occurs with bronchial and ovarian carcinoids, because their venous drainage does not enter the hepatic portal vein system. Most carcinoids that produce the carcinoid syndrome originate in the intestine, and the syndrome usually does not appear until there is extensive metastasis by the carcinoid to the liver. However, the syndrome may occur without liver metastasis, especially when the primary site is the ovary. Conversely, in one third to two thirds of patients, liver metastases develop without the carcinoid syndrome.

Urine 5-Hydroxyindoleacetic Acid Assay.—Diagnosis of carcinoid syndrome can usually be made by testing for abnormal urine levels of 5-hydroxyindoleacetic acid (5-HIAA), the chief metabolic breakdown product of serotonin. Interestingly, there is very little specific information in the literature regarding the incidence of 5-HIAA elevation in either the carcinoid syndrome or in carcinoid patients without the carcinoid syndrome. In three studies of carcinoid patients (some with and some without the carcinoid syndrome), incidence of elevated urine 5-HIAA levels in those patients assayed was about 65% (range, 60%–87%). References that mention incidence of elevated 5-HIAA levels usually state that most patients with the malignant carcinoid syndrome have elevated 5-HIAA levels. However, some patients do not have continually elevated values; and in some cases repeated specimens may be necessary. Some patients with carcinoid may have elevated urine 5-HIAA levels without

TABLE 32–4.
Carcinoid Syndrome

Carcinoid Syndrome	Approximate %
Acute	
Cutaneous flush (red or cyanosis)	80
Diarrhea	75
Asthma	25
Abdominal "crisis"	Uncommon
Chronic	
Hepatomegaly	70
Cardiac lesions (right-sided valve fibrosis)	50
Spontaneous fibrosis	Uncommon
Pellagra	Uncommon

manifestations of the carcinoid syndrome; how often this happens is not known. Certain foods may elevate urine 5-HIAA levels (see chapter 36). A few conditions, such as nontropical sprue and Whipple's disease may produce mildly elevated urinary 5-HIAA in some patients. One study found that a few carcinoid patients with normal or only slightly elevated urine 5-HIAA had elevated urine serotonin (5-hydroxytryptamine). However, serotonin assay is difficult and expensive.

BREAST

Mammography.—Until 1960 diagnosis of mammary carcinoma depended on discovery of a breast mass by physical examination, followed by a biopsy of the lesion. It has been said that, with experience, carcinoma as small as 1 cm may be regularly detected by palpation. After 1960, x-ray study of the breast (mammography) began to receive considerable attention. Several favorable reports have been published, and several mass screening surveys have been attempted. To date, available information on the status of mammography includes the following:

1. Breast carcinoma can be visualized on mammography in some cases (23%–42%) in which it is not palpable. Reports indicate that 9%–42% of visualized nonpalpable lesions are malignant, with an incidence of lymph node metastasis of 0%–38%.
2. Screening surveys utilizing mammography are reporting detection of two–three times the expected rate of breast carcinoma.
3. Proper technique is of the utmost importance; this calls for special training and conscientious technicians.
4. Mammography is definitely not infallible. The average good radiologist will probably miss a malignant diagnosis in about 15% of cases (range, 4%–44%) and call a benign lesion malignant in about 5%–10% (range, 4%–15%). Reported incidence of palpable lesions not visualized on mammography ranges from 5%–20%. Biopsy or some other type of tissue diagnosis is still essential for all breast lesions.
5. Mammography is best in the postmenopausal or large breast where fatty tissue predominates. In these circumstances, probably 80%–90% of malignant tumors can be diagnosed correctly, whereas the figure decreases to 55% for women under age 45 years.
6. Mammography is useful for indicating the site for biopsy when several breast masses are present, for demonstrating unexpected additional foci of tumor elsewhere in the breast, and for detecting unsuspected tumor in the opposite (contralateral) breast. Mammography has demonstrated simultaneous tumor in the contralateral breast in 2%–3% of patients and eventual development of contralateral breast carcinoma in 6%–8% of patients. However, not all such tumors are detected by mammography. Pathology studies on mastectomy specimens have disclosed multiple foci of carcinoma in the same breast in 20%–30% of cases (literature range, 13%–75%), and biopsies of the contralateral breast have detected invasive carcinoma in about 1%–2% (0.5%–16%) and lobular carcinoma in situ in about 20%–30% (10%–53%).
7. At present, mammography is not an ideal screening procedure, because only a limited number of satisfactory studies can be performed daily under present conditions in the average radiology office.

Radionuclide Bone Scan.—When the diagnosis of breast cancer is first made or suspected, the question may arise as to which tests provide useful information that might influence type or extent of treatment. Bone scan detects lesions on initial workup in about 5% of clinical stage I lesions (literature range, 0%–30%), about 10% of clinical stage II lesions (0%–43%), about 8% of combined stage I and II lesions (1%–40%), about 25% of clinical stage III lesions (0%–62%), and about 15% of all lesions (4%–48%). Also, about one half of patients with solitary bone scan abnormalities have no demonstrable tumor at the abnormal site, the scan changes being due to benign abnormalities of bone. The incidence of overall false positive scan findings in patients with breast carcinoma is about 10% (3%–57%). About 10% (4%–33%) of breast carcinoma metastases to bone seen on x-ray film will be missed by bone scan, because breast carcinoma produces a relatively high number of osteolytic lesions, which are not as frequently seen with radionuclides as osteoblastic lesions. Bone scan detects about 20% (10%–40%) of metastases not seen on x-ray film. The small amount of information available on results of initial-visit brain scanning suggests that fewer than 5% will be abnormal if there are no neurologic signs or symptoms. Surprisingly few data are available on the contribution of liver scan to initial (pretherapy) workup, but one study found that liver scan yielded only 1% true positive results.

Fine-Needle Aspiration.—Another diagnostic modality is fine-needle (22-gauge) aspiration of breast masses with cytologic examination of the aspirate. Studies have shown about 1% (range, 0%–3%) false positive results and about 5%–10% (range, 0%–24%) false negative results. The procedure gives excellent results when the person doing the aspiration and the cytologist are experienced. Reliable interpretation requires special training. A definite cytologic diagnosis of malignancy is much more helpful than a diagnosis of benignity due to the significant rate of false negative results. Whether this procedure should replace surgical biopsy with frozen section is controversial. In cases where the patient refuses biopsy, when surgery cannot be performed, or when the lesion is cystic, there is not the same controversy.

Estrogen Receptor Assay.—Estrogen receptor assay (ERA) is widely used as an aid in selection of breast cancer therapy. It has been shown that approximately 30%–40% of postmenopausal breast cancer patients respond to ovariectomy, adrenalectomy, hypophysectomy, or estrogen therapy. Premenopausal patients respond less frequently. Certain tissues, such as endometrium, vagina, and breast, have been shown to respond to estrogen stimulation of estrogen receptor sites within their epithelial cells. Estrogen receptor assay techniques most frequently used involve tissue slices or cytoplasm (cytosol) extracts from the tumor to be evaluated. Radioactive estradiol and another estrogen-binding substance are added, and the tumor estrogen receptors compete with the estrogen binder for the labeled estradiol. The amount of labeled estradiol bound by the tumor estrogen receptors can then be determined. This type of assay is an estimate of the number of unoccupied ("active") estrogen-binding sites. Immunoassays of several types are also becoming available. This technique estimates total quantity of estrogen receptors, including both active and inactive receptors. According to current information, about 60%–65% (literature range, 30%–80%) of primary breast carcinomas and about 45%–50% of breast carcinoma metastases have tumor cells with estrogen receptors that bind sufficient estrogen per unit of cancer tissue to be considered estrogen receptive, or "positive." Estrogen receptor assay positivity does not show satisfactory correlation with presence or absence of lymph node involvement or the degree of differentiation of the tumor. Breast carcinomas in postmenopausal women are more likely to have estrogen receptors than those in premenopausal women. About 60%–70% of women whose tumors are estrogen-receptor positive respond to hormonal manipulation (estrogens, antiestrogens, endocrine ablation, or androgens). About 5%–10% of those considered ERA negative will respond (some laboratories report < 5%). Thus, a negative ERA result is interpreted by many as an indication that chemotherapy is more likely to be effective than endocrine therapy. In general, metastases tend to share the same type of receptor status as the primary tumor. However, some investigators report that metastases from estrogen-treated primary tumors are frequently receptor negative.

Certain laboratory aspects of the test are important. There are several techniques for preparing tissue for the receptor assay, and some of the techniques differ significantly in the number of patient tumors that demonstrate apparently increased receptors. At present, it is necessary to secure at least 1 gm of tumor after eliminating all fat and normal breast tissue. The tumor must be fresh and must be frozen by dry ice within a short time (preferably within 15 minutes) after excision. The specimen must be kept on dry ice and sent to the reference laboratory on dry ice. The estrogen receptors are very labile, and failure to quick-freeze and provide adequate low temperatures produces false negative results. In addition, quality control surveys have shown considerable variation among laboratories in ability to detect low concentrations of estrogen receptors.

As the description of this test indicates, with present-day techniques the procedure is partially a bioassay and therefore is available only at larger institutions or reference laboratories.

Progesterone Receptor Assay.—Progesterone receptors can be assayed (PRA) on the same tumor tissue in a manner similar to estrogen receptors. In general, demonstration that a breast carcinoma is PRA positive adds about

10%–15% more likelihood to ERA positivity that the tumor will respond to hormonal manipulation. Thus, tumors that are both estrogen- and progesterone-receptor positive have about a 70%–80% chance of responding to hormonal therapy. Those negative for both receptors have less than a 10% chance of responding to hormones or antihormones. Eighteen percent to 49% of patients are ERA positive but PRA negative and have about a 30% chance of responding. Three percent to 13% of patients are ERA negative and PRA positive.

Immunocytochemical Estrogen Receptor Methods.—Several investigators have developed immunologic methods to visually demonstrate presence or absence of estrogen receptors in cells within fixed tissue microscopic sections or cytology smears. Although true receptor quantitation cannot be done, this technique permits visualization of receptor distribution; that is, how many tumor cells are visually positive or negative. Many carcinomas do not have a cell population that is uniformly estrogen receptor positive or negative. Studies to date have reported about 80%–85% (range, 60%–90%) correlation with standard ERA results.

UTERUS

Cervix.—The mainstay of screening for uterine carcinoma is the Papanicolaou smear. For Papanicolaou examination of the cervix, material is best obtained directly from the cervix by some type of scraping technique. Vaginal irrigation or vaginal pool smears are reported to be only 50%–75% as accurate as cervical scrape for detection of cervical carcinoma. A single scrape smear has a false negative rate of about 30% (literature range, 5%–50%). Some reports indicate that the false negative rate can be reduced by one half or more by obtaining two successive cervical scrape specimens at the same examination or by obtaining both a cervical scrape specimen and an endocervical aspiration or endocervical swab specimen (making another smear with the endocervical specimen, either on the same slide as the scrape material or on another slide). Care should be taken not to contaminate the cervix area with water or lubricating jelly, both of which distort the tissue cells.

The most significant changes in cervix cytology in the 1980s are the histologic classification of cervix abnormality using the cervical intraepithelial neoplasia (CIN) system instead of degrees of dysplasia, and the change in management of Papanicolaou smears formerly classified as class II (on a scale of I–V). The CIN classification is similar to the previous dysplasia system but avoids having to differentiate severe dysplasia from carcinoma in situ (by combining both into the category CIN III) and by putting more emphasis on treatment of lesser degrees of involvement of cervical epithelium (CIN I). Class II Papanicolaou smears were originally defined as containing one or more cells with "atypical cytology, but not suspicious for malignancy" (i.e., only small or minor atypical nuclear changes). Some of these changes were often associated with inflammation. For a long time the class II "nonspecific inflammatory" Papanicolaou smears were thought to be benign and were often disregarded. Reevaluation of this category by culposcopic biopsy has disclosed a substantial number of patients (12%–25%) with CIN of varying degree, including CIN III. Papanicolaou findings of mild or borderline atypia or dyskaryosis, some of which would have been included in class II Papanicolaou category, have an even higher incidence of cervical CIN abnormality. In the past, if a patient had a class II Papanicolaou smear, the physician would follow the patient with periodic cytology specimens. However, an increasing number of investigators point toward substantial false negative rates on repeat cytology (similar to false negative inital cytology, noted earlier) and recommend culposcopy after the first abnormal Papanicolaou result regardless of the degree of abnormality.

Considerable evidence has accumulated linking cervical infection by human papillomavirus, predominantly types 16 and 18, with cervical epithelial cell atypia, premalignant changes, and progression to carcinoma.

Endometrium.—Screening for endometrial carcinoma can be done using endometrial suction biopsy, endometrial aspiration for cytology, endometrial washing methods, endometrial brushing, and cytology specimens taken from the endocervix or vaginal pool. Endometrial sampling methods are somewhat difficult to evaluate due to a considerable number of methods that can vary in detection rate but that are frequently lumped together in the literature. Endometrial biopsy using the Vabra aspirator generally is reported to detect about 96% (literature range, 80%–100%) of endometrial carcinomas. Endometrial biopsy with the Novak suction curette has been reported to detect about 91% of cases (range, 77%–94%). Endometrial cavity aspiration for cytology with a device known as the Isaacs cell sampler detects about 92%–94% of cases (range, 78%–100%). The Gravlee cell wash (endometrial lavage) technique detects about 80%–85% of cases (range, 66%–100%). Endometrial mechanical cell dislodgement methods, such as the MiMark and Endopap devices, are reported to detect more than 90% of carcinomas. Endometrial brush methods (another way to dislodge cells mechanically) are reported to detect 57%–92% of cases. In methods depending predominantly on cytology, hyperplasias and abnormalities other than tumor are not as easily identified as they can be with tissue specimens provided by biopsy. Endocervical aspiration detects endometrial carcinoma in about 70% of cases (range, 14%–90%). Smears from the vaginal pool in the posterior fornix of the vagina detect 30%–50% of cases (range, 18%–90%). Specimens from the cervix detect only about 35% (range, 25%–55%) of advanced endometrial carcinoma.

Follow-up of Abnormal Papanicolaou Smear.—Abnormal or definitely positive Papanicolaou smears should be followed up with a biopsy of the site indicated to confirm the diagnosis and determine the extent and histologic characteristics of the neoplasm. For the cervix, colposcopic examination with biopsy is becoming the most widely used technique. For the endometrium, dilation and curettage should be done.

Placental Neoplasms.—Hydatidiform mole and choriocarcinoma were discussed in the section on tests in obstetrics in chapter 30.

OVARY

Cancer Antigen 125.—The cancer antigen 125 (CA 125) test uses an antibody against antigen from tissue culture of an ovarian tumor cell line. Various published evaluations report sensitivity of about 75%–80% in patients with ovarian carcinoma. There is also an appreciable incidence of elevated values in nonovarian malignancies and in certain benign conditions (Table 32–5). Test values may transiently increase during chemotherapy.

TABLE 32–5.
CA 125 in Various Conditions

Malignant
Epithelial ovarian carcinoma, 75%–80% (range, 25%–92%) (better in serous than mucinous cystadenocarcinoma)
Endometrial carcinoma, 25%–48% (2%–90%)
Pancreatic carcinoma, 59%
Colorectal carcinoma, 20% (15%–56%)
Endocervical adenocarcinoma, 83%
Squamous cervical or vaginal carcinoma, 7%–14%
Lung carcinoma, 32%
Breast carcinoma, 12%–40%
Lymphoma, 35%
Benign
Cirrhosis, 40%–80%
Acute pancreatitis, 38%
Acute peritonitis, 75%
Endometriosis, 88%
Acute PID, 33%
Pregnancy 1st trimester, 2%–24%
During menstruation (occasionally)
Renal failure (? frequency)
Normal persons, 0.6%–1.4%

Cancer antigen 125 has been advocated to monitor patients for recurrence of ovarian carcinoma after initial surgery, similar to the use of carcinoembryonic antigen (CEA) after surgery for colon carcinoma. With both CA 125 and CEA there are sufficient normal results (at least 20%) in patients with cancer and sufficient abnormal results in other tumors and in benign conditions to preclude use of the test to screen for tumor under most circumstances. Studies in patients after therapy showed that up to 90% of patients with persistent CA 125 elevation after surgery had residual tumor, and that nearly all patients with rising titers had recurrent disease, but 50%–61% of patients with normal levels also had recurrent or persistent tumor. Therefore, only a change from normal to abnormal or a rising titer is significant. In one study an increase in titer preceded clinical evidence of metastasis or recurrence by an average of 3 months (range, 1–11 months).

LUNG

Chest X-ray Films.—Chest x-ray films have been the usual means of detecting lung cancer. Unfortunately, best results are obtained from the less common peripheral lesions rather than the more usual bronchogenic carcinomas arising in major bronchi. In general, chest x-ray films are not an efficient means of early diagnosis, and this is especially true for the miniature films used in mass survey work.

Sputum Cytology.—Sputum cytology is generally considered more sensitive than x-ray films, although some studies detected about equal numbers of asymptomatic tumor with either technique. Sputum cytology yield increases if the patient is a smoker and has symptoms such as chronic cough, hemoptysis, or recurrent pneumonia. Sputum samples for cytology should be obtained once daily (before breakfast and after rinsing the mouth with water) for at least 3 days. The material should be from a "deep cough"; saliva is not adequate. Many cytopathologists recommend expectoration directly into a bottle containing a special fixative (e.g., 50% ethanol, with or without additives). This type of specimen cannot be used for bacterial culture. In patients who do not have a productive (sputum-producing) cough, aerosol induction of sputum has been recommended. Some investigators achieved better results with a 3-day collection period than with aerosol inducement when several deep-cough specimens per day were expectorated directly into sputum cytology fixative. Twenty-four-hour collections without fixative are not recommended due to cell disintegration. A good specimen is the key to success in pulmonary cytology, because tumor cells may not be present continuously, because upper respiratory tract material usually does not reflect lower respiratory tract disease, and because pulmonary cytologic interpretation is more difficult than with uterine material.

Sensitivity of various diagnostic methods for lung cancer is not always easy to determine from the literature. The detection rate of carcinoma in asymptomatic persons (occult carcinoma) is naturally lower than in patients who have symptoms. For sputum cytology, better results are found if detection rates are used ("definitely positive" plus "suspicious" diagnoses) rather than only positive diagnoses. Unfortunately, it is often not clear which reporting method is being used. There is no question that more than one sputum sample, each sample being obtained on different days, significantly increases diagnostic yield (Table 32–6). Aerosol inducement of sputum also increases diagnostic yield (by about 20%–30%). There is a difference in detectability of central lesions (higher sputum cytology sensitivity) vs. peripheral lung lesions (lower sputum sensitivity). For that reason, squamous cell carcinoma is more readily detectable by sputum cytology (literature range, 58%–85%), due to its tendency for proximal bronchus origin, than adenocarcinoma (10%–57%), which tends to be peripherally located. Small cell undifferentiated carcinoma has intermediate detectability (30%–70%).

Bronchoscopy.—Bronchoscopy is reported to detect about 70%–80% of cases (45%–90%), with better detection of central vs. peripheral lesions and with better results from direct biopsy of visible lesions vs. bronchial washings, brushings, or blind biopsy. Percutaneous needle biopsy of lung tumors visible on x-ray film is reported to verify about 65%–70% of cases (48%–90%). Scalene node biopsy detects about 10% of cases (5%–21%). Mediastinoscopy with mediastinal node biopsy is reported to provide the only preoperative tissue evidence of carcinoma in 7%–20% of cases.

When cytologic material is obtained by bronchoscopy, saline is often used for bronchial washings. It is essential to use some type of "physiologic" saline rather than "normal" saline; contrary to common belief, the two are not identical. Normal saline (0.85% sodium chloride [NaCl]) can produce cellular artifact if the slides are not prepared within 5 minutes after collection. Physiologic saline is a bal

TABLE 32–6.

Sensitivity of Sputum Cytology in Primary Lung Carcinoma

No. of Specimens	Approximate % Detected
1	40–45
2	55
3	70–80
5	80–85
Overall literature range for sputum cytology	55–65 (40–95)

anced salt preparation with other minerals besides NaCl.

Radionuclide Scans.—When the diagnosis of lung cancer is first made, the question frequently arises as to which tests might help delineate extent of disease and thus establish operability. Bone scan is reported to detect lesions in approximately 35%–45% of patients, the frequency correlating roughly with clinical stage of the disease. However, a smaller number of those who are asymptomatic have an abnormal bone scan (14%–36%) and some of these abnormalities may not be due to metastasis. Brain scans have produced as many as 14%–20% positive results, but most studies found less than 6% were positive if there were no neurologic signs or symptoms. Initial workup liver scans disclose 13%–19% of abnormal results but less than 6% when there is no laboratory or physical examination evidence of liver metastases.

Computerized Tomography.—Computerized tomography has been very useful to determine operability by visualizing the size and location of the lesion, the presence of thoracic metastases, and the size of the mediastinal lymph nodes.

PANCREAS

The three most important pancreatic tumors are carcinoma of the exocrine pancreas (pancreatic adenocarcinoma of duct origin), islet cell tumors producing insulin (insulinoma), and islet cell tumors producing gastrin (gastrinoma) associated with the Zollinger-Ellison (Z-E) syndrome. Of these, insulinoma is discussed in chapter 27.

Exocrine Adenocarcinoma.—Carcinoma of the pancreas as a descriptive term usually refers to an adenocarcinoma of the exocrine pancreatic ducts, which comprises 90%–95% of pancreatic carcinomas. At the time of diagnosis about 65% are located in the head of the pancreas, about 20% in the body, about 5% in the tail, and about 10% are relatively diffuse. At the time of initial diagnosis, pain (usually abdominal) is present in about 75% of patients, weight loss in 50%–60%, bowel symptoms in 20%–30%, an abdominal mass in 5%–50%, and thrombophlebitis or thromboembolism (traditionally highly associated with pancreatic carcinoma) in 5%–10% (more common with body or tail lesions). At the time of diagnosis there is said to be local invasion or lymph node spread in about 25% of cases and distant metastases in about 60% (although literature ranges for distant metastases vary widely, depending on whether the metastases are overt or occult).

Laboratory findings include anemia in 25%–50% of cases, stool occult blood in as many as 50% of tumors in the pancreatic head, fasting hyperglycemia in about 20%, and oral glucose tolerance test abnormality in about 50% (literature range, 20%–81%, depending on criteria used). Jaundice is present in about 65% (seen in 45%–95% of pancreatic head tumors but much less common in those from the body and tail). Alkaline phosphatase level is elevated in most patients with jaundice and about one third of those without jaundice. Serum amylase level is elevated in only about 10% of patients.

Cancer antigen 19-9 (CA 19-9) and CEA levels are elevated in a substantial percentage of patients with pancreatic carcinoma. However, at least 10%–20% of patients have normal levels of these tumor markers, and levels of both markers are elevated in a significant percentage of other tumors and nonmalignant conditions. Therefore, neither test is currently being widely used for screening, diagnosis, or therapy of pancreatic carcinoma. Additional information is located in chapter 35.

Upper GI series is reported to be about 50% sensitive alone and about 80% sensitive with hypotonic duodenography for detecting carcinoma of the pancreas head. Duodenal tube drainage with secretin stimulation has an overall sensitivity of 30% (literature range, 10%–90%), which is increased to 50% (20%–84%) when cytologic study is performed on the pancreatic duodenal secretions. Ultrasound has overall sensitivity of 80% (68%–94%), with about 10%–15% of the studies attempted being technically unsatisfactory. Computerized tomography scan averages about 80% overall sensitivity (60%–92%), with average sensitivity probably even better with the newest-generation scanners. Endoscopic retrograde choledochopancreatography (ERCP, chapter 26) is 80% sensitive (54%–96%), whereas ERCP combined with duct aspiration cytology is reported to be 85% sensitive. Endoscopic retrograde choledochopancreatography technical failures occur in about 15%–20% of cases. Selective angiography (celiac and superior mesenteric artery) detects 60% of carcinomas, whereas catheterization of pancreatic vessels ("superselective angiography") may detect about 90%. Percutaneous transhepatic cholangiography is occasionally needed when jaundice is present and the other methods fail to yield a diagnosis or cannot be used.

Zollinger-Ellison Syndrome.—The Z-E syndrome is caused by a gastrin-producing nonbeta islet cell (G-cell) tumor of the pancreas (gastrinoma). There are multiple tumors in 70% of cases (literature range, 55%–80%). Two thirds (range, 60%–100%) of the tumors are malignant. Most gastrinomas originate in the pancreas, but occasionally they are found in an "ectopic" location (alone or in addition to the pancreas). Thus, about 10%–13% occur in the duodenum, and, rarely, they may arise in the stomach. Within the pancreas, the majority are in the head or the tail. Their microscopic appearance is similar to that of an insulinoma or carcinoid. About 10%–40% of patients with gastrinomas also have other endocrine tumors (most commonly a parathyroid adenoma); and association with the MEN I syndrome is fairly common.

The major components of the Z-E syndrome are listed in Table 32–7. Approximately 50%–60% of Z-E syndrome ulcers (31%–75%) are located in the proximal duodenum, which is the usual site for peptic ulcers; 25% (range, 20%–42%) are found in the distal duodenum or the jejunum; and 10% (range, 8%–15%) are found in the stomach. Multiple ulcers occur in 10%–20% of patients. About 10% (range, 7%–15%) have no ulcer. Diarrhea is found in 30%–35% of patients (range, 16%–75%). The degree of diarrhea is variable, but severe chronic diarrhea with hypokalemia is typical. Diarrhea is the only symptom of the Z-E syndrome in 7%–10% of cases. Steatorrhea occurs in 40% of cases (range, 38%–66%). However, many patients initially present with symptoms very similar to ordinary peptic ulcer without the classic features of Z-E syndrome.

The Z-E syndrome has been divided into two types. Type I is caused by so-called G-cell hyperplasia, an increase in number or activity of gastric antrum G cells without gastrinoma tumor. Type II is due to gastrinoma of the pancreas or duodenum.

TABLE 32–7.
Signs and Symptoms Suggestive of the Zollinger-Ellison Syndrome

Intractable or recurrent peptic ulcer(s)
Multiple peptic ulcers or ulcers in unusual locations
Recurrent or marginal ulcer after complete vagotomy or partial gastric resection
Chronic diarrhea
Gastric acid hypersecretion

Gastric Analysis.—The Z-E syndrome is usually accompanied by gastric hypersecretion and hyperacidity, which some consider an integral part of the syndrome. According to the old gastric analysis method using Topfer's reagent as a pH indicator, now considered outmoded, basal gastric secretion quantity more than 200 ml/hour and basal gastric acid secretion more than 100 mEq/L/12 hours were considered suggestive of Z-E syndrome. According to the currently recommended gastric analysis methods using a pH meter or methyl red pH indicator, basal (1-hour) acid secretion greater than 10 mEq of hydrochloric acid (HCl)/hour and a ratio of basal acid output (BAO) to maximal acid output (MAO) of 0.4 or greater raise the question of Z-E syndrome; a BAO of 15 mEq/hour and a BAO/MAO ratio of 0.6 or greater are very suggestive of Z-E syndrome (although not pathognomonic) (Table 32–8).

Serum Gastrin.—Serum gastrin assay is the method of choice for diagnosis. Gastrin levels are elevated in more than 95% of gastrinomas. Serum gastrin levels more than five times the upper limit of the reference range are virtually diagnostic of Z-E syndrome. Some believe that gastric analysis can therefore be omitted in these patients. However, a few patients with gastrinoma have basal gastrin levels that are within reference range, and some have levels that are only mildly or moderately elevated and overlap with values found in certain other conditions associated with elevated serum gastrin levels. These other conditions include diseases associated with hypochlorhydria or achlorhydria, such as atrophic gastritis and pernicious anemia (if the antrum is not severely affected), after vagotomy, in patients with retained antrum following gastrojejunostomy, in uremia, and possibly in chronic hypercalcemia. In one series, about 60% of patients with elevated serum gastrin level had hypochlorhydria or achlorhydria as the cause of the elevated gastrin level. Because of this, some investigators recommend gastric analysis in patients with mild or moderate gastrin elevations. Food ingestion has also been reported to produce a significant temporary increase in serum gastrin level. A high-protein meal is said to increase serum gastrin levels two–five times baseline values. In addition, some patients with peptic ulcer have mild or moderate serum gastrin elevation that overlaps with those occasional gastrinoma patients who have values that are not markedly elevated.

Gastrin Stimulation Tests.—Since overlap in gastrin values may occur between gastrinoma and other conditions, stimulation tests have been devised to assist differentiation. The original standard procedure was calcium infusion. Patients with gastrinomas more than double baseline values, whereas ulcer patients fail to do so. Patients with pernicious anemia, however, frequently respond to calcium. Secretin stimulation appears to be replacing calcium as the confirmatory procedure of choice, as secretin seems a little more sensitive than calcium and appears to differentiate better between gastrinomas and other etiologies of elevated serum gastrin. It has been reported that achlorhydric patients do not respond to secretin (Table 32–9).

Primary Gastrinoma Localization.—Ultrasound is reported to demonstrate 21%–28% of gastrinomas, CT is said to detect 35%–60% (range, 18%–80%), and selective angiography can locate 35%–68%.

TABLE 32–8.
Gastric Analysis in Zollinger-Ellison Syndrome*

Values	Z-E (%)	Duodenal Ulcer (%)
BAO ≥15 mEq/hr (intact stomach); normal = 1–6 mEq/hr)	70 (50–82)	8 (2–10)
BAO ≥5 mEq/hr (after gastric operation)	55	6
BAO-MAO ratio >0.4	70 (60–75)	3 (2–5)
BAO-MAO ratio >0.5	60 (41–75)	3 (2–3.5)
BAO-MAO ratio >0.6	55 (35–75)	2 (1–5)

*Data indicate approximate number of patients; parentheses enclose range found in the literature.

TABLE 32–9.
Gastrin Stimulation Tests in Zollinger-Ellison Syndrome

Secretin (2 units/kg intravenously): Peak response (2, 5, or 10 min) of >200 pg/ml over baseline occurs in >90% of Z-E syndrome patients.
Calcium infusion: Increase over twice baseline occurs in ≥95% Z-E syndrome patients; increase over three times baseline occurs in ≥85%. Response to calcium is less specific than response to secretin.

LIVER

Tumor in the liver is most often metastatic. The liver receives metastases more frequently than any other organ, since 25%–50% of all metastasizing cancers reach the liver. The GI tract (including the pancreas), breast, kidney, lung, melanomas, and sarcomas are especially apt to produce hepatic metastases.

Tests for detection include alkaline phosphatase, γ-glutamyltransferase, liver scan (radionuclide, ultrasound, CT), and liver biopsy (see chapter 19). Primary liver cell carcinoma (hepatoma) is more common in cirrhosis. On liver scan, it typically appears as a large, dominant, space-occupying lesion. The alpha-fetoprotein (AFP) result (chapter 19) is often positive. Liver biopsy is essential to verify a diagnosis of cancer in the liver, since non-neoplastic diseases may produce abnormalities identical to those of neoplasia in any of the tests.

CENTRAL NERVOUS SYSTEM

In primary brain tumor, cerebrospinal fluid protein level is elevated in up to 70% of patients and cell count in about 30% of cases. One or the other is abnormal in 65%–80% of cases. Electroencephalogram (EEG) is abnormal in about 70%–75% of patients (literature range, 70%–92%), brain scan in about 80%–85% (65%–96%), and CT in about 90%–95% (85%–100%). Therefore, CT scan is clearly the best single test for primary brain tumor (or any space-occupying brain lesion), whereas EEG adds little, if anything, to CT or brain scan information.

SYMPATHETIC NERVOUS SYSTEM

Neuroblastoma is one of the most frequent tumors of childhood, during which it is the most frequent abdominal neoplasm except for Wilms' tumor of infancy. Treatment by combined radiation and chemotherapy is beginning to produce worthwhile results, so diagnosis has become of more than academic interest. It usually presents as an abdominal mass, and frequently the only method of definitive diagnosis is abdominal exploration with biopsy. Urine vanillylmandelic acid (VMA) levels have been found elevated in more than 90% of patients (literature range, 61%–100%), although some elevations were not present on initial specimens. Homovanillic acid (HVA) values, a metabolic product of the catecholamine precursor dopamine, are reported to be abnormal in about 80% (53%–93%) of patients. Combined VMA and HVA positive results include nearly 100% of patients. Bone marrow aspiration has been reported abnormal in up to 50% of patients. Therefore, some investigators recommend that bone marrow aspiration be done on all patients, since the finding of marrow metastases rules out surgery alone as a curative procedure.

Pheochromocytoma has been discussed in chapter 29.

TESTIS

Alpha-fetoprotein and beta subunit chorionic gonadotropin (hCG) levels by RIA methods are elevated in certain gonadal tumors. In general, pure seminomas fail to produce AFP, whereas hCG production in seminoma ranges from 0%–37%. Some 70% or more of patients with embryonal cell carcinoma and malignant teratoma have elevated AFP levels, and 40%–60% or more have elevated hCG levels. Eighty-five percent or more patients have elevated levels of one or both. Elevation of AFP levels by RIA occurs in hepatoma (70%–90%, chapter 19) and has also been reported in up to 18% of patients with gastric carcinoma, up to 23% of those with pancreatic carcinoma, and in occasional patients with lung carcinoma or other tumors, mostly in low titer. Elevated AFP level is also reported in up to 30% of patients with acute and chronic active hepatitis. Elevated hCG level is found in choriocarcinoma or hydatidiform mole (chapter 30) and has also been reported in low titer with a small number of various other neoplasms, notably gastric, hepatic, pancreatic, and breast carcinoma. It has even been detected in a few patients with melanoma and myeloma (again, usually in very low titer).

THYROID

Thyroid carcinoma seems to have generated a considerable number of misconceptions. About 20% of these tumors are "pure" papillary, about 10% pure follicular, about 50% mixed papillary and follicular, and about 10% are called medullary. However, the pure papillary carcinoma usually has a few follicular elements if enough histologic sections are made, and the reverse is sometimes true in follicular tumors. In addition, some pathologists classify the tumors according to the predominant element unless the proportions of each element are very similar. If this were done, about 65% would be called papillary and about 20% follicular. There is enough diversity in classification methods to create difficulty in relating pathology reports to statistics in the literature. Papillary and most mixed papillary-follicular carcinomas metastasize primarily to regional lymph nodes. Prognosis is excellent in young adults but less so in older persons. Follicular carcinoma tends to produce hematogenous metastases, most often to lungs and bone.

Thyroid Radionuclide Scan.—The major screening test is the thyroid scan. The characteristic appearance of thyroid carcinoma is a single nonfunctioning nodule. A gland that is multinodular on scan has less chance of containing carcinoma than one with a solitary nodule. On occasion, a palpable nodule may represent metastatic carcinoma from another primary site in a lymph node close to the thyroid.

Radionuclide scanning of thyroid nodules can be performed with radioactive iodine or technetium 99m pertechnetate. Results from comparison studies usually agree, but occasional carcinomas that appear to have some function on technetium scan but not on iodine scan have been found. About 20%–30% of single thyroid nodules without demonstrable function on scan are malignant (literature range, 3%–58%). About 6% of nodules with some function (reduced, but present) and about 6%–8% of nodules with apparent normal function (literature range, 0%–38%) are reported to be malignant. In some of these cases, normal thyroid tissue above or below the nodule creates a false impression of nodule function. Hyperactive nodules are very rarely malignant, although occasionally a malignancy is found unexpectedly in the same gland.

A minority of investigators believe that radioiodine or technetium scanning is not helpful in evaluation of thyroid nodules for possible malignancy. As noted previously, a single nodule without demonstrable function on scan has a 20%–30% chance of malignancy, which means that 70%–80% of such nodules will be falsely positive for malignancy. On the other hand, some reports indicate that 6%–8% of nodules with apparently normal function may actually be malignant and thus represent false negative results. Therefore, some investigators rely on criteria other than thyroid scan to determine which patients with thyroid nodules should receive operative therapy. The criteria that have been used include patient history, characteristics of the nodule on physical examination, fine needle aspiration, or response of the nodule to thyroid hormone suppression. In the suppression test, failure of the nodule to diminish at least 50% in size during 3 months of suppression would increase the chance of malignancy.

A significant number of patients are referred for thyroid scan while thyroid uptake of radionuclide is being suppressed by administration of thyroid hormone or by x-ray contrast media. This frequently produces unsatisfactory or even misleading results.

Thyroid Scan to Detect Thyroid Carcinoma Metastases.—A different problem may arise when thyroid cancer is discovered and patients are referred for scanning to detect metastases, either before or after initial therapy. Unless all of the normal thyroid tissue is removed or is ablated by radioiodine therapy, enough of the scanning dose will be taken up by normal tissue to make such attempts useless in most cases. In addition, replacement thyroid hormone administration must cease for 2–4 weeks prior to scanning, so that the pituitary will once again produce thyroid-stimulating hormone (TSH), which, in turn, will help stimulate the tumor to take up the radioiodine. The dose of radioactive iodine (1–5 mCi) for a metastatic tumor scan is more than 10 times the usual thyroid scan dose, and the optimal time to scan is 72 hours after administration of the dose. Some prefer a technetium phosphate bone scan to an iodine 131 tumor scan. Most bone metastases detected by iodine are also detected by technetium phosphate, and the remaining thyroid tissue does not have to be ablated. However, a few bone metastases are detected by radioiodine and not by technetium. Lung metastases or recurrent neck tumor would be missed using technetium bone scan agents.

Serum Thyroglobulin Assay.—The serum thyroglobulin (TG) assay has been advocated to follow patients after treatment of thyroid carcinoma. Thyroglobulin is synthesized by thyroid epithelial cells. It is present in measurable amounts in the serum of normal persons on immunoassay (using antibodies against thyroglobulin) and is increased following TSH stimulation. Elevated values are found in active thyrotoxicosis (diffuse or nodular), thyroiditis, iodine deficiency, benign thyroid adenomas, and differentiated thyroid carcinomas. Therefore, TG elevation is too nonspecific to use for diagnosis of thyroid carcinoma. In thyroid carcinoma, the TG level is usually elevated in papillary, follicular, and mixed papillary-follicular neoplasms. Some anaplastic thyroid carcinomas produce elevated values and some do not. Medullary carcinomas do not produce TG. The TG assay can be used to monitor the progress of differentiated thyroid carcinomas after treatment. The half-life of circulating TG is said to be 8–22 hours, so circulating levels should be absent in 7–14 days after total destruction of all normal thyroid tissue and tumor tissue by surgery. Ablation by radioactive iodine is much more gradual and variable. Thyroglobulin values that are nondetectable or nearly so following therapy signify that no residual thyroid or tumor remains, and future elevations mean tumor recurrence or metastasis. Thyroglobulin values that are within the reference range following therapy could either be tumor or could be remnants of normal thyroid, and a thyroid tumor scan with ^{131}I is required to differentiate these possibilities.

One advantage of TG monitoring is less need for ^{131}I scanning. This avoids both additional radiation and the need to temporarily stop thyroxine replacement therapy to perform the scan. Also, occasional patients with metastases associated with elevated TG levels but not detected on ^{131}I tumor scan have been reported. Disadvantages include a small number of patients with metastases detected on ^{131}I tumor scan but TG values within the reference range. This occurs in about 4% of cases (literature range, 0%–63%). Thyroglobulin levels are more likely to be normal with pure papillary tumors or those with only lung metastases. Also, the presence of patient anti-TG autoantibodies may interfere with the TG assay.

Fine-Needle Aspiration Cytology.—Fine-needle aspiration of thyroid nodules with cytologic smear examination of the aspirate has been advocated to aid diagnosis and, when possible, to replace surgical biopsy. Results in the literature vary rather widely, partially depending on experience with the technique, patient selection, and method of reporting positive results (for example,"definitely malignant" would detect fewer cases of carcinoma than the combination of "malignant" and "suspicious for malignancy"). Some centers report a false negative rate of less than 5% and a false positive rate of less than 2%. Most hospitals could not expect to achieve such good results. The average false negative rate for malignancy with experienced cytologists is about 5%–10%, and the average reported rate overall is about 10%–15% (literature range, 0%–50%). Follicular carcinoma is more difficult to diagnose than papillary carcinoma. The average false positive rate for experienced cytologists is about 2%–4%, and the average reported rate overall is about 5% (range, 0%–14%). Most pathologists without special interest or extensive experience in fine-needle aspiration cytology are better able to interpret needle tissue biopsy material than thyroid aspiration cytology, because thyroid cytology takes special training and experience. However, well-differentiated follicular carcinoma is difficult to diagnose on needle biopsy as well as on aspiration. Needle biopsy is also useful to diagnose thyroiditis.

Thermography and B-mode Ultrasound have been used to help evaluate thyroid nodules for malignancy. Results of thermography to date have been rather disappointing. Ultrasound has been used to differentiate cystic thyroid lesions from solid ones. About 15%–20% of thyroid nodules that fail to concentrate radioactive iodine are cystic. Typical completely cystic lesions are rarely malignant (about 2%; literature range, 0%–14%). Ultrasound accuracy in differentiating pure cystic lesions from solid or mixed cystic-solid lesions is usually quoted as about 95% (80%–100%). The procedure in many clinics is to perform aspiration with cytology on ultrasonically pure cysts.

Medullary Carcinoma of the Thyroid.—Medullary carcinoma constitutes 3%–10% of thyroid carcinomas. It is derived from certain stromal cells known as "C cells." The tumor has an intermediate degree of malignancy. It may occur sporadically or in a hereditary form. The familial variety is transmitted as an autosomal dominant trait, is usually present in both thyroid lobes, and is frequently associated with other neoplasms (pheochromocytoma, mucosal neuromas) as part of the Sipple syndrome (MEN II). This also includes some degree of association with other endocrine abnormalities, such as parathyroid adenoma and Cushing's syndrome. The tumor may present in a variety of histologic patterns, but the classic form is solid nests of cells that are separated by a stroma containing amyloid. These tumors have aroused great interest, since most secrete abnormal amounts of the hormone calcitonin (thyrocalcitonin). Calcitonin has a calcium-lowering action derived from inhibition of bone resorption; therefore, calcitonin acts as an antagonist to parathyroid hormone. Thyroid C cells produce calcitonin as a normal reaction to the stimulus of hypercalcemia. About 70%–75% of medullary carcinomas produce elevated levels of serum calcitonin. In those that do not, elevated calcitonin levels can be induced by stimulation with calcium infusion or pentagastrin. Glucagon also stimulates calcitonin secretion but not as effectively. A few medullary carcinomas are reported to secrete serotonin or prostaglandins. About 30% of patients experience diarrhea. Besides medullary thyroid carcinoma, calcitonin secretion has been reported in as many as 60% of patients with bronchogenic carcinoma (small-cell and adenocarcinoma tumor types)

METASTATIC CARCINOMA TO BONE

Any carcinoma, lymphoma, or sarcoma may metastasize to bone, although those primary in certain organs do so much more frequently than others. Breast, prostate, lung, kidney, and thyroid are the most common carcinomas. Once in bone they may cause local destruction that is manifested on x-ray film by an osteolytic lesion. In many cases there is osseous reaction surrounding the tumor with the formation of new bone or osteoid, and with sufficient degree of reaction this appears on x-ray films as an osteoblastic lesion. Prostate carcinoma is usually osteoblastic on x-ray film. Breast and lung carcinomas are more commonly osteolytic, but a significant number are osteoblastic. The others usually have an osteolytic appearance.

Hematologic.—About one half of the carcinomas metastatic to bone replace or at least injure bone marrow to such an extent as to give hematologic symptoms. This must be distinguished from the anemia of neoplasia, which appears in a considerable number of patients without direct marrow involvement and whose mechanism may be hemolytic, toxic depression of marrow production, or unknown. The degree of actual bone marrow replacement is often relatively small in relation to the total amount of bone marrow, and some sort of toxic influence of the cancer on the blood-forming elements has been postulated. Whatever the mechanism, about one half of patients with metastatic carcinoma to bone have anemia when first seen (i.e., a hemoglobin value at least 2 gm/100 ml (20 g/L) below the lower limit of the reference range). When the hemoglobin value is less than 8 gm/100 ml (80 g/L), nucleated red blood cells (RBCs) and immature white blood cells (WBCs) may appear in the peripheral blood, and thrombocytopenia may be present. By this time there is often extensive marrow replacement.

Therefore, one peripheral blood finding that is always suspicious of extensive marrow replacement is the presence of thrombocytopenia in a patient with known cancer (unless the patient is on cytotoxic therapy). Another is the appearance of nucleated RBCs in the peripheral blood, sometimes in addition to slightly more immature WBCs. This does not occur in multiple myeloma, even though this disease often produces discrete bone lesions on x-ray film and the malignant plasma cells may replace much of the bone marrow.

Alkaline Phosphatase.—Because of bone destruction and local attempts at repair, the serum alkaline phosphatase level is often elevated. Roughly one third of patients with metastatic carcinomas to bone from lung, kidney, or thyroid have elevated alkaline phosphatase levels on first examination. For breast carcinoma this may be true in up to 50% of patients, whereas for the prostate, reports vary from 70%–90%.

Bone X-ray Film.—If an x-ray skeletal survey is done, bone lesions will be seen in approximately 50% of patients with actual bone metastases. More are not detected on first examination because lesions must be more than 1.5 cm to be seen on x-ray films, because parts of the bone are obscured by overlying structures, and because the tumor spread may be concealed by new bone formation. Almost any bone may be affected, but the vertebral column is by far the most frequent.

Bone Radionuclide Scan.—Bone scanning for metastases is available in most sizable institutions using radioactive isotopes of elements that take part in bone metabolism (see chapter 22). Bone scanning detects 10%–40% more foci of metastatic carcinoma than x-ray film and is the method of choice in screening for bone metastases. A possible exception is breast carcinoma. Although bone scan is more sensitive for breast carcinoma metastasis than x-ray film, sufficient additional lesions are found by x-ray film to make skeletal surveys useful in addition to bone scanning. Also, in cases in which a single lesion or only a few lesions are detected by scan, x-ray film of the focal areas involved should be done since scans detect benign as well as malignant processes that alter bone (as long as osteoblastic activity is taking place), and the x-ray appearance may help to differentiate benign from malignant etiology. Bone scan is much more sensitive than bone marrow examination in patients with most types of metastatic carcinoma. However, tumors that seed in a more diffuse fashion, such as small-cell lung carcinoma, neuroblastoma, and malignant lymphoma, are exceptions to this rule and could benefit from marrow biopsy in addition to scan.

Bone Marrow Examination.—Bone marrow aspiration will demonstrate tumor cells in a certain number of patients with metastatic carcinoma to bone. Reports do not agree on whether there is any difference in positive yield between the sternum and iliac crest. Between 7% and 40% of the patients with tumor in the bone have been said to have a positive bone marrow result. This varies with the site of primary tumor, whether the marrow is tested early or late in the disease, and whether random aspiration or aspiration from x-ray lesions is performed. The true incidence of positive marrow results is probably about 15%. Prostatic carcinoma has the highest rate of yield, since this tumor metastasizes to bone the most frequently, mostly to the vertebral column and pelvic bones. Lung small cell (oat cell) carcinoma, neuroblastoma, and malignant lymphoma also have a reasonable chance of detection by bone marrow aspiration.

Several studies have shown that marrow aspiration clot sections detect more tumor than marrow smears and that needle biopsy locates tumor more often than clot section. Two needle biopsies are said to produce approximately 30% more positive results than only one.

The question often arises as to the value of bone marrow aspiration in suspected metastatic carcinoma to bone. In this regard, the following statements seem valid:

1. It usually is difficult or often impossible to determine either the exact tumor type or the origin (primary site) of tumor cells from marrow aspiration.
2. If localized bone lesions exist on x-ray film and it becomes essential to determine their nature, a direct bone biopsy of these lesions using a special needle is much better than random marrow aspiration or even aspiration of the lesion area. In this way, a histologic tissue pattern may be obtained.
3. If a patient has a normal alkaline phosphatase level, no anemia, and no bone lesions on bone scan (or skeletal x-ray survey, if bone scan is not available), and in addition has a normal acid phosphatase level in cases of prostatic carcinoma, the chances of obtaining a positive bone marrow aspirate are less than 5% (exceptions are small-cell lung carcinoma, lymphoma, and neuroblastoma).
4. If a patient has known carcinoma or definite evidence of carcinoma and x-ray lesions of bone, chemical studies or bone marrow aspiration usually have little practical value except in certain special situations in which anemia or thrombocytopenia may be caused by a disease that the patient has in addition to the carcinoma.

EFFUSIONS AND TESTS FOR CANCER

In general, when an effusion occurs, the problem is differentiation among neoplastic, infectious, and fluid leakage etiologies. Effusions due to neoplasms or infection are frequently termed exudates and those due to hydrostatic leakage from vessels are called transudates. Several criteria have been proposed to separate transudates and exudates and to differentiate among the three major diagnostic categories. Most work has been done on pleural fluids.

Etiology.—The two most common causes of pleural effusions are congestive heart failure and neoplasm. Infection (tuberculosis or pneumonia) is the third most frequent etiology. In some cases it is necessary to establish the diagnosis of chylous effusion. Chylous effusions usually have a triglyceride content of 110 mg/100 ml (1.2 mmol/L) or greater and are usually more than twice the serum triglyceride value. Centrifugation does not clear a supernate area, and it may be possible to demonstrate fat droplets with a fat stain such as Sudan III. Another problem that occasionally arises is to differentiate urine from effusion fluid. Urine almost always has a creatinine concentration twice that of serum or more, whereas effusion fluid usually has the same creatinine concentration as the patient's serum or at least is not elevated as much as twice the serum level.

Specific Gravity.—Exudates typically have a specific gravity of 1.016 or more and transudates less than 1.015. One study found about 25% error in misclassification of either transudates or exudates.

Protein Content.—Total protein levels

higher than 3 gm/100 ml (30 g/L) are characteristic of exudates. Transudates have total protein content of less than 3 and usually less than 2 gm. Two studies found that 8% of exudates and 11%–15% of transudates would be misdiagnosed if 3 gm/100 ml were used as the dividing line. Most exudates that were misdiagnosed as transudates were neoplastic. A pleural fluid/serum protein ratio of 0.5 may be a slightly better dividing line; exudates usually have a ratio greater than 0.5. With this criterion, accuracy in identifying transudates improved; but 10% of the exudates, mostly of malignant origin, were incorrectly classified as transudates. Pulmonary infarct, rheumatoid-collagen diseases, acute pancreatitis, cirrhosis with high-protein ascites (12%–19% of cases), and other conditions may produce effusions with protein content compatible with exudates.

Several investigators report that the albumin gradient between serum and ascitic fluid differentiates between transudate or exudate nature of ascites better than total protein content. In one study, total protein ascitic values produced 64% overlap between etiologies of the exudate and transudate groups, whereas the serum albumin–ascitic fluid albumin gradient (SA-AFAG) produced 38% overlap. Another study produced only 7% overlap. The SA-AFAG consists of subtracting the ascitic albumin value from the serum albumin value. A SA-AFAG value of 1.1 gm/100 ml (11 g/L) or more suggests a transudate, usually due to cirrhosis. A SA-AFAG value less than 1.1 gm suggests an exudate but will not differentiate malignancy from infection or inflammation. Another problem may arise when two conditions, such as liver metastases in a patient with cirrhotic ascites, coexist.

Effusion Lactic Dehydrogenase.—A pleural fluid to serum lactic dehydrogenase (LDH) ratio greater than 0.6 is reported to be typical of exudates. One study found that most transudates were correctly identified but that nearly 30% of exudates were misclassified.

Combinations of Criteria.—The more criteria that favor one category as opposed to the other, the more accurate the results become. One study found that the combination of pleural fluid/serum protein ratio and pleural fluid/serum LDH ratio correctly identified most transudates and exudates.

pH.—An effusion fluid pH higher than 7.40 usually is associated with a transudate, whereas a pH of less than 7.40 is more likely to be an exudate caused by infection, inflammation, or tumor.

Glucose.—A pleural fluid glucose level more than 10 mg/100 ml below lower limits of normal for serum, especially when the actual pleural fluid value is less than 20 mg/100 ml, is reported to be suggestive of neoplasm or infection. Possibly 15%–20% of malignant effusions have decreased glucose levels. Patient hypoglycemia, rheumatoid arthritis, and infection are other etiologies.

Cell Count and Differential.—In ascites, a total WBC count of 500/cu mm or more suggests infection, especially when neutrophils exceed 50% of total cells. Patients with cirrhotic ascites develop bacterial ascitic fluid infection ("spontaneous bacterial peritonitis") in 4%–15% of cases. In any body fluid, presence of many segmented granulocytes suggests infection (empyema); many mononuclear cells raise the question of lymphoid malignancy, carcinoma, or tuberculosis. Several investigators state that sufficient exceptions occur to severely limit the usefulness of differential counts in the diagnosis of individual patients.

Culture.—Culture is frequently performed for tuberculosis, fungus, and ordinary bacteria. Pleural fluid culture for tuberculosis is said to be positive only in approximately 25% of known cases of tuberculosis effusion. Some believe that tuberculosis culture should be limited to high-risk patients or patients who have a positive skin test result. Whereas tuberculosis is an important cause of idiopathic pleural effusion, although less common in the United States than in the past, fungus is an uncommon cause of pulmonary infection except in patient groups with compromised immunologic defenses.

Cytology.—About 30%–40% (literature range, 25%–52%) of all pleural effusions are associated with neoplasms. About 35%–40% are caused by lung carcinoma (most often adenocarcinoma), and about 20%–25% are due to breast carcinoma, with lymphoma or leukemia, ovary, or unknown primary in third place. Cytologic study is reported to detect tumor cells in about 50%–65% (literature range, 30%–98%) of patients with malignant effusions. One problem that sometimes occurs is poor cytologic preparations due to blood in the pleural fluid. We have obtained better results by using cytologic spray fixative when the cytologic slides are prepared rather than fixing the slides by the usual technique of dipping them in alcohol.

Pleural Effusion Carcinoembryonic Antigen.—Carcinoembryonic antigen (CEA) is discussed in detail later in this chapter. Pleural fluid CEA levels may be elevated in various malignant and some benign conditions. When a cutoff level approximately four times the upper reference limit (corresponding to 10 ng/ml with the Hansen technique, whose upper normal limit is 2.5 ng/ml) is used, most elevations due to nonmalignant cause are eliminated (< 5% false positive results; literature range, 1%–12%). About 35%–50% of malignancies are detected (25%–89%). Therefore, CEA by itself is less sensitive than cytology. Addition of CEA to cytology (using a CEA cutoff value sufficient to exclude benign disease) improves detection of malignancy about 10%–15% over cytology alone. Carcinoembryonic antigen assay can also be used for ascitic fluid.

Peritoneal Lavage for Traumatic Injury.—Although this subject does not involve cancer, it does fit with discussions on tests for effusions, and thus it is included here. The standard criteria leading to high expectation of intra-abdominal bleeding are one or more of the following: aspiration of gross blood (the quantity required is not uniform, but at least 10 ml or 20 ml are most often mentioned), fluid with an RBC count greater than 100,000/cu mm, or a WBC count greater than 500/cu mm. Other criteria that have been proposed but that are not widely accepted are abdominal fluid bilirubin or creatinine values higher than serum values or elevated effusion amylase. In most series the standard criteria detect significant intra-abdominal bleeding in about 90% of cases and falsely suggest significant bleeding in about 10%–15% of cases (some of these patients may have bleeding that retrospectively is not considered sufficient to warrant laparotomy). Computerized tomography scanning has proved extremely useful in trauma patients, with a sensitivity equal to that of lavage and a false positive rate significantly less than that of lavage. In addition, CT can demonstrate what organs are affected.

General Considerations.—Three anticoagulated tubes of effusion fluid should be sent to the laboratory, one tube containing ethylenediamine tetraacetic acid (EDTA) anticoagulant, one tube containing 0.05% sodium polyanetholesulfonate (SPS; Liquoid), and the third containing heparin. The EDTA tube is used for cell count and differential; the SPS tube for culture, and the heparinized tube for cytology. Without anticoagulant there may be sufficient protein in the specimen to induce spontaneous clotting, which can trap WBCs and bacteria and produce erroneous cell counts and falsely negative cultures. Some use the heparinized tube both for culture and for cytology, but too much heparin may inhibit bacterial growth. Nonanticoagulated effusion fluid should also be sent to perform biochemical tests.

MISCELLANEOUS TESTS FOR CANCER

Serum Lactic Dehydrogenase.—Serum LDH levels are sometimes elevated in extensive carcinomatosis, often without any obvious reason. This is especially true in lymphoma, where it may be abnormal in up to 50% cases. However, LDH levels can be elevated in many conditions, which considerably lessens its usefulness in cancer diagnosis.

Carcinoembryonic Antigen.—Gastrointestinal tract epithelium in early fetal life contains CEA, an antigen that has also been found in extracts from tumors in the adult GI tract. Immunologic tests have been based on antibodies against CEA. The procedure was originally thought to be specific for colon adenocarcinoma, but as more experience was obtained and modifications of the original technique were developed, it became evident that abnormal results could be obtained in persons with malignancies of various organs, in certain benign diseases (usually involving tissue inflammation or destruction), in occasional benign tumors, and in persons who smoke cigarettes.

Several basic RIA techniques have been

published. The most frequently used method for many years was the Hansen procedure, in which Z-gel is used as a radioactivity separation agent. More recently, many laboratories have changed to shorter and more simple immunoassay methods, frequently using a sandwich antigen-antibody technique. Reference values for both of these techniques are approximately 0–2.5 ng/ml. Although values for the two methods generally are similar when performed on the same specimens, there are a moderate number of discrepancies, sufficient that serial tests on the same patient should be performed by the same method.

Test Results in Colon Cancer and Other Conditions.—In colon carcinoma, different investigators have published widely divergent results, with about 75% average detection of carcinoma, but with reported detection rates ranging from 59%–97% (see Table 25–3). The smaller and earlier-stage tumors are less likely to give positive results. Among noncolonic tumors, using the Hansen method, more than one investigator has reported that 70%–90% of lung, 85%–100% of pancreatic, and 45%–60% of breast and gastric carcinomas produce abnormal results. Normal persons who smoke were CEA reactive in nearly 20% of cases, and conditions associated with elevation in more than 10% of patients include pulmonary emphysema, benign rectal polyps, benign breast diseases, cholecystitis or extrahepatic biliary duct obstruction, alcoholic cirrhosis, and ulcerative colitis. At CEA levels more than 5 ng/ml (twice upper limits), abnormal results in colorectal, lung, and pancreatic carcinoma decreased to 50%–60% and decreased to 30% in breast and gastric carcinoma. Most other conditions were reduced to 5% abnormality or less, except for alcoholic cirrhosis (about 25%), common bile duct obstruction (17%), active ulcerative colitis (13%), and emphysema (20%). At CEA levels greater than 10 ng/ml (four times the upper normal limit), abnormal results were found in 35% of colorectal, 25% of lung, 35% of pancreatic, and 15%–30% of gastric and breast carcinoma. All the benign conditions were less than 1% reactive except for emphysema (4%), active ulcerative colitis (5%), and alcoholic cirrhosis (2%).

These data indicate that CEA results greater than 10 ng/ml are strongly suggestive of tumor. Results in the 5–10 ng/ml range are suspicious for tumor, and results less than 5 ng/ml are either equivocal or not helpful. However, since a substantial minority of colon cancers are not detected, since a varying number of patients with other tumors are detected, and since certain benign conditions may produce elevated values, most investigators do not recommend CEA as a screening test either for colon cancer or in most circumstances for cancer in general.

Prognostic Value of Carcinoembryonic Antigen Level in Colon Cancer.—In general, CEA titers greater than 10 ng/ml (four times the upper reference limit) in colorectal carcinoma most often occur in more advanced tumor stages and imply a worse prognosis. However, about 5%–10% (literature range, 0%–18%) of Dukes' A lesions (tumor confined to the colon wall) and about 50% of Dukes' B and C (local tumor extension with or without local node involvement) have CEA titers of 10 ng/ml or more, while about 10% (0%–16%) of Dukes' D (distant metastases) have normal CEA levels. Therefore, a normal CEA level does not exclude far-advanced tumor, and high CEA titers do not mean that a colorectal carcinoma is unresectable, although high CEA titers are reasonable (but not conclusive) evidence against an early (Dukes' A) tumor stage.

Use of Carcinoembryonic Antigen to Detect Recurrent Tumor.—The major currently recommended use for CEA is to follow the results of tumor therapy. For this, a pretherapy baseline assay is needed to determine if the CEA level is elevated. After surgical treatment, at least 4 weeks should elapse before follow-up CEA assay is performed (some cases have been reported in which CEA levels did not return to normal for 2–6 months). Another problem associated with interpretation of CEA response to therapy is a transient elevation above baseline after the start of chemotherapy or radiation therapy in some patients, probably related to the destructive effect of therapy on the tumor. Return of CEA titer to the reference range or nondetectable level is fairly reliable evidence that most of the tumor has been removed. This does not guarantee that all tumor has been eliminated. Future elevation of CEA levels suggests recurrence (either local disease or metastasis). This may develop as much as 6 months before clinical evidence of recurrence. However, numerous reports indicate that sporadic nonsustained CEA elevations that are not due to neoplasia may occur; sometimes they are associated with nonmalignant illness, but often there is no apparent cause. These elevations are usually less than 5 ng/ml. The most reliable indicator of recurrence is a sustained (on at least two occasions) elevation of at least 5 ng/ml. Even this conservative criterion is associated with about a 10% false positive rate, based on "second-look" operations. However, in some cases where tumor was not found, recurrences developed later.

MULTIPLE ENDOCRINE NEOPLASIA SYNDROMES

These syndromes have been mentioned in the discussion of certain tumors that may be associated with MEN. A summary of the MEN syndromes is presented in Table 32–10. These syndromes are familial, with types I and II being inherited as an autosomal dominant disorder. About one half of type III cases are sporadic. Some cases of incomplete or overlapping organ tumor patterns have been reported.

Although carcinoid tumors are not considered part of the MEN syndromes, carcinoids of foregut origin (bronchial and gastric) may be associated with MEN I. Gastrinomas of the Z-E syndrome may be associated with MEN I, which includes pancreatic islet cell tumors (these tumors may produce insulin, gastrin, or vasoactive intestinal polypeptide). About 5%–10% of pheochromocytomas are associated with MEN types II and III.

Many patients with the MEN syndromes do not have all the tumor types included with the syndromes.

TUMOR-SEEKING RADIOPHARMACEUTICALS

Certain compounds have been found empirically to localize in neoplasms. These can be tagged with a radioisotope and used to detect tumor by scanning. Currently, gallium 67 citrate is the most widely used. Labeled bleomycin may be used more frequently in the future. Both are not specific tumor markers; both may appear in certain organs or tissues (liver, spleen, and bone, and in the case of gallium, in areas of localized infection). Tagged monoclonal antibodies are currently in the experimental stage.

Gallium scan abnormality has been reported in approximately 90% of primary site lung carcinomas, 85% of Hodgkin's disease, 60%–75% of non-Hodgkin's lymphomas (depending on cell type), 55% of acute leukemia lymph nodes, 75%–85% of brain tumors, 75% of hypernephromas, 65% of breast carcinomas, 45% of melanomas, and about 30%–35% of adenocarcinomas from GI tract, pancreas, and ovary. Gallium is less sensitive than ordinary

TABLE 32–10.
Multiple Endocrine Neoplasias

Organ	Tumor	Approximate % of Cases
	Type I (Wermer's syndrome)	
Parathyroid	Adenoma or hyperplasia	65–90
Pancreas	Islet cell tumor	80
Pituitary	Adenoma	
	Type II (type IIA, Sipple syndrome)	
Parathyroid	Adenoma or hyperplasia	≤50
Thyroid	Medullary carcinoma	>90
Adrenal	Pheochromocytoma	50–90, usually bilateral
	Type III (type IIB)	
Thyroid	Medullary carcinoma	90
Adrenal	Pheochromocytoma	
Neural tissue	Neural tumors (mucosal neuromas, intestinal ganglioneuromas)	
	Hyperplastic corneal nerves	
Somatic	Marfanoid habitus	

bone scan agents for detection of skeletal metastases. After 24 hours, gallium is excreted in the feces, so colon activity may interfere unless adequate bowel cleansing is performed.

TUMOR HORMONE PRODUCTION

Some tumors produce hormones. In some cases, detection of these hormones is useful for diagnosis or therapy. This topic is mentioned when the individual tumor is discussed. Some tumors secrete hormones not normally expected from tumor in that location (e.g., adrenocorticotropic hormone secretion by small cell lung carcinoma). This type of tumor hormone secretion is considered ectopic. Table 36–32 contains some data on ectopic tumor hormone production additional to those included in discussion of various hormones in the text.

Additional tests relevant to this chapter are discussed in chapter 35.

BIBLIOGRAPHY

Bolin S, et al: Carcinoma of the colon and rectum: Tumors missed by radiologic examination in 61 patients. *Cancer* 1988; 61:1999.

Roberts LJ: Carxcinoid syndrome and disorders of systemic mast-cell activation including systemic mastocytosis. *Endocrinol Metab Clin North Am* 1988; 17:415.

Feldman JM: Detection and treatment of carcinoid tumors. *Hosp Pract* 1988; 23(2):219.

Cahn DW: PSA as a marker for prostate carcinoma. *Lab Mgmt* 1988; 26(1):35.

Virgi MA, et al: Tumor markers in cancer diagnosis and prognosis. *CA* 1988; 38:104.

Panza N, et al: Cancer antigen 125, tissue polypeptide antigen, carcinoembryonic antigen, and beta-chain human chorionic gonadotropin as serum markers of epithelial ovarian carcinoma. *Cancer* 1988; 61:76.

Hoie J, et al: Distant metastases in papillary thyroid cancer. *Cancer* 1988; 61:1.

Bakke AC, et al: Application of flow cytometry in surgical pathology. *Lab Med* 1987; 18:590.

Houston MC: Pleural fluid pH. *Am J Surg* 1987; 154:333.

Silverstein MJ, et al: Hooked-wire-directed breast biopsy and overpenetrated mammography. *Cancer* 1987; 59:715.

Sheikh FA, et al: Final diagnosis by fine-needle aspiration biopsy for definitive operation in breast cancer. *Am J Surg* 1987; 154:470.

Hermansen C, et al: Diagnostic reliability of combined physical examination, mammography, and fine-needle puncture ("triple-test") in breast tumors. *Cancer* 1987; 60:1866.

Estaban JM, et al: Intraoperative diagnosis of breast lesions: Comparison of cytologic with frozen section techniques. *Am J Clin Pathol* 1987; 88:681.

Fisher ER, et al: Pathologic findings from the national surgical adjuvant breast project: Correlation with concordant and discordant estrogen and progesterone receptors. *Cancer* 1987; 59:1554.

Masood S, Johnson H: The value of imprint cytology in cytochemical detection of steroid hormone receptors in breast cancer. *Am J Clin Pathol* 1987; 87:30.

Chomet J: Screening for cervical cancer: A new scope for general practitioners? *Br Med J* 1987; 294:1326.

Wolfe MM, Jensen RT: Zollinger-Ellison syndrome. *N Engl J Med* 1987; 317:1200.

Richart RM: Causes and management of cervical intraepithelial neoplasia. *Cancer* 1987; 60:1951.

Koss LG: Cytologic and histologic manifestations of human papillomavirus infection of the female genital tract and their clinical significance. *Cancer* 1987; 60:1942.

Hamburger JI: Consistency of sequential needle biopsy findings for thyroid nodules. *Arch Intern Med* 1987; 147:97.

Rector WG: An improved diagnostic approach to ascites. *Arch Intern Med* 1987; 147:215.

Alvarez RD, et al: CA 125 as a serum marker for poor prognosis in ovarian malignancies. *Gynecol Oncol* 1987; 26:284.

Mundy GR: Ectopic hormonal syndromes in neoplastic disease. *Hosp Pract* 1987; 22:179.

Gharib H, et al: Determination of silica-purified plasma calcitonin for the detection and management of medullary thyroid carcinoma: Comparison of two provocative tests. *Mayo Clin Proc* 1987; 62:373.

Gibb I, et al: Immunological and colorimetric determination of prostatic acid phosphatase. *Clin Chem* 1986; 32:1760.

Barrows GH, et al: Fine-needle aspiration of breast cancer. *Cancer* 1986; 58:1493.

Vollenweider-Zerargui L, et al: The predictive value of estrogen and progesterone receptors' concentrations on the clinical behavior of breast cancer in women. *Cancer* 1986; 57:1171.

Jensen EV, et al: The estrogen-receptor immunoassay in the prognosis and treatment of breast cancer. *Lab Mgmt* 1986; 24(9):25.

Feldman JG, et al: Histochemical estrogen binding. *Cancer* 1986; 57:911.

Toon PG, et al: Human papillomavirus infection of the uterine cervix of women without cytological signs of neoplasia. *Br Med J* 1986; 293:1261.

Jones WB, Saigo PE: The "atypical" Papanicolaou smear. *CA* 1986; 36:237.

Spindel E, et al: Decision analysis in evaluation of hypergastrinemia. *Am J Med* 1986; 80:11.

Dugan JM, Atkinson BF: Endometrial neoplasia: Screening and diagnostic methods. *Lab Mgmt* 1986; 24(8):37.

Fritsche HA: Some new and prospective tumor markers. *Lab Mgmt* 1986; 24(12):25.

Ryff-de Leche A, et al: Thyroglobulin production by malignant thyroid tumors. *Cancer* 1986; 57:1145.

Berry RB, Light R: When thoracentesis yields blood pleural fluid. *J Respir Dis* 1986; 7(6):18.

Jay SJ: Pleural effusions. *Postgrad Med* 1986; 80:164.

Varkey B: Pleural effusions caused by infection. *Postgrad Med* 1986; 80:213.

Kaplan LA, et al: Cinical utility of serum prostatic acid phosphatase measurements for detection (screening), diagnosis, and therapeutic monitoring of prostatic carcinoma. *Am J Clin Pathol* 1985; 84:334.

Lieber MM: Renal cell carcinoma: New developments. *Mayo Clin Proc* 1985; 60:715.

Zucker PK: The validity of Pap smear parameters as predictors of endometrial pathology in menopausal women. *Cancer* 1985; 56:2256.

Schumann GB, Genack L: Quality assurance system for gynecologic cytology. *Lab Med* 1985; 16:169.

De Bustros A, Baylin SB: Hormone production by tumours: Biological and clinical aspects. *Clin Endocrinol Metab* 1985; 14:221.

Stefanini M: Enzymes, isozymes, and enzyme variants in the diagnosis of cancer. *Cancer* 1985; 55:1931.

McLellan BA, et al: Analysis of peritoneal lavage parameters in blunt abdominal trauma. *J Trauma* 1985; 25:393.

Ramanna L, et al: Correlation of thyroglobulin measurements and radioiodine scans in the follow-up of patients with differentiated thyroid cancer. *Cancer* 1985; 55:1525.

American College of Physicians: Diagnostic thoracentesis and pleural biopsy in pleural effusions. *Ann Intern Med* 1985; 103:799.

Mushlin AI: Diagnostic tests in breast cancer. *Ann Intern Med* 1984; 103:79.

Bakerman S: Tumor markers: Types and applications. *Lab Mgmt* 1984; 22(3):19.

Ramacciotti CE, et al: Diagnostic accuracy and use of aspiration biopsy in the management of thyroid nodules. *Arch Intern Med* 1984; 144:1169.

Holland R, et al: Mammographically occult breast cancer. *Cancer* 1983; 52:1810.

Jensen RT, et al: Zollinger-Ellison syndrome: Current concepts and management. *Ann Intern Med* 1983; 98:59.

Muggia FM: Advances in the management of testicular cancer. *Curr Concepts Oncol* 1983; 5(4):3.

Deitch EA: Peritoneal lavage and abdominal trauma. *JAMA* 1983; 249:640.

Mendelsohn G, Baylin SB: Medullary thyroid carcinoma: Diagnostic and clinical features. *Lab Mgmt* 1983; 21(8):21.

Pare P, et al: Serum-ascites albumin concentration: A physiologic approach to the differential diagnosis of ascites. *Gastroenterology* 1983; 85:240.

Wareing TH, Sawyers JL: Carcinoids and the carcinoid syndrome. *Am J Surg* 1983; 145:769.

Koss LG: Cytologic evaluation of the uterine cervix—factors influencing its accuracy. *Pathologist* 1982; 36:401.

Haagensen DE: Tumor markers for breast carcinoma. *Clin Lab Med* 1982; 2:543.

Foley DV, Masukawa T: Endometrial monitoring of high-risk women. *Cancer* 1981; 48:511.

Javadpour N: The role of biologic tumor markers in testicular cancer. *Cancer* 1980; 45:1755.

Smalley RV, et al: Preoperative scanning: Evaluation for metastatic disease in carcinoma of the breast, lung, colon, bladder, and prostate. *Semin Oncol* 1980; 7:358.

Hoffer P: Status of gallium-67 in tumor detection. *J Nucl Med* 1980; 21:394.

33 Genetic Disorders

Genetic disorders will be considered as clinical conditions resulting from a genetically determined abnormality. Such a category includes a wide variety of unrelated disorders. Although a great many syndromes and diseases are known, only selected conditions among those for which adequate laboratory diagnostic tests are available will be discussed in this chapter.

DIAGNOSTIC METHODS

Various diagnostic modalities are available. Some disorders call for chromosome studies. Others are due to a defective or a missing enzyme and are diagnosed by measurement of the enzyme responsible. Sometimes it is necessary to demonstrate that the enzyme does not produce its expected degree of activity. Finally, genetic abnormalities may be due to a gene defect not shown by standard chromosome analysis. In some of these cases, diagnosis can be made by methods using "gene probes." This technique is described in chapter 14. Briefly, a specific amino acid sequence is obtained from RNA or DNA using an enzyme known as "restriction endonuclease." This probe fragment is spliced into a DNA strand (recombinant DNA) using an enzyme called "reverse transcriptase." The probe is then used to identify patient DNA that contains the same amino acid sequence as the probe. It is also possible to construct a probe for certain gene deletions (chromosome regions where part of a gene area has been deleted) and for certain mutations (if the mutation has eliminated a restriction endonuclease cleavage site).

Genetic diagnosis has recently been extended to the fetus by means of amniotic cells obtained through amniocentesis. This is usually carried out at 16–18 weeks' gestation. It is possible to obtain a small sample of chorionic villi from the placenta at 9–11 weeks' gestation (before the amniotic sac completely fills the uterine cavity) using suction from a catheter introduced through the cervix into the uterine cavity and then into the placenta with the guidance of ultrasound. There appears to be about a 2%–4% (range, 1%–6.4%) incidence of fetal death after the procedure. An impressive and continually increasing number of conditions can be diagnosed prenatally.

Neonatal genetic diagnosis is being increasingly mandated by state governments. Currently, for example, the state of Illinois requires neonatal screening for phenylketonuria (PKU), galactosemia, biotinidase deficiency, congenital adrenal hyperplasia, and hypothyroidism. All of these disorders can be diagnosed using heelstick blood spotted on filter paper.

HEMATOLOGIC DISEASES

Hematologic diseases include principally the hemoglobinopathies and thalassemias (chapter 5), red blood cell (RBC) glucose-6-phosphate dehydrogenase deficiency (chapter 5), and the hemophilias (chapter 8). These diseases were discussed in the appropriate sections on hematology. Sickle cell disease and various thalassemias can be diagnosed prenatally, and possibly also hemophilia A. The Philadelphia chromosome abnormality found in chronic myelogenous leukemia was noted when that disease was reviewed (chapter 7).

DISEASES OF CARBOHYDRATE METABOLISM

Renal Glucosuria.—Renal glucosuria is a disorder of the renal tubule glucose transport mechanism that was discussed in chapter 27.

Galactosemia.—Galactosemia results from congenital inability to metabolize galactose to glucose. The most common source of galactose is milk, which contains lactose. Lactose is converted to glucose and galactose in the gastrointestinal (GI) tract by the enzyme lactase. There are three forms of galactosemia, each with autosomal recessive inheritance, and each caused by an enzyme defect in the galactose-glucose metabolic pathway. This enzyme system is located primarily in RBCs. The classic and most common type of abnormality is found in 1 in 62,000 infants and is due to deficiency of the enzyme galactose-1-phosphate uridyltransferase (Gal-1-PUT); the defect is called transferase deficiency galactosemia (T-D-galactosemia). Normally, galactose is metabolized to galactose-1-phosphate, and Gal-1-PUT mediates conversion to the next step in the sequence toward glucose-1-phosphate.

Transferase deficiency galactosemia is not clinically evident at birth, but symptoms commence within a few days after the infant starts a milk diet. Failure to thrive occurs in 50%–95% of patients. Vomiting (about 50% of cases), diarrhea (about 30%), or both occur in nearly 90% of patients. Evidence of liver dysfunction develops in about 90% of patients, consisting of hepatomegaly (about 70%), jaundice (about 60%), or both. Physiologic jaundice may seem to persist, or jaundice may develop later. Splenomegaly may appear in 10%–30% of patients. Individual signs and symptoms are sufficiently variable that a complete full-blown classic picture does not appear in a substantial number of affected infants. Cataracts develop in several weeks in about 50%, and mental retardation is a sequel in about one third of the patients. The disease is treatable with a lactose-free diet, if the diet is begun early enough.

Laboratory Abnormalities.—Transferase deficiency galactosemia has multiple laboratory test abnormalities. Urinalysis typically reveals protein and galactose, although in one series only two thirds of patients demonstrated urine galactose. Urine galactose excretion depends on lactose ingestion and may be absent if the infant refuses milk or vomits persistently. Galactose in urine can be detected by a positive copper sulfate–reducing substance test (e.g., Clinitest) plus a negative test specific for glucose (such as glucose oxidase test strips). A nonglucose reducing substance must be identified by more specific tests, because lactose and various other sugars can produce the same reaction as galactose on the screening procedure. There is also abnormal amino acid urine excretion that can be detected by chromatography, although such information adds little to the diagnosis. Positive urine galactose test results do not mean that the infant has galactosemia, since occasional normal newborns have transient galactosuria. However, urine screening is important, because detection of galactose enables a tentative diagnosis to be made and treatment started, pending results of confirmatory tests.

Other nonspecific abnormalities in classic transferase-deficient galactosemia include hepatomegaly and jaundice, although jaundice may not be present. Liver function test results are variable, although the aspartate aminotransferase (AST, formerly serum glutamate oxaloacetate) and possibly alkaline phosphatase levels are frequently elevated. Liver function test results must be interpreted with knowledge that the reference ranges are different in the neonate than in adults. Liver biopsy has been used in certain problematic patients (mostly before Gal-1-PUT assays were available). The histologic changes are suggestive but not conclusive and consist of early fatty metamorphosis, with a type of cirrhosis pattern often developing after about 3 months of age.

Diagnosis.—Diagnosis of classic T-D-galactosemia depends on assay of Gal-1-PUT in the RBCs of the infant. Several methods have been described, all of which are sufficiently difficult that the test is available only in university centers and a few large reference laboratories. The specimen presents certain problems. Red blood cells from anticoagulated whole blood are tested, so the specimen cannot be frozen. On the other hand, one report indicates that 25% of the enzyme activity is lost after 24 hours at either room temperature or refrigerator temperature. For this and other reasons, many physicians rely on screening tests for transferase enzyme deficiency and, after starting therapy, refer the patient to a specialized center for definitive diagnosis.

The galactose tolerance test was once the most widely used method for confirmation of galactosemia. However, there is considerable danger of hypoglycemia and hypokalemia during the test, and it has been replaced by chromatography and RBC enzyme assay.

Screening Tests.—Several screening tests are available. The most popular are a bacterial inhibition method (Paigen assay, roughly similar to the PKU Guthrie test) and the Beutler fluorometric method. The Paigen assay measures elevated blood galactose (or galactose-6-phosphate) levels, and the Beutler assay measures Gal-1-PUT activity. Both can be performed on filter paper blood spots. The Paigen test depends on elevated blood galactose levels, and therefore milk feeding is necessary. Specimens from patients not receiving milk or specimens drawn several hours after a milk feeding may yield false negative (normal) results. If the Paigen test is adapted to detect galactose-1-phosphate rather than galactose, length of time after feeding is not a problem, and even most cases in patients on a galactose-free diet are reportedly detected. The Paigen test (either type) detects galactokinase deficiency as well as transferase deficiency. The Beutler test does not depend on milk feeding. However, the test does not detect galactokinase deficiency and is more subject to effects of heat and humidity on the filter paper specimen. The Beutler test also can detect certain nonpathologic variants of transferase enzyme such as the Duarte variant.

Variants.—There are at least four variants of the transferase enzyme. The Duarte variant is the most frequent. Patients with this disorder exhibit about 50% of normal Gal-1-PUT activity on RBC assay and are clinically asymptomatic. In classic (homozygous) transferase deficiency there is almost no Gal-1-PUT activity on assay.

Other Forms of Galactosemia.—There are two other forms of galactosemia. One consists of deficiency in the enzyme galactokinase. Development of cataracts is the only symptom. The incidence of galactokinase deficiency has been variously reported as equal to that of transferase deficiency or less. The third type is deficiency of the enzyme erythrocyte epimerase, of which very few cases have been reported. These patients seem to be completely asymptomatic.

Disaccharide Malabsorption.—Certain enzymes are present in the lumen border of small intestinal mucosal cells that aid in absorption of various complex sugars by preliminary hydrolyzation. Deficiency of one or more of these enzymes may impair absorption of the affected sugar, depending on the degree of enzyme deficiency. The most common deficiency affects the disaccharide sugar lactose. Lactose is present in milk or milk products such as ice cream, yogurt, and many types of cheese. Northern Europeans as a group usually have normal intestinal lactase throughout life. Many other ethnic populations have a high incidence of lactase deficiency. The highest incidences are reported in Asians such as Chinese and Japanese, American Indians, and Eastern European (Ashkenazic) Jews. American blacks and persons of Mediterranean or South American ancestry have a high rate of deficiency. Besides primary (genetic) lactase deficiency, secondary deficiency may be induced, more or less temporarily, by certain diseases affecting the small intestine. These include primary small intestine mucosal disease (sprue), short bowel syndrome, severe acute gastroenteritis, prolonged protein-calorie malnutrition, and certain antibiotics (e.g., neomycin and kanamycin). Lactase deficiency may also occur due to prematurity. Between 26 and 34 weeks of gestation there is only about one third of full-term lactase activity present. This increases to about 70% between 35 and 38 weeks. Full activity levels are attained by birth at 40 weeks.

Persons who inherit the trait for lactase deficiency usually have normal lactase activity levels at (full-term) birth. However, at about age 3–5 years there is a fall in lactase activity. After this time there is some individual variation in degree of clinical tolerance to milk, even when intestinal lactase activity measurement is low.

Symptoms of lactase intolerance include some combination of abdominal cramps, diarrhea, bloating, and flatulence, usually occurring at or becoming worse after meals. One study involving children from age 4 years to teen-age years who had intermittent abdominal pain found their symptoms could be explained by lactose malabsorption in a high proportion of those from ethnic groups with a high incidence of lactase deficiency. Lactase deficiency in full-term newborns or young children is thought to be rare. Milk allergy may produce similar symptoms but is uncommon, usually includes allergy symptoms such as asthma with any GI symptoms, and the parents usually have a history of allergy.

Screening tests for lactase deficiency include testing of stool for pH and sugar at a time when the patient is symptomatic. Normal stool pH is 7.0–8.0. A stool pH below 6.0 raises the question of lactase deficiency. The stool can be tested for sugar by either a reducing substance method or a glucose oxidase paper strip method. The presence of glucose in the stool suggests lactase deficiency. However, in one study, parenteral antibiotics administered to neonates caused an increase in fecal reducing substances beginning within 48 hours after starting the antibiotics. Negative test results for pH and sugar do not exclude the diagnosis, and positive test results do not conclusively establish the diagnosis. Acidic stool pH can be found in certain other conditions associated with diarrhea, especially steatorrhea.

Diagnostic tests for lactase deficiency include the lactose tolerance test, hydrogen breath test, and small intestine biopsy with tissue assay for lactase. The lactose tolerance test is performed in a similar manner to the oral glucose tolerance test. After overnight fasting, 50 gm of oral lactose (in children, 1–2 gm of lactose/kg of body weight) is given in some type of flavored liquid. Serum glucose levels are assayed before lactose administration and 15, 30, 60, and 90 minutes afterward (some investigators use different time intervals; some beginning at 30 minutes instead of 15 and some ending at 120 minutes instead of 90 minutes). Normal lactase activity results in a postdose glucose elevation more than 20 mg/100 ml (1.1 mmol/L) over baseline. This assumes that malabsorption from some other cause is excluded. Some investigators measure galactose instead of glucose; 150 mg of ethanol/kg of body weight is administered with the lactose dose to inhibit liver conversion of galactose to glucose. A single blood or urine sample is obtained 40 minutes after the test dose and is assayed for galactose. The advantage of this procedure is need for only one test specimen. However, this method has not been evaluated as thoroughly as the standard lactose tolerance procedure. The hydrogen breath test is currently considered the most accurate of the tolerance tests. This is described in detail in chapter 25. Briefly, it consists of analysis of expiratory breath for hydrogen, followed by administration of oral lactose and retesting of breath samples at either 30- or 60-minute intervals for 2–4 hours. Lactase deficiency results in deposition of excess lactose into the colon, where bacterial fermentation produces excess hydrogen, which is excreted through the lungs. The hydrogen breath test can be performed only by specialized medical centers. Small intestine biopsy with quantitation of tissue levels of intestinal lactase is performed during an endoscopy procedure. Tissue biopsy has the added advantage that some of the secondary causes of lactase deficiency (e.g., sprue) can be detected. However, intestinal lactase measurement is available only at specialized medical centers.

Lactosuria.—Some patients with lactase deficiency absorb lactose from the GI tract after oral intake of lactose and excrete the lactose in the urine. However, other lactase-deficient persons do not exhibit lactosuria. Premature infants are said to be predisposed to temporary lactosuria (presumably due to their relatively lactase-deficient state). Lactosuria is apparently not uncommon in the last trimester of pregnancy and for several days following delivery.

Sucrase Enzyme Deficiency.—The disaccharide sugar sucrose is commonly used as a carbohydrate supplement. Sucrose is hydrolyzed by the enzyme sucrase in small intestine mucosa cells. Congenital sucrase deficiency has been reported but is not common. Most cases became clinically manifest within the first year of life, with symptoms predominantly of failure to thrive, diarrhea, or both. Stool pH is usually acidic. Reducing substance sugar test methods are not accurate for stool testing, since sucrose is not a biochemical reducing substance. Definitive diagnosis usually requires small intestine biopsy with tissue assay for sucrase activity.

Glycogen Storage Disease.—Glycogen storage disease includes a spectrum of syndromes resulting from defective synthesis or utilization of glycogen. Clinical manifestations depend on the organ or tissue primarily affected and the specific enzyme involved. The disease in one or another of its clinical syndromes may affect the liver, heart, or skeletal muscle. The most common is von Gierke's disease, whose clinical manifestations primarily involve the liver.

Diagnosis.—Diagnosis of the various forms of glycogen storage disease requires biopsy of liver or muscle (depending on the particular disease variant) for glycogen and enzyme analysis (see Table 36–33). In some cases, enzyme assay can be performed on other tissues. These are specialized tests, and it is best to contact a pediatric research center rather than expose the patient to inappropriate or incomplete diagnostic procedures.

LYSOSOMAL STORAGE DISEASES

Lysosomal storage diseases are the result of genetic deficiency in certain enzymes found in tissue cell cytoplasmic lysosomes. These enzymes help metabolize certain glycoproteins, glycolipids, and mucopolysaccharides. The substance normally altered by the deficient enzyme accumulates in the cell lysosome area, and a storage disease results. The nonmetabolized substance either is stored in the tissue cell cytoplasm or is taken up by phagocytes. Most of these conditions can be diagnosed by rather sophisticated assays for the enzyme that is deficient. In some instances the assay can be carried out on plasma or serum; in other cases, on peripheral blood white blood cells (WBCs); and for some enzymes, it is necessary to use patient fibroblasts obtained by skin biopsy and grown in tissue culture. In some cases the diagnosis can be made from fetal cells obtained by amniocentesis and grown in tissue culture. In most cases the assays are available only at university medical centers or specialized clinics. A few are available at certain large reference laboratories. It is recommended that a university medical center specializing in such problems or the Neurological Diseases branch of the National Institutes of Health be contacted for details on how to proceed with any patient suspected of having a lipid storage disease. It is highly preferable that the patient be sent directly to the center for biopsy or required specimen collection to avoid unnecessary and costly delays and to prevent damage to the specimen in transport.

The lysosomal storage diseases can be divided into two major categories: the sphingolipidoses and the mucopolysaccharidoses. A short summary of these conditions is presented in Table 36–36. Several are described below in more detail. Many of these disorders can be diagnosed in the first trimester of pregnancy by chorionic villus biopsy.

Sphingolipidoses (Disordered Lipid Metabolism)

The best known of this group are glycolipid storage diseases, including ganglioside storage (Tay-Sachs disease and metachromatic leukodystrophy) and ceramide storage diseases (Gaucher's disease and Niemann-Pick disease).

Tay-Sachs Disease.—This condition is due to accumulation of the ganglioside GM_2 in various tissues but most notably in the brain. The defective enzyme responsible is known as "hexaminidase." There are two forms (similar to isoenzymes) of hexaminidase, commonly abbreviated as hex-A and hex-B. The ethnic groups most often affected by classic Tay-Sachs disease are Askenazim (Central or Eastern European) Jews and, to a lesser extent, other Jews and inhabitants of the Middle East country of Yemen. There are several other very similar disorders involving hexaminidase deficiency that are generally considered variants of Tay-Sachs disease and are not commoner in Jews. In the classic and commonest form of Tay-Sachs disease, the infant appears normal at birth and for the first 5–6 months but then fails to develop any further mentally, loses some motor ability, and develops a "cherry-red spot" on the macula of the eye. The disease proceeds to dementia, flaccid muscles followed by spastic muscles, blindness, and death by age 3 years. There are less common variants that proceed more swiftly or in a somewhat more prolonged fashion.

Diagnosis.—The classic form of Tay-Sachs disease is due to deficiency in hex-A enzyme. The hex-A enzyme can be assayed in serum; peripheral blood WBCs and patient fibroblasts can also be used. The diagnosis can be established in the fetus by amniocentesis. The hex-A assay can be used to detect carriers of the Tay-Sachs gene. The disease is transmitted as an autosomal recessive trait, so that if one parent is tested and has normal hex-A levels, the infant will not be homozygous. Therefore, the infant will not be clinically affected, even if the other parent has the gene. Tay-Sachs screening on the fetus in utero can be performed by chorionic villus biopsy in the first trimester.

Gaucher's Disease.—Gaucher's disease is a disorder in which the glycolipid cerebroside compound kerasin is phagocytized by the reticuloendothelial system. There seem to be two subgroups of this disorder—a fatal disease of relatively short duration in infancy accompanied by mental retardation, and a more slowly progressive disease found in older children and young adults and not accompanied by mental retardation. Splenomegaly is the most characteristic finding, but the liver and occasionally the lymph nodes also may become enlarged. The most characteristic x-ray findings are aseptic necrosis of the femoral heads and widening of the femoral marrow cavities; although typical, these findings may be absent. Anemia is frequent, and there may be leukopenia and thrombocytopenia due to hypersplenism. The serum acid phosphatase level usually is elevated if the chemical method used is not reasonably specific for prostatic acid phosphatase. (There are several widely used chemical methods, and although none is completely specific for prostatic acid phosphatase, some are considerably more so than others.)

Before the late 1970s, diagnosis was made by bone marrow aspiration. Wright-stained bone marrow smears frequently would contain characteristic Gaucher's cells, which are large mononuclear phagocytes whose cytoplasm is filled with a peculiar linear or fibrillar material. Splenic aspiration or liver biopsy was also done in problematic cases. The diagnosis is now made by assay of peripheral blood leukocytes for beta-glucosidase, the enzyme whose deficiency is the cause of the disease. Skin biopsy with tissue culture of skin fibroblasts followed by beta-glucosidase assay is also possible.

Niemann-Pick Disease.—Niemann-Pick disease is similar clinically and pathologically to the fatal early childhood form of Gaucher's disease, except that the abnormal lipid involved is the phospholipid sphingomyelin. As in Gaucher's disease, diagnosis used to be made by bone marrow aspiration, although the phagocytic cells are not as characteristic as those of Gaucher's disease. Splenic biopsy with tissue lipid analysis was also done. The diagnosis is now made by skin biopsy with tissue culture of the fibroblasts and assay of the fibroblasts for sphingomyelinase, the enzyme whose deficiency is the cause of the disease.

Mucopolysaccharidoses (Disorders of Connective Tissue and Bone)

The best known of this group are Hunter's and Hurler's syndromes. In these conditions there is inability to metabolize certain mucopolysaccharides, resulting in accumulation and storage of these substances in various body organs and tissues and excretion of some stored material in the urine (see Table 36–37).

Hurler's Syndrome.—Hurler's syndrome is caused by deficiency of the enzyme alpha-L-iduronase. Affected infants appear normal for the first 6–8 months of life but then develop skeletal abnormalities (short stature, kyphosis, broad hands, saddle-shaped deformity of the bridge of the nose), clouding of the cornea leading to severe loss of vision, a tendency toward umbilical and inguinal hernias, hepatosplenomegaly, thick tongue, and mental retardation. Diagnosis of Hurler's syndrome (or any of the mucopolysaccharide disorders) can be made by chromatographic identification of the mucopolysaccharide excreted in the urine. A more conclusive diagnosis can be established by tissue culture of skin biopsy fibroblasts with assay for the specific enzyme involved.

Other Connective Tissue Disorders.—There is an important group of hereditary connective tissue disorders, including Marfan's syndrome, Ehlers-Danlos syndrome, and osteogenesis imperfecta, for which no laboratory screening test or specific diagnostic biochemical test is available. Diagnosis is made by clinical criteria, in some cases supported by x-ray findings.

DEFECTS IN AMINO ACID METABOLISM (AMINOACIDOPATHIES)

Primary (Metabolic) Aminoacidopathies

Phenylketonuria (PKU).—Classic PKU is inherited as an autosomal recessive trait. It is uncommon in Asians and blacks. The disease is due to deficiency of a liver enzyme known as "phenylalanine hydroxylase," which is needed to convert the amino acid phenylalanine to tyrosine. With its major utilization pathway blocked, phenylalanine accumulates in the blood and leads to early onset of progressive mental deficiency. This disease is one of the more common causes of hereditary mental deficiency and one of the few whose bad effects can be prevented by early treatment of the infant. At birth the infant usually has normal serum levels of phenylalanine (< 2 mg/100 ml) due to maternal enzyme activity, although some instances of mental damage in utero occur. In the neonatal period, after beginning a diet containing phenylalanine (e.g., milk), serum phenylalanine levels begin to rise. When the phenylalanine to tyrosine pathway is blocked, some phenylalanine metabolism is shunted to ordinarily little-used systems such as transamination to phenylpyruvic acid.

Urine Screening Tests.—When the serum phenylalanine level reaches 12–15 mg/100 ml, sufficient phenylpyruvic acid is produced that it begins to appear in the urine. This becomes detectable by urine screening tests (Phenistix or the older ferric chloride test) at some time between ages 3 and 6 weeks. Unfortunately, by then some degree of irreversible mental damage may have occurred. Therefore, it is highly desirable to make an earlier diagnosis to begin treatment as soon as possible after birth.

Blood Screening Tests.—The most widely used screening test for elevated serum phenylalanine levels is the Guthrie test. This is a bacterial inhibition procedure. A certain substance that competes with phenylalanine in *Bacillus subtilis* metabolism is incorporated into culture medium; this essentially provides a phenylalanine-deficient culture medium. *Bacillus subtilis* spores are seeded into this medium; but to produce significant bacterial growth, a quantity of phenylalanine equivalent to more than normal blood levels must be furnished. Next, a sample of the patient's blood is added, and the presence of abnormal quantities of serum phenylalanine is reflected by bacterial growth in the area where the specimen was applied. The Guthrie test, if properly done, is adequately sensitive and accurate and reliably detects definitely abnormal levels of serum phenylalanine (≥ 4 mg/100 ml). It also fulfills the requirements for an acceptable screening method. However, there are two controversial aspects to this test. First, the standard practice is to obtain a blood specimen from the infant (usually as a filter paper blood spot using a heel puncture) before discharge from the hospital. In some cases this may result in the specimen being obtained 48 hours or less after birth, with an even shorter duration of phenylalanine intake if milk feeding is not begun soon after birth. There is some controversy in the literature as to whether a significant percentage (about 5%–10%) of infants with PKU will be missed if the specimen is obtained in the first 48 hours of life. A few studies indicate that this is unlikely, but the number of patients was not large enough to conclusively establish this point. Some screening programs recommend second testing of infants discharged before 48 hours of life, and most authorities recommend retesting if the initial test specimen was obtained before 24 hours of life.

Second, PKU is not the only cause of elevated serum phenylalanine levels in the neonate. In fact, more positive (abnormally elevated) Guthrie test results are reportedly caused by non-PKU etiologies than by PKU. A major etiology is temporary ("late enzyme development") hypertyrosinemia associated with low birth weight, high-protein formulas, and vitamin C deficiency. Some infants with severe liver disease and some with galactosemia have been reported to have elevated serum phenylalanine levels. Since hyperphenylalaninemia is not diagnostic of PKU, and since a long-term low-phenylalanine diet could be harmful to some persons who do not have PKU, an abnormal Guthrie test result should be followed up by more detailed investigation, including, as a minimum, both the serum phenylalanine and tyrosine levels. The typical PKU patient has a serum phenylalanine level greater than 15 mg/100 ml, with a serum tyrosine level less than 5 mg/100 ml. The tests may have to be repeated in 1–2 weeks if values have not reached these levels.

Phenylketonuria Variants.—About 10% of infants with apparent PKU have been found to have a PKU variant. The enzyme system for alteration of phenylalanine to tyrosine is actually a group of at least four enzymes and coenzymes. Deficiency in the hydroxylase enzyme produces classic PKU. Deficiency in one of the other components of the system produces variant PKU. In particular, the variant caused by deficiency of the co-factor tetrahydrobiopterin (estimated to account for 0.5%–3.0% of persistent hyperphenylalaninemias) requires therapy in addition to a phenylalanine-deficient diet. Some patients with other variants of PKU do not require a phenylalanine-free diet.

Diagnosis of PKU variants was originally made with a tolerance test using oral phenylalanine (in milk or other materials). Persistence of elevated blood phenylalanine levels greater than 20 mg/100 ml for more than 72 hours was considered indicative of classic PKU, whereas a decrease below the 20-ml level before 72 hours was considered indicative of variant PKU. This association has been challenged by others, and sophisticated tests have been devised to determine the exact etiology of the different forms of persistent hyperphenylalaninemia. Some of these procedures are available only in pediatric research centers. It would seem reasonable to recommend that an abnormal Guthrie test result be immediately followed up with a blood specimen for assay of phenylalanine and tyrosine levels. Afterward, pending results, the infant should be placed on a low-phenylalanine diet. If both phenylalanine and tyrosine levels are high, the patient probably does not have PKU. If only the phenylalanine level is high, and especially if it is greater than 15 mg/100 ml, the infant should be referred to a specialized PKU center for additional studies while the low-phenylalanine diet is continued.

Alkaptonuria (Ochronosis).—The typical manifestations of this uncommon disease are the triad of arthritis, black pigmentation of cartilage (ochronosis), and excretion of homogentisic acid in the urine. Arthritis usually begins in middle age and typically involves the spine and the large joints. Black pigmentation of cartilage is most apparent in the ears but may be noticed in cartilage elsewhere or may even appear in tendons. The intervertebral disks often become heavily calcified and thus provide a characteristic x-ray picture. The disease is caused by abnormal accumulation of homogentisic acid, an intermediate metabolic product of tyrosine; this, in turn, is caused by a deficiency of the liver enzyme homogentisic acid oxidase, which mediates the further breakdown of the acid. Most of the hemogentisic acid is excreted in the urine, but enough slowly accumulates in cartilage and surrounding tissues to cause the characteristic changes previously described. Diagnosis is established by demonstration of homogentisic acid in the urine. Addition of 10% sodium hydroxide turns the urine black or gray-black. A false positive urine glucose test result is produced by copper reduction methods such as Benedict's test or Clinitest, whereas glucose oxidase dipstick methods are negative.

Other Primary Aminoacidopathies.—These are numerous, varied, and rare. They are mostly diagnosed by paper chromatography of urine (or serum), looking for abnormal quantities of the particular amino acid involved whose metabolic pathway has been blocked. The most widely known diseases (apart from PKU and alkaptonuria) are maple syrup disease and histidinemia. The most common is homocystinuria. Many of the primary aminoacidopathies can be diagnosed in the first trimester of pregnancy by means of chorionic villus biopsy.

Secondary Aminoacidopathies.—Secondary aminoacidopathies are associated with a renal defect, usually of reabsorption, rather than a primary defect in the metabolic pathway of the amino acid in question. The serum levels are normal. The most common cause is a systemic disease such as Wilson's disease, lead poisoning, or Fanconi's syndrome. In such cases, several amino acids usually are found in the urine. Aminoaciduria may occur normally in the first week of life, especially in premature infants. A much smaller number of patients have a more specific amino acid renal defect with one or more specific amino acids excreted; the most common of these diseases is cystinuria. Patients with cystinuria develop cystine renal calculi. Cystine crystals may be identified in acidified urine, proving the diagnosis. Otherwise, combined urine and serum paper chromatography is the diagnostic method of choice.

CHROMOSOMAL ABNORMALITIES

Chromosome Analysis.—There are several conditions, some relatively common and some rare, that result from either abnormal numbers of chromosomes, defects in size or configuration of certain single chromosomes, or abnormal composition of the chromosome group that determines sexual characteristics. Laboratory diagnosis, at present, takes two forms. First, chromosome charts may be prepared on any individual by culturing certain body cells, such as WBCs from peripheral blood or bone marrow, and by introducing a chemical such as colchicine, which kills the cells at a specific stage in mitosis when the chromosomes become organized and separated, and then photographing and separating the individual chromosomes into specific groups according to similarity in size and configuration. The most widely used system is the Denver classification. The 46 human chromosomes are composed of 22 chromosome pairs and, in addition, 2 unpaired chromosomes, the sex chromosomes (XX in the female and XY in the male). In a Denver chromosome chart (karyotype) the 22 paired chromosomes are separated into 7 groups, each containing 2 or more individually identified and numbered chromosomes. For example, the first group contains chromosomes 1 to 3, the seventh group contains chromosomes 21 to 22. In addition, there is an eighth group for the two unpaired sex chromosomes. Chromosome culture requires substantial experience and care in preparation and interpretation. Material for chromosome analysis can be obtained in the first trimester of pregnancy by means of chorionic villus biopsy.

Barr Body Test.—The other, more widely used technique provides certain useful information about the composition of the sex chromosome group. Barr found that the nuclei of various body cells contain a certain stainable sex chromatin mass (Barr body) that appears for each X chromosome more than one that the cell possesses. Therefore, a normal male (XY) cell has no Barr body because there is only one X chromosome, a normal female (XX) cell has one Barr body, and a person with the abnormal configuration XXX has two Barr bodies. The most convenient method for Barr body detection at present is the buccal smear. This is obtained by scraping the oral mucosa, smearing the epithelial cells thus collected onto a glass slide in a monolayer, and, after immediate chemical fixation, staining with special stains. Comparison of the results, together with the secondary sex characteristics and genitalia of the patient, allows presumptive diagnosis of certain sex chromosome abnormalities. The results may be confirmed, if necessary, by chromosome karyotyping.

Specimens for buccal smear should not be obtained during the first week of life or during adrenocorticosteroid or estrogen therapy, because these situations falsely lower the incidence of sex chromatin Barr bodies. Certain artifacts may be confused with the nuclear Barr bodies. Poor slide preparations may obscure the sex chromatin mass and lead to false negative appearances. Also, only about 40%–60% of normal female cells contain an identifiable Barr body. The buccal smear by itself does not reveal the true genetic sex; it is only an indication of the number of female (X) chromosomes present.

Klinefelter's Syndrome.—In this condition the patient looks outwardly like a male, but the sex chromosome makeup is XXY instead of XY. The external genitalia are usually normal, except for small testes. There is a tendency toward androgen deficiency and thus toward gynecomastia and decreased body hair, but these findings may be slight or not evident. There also is a tendency toward mental deficiency, but most affected persons have perfectly normal intelligence. Patients with Klinefelter's syndrome are almost always sterile. Testicular biopsy used to be the main diagnostic method, with histologic specimens showing marked atrophy of the seminiferous tubules. At present, a buccal smear is the procedure of choice; it shows a "normal female" configuration with one Barr body (due to the two XX chromosomes). In the presence of unmistakably male genitalia, this usually is sufficient for clinical diagnosis. Chromosome karyotyping may be necessary to confirm the diagnosis in doubtful cases.

Turner's Syndrome (Ovarian Agenesis).—Turner's syndrome is the most frequent chromosomal sexual abnormality in females, just as Klinefelter's syndrome is in males. In Turner's syndrome there is a deletion of 1 female (X) chromosome so that the patient has only 45 chromosomes instead of 46 and only 1 female sex chromosome instead of 2. Typically the affected female has relatively short stature but normal body proportions. There is deficient development of secondary sex characteristics and small genitalia, although body hair usually is female in distribution. Some affected persons have associated anomalies such as webbing of the neck, coarctation of the aorta, and short fingers. They do not menstruate and actually lack ovaries. Diagnosis may be made in most cases by buccal smear; this should be "sex-chromatin negative," since Barr bodies appear only when the female sex chromosomes number more than one. If the buccal smear is "chromatin positive," a chromosome karyotype should be ordered, because some patients with Turner's syndrome have mixtures of normal cells and defective cells (mosaicism). Some investigators believe that if the patient does not have definite clinical (physical) evidence of Turner's syndrome except for short stature, chromosome karyotyping should be done without a buccal smear, since most of the "nonphenotypic" Turner's syndrome patients have mosaicism rather than XO genotype.

Mongolism (Down's Syndrome).—Down's syndrome is a relatively frequent disorder associated with two different chromosome abnormalities. Most patients (about 92%) have an extra number 21 chromosome in the number 21–22 chromosome group (therefore having 3 chromosomes in this group instead of 2, a condition known as trisomy 21). These patients have a total of 47 chromosomes instead of 46. The chromosome abnormality has nothing to do with the sex chromosomes, which are normal. This type of mongolism apparently is spontaneous, not inherited (i.e., there is no family history of mongolism, and there is very little risk the parents will produce another affected child). This type of Down's syndrome occurs with increased frequency when the mother is over age 35. About 5% of patients with Down's syndrome have an extra 21-type chromosome, but it is attached to one of the other chromosomes, most often in the 13–15 group (called the "D group" in some nomenclatures). This type of arrangement is called a "translocation." The translocation attachment is most frequent on the number 14 chromosome, but it may attach elsewhere. The translocation abnormality can be inherited; it means that one parent has a normal total number of chromosomes, but one of the pair of number 21 chromosomes was attached to one of the number 14 chromosomes. The other number 21 and the other number 14 chromosome are normal. The two-chromosome (14 + 21) cluster behaves in meiosis as though it were a single number 14 chromosome. If the abnormal chromosome cluster is passed to a child, two situations could result: a child with clinical Down's syndrome who received the translocated 14 + 21 chromosome plus the normal number 21 chromosome from one parent (and another number 21 chromosome from the other parent, making a total of three number 21 chromosomes), or a carrier who received the translocated 14 + 21 chromosome but did not receive the other (normal) number 21 chromosome from the same parent (the translocated 14 + 21 chromosome plus a number 21 chromosome from the other parent make a total of two number 21 chromosomes). The translocation Down's syndrome patient has a total of 46 chromosomes (the two-chromosome unit counts as a single chromosome).

Clinically, an infant or child with Down's syndrome usually has some combination of the following: prominent epicanthal folds at the medial aspect of the eyes, flattened facies, flat bridge of the nose, slanted lateral aspect of the eyes, mental retardation or deficiency, broad hands and feet, and a single long transverse crease on the palm instead of several shorter transverse creases. Other frequent but still less common associated abnormalities are umbilical hernia, webbing of the toes, and certain types of congenital heart disease. There also is an increased incidence of acute leukemia.

Diagnosis usually can be made clinically, but chromosome karyotyping is a valuable means of confirmation and of diagnosis in equivocal cases. It probably is advisable to do chromosome karyotyping in most children with mongolism, because the type of chromosome pattern gives an indication of the prognosis for future children.

Prenatal diagnosis can be made in the first trimester by chorionic villus biopsy. Maternal alpha-fetoprotein blood levels lower than normal in the 16th to 18th week of gestation suggest possible Down's syndrome. This would have to be confirmed with fetal cells obtained by amniocentesis.

Fragile X Chromosome.—The fragile X chromosome refers to a narrowing in the X chromosome, at which point the chromosome breaks more easily than usual when cultured in a medium that is deficient in thymidine and folic acid. The syndrome is said to be second only to Down's syndrome as a cause of hereditary mental retardation. The fragile X abnormality is reported to be associated with 30%–50% of cases of X-linked mental retardation as part of a syndrome which also includes certain mild facial changes. About 30% of female carriers may have mild mental retardation, which is unusual for heterozygotic status in most illnesses. Male offspring of a (heterozygous) carrier female would have a 50% chance of developing the syndrome. Unfortunately, only about 30%–56% of heterozygotic females demonstrate the fragile X defect using current laboratory methods. Sensitivity of these methods is age dependent, and best detection rates occur testing women less than 30 years old. There have also been reports of some affected men with normal range IQ who would qualify as carriers. It has been estimated that as many as 20% of male offspring with normal IQs born to female carriers actually are themselves carriers.

Other Chromosomal Disorders.—A wide variety of syndromes, usually consisting of multiple congenital deformities and anomalies, are now found to be due to specific chromosomal abnormalities. The most common of these involve trisomy in the 13–15 (D) group and in the 16–18 (E) group. Some patients with repeated spontaneous abortions have abnormal karyotypes. Various tumors have yielded abnormal chromosome patterns, but no one type of tumor is associated with any consistent pattern (except for chronic myelogenous leukemia).

Commonly Accepted Indications for Buccal Smear.—These include the following:

1. Ambiguous or abnormal genitalia
2. Male or female infertility without other known cause
3. Symptoms suggestive of Turner's syndrome or Klinefelter's syndrome, such as primary amenorrhea

Indications for Chromosome Karyotyping.—These include selected patients in the buccal smear groups just described for confirmation or initial diagnosis and:

1. Mongoloid infants; also, possible carriers
2. Mentally defective persons
3. Persons with multiple congenital anomalies

CONGENITAL DISEASES OF SKELETAL MUSCLE

Several well-known disorders affecting skeletal muscle either are not congenital or do not as yet have any conspicuously useful laboratory test. Among these are disorders whose primary defect is located in the central nervous system or peripheral nervous system rather than in skeletal muscle itself. In this group are various neurologic diseases that secondarily result in symptoms of muscle weakness. The following discussion involves inherited disorders. Some can be diagnosed in the first trimester of pregnancy by means of amniotic villus biopsy.

Muscular Dystrophies.—The muscular dystrophies can be divided into several subgroups (see Table 36–34). The most common is Duchenne's (pseudohypertrophic) dystrophy. Duchenne's dystrophy is usually transmitted as a sex-linked recessive disorder, although sporadic instances have been reported. The patient is clinically normal for the first few months of life; symptoms develop usually between ages 1 and 6 years. The most frequent symptoms are lower extremity and pelvic muscle weakness. There is spotty but progressive muscle fiber dissolution, with excessive replacement by fat and fibrous tissue. The latter process leads to the most characteristic physical finding of the disease, pseudohypertrophy of the calf muscles.

Laboratory Tests.—The usefulness of laboratory tests is based on the fact that certain enzymes are found in relatively high concentrations in normal skeletal muscle. These include creatine phosphokinase, aldolase, AST, and lactic dehydrogenase (LDH). Despite external pseudohypertrophy, the dystrophic muscles actually undergo individual fiber dissolution and loss of skeletal muscle substance, accompanied by release of muscle enzymes into the bloodstream. In many tissues AST, LDH, and aldolase are found together. Pulmonary infarction, myocardial infarction, and acute liver cell damage among other conditions cause elevated serum levels of these enzymes. Aldolase follows a pattern similar to AST in liver disease and to LDH otherwise. Creatine phosphokinase (CPK) is found in significant concentration only in brain, heart muscle, and skeletal muscle.

The two most helpful tests in Duchenne's muscular dystrophy are CPK and aldolase assays. Aldolase and CPK values are elevated very early in the disease, well before clinical symptoms become manifest, and the elevations usually are more than 10 times normal, at least for CPK. This marked elevation persists as symptoms develop. Eventually, after replacement of muscle substance has become chronic and extensive, the aldolase level often becomes normal and the CPK level may be either normal or only mildly elevated (less than five times normal). In the hereditary type of Duchenne's dystrophy, borderline or elevated CPK values have been reported in variable numbers of carrier females (in one study, up to 80%). Aldolase values are much less frequently abnormal; AST and LDH values tend to parallel CPK and aldolase values but at a much lower level. Therefore, these enzyme values frequently are normal in the later stages of the disease, when the more sensitive tests are still considerably abnormal, and so are not of much use in detecting carriers. Even with CPK, a normal result does not exclude carrier status.

The CPK isoenzyme pattern in Duchenne's dystrophy may show an increased MB isoenzyme as well as MM fraction, especially in the earlier phases of the illness.

In fascioscapulohumeral dystrophy and limbgirdle dystrophy, conditions that resemble Duchenne's dystrophy in many respects, CPK and aldolase levels are variable but frequently are normal.

Other muscular disorders in which the serum enzyme levels may be elevated are trauma, dermatomyositis, and polymyositis. The levels of elevation are said to be considerably below those seen in early cases of Duchenne's dystrophy. Neurologic disease is usually not associated with elevated levels, even when there is marked secondary muscular atrophy.

Definitive Diagnosis.—Diagnosis of the muscular dystrophies may sometimes be made on the basis of the clinical picture and enzyme values. A more definitive diagnosis can be made with the addition of muscle biopsy. This becomes essential when the findings are not clear cut. The biceps or quadriceps muscles are the preferred biopsy location. The biopsy is best done at a pediatric or congenital disease research center where special studies (e.g., histochemical staining or electron microscopy) can be performed and the proper specimen secured for this purpose (these special studies provide additional information and are essential when biopsy results are atypical or yield unexpected findings). Diagnosis in the first trimester of pregnancy can be done using DNA probe techniques on a chorionic villus biopsy specimen.

Malignant Hyperpyrexia (Malignant Hyperthermia.—Malignant hyperpyrexia (MH) is a rare complication of anesthesia triggered by various conduction and inhalation agents (most commonly succinylcholine) that produces a marked increase in both aerobic and anaerobic skeletal muscle metabolism. This results in greatly increased production of carbon dioxide, lactic acid, and heat. Such overproduction, in turn, is clinically manifested by a marked increase in body temperature, tachycardia, muscle rigidity, tachypnea, and finally shock. The first clinical sign is said to be muscle rigidity, which occurs in about 70%–75% of patients. The next clinical evidence of developing MH is tachycardia or cardiac ventricular multifocal arrhythmias. A rise in temperature eventually occurs in nearly all patients (some cases have been reported without temperature elevation), first slowly and then rapidly. The characteristic temperature elevation may not be present in the early stages, or the initial elevation may be gradual. A defect in muscle cell membrane transport has been postulated. The majority of cases have been familial.

Laboratory Tests.—Biochemical abnormalities include metabolic acidosis (markedly elevated lactic acid value) and respiratory acidosis (increased partial pressure of carbon dioxide [PCO_2] due to muscle CO_2 production). The anion gap is increased due to the lactic acid. In the early phases, venous PCO_2 is markedly increased, whereas arterial PCO_2 may be normal or only mildly increased (widening of the normal arteriovenous [AV] CO_2 dissociation). The same accentuation of normal AV differences also occurs with the PO_2 values. Later, arterial blood gas values also show increased PCO_2, decreased pH, and decreased PO_2. In addition to blood gas changes there typically is greatly increased CPK levels (from muscle contraction), and myoglobin appears in the urine. In the later stages there may be hyperkalemia, hypernatremia, muscle edema, pulmonary edema, renal failure, disseminated intravascular coagulation, and shock. The serum calcium level may be normal or increased, but the ionized calcium level is increased.

Diagnosis.—Creatine phosphokinase elevation without known cause has been proposed as a screening test; there is marked difference of opinion among investigators as to the usefulness of the procedure, either in screening for surgery or in family studies (30%–40% of MH patients without active MH have been reported to have normal CPK values). Likewise, disagreement exists as to the CPK isoenzyme associated with abnormality; BB has been reported by some, although the majority found MM to be responsible. However, CPK assay is still the most widely used screening test. Muscle biopsy with special in vitro testing of muscle fiber sensitivity to such agents as caffeine and halothane is considered a definitive diagnostic procedure but is available only in a few research centers. Microscopic examination of muscle biopsy specimens shows only nonspecific abnormalities, most often described as compatible with myopathy. Several other tests such as halothane-stimulated platelet bioassay for certain nucleotides and muscle assay for increased myophosphorylase A have been proposed, but these have not yet been sufficiently evaluated.

DISEASES OF MINERAL METABOLISM

Wilson's Disease (Hepatolenticular Degeneration).—Wilson's disease most often becomes manifest between ages 8 and 30 years. It is uncommon for symptoms to develop before age 6 years. About 40%–50% of patients initially develop hepatic symptoms, about 40% begin with neurologic symptoms, and about 20% initially are said to have psychiatric abnormalities, such as schizophrenia. A few patients develop a Coombs-negative hemolytic anemia. Hepatic symptoms are more typically seen in children, although they may occur at any age. In children, this most commonly takes the form of chronic hepatitis, although in some patients the test results may resemble acute hepatitis virus hepatitis. A macronodular type of cirrhosis develops later and is usually present in patients with late-stage Wilson's disease, whether or not there were symptoms of active liver disease. Some patients present with minimally active or with nonactive cirrhosis. Neurologic symptoms typically originate in the basal ganglia area (lentiform nucleus) of the brain and consist of varying degrees of incoordination, tremor, spasticity, rigidity, and dysarthria. There may also be a peculiar flapping tremor.

Wilson's disease is characterized by inability of the liver to manufacture normal quantities of the alpha-2 globulin ceruloplasmin, which is the plasma transport agent for copper. For reasons not entirely understood, excessive copper is deposited in various tissues, eventually producing damage to the basal ganglia of the brain and to the liver. The kidney is also affected, leading to aminoaciduria, and copper is deposited in the cornea, producing a zone of discoloration called the Kayser-Fleischer ring.

Clinical Diagnosis.—The triad of typical basal ganglia symptoms, Kayser-Fleischer ring, and hepatic cirrhosis, is virtually diagnostic. However, many patients do not have the textbook picture, especially in the early stages. The Kayser-Fleischer ring is often grossly visible but in many cases can be seen only by slit lamp examination. All patients with neurologic symptoms are said to have the Kayser-Fleischer ring as well as the majority of those with hepatic symptoms. The Kayser-Fleischer ring may not be present in some asymptomatic patients detected during family study investigation or at the beginning of symptoms from hepatic disease without neurologic findings. In one series, about 15% of patients did not have a demonstrable Kayser-Fleischer ring at the time of diagnosis. Patients with primary biliary cirrhosis may also develop a corneal abnormality identical to the Kayser-Fleischer ring.

Plasma Ceruloplasmin Assay.—Laboratory studies may be of value in diagnosis, especially in the preclinical or early stages. The plasma ceruloplasmin level is low from birth in 95% of patients, and is considered the best screening test for Wilson's disease. However, normal newborn infants may have decreased ceruloplasmin levels, and the test is not considered reliable until about 3 months of age. Although a normal ceruloplasmin level (> 20 mg/100 ml; 200 mg/L) is usually interpreted as excluding Wilson's disease, about 5% (range, 4%–10%) of Wilson's disease patients have values greater than 20 mg/100 ml. Estrogen therapy can raise ceruloplasmin levels. Smoking is reported to raise ceruloplasmin levels about 30%. Although a decreased ceruloplasmin level is usually considered suggestive of Wilson's disease, about 5% of normal persons may have values less than 20 mg/100 ml (200 mg/L), and values may be decreased in the nephrotic syndrome, malabsorption syndromes such as sprue, and in various liver diseases (about 20% of cases in one study). However, it is possible that some patients with liver disease and decreased ceruloplasmin levels have Wilson's disease.

Liver biopsy has also been used for diagnosis. The microscopic findings are not specific, and most often consist of either macronodular cirrhosis (often with some fatty change and occasionally with Mallory bodies) or chronic active hepatitis (10%–15% of patients with Wilson's disease). The most typical finding is increased hepatic copper content by special stains (or tissue analysis, if available). For histologic staining of copper, fixation of the biopsy specimen in alcohol rather than the routine fixatives is recommended. Here again, it is advisable to wait 6–12 weeks after birth. Increased hepatic copper content is not specific for Wilson's disease, since some degree of copper increase has been reported to occur in some patients with postnecrotic cirrhosis due to hepatitis virus hepatitis, in patients with primary biliary cirrhosis, and occasionally in patients with other chronic cholestatic syndromes. Also, increased hepatic copper content is not present in all patients with Wilson's disease, especially in small-needle biopsy specimens.

Serum and Urine Copper.—Serum copper levels are usually normal or increased in contrast to decreased plasma ceruloplasmin levels. Urine copper level in symptomatic Wilson's disease is almost always considerably increased (more than twice normal in a 24-hour urine specimen). Increased urine copper excretion is not specific for Wilson's disease and may be found in various liver diseases, especially those with some degree of cholestasis. However, these conditions usually have normal or elevated plasma ceruloplasmin levels.

Other Laboratory Abnormalities.—Besides abnormalities in copper metabolism, many patients have a low serum uric acid level, a finding that should arouse suspicion of Wilson's disease if supporting evidence is present. Other laboratory findings that may be encountered in some patients are low serum phosphorus levels, thrombocytopenia, aminoaciduria, glucosuria, and uricosuria. A Coombs-negative hemolytic anemia occurs in a few patients.

Hemochromatosis.—Hemochromatosis is an uncommon disease produced by idiopathic excess iron absorption from the GI tract, which leads to excess deposition of iron in various tissues, especially the liver. There still is dispute as to which iron storage diseases should be included within the term hemochromatosis. In this discussion, hemochromatosis refers to the hereditary iron storage disorder and hemosiderosis to nonhereditary (secondary) forms. Hemochromatosis is transmitted as an autosomal recessive trait. Males are affected more often than females (3:2 in one series), and males seem overall to have more severe disease than females.

Clinical onset of the disease is usually between ages 40 and 60 years. Signs, symptoms, and laboratory abnormalities depend on the stage of disease and (probably) whether there is also a significant degree of alcohol intake. Cirrhosis, diabetes mellitus, and bronze skin pigmentation form a classic triad diagnostic of hemochromatosis. However, this triad is a late manifestation, and in one study including more early cases it was present in less than 10% of the patients. The most frequent symptom is joint pain (47%–57% of patients), which can be confused with rheumatoid arthritis. Hepatomegaly is present in 54%–93% of patients, cirrhosis on liver biopsy in 57%–94%, heart failure in 0%–35%, hypogonadism (in males) in 18%–61%, skin pigmentation in 51%–85% (not really noticeable in many patients), and clinically evident diabetes in 6%–72%. Alcoholism (15%–50%) or poor nutrition was frequent in some series. Hepatoma has been reported to develop in 15%–30% of patients.

Laboratory findings include the expected blood glucose abnormalities of diabetes (chapter 27) in those patients with overt diabetes, and decreased glucose tolerance in some of those without clinical diabetes. Aspartate aminotransferase levels are elevated in 46%–54% of cases, reflecting active liver cell involvement.

Laboratory Iron Studies.—The body iron abnormality is manifested by actual or relative increase in serum iron levels and decrease in total iron–binding capacity (TIBC), producing increased saturation (% saturation) of the TIBC. In addition, hemosiderin very often can be demonstrated in the urine sediment by iron stains. The most sensitive laboratory test for hemochromatosis is % saturation of TIBC (or of transferrin), which is greater than 60% (reference range, 16%–50%) in nearly all patients. Serum iron level is increased in more than 80% of patients and serum ferritin level is increased in more than 72% of patients; both of these tests are usually abnormal in affected males but much more variable in females. Liver biopsy demonstrates marked deposition of iron in parenchymal cells and frequently reveals cirrhosis.

The most widely used screening test is serum iron. Elevated values raise the question of hemochromatosis. About 2.4% of normal persons are reported to have elevated serum iron values that spontaneously return to the reference range within 1–2 days. Serum iron levels can also be increased in hemosiderosis (nonhereditary iron overload), due to blood transfusion, chronic severe hemolytic anemias, sideroblastic anemias, alcoholic cirrhosis, parenteral iron therapy, and considerably increased iron intake. Several other conditions that may be associated with increased serum iron levels are listed in chapter 36. Various diseases (see chaptere 3) can lower the serum iron level, and if one of these conditions is superimposed on hemochromatosis, the serum iron level might be decreased sufficiently to reach the reference range area.

As noted earlier, the best screening procedure is percent saturation of transferrin. This is calculated by dividing the serum iron value by the TIBC value. However, like serum iron, increase in % transferrin saturation is not specific for hemochromatosis, since there are other conditions that decrease percent saturation (see chapter 36). Even liver biopsy iron may not differentiate hemochromatosis from hemosiderosis in some cases, and the liver cells of cirrhosis without abnormality of iron metabolism may display some degree of increased iron levels.

Family Member Screening.—Hemochromatosis rarely becomes clinically evident before age 30, so that screening family members of patients has been advocated to detect unrecognized homozygotes to begin therapy before clinical symptoms develop. One study found that % transferrin saturation detected about 90% of occult homozygotes, whereas assay of serum iron levels detected about 85% and assay of serum ferritin levels detected about 50%.

ABNORMALITIES OF GLANDULAR SECRETION

Cystic Fibrosis.—Cystic fibrosis (mucoviscidosis, or fibrocystic disease of the pancreas) is the most common eventually lethal autosomal recessive inherited disorder in whites, with an estimated gene frequency of 1 in 2,000 live births. The incidence in blacks is about 2% of that in whites; the disorder is rare in Asians. Symptoms result predominantly from damage to mucus-producing exocrine glands, although non–mucus-producing exocrine glands can also be affected. The mucus glands produce abnormally viscid secretions that may inspissate, plug the gland ducts, and generate obstructive complications. In the lungs, this may lead to recurrent bronchopneumonia, the most frequent and most dangerous complication of cystic fibrosis. *Pseudomonas aeruginosa* and *Staphylococcus aureus* are the most frequent pathogens. The next most common abnormality is complete or partial destruction of the exocrine portions of the pancreas, leading to various degrees of malabsorption, steatorrhea, digestive disturbances, and malnutrition. This manifestation varies in severity, and about 15% of patients have only a minimal disorder or even a normal pancreatic exocrine function. Less common findings are biliary cirrhosis, most often focal, due to obstruction of bile ductules; and intestinal obstruction by inspissated meconium (meconium ileus), found in 10%–15% of newborns with cystic fibrosis.

Sweat Test for Screening.—Non–mucus-producing exocrine glands such as the sweat glands do not ordinarily cause symptoms. However, they are also affected, because the sodium and chloride concentration in sweat is higher than normal in patients with cystic fibrosis, even though the volume of sweat is not abnormally increased. Therefore, unusually high quantities of sodium and chloride are lost in sweat, and this fact is utilized for diagnosis. Screening tests (silver nitrate or Schwachman test) that depend on the incorporation of silver nitrate into agar plates or special paper have been devised. The patient's hand is carefully washed and dried, since previously dried sweat will leave a concentrated chloride residue on the skin and give a false positive result. After an extended period or after exercise to increase secretions, the palm or fingers are placed on the silver nitrate surface. Excess chlorides will combine with the silver nitrate to form visible silver chloride. However, this method is not accurate in patients less than 2 months old.

Sweat Test for Diagnosis.—For definitive diagnosis, sweat is collected by plastic bag or by a technique known as iontophoresis. Iontophoresis using the Gibson-Cooke method is the current standard procedure. Sweat is induced by sweat stimulants such as pilocarpine. The iontophoresis apparatus consists of two small electrodes that create a tiny electric current to transport the stimulating drug into the sweat glands of the skin. The sweat is collected in small gauze pads. The procedure is painless. Modifications of the equipment and collection system have been devised and are commercially available.

In children, a sweat chloride content greater than 60 mEq/L (60 mmol/L) or a sweat sodium content greater than 70 mEq/L (70 mmol/L) is considered definitely abnormal. Sodium and chloride values may be higher (75–80 mEq/L) during the first 3 days of life, decreasing to childhood values by the fourth day. In children there is an equivocal zone (50–80 mEq/L chloride, possibly even up to 90 mEq/L) in which the diagnosis should be considered unproved. Repeated determinations using good technique and acquiring an adequate quantity of sweat are needed. Volumes of sweat weighing less than 50 mg are not considered reliable for analysis. For diagnostic sweat collection it is recommended that the hand not be used, because the concentration of electrolytes in the palm is significantly greater than elsewhere. A further caution pertains to reference values in persons over age 15 years. Whereas in one study there were only 5% of children with cystic fibrosis who had sweat chloride values less than 50 mEq/L and 3% of controls with values of 60–70 mEq/L, 34% of a group of normal adults were found to have sweat sodium concentration greater than 60 mEq/L and in 4% values were more than 90 mEq/L. Another report did not verify these data; therefore, the diagnosis may be more difficult in adults.

One might gather from this discussion that sweat electrolyte analysis is no more difficult than standard laboratory tests such as blood gas analysis or serum protein electrophoresis. Unfortunately, surveys have shown that the majority of laboratories have a relatively low level of accuracy for sweat testing. The newer commercially available iontophoresis modifications have not shown that they can consistently achieve the accuracy of a carefully performed Gibson-Cooke analysis, although some evaluations have been very favorable. Authorities in cystic fibrosis strongly recommend that the diagnosis of cystic fibrosis should not be made, nor should the diagnosis be excluded with certainty, on the basis of a single sweat analysis. A minimum of two tests showing unequivocal results with adequate control results are necessary. It is preferable to refer a patient with symptoms suggestive of cystic fibrosis to a specialized cystic fibrosis center experienced in the Gibson-Cooke technique to obtain a definitive diagnosis.

Clinically normal heterozygotes and relatives of patients with cystic fibrosis have been reported to have abnormal sweat electrolytes in 5%–20% of instances, although some investigators dispute these findings.

Some investigators feel that sweat chloride provides better separation of normal persons from persons with cystic fibrosis than sweat sodium.

DNA Linkage Analysis.—DNA probe techniques using the indirect linkage analysis method are now becoming available for diagnosis of cystic fibrosis and reportedly have an accuracy of 80%–99%, depending on the particular medical center. This technique can be applied to prenatal diagnosis in the first trimester using a chorionic villus biopsy specimen.

Other Screening Tests.—Other tests have

been suggested to screen for cystic fibrosis. Trypsin is an enzyme produced only in the pancreas. Serum trypsin is elevated in the first months or years of the disease (as the pancreatic cells are destroyed) but eventually decreases below the reference range. However, this leads to considerable overlap with normal persons (in the transition stage between elevated values and decreased values), so that only unequivocally high or low values are significant. Other methods involve testing meconium in the first stools produced by newborns. One technique tests for increased protein levels (which are predominantly albumin) using a paper dipstick that detects elevated levels of albumin. Since 15%–25% of infants with cystic fibrosis have normal degrees of pancreatic enzyme activity, the test yields at least that number of false negative results. In addition, it yields a considerable number of false positive results. The greatest number of false positives (about 50% of all positive specimens in one study) comes from low birth weight infants. Other causes for false positive results include contamination by blood, protein from infant formula, and protein in baby cream. Another approach involves a test for glucose on the meconium stools, which is supposed to reflect the presence or absence of lactase activity. In one study, about one third of cystic fibrosis cases were missed by both the albumin and the glucose (lactose activity) tests.

ENZYME DEFICIENCY DISEASES

Congenital Cholinesterase Deficiency (Succinylcholine Apnea).—Cholinesterase is an enzyme best known for its role in regulation of nerve impulse transmission via breakdown of acetylcholine at the nerve synapse and neuromuscular junction. There are two categories of cholinesterase: acetylcholinesterase ("true cholinesterase"), found in RBCs and nerve tissue, and serum cholinesterase ("pseudocholinesterase"). Cholinesterase deficiency became important when it was noted that such patients were predisposed to prolonged periods of apnea after administration of succinylcholine, a competitor to acetylcholine. Serum cholinesterase inactivates succinylcholine, but acetylcholinesterase does not. Serum cholinesterase deficiency may be congenital or acquired; the congenital type is uncommon but is responsible for most of the cases of prolonged apnea. The patient with congenital deficiency seems to have an abnormal ("atypical") cholinesterase, of which several genetic variants have been reported.

Laboratory Diagnosis.—Serum cholinesterase assay is currently the best screening test for cholinesterase deficiency. If abnormally low values are found, it is necessary to perform inhibition procedures with dibucaine and fluoride to distinguish congenital deficiency (atypical cholinesterase) from acquired deficiency of the normal enzyme. Deficiency of normal enzyme may cause prolonged succinylcholine apnea but not predictably and usually only in very severe deficiency. Acute or chronic liver disease is the most frequent etiology for acquired deficiency. Hypoalbuminemia is frequently associated in hepatic or nonhepatic etiologies. A considerable number of drugs lower serum cholinesterase levels and thus might potentiate the action of succinylcholine.

Cholinesterase levels are also decreased in organic phosphate poisoning (chapter 34); this affects both RBC and plasma enzyme levels. Screening tests have been devised using "dip-and-read" paper strips. These are probably satisfactory for ruling out phosphate insecticide poisoning but are not accurate in diagnosis of potential for succinylcholine apnea.

Alpha-1 Antitrypsin Deficiency.—Alpha-1 antitrypsin deficiency has been associated with two different diseases: pulmonary emphysema in adults (relatively common) and cirrhosis in children (rare). This type of emphysema is characteristically, although not invariably, more severe in the lower lobes. A substantial number of those with homozygous antitrypsin deficiency are affected; reports differ on whether heterozygotes have an increased predisposition to emphysema or to pulmonary disease.

Laboratory Diagnosis.—The most useful screening test at present is serum protein electrophoresis; the alpha-1 globulin peak is absent or nearly absent in homozygotes. More definitive diagnosis, as well as separation of severe from intermediate degrees of deficiency, may be accomplished by quantitation of alpha-1 antitrypsin using immunoassay methods such as immunonephelometry or immunodiffusion. Estrogen therapy (birth control pills) may elevate alpha-1 antitrypsin levels. Since this protein is one of the acute-phase reactants involving the alpha-1 and alpha-2 globulin group on electrophoresis, values are frequently elevated in acute or severe chronic infections, sarcoidosis, inflammation, active rheumatoid-collagen disease, steroid therapy, tissue destruction, and some cases of malignancy. In some cases, measurement of other acute-phase reactants, such as C-reactive protein or serum haptoglobin, might help decide whether alpha-1 antitrypsin might be elevated for this reason. Conditions besides congenital deficiency that reduce alpha-1 antitrypsin activity include severe protein loss, severe renal disease, malabsorption, and thyroiditis.

Biotinidase Deficiency.—Biotin is a water-soluble vitamin that is present in most common foods and, in addition, can be synthesized by GI tract bacteria. Biotin is a cofactor for activity of several carboxylase enzymes that are found in the carboxylic acid cycle, leucine metabolism, and proprionic acid metabolism. Biotinidase converts the precursor substance biocytin to biotin. Biotinidase deficiency prevents conversion of biocytin from dietary sources and forces dependence on biotin produced by GI tract bacteria. Suppression of these bacteria or inactivation of biotin by certain substances such as the glycoprotein avidin in egg white (most commonly caused by eating large quantities of raw eggs) can precipitate biotin deficiency. Other possible causes of biotin deficiency include chronic hemodialysis, long-term total parenteral nutrition without biotin supplement, and occasionally long-term anticonvulsant therapy. Symptoms include retarded growth, weakness, ataxia, hair loss, skin rash, metabolic acidosis, and sometimes convulsions.

Laboratory Diagnosis.—Neonatal screening for biotinidase deficiency can be done on heelstick blood spotted on filter paper using a variety of assay methods. The same methods can be used on venous blood.

BIBLIOGRAPHY

Buffone GJ, et al: Prenatal diagnosis of cystic fibrosis: Microvillar enzymes and DNA compared. *Clin Chem* 1988; 34:933.

Pierce JA: Antitrypsin and emphysema. *JAMA* 1988; 529:2890.

Knight JA, Wu JT: Alpha-fetoprotein: Its role in the prenatal diagnosis of congenital anomalies. *Lab Med* 1988; 19:219.

Buist NRM: Laboratory aspects of newborn screening for metabolic disorders. *Lab Med* 1988; 19:145.

Darras BT, et al: Prenatal diagnosis and detection of carriers with DNA probes in Duchenne's muscular dystrophy. *N Engl J Med* 1987; 316:985.

Littman A: Lactase deficiency. *Hosp. Pract* 1987; 120:111.

Newcomer AD, McGill DB: Clinical significance of lactase deficiency. *Intern Med Specialist* 1987; 8:116.

Bates HM: Biotinidase deficiency: Screening and treatment. *Lab Mgmt* 1987; 25(4):15.

Crosby WH: Hemochromatosis: Current concepts and management. *Hosp Pract* 1987; 22:173.

Le Grys VA: Cystic Fibrosis: Recent diagnostic developments. *Lab Mgmt* 1986; 24(11):43.

Whang-Peng J, Knutsen T: Cytogenetics: Methods and findings in hematologic disease. *Lab Mgmt* 1986; 24(4):19.

High KA, Benz EJ: Recombinant DNA technology in antenatal diagnosis. *Lab Mgmt* 1986; 24(3):31.

Turley CP: Fibroblast culture: A tool for identifying metabolic disease. *Lab Mgmt* 1986; 24(5):52.

Fairbanks VF, Baldus WP: Hemochromatosis: The neglected diagnosis. *Mayo Clin Proc* 1986; 61:296.

Seiler J, Bope ET: The muscular dystrophies. *Am Fam Pract* 1986; 34:123.

Pyeritz RE: The Marfan syndrome. *Am Fam Pract* 1986; 34:83.

Young RS, et al: Fragile-X mental retardation syndrome transmitted through intellectually normal males. *South Med J* 1986; 79:405.

Hammond K: Problems in diagnosing cystic fibrosis. *Diagn Med* 1985; 8(4):35.

Bird SJ: Presymptomatic testing for Huntington's disease. *JAMA* 1985; 253:3286.

Jackson LG: First-trimester diagnosis of fetal genetic disorders. *Hosp Pract* 1985; 20:39.

Kazazian HH: Gene probes: Application to prenatal and postnatal diagnosis of genetic disease. *Clin Chem* 1985; 31:1509.

Berry HK: Screening newborns for genetic disease: The PKU model. *Diagn Med* 1984; 7(1):50.

Berry HK: The spectrum of metabolic disorders. *Diagn Med* 1984; 7(3):39.

Joseph F, Thurmon TF: Amino acid screening—an objective approach. *Lab Med* 1984; 14:427.

Newcomer AD, McGill DB: Irritable bowel syndrome: Role of lactase deficiency. *Mayo Clin Proc* 1983; 58:339.

Solomons NW: The use of H2 breath-analysis tests in gastrointestinal diagnosis. *Curr Concepts Gastroenterol* 1983; 8:30.

Masoero G, et al: Serum trypsinlike immunoreactivity in cystic fibrosis. *Am J Dis Child* 1983; 137:167.

Knight JA, Wu JT: Screening profile for detection of inherited metabolic disorders. *Lab Med* 1982; 13:681.

Dadone MM, et al: Hereditary hemochromatosis. *Am J Clin Pathol* 1982; 78:196.

Brady RO, Kolodney EH: The sphingolipid storage disorder: Diagnosis and detection. *Lab Mgmt* 1982; 20:27.

Halliday JW, Powell LW: Iron overload. *Semin Hematol* 1982; 19:42.

Wills JH: Blood cholinesterase: Assay methods and considerations. *Lab Mgmt* 1982; 20:53.

Milbeck R: Cytogenetic examination: Specimen acquisition and handling. *Lab Med* 1982; 13:416.

Lorincz AE, et al: The early laboratory diagnosis of mucopolysaccharidoses. *Ann Clin Lab Sci* 1982; 12:258.

Thompson JN: The human genetic mucopolysaccharidoses. *Ala J Med Sci* 1982; 19:168.

Arola H, et al: Simple urinary test for lactose malabsorption. *Lancet* 1982; 2:524.

Berry HK: The diagnosis of phenylketonuria. *Am J Dis Child* 1981; 135:211.

Stephenson SR, Weaver DD: Prenatal diagnosis: A compilation of diagnosed conditions. *Am J Obstet Gynecol* 1981; 141:319.

Lee RE: Gaucher's disease. *Arch Pathol Lab Med* 1981; 105:102.

Potter JL, Robinson HB: Screening for the Tay-Sachs Carrier. *Clin Chem* 1981; 27:523.

Brewster MA: Leukocyte enzymes in birth defects—a review. *Ann Clin Lab Sci* 1981; 11:146.

Gronert GA: Malignant hyperthermia. *Anesthesiology* 1980; 53:395.

O'Flynn ME, et al: The diagnosis of phenylketonuria. *Am J Dis Child* 1980; 134:769.

Pesce MA, Bodourian SH: Pitfalls in the diagnosis of transferase and galactokinase deficient galactosemia. *Ann Clin Lab Sci* 1979; 10:26.

Dobyns WB: Clinical spectrum of Wilson's disease (hepatolenticular degeneration). *Mayo Clin Proc* 1979; 54:35.

34 Laboratory Analysis of Therapeutic and Toxic Substances

THERAPEUTIC DRUG MONITORING

Various studies have shown that therapy guided by drug blood levels (therapeutic drug monitoring, TDM) has a considerably better chance of achieving therapeutic effect and avoiding toxicity than therapy using empiric drug dosage. Therapeutic drug monitoring can be helpful in a variety of circumstances, as can be seen in the following discussion.

Why Obtain Therapeutic Drug Blood Levels?

1. To be certain that adequate blood concentrations are reached. This is especially important when therapeutic effect must be achieved immediately but therapeutic results are not evident immediately, as might happen when aminoglycoside antibiotics are used.

2. When effective blood levels are close to toxic levels ("narrow therapeutic window"). It is useful to know what margin of safety is permitted by the current medication dose. If blood levels are close to toxic values, a decrease in the dose might be attempted.

3. If expected therapeutic effect is not achieved with standard dosage. It is important to know whether the fault is due to insufficient blood levels or is attributable to some other factor (e.g., patient tolerance to the medication effect or interference with the therapeutic effect by other drugs).

4. If symptoms of toxicity appear with standard dosage. The problem might be one of excessive blood levels, enhancement of effect by other medications, an increase in free as opposed to total drug blood levels, or symptoms that are not due to toxicity from the drug in question.

5. If a disease is present that is known to affect drug absorption, protein binding, metabolism, or excretion.

6. Possible drug interaction. It is safer to know in advance whether other medications have altered the expected blood levels of a drug before symptoms appear of toxicity or of insufficient therapeutic effect.

7. Combination drug therapy. If multiple drugs are used simultaneously for the same purpose (e.g., control of convulsions), knowledge of baseline blood levels for each drug would be helpful should problems develop and the question arise as to which drug is responsible.

8. Possible patient noncompliance. Patients may decrease the dosage or cease taking medication altogether if symptoms improve or may simply forget to take doses.

9. Possible medicolegal considerations. An example is the aminoglycoside antibiotic group, whose use is known to be associated with renal failure in a certain percentage of cases. If a patient develops renal failure while taking one of these antibiotics, the renal failure could be due either to drug toxicity or to the underlying disease. If previous and current antibiotic blood levels are within an established range that is not associated with toxicity, the presumptive

cause of renal failure is shifted toward the disease rather than the therapy.

10. Change in dosage or patient status to establish a new baseline for future references.

What Factors Influence Therapeutic Drug Blood Levels?

A great many factors influence TDM blood levels. Discussion of some of the more important follows.

Route of Administration.—Intravenous (IV) administration places medication into the blood faster than intramuscular injection, which, in turn, is usually faster than oral intake. Oral medication may be influenced by malabsorption.

Drug Absorption.—This may be altered by gastrointestinal (GI) tract motility variations, changes of intestinal acidity, malabsorption disorders, and in some cases interference from food or laxatives.

Drug Transport.—Many drugs have a substantial fraction that is bound to plasma proteins. Acidic drugs bind predominantly to albumin, and basic drugs bind predominantly to alpha-1 glycoproteins. Protein-bound drug molecules are not metabolically active. Therapeutic drug monitoring using total drug concentration is based on the assumption that the ratio between bound and unbound ("free") drug remains constant, and therefore alterations in the total drug level mirror alterations in the free drug level. In most cases this is true. However, when 80% or more of a drug is protein bound, there may be circumstances in which alterations in the ratio of bound to free drug may occur. These alterations may consist of either a free drug concentration within toxic range coupled with a total drug concentration within therapeutic range or a free drug concentration within therapeutic range coincident with a total drug concentration within toxic range. This may happen when the quantity of binding protein is reduced (e.g., in hypoalbuminemia) and the dose rate is not changed from that used with normal protein levels. Problems may also arise when the quantity of binding protein is normal but the degree of binding is reduced (in neonatal life and in uremia) or when competition from other drugs displaces some of the bound fraction, interaction between acidic drugs with a high percentage of protein binding (e.g., valproic acid and phenytoin); if metabolism of free drug decreases (severe liver disease); or if excretion of free drug decreases (renal failure). Although an increase in free drug quantity may explain toxic symptoms, it is helpful also to know the total drug concentration to deduce what has happened. In routine TDM, total drug concentration is usually sufficient. If toxicity occurs with total drug levels within the therapeutic range, free drug levels may provide an explanation and a better guideline for therapy. Free drug assays currently are done only by large reference laboratories. The introduction of relatively simple techniques to separate bound from free drug (e.g., membrane filtration) may permit wider availability of free drug assay.

Drug Uptake by Target Tissues.—Drug molecules must reach target tissue and penetrate into tissue cells. Conditions such as congestive heart failure can decrease tissue perfusion and thereby delay tissue uptake of the drug.

Extent of Drug Distribution (Volume of Distribution).—Lipid-soluble drugs penetrate tissues easily and have a much greater diffusion or dispersal throughout the body than non-lipid-soluble drugs. Dispersal away from the blood or target organ decreases blood levels or target tissue levels. The tendency to diffuse throughout the body is measured by dividing the administered drug dose by the plasma concentration of the drug (at equilibrium). This results in the theoretical volume of body fluid within which the drug is diffused to produce the measured serum concentration, which, in turn, indicates the extent of extravascular distribution of the drug.

Drug Tissue Utilization.—Various conditions may alter this parameter, such as disease of the target organ, electrolyte or metabolic derangements, and effect of other medications.

Drug Metabolism.—Most drugs for which TDM is employed are wholly or partially inactivated ("detoxified") within the liver. Liver function becomes a critical factor when severe liver damage occurs. Also, some persons metabolize a drug faster than average ("fast metabolizer"), and some metabolize drugs slower ("slow metabolizer"). Certain drugs such as digoxin and lithium carbonate are not metabolized in the liver. The rate of drug metabolism plus the rate of excretion are major determinants of two important TDM parameters. **Half-life** (biologic half-life) refers to the time required to decrease drug blood concentration by 50%. It is usually measured after absorption has been completed. **Steady state** refers to drug blood level equilibrium between drug intake and elimination. Before steady state is achieved, drug blood values typically are lower than the level that they eventually attain. As a general rule it takes five half-lives before steady state is reached. Loading doses can decrease this time span considerably. A few investigators use three half-lives as the basis for steady-state measurements.

Drug Excretion.—Nearly all TDM drugs are excreted predominantly through the kidneys (the major exception is theophylline). Markedly decreased renal function obviously leads to drug retention. The creatinine clearance rate is commonly used to estimate the degree of residual kidney function. When the serum creatinine is more than twice reference upper limits, creatinine clearance is usually less than 25% of normal and measurement is less accurate. In addition, creatinine clearance is somewhat reduced in the elderly, and some maintain that clearance reference ranges should be adjusted for old age.

Dosage.—Size and frequency of dose obviously affect drug blood levels.

Age.—Infants in general receive the same dose per unit weight as adults; children receive twice the dose, and the elderly receive less. A very troublesome period is the transition between childhood and puberty (approximately ages 10–13 years) since dosage requirements may change considerably and without warning within a few months.

Weight.—Dosage based on weight yields desirable drug blood levels more frequently than arbitrary, fixed dose schedules. One assumes that a larger person has a larger total blood volume and extracellular fluid space within which the drug is distributed and a larger liver to metabolize the drug.

Interference From Other Medications.—Such interference may become manifest at any point in drug intake, metabolism, tissue therapeutic effect, and excretion, as well as lead to possible artifact in technical aspects of drug assay.

Effect of Disease on any Previously Mentioned Factors.—This most frequently involves considerable loss of renal or hepatic function.

Assay of Peak or Residual Level.—In general, peak levels correlate with toxicity, whereas residual (trough) levels are more an indication of proper therapeutic range (i.e., whether the blood level remains within the therapeutic range). Of course, if the residual level is in the toxic range this is an even stronger indication of toxicity. An exception to the general rule is the aminoglycoside antibiotic group, in which the peak level is used to indicate whether therapeutic levels are being reached and the residual level is considered (some disagreement exists on this point) to correlate best with nephrotoxicity. For most drugs, the residual level should be kept within the therapeutic range and the peak level should be kept out of the toxic range. To avoid large fluctuations, some have recommended that the dose interval be one half of the drug half-life; in other words, the drug should be administered at least once during each half-life.

One of the most important laboratory problems of drug level monitoring is the proper time in relationship to dose administration at which to obtain the specimen. There are two guidelines. First, the drug blood level should have reached steady state or equilibrium, which as a rule of thumb takes five drug half-lives. Second, the drug blood level should be at a true peak or residual level. Peak levels are usually reached about 1–2 hours after oral intake, about 1 hour after intramuscular administration, or about 30 minutes after IV medication. Residual levels are usually reached shortly (0–15 minutes) before the next scheduled dose. The greatest problem is being certain when the drug was actually given. I have had best results by first learning when the drug is supposed to be given. If a residual level is needed, the nursing service is then instructed to withhold the dose. The blood specimen is drawn approximately 15 minutes before the scheduled dose time, and the nursing service is then told to administer the dose. If a peak level is needed, the laboratory technologist should make arrangements to have the nursing service record the exact minute that the dose is given and telephone the laboratory. Unless the exact time the specimen was obtained and the exact time the drug dose was given are both known with certainty, drug blood level results cannot be properly interpreted and may be greatly misleading.

Laboratory Technical Factors.—These include the inherent technical variability of any drug assay method (expressed as a coefficient of variation) as well as the other sources of error discussed in chapter 1. Therapeutic drug monitoring assays in general have shown greater differences between laboratories than found with simple well-established tests such as blood urea nitrogen or serum glucose levels.

Patient Compliance.—Various studies have shown astonishingly high rates of patient noncompliance with dose instructions, including failure to take any medication at all. Possibly 20%–80% of all patients may be involved. Noncompliance results in subtherapeutic medication blood levels. Some believe that noncompliance is the most frequent cause of problems in patients on long-term therapy.

TABLE 34–1.
Some Conditions That Produce Unexpected Therapeutic Drug Monitoring Results

High plasma concentration on normal or low prescribed dose
Patient accidental overdose
Slow metabolizer
Drug interaction that blocks original drug metabolism in liver or injures the liver
Poor liver function (severe damage)
Drug excretion block
Increased binding proteins
Residual level determined on sample drawn after dose was administered instead of before
Laboratory technical factors
Low plasma concentration on normal or high prescribed dose
Poor drug absorption (oral dose)
Interference by another drug
Patient noncompliance
Fast metabolizer
Decreased binding proteins
Peak level determined on sample drawn at incorrect time
Laboratory technical factors
Toxic symptoms with blood levels in therapeutic range
Drug released from proteins (free drug increased)
Drug effect enhanced at tissue level by some other drug or condition
Blood level obtained at incorrect time
Laboratory technical factors
Symptoms may not be due to toxicity of that drug

Therapeutic and Toxic Ranges

Therapeutic ranges are drug blood levels that have been empirically observed to correlate with desired therapeutic effects in most patients being treated for an uncomplicated disease. The same relationship is true for toxicity and toxic ranges. However, these ranges are not absolute and do not cover the response to a drug in all individual patients or the response when some unexpected factor (e.g., other diseases or other drugs) is superimposed. The primary guide to therapy is a good therapeutic response without evidence of toxicity. Most of the time this will correspond with a drug blood level within the therapeutic range, so the therapeutic range can be used as a general guideline for therapy. In some cases a good response does not correlate with the therapeutic range. In such cases the assay should be repeated on a new specimen to exclude technical error or specimens drawn at the wrong time in relation to dose. If the redrawn result is unchanged, clinical judgment should prevail. Some attempt should be made, however, to see if there is some factor (Table 34–1) that is superimposed on the disease being treated that could explain the discrepancy. Removal or increase of such a factor could affect the result of therapy at a later date. The same general statements are true for toxicity and toxic ranges. Some patients may develop toxicity at blood levels below the statistically defined toxic range and some may be asymptomatic at blood levels within the toxic range. However, the further the values enter into the toxic range, the more likely it is that toxicity will develop. Thus, patient response and drug level data are both important, and both are often necessary to interpret the total picture.

When to Obtain Specimens for Therapeutic Drug Monitoring

If a patient develops symptoms that might be caused by a drug, the best time to obtain a specimen for TDM is during the period when the patient has the symptoms (if this is not possible, within a short time afterward). One possible exception, however, is digoxin, whose blood level does not equilibrate with tissue levels until at least 6–8 hours after the dose is given. Therefore, specimens for digoxin TDM should not be drawn less than 6 hours after administration of the previous dose, even if toxic symptoms occur earlier. It should be ascertained how much time elapsed between the onset of toxic symptoms and the time of the last previous medication dose. This information is necessary to determine if there is a relationship of the symptoms to the peak blood level of the drug. If the specimen cannot be drawn during symptoms, the next best alternative is to deliberately obtain a specimen at the peak of the drug blood level. This will indicate if the peak level is within the toxic range. In some instances it may be useful to obtain a blood specimen for TDM at a drug peak level even without toxic symptoms, to be certain that the drug dosage is not too high.

In some cases the question is not drug toxicity but whether dosage is adequate to achieve the desired therapeutic effect. In that case, the best specimen for TDM is one drawn at the residual (valley or trough) drug level, shortly before the next medication dose is given. The major exception to this rule is theophylline, for which a peak level is more helpful than a residual level.

For most drugs, both peak and residual levels should be within the therapeutic range. The peak value should not enter the toxic range and the residual value should not fall to therapeutically inadequate levels.

Information on some of the medications for which TDM is currently being used is given in Table 36–39. Table 34–1 lists some conditions that produce unexpected TDM results.

Summary

Therapeutic drug monitoring can be extremely helpful in establishing drug levels that are both therapeutically adequate and nontoxic. To interpret TDM results, the clinician should know the pharmacodynamics of the medication, ascertain that steady-state levels have been achieved before ordering TDM assays, try to ensure that specimens are drawn at the correct time in relation to dose administration, be aware of effects from other medication, and view TDM results as one component in the overall clinical picture rather than the sole basis for deciding whether drug dosages are correct. Drug monitoring is carried out in two basic situations: (1) in an isolated attempt to find the reason for therapeutic failure (either toxic symptoms or nonresponse to therapy) and (2) to obtain a baseline value after sufficient time has elapsed for stabilization. Baseline values are needed for comparison with future values if trouble develops and to establish the relationship of a patient's drug blood level to accepted therapeutic range. This information can be invaluable in future emergencies.

Comments on Therapeutic Drug Monitoring Assay

To receive adequate service, the physician must provide the laboratory with certain information as well as the patient specimen. This information includes the exact drug or drugs to be assayed, patient age, time elapsed from the last dose until the specimen was obtained, drug dose, and route of administration. All of these factors affect normal values. It is also desirable to state the reason for the assay (i.e., what is the question that the clinician wants answered) and provide a list of medications the patient is receiving.

Some (not all) of the methods used in drug assay include gas-liquid chromatography (technically difficult but especially useful when several drugs are being administered simultaneously, as frequently occurs in epileptics), thin-layer chromatography (TLC; more frequently used for the hypnotic drugs), radioimmunoassay (RIA); fluorescence-polarization immunoassay, and enzyme-multiplied immunoassay (EMIT).

One of the major reasons why TDM has not achieved wider acceptance is that reliable results are frequently not obtainable. Even when they are, the time needed to obtain a report may be several days rather than several hours. It is essential that the physician be certain that the reference laboratory, whether local or not, is providing reliable results. Reliability can be investigated in several ways: by splitting patient samples to be evaluated between the laboratory and a reference laboratory whose work is known to be good (but if isolated values are discrepant, a question may arise as to whose is correct), by splitting samples and sending one portion 1 week and the remainder the next week; or by obtaining standards from commercial companies and submitting these as unknowns. Most good reference laboratories will do a reasonable amount of such testing without charge if requested to do so beforehand.

In some situations, assay results may be misleading without additional information. In certain drugs, such as phenytoin (Dilantin), digitoxin, and quinidine, a high percentage is bound to serum albumin and only the nonbound fraction is metabolically active. This is similar to thyroid hormone protein binding, discussed in chapter 28. The free (nonbound) fraction may be increased in hypoalbuminemia or in conditions that change protein binding, such as uremia or administration of drugs that block binding or compete for binding sites. Drug level assays measure total drug and do not reflect changes in protein binding. In addition, some drugs, diseases, or metabolic states may potentiate or inhibit the action of certain therapeutic agents without altering blood levels or protein binding. An example is digoxin toxicity induced by hypokalemia.

SELECTED DRUGS AND DRUG GROUPS

Anticonvulsants

Most epileptics can be controlled with phenytoin (Dilantin), primidone (Mysoline), phenobarbital, or other agents. Frequently drug combinations are required. Therapy is usually a long-term project. When toxicity develops, many of these therapeutic agents produce symptoms that could also be caused by central nervous system (CNS) disease, such as confusion, somnolence, and various changes in mental behavior. Some drugs, such as primidone, must be carefully brought to a therapeutic level by stages rather than in a single dose. Most antiepileptic drugs are administered to control seizures; but if seizures are infrequent, it is difficult to be certain that the medication is sufficient to prevent future episodes. When drug combinations are used, levels for all the agents should be obtained so that if only one drug is involved in toxicity or therapeutic failure, it can be identified.

When specimens are sent to the laboratory for drug assay, the physician should list all drugs being administered. Some are metabolized to substances that themselves have antiepileptic activity (e.g., primidone is partially metabolized to phenobarbital), and the laboratory then must assay both the parent drug and its metabolite. Without a complete list of medications, there is a good chance that one or more drugs will be overlooked. Once drug blood levels have been obtained, the physician should remember that they are often not linear in relation to dose, so that a percentage change in dose may not result in the same percentage change in blood level. Repeated assays may be needed to guide dosage to achieve desired blood levels. Finally, published therapeutic ranges may not predict the individual response of some patients to the drug. Clinical judgments as well as laboratory values must be used.

Phenytoin.—Phenytoin is about 90% bound to serum proteins. About 70% is metabolized in the liver, although only 5% or less is excreted unchanged through the kidneys. Peak phenytoin levels are reached 4–8 hours after an oral dose and within 15 minutes after IV administration. Serum half-life is about 18–30 hours (literature range, 10–95 hours), with an average of about 24 hours. This variation occurs in part because higher doses saturate the liver metabolic pathway and thus increase the half-life with nonmetabolized drug. The serum dose-response curve is not linear, so that relatively small increases in dose may generate relatively large changes in serum levels. Time to reach steady state is usually 4–6 days but may take as long as 5 weeks. Administration by intramuscular injection rather than oral intake is said to reduce blood levels about 50%. The therapeutic range is 10–20 μg/ml. Specimens for TDM are usually drawn just before the next scheduled dose to evaluate adequacy of dosage. Specimens drawn during symptoms or peak levels are needed to investigate toxic symptoms.

Certain drugs or diseases may affect phenytoin blood levels (see Table 36–2). Severe chronic liver disease, hepatic immaturity in premature infants, or disulfiram (Antabuse) therapy often increase phenytoin levels. Certain other drugs, such as coumarin anticoagulants, chloramphenicol (Chloromycetin), methylphenidate (Ritalin), and certain benzodiazepine tranquilizers such as diazepam (Valium) and chlordiazepoxide (Librium) have caused significant elevations in a minority of patients. Acute alcohol intake may also elevate plasma levels. On the other hand, pregnancy, acute hepatitis, low doses of phenobarbital, carbamazepine (Tegretol), and chronic alcoholism may decrease phenytoin plasma levels, and they may also be decreased in full-term infants up to age 12 weeks and in some patients with renal disease. As noted previously, there may be disproportionate changes in either bound or free phenytoin in certain circumstances. About 10% of total phenytoin is theoretically free, but in one study only about 30% of patients who had free phenytoin measured conformed to this level with the remainder showing considerable variation. Certain clinical conditions or acidic highly protein-bound drugs may displace some phenytoin from albumin, causing the unbound (free) fraction of serum phenytoin to rise. Initially, total serum concentration may be decreased somewhat if the liver metabolizes the newly released free drug. However, the hepatic metabolic pathway may become saturated, with resulting persistent increase in the unbound fraction and return of the total phenytoin level into the reference range. At this time the usual phenytoin assay (total drug) could be normal while the free drug level is increased. Drugs that can displace phenytoin from albumin include valproic acid (Depakene), salicylates, and phenylbutasone. Large quantities of urea or bilirubin have a similar effect. Infants aged 0–12 weeks have reduced phenytoin protein binding. On the other hand, hypoalbuminemia means less binding protein is available and may result in increased free phenytoin levels coincident with decreased total phenytoin levels.

Phenytoin has some interesting side effects in a minority of patients, among which are megaloblastic anemia and a type of benign lymphoid hyperplasia that clinically can suggest malignant lymphoma. Occasional patients develop gum hypertrophy or hirsutism. Phenytoin also can decrease blood levels of cortisol-type drugs, digitoxin, and primidone, and can increase the effect of coumadin and the serum levels of the enzymes γ-glutamyltransferase and alkaline phosphatase. Phenytoin produces its effects on drugs by competing for binding sites on protein or by stimulating liver microsome activity (see Table 36–3). Phenytoin alters the serum enzymes by its effect on the liver microsome system.

Primidone.—Primidone is not significantly bound to serum proteins and is about 50% metabolized in the liver. About 50% is excreted unchanged by the kidneys. Its major metabolites are phenobarbital (about 20%) and phenylethylmalonamide (about 20%), both of which have anticonvulsant activity of their own and both of which accumulate with long-term primidone administration. Phenobarbital is usually not detectable for 5–7 days after beginning primidone therapy. The ratio of phenobarbital to primidone has been variously reported as 1.0–3.0 after steady state of both drugs has been reached (unless phenobarbital is administered in addition to primidone). If phenytoin is given in addition to primidone, primidone conversion to phenobarbital is increased and the phenobarbital/primidone ratio is therefore increased. Peak serum concentration of primidone occurs in 1–3 hours, although this is somewhat variable. Serum half-life in adults is about 6–12 hours (literature range, 3.3–18 hours). Steady state is reached in about 50 hours (range, 16–60 hours). The therapeutic range is 5–12 μg/ml. It is usually recommended that both primidone and phenobarbital levels be assayed when primidone is used, rather than primidone levels only. If this is done, one must wait until steady state for phenobarbital is reached, which takes a much longer time (8–15 days for children, 10–25 days for adults) than steady state for primidone. Specimens for TDM are usually drawn just before the next scheduled dose to evaluate adequacy of dosage. Specimens drawn during symptoms or peak levels are needed to investigate toxic symptoms.

Phenobarbital.—Phenobarbital is about 50% bound to serum protein. It has a very long half-life of 2–5 days (50–120 hours) and takes 2–3 weeks (8–15 days in children, 10–25 days in adults) to reach steady state. About 70%–80% is metabolized by the liver and about 10%–30% is excreted unchanged by the kidneys. Phenobarbital, as well as phenytoin, carbamazepine, and phenylbutasone, has the interesting ability to activate hepatic microsome activity. Thus, phenobarbital increases the activation of the phenytoin liver metabolic pathway and also competes with phenytoin for that pathway. Phenobarbital incidentally increases degradation of other drugs that are metabolized by hepatic microsome activity, such as coumarin anticoagulants, adrenocorticosteroids, quinidine, tetracycline, and tricyclic antidepressants. Acute alcoholism increases patient response to phenobarbital and chronic alcoholism is said to decrease response. Specimens for TDM are usually drawn just before the next scheduled dose to evaluate adequacy of dosage. Specimens drawn during symptoms or peak levels are needed to investigate toxic symptoms.

Valproic Acid.—Valproic acid has been used to treat petit mal "absence" seizures and, in some cases, tonic-clonic generalized seizures and myoclonic disorders. About 90% is bound to plasma proteins. There is a relatively small volume of distribution, because most of the drug remains in the vascular system. More than 90% is metabolized in the liver, with 5% or less excreted unchanged by the kidneys. Time to peak after oral dose is 1–3 hours. Food intake may delay the peak. Serum half-life is relatively short (about 12 hours; range, 8–15 hours), and steady state (oral dose) is reached in 2–3 days (range, 30–85 hours in adults; 20–70 hours in children). Liver disease may prolong the interval before steady state. Interestingly, therapeutic effect usually does not appear until several weeks have elapsed. There is some fluctuation in serum values (said to be 20%–50%) even at steady state. Hepatic enzyme–inducing drugs such as phenytoin, phenobarbital, carbamazepine, and primadone increase the rate of valproic acid degradation and thus its rate of excretion, and therefore tend to decrease the serum levels. Hypoalbuminemia or displacement of valproic acid from albumin by acidic strongly protein-bound drugs such as salicylates decrease total valproic acid blood levels. Valproic acid can affect phenytoin and primidone levels, but the effect is variable. Phenobarbital levels are increased due to interference with liver metabolism. One report indicates that ethosuximide levels may also be increased. Specimens for TDM are usually drawn just before the next scheduled dose to evaluate adequacy of dosage. Specimens drawn during symptoms or peak levels are needed to investigate toxic symptoms.

Rarely, valproic acid may produce liver failure. Two types have been described. The more common type appears after months of therapy, with gradual and potentially reversible progression signaled by rising AST levels. Periodic AST measurement has been advocated to prevent this complication. The other type is sudden, is nonreversible, and appears soon after therapy is started.

Carbamazepine.—Carbamazepine is used for treatment of grand mal and psychomotor epilepsy. About 70% (range, 65%–85%) is protein bound, not enough to make binding a frequent problem. Carbamazepine is metabolized by the liver. It speeds its own metabolism by activation of the liver microsome system. Only 1% is excreted unchanged in the urine. The major metabolites are the epoxide form, which is metabolically active, and the dihydroxide form, which is derived from the epoxide form. The metabolites are excreted in urine. Carbamazepine absorption after oral dose in tablet form is slow, incomplete (70%–80%), and variable. Pharmacologic data in the literature are likewise quite variable. Dosage with tablets results in a peak level that is reached in about 6–8 hours (range, 2–24 hours). Dosage as a suspension or solution or ingestion of tablets with food results in peak levels at about 3 hours. Serum half-life is about 10–30 hours (range, 8–35 hours) when therapy is begun. But after several days the liver microsome system becomes fully activated, and when this occurs the half-life for a dose change may be reduced to about 12 hours (range, 5–27 hours). Phenytoin, phenobarbital, or primidone also activate the liver microsome system, thereby increasing carbamazepine metabolism and reducing its half-life. The time to steady state is about 2 weeks (range, 2–4 weeks) during initial therapy. Later on, time to steady state for dose changes is about 3–4 days (range, 2–6 days). Transient leukopenia has been reported in about 10% of patients (range, 2%–60%) and persistent leukopenia in about 2% (range, 0%–8%). Thrombocytopenia has been reported in about 2%. Aplastic anemia may occur, but it has been rare.

Psychiatric Medications

Lithium Carbonate.—Lithium is used for control of the manic phase of manic-depressive psychiatric illness. Peak levels are reached in 1–3 hours, and plasma half-life (in young adults) is about 24 hours (range, 8–35 hours). Time to steady state is about 5 days (range, 2–7 days). Most excretion is through the kidneys, where there is both excretion and reabsorption. Excretion is decreased (tending to increase half-life and blood levels) with poor renal function and also with sodium deficiency. Methyldopa also tends to delay lithium excretion. More rapid excretion occurs with salt loading or sodium retention. Interesting side effects are reversible hypothyroidism (about 5% of cases, with some thyroid-stimulating hormone elevation in up to 30% of cases) and neutrophilic leukocytosis. Therapeutic drug monitoring assays are usually performed 12 hours after the last dose (before administration of the next dose). The usual laboratory method is flame photometry, although other methods are becoming available. The therapeutic range is somewhat narrow (approximately 0.5–1.5 mEq/L). Values higher than 2.0 mEq/L are usually considered to be in the toxic range. Maintenance therapy is customarily monitored once a month. Some interest has been shown in RBC lithium analysis, especially when lack of patient compliance is suspected. Red blood cell lithium levels are more stable over periods of time than serum lithium levels due to the relatively short half-life of serum lithium. Low RBC lithium levels in the presence of normal or elevated serum lithium levels suggest that the patient is noncompliant but took a lithium dose shortly before coming to have the specimen drawn.

Tricyclic Antidepressants.—The group name of these medications refers to their three-ring structure. They are widely used to treat unipolar psychiatric depression (i.e., depression without a manic phase). About 70% of these patients show some improvement. The tricyclics are thought to act through blocking one of the deactivation pathways of norepinephrine and serotonin at the brain nerve endings, thereby increasing the availability of these neurotransmitter agents in the synapse area. The different drugs differ in their effect on norepinephrine, serotonin, or both. Currently, the most commonly used tricyclics are imipramine (Tofranil), amitriptyline (Elavil), protrypyline (Vivactil), and doxepin (Sinequan). Of these, imipramine is metabolized to desipramine, and amitriptyline is metabolized to nortriptyline; in both cases the metabolites have pharmacologic activity and are actually marketed themselves under different trade names. Doxepin is also metabolized to the active compound desmethyldoxepin. If these parent compounds are assayed, their major metabolite must also be assayed as well as the parent. Other tricyclics are available, and still others are being introduced.

Oral doses are fairly completely absorbed from the GI tract. Once absorbed, there is 70%–96% binding to plasma proteins and considerable first-pass metabolism in the liver. By 6–8 days 60%–85% of the dose is excreted in the urine in the form of metabolites. Peak serum levels are generally attained 2–6 hours (range, 2–8 hours) after an oral dose. There is variation in peak level depending on the drug formula. There is considerable variation in metabolism between individuals, with variation of 5- to 10-fold in steady-state levels being common and sometimes differences reported as great as 30-fold. The half-life averages 20–30 hours (range, 15–93 hours), and steady state is reached on the average in about 7–10 days (range, 2–19 days). Imipramine has a somewhat shorter half-life (6–24 hours) and time to steady state (about 2-5 days) than the other tricyclics. However, there is variation between the various drugs and between individuals taking the same drug. It is reported that 30% or more patients have serum assay values outside the standard therapeutic range. Blacks may reach higher steady-state serum levels than whites.

Currently, high-performance liquid chromatography (HPLC) is considered the best assay method. Immunoassay (EMIT method) is also used but is not as specific. For example, thioridizine (Melloril) and possibly other phenothiazines may produce a reaction in the EMIT tricyclic test. When tricyclics are given once daily, TDM specimens are usually drawn 10–14 hours after the last dose (if the dose is given at bedtime, the specimen is drawn in the morning about 12 hours later). If the patient is on divided doses, the specimen should be drawn 4–6 hours after the last dose (this usually means that the specimen is drawn just before the next dose). The literature warns that some collection tube stoppers contain interfering substances and that certain serum separation devices using gels or filtration also might interfere. It is obviously necessary to select a collection and processing method that is known to be safe. Serum should be refrigerated rather than frozen. Quality control studies have shown variation within laboratories and between laboratories that is greater than the level of variation for routine chemistry tests.

Antiarrythmic Drugs

There is a large and ever-growing list of these medications, too many to include here. Therapeutic drug monitoring data for some members of this group are summarized in Table 36–39. Several have been selected for more detailed discussion here.

Procainamide.—Procainamide is used to control certain ventricular arrhythmias and can be given orally or intravenously. Only about 10% is bound to serum protein. Maintenance is usually achieved by oral medication. About 85% of the oral dose is absorbed, mostly in the small intestine. About 50% of the drug is excreted unchanged by the kidneys. About 50% is metabolized, predominantly by the liver. The major metabolite of procainamide is N-acetylprocainamide (NAPA), which constitutes about 25%–30% of the original dose (7%–40%). N-acetylprocainamide is produced in the liver by a process known as N-acetylation. It has antiarrhythmic properties about equal to that of its parent compound. About 10% is bound to serum protein and about 85% is excreted unchanged by the kidneys. It has a serum half-life about twice that of procainamide. Therefore, NAPA levels continue to rise for a time after procainamide levels have stabilized. There is approximately a 1:1 ratio of procainamide to NAPA after both have equilibrated. Poor liver function may decrease NAPA formation and produce a high ratio (> 1.0) of procainamide to NAPA (i.e., less NAPA relative to the amount of procainamide). Even though procainamide degradation may be decreased, it is only 25%–30% metabolized in the liver, so that it is not affected as much as NAPA. On the other hand, poor renal function decreases NAPA excretion and decreases the procainamide/NAPA ratio to less than 1.0 (i.e., more NAPA relative to procainamide). Even though procainamide excretion may also be decreased, the amount of NAPA excreted through the kidneys is much higher than the amount of procainamide, so that poor renal function affects NAPA proportionally more than procainamide. Another factor is the acetylating process of the liver, which is an inherited characteristic. Isoniazid and hydralazine are also metabolized by this system. About one half of the population are slow acetylators and about one half are fast acetylators. Fast acetylation produces more NAPA (tending to produce a procainamide/NAPA ratio < 1.0), and slow acetylation produces less NAPA (procainamide/NAPA ratio > 1.0). Assessment of acetylation status is dependent on adequate renal function, since poor renal function can affect the procainamide-NAPA ratio. About 50% of patients on long-term procainamide therapy develop antinuclear antibodies, and up to 30% may develop a syndrome very similar to systemic lupus erythematosus. Slow acetylators are more likely to develop these conditions than fast acetylators.

Since both procainamide and NAPA have antiarrhythmic action and since several factors influence their levels and their relationship to each other, most authorities recommend that both be assayed and that therapeutic decisions be based on the sum of both rather than on either one alone. Therapeutic range for the combination of procainamide and NAPA is 10–30 μg/ml (42.50–127.47 μmol/L). Specimens for TDM are usually obtained just before the next scheduled dose to evaluate adequacy of dosage. Peak levels or specimens drawn during symptoms are needed to investigate toxic symptoms.

There are two types of procainamide oral preparations, standard (relatively short acting) and sustained release (SR). For the standard type, peak absorption levels are usually reached in about 1.5 hours (range, 1–2 hours) after an oral dose. However, some persons absorb procainamide relatively slowly, and the peak may be delayed up to 4 hours after the dose, close to the time one would expect a trough level. In one study, this occurred about one third of the time. Therefore, some investigators recommend both peak and trough for initial evaluation. Patients with acute myocardial infarction or cardiac failure are more likely to have delayed absorption. Serum half-life is about 3 hours (2–4 hours). Time to steady state is about 18 hours (11–20 hours). Therefore, the half-life is considered a short one, and there is a greater fluctuation in serum values compared with an agent with a long half-life. The peak level after oral SR procainamide occurs about 2 hours after the dose (range, 1–3 hours) but may not occur until later in patients with slow absorption. Time to steady state is about 24–30 hours.

Lidocaine.—Lidocaine (Xylocaine) hydrochloride is a local anesthetic that has antiarrhythmic properties. Used as an antiarrhythmic, it is generally given intravenously to patients who are seriously ill. Lidocaine is lipid soluble and distributes rapidly to many tissues. When it is given as a single bolus, plasma levels fall rapidly, with perhaps as much as a 50% decrease in about 20 minutes. On the other hand, drug given by IV infusion reaches a plateau rather slowly because so much of the drug is distributed to peripheral tissues. Therefore, administration is usually done with one or more bolus loading dose injections followed by IV infusion. The half-life of lidocaine is 1–2 hours, and time to steady state is 5–10 hours (5–12 hours). About 70% is protein bound; of the total that is protein bound, about 30% is bound to albumin and 70% to alpha-1 acid glycoprotein. Lidocaine is about 90% metabolized in the liver, with 5%–10% excreted unchanged by the kidneys. The major hepatic metabolites of lidocaine also have some antiarrhythmic effect. The primary metabolites are themselves further metabolized in the liver, with less than 10% of the primary metabolites being excreted unchanged in urine.

Conditions that produce an increase in plasma lidocaine levels are severe chronic liver disease (decreased drug inactivation), chronic renal disease (decreased excretion), and congestive heart failure (reduced volume of distribution). In acute myocardial infarction, there is increase in the binding protein alpha-1 acid glycoprotein and a subsequent increase in plasma total lidocaine values; however, bound drug is pharmacologically inactive, and the nonbound active fraction often does not increase. Propranolol has been reported to decrease lidocaine clearance, producing higher plasma values.

Complications related to lidocaine therapy have been reported in 6%–20% of cases. Therapeutic drug monitoring requires a method that is fast and that can be performed without much delay. High-performance liquid chromatography and EMIT are the two most frequently used methods. Colorimetric methods are also available. It has been recommended that lidocaine specimens be drawn 12 hours after beginning therapy and then daily. In seriously ill patients, in those whose arrhythmias persist in spite of lidocaine, and when lidocaine toxicity is suspected, assay every 12 hours could be helpful. The therapeutic range is 1.5–5 μg/ml.

Tocainide.—Tocainide (Tonocard) is an analog of lidocaine that also is used to treat ventricular arrythmias. Tocainide has some advantages over lidocaine since tocainide can be given orally and has a longer half-life (about 15 hours; range, 12–18 hours) due to much less first-pass hepatic metabolism. The half-life may be increased with severe liver disease or chronic renal failure. About 10% is bound to serum protein. The metabolites of tocainide are excreted in the urine and do not have antiarrythmic activity. Peak serum levels are reached 1.5–2.0 hours after an oral dose. Steady state is reached in 3 days. Therapeutic range is 4–10 μg/ml. Assay is usually done by HPLC.

Quinidine.—Quinidine has been used for treating both atrial and ventricular arrhythmias. There are two forms of quinidine: the sulfate and the gluconate. Both are available for oral administration in both regular and long-acting (SR) preparations. The gluconate form can be given intravenously. Oral regular quinidine sulfate has a time to peak value of about 2 hours (range, 1–3 hours), a serum half-life of about 6 hours (range, 5–8 hours), and a time to steady state of about 24 hours. Regular oral quinidine gluconate has a time to peak value of about 4 hours. Sustained-release quinidine sulfate (Quinidex) has a time to peak value of about 2 hours, a serum half-life of about 20 hours, and a time to steady state of about 4 days. Sustained-release quinidine gluconate (Quiniglute, Duraquin) has a time to peak value of about 4 hours and a half-life of about 10 hours. However, when the SR preparations are used, there is relatively little fall in serum levels after the initial dose before subsequent doses. About 80% of quinidine (literature range, 60%–90%) is bound to serum proteins. Quinidine is metabolized by the liver, with about 10%–20% excreted unchanged in urine by glomerular filtration. Urine excretion is influenced by urine pH.

Factors that may decrease quinidine levels include hypoalbuminemia, drugs that compete for albumin binding, and drugs that activate hepatic enzyme activity, such as phenytoin and phenobarbital. Factors that tend to increase quinidine levels include congestive heart failure, poor renal function (prerenal or intrinsic renal disease), and possibly severe liver disease. Renal excretion is increased by acidification of the urine and decreased by urine alkalinization.

Several methods are available for quinidine assay. The most commonly used are fluorometric procedures, with or without preliminary extraction steps. These measurements include quinidine and several of its metabolites. Certain other fluorescing compounds may interfere. Extraction eliminates some but not all of the metabolites. More specific methods include HPLC and EMIT. Values for the direct (nonextracted) fluorescent methods are about 50% higher than those using HPLC or EMIT (i.e., the therapeutic range with the nonextracted fluorometric method is about 3–8 μg/ml [9.25–24.66 μmol/L], whereas the range using the double-extracted fluorometric method or HPLC is 2.3–5 μg/ml [7.09–15.41 μmol/L]). The specimen for TDM should be drawn just before the next dose is to be given (residual or trough level).

Reasons for TDM of quinidine include the following:

1. Various quinidine commercial products differ considerably in absorption.
2. Toxic levels of quinidine can produce certain arrhythmias that could be due to patient disease (either from noncontrol or noncompliance).
3. There is a possibility of drug interaction, because patients taking quinidine are likely to be taking several drugs or to receive additional drugs in the future.
4. Patient disease may modify quinidine metabolism or excretion (old age frequently is associated with reduced renal function, which modifies renal excretion of quinidine).

Flecainide.—Flecainide (Tambocor) is another drug used for ventricular arrythmias, including premature ventricular contractions and ventricular tachycardia or fibrillation. About 95% is absorbed. Food or antacids do not affect absorption. After absorption, roughly 40% is bound to serum proteins. About 30% (range, 10%–50%) is excreted unchanged in the urine. The major metabolites have no antiarrythmic activity. Peak plasma levels after oral dosage are reached in about 3 hours (range, 1–6 hours). Serum half-life averages 20 hours (range, 7–27 hours) and may be longer in patients with severe renal disease or congestive failure. Steady state is reached in 3–5 days. Propranolol increases flecainide serum levels approximately 20%. Hypokalemia or hyperkalemia may affect the therapeutic action of flecainide. Flecainide paradoxically aggravates ventricular arrythmias in about 7% of patients, especially in the presence of congestive heart failure.

Digoxin.—Digoxin could be included in the section on toxicology, since most serum assay requests are for the purpose of investigating possible digoxin toxicity. However, an increasing number of studies have demonstrated unsuspected overdosage or underdosage (30% toxicity and 11% underdigitalization in one study), and requests for baseline levels are becoming more frequent. The volume of requests and the relative ease of performance (by RIA or EMIT) make this assay readily available, even in smaller laboratories. The widespread use of digoxin, the narrow borderline between therapeutic range and toxicity, and the nonspecific nature of mild or moderate toxic signs and symptoms that mimic a variety of common disorders (diarrhea, nausea, arrhythmias, and ECG changes) contribute to the need for serum assay.

Digoxin Therapeutic Drug Monitoring Data.—About 20%–30% of digoxin is bound to serum albumin. About 80% (range, 60%–90%) is excreted unchanged by the kidneys. About 20% is metabolized in the liver, with most of this being excreted as digoxin metabolites. About 10% of the adult population metabolizes a greater percentage of digoxin (which may be as high as 55%). After an oral dose is given, serum levels rise to a peak at 30–90 minutes and then slowly decline until a plateau is reached about 6–8 hours after administration. Digoxin assay specimens must be drawn at least 6 hours (preferably at least 8 hours) after the last dose in either oral or IV administration, to avoid blood levels that are significantly higher than would be the case when tissue levels have equilibrated. The 6- to 8-hour time span mentioned is minimum elapsed time; specimens may be drawn later. In many cases more information is obtained from a sample drawn shortly before the next scheduled dose. Serum half-life is approximately 36-38 hours. Normal therapeutic range is 0.5–2.0 μg/100 ml (0.6–2.56 nmol/L).

Various metabolic disorders and medications may alter body concentration or serum levels of digoxin or may affect myocardial response to usual dosage. The kidney is the major route of excretion, and a decrease in renal function sufficient to raise serum creatinine levels will elevate serum digoxin levels as well. Hypothyroidism also increases digoxin serum values. On the other hand, certain conditions affect patient response to digitalis without affecting blood levels. Myocardial sensitivity to digoxin, regardless of dose, is increased by acute myocardial damage, hypokalemia, hypercalcemia, hypermagnesemia or hypomagnesemia, alkalosis, tissue anoxia, and glucagon. Drugs that produce hypokalemia (including various diuretics, amphotericin B, corticosteroids, or glucose infusion) thus predispose to toxicity. Other medications, such as phenylbutasone, phenytoin, and barbiturates (which activate hepatic degradation mechanisms), or kaolin (Kaopectate), antacids, cholestyramine, and certain oral antibiotics such as neomycin (which interfere with absorption) tend to be antagonistic to the effect of digitalis. Quinidine elevates digoxin levels in about 90% of patients by 50%–100% (range, 30%–330%). The effect on digoxin levels begins within 24 hours, with peak effect in 4–5 days. Certain other medications can increase serum digoxin levels to some extent (Table 36–2, X).

Interfering Substances.—Digoxin can be measured by a variety of immunoassay methods. Digoxin-like cross-reacting substances have been reported in many patients (not all) in the third trimester of pregnancy, infants up to 6 months of age (the effect peaking at 1 week of age), patients with renal failure, and patients with severe liver disease. Different kits are affected to different extents. Some investigators report that the cross-reacting substances bind to serum proteins. In most cases the cross-reaction increases serum digoxin less than 1.0 μg/100 ml, but sometimes the effect may be greater.

Anti-Digoxin Antibody Therapy.—Another analytical problem occurs when digitalis toxicity is treated with fragments of antidigoxin antibodies (Fab, "antigen-binding fragments"). These fragments are prepared by first producing anti-digoxin IgG class antibody in animals, then enzymatically splitting off the antigen-binding variable regions ("Fab" portion) of the IgG molecule. This eliminates the "constant" region of the IgG molecule, which is the most antigenic portion of the molecule. The anti-digoxin antibody Fab fragments bind to plasma and extracellular fluid digoxin. This creates a disturbance in equilibrium between free (unbound) digoxin within cells and within the extracellular compartments, so that some intracellular digoxin moves out of body cells to restore the equilibrium. The digoxin-Fab bound complexes are excreted in the urine by glomerular filtration. Their elimination half-life with normal renal function is about 15–20 hours (range, 14–25 hours).

Laboratory digoxin assay is involved for two reasons. First, a pretherapy baseline is required to help establish the diagnosis of digoxin toxicity and to help estimate the dose of Fab fragments needed. Second, after injection of the Fab dose, another assay is helpful to determine if adequate therapy was given, either because pretreatment digoxin tissue levels were higher than estimated or too much of the Fab fragment dose was lost in urine before sufficient digoxin had diffused out of the body cells. It is necessary to wait at least 6–8 hours after therapy for a postdose assay, to allow for equilibration time between cells and extracellular fluid. An assay system specific for free digoxin is necessary (usually done by a technique such as microfiltration, which separates unbound from Fab-bound digoxin), because the Fab-digoxin bound complexes are included with unbound ("free") digoxin in total digoxin assays. Soon after therapy begins there is greatly increased Fab-digoxin bound complex formation in plasma (and, therefore, elevated total digoxin levels, sometimes as high as 20 times pretreatment levels), whereas free digoxin levels are low. Later, 12–20 hours after the initial therapeutic dose, plasma free digoxin re-equilibrates, and may reach toxic levels again if sufficient intracellular digoxin has not been captured. It may take several days to excrete all the Fab-digoxin bound complexes, and the serum total digoxin level may remain elevated more than 1 week if there is poor renal function.

Digoxin Assay Clinical Correlation.—In various studies, there is a certain amount of overlap in the area that statistically separates normally digitalized patients from those with toxicity. This overlap exists because it is difficult to recognize mild degrees of toxicity, because patient sensitivity to digitalis varies, and because the assay technique itself, no matter how well done, like all laboratory tests displays a certain amount of variation when repeated determinations are performed on the same specimen. Regardless of these problems, if the clinical picture does not agree with the level of toxicity predicted by digoxin assay values, and laboratory quality control is adequate, the physician should not dismiss or ignore the assay results but should investigate the possibility of interference by improper specimen collection time interval, drug interaction, or metabolic alterations. However, the assay should be repeated first, to verify that a problem exists.

Digitoxin.—Digitoxin is more than 95% bound to serum albumin. Serum half-life is about 8 days (2.5–16.5 days). Digitoxin is about 90% metabolized in the liver. About 5%–10% is excreted unchanged through the kidneys. Drugs that activate hepatic enzyme systems, such as phenytoin and barbiturates, increase metabolism of digitoxin and decrease serum levels. Hypoalbuminemia and drugs that compete for binding sites on albumin also tend to decrease digitoxin serum levels. The long half-life of the drug means that toxicity is difficult to overcome, so digoxin has mostly replaced digitoxin in the United States. The therapeutic range of digitoxin is 15–25 ng/ml.

Theophylline (Aminophylline)

Theophylline is used primarily as a bronchodilating agent for therapy of asthma. Over the therapeutic range there is a reasonably linear correlation between dosage and therapeutic effect. The drug is administered intravenously and orally. Oral medication is available in regular (noncoated or liquid) and slow-release (SR) forms. SR forms are available in twice-daily, and even once-daily, dosages. For most (but not all) regular oral preparations, absorption takes place predominantly in the small intestine, absorption is essentially complete, and food usually does not interfere significantly. Absorption rates are more apt to vary and time to serum peak is less predictable among the different slow-release preparations. In addition, food (especially a high-fat meal) is more likely to interfere with absorption of some SR preparations. One investigator recommends dose intake 1 hour before or 2 hours after meals when using SR preparations influenced by food. For the regular oral medication, time to peak (for adults) is about 2–3 hours, half-life is 4–6 hours (range, 3–8 hours), and time to steady state is about 15–20 hours. For children, half-life is more variable (1–8 hours) and time to steady state is also more variable (5–40 hours). Time to peak for the oral SR preparation is about 5 hours. About 50%–60% (range, 40%–65%) of theophylline is bound to serum albumin. Binding is less in neonates and at lower pH (acidosis). About 90% is metabolized in the liver, and most of the metabolites, plus about 10%–15% of unchanged theophylline, is excreted by the kidneys. Therefore, except in the first several months of life, renal function is not a major factor in theophylline serum concentration. Adults who smoke tobacco or marijuana and children excrete theophylline somewhat more rapidly (decreased serum half-life) than nonsmoking adults. Factors that reduce theophylline clearance (increased serum half-life) include young infants (ages 0–8 months), congestive heart failure, cor pulmonale, severe liver dysfunction, sustained fever, pneumonia, obesity, cessation of smoking, cimetidine, ciprofloxacin, and erythromycin family antibiotics. Some theophylline assay methods may show partial interference (some false increase in values) from substances present in uremia. Children show more individual differences in theophylline clearance and as a group eliminate theophylline more rapidly than adults. In addition, one report indicated that in children on a high-protein diet increased theophylline elimination and a high-carbohydrate diet decreased it.

Besides the factors just mentioned, therapy is complicated by the many theophylline preparations available, many of which vary significantly in theophylline content and the rate it is absorbed. Noncompliance is a constant problem in therapy and in the interpretation of theophylline blood levels, because low levels due to noncompliance may be misinterpreted as due to rapid metabolism or excretion. The reverse mistake can also be made. Another difficulty is the asthmatic who may already have taken one or more extra doses of theophylline prior to being seen by the physician.

There is a relatively narrow zone between therapeutic range (10–20 μg/ml; 55–110 μmol/L) and values associated with toxicity. The degree of elevation over reference range is not a reliable predictor of toxicity risk except in a very general way, since severe toxicity can develop in some patients at less than twice the upper limit of the reference range. Although there are mild toxic symptoms, severe toxicity may develop without warning. If there is a question about previous drug intake, a specimen for theophylline assay should be obtained before therapy is begun. Therapy can then be started and the dosage modified when assay results become available. Thereafter, when steady state is achieved, serum peak concentration should be measured (30 minutes after the dose for IV theophylline, 2 hours after the dose for regular theophylline, and about 5 hours (range, 3–7 hours, depending on the particular medication) after the dose for sustained-release forms). Theophylline is thus an exception to the general rule that the residual (trough) level is better than the peak level to monitor therapy.

Antibiotics

Gentamicin.—Methods of estimating antibiotic therapeutic effectiveness have been discussed elsewhere (chapter 14). Several antibiotics possess therapeutic ranges whose upper limits border on toxicity. Serum assays for several of these have been developed, most commonly using some type of immunoassay. One example will be used to illustrate general principles. Gentamicin (Garamycin) is one of the aminoglycoside antibiotics that is active against gram-negative organisms, including *Pseudomonas aeruginosa*. Unfortunately, side effects include ototoxicity and nephrotoxicity. Drug excretion is mainly through renal glomerular filtration. Serum peak levels and residual (trough) levels both provide valuable information. Residual levels are measured just prior to the next dose. Values at this time correlate best with nephrotoxicity, especially when serum levels are greater than 2 μg/ml. Specimens for peak level determination are obtained approximately 30 minutes after the end of IV infusion and 1 hour after intramuscular injection. Peak levels correlate best with therapeutic effectiveness (i.e., whether adequate serum levels are present) and possibly with ototoxicity. Normal peak values are usually considered 4–8 μg/ml. Values less than 4μg/ml may be ineffective, whereas those greater than 10 μg/ml predispose to toxicity. Gentamicin assay is desirable because serum levels differ considerably among patients receiving the same dose, and serum gentamicin half-life is equally variable. Standard doses or nomograms based on serum creatinine level fail to predict blood concentration accurately for peak or residual levels in a substantial number of patients even with adequate renal function. When renal function is impaired or when nephrotoxic antibiotics have previously been administered, serum assay becomes essential. It should be mentioned that peak or residual levels within accepted reference limits do not guarantee safety, since some studies have shown onset of renal function decrease in the presence of acceptable serum values.

Vancomycin.—Only a small mount of oral vancomycin is absorbed, so that the oral form is used to kill GI tract bacteria such as *Clostridium difficile* (chapter 16). Intravenous medication is used for other infections. Intravenous vancomycin is about 50%–60% bound to serum albumin, and 80%–90% is excreted unchanged in the urine. The serum half-life is 2–3 hours in children and 4–8 hours in adults with normal renal function. In renal failure, the serum half-life becomes 7–8 days (range, 4–9 days), and instead of the usual adult IV dose of 500 mg every 6 hours, only 500–1,000 mg once per week is sufficient. Peak and residual (trough) levels are usually recommended. Residual levels are usually obtained just before a dose is given; the reference values are 5–10 mg/100 ml. Unfortunately, different investigators do not agree when to draw specimens after the end of IV infusion for peak values, with times suggested including immediately, 15 minutes, 30 minutes, and 2 hours after the infusion. Vancomycin serum levels apparently fall rapidly for a time after the end of IV infusion and then more slowly. At 15 minutes after the end of infusion, serum values of 25–30 mg/100 ml are equivalent to 30–40 mg/100 ml levels (the most commonly accepted peak value range) at the end of infusion.

Cyclosporine

Cyclosporine (previously called "cyclosporin A") is a compound derived from a soil fungus that has strong immunosuppressive activity and is widely used to prevent transplant rejection. Cyclosporine is thought to inhibit helper T-cell function with minimal effect on B-cell function. Cyclosporine can be administered orally or intravenously. If given orally, it is absorbed through the lymphatics of the distal ileum, with considerable variability in time and degree of absorption. During the immediate postoperative period, 8%–60% of the dose is absorbed, although later absorption may improve somewhat. After an oral dose, peak serum levels are reached in about 2.5 hours, and subsequent body elimination half-life is about 4 hours. There is wide variation of these two parameters between individual patients (e.g., elimination time variation of 4.3–53 hours in renal transplant patients). About 50%–60% of the absorbed dose is bound to RBCs, 25%–35% is in plasma, and about 10%–15% is bound to leukocytes. The plasma component is about 60% bound to high-density lipoproteins, about 25% to low-density lipoproteins, and about 10% to other plasma proteins, leaving about 5% unbound. Almost all of the drug is metabolized by the liver microsome system into various derivatives that are excreted in bile and feces, with only 1%–6% of the metabolites excreted in urine. There are several serious side effects. About 25% of transplant patients show some degree of renal toxicity. Lesser numbers develop hypertension or liver toxicity.

Cyclosporine Assay.—The blood concentration of cyclosporine cannot be predicted from an oral dose. In addition, there is a narrow balance between insufficient immunosuppression with too little drug and inducement of toxicity with too much. Therefore, TDM is considered essential. However, there is considerable controversy in the literature regarding the technical details of cyclosporine TDM. Either whole blood or plasma can be analyzed. Distribution of the drug between plasma and RBCs is temperature dependent, with decrease in serum concentration as temperature decreases. Therefore, to obtain plasma, one must equilibrate the blood at a fixed temperature, and this temperature will influence the assay value. On the other hand, whole blood assay results are affected by the patient hematocrit. Whole blood assay is recommended by the AACC Task Force on Cyclosporine Monitoring (1987). The two widely used assay methods are HPLC and RIA. Radioimmunoassay produces higher values than HPLC and includes some cross-reacting metabolites with the cyclosporine measurement. The HPLC assay is more specific since it does not include metabolites. However, there are many published HPLC procedures that vary in one or more technical details. At present, there is no consensus on a single analytic protocol, and since different methods and technical variations produce different results, an exact therapeutic range has not been established. Average values from the literature are 250–1,000 μg/L using whole blood by RIA, 50–200 μg/L using plasma by RIA, and 100–500 μg/L using whole blood by HPLC. Trough levels are usually obtained. Certain medications affect cyclosporine assay, such as phenytoin, which activates the liver microsome system.

Drugs of Abuse

Testing for drugs of abuse usually occurs in two circumstances: possible or known overdose or testing of clinically well persons to detect drug use. Overdose will be discussed in the section on toxicology. Drug screening has its own unique problems. For example, it is necessary to provide legal chain of custody protection to specimens so that each time a specimen changes hands the person receiving it documents this fact and thereby becomes the theoretical protector of the specimen. Another difficulty is attempts by some patients to invalidate the tests if the tests are performed on urine. This may involve diluting the urine specimen, adding substances that might interfere with the test, or substituting someone else's specimen. Possible dilution can be suspected or detected by specimen appearance (appearance suggesting water), very low specific gravity, or specimen temperature less than or more than body temperature. One investigator has found normal urine temperature immediately after voiding to be 97%–100°F (36°–38°C); the National Institute of Drug Abuse (NIDA) current guidelines are 90.5°–99.8°F (32.5°–37.7°C). Addition of foreign substances may be detected by unusual color or other appearance, low specimen temperature, or by unusually low or high specimen pH (normal urine pH is generally considered to be 4.5–8.0). Sometimes there may be an unusual smell. Specimen substitution by the patient may be suspected by specimen temperature lower than body temperature. A fluid without creatinine is probably not urine. Patient identity should be verified, by photograph if possible, to prevent a substitute from providing the specimen.

A variety of methods can be used for initial

screening. Currently, the two most popular are TLC and some form of immunoassay. The Syva Company EMIT immunoassay was one of the first to be introduced and remains the most popular. Due to the possibility of cross-reacting substances and the implications of a positive test result to the patient, as well as legal considerations, positive screening test results should be confirmed by a method that uses a different detection principle. Currently, the method of choice is gas chromatography followed by mass spectrometry (GC/MS). Instruments are available that combine both components. Gas chromatography separates the various substances in the mixture and the mass spectrometer bombards each substance from the chromatographic separation with electrons to ionize the constituents. The constituents are separated on the basis of mass/charge ratio, and a mass spectrum peak is calculated for each by comparing the mass to the number of ions of that mass that are present. The spectrum peak is a fingerprint that identifies the compound. Therefore, the gas chromatography element separates the constituents, and the mass spectrometry component identifies them.

Marijuana *(Cannabis)*.—The most important active component of marijuana is δ-9-tetrahydrocannabinol (δ-9-THC, usually, although incorrect technically, abbreviated as THC). After inhalation of marijuana, THC can be detected in blood in about 1–2 minutes and reaches a peak in about 7 minutes. The sensation attributed to THC, however, does not appear until about 20–30 minutes after the serum peak, at a time when the serum level of THC is considerably lower. It is fat soluble and is quickly deposited into many tissues, including the brain. At the same time, the THC that reaches the liver is metabolized to a compound with psychogenic properties called "11-hydroxy-THC," which then itself is rapidly metabolized to various compounds, the principle metabolite being a nonpsychogenic water-soluble compound conjugated to glucuronide molecules called "carboxy-THC." About 30 minutes after absorption into tissues, THC is slowly released back into the blood, where liver metabolism continually reduces its body availability. If more marijuana is smoked before the previous amount has been eliminated, more THC will be deposited in tissues (up to a saturation point), and total elimination takes longer. Shortly after reaching the serum peak, the serum level of THC begins to fall due to tissue absorption and liver metabolism even if smoking continues, reaching only 10% of the peak levels in 1–2 hours. The serum half-life of THC after inhalation is about 0.5–1.5 hours. Carboxy-THC reaches a serum peak at about 20–30 minutes, at which time it begins to exceed THC. At 1 hour after inhalation, about 15% of plasma cannabinoids is THC and about 40% is carboxy-THC. Both THC and carboxy-THC are nearly all bound to plasma proteins (predominantly lipoproteins), and their concentration in plasma is about twice that of whole blood. About two thirds of the cannabinoid metabolites are excreted in feces and about one third in urine. The body elimination half-life of THC is about 24 hours (range, 18–30 hours), and the elimination half-life of carboxy-THC, the principle metabolite, is 3–6 days. Since the elimination half-life of THC is about 1 day and since steady state is reached after five half-lives, if the individual smokes roughly the same number of marijuana cigarettes each day, there will be equilibrium between intake and elimination of THC in about 5 days. Carboxy-THC has a longer elimination half-life, so that constant or heavy use of marijuana greatly prolongs the time that carboxy-THC will be detectable in the urine. Marijuana can be eaten as well as smoked. Absorption from the GI tract is slower and less predictable than through the lungs. Onset of the psychogenic effect occurs about 1–3 hours after ingestion of marijuana. Serum levels of 11-hydroxy-THC are considerably higher after oral intake of cannabis than levels after smoking.

Urine Assay.—Carboxy-THC is the major metabolite of THC and is the one usually assayed in urine. Length of detectable urinary excretion varies with the amount of marijuana used per day, which, in turn, depends on the type of material (e.g., ordinary marijuana, hashish, or other forms) and the number of times per day of administration. There is also some effect from the route of use (smoking or ingestion) and individual tolerance or variation in the rate of metabolism. There are also assay technical factors. Most investigation of urine carboxy-THC detection has used detection cutoff levels of either 20 ng/ml or 100 ng/ml. The 100 ng/ml cutoff point was used in order to avoid claims that inhaling smoke from someone else's marijuana cigarette might produce a positive urine test result. Actually, several studies have tested persons exposed to prolonged inhalation from cigarettes of other persons in small, confined areas (severe passive inhalation), and found that only a few persons had positive urine tests at the 20 ng/ml cutoff level. The longest time interval for a positive test was 3 days. Under ordinary experimental conditions of passive exposure, only a few individuals had detectable urine levels at the 20 ng/ml cutoff; detectability usually disappeared in less than 24 hours and almost always by 48 hours. Urine specimens should be frozen if testing is delayed, to preserve carboxy-THC values.

Saliva Assay.—It has been reported that THC remains in saliva up to 5 hours after cannabis inhalation. Therefore, detection of THC in saliva theoretically might indicate recent use of marijuana. To date, saliva assay has not been widely used.

Time Period After Use That Marijuana Presence Can Be Detected.—After a single cigarette containing usual amounts of THC is smoked, urine levels become detectable after about 1 hour and remain detectable at the 100 ng/ml cutoff level for 1–3 days and at the 20 ng/ml cutoff level for 2–7 days (therefore, the total detectable time period at the 20 ng/ml level is about 5–7 days, with a range of 2–10 days). For example, in one study those patients tested after smoking a single cigarette showed urine results more than 100 ng/ml for up to 3 days and results more than 20 ng/ml for an additional 5–8 days. Smoking more than one cigarette on the same day for 1 day only extends the detectability time about 2 days. In chronic heavy users, after smoking is prevented, urine results can remain positive at the 20 ng/ml level in some individuals up to 30–40 days. In one report, chronic marijuana users with recent heavy intake had urine assays more than 100 ng/ml for 7–14 days, followed by assays greater than 20 ng/ml for an additional 7–14 days. However, in another study of chronic marijuana smokers, results of about 25% of those who had smoked within 2 days of testing were negative at the 100 ng/ml level.

Interpretation of Test Results.—Carboxy-THC is not psychotropically active, and because of the variability of excretion due to the different factors just noted, detection of this substance in urine (if confirmed) indicates only that the patient has used marijuana in the recent past without providing evidence that correlates with physical or mental effects of marijuana. Serum levels of THC greater than 2 ng/ml is thought to indicate probability that an individual would have some undesirable effects. In some circumstances, such as patient actions that may have been influenced by marijuana, it might be useful to obtain a THC serum level immediately as an indicator of current status and to compare with the urine carboxy-THC level. If the question arises whether marijuana use is ongoing, monitoring the urine periodically (e.g., every 4–5 days) should demonstrate a progressive downward trend in the values if smoking has indeed stopped, although there may be some fluctuations during this time. Initially positive test results with any screening procedure must be verified by a confirmatory procedure (such as GC/MS) if the positive results will lead to some significant action. The different sensitivity levels of different tests must also be kept in mind, as well as the effect of urine concentration or dilution.

Cocaine.—Cocaine can be self-administered intranasally, by smoking, or intravenously. It may also be taken orally, but this is not common since gastric juice inactivates most of the drug. Intranasal administration produces peak blood levels in 30–40 minutes (range, 15–60 minutes). About 80% of the dose reaches the bloodstream. Intravenous administration produces peak levels in 3–5 minutes. Smoking pharmacokinetics are similar to those of IV use, with peak levels reached in about 5 minutes, although only an average of about 45% of the dose reaches the bloodstream. The most common form used for smoking is known as "freebase," which is derived from the active ingredient cocaine hydrochloride by separating the cocaine base from the hydrochloride ions, usually by extracting the cocaine base in a solvent. Already processed cocaine base is often called "crack." This is the most potent form of cocaine. Cocaine is very lipophilic and is rapidly taken up by tissues containing lipid, such as the brain. The half-life of cocaine in the body after the serum peak is about 1.5 hours (range, 0.5–2 hours) for all methods of drug intake. About 25%–40% of the dose that reaches the bloodstream is converted to the major metabolite benzoylecgonine by hydrolysis in fluids and peripheral tissues and excreted in the urine. Benzoylecgonine has a body half-life of 7–9 hours, which is about six times as long as that of cocaine. About 20%–25% of serum cocaine is converted to other metabolites, with roughly equal contribution by the liver and by serum cholinesterase. About 1% is excreted unchanged in the urine.

Detection of Cocaine.—Cocaine or its metabolites can be measured in serum or in urine. The serum half-life of cocaine is short, and cocaine from a single dose is usually nondetectable in 6–10 hours, although it may be detectable longer with very sensitive methodology. Multiple doses may prolong serum detectability. Cocaine in urine is detectable for only about 8–12 hours after a single dose. Cocaine is usually investigated in urine through detection of its metabolite benzoylecgonine. This is detectable in urine beginning 1–4 hours after a cocaine dose. How long it will remain detectable depends on the quantity ingested, whether dosage is single or multiple, individual patient variation, and the sensitivity of the detection method. Radioimmunoassay is the most sensitive of the screening methods (5 μg/L) and may detect cocaine metabolites as long as 7 days after a large dose. Enzyme immunoassay (EIA, an EMIT variant) is less sensitive (300 μg/L) and would detect the presence of the same dose for about 2–3 days. Since some false positive results can be obtained with any of the screening tests, a positive result must be verified by a confirmatory method such as gas chromatography plus mass spectrometry. The screening methods are designed to detect benzoylecgonine, which remains detectable considerably longer than cocaine, so that a positive urine screening test result does not mean the patient was under the influence of cocaine at the time he or she produced the urine specimen, and the result usually will not predict (except as an estimate involving considerable time variation) when the last dose was taken. Proof of use at a specific time requires detection of cocaine itself in serum or other body tissue. This is usually done by gas chromatography plus mass spectrometry. Specimens should be placed in ice and the serum frozen to prevent hydrolysis of cocaine to its metabolites.

Phencyclidine.—Phencyclidine (PCP) effects are frequently not recognized; in one study, only 29% of patients were correctly diagnosed on admission. Phencyclidine is a water-soluble powder that is administered by smoking water-dissolved drug applied to some smoking material or by ingestion. About 70% of the dose reaches the bloodstream by either route. Peak serum levels are reached 5–15 minutes after smoking. Peak levels after oral intake are reached after about 2 hours. The body half-life of PCP after serum peak levels are reached varies considerably, averaging about 18 hours with a range of 8–55 hours, and are somewhat dependent on the dose. About 10% of the dose is excreted in the urine unchanged, and the remainder as various metabolites without one of them being greatly predominant. Phencyclidine or its metabolites are often detected in urine for about 1 week. In some cases it may be detected for several days to several weeks, again depending on the quantity administered, whether administration was acute or chronic, and the sensitivity of the detection method. Drug excretion can be increased by urine acidification. Serum or urine levels do not correlate well with severity of symptoms. Phencyclidine or some of its metabolites can be detected by RIA, EIA, TLC, and other techniques. These methods differ in sensitivity and each method has some substances that may cross-react. Gas chromatography plus mass spectrometry is the best confirmatory method.

Amphetamines.—Metamphetamine is used more frequently than the other amphetamines. Amphetamines can be administered orally, intravenously, or by smoking. Tolerance frequently develops, necessitating larger doses to achieve desired effects. Other drugs are frequently used at the same time. Absorption from the GI tract is fairly rapid. Body half-life is 4–24 hours. About half the dose is metabolized in the liver. About 45% of the metamphetamine dose is excreted in urine unchanged, about 5% as amphetamine, and the remainder as other metabolites. Amphetamines are usually detectable in urine by 3 hours after administration of a single dose, and screening test results can be positive for 24–48 hours (dependent to some extent on the size of the dose and the sensitivity of the method). A positive result for amphetamines in urine generally means use in the last 24–48 hours. Screening methods include RIA, EIA, TLC, and other techniques. A substantial number of over-the-counter medications for colds or for weight reduction contain amphetamines or amphetamine analogs that may cross-react in one or more screening tests. Other medications may also interfere. Gas chromatography plus mass spectrometry is the best confirmatory method.

Morphine and Related Alkaloids.—Morphine and codeine are made from seed pods of the opium poppy. Heroin is made from morphine. Morphine and heroin are usually injected intravenously. About 10% (range 2%–12%) of a morphine dose is excreted unchanged in the urine, and about 60%–80% of the dose is excreted in urine as conjugated glucuronides. The body half-life is 1.7–4.5 hours. Heroin is rapidly metabolized to morphine, with about 7% of the dose excreted as morphine and 50%–60% excreted as conjugated morphine glucuronides. Codeine is excreted primarily as conjugated codeine glucuronides in the urine, but a small amount (< 10%) is metabolized to morphine and morphine conjugated glucuronides, which appear in the urine. Poppy seeds are used as a filling for baked goods and also are used unprocessed; they are sold legally even though they contain some natural morphine and codeine. The amount of opiate alkaloids in poppy seeds is not sufficient to produce any symptoms or noticeable sensation, but consumption of a moderate amount of this material can result in detectable concentrations of morphine in the urine that can last as long as 36–60 hours.

Screening tests for morphine and other opiates are similar to those for other drugs of abuse: RIA, EIA (EMIT and others), TLC, and in addition a hemagglutination inhibition assay. Most of these methods cannot differentiate between codeine and morphine. Also, since codeine metabolism results in a small but measurable amount of morphine conjugates, prescription medications containing codeine for pain relief or cough suppressive effects may produce positive test results for morphine. In general, if the concentration of codeine greatly exceeds that of morphine, the parent drug is probably codeine. In general, excluding prescription drugs, the presence of morphine in the urine indicates nonlegal use of morphine, heroin, or codeine in the past 1–2 days. Detection of these compounds should be confirmed, and the compound identified, using gas chromatography plus mass spectrometry. In addition, GC/MS can differentiate between poppy seed ingestion and heroin intake by detecting and measuring 6-monoacetylmorphine, a metabolite of heroin that is not present in poppy seeds or in the urine of persons who ingest poppy seeds.

TOXICOLOGY

This section includes a selected list of conditions that seem especially important in drug detection, overdose, or poisoning. Treatment of drug overdose by dialysis or other means can often be assisted with the objective information derived from drug levels. In some cases, drug screening of urine and serum may reveal additional drugs or substances, such as alcohol, which affect management or clinical response.

Lead.—Lead exposure in adults is most often due to occupational hazard (e.g., exposure to lead in manufacture or use of gasoline additives and in smelting) or to homemade "moonshine" whiskey distilled in lead-containing equipment. When children are severely affected, it is usually from eating old lead-containing paint chips. One group found some indications of chronic lead exposure in about one half of those persons examined who had lived for more than 5 years near a busy automobile expressway in a major city. Fertilization of crops with city sewage sludge is reported to increase the lead content of the crops.

Symptoms.—Acute lead poisoning is uncommon. Symptoms may include "lead colic" (crampy abdominal pain, constipation, occasional bloody diarrhea) and, in 50% of patients, hypertensive encephalopathy. Chronic poisoning is more common. Its varying symptoms may include lead colic, constipation with anorexia (85% of patients), and peripheral neuritis (wrist drop) in adults and lead encephalopathy (headache, convulsions) in children. A "lead line" is frequently present just below the epiphyses (in approximately 70% of patients with clinical symptoms and 20%–40% of persons with abnormal exposure but no symptoms).

Hematologic Findings.—Most patients develop slight to moderate anemia, usually hypochromic but sometimes normochromic. Red blood cells with basophilic stippling is the most characteristic peripheral blood finding. Some authors claim stippling is invariably present; others report that stippling is present in only 20%–30% of cases. Normal persons may have as many as 500 stippled cells/1 million RBCs. The reticulocyte count is usually greater than 4%.

δ-Aminolevulinic Acid Dehydrase.—Body intake of lead produces biochemical effects on heme synthesis (see Fig 20–2). The level of δ-aminolevulinic acid dehydrase (ALA-D), which converts ALA to porphobilinogen, is decreased as early as the fourth day after exposure begins. Once the ALA-D level is reduced, persistence of abnormality correlates with the amount of lead in body tissues (body burden), so that the ALA-D level remains reduced as long as significant quantities of lead remain. Therefore, after chronic lead exposure, low ALA-D values may persist for years even though exposure has ceased. The level of ALA-D is also a very sensitive indicator of lead toxicity and is usually reduced to 50% or less of normal activity when blood lead values are in the 30–50 μg/100 ml range. Unfortunately, the ALA-D level reaches a plateau when marked reduction takes place, so it cannot be used to quantitate degree of exposure. In addition, this enzyme must be assayed within 24 hours after the blood specimen is secured. Relatively few laboratories perform the test, although it has only a moderate degree of technical difficulty.

Blood Lead Assay.—Intake of lead ordinarily results in rapid urinary lead excretion. If excessive lead exposure continues, lead is stored in bone. If bone storage capacity is exceeded, lead accumulates in soft tissues. Blood lead levels depend on the relationship between intake, storage, and excretion. The blood lead level is primarily an indication of acute (current) exposure but is also influenced by previous storage. Blood lead values of 10–20 μg/100 ml (whole blood) (0.48–0.96 μmol/L) are considered normal. Values higher than 25 μg/100 ml (1.21 μmol/L) are considered abnormal in children. Values higher than 40 μg/100 ml (1.93 μmol/L) are generally considered abnormal in adults, although the cutoff point for children may also be valid for adults. Symptoms of lead poisoning are associated with levels higher than 80 μg/100 ml (3.86 μmol/L), although mild symptoms may occur at 50 μg/100 ml (2.41 μmol/L) in children. Blood lead assay takes considerable experience and dedication to perform accurately. Contamination is a major headache—in drawing the specimen, in sample tubes, in laboratory glassware, and in the assay procedure itself. Special Vacutainer-type tubes for trace metal determination are commercially available and are strongly recommended.

Urine δ-Aminolevulinic Acid (ALA) Assay.—Another procedure frequently used is urine ALA assay. Blood and urine ALA levels increase when the blood ALA-D level is considerably reduced. Therefore, ALA also becomes an indicator of body lead burden, and urine ALA begins to increase when blood lead values are higher than 40 μg/100 ml (1.93 μmol/L). Disadvantages of urine ALA assay are difficulties with 24-hour urine collection or, if random specimens are used, the effects of urine concentration or dilution on apparent ALA concentration. In addition, at least one investigator found that the urine ALA level was normal in a significant number of cases when the blood lead level was in the 40–80 μg/100 ml (1.93–3.86 μmol/L) (mildly to moderately abnormal) range. Light, room temperature, and alkaline pH all decrease ALA levels. If ALA determination is not done immediately, the specimen must be refrigerated and kept in the dark (the collection bottle wrapped in paper or foil) with the specimen acidified, using glacial acetic or tartaric acid.

Detecting Lead Exposure.—If a patient is subjected to continuous lead exposure of sufficient magnitude, blood lead level, urine lead excretion, ALA-D level, and urine ALA level all correlate well. If the exposure ceases before laboratory tests are made, blood lead level (and sometimes even urine lead level) may decrease relative to ALA-D or urine ALA. Assay of ALA-D is the most sensitive of these tests. In fact, certain patients whose urine ALA and blood lead levels are within normal limits may display a mild to moderate decrease in ALA-D levels. It remains to be determined whether this reflects previous toxicity in all cases or simply means that ALA-D levels between 50% and

100% of normal are too easily produced to mean truly abnormal lead exposure.

Urine lead excretion has also been employed as an index of exposure, since blood lead values change more rapidly than urine lead excretion. However, excretion values depend on 24-hour urine specimens, with the usual difficulty in complete collection. A further problem is that excretion values may be normal in borderline cases or in cases of previous exposure. Urine lead has been measured after administration of a chelating agent such as ethylenediamine tetraacetic acid (EDTA), which mobilizes body stores of lead. This is a more satisfactory technique than ordinary urine excretion for determining body burden (i.e., previous exposure). Abnormal exposure is suggested when the 24-hour urine lead excretion is greater than 1 μg for each milligram of calcium-EDTA administered. Disadvantages are those of incomplete urine collection, difficulty in accurate lead measurement, and occasional cases of EDTA toxicity.

Erythrocyte protoporphyrin (zinc protoporphyrin, or ZPP) is still another indicator of lead exposure. Lead inhibits ferrochelatase (heme synthetase), an enzyme that incorporates iron into protoporphyrin IX (erythrocyte protoporphyrin) to form heme. Decreased erythrocyte protoporphyrin conversion leads to increased erythrocyte protoporphyrin levels. The standard assay for erythrocyte protoporphyrin involved extraction of a mixture of porphyrins, including protoporphyrin IX, from blood, and measurement of protoporphyrin using fluorescent wavelengths. In normal persons, protoporphyrin IX is not complexed to metal ions. Under the conditions of measurement it was thought that the protoporphyrin being measured was metal free, since iron-complexed protoporphyrin did not fluoresce, so that what was being measured was called "free erythrocyte protoporphyrin." However, in lead poisoning, protoporphyrin IX becomes complexed to zinc; hence, the term ZPP. The protoporphyrin-zinc complex will fluoresce although the protoporphyrin-iron complex will not. Therefore, most laboratory analytic techniques for ZPP involve fluorescent methods. In fact, some have used visual RBC fluorescence (in a heparinized wet preparation using a microscope equipped with ultraviolet light) as a rapid screening test for lead poisoning. Zinc protoporphyrin levels are elevated in about 50%–75% of those who have a subclinical increase in blood lead levels (40–60 μg/100 ml) and are almost always elevated in symptomatic lead poisoning. An instrument called the "hematofluorometer" is available from several manufacturers and can analyze a single drop of whole blood for ZPP. The reading is affected by the number of RBCs present and must be corrected for hematocrit level. The ZPP test results are abnormal in chronic iron deficiency and hemolytic anemia as well as in lead poisoning. The ZPP level is also elevated in erythropoietic protoporphyria (a rare congenital porphyria variant) and in chronic febrile illness. An increased serum bilirubin level falsely increases ZPP readings, and fluorescing drugs or other substances in plasma may interfere.

Urinary coproporphyrin III excretion is usually, although not invariably, increased in clinically evident lead poisoning. Since this compound fluoresces under Wood's light, simple screening tests based on fluorescence of coproporphyrin III in urine specimens under ultraviolet light have been devised.

Diagnosis of Lead Poisoning.—The question arises as to which test should be used to detect or diagnose lead poisoning. The ALA-D assay is the most sensitive current test, and ALA-D levels may be abnormal (decreased) when all other test results are still normal. Disadvantages are the long-term persistence of abnormality once it is established, which may represent past instead of recent exposure. The specimen is unstable, and few laboratories perform the test. Zinc protoporphyrin is sensitive for lead poisoning and detects 50%–70% of cases of subclinical lead exposures. The hematofluorometer can assay microsamples of blood and is a good screening method. Disadvantages are the irreversible change induced in the RBCs, which remains throughout the 120-day life span of the RBCs. Thus, ZPP represents biologic effects of lead averaged over 3–4 months' time. Also, the test is not specific for lead exposure. Blood lead assay is considered the best diagnostic test for actual lead poisoning. Blood lead indicates either acute or current exposure; levels in single short exposures rise and fall fairly quickly. However, small elevations (in the 40–60 μg/100 ml range), especially in single determinations, may be difficult to interpret because of laboratory variation in the assay. Some investigators recommend assay of blood lead together with ZPP, since elevation of ZPP values would suggest that exposure to lead must have been more than a few days' duration.

Heavy Metals.—Mercury, arsenic, bismuth, and antimony are included. Urine samples are preferred to blood samples. Hair and nails are useful for detection or documentation of long-term exposure to arsenic or mercury.

Organic Phosphates (Cholinesterase Inhibitors).—Certain insecticides such as parathion and the less powerful malathion are inhibitors of the enzyme acetylcholinesterase. Acetylcholinesterase inactivates excess acetylcholine at nerve endings. Inhibition or inactivation of acetylcholinesterase permits overproduction of acetylcholine at nerve-muscle junctions. Symptoms include muscle twitching, cramps, and weakness; parasympathetic effects such as pinpoint pupils, nausea, sweating, diarrhea, and salivation; and various CNS aberrations. Organic phosphate poisons inactivate not only acetylcholinesterase (which is found in RBCs as well as at nerve endings) but also pseudocholinesterase, which is found in plasma. Therefore, laboratory diagnosis of organophosphate poisoning is based on finding decreased acetylcholinesterase levels in RBCs or pseudocholinesterase in plasma (these two cholinesterase types are frequently referred to in the laboratory simply as "cholinesterase" with either RBCs or plasma specified). Levels in RBCs reflect poisoning more accurately than plasma values, since plasma levels are reduced by many conditions and drugs. However, plasma measurement is much easier, so that screening tests are generally based on plasma measurement (chapter 33). In acute poisoning, RBC or plasma cholinesterase activity is less than 50% of normal. In most cases, a normal result rules out severe acute anticholinesterase toxicity. However, the population reference range is fairly wide, so that a person with a preexposure value in the upper end of the population range might have his or her value decreased 50% and still be within the population reference range. Therefore, low normal values do not exclude the possibility of organophosphate toxicity. It is strongly recommended that persons who may be occupationally exposed to the organophosphates should have their baseline plasma cholinesterase (pseudocholinesterase) value established. Once this is done, periodic monitoring could be done to detect subclinical toxicity.

Barbiturates and Glutethimide .—Barbiturates and glutethimide (Doriden) are the most common vehicles of drug-overdose suicide. In testing, either anticoagulated (not heparinized) whole blood or urine can be used; blood is preferred. Thin-layer chromatography is used both for screening and to identify the individual substance involved. Chemical screening tests are also available. It is preferable to secure both blood and urine specimens plus gastric contents, if available. Many of the larger laboratories can perform quantitative assay of serum phenobarbital.

Phenothiazine Tranquilizers.—Urine can be screened with the dipstick Phenistix or the ferric chloride procedure. Thin-layer chromatography, gas chromatography, and other techniques are available for detection and quantitation.

Acetaminophen.—Acetaminophen (Paracetamol; many different brand names) has been replacing aspirin for headache and minor pain because of the gastric irritant and anticoagulant side effects of aspirin. With greater use of acetaminophen has come occasional cases of overdose. Acetaminophen is rapidly absorbed from the small intestine. Peak serum concentration is reached in 0.5–2 hours, and the serum half-life is 1–4 hours. About 15%–50% is bound to serum albumin. Acetaminophen is 80%–90% metabolized by the liver microsome pathway, 4%–14% is excreted unchanged by the kidneys, and a small amount is degraded by other mechanisms.

Liver Toxicity.—The usual adult dose is 0.5 gm every 3–4 hours. In adults, liver toxicity is unlikely to occur if the ingested dose is less than 10 gm at one time, and death is unlikely if less than 15 gm is ingested. However, 10 gm or more at one time may produce liver damage, and 25 gm can be fatal. Children under age 5 years are less likely to develop liver injury. The toxic symptoms of overdose usually subside in 24 hours after the overdose, even in persons who subsequently develop liver injury. Liver function test results are typical of acute hepatocellular injury, with AST (SGOT) levels similar to those of acute hepatitis virus hepatitis. The peak of AST elevation most often occurs 4–6 days after onset. The liver completely recovers in about 3 months if the patient survives.

Laboratory Evaluation.—Serum acetaminophen levels are helpful to estimate the likelihood of hepatic damage. These levels are used as a guide to continue or discontinue therapy. Peak acetaminophen levels provide the best correlation with toxicity. Current recommendations are that the assay specimen should be drawn 4 hours after ingestion of the dose—not earlier—to be certain that the peak has been reached. A serum level greater than 200 μg/ml (13.2 μmol/L) at 4 hours is considered potentially toxic, and a level less than 150 μg/ml (9.9 μmol/L) is considered nontoxic. The assay should be repeated 12 hours after ingestion. A value greater than 50 μg/ml (3.3 μmol/L) is considered toxic, and a value less than 35 μg/ml (2.3 μmol/L) is considered nontoxic. Colorimetric assay methods are available in kit form that are technically simple and reasonably accurate. However, inexperienced persons can obtain misleading results, so the amount of drug ingested and other factors should also be considered before therapy is terminated. Salicylates, ketones, and ascorbic acid (vitamin C) in high concentration interfere in some assay methods. Either AST or alanine aminotransferase levels should be determined daily for at least 4 days as a further check on liver function.

Acetylsalicylic Acid (Aspirin).—Absorption of aspirin takes place in the stomach and small intestine. Absorption is influenced by rate of tablet dissolution and by pH (acid pH assists absorption and alkaline pH retards it). Peak plasma concentration from ordinary aspirin doses is reached in about 2 hours (1–4 hours), with the peak from enteric-coated aspirin about 4–6 hours later. In some cases of overdose serum values from ordinary aspirin may take several hours to reach their maximum level due to pylorospasm. Aspirin is rapidly metabolized to salicylic acid in GI tract mucosa and liver; it is further metabolized by the liver to metabolically inactive salicyluric acid. Of the original dose, 10%–80% is excreted by the kidneys as salicylate, 5%–15% as salicylic acid, and 15%–40% as salicyluric acid. The half-life of salicylate or its active metabolites in serum at usual drug doses is 2–4.5 hours. The half-life is dose dependent, since the degradation pathways can be saturated. At high doses the half-life may be 15–30 hours. Also, steady-state serum concentration is not linear with respect to dose, with disproportionate serum levels being produced by much smaller increments in dose.

Laboratory Tests.—Mild toxicity (tinnitus, visual disturbances, GI tract disturbances) correlates with serum salicylate levels more than 30 mg/100 ml (300 μg/ml), and severe toxicity (CNS symptoms) is associated with levels more than 50 mg/100 ml (500 μg/ml). In younger children, severe toxicity is often associated with ketosis and metabolic acidosis, whereas in older children and adults, respiratory alkalosis or mixed acidosis-alkalosis is more frequent. Peak serum salicylate values correlate best with toxicity. It is recommended that these be drawn at least 6 hours after the overdose to avoid serum values falsely below peak levels due to delayed absorption. Enteric-coated aspirin delays absorption an additional 4–6 hours. Screening tests for salicylates include urine testing with a ferric chloride reagent or Phenistix (both of these tests are also used in the diagnosis of phenylketonuria). The most commonly used quantitative test is a colorimetric procedure based on ferric chloride. Ketone bodies and phenothiazine tranquilizers can interfere.

Carbon Monoxide.—Carbon monoxide combines with hemoglobin to form carboxyhemoglobin. While doing this it occupies oxygen-binding sites and also produces a change in the hemoglobin molecule that binds the remaining oxygen more tightly, with less being available for tissue cell respiration. Headache, fatigue, and lightheadedness are the most frequent symptoms.

Laboratory Diagnosis.—Carbon monoxide poisoning is detected by hemoglobin analysis for carboxyhemoglobin. This is most readily done on an instrument called a CO-Oximeter. A 30%–40% carboxyhemoglobin content is associated with severe symptoms, and more than 50% is associated with coma. Cigarette smoking may produce levels as high as 10%–15%. Carboxyhemoglobin is stable for more than 1 week at room temperature in EDTA anticoagulant. The specimen should be drawn as soon as possible after exposure, since carbon monoxide is rapidly cleared from hemoglobin by breathing normal air.

Carbon monoxide poisoning can be suspected from an arterial blood gas specimen when a measured oxygen saturation (percent O_2 saturation of hemoglobin) value is found to be significantly below what would be expected if oxygen saturation were calculated from the PO_2 and pH values. For this screening procedure to be valid, the O_2 saturation must be measured directly, not calculated. Some blood gas machines measure O_2 saturation, but the majority calculate it from the PO_2 and pH values.

Ethyl Alcohol (Ethanol).—Ethanol is absorbed from the small intestine and, to a lesser extent, from the stomach. Factors that influence absorption are (1) whether food is also ingested, since food delays absorption, and if so, the amount and kind of food; (2) the rate of gastric emptying; and (3) the type of alcoholic beverage ingested. Without food, the absorptive phase (time period during which alcohol is being absorbed until the peak blood value is reached) may be as short as 15 minutes or as long as 2 hours. In one study, peak values occurred at 30 minutes after ingestion in nearly 50% of experimental subjects and in about 75% by 1 hour; but 6% peaked as late as 2 hours. With food, absorption is delayed to varying degrees. Once absorbed, ethanol rapidly equilibrates throughout most body tissues. The liver metabolizes about 75% of absorbed ethanol. The predominant liver cell metabolic pathway of ethanol is the alcohol dehydrogenase enzyme system, whose product is acetaldehyde. Acetaldehyde, in turn, is metabolized by the hepatic microsome system. About 10%–15% of absorbed ethanol is excreted unchanged through the kidneys and through the lungs.

Ethanol Measurement.—There are several methods for patient alcohol measurement. The legal system generally recognizes whole blood as the gold standard specimen. Arterial blood ethanol is somewhat higher than venous blood levels, especially in the active absorption phase. Capillary blood (fingerstick or ear lobe blood) is about 70%–85% of the arterial concentration. The major problems with whole blood are that values are influenced by the hematocrit, and most present-day chemistry analyzers must use serum. Serum is the usual specimen analyzed in routine laboratories. A serum value is higher than a whole blood value obtained on the same specimen, whereas blood levels correlated by law to degrees of physical and mental impairment are defined by whole blood assay. Serum values can be converted to equivalent whole blood values by means of a conversion ratio. Unfortunately, there is significant disagreement in the literature on which ratio to use; different investigators report serum/whole blood ratios varying between 1.03 and 1.25. Enzymatic methods using alcohol dehydrogenase or alcohol oxidase are replacing the classic potassium dicromate methods. There is some dispute in the literature whether or not alcohol dehydrogenase methods are affected by isopropanol (commonly used for venipuncture skin cleansing). In experiments performed in my laboratory, no cross-reaction was found in dilutions stronger than what should be encountered from skin cleansing. Nevertheless, because of legal considerations, specimens for ethanol should be drawn without using any type of alcohol as a skin-cleansing agent. Increased blood ketones, as found in diabetic ketoacidosis, can falsely elevate either blood or breath alcohol test results. Urine is not recommended for analysis, because the blood/urine ratio is highly variable and there may be stasis of the specimen in the bladder. However, urine can be used to screen for the presence of alcohol. Breath analyzers are the assay method most commonly used for police work since the measurement can be done wherever or whenever it is desirable. Breath analyzers measure the ethanol content at the end of expiration following a deep inspiration. The measurement is then correlated to whole blood by multiplying the measured breath ethanol level by the factor 2,100. On the average, breath alcohol concentration correlates reasonably well with whole blood alcohol concentration using this factor. However, there is significant variation between correlation factors reported in different individuals and average factors in different groups, so that use of any single "universal" factor will underestimate the blood ethanol concentration in some persons and overestimate it in others. Also, correlation with blood ethanol levels is better when breath ethanol is measured in the postabsorptive state than in the absorptive state. When breath analyzers are used, it is important that there be a time period of at least 15 minutes prior to testing during which no alcohol ingestion, smoking, food or drink consumption, or vomiting has taken place to avoid contamination of the breath specimen by alcohol in the mouth. Ketone bodies in patients with diabetic acidosis may interfere with breath ethanol measurement. One further advantage of breath testing in the field is the usefulness of a negative test for ethanol in a person whose behavior suggests effects of alcohol; this result could mean a serious acute medical problem that needs immediate attention.

Legal Use of Blood Alcohol Assay.—Most courts of law follow the recommendations of the National Safety Council on alcohol and drugs (the following ethanol values are whole blood values):

- Below 0.05% (50 mg/100 ml): No influence by alcohol within the meaning of the law.
- Between 0.05% and 0.10% (50–100 mg/100 ml): A liberal, wide zone in which alcohol influence usually is present, but courts of law are advised to consider the person's behavior and circumstances leading to the arrest in making their decision.
- Above 0.10% (100 mg/100 ml): Definite evidence of being "under the influence," since most persons with this concentration will have lost, to a measurable extent, some of the clearness of intellect and self-control they would normally possess.

Some organizations, including the AMA Council on Scientific Affairs (1986), suggest adopting 0.05% blood alcohol content as per se evidence of alcohol-impaired driving.

Estimating Previous Blood Alcohol Levels.—In certain situations it would be desirable to estimate the blood alcohol level at some previous time from the results of a subsequent alcohol level. The usual method for this is the Widmark equation: $P = A + (F \times T)$, when P is the concentration of blood alcohol (in milligrams per liter) at the previous time, A is the concentration of blood alcohol (in milligrams per liter) when it was measured, F is a factor (or constant) whose value is 130 (in milligrams per kilogram per hour), and T is the time (in hours) elapsed between the time the blood alcohol was measured and the previous time that the blood alcohol value must be estimated.

There is considerable controversy regarding the usefulness of the Widmark equation. The equation is valid for a person only in the postabsorptive state (i.e., after the peak blood alcohol level is reached). Time to peak is most often considered to be 0.5–2.0 hours, so that the blood specimen must be drawn no earlier than 2 hours after the beginning of alcohol intake. The Widmark equation is based on kinetics of alcohol taken during fasting. Food increases alcohol elimination, so that food would cause the Widmark equation to overestimate the previous alcohol level. The factor (constant) of 130 is not necessarily applicable to any individual person, since a range of experimentally measured individual values from 100–340 has been reported.

Clinical and Laboratory Effects of Alcohol.—Alcohol has a considerable number of metabolic and toxic effects that may directly or indirectly involve the clinical laboratory. Liver manifestations include γ-glutamyltransferase (GGT; formerly γ-glutamyl transpeptidase) elevation, fatty liver, acute alcoholic hepatitis ("active cirrhosis"), or Laennec's cirrhosis, and may lead indirectly to bleeding from esophageal varices or to cytopenia either from hypersplenism or through other mechanisms. Red blood cell macrocytosis is frequently associated with chronic alcoholism, and nutritional anemia such as that due to folic acid may be present. Other frequently associated conditions include acute pancreatitis, hypertriglyceridemia, alcoholic gastritis, alcoholic hypoglycemia, various neurologic abnormalities, and subdural hematoma. The chronic alcoholic is more susceptible to infection. Finally, alcohol interacts with a variety of medications. It potentiates many of the CNS depressants, such as various sedatives, narcotics, hypnotics, and tranquilizers (especially chlordiazepoxide and diazepam. Alcohol is a factor in many cases of overdose, even when the patient has no history of alcohol intake or denies intake. The presence of alcohol should be suspected when toxicity symptoms from barbiturates or other medications are associated with blood levels that normally would be considered safe. Alcohol may antagonize the action of various other medications, such as coumarin and phenytoin. Alcohol intake in pregnancy has been reported to produce increased rates of stillbirth and infant growth deficiency as well as a specific "fetal alcohol syndrome." Fetal alcohol syndrome includes a particular pattern of facial appearance, postnatal growth deficiency with normal bone age, various skeletal and organ malformations, and various neurologic abnormalities (including average IQ below normal).

Ethanol is one of a number of substances (other alcohols, lactic acid, etc.) that elevate serum osmolality using freezing point depression methods. This creates a gap between measured osmolality and calculated osmolality. Osmolality using vapor pressure instruments is not affected by ethanol.

Laboratory Screening for Alcoholism.— Various tests have been used to screen for chronic alcoholism. Of these, the most commonly advocated is the GGT. This test and the AST reflect the effect of alcohol on the liver. A third possibility is mean corpuscular volume (MCV), the average size of the patient RBC. This reflects macrocytosis induced by liver disease and possibly also by folic acid deficiency in alcoholics. In heavy drinkers or alcoholics, GGT has a sensitivity of about 70% (literature range, 63%–81%), MCV detects about 60% (26%–90%), and the AST value is elevated in about 50% (27%–77%). Most (but not all) reports indicate some correlation in likelihood and degree of GGT elevation with the amount and frequency of alcohol consumption. Thus, heavy drinkers are more likely to have GGT elevations, and these elevations are (on the average) higher than those of less heavy drinkers. However, there are many exceptions. There is some disagreement as to whether so-called social drinkers have a significant incidence of elevated GGT levels. The majority of investigators seem to believe that they do not.

Other biochemical abnormalities associated with alcoholism (but found in < 40% of cases) include hypophosphatemia, hypomagnesemia, hyponatremia, hypertriglyceridemia, and hyperuricemia.

Additional tests relevant to this chapter are discussed in chapter 35.

BIBLIOGRAPHY

Mule SJ, Casella GA: Rendering the "poppy-seed defense" defenseless: Identification of 6-monoacetylmorphine in urine by gas chromatography/mass spectrometry. *Clin Chem* 1988; 34:1427.

Simpson G: Medicolegal alcohol determination: Widmark revisited. *Clin Chem* 1988; 34:888.

American Association of Clinical Chemistry: Critical issues in urinalysis of abused substances: Report of the Substance Abuse Testing Committee. *Clin Chem* 1988; 34:605.

Preskorn SH, et al: Therapeutic drug monitoring of tricyclic antidepressants. *Clin Chem* 1988; 34:882.

Chisolm JJ: Mobilization of lead by calcium disodium edetate. *Am J Dis Child* 1987; 141:1256.

Simpson G: Accuracy and precision of breath alcohol measurements for subjects in the absorptive state. *Clin Chem* 1987; 33:753.

Jones AW: Concerning accuracy and precision of breath-alcohol measurements. *Clin Chem* 1987; 33:1701.

Schwartz RH, et al: Urinary cannabinoids in monitoring abstinence in a drug abuse treatment program. *Arch Pathol Lab Med* 1987; 111:708.

Hursting MJ: Drug-specific Fab therapy in drug overdose. *Arch Pathol Lab Med* 1987; 111:693.

Mooradian AD, Wynn EM: Pharmacokinetic prediction of serum digoxin concentration in the elderly. *Arch Intern Med* 1987; 147:650.

Bertino JS, Walker JW: Reassessment of theophylline toxicity. *Arch Intern Med* 1987; 147:757.

Jones AW, Neri A: Reinvestigation of Widmark's method for quantitative evaluation of blood-ethanol profiles: Influence of alcohol dose and mode of drinking. *Clin Chem* 1987; 33:1469.

Smith BR, Lefrock JL: Vancomycin update. *Am Fam Phys* 1987; 35:223.

Fogerson R: Adulterated urine samples. *Syva Monitor* 1987; 5(2):1.

Dowling GP, et al: "Eve" and "Ecstasy": A report of five deaths associated with the use of MDEA and MDMA. *JAMA* 1987; 257:1615.

Syva Corporation: About amphetamines. *Syva Monitor* 1987; 5(1):8.

Pettitt BC, et al: Opiates in poppy seed: Effect on urinalysis results after consumption of poppy seed cakefilling. *Clin Chem* 1987; 33:1251.

American Association of Clinical Chemistry Task Force on Cyclosporine Monitoring: Critical issues in cyclosporine monitoring. *Clin Chem* 1987; 33:1269.

Tackett SL: Lead in the environment: Effects of human exposure. *Am Clin Prod Rev* 1987; 6(5):14.

Coye MJ: Clinical confirmation of organophosphate poisoning by serial cholinesterase analyses. *Arch Intern Med* 1987; 147:438.

Friedman H, Greenblatt DJ: Rational therapeutic drug monitoring. *JAMA* 1986; 256:2227.

Wilson F: Therapeutic drug monitoring in the physician's office laboratory. *Lab Mgmt* 1986; 24(10):51.

Singh SN, Tortosa L: New antiarrhythmic agents: Part IX. Pharmacology and clinical use of Flecainide Acetate. *Pract Cardiol* 1986; 12(13):80.

Witherspoon L, et al: Digoxin-like substance in term pregnancy, newborns, and renal failure. *J Nucl Med* 1986; 27:1418.

Soldin SJ: Digoxin—issues and controversies. *Clin Chem* 1986; 32:5.

Orsulak PJ: The antidepressant drugs: developments in therapeutic monitoring. *Lab Mgmt* 1986; 24(12):43.

Willette RE: Interpreting cannabinoid assay results. *Syva Monitor* 1986; 4(1):1.

Boeckx RL: Therapeutic drug monitoring in infants and children. *Med Lab Prod* 1986; 1(1):19.

Haddad LM: Cocaine abuse. *Intern Med Specialist* 1986; 7(9):67.

Nelson TC, Burritt MF: Pesticide poisoning, succinylcholine-induced apnea, and pseudocholinesterase. *Mayo Clin Proc* 1986; 61:750.

Marzella L, Myers RAM: Carbon monoxide poisoning. *Am Fam Phys* 1986; 34:186.

Spiehler V: Cocaine and metabolites. *Clin Chem Newslett* 1986; 12(7):24.

Hawks RL, Chiang CN (ed): *Urine Testing for Drugs of Abuse.* NIDA Research Monograph 73, 1986.

AMA Council on Scientific Affairs: Alcohol and the driver. *JAMA* 1986; 255:522.

Orsulak PJ: *Tricyclic Antidepressants: Considerations for Therapeutic Drug Monitoring.* Syva Company Monograph, 1985.

Flint LM: Serum level monitoring of aminoglycoside antibiotics. *Arch Surg* 1985; 120:99.

Collin DP, Vine W: Controversy continues to surround methods of monitoring cyclosporine. *Clin Chem Newslett* 1985; 11(4):15.

Lake KD, Peterson CD: A simplified dosing method for initiating vancomycin therapy. *Pharmacotherapy* 1985; 5:340.

Schwartz RH, Hawks R: Laboratory detection of marijuana use. *JAMA* 1985; 254:788.

Kwong TC: Salicylates. *Clin Chem Newslett* 1985; 11(1):14.

Di Maio VJM, Garriott JC: How valid is the 0.10 percent alcohol level as an indicator of intoxication? *Pathologist* 1985; 39(3):32.

Jones AW: Interindividual variations in the disposition and metabolism of ethanol in healthy men. *Alcohol* 1984; 1:385.

Pippenger CE: Therapeutic drug monitoring: Pharmacologic principles. *Diagn Med* 1983; 6(4):28.

DeMonaco HJ, Lawless LM: Variability of phenytoin protein binding in epileptic patients. *Arch Neurol* 1983; 40:481.

Hendeles L, Weinberger M: Theophylline: A "state of the art" review. *Pharmacotherapy* 1983; 3:2.

Aniline O, Allen RE: Most PCP intoxication is missed. *Cont Ed Fam Phys* 1983; 18:367.

Cullen MR, et al: Adult inorganic lead intoxication. *Medicine* (Baltimore) 1983; 62:221.

Sterling GH: Poisoning by cholinesterase-inhibiting insecticides. *Am Fam Phys* 1983; 27:159.

Lesar TS: Gentamicin dosing errors with four commonly used nomograms. *JAMA* 1982; 248:1190.

Dubowski KM: Alcohol analysis: Clinical laboratory aspects: Parts I and II. *Lab Mgmt* 1982; 20(3):43; 20(4):27.

Holt S, et al: Early identification of alcohol abuse: 2. Clinical and laboratory indicators. *Can Med Assoc J* 1981; 124:1279.

Taylor WJ, Finn AL (eds): *Individualizing Drug Therapy.* New York, Gross, Townsend, Frank, 1981, vol. 1–3.

Kaye S: The collection and handling of the blood alcohol specimen. *Am J Clin Pathol* 1980; 74:743.

Schoolmeester WL, White DR: Arsenic poisoning. *South Med J* 1980; 73:198.

Dito WR: Therapeutic drug monitoring: Lithium. *Diagn Med* 1980; 3(1):39.

35 Special Category Tests

This chapter includes tests that should be mentioned for special reasons but have been left out of the main text for the sake of succinctness. Some are too new and initial reports need independent confirmation, some have generated highly favorable evaluations that have not been confirmed by the experience of others, some are older tests that are being replaced but occupy a prominent place in the older medical literature, and others are rarely used procedures that might be useful in unusual circumstances. The tests are listed by the chapters in which they could have been placed.

CHAPTER 1. INTERPRETATION OF LABORATORY TEST DATA

Nonparametric Calculation of the Reference Range.—The current standard method for determining reference ranges assumes that the data have a gaussian (homogeneous symmetric) value distribution. In fact, many population sample results are not gaussian. In a gaussian value distribution, the mean value (average sample value) and the median value (value in the center of the range) coincide. In nongaussian distributions, the mean value and the median value are not the same, thus indicating skewness (asymmetric distribution). In these cases, statisticians recommend some type of nonparametric statistical method. Nonparametric formulas do not make any assumption regarding data symmetry. Unfortunately, nonparametric methods are much more cumbersome to use and require a larger value sample (e.g., ≥ 120 values) than do gaussian distributions (e.g., ≥ 20 values). One such nonparametric approach is to rank the values obtained in ascending order and then apply the nonparametric percentile estimate formula.

Other Reference Range Methods or Interpretive Systems.—Some investigators have responded to the problems inherent in basing medical action on reference range limits by proposing alternate or supplementary systems. One example is a percentile system that ranks patient laboratory values in the normal and mildly abnormal areas according to what fraction of the normal (reference) population would be expected to have that value (e.g., a value in the 98th percentile means that only 2% of the reference population should have values above that level; a value in the 5th percentile means that 95% of the reference population should have values above that level). Another example is establishment of "decision levels" ("action levels"), which are empirical cutoff values beyond which some type of physician action is suggested. These values are based primarily on the particular disease or clinical condition entering the differential diagnosis of results from a particular test. For example, an aspartate aminotransferase (AST, formerly SGOT) level 20 times the upper normal limit strongly suggests acute hepatitis virus hepatitis, so that value (20 times upper limit) represents a decision level for additional workup or other action based on the strong degree of suspicion for hepatitis virus hepatitis. A blood urea nitrogen value more than 50% below the lower limit of normal range might be a decision level for possible severe liver disease and so on. Decision levels may also be established to exclude a disease. The physician action in that case would be to eliminate the disease from consideration.

BIBLIOGRAPHY

Butts WC, Lilje DJ: Clinical significant reference intervals. *Am J Med Technol* 1982; 48:587.

Massod MF: Nonparametric percentile estimate of clinical normal ranges. *Am J Med Technol* 1977; 43:243.

CHAPTER 3. FACTOR DEFICIENCY ANEMIA

Formiminoglutamic Acid and Methylmalonic Acid.—Formiminoglutamic acid (FIGLU) is a compound that is derived from the amino acid histidine and requires active folic acid (tetrahydrofolic acid) for normal metabolism to glutamic acid. In significant folic acid deficiency, FIGLU cannot be properly utilized and is excreted into the urine in abnormal quantities. Vitamin B12 deficiency also influences FIGLU metabolism to some extent, because B12 is necessary for the conversion of folic acid to metabolically active tetrahydrofolic acid. Urine assay for FIGLU has proved rather difficult, and several techniques are available. Some of these have poor sensitivity, others are not sufficiently specific, and others are technically difficult. To circumvent some of the problems of sensitivity and specificity, a loading dose of oral histidine (15 gm in three divided doses, given over 12 hours) with a 24-hour urine collection for FIGLU has proved helpful. Challenge with a loading dose of histidine augments FIGLU excretion in folic acid–deficient states. Excretion of FIGLU after histidine loading is reported to be a reasonably accurate parameter of folic acid deficiency. However, FIGLU measurement is not widely available. Histidine may produce a reticulocyte response in megaloblastic anemia. Collection of urine must be done using a container with acid as a preservative. Many diseases produce elevated FIGLU excretion, so false positive results are common. Treatment of megaloblastic anemia returns FIGLU levels to normal.

Methylmalonic acid (MMA) excretion has been proposed as a specific test for vitamin B12 deficiency. However, the assay is difficult and not always reliable. Patients with mild serum B12 decrease and mild megaloblastosis may still have normal MMA values, and some patients with folic acid deficiency anemia are reported to have elevated urine MMA levels because of coexisting B12 deficiency. Treatment of B12 deficiency restores MMA levels to normal.

With the availability of serum B12 and folic acid assays, there seems little use for routine FIGLU or MMA determination.

The Therapeutic Trial.—In deficiency diseases, treatment with the specific agent that is lacking will result in a characteristic response in certain laboratory tests. This response may be used as a confirmation of the original diagnosis. Failure to obtain the expected response casts doubt on the original diagnosis; suggests that treatment has been inadequate in dosage, absorption, utilization, or type of agent used; or suggests that some other condition is present that is interfering with treatment or possibly is superimposed on the more obvious deficiency problem. The two usual deficiency diseases are chronic iron deficiency and vitamin B12 or folic acid deficiency. When a test agent such as iron is given in a therapeutic dose, a reticulocyte response should be manifested in 3–7 days, with values at least twice normal (or significantly elevated over baseline values if the baseline is already elevated). Usually, the reticulocyte count is normal or only slightly elevated in uncomplicated hematologic deficiency diseases. If the baseline reticulocyte values are already significantly elevated over normal range in a suspected deficiency disease, this suggests either previous treatment (or, in some cases, a response to hospital diet), wrong diagnosis, or some other superimposed factor (e.g., recent acute blood loss superimposed on chronic iron deficiency anemia). If the baseline values are already more than twice normal, it may not be possible to document a response. Once the correct replacement substance is given in adequate dosage, hemoglobin values usually rise toward normal at a rate of approximately 1 gm/100 ml/week.

Two major cautions must be made regarding the therapeutic trial: (1) it never takes the place of a careful, systematic search for the etiology of a suspected deficiency state, and (2) the patient may respond to one agent and at the same time have another factor deficiency or more serious underlying disease.

A therapeutic trial usually is initiated with therapeutic doses of the test agent. This standard procedure does not differentiate vitamin B12 deficiency from folic acid deficiency, since therapeutic doses of either will evoke a reticulocyte response in cases of deficiency due to the other. If a therapeutic trial is desired in these circumstances, a small physiologic dose should be used, such as 1 μg of vitamin B12/day for 10 days, or 100 μg of folic acid/day for 10 days. At least 10 days should elapse between completion of one trial agent and beginning of another. Also, the patient should be on a diet deficient in folic acid or B12, and baseline reticulocyte studies should be performed for 1 week with the patient on this diet before initiation of the actual trial. Generally, in vitamin B12 deficiency, the Schilling test (without intrinsic factor) gives the same information and can be repeated with the addition of intrinsic factor to pinpoint the etiology. In folic acid deficiency, a therapeutic trial may be helpful in establishing the diagnosis. The main drawback to using the therapeutic trial in diagnosis is the time involved.

Assay for Intrinsic Factor and for Antibody to Intrinsic Factor.—In vitro techniques have been described for assay of these substances. For assay of intrinsic factor, aspiration of gastric juice is necessary. The specimens from routine gastric analysis are satisfactory. Antibody to intrinsic factor is said to be present in the serum of 50%–75% of patients with pernicious anemia. Actually, two different antibodies have been found. Type I is a blocking antibody that prevents binding of B12 to intrinsic factor. This is the antibody usually present in pernicious anemia patients. The type II antibody is a binding-type antibody that binds to intrinsic factor or to the intrinsic factor–vitamin B12 complex. This antibody is uncommon in serum from patients with pernicious anemia. Presence of the type I antibody is considered by some to be almost diagnostic of pernicious anemia. However, presently available kits have been reported to give false positive results when serum B12 levels are very high (most commonly, within 24 hours after a B12 dose injection. One institution obtained false results as long as 1 week). False positive results have also been reported in a small number of patients with diabetes mellitus, adrenal insufficiency, thyroid diseases, and various gastric abnormalities. The test is available at present only in some medical centers and a few large reference laboratories. More work should be done with commercial kits to ascertain their level of performance and what false results can be expected. Intrinsic factor antibody assay, if positive, may be useful to help confirm a diagnosis of pernicious anemia in equivocal cases.

Neutrophil Hypersegmentation.—Hypersegmentation is defined as a segmented neutrophil with 5 or more lobes. An elevated neutrophil lobe count (defined as 5 or more lobes in more than 5% of all neutrophils) is reported to be more sensitive and reliable than elevated MCV or peripheral smear macrocytosis in detecting megaloblastic anemia, and also is not affected by coexisting iron deficiency.

BIBLIOGRAPHY

Bates HM: Pernicious anemia: The IF blocking antibody assay. *Lab Mgmt* 1982; 20(9):17.

Herbert V: The nutritional anemias. *Hosp Pract* 1980; 15:65.

Chanerin I: *The Megaloblastic Anaemias*, ed 2. Boston, Blackwell Scientific Publications, 1980.

CHAPTER 7. LEUKEMIA, LYMPHOMAS, AND MYELOPROLIFERATIVE SYNDROMES

Vitamin B12 and Unsaturated Vitamin B12–Binding Capacity.—Serum vitamin B12 levels are increased above reference range in about 40% of patients with polycythemia vera, about 7% of normal persons, about 10% of patients with relative or secondary polycythemia, and about 66% of patients with myeloid metaplasia.

Unsaturated vitamin B12–binding capacity (UBBC) tends to increase roughly in proportion to white blood cell (WBC) mass. Thus, various conditions that produce significantly increased WBC counts may be associated with increased UBBC values. The UBBC is elevated in up to 85% of patients with untreated polycythemia vera. More important, about one third of polycythemia vera patients with WBC counts less than 12,000/cu mm have an increased UBBC. However, about 4% of normal persons and 13% of patients with relative or secondary polycythemia also are reported to have elevated UBBC values. In addition, more than 50% of patients with myeloproliferative diseases other than polycythemia vera (e.g., myeloid metaplasia) have an elevated UBBC. The greatest increases in UBBC tend to occur in conditions with higher WBC counts, such as chronic myelogenous leukemia.

Classification of Non-Hodgkin's Lymphoma.—Although the Rappaport classification is currently the one most widely used in the United States, several others have been proposed. These include the classification of Lukes and Collins, the Palo Alto Expert Panel (both discussed in chapter 7), Dorfman's, the classification of a British pathology group (Bennett and colleagues), and the Kiel classification (Lennert, Gerard-Marchant, and colleagues). Although certain categories in each format roughly correspond to categories in the Rappaport system, exact correlation does not seem possible, and in some instances it is difficult to determine precisely what morphologic criteria are being used to classify groups and subgroups.

Chromosome Analysis in Leukemia.—Chromosome analysis may be helpful in certain situations involving leukemia. Material from the long arm of chromosome 9 that is translocated to the long arm of chromosome 22 is the Philadelphia chromosome abnormality of chronic granulocytic leukemia discussed in chapter 7. Translocation of material from the long arm of chromosome 4 to the long arm of chromosome 11 is said to be specific for acute heterogenous lymphoblastic leukemia (FAB L2). Translocation of material from the long arm of chromosome 8 to the long arm of chromosome 21 is said to be specific for acute myelocytic leukemia with differentiation (FAB M2); however, only a relatively small number of cases have this chromosome marker. Translocation of material from the long arm of chromosome 15 to the long arm of chromosome 17 is found in 40%–50% of patients with acute promyelocytic leukemia (FAB M3), both in the heavy granular and the microgranular variants. An inversion in the long arm of chromosome 16 is said to be specific for acute myelomonocytic leukemia (FAB M4). Deletion of the long arm of chromosome 5 (5q-) is commonly associated with the myelodysplastic syndromes, where it occurs in about 65% of refractory anemia and in about 35% of refractory anemia with excess blasts. It can also be found in 15%–40% of patients with acute nonlymphocytic leukemia, occurring in varying percentages of all the acute nonlymphocytic leukemia FAB subtypes except FAB 3 and 7.

There is some evidence that if chromosome abnormalities are found in a patient with bone marrow findings compatible with the myelodysplastic syndromes, the patient is more likely to develop leukemia.

BIBLIOGRAPHY

Koeffler HP: Syndromes of acute nonlymphocytic leukemia. *Ann Intern Med* 1987; 107:748.

Bunn HF: 5q- and disordered haematopoiesis. *Clin Haematol* 1986; 15:1023.

Bennett MH, et al.: Classification of non-Hodgkin's lymphomas. *Lancet* 1974; 2:405.

Carmel R: Vitamin B12-binding proteins in serum and plasma in various disorders. *Am J Clin Pathol* 1978; 69:319.

Dorfman RF: Classification of non-Hodgkin's lymphomas. *Lancet* 1974; 1:1295.

Gerard-Marchant R, et al: Classification of non-Hodgkin's lymphomas. *Lancet* 1974; 2:406.

CHAPTER 8. BLOOD COAGULATION

Thromboplastin Generation Time.—Thromboplastin generation time (TGT) is the basic reference test for pinpointing defects of intrinsic pathway factors and can be used to assay the degree of defect. This procedure tests the ability of the patient to generate adequate prothrombin activation through the intrinsic system pathway. If the patient's platelets are used in the TGT instead of a platelet substitute, the test then provides a sensitive assay system for defects in platelet number or function. The TGT is quite complicated and time-consuming and demands an expert technologist with strict attention to a considerable number of technical details to provide reliable results. Therefore, only a relatively few research laboratories perform the test. The TGT is extremely sensitive to intrinsic system factor deficiency, detecting abnormality when 30% or less of the factor in question is present. The TGT can also pinpoint which factor of the intrinsic system is deficient. Prothrombin and fibrinogen/fibrin abnormalities can be found but are more easily detected by other tests.

Tests for Fibrinolysin.—The following tests are in limited use and merit some attention.

Clot Lysis Test.—The clot lysis test is a simple, moderately sensitive, and reliable test for circulating fibrinolysins. Normally a blood clot retracts and forms a solid, firm, hard mass. Circulating fibrinolysin in sufficient quantity attacks and dissolves the clot. This is different from the clot retraction defect of thrombocytopenia, in which the clot forms and simply does not retract well but does not dissolve. In mild cases of circulating fibrinolysins, the patient's own blood will clot, followed by clot lysis. However, if the fibrinolysin is potent, fibrinogen may be inactivated and the blood will not clot. In these cases, plasma fibrinogen level determinations will show a falsely low level, as previously noted. The clot lysis test should then be done by adding the patient's plasma to a fresh blood clot from a normal person. The euglobulin lysis test, a variation of the clot lysis procedure, is considered more sensitive and accurate. However, it is not widely available. The clot lysis test is no longer widely used because of the length of time needed to obtain results.

Ethanol Gelation.—It is postulated that certain concentrations of ethyl alcohol allow breakup of abnormal complexes formed by fibrinogen and fibrin monomer, with subsequent gel formation by the fibrin monomer. With certain modifications, the procedure has been praised in some reports, but the majority of investigators currently believe that it is not adequately sensitive.

Screening Test for Fletcher Factor.—One report indicates that Fletcher factor deficiency increased the activated partial thromboplastin (PT) time (APTT) when kaolin (but not ellagic acid) was used as the activator and 3 minutes was the duration of activation permitted, whereas the kaolin APTT became normal when duration of activation was increased to 10 minutes. Some patients had mild rather than marked prolongation of the 3-minute APTT, and some of these were found to have partial Fletcher factor deficiency. More data are needed.

Tests for Heparin Therapy Monitoring.—***Whole Blood Recalcification Time.***—Whole blood is drawn into a tube with citrate anticoagulant. Calcium chloride is added to an aliquot of the whole blood to begin the clotting process. The reference range upper limit for clotting is about 2 minutes at 37°C or 5 minutes at room temperature. Test results are said to be adequately reproducible. The whole blood recalcification time (WBRT) is used primarily to monitor heparin therapy. Its advantage is that whole blood clotting may be a more truthful representation of the varied effects of heparin than tests that circumvent part of the normal clotting process. Only one very cheap reagent is needed. The WBRT is sensitive to platelet variations and is more linear than the APTT at greater heparin effects. The major disadvantage is that the test cannot be automated. One report states that the test must be performed within 1 hour after venipuncture.

Whole Blood Activated Recalcification Time.—This test is similar to the WBRT except that a contact factor activator is added to the anticoagulant tube. The reference range upper limit is about 90 seconds. The test is said to be linear at all heparin concentrations. Platelets will affect results. The test can be automated.

Whole Blood Activated Partial Thromboplastin Time.—Two milliliters of nonanticoagulated whole blood is added to an APTT reagent at the bedside. The tube is tilted every 15 seconds at room temperature until a clot begins. The reference range upper limit is about 2.5 minutes. The test is said to have a good correlation with the Lee-White clotting time in all ranges of heparin effect and to be more sensitive to heparin than the APTT.

Plasma Recalcification Time.—Anticoagulated blood is obtained, the specimen is centrifuged at low speed to obtain platelet-rich plasma, and calcium is added to an aliquot of the plasma to begin the clotting process. The reference range upper limit is approximately 130 seconds. The test is used to monitor heparin therapy and yields results similar to those of whole blood recalcification methods. Values are reasonably linear at higher concentrations of heparin. Platelets affect the results when platelet-rich plasma is used.

Thrombin Time.—One aliquot of diluted thrombin is added to 1 aliquot of patient plasma. Clotting time upper limit is approximately 20 seconds. The test is simple and said to be very sensitive to heparin effect. It is not affected by sodium warfarin (Coumadin). As originally performed, the method was nonlinear and, like the APTT, was greatly prolonged in higher degrees of heparin effect. Certain modifications may have partially corrected this problem. Reagent source and composition may affect results considerably.

Hexadimethrine Bromide Neutralization Test.—Hexadimethrine bromide (Polybrene), like protamine, is a substance that neutralizes heparin. The test entails adding thrombin to aliquots of patient platelet-rich plasma, then adding increasing concentrations of hexadimethrine bromide. The hexadimethrine bromide concentration that neutralizes the heparin present (indicated by clot formation) can be related to heparin concentration by a standard curve. A major advantage is freedom from interference by sodium warfarin.

Tests for Monitoring Sodium Warfarin Therapy.—***Thrombotest (Owren).***—This test uses a special thromboplastin reagent designed to measure factor IX in addition to factors that affect the Quick one-stage PT test (prothrombin, VII and X). However, there is controversy as to whether the thrombotest responds adequately to severe factor IX deficiency, since it has been reported that factor IX must be reduced below 10% of normal to affect the test. In a significant minority of patients the results are below the recommended therapeutic range of 25% of normal (corresponding to a PT of about 1.5 times normal) when the PT is within therapeutic range.

P&P Test (Ware and Stragnell Modification).—The name relates to early experiments indicating that the test measured only prothrombin and proconvertin (factor VII). Actually, the procedure is similar to the PT test except that patient plasma is diluted 1:10 and extra factor V and fibrinogen are added. The main advantage is said to be increased sensitivity to changes in factor VII. However, increased sensitivity may lead to more fluctuation in test values, and the sodium warfarin dose may have to be adjusted more often.

Thrombocytosis.—Most attention given to blood platelets is focused on disorders of platelet function or decreased platelet number. However, thrombocytosis may sometimes occur. If the platelet count is greater than 900,000 or 1,000,000/cu mm, there is concern for the possibility of hypercoagulability leading to venous thrombosis. In one report, about 25% of patients with thrombocytosis (platelet count > 900,000/cu mm) had a hematologic disorder (myeloproliferative syndrome, idiopathic thrombocythemia, severe hemolytic anemia, posthemorrhage, etc.), about 25% had cancer, about 20% were postsplenectomy, about 20% had acute or chronic inflammatory conditions, and about 10% had collagen disease.

Mean Platelet Volume.—Certain automatic particle counters that count platelets also calculate the mean platelet volume (MPV). The reference range apparently varies inversely with the platelet count, unless a wide reference range is established to include all patients with platelet counts within the platelet count reference range. The MPV is said to be increased in immune thrombocytopenic purpura (which could in part be due to the thrombocytopenia) and is decreased in some patients with acute leukemia or hypersplenism. Occasionally, RBC fragments may be counted as platelets producing artifactual increase in the platelet count. However, MPV is also increased in these patients.

BIBLIOGRAPHY

Baden JP: The precise management of heparin therapy. *Am J Surg* 1972; 124:777.

Belko JS, Warren R: The recalcification time of blood. *Arch Surg* 1958; 76:210.

Bessman JD, et al: The inverse relation of platelet size and count in normal subjects, and an artifact of other particles. *Am J Clin Pathol* 1981; 76:289.

Jones MJ, Pierre RV: The clinician's heed to platelet counts is evaluated. *Am Fam Phys* 1981; 23:198.

CHAPTER 12. URINALYSIS

Red Blood Cell Casts in Diabetic Nephropathy.—Diabetic glomerulosclerosis typically does not produce hematuria; and if hematuria occurs, RBC casts are not present. Hematuria and RBC casts are usually ascribed to another superimposed disease. However, one report detected hematuria in 30% of diabetic nephropathy patients and RBC casts in 13%. Of those with RBC casts, about 40% had diabetic changes plus some type of superimposed glomerulitis on renal biopsy, but nearly 60% had no changes other than diabetic nephropathy.

Laboratory Evaluation of Urinary Tract Calculi.—Laboratory evaluation consists of (1) stone universal analysis, and (2) investigation of stone-formation etiology. Stone mineral analysis is performed by x-ray diffraction, infrared spectroscopy, optical crystallography (polarization microscopy), or some combination of these techniques. Standard chemical analysis of crushed stone material is no longer recommended, due to fragment inaccuracies, interferences, lack of sensitivity, and problems with sufficient specimen if the stone is small. There is no universally accepted standard workup protocol to investigate pathogenesis. However, the majority of investigators require both a 24-hour urine specimen and a fasting serum specimen obtained on the same day, on three separate occasions. The urine specimen should be kept on ice or in the refrigerator during collection. In the laboratory, the specimen is preserved in the refrigerator if necessary tests are performed in house; if the specimen is sent to an outside laboratory, appropriate preservatives should be added. The patient is usually on his/her regular diet (at least initially). The substances measured vary somewhat among investigators, but measurements most often include calcium, phosphate, uric acid, oxalate, urine pH, and urine volumes. Citrate and cystine are also frequently assayed.

Representative reference ranges (24-hour urine) are as follows: calcium, <250 mg (6.24 mmol)/day on normal diet and <150 mg/(6.24 mmol)/day on low-calcium diet; uric acid, 250–800 mg (1.49–4.76 mmol)/day on normal diet and <600 mg (3.57 mmol)/day on low-purine diet; phosphate, 400–1,300 mg (12.9–42 mmol)/day; and oxalate, 10–40 mg (0.11–0.44 mmol)/day.

BIBLIOGRAPHY

Coe FL, Parks JH: Pathophysiology of kidney stones and strategies for treatment. *Hosp Pract* 1988; 23(3):815.

Nicar MJ, et al: The preservation of urine samples for determination of renal stone risk factors. *Lab Med* 1987; 18:382.

Mandel N: Urinary tract calculi. *Lab Med* 1986; 17:449.

Blath RA: Renal calculi. *Consultant* 1984; 24(11):54.

O'Neill WM, et al: Hematuria and red cell casts in typical diabetic nephropathy. *Am J Med* 1983; 74:389.

CHAPTER 13. RENAL FUNCTION TESTS

Phenolsulfonphthalein Excretion Test.— More than 85% of phenolsulfonphthalein (PSP) is actively excreted by the renal proximal tubular epithelium, less than 5% is filtered at the glomerulus, and the remainder is excreted by the liver. Thus, PSP excretion is a measure of one tubular "function" and indirectly of tubular health. A measured dose of PSP is given intravenously, and urine specimens are obtained 15, 60, and 120 minutes after injection. The specimens are analyzed for PSP content. The 15-minute measurement provides the most information. It is very important to hydrate the patient beforehand and to have some urine in the bladder when dye is injected. This volume of urine is not a factor in the results but helps to recover all the excreted dye. Also essential are accurately timed specimen collection and care taken to ensure complete bladder emptying at the collection periods, even if catheterization is necessary (however, catheterization for this test alone is not justified clinically because of the risk of introducing infection). Normal values are 25% or greater excretion at 15 minutes, 40%–60% at 1 hour, and 60%–80% at 2 hours. The importance of the 15-minute specimen lies in the fact that relatively early or mild bilateral renal disease may decrease function enough to influence the early collection specimen, whereas the later specimens may still fall within the normal range, since they represent an additive or cumulative effect over the longer time intervals.

The PSP gives similar information to clearance procedures over much of the same renal function area. It is not quite as dependent on renal blood flow, although this is a factor; also, it takes a total of 2 hours, during which most patients can hold their urine. Disadvantages are that the patient is not always able to void accurately for the 15-minute specimen, which is often the most important value, or even for the other specimens. A certain constant percentage of the PSP dye is excreted into the urine on each cycle of blood flow to the kidney. Therefore, the 15-minute value may be low, although over a prolonged period the total values for 2 hours when added together may be almost within normal range, as noted previously. However, when kidney function is moderately to considerably decreased, the 2-hour value also starts falling. Obviously, it is necessary to be sure that the urine collection is complete so that all the PSP dye is recovered. If the patient has significant residual urine, the results may be falsely low.

In the usual case of chronic diffuse bilateral renal disease, the first demonstrable abnormality is impairment of the concentration test. As the disease progresses, the creatinine clearance and 15-minute PSP value start to become reduced. Then the specific gravity becomes fixed, and the creatinine clearance, followed by the 2-hour PSP value, shows considerable decrease. Finally, results of both of these tests show a marked decrease and the BUN starts to rise, followed shortly by the serum creatinine value (Fig 35–1).

Beta-2 Microglobulin Assay.—This test is discussed in chapter 16. Beta-2 microglobulin (B2M) has been used to estimate glomerular filtration rate (GFR). In addition, if the measured GFR is normal and the urine B2M level is elevated, this suggests inability of the renal tubules to metabolize B2M, and this, in turn, suggests damage localized to the renal tubules. However, in chronic azotemia (serum creatinine values > 4 mg/100 ml), urine B2M excretion no longer differentiates primary tubule disease from glomerular disease. Also, there is disagreement about the reliability of B2M urinary measurement in differentiating glomerular from tubular injury.

Tests Used to Differentiate Prerenal Azotemia From Acute Tubular Necrosis.—The selection of tests listed here rather than discussed in the main text is arbitrary, based on my experience as well as reports in the literature. The reference values used are composites from the literature, designed to provide reasonably good differentiation between prerenal azotemia (PRA) and acute tubular necrosis (ATN) in most instances. However, this leaves a considerable number of cases in the overlap zone between the cutoff points for PRA and ATN.

Although some of the older indices contain the word plasma, serum is used today instead of plasma.

1. Urine osmolality
   PRA = More than 600 mOsm
2. Urine to plasma osmolality ratio
   PRA = Greater than 2
   ATN = Less than 1.2
   $$\frac{\text{Urine (mOsm)}}{\text{Plasma (mOsm)}}$$
3. Urine to plasma urea ratio
   PRA = Greater than 10
   ATN = Less than 10
   $$\frac{\text{Urine urea}}{\text{Plasma urea}}$$
4. Urine to plasma creatinine ratio
   PRA = Over 40
   ATN = Less than 10
   $$\frac{\text{Urine creatinine}}{\text{Plasma creatinine}}$$
5. BUN to plasma creatinine ratio*
   PRA = Over 10
   ATN = Under 10
   $$\frac{\text{BUN}}{\text{Plasma creatinine}}$$
6. Renal failure index
   PRA = Less than 1
   ATN = Greater than 2
   $$\frac{\text{Urine sodium}}{\text{Urine creatinine/Plasma creatinine}}$$
7. Fractional excretion of sodium (FE_{Na})
   PRA = Less than 1
   ATN = More than 3
   $$\frac{\text{Urine sodium/Serum sodium}}{\text{Urine creatinine/Serum creatinine}}$$
8. Free water clearance
   Free water clearance (ml/hr) = Urine volume (ml/hr) − Osmolar clearance/hr.
   $$\text{Osmolar clearance/hr} = \frac{\text{Urine osmolality} \times \text{Urine volume (ml/hr)}}{\text{Serum osmolality}}$$
   PRA = −20 to −100
   ATN = −10 to positive (+) number
9. Urine sodium excretion
   PRA = Less than 15 mEq/L

*The BUN/PCR ratio is also elevated in postrenal urinary tract obstruction and in gastrointestinal tract bleeding. The ratio may be decreased in pregnancy, during low-calorie diets, and after renal dialysis.

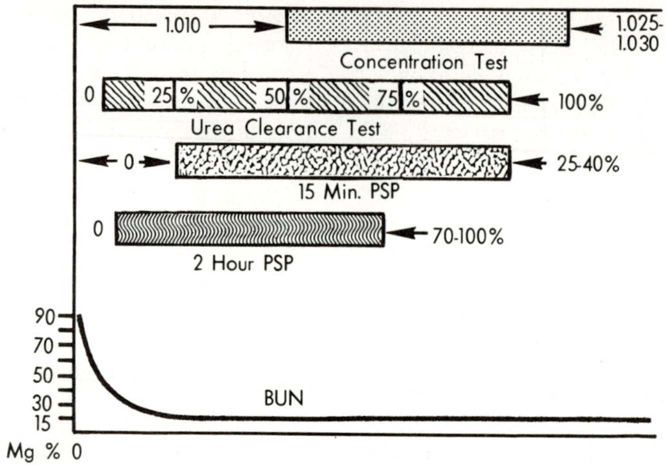

FIG 35–1.
Comparison of renal function tests in chronic diffuse bilateral renal disease.

BIBLIOGRAPHY

Brown R, et al: Renal function in critically ill postoperative patients: Sequential assessment of creatinine, osmolar, and free water clearance. *Crit Care Med* 1980; 8:68.

Crowe LR, Hatch FE: Evaluating renal function. *Postgrad Med* 1977; 62:58.

Miller TR, et al: Urinary diagnostic indices in acute renal failure. *Ann Intern Med* 1978; 89:47.

Oken DE: On the differential diagnosis of acute renal failure. *Am J Med* 1981; 71:916.

Schrier RW: Acute renal failure: Pathogenesis, diagnosis, and management. *Hosp Pract* 1981; 16:93.

Vacca CV: A simple diagnostic test of renal disease. *Am J Clin Pathol* 1974; 62:134.

CHAPTER 14. BACTERIAL INFECTIOUS DISEASES

Hemolytic Reactions of Bacteria on Blood Agar.—These hemolytic reactions may be altered by the type of blood used. Alpha streptococci produce green alpha hemolysis on human blood or sheep blood agar but not on rabbit blood. *Haemophilus* species do not grow well on sheep blood agar.

The type of agar base and other conditions of culture technique can also influence hemolysis in group A streptococci. Failure to incubate isolation plates under reduced oxygen tension (carbon dioxide [CO_2] atmosphere or stab technique) may result in failure to produce recognizable beta hemolysis.

Counterimmunoelectrophoresis.—The counterimmunoelectrophoresis (CIE) technique has been applied to the diagnosis of infectious disease through detection of specific bacterial antigens. It entails placing an antibody specific against a certain antigen into a small circular hole cut into agar and applying the substance to be tested (cerebrospinal fluid [CSF], serum, urine, etc.) into a second hole nearby. The agar is then submitted to electrophoresis in such a way as to force the contents of the two wells toward each other. If specific antigen to the antibody is present, a visible precipitin line will result when antigen and antibody meet. The method is relatively easy to perform and takes less than 1 hour to complete. Thus far, the most widely used application is in the diagnosis of bacterial meningitis. Antibodies against the most common infectious agents (*Haemophilus influenzae*, meningococcus, pneumococcus, and *Streptococcus* B) are available. Detection rate is said to be about 85% (literature range, 60%–100%). Presently available antisera are more sensitive for *H. influenzae* and meningococcus than for pneumococcus. Other body fluids or even nonfluid material may be subjected to the same procedure, although results to date are less impressive than with CSF. The major technical difficulty has been variation in potency of commercial antisera. CIE is being replaced by latex agglutination methods, which are faster, easier, and equally as sensitive (discussed in the section on CSF).

Counterimmunoelectrophoresis has proved useful in the diagnosis of systemic *Candida* infection, although there has been some overlap between patient groups who are colonized by *Candida* and those with actual infection.

Antibody-Coated Bacteria Test.—One of the problems encountered in urinary tract infection is finding the exact location of the infection. Renal and prostatic infections require more prolonged and intensive therapy than does uncomplicated bladder infection. At present, the Fairly bladder washout test is the standard reference procedure. A Foley catheter is inserted, and the bladder is drained. The bladder is then washed with saline. Some protocols also use a proteolytic enzyme solution with antibiotics to eliminate any material coating the bladder mucosa. Then a diuretic (furosemide) is administered, and urine specimens are obtained from the catheter for culture 10, 20, and 30 minutes later. A bladder infection should demonstrate no appreciable rise in specimen colony count, whereas an upper urinary tract infection places infected urine into the bladder and results in considerable increase in colony counts soon after irrigation and drainage. Recently it was found that bacteria in urine from kidney and prostate infections usually become coated with antibody by the time they reach the bladder. A simple direct immunofluorescence procedure using one drop of centrifuged urine sediment dried on a slide to which some fluorescein-tagged antihuman globulin antiserum is added can visualize those bacteria that are coated with antibody.

There have been several highly favorable reports regarding sensitivity and accuracy. However, other reports have not been enthusiastic. Detection rate of upper urinary tract infection is about 85% (literature range, 54%–100%), and the false positive rate (positive test result in bladder infection) is about 25% (0%–50%).

***Streptococcus* MG.**—This is a test for the *Mycoplasma*-induced antibodies of primary atypical pneumonia. The test is based on the unusual reactivity of these antibodies for material from this strain of the streptococcal organism. Most investigators believe the test is not as sensitive as cold agglutinins. It gives positive results in less than 40% of cases, although reports range from 10%–80%.

BIBLIOGRAPHY

Pifer LL: Rapid assays for pediatric infectious disease. *Lab Mgmt* 1983; 21(2):35.

Matuscak RR, Albert AC: Detection of antibody-coated bacteria in urine sediments: A review. *Am J Med Technol* 1982; 48:191.

Bates HM: The ACB test in urinary tract infection. *Lab Mgmt* 1982; 20(5):17.

Montplaiser S, et al: Limitations of the direct immunofluorescence test for antibody-coated bacteria in determining the site of urinary tract infection in children. *Can Med Assoc J* 1981; 125:993.

Hellerstein S, et al: Urinary tract infection localization in women. *JAMA* 1979; 241:789.

Kaplan SL, Feigin RD: Rapid identification of the invading microorganism. *Pediatr Clin North Am* 1980; 27:783.

Rytel MW: Counterimmunoelectrophoresis: A diagnostic adjunct in clinical microbiology. *Lab Med* 1980; 11:655.

Kozinin PJ, et al: The precipitin test in systemic candidiasis. *JAMA* 1976; 235:628.

Purcell RH, Chanock RM: Role of mycoplasmas in human respiratory disease. *Med Clin North Am* 1967; 51:791.

CHAPTER 16. VIRAL AND RICKETTSIAL INFECTIOUS DISEASES

Diagnosis of Rubella Infection.—In chapter 16, diagnosis of rubella by means of serologic tests was discussed. Since there appears to be confusion regarding test use and interpretation in various clinical situations, I have chosen to repeat this information here, using a different format. Part of the confusion is caused by tests that detect both IgM and IgG antibodies against rubella but do not differentiate between them. Frequently, this is not made clear to the physician. In rubella testing, a test that detects both IgM and IgG together is used and interpreted as though it detected only IgG. Also, some procedures are reported as a titer and some as positive or negative for rubella antibody. Specific tests for rubella IgM and IgG antibodies are available in medical centers and large reference laboratories. Interpretation of these tests may be summarized as follows:

1. If a serum specimen is obtained 7 days or less after exposure (before a rash develops):
   a. A significantly elevated rubella IgM titer means acute rubella infection.
   b. If the rubella IgM result is negative, a new specimen would have to be obtained 2–3 weeks later. If results are still negative, this rules out acute primary rubella infection.
   c. If IgM tests are not available, an IgG test can be done and a second specimen must be obtained 2–3 weeks later. A fourfold increase in titer confirms acute rubella. If the initial specimen was nonreactive, a fourfold increase in titer means acute primary rubella infection. If the first specimen had detectable titer, a fourfold increase in titer could mean either acute primary rubella or (less frequently) acute stage of rubella reinfection. A stable (nonrising) titer indicates previous infection at some undetermined time.
2. If the serum specimen is obtained after development of a rash or other symptoms of possible rubella:
   a. A significantly elevated rubella IgM titer means acute primary rubella infection.
   b. If the rubella IgM test result is negative, a new specimen would have to be obtained 2–3 weeks later. If the result is still negative, this rules out acute rubella infection.
   c. If IgM tests are not available, an IgG test can be done. Whether or not the IgG test shows a significantly elevated titer, another specimen must be obtained 2–3 weeks later. A rising titer means either acute primary rubella or (less frequently) acute stage of rubella reinfection. A stable (nonrising) titer could mean either infection at some previous time or an acute infection in which the first specimen was drawn after the peak titer was reached (too late to detect a fourfold rising titer). Only an IgM test on the first specimen (and, if the findings of the first specimen were negative, on the second specimen also) could resolve this problem. However, if the first specimen were obtained more than 3 weeks after appearance of the rash, the IgM titer could have fallen to nondetectable levels. If both the original and the repeat IgG test results are negative, this indicates no rubella infection. If the first IgG specimen was obtained 4 weeks or more after onset of the rash and the result is negative, this indicates no acute infection and a second specimen is not necessary.

There are four major difficulties with interpretation of rubella data:

1. Laboratory variation or error. Both the acute and the convalescent sera should be tested at the same time to minimize technical variation.

2. If only a single specimen is obtained, it may be obtained too early for IgM or IgG antibodies to appear. A single specimen is useful only if IgM antibodies are present (signifying acute primary rubella infection) or if the only question is whether or not the patient is immune to a future rubella infection (in which case a significantly elevated titer of rubella antibodies means past or current infection and therefore immunity to future infection).

3. The initial IgM specimen may be obtained too late, when the IgM titer has already returned to nondetectable levels; or the initial IgG specimen may be obtained too late, when the IgG titer has already reached its peak (possibly simulating old infection).

4. Reinfection may further elevate a preexisting elevated IgG titer, simulating the fourfold rising titer of a first infection. However, the IgM titer does not become elevated. Reinfection by rubella is not thought to produce clinical symptoms, infect other people, or injure the fetus.

Parvovirus B19.—Parvovirus B19 belongs to a genus that infects both animals and man. These are small viruses without an outer envelope. Replication appears to take place in erythroid precursors of the bone marrow. The two most common diseases produced are erythema infectiosum ("fifth disease"), a condition somewhat resembling rubella, but with a rash that has a somewhat different body distribution; and transient aplastic crises. Both are more frequent in children. In both conditions, the incubation period is about 5–15 days, but may be as long as 20 days. In both conditions there may be a viral-type prodrome with fever, malaise, and other symptoms. Most patients with aplastic crises due to B19 already have some type of hemolytic anemia, either congenital or acquired. It is thought that B19 infection is responsible for 90% of aplastic crises in these patients.

Tests for Non-A, Non-B Hepatitis.—Recent reports indicate that a commercial company has succeeded in cloning certain protein sequences from non-A, non-B hepatitis virus obtained from serum of infected patients. An immunoassay based on these antigens that detects antibody response has been developed and is being tested.

Transfusion-Acquired Neonatal Cytomegalovirus Infection.—One report reviewed several studies that showed considerably less infection rate, morbidity, and mortality than studies reported previously (i.e., infection rates of 0.8%–8.7% compared to previously reported infection rates of 10%–30%).

Skin Biopsy With Immunofluorescence for Diagnosis of Rocky Mountain Spotted Fever.—A punch biopsy specimen of a skin rash area is obtained, prepared by frozen section, and stained with immunofluorescent antibody against *Rickettsia*. The technique can provide a diagnosis the same day, and results may be positive as early as the fourth day of illness. However, in one study only about one half of the patients had positive results. Antibiotic therapy reduces the number of rickettsiae in skin lesions, further reducing the sensitivity of the test. This test would be available in only a few medical centers or reference laboratories.

BIBLIOGRAPHY

Young C: Hepatitis non-A, non-B virus cloned. *Lab Mgmt* 1988; 26(7):8.

Preiksaitis JK, et al: Transfusion-acquired cytomegalovirus infection in neonates. *Transfusion* 1988; 28:205.

Anderson LJ; Role of parvovirus B19 in human disease. *Pediatr Infect Dis J* 1987; 6:711.

Hechemy KE, Michaelson EE: Rocky Mountain spotted fever: A resurgent problem. *Lab Mgmt* 1981; 4:29.

Oster CN: Early diagnosis of Rocky Mountain spotted fever. *Arch Intern Med* 1979; 134:400.

CHAPTER 18. CEREBROSPINAL FLUID EXAMINATION

Colloidal Gold Reaction.—In certain pathologic central nervous system conditions, a suspension of colloidal gold in sodium chloride is precipitated, giving characteristic color changes in standard dilutions. The color normally is wine red but may change to blue and even to a clear color, depending on the degree of precipitation. Each dilution tube is given a number from 0–5, depending on the degree of color change. There are 10 tubes, each with a different dilution, so results are reported as a series of 10 numbers.

A reading of 1 in all tubes is within normal limits. A reading of 2 is of doubtful significance, and to be significant, at least 1 of the 10 tubes must read 3 or over. According to classic theories, globulin tends to precipitate the gold particles in the solution, whereas albumin tends to "protect" the finely dispersed colloidal state. More recent work indicates that the gamma globulins have the strongest precipitating action, whereas most, but not all, of the protective function seems to be in the albumin and alpha globulins. When gamma globulin is increased without significant increases in albumin or alpha globulin, color changes are mostly in the lower dilution tubes, producing a "first-zone" curve (e.g., 5553211111). This pattern is characteristically found in syphilitic general paresis and in multiple sclerosis but not always in either. When both the albumin and the globulin values are increased in the same general proportions but only moderately, or when the gamma globulin value is only very slightly increased, a "second-zone" curve is produced in which the middle dilution tubes show precipitation and thus have color change (e.g., 1113321111). Theoretically, the albumin or alpha globulin was present in sufficient quantities to prevent precipitation in the first zone but was diluted out after the first few tubes. Due to the relatively mild gamma-globulin increase, this globulin also is supposed to be diluted out but not until the last tubes. A second-zone curve is classically found in tabes dorsalis; again, many other conditions occasionally produce a similar effect. In patients with high CSF total protein levels, the precipitating action of the gamma globulin may not appear until the last dilution tubes, by which time the albumin and alpha globulin are diluted enough to unmask the gamma globulin effect. This is called a "third-zone," or "end-zone," curve and classically is found in acute bacterial meningitis.

The colloidal gold curve, however, is not nearly as specific as one would gather from this simplified account, since, for example, acute bacterial meningitis can give any of three types of curves as well as no curve at all, and many other diseases can occasionally give one or the other type of curve. The classic pattern associated with multiple sclerosis is a "first-zone" curve; however, only about 25% of patients actually displayed a first-zone curve, whereas about 25% had a second-zone pattern. Therefore, fewer than 50% had an abnormal colloidal gold curve. The typical "multiple sclerosis pattern" was found in a distinct minority of cases, and the pattern is actually not specific, since it is also found in general paresis and occasionally in a variety of other disorders. Immunoglobulin quantitation by CSF electrophoresis or immunodiffusion, oligoclonal band testing, and other procedures are replacing the colloidal gold test.

CSF Oligoclonal Bands vs. Serum Bands.—Many investigators believe that CSF oligoclonal bands should not be interpreted without electrophoresis of the patient's serum to exclude possible serum bands. If serum also contains oligoclonal bands, only CSF bands not found in the serum would be considered a significant abnormality.

Radioisotope Studies in Various Central Nervous System Conditions.—Radioisotope studies include brain scan, cerebral blood flow study, and isotope cisternography. Scanning the brain is similar to scanning any other organ. An appropriate compound labeled with a radioactive isotope is injected. Later, a radioactivity counting device surveys ("scans") various areas of the brain, producing an overall pattern of radioactivity in those areas. A special device translates focal variations in cerebral radioactivity into a visual picture of light and dark areas.

The brain scan has become an important screening technique in certain brain disorders. Brain scanning originated with the observation that certain radioactive isotopes seemed to localize in brain tumors. It is not certain whether this phenomenon is due to focal alterations of cerebral vascular permeability (blood-brain barrier), to the increased vascularity of most tumors, or to both. In subsequent experience, it was shown that subdural hematomas and cerebral infarctions could also display increased isotope accumulation compared with normal brain tissue, so that brain scanning was useful for diagnosis of these conditions. Unfortunately, brain scanning cannot differentiate with certainty between tumor and cerebral infarct. Brain scanning is also helpful in diagnosis of brain abscess.

In brain tumors, best results are obtained with meningiomas and the higher-grade (more poorly differentiated) astrocytomas. Grade I astrocytomas, histologically very similar to normal cerebral tissue, often do not concentrate the isotopes enough to stand out from normal surrounding tissue. In addition, scanning with present-day equipment will miss the majority of tumors less than 2 cm, regardless of type. Posterior fossa tumors are difficult to detect and require special techniques. Pituitary tumors frequently are not detected because of high vascularity in surrounding structures. Scanning is less useful for spinal cord tumors. Despite these limitations, brain scanning is a good screening test for either primary or metastatic brain tumors, since it can be done with negligible risk on an outpatient basis. Accuracy in diagnosis is quoted as 80%–90%. Cerebral arteriography can have a similar success rate but requires a neuroradiologist for best results and is more complicated and dangerous to perform. If both cerebral arteriography and brain scanning are to be done, the brain scan should be performed first. Angiography causes cerebral vessel dilation and may produce a false positive brain scan. It is necessary to wait at least 48 hours after cerebral arteriography to do a brain scan.

Fewer than one half of patients with cerebral infarction have a positive brain scan if the scan is done before the end of the second week after cerebral damage occurs. In the second to fourth weeks after infarction, 75% or more of patients have abnormal scans. After 6 weeks, the abnormal findings often disappear. The optimal time for scanning to detect cerebral infarction is during the third week after onset of symptoms. Cerebral arteriography can detect lesions soon after damage occurs, but it carries a definite risk.

A helpful alternative to angiography is available to those institutions that possess a stationary radioactive imaging device, such as the Anger scintillation camera. Certain isotopes can be injected intravenously and followed through major arteries by means of rapid-sequence photography or magnetic tape playback. Results do not have the same degree of detail as x-ray angiography, but complete or nearly complete large-vessel occlusion can be visualized.

Cerebral isotope angiography ("flow study") of the carotid and major cerebral vessels is frequently abnormal in the early stage of a cerebral vascular accident or subdural hematoma, when brain scan is normal. Both of these lesions very often give a similar pattern; occasionally a subdural does have characteristic features. Arteriovenous malformations are frequently diagnosable.

Subdural hematoma is often a diagnostic problem. According to one study, 20% of patients did not have any history of head trauma, and 30% had no localizing neurologic signs. Textbook CSF findings of protein increase and xanthochromia were present in only 50% of subacute and chronic cases. In subdural hematoma, cerebral isotope dynamic flow study is a good screening procedure, although computerized tomography (CT) or arteriography is the procedure of choice for diagnosis in the first 2 weeks after onset. Brain scans most often do not become abnormal until after 2 weeks. It is thought that increased isotope pickup is not due to the hematoma itself but to the "membrane" that develops around the hematoma, consisting of highly vascular granulation tissue. Therefore, brain scanning is not very accurate for diagnosis of acute subdural hematoma but is very useful in detecting chronic subdural hematoma. The blood flow study increases accuracy in detection of the chronic form and, in addition, is more sensitive than the scan in acute subdural hematoma.

An abnormal scan must be interpreted with the aid of skull x-ray studies, since lesions of bone (e.g., as hyperostosis and Paget's disease) or scalp (hematoma or laceration) may concentrate the isotope.

Intracerebral abscess can be seen on brain scans in 80%–100% of cases. Although lesions may be detected soon after onset of symptoms, some believe that the sensitivity of the scan is increased after an additional several days. A gallium scan may improve detection in early or equivocal cases.

Brain scanning can aid the diagnosis and management of hydrocephalus. A small amount of special isotope-tagged material can be injected into the lumbar spinal fluid, and sequential scans can follow the distribution of this material throughout the cerebrospinal fluid (CSF) ("cisternogram"). This is especially valuable in patients with normal-pressure hydrocephalus (Hakim's syndrome). These are predominantly older patients with progressive dementia. The classic triad is dementia, incontinence, and lower extremity weakness. When cisternography reveals classic findings of lateral ventricle filling plus inability of CSF to reach the superior sagittal sinus by 48 hours, ventricular shunting frequently produces dramatic improvement.

In spite of the versatility and acceptable degree of accuracy of central nervous system (CNS) radionuclide studies, CT is replacing brain scanning in those institutions with access to a CT scanner. Computerized tomography, in general, provides better anatomical orientation and is about 10%–15% more sensitive for space-occupying lesions and subdural hematomas.

BIBLIOGRAPHY

Tate J: Campbell B: Must CSF oligoclonal bands be unique to cerebrospinal fluid and absent from serum to support the diagnosis of multiple sclerosis? *Clin Chem* 1988; 34:1521.

Prusiner SB: Prion disease and central nervous system degeneration. *Clin Res* 1987; 35:177.

CHAPTER 19. LIVER AND BILIARY TRACT TESTS

Ornithine Carbamyl Transferase.—The ornithine carbamyltransferase (OCT) enzyme is found mainly in liver and, to a much lesser extent, within intestinal mucosa. Since it takes extensive intestinal infarction to provoke significant OCT elevation, this enzyme is nearly specific for liver cell disease. It is even more sensitive than aspartate aminotransferase (AST formerly serum glutamate oxaloacetate transaminase) to hepatocellular injury and reportedly may be elevated in some cases without histologic cell changes.

Isocitric Dehydrogenase.—The isocitric dehydrogenase (ICD) enzyme behaves like the AST in liver disease. Although ICD is found in cardiac muscle and several tissues besides liver, it is not elevated in myocardial infarction (MI) and usually is abnormal only in liver disease.

Alkaline Phosphatase Isoenzymes.—Alkaline phosphatase can be separated into single enzymes that are relatively specific for bone, liver, placenta, and intestine. The easiest method is heat fractionation; bone isoenzyme is heat inactivated, whereas liver is heat stable. Placenta has the greatest heat stability. More than 30% heat stable suggests liver origin; less than 30% heat stable suggests bone. This method has not been reliable in my laboratory. Chemical fractionation is possible but has not become popular. Electrophoretic separation methods that have the added advantage that both the liver and the bone fraction can be visually inspected are available. However, separation of liver from bone is not clear cut with many systems, making it difficult to interpret small degrees of abnormality. Enzymatic methods using wheat germ have been described and are becoming available. Wheat germ inactivates bone isoenzyme.

Besides the major alkaline phosphatase isoenzymes, ALP isoenzyme electrophoresis may sometimes demonstrate other isoenzymes. One of these is the so-called "fast liver" band that appears anodal to the liver band, corresponding to the alpha-1 area of serum. This band is most frequently associated with metastatic carcinoma in the liver (44%–96% of patients), but in several small series of patients has also been associated with alcoholic active cirrhosis (33%–36% of patients), hepatitis virus hepatitis (12%–50%), common bile duct stones (53%–63%), and cancer not metastatic to the liver (16%–33%). It rarely appears in normal persons. Another isoenzyme is called the Regan isoenzyme. This migrates in the placenta (fast beta) area. This is reported in 3%–15% of patients with cancer (although some investigators had to concentrate the patient serum); 2%–4% of apparently normal persons; and occasional persons with nonmalignant disease, especially active cirrhosis and inflammatory bowel disease.

5-Nucleotidase.—This enzyme is a member of the alkaline phosphatase group but is thought to be more specific (and possibly more sensitive) than alkaline phosphatase for hepatobiliary tract disease. However, one study suggests elevated levels in some patients with bone lesions.

Leucine Amino Peptidase.—Leucine amino peptidase (LAP) is an enzyme produced exclusively by the liver. In general, its level tends to parallel the alkaline phosphatase level, although it is not as sensitive. Bone lesions do not affect this test. When originally reported, LAP elevation was thought to indicate pancreatic carcinoma, but all agree now that this theory was wrong and that the only association occurs when pancreatic carcinoma causes biliary obstruction, just as alkaline phosphatase values are elevated in the same situation.

Immunoglobulin Levels.—Marked IgM increase has been reported in 80% of patients with biliary cirrhosis, but elevated levels may occur in extrahepatic obstruction and other diseases. Immunoglobulin A levels are increased in about 45% of patients with alcoholic cirrhosis, but IgA may be increased in various other liver diseases. Immunoglobulins have not, therefore, been very helpful.

Cholesterol and Cholesterol Esters.—Cholesterol is synthesized in several tissues, but the liver is the chief organ in its manufacture, alteration, and degradation. Normally about 70% is esterified, and about 30% exists in the free form. Esterification is affected much more than total cholesterol by liver damage. In moderate degrees of acute or chronic liver damage, the percentage of cholesterol esters may decrease to the 40%–50% range. They usually do not fall below 20% without severe liver parenchymal destruction. The total cholesterol level is reduced below reference ranges (150–240 mg/100 ml) only in severe damage, most often chronic. However, the usefulness of cholesterol as an index of liver function is severely handicapped by the technical difficulties of the test itself. Laboratories have considerable variation in accuracy even from day to day, so it is difficult to know if a slightly or moderately reduced value is genuine or not. Also, the normal range is so wide that a patient may have a one-third or more decrease in his or her usual normal value and still be within population reference ranges. Other diseases such as hyperthyroidism, severe infections, and malnutrition will lower serum cholesterol levels. On the other hand, certain types of liver diseases are associated with increased cholesterol levels; these include biliary cirrhosis, chronic biliary obstruction, and many cases of cholangitis. Nonhepatic diseases that cause elevated values are hypothyroidism, nephrotic syndrome, idiopathic hypercholesterolemia, and often diabetes.

Bromsulphalein Test.—The liver excretes bilirubin by conjugating it with glucuronide molecules and then releasing it into the bile. It has been found that certain synthetic substances such as bromsulphalein (BSP) dye are handled by the liver in a similar manner. On injection into the bloodstream, the dye is mostly bound to serum albumin. As it passes through the intrahepatic sinusoidal circulation, BSP is taken into the hepatic cells. Once there, some of the dye is conjugated with glutathione molecules, and all of the absorbed BSP, whether conjugated or free, is excreted into the bile. About 1% is excreted in urine without liver involvement, and a small percentage seems to be removed by other tissues. The rate of hepatic uptake is proportional to the amount of BSP in the plasma, meaning that a fairly constant percentage is removed by the liver on each passage through it. Therefore, the great bulk of the dye is removed from plasma relatively early, with the remaining amount getting progressively less as time passes. The four variables concerned in the test may be summarized as follows: (1) the amount of dye injected, (2) the plasma volume in which it is diluted, (3) the ability of the hepatic parenchymal cell mass to remove the BSP, and (4) the patency of the bile ducts through which the excreted final products must pass to the duodenum.

Although BSP excretion is normal in uncomplicated hyperbilirubinemia due to hemolytic anemia, most other etiologies of jaundice are associated with elevated BSP excretion, whether due to intrahepatic or to extrahepatic disease. Most disorders that produce a significant degree of injury to hepatic cells, even without jaundice, usually produce some degree of BSP abnormality. These include space-occupying lesions such as metastatic tumor or granulomatous diseases, in which the BSP excretion is abnormal more frequently than other standard biochemical liver function tests (sensitivity about 80%). In addition to diseases of liver cells and bile ducts, liver passive congestion or shock elevates BSP results due to decrease and stasis of hepatic blood flow. Transient degrees of BSP elevation have been reported in some cases of acute pancreatitis, high fever, severe stress such as trauma, and acute severe upper gastrointestinal (GI) tract hemorrhage.

Despite excellent characteristics as a screening test for liver disease compared with other liver function tests, use of BSP is discouraged by many authorities because of patient reactions to BSP that, although rare, may be severe or even fatal. In most cases it is being replaced by indocyanine green (Cardio-Green). Other considerations include (1) the test seldom provides information that is not obtainable in other ways, (2) the test shows only nonspecific abnormality in a wide variety of liver conditions that include any cause of jaundice, and (3) false results are often obtained when opiates or gallbladder x-ray contrast media are present in the blood or when a patient is obese.

Indocyanine green is a dye that is metabolized by liver cells in a manner similar to BSP. Evaluations suggest results equivalent to BSP, although the dye is slightly less sensitive for inactive cirrhosis. Indocyanine green has one advantage: no tissue toxicity or hypersensitivity reactions have been reported. The dye is five times more expensive than BSP and has not had the same degree of clinical evaluation and publicity.

Congenital Hyperbilirubinemias

There are five major groups of inherited defects in bilirubin metabolism: (1) Gilbert's syndrome, (2) Crigler-Najjar syndrome (type I), (3) Arias syndrome (Crigler-Najjar syndrome type II), (4) Dubin-Johnson syndrome, and (5) Rotor syndrome.

Gilbert's Syndrome.—Unconjugated bilirubin values are increased due to a deficiency in hepatic cell membrane transglucuronidation enzyme that adds the second glucuronide molecule to bilirubin monoglucuronide. Increase in bilirubin value is mild (usually < 3.0 mg/100 ml) but may be enhanced by fasting or illness. Jaundice frequently does not occur until after puberty. Serum AST and serum bile acid levels are normal.

Crigler-Najjar Syndrome (Type I).—Unconjugated bilirubin is increased due to absence of the liver cell microsomal enzyme bilirubin uridine diphosphate-glucuronate glucuronyl transferase (UDP-GT), which adds glucuronide to unconjugated bilirubin to form bilirubin monoglucuronide. Newborns and infants display marked hyperbilirubinemia with jaundice, and death may occur. There is autosomal recessive inheritance. The jaundice does not respond to phenobarbital therapy.

Arias Syndrome (Crigler-Najjar Type II).—Unconjugated bilirubin level is increased, but the defect is still somewhat uncertain. The usual stated etiology is partial defect of liver cell microsomal enzyme UDP-GT, but others believe it may be due to a deficiency in hepatic cell wall transglucuronide enzyme. Patients have moderate hyperbilirubinemia (6–20 mg/100 ml), and the jaundice responds well to phenobarbital therapy.

Dubin-Johnson Syndrome.—Both conjugated and unconjugated bilirubin levels are increased, with conjugated type predominating, due to a defect in transport of bilirubin from the liver cells to the bile ducts. Hyperbilirubinemia is usually mild, and jaundice may be precipitated by other illness or by pregnancy. Inheritance is autosomal recessive. Serum BSP excretion levels are normal 45 minutes after injection but characteristically become elevated 90–120 minutes after injection. Serum bile acid levels are normal. The gallbladder usually does not visualize on oral cholecystography.

Urine coproporphyrin analysis may be helpful for diagnosis. Normally, urine coproporphyrin is predominantly (about two thirds) type III. In Dubin-Johnson syndrome, the predominant isomer in urine becomes type I, even though total urinary coproporphyrin excretion levels are frequently normal. Some (not all) asymptomatic carriers may also have predominantly type I.

Rotor Syndrome.—This condition is associated with an increase in conjugated bilirubin levels due to defect in liver cell excretion of bilirubin. Inheritance is autosomal recessive. There usually is mild hyperbilirubinemia; jaundice may be induced by other illness. Liver uptake and storage of BSP is decreased (BSP retention in serum at 45 minutes after injection is increased), and serum bile acid levels are increased.

BIBLIOGRAPHY

Desoize B, et al: Alkaline phosphatase isoenzyme reactivity with wheat germ agglutinin. *Clin Chem* 1986; 32:402.

Viot M, et al: Alpha-1 isoenzyme of alkaline phosphatases. *Cancer* 1983; 52:140.

Hindmarsh JT: Clinical disorders of porphyrin metabolism. *Clin Biochem* 1983; 16:209.

Hollander IJ: Nonhemolytic hyperbilirubinemias. *Ann Clin Lab Sci* 1980; 10:204.

Berk PD, et al: Inborn errors of bilirubin metabolism. *Med Clin North Am* 1975; 59:803.

Breen KJ, Schenker S: Liver function tests. *CRC Crit Rev Clin Lab Sci* 1971; 2:573.

Fitzgerald MXM, et al: Value of differential alkaline phosphatase thermostability in clinical diagnosis. *Am J Clin Pathol* 1969; 51:194.

CHAPTER 20. CARDIAC, PULMONARY, PSYCHIATRIC, AND MISCELLANEOUS DIAGNOSTIC PROCEDURES

Myoglobin in Diagnosis of Myocardial Infarct.—Myoglobin is found in cardiac and skeletal muscle and is measured by immunoassay. The studies so far available indicate that serum myoglobin levels after myocardial infarct reach a peak in approximately 8–12 hours. During this time, serum myoglobin values are abnormal in approximately 90% of patients (literature range, 77%–100%). By 12 hours after admission, serum levels in a few patients may already have returned to normal range. By 12–24 hours after admission, levels remain elevated in fewer than 50% of patients. Another investigator found that myoglobin appeared intermittently and that serial determinations within the first 6–18 hours increased the chances of detecting abnormality.

Myoglobin is excreted in urine by renal

glomerular filtration. There is evidence that myoglobinuria may appear as early as 3 hours after onset of infarct symptoms. In several patients, urine values returned to upper normal limits by 30 hours but remained elevated longer in most cases. Another study recorded 90% sensitivity 24 and 48 hours after hospital admission, diminishing to 76% by 72 hours.

Besides cardiac muscle injury, skeletal muscle injury due to trauma, ischemia, or inflammation may release myoglobin. Nondestructive conditions affecting muscle such as delirium tremens and severe exertion also may produce myoglobinuria, and it has also been reported in some patients with diabetic acidosis, hypokalemia, systemic infection with fever, barbiturate poisoning, and certain more uncommon etiologies (see Table 36–15). Since myoglobin is excreted through the kidneys, renal function might also influence results. The serum myoglobin "false positive" rate in patients without acute myocardial infarct has been reported to range from 0%–22%.

Enzymatic Estimation of Myocardial Infarct Size.—Several investigators reported that there was a reasonably good correlation between infarct size and the peak value of either total creatine phosphokinase (CPK) or CPK-MB (isoenzyme of creatine kinase containing M and B subunits). Most investigators favor CPK-MB because of its greater specificity for myocardium (e.g., the problem of intramuscular injection interference with total CPK). However, some reports indicate that infarct location is as important as size, and other reports did not find consistent clear-cut differences in prognosis between a considerable number of infarcts with moderate differences in CPK-MB values.

Creatine Phosphokinase–MB Isoforms in Acute Myocardial Infarction.—There are three major CPK isoenzymes, but each of the three has now been shown to exist in subforms (isoforms). MM-CK in myocardium is a dimer of two identical M chains, each with a terminal lysine amino acid (this M chain is designated MMa by some and MM3 by others). When myocardial muscle fiber injury occurs, MMa (MM3) is released into the blood. The terminal lysine group from one of the two M chains is rapidly removed, yielding MMb (MM2). Subsequently, there is cleavage of the terminal lysine molecule from the other M chain, a configuration known as MMc (MM1), that is relatively long lived. The three MM isoforms can be separated by physical methods such as high-voltage electrophoresis or isoelectric focusing and by other techniques. Since MM1 (MMc) is stable in serum and since the first isoform released from damaged muscle is MM3 (MMa) which is short lived, most investigators are using the MM3/MM1 (MMa/MMc) ratio instead of an individual isoform. The MM3/MM1 ratio is said to become abnormal 2–4 hours (or even earlier) after onset of acute MI and peaks about 6–9 hours after onset of acute MI. In both cases the MM isoform abnormality precedes corresponding CPK-MB abnormality. For example, in one study the MM3/MM1 ratio was abnormal in 90% of acute MI patients by 6–9 hours, whereas CPK-MB values were elevated in 79% of the patients. In another study, the ratio detected 86% of acute MI on the first sample, obtained less than 4 hours after onset of chest pain. Therefore, the isoform measurement is similar to myoglobin regarding early abnormality but is more specific for myocardial damage. Isoform measurement can be used to obtain an earlier confirmation of acute MI than standard laboratory tests can provide and has been proposed for use to assist decisions whether to begin interventional therapy such as intracoronary thrombolytic agents or balloon angioplasty.

Like all laboratory tests, the isoform ratio has drawbacks. At present, assay of the isoforms requires special techniques not available in most laboratories; and even if available, results cannot be obtained in less than 1 hour (or more). False negative results may occur in 10%–15% of patients before 6–9 hours after onset of chest pain. As time passes, MM3 is converted to MM1, and the isoform ratio decreases. Not all patients seek medical attention immediately after onset of chest pain, and even with those who do, it takes time before a blood specimen is obtained. In the study mentioned previously, if the specimen was not drawn before 9–12 hours after onset of chest pain, the isoform ratio detected 88% of acute MI and CPK–MB detected 87%. After 12–15 hours, the isoform ratio detected 79% and CPK-MB detected 90%. Therefore, after about 10 hours following onset of acute MI, CPK-MB sensitivity becomes equal to or greater than the isoform ratio.

Detection of Reperfusion After Thrombolytic Agents.—After interventional therapy for acute MI, not all patients obtain reopening of the affected coronary artery. This information would be useful to assess the need for additional therapy or perhaps for more invasive measures such as balloon angioplasty or coronary artery bypass. Several investigators have found that enzymes released after myocardial fiber damage reach their peak earlier than would be the case if reperfusion did not take place. This is explained on the basis of release of accumulated enzyme after reperfusion occurs ("washout phenomenon"). The reperfusion peak for CPK-MB was reached at an average of about 13 hours, whereas the peak for nonreperfused patients was reached at an average of about 18–22 hours. There is disagreement in the reports whether peak enzyme values are greater in the reperfused patients. In addition, although there is clear separation between the mean time duration before the peak in the two groups, in most reports there is overlap between the two groups regarding the time duration of individual patients, with some nonreperfused patients reaching a peak in the same time range as that of some reperfused patients. However, some of the overlap may be due to spontaneous reopening of coronary occlusion or arterial spasm in some nontreated patients. At least partially because of the overlap between patient values, early CPK-MB peaking in one study showed a sensitivity of only 69% in detection of reperfusion. Since most of the reports to date have included only relatively small groups of patients, more definitive studies are needed.

Radioisotope Pulmonary Function Tests.—Radioactive xenon is a gas that can be either inhaled or injected intravenously. Inhalation fills the alveoli for a few moments before the gas is exhaled. If injected intravenously, xenon quickly diffuses into the alveoli and then is exhaled. In either case a stationary rapid imaging device such as the Anger scintillation camera can photograph alveolar distribution of the gas. Conditions that alter ventilatory distribution, such as emphysema or space-occupying lesions, produce various abnormalities in the distribution of xenon. In pulmonary embolization the xenon inhalation scan typically is normal in areas of defects seen on perfusion scans with isotope-labeled particles that outline pulmonary blood distribution. However, if emphysema is present, both the ventilation and the perfusion scan will be abnormal, and this provides a way to differentiate embolization from emphysema. Unfortunately, emboli sometimes occur in areas with preexisting severe emphysema. Xenon tests are available at present only in large hospitals. The gas is very expensive and necessitates special apparatus to avoid contamination of the room.

Isotope-labeled particles can be inhaled via aerosol; this allows visualization of the pattern of the major bronchi. It is claimed that this method can distinguish pure emphysema from that secondary to bronchitis. The technique is not widely used.

BIBLIOGRAPHY

Kondo M, et al: Comparison of early myocardial technetium-99m pyrophosphate uptake to early peaking of creatine kinase and creatine kinase-MB as indicators of early reperfusion in acute myocardial infarction. *Am J Cardiol* 1987; 60:762.

Wu AHB, et al: Early diagnosis of acute myocardial infarction by rapid analysis of creatine kinase isoenzyme-3 (CK-MM) subtypes. *Clin Chem* 1987; 33:358.

Gibler WB: Myoglobin as an early indicator of acute myocardial infarction. *Ann Emerg Med* 1987; 16:851.

Jaffe AS, et al: Diagnostic changes in plasma creatine kinase isoforms early after the onset of acute myocardial infarction. *Circulation* 1986; 74:105.

Hindman N, et al: Relation between electrocardiographic and enzymatic methods of estimating acute myocardial infarct size. *Am J Cardiol* 1986; 58:31.

Lee TH, Goldman L: Serum enzyme assays in the diagnosis of acute myocardial infarction. *Ann Intern Med* 1986; 105:221.

Hands, M.E. et al: Prognostic significance of electrocardiographic site of infarction after correction for enzymatic size of infarction. *Circulation* 1986; 73:885.

Wei JY, et al: Time course of serum cardiac enzymes after intracoronary thrombolytic therapy. *Arch Intern Med* 1985; 145:1596.

Kwong TC, et al: Activities of some enzymes in serum after therapy with intracoronary streptokinase in acute myocardial infarction. *Clin Chem* 1984; 30:731.

Fiolet JWT, et al: Infarct size estimation from serial CK-MB determinations. *Br Heart J* 1983; 9:373.

McNeil BM: Ventilation-perfusion studies and the diagnosis of pulmonary embolism. *J Nucl Med* 1980; 21:319.
Oxley DK, et al: Myoglobin in myocardial infarction. *Am J Clin Pathol* 1979; 72:137.
Reese L, Uksik P: Radioimmunoassay of serum myoglobin in screening for acute myocardial infarction. *Can Med Assoc J* 1981; 124:1585.

CHAPTER 21. SERUM PROTEINS

IgM Monoclonal Proteins.—In one series of 430 patients who had monoclonal IgM detected, 56% had idiopathic IgM at the time of diagnosis, 17% had Waldenström's macroglobulinemia, 7% had malignant lymphoma, 5% had chronic lymphocytic leukemia, 14% had other malignant leukemias or lymphomas, and 17% had amyloidosis. About 20% of those who had idiopathic IgM eventually developed lymphocytic leukemia or lymphoma.

BIBLIOGRAPHY

Kyle RA, Garton JP: The spectrum of IgM monoclonal gammopthay in 430 cases. *Mayo Clin Proc* 1987; 62:719.

CHAPTER 24. SERUM ELECTROLYTES AND PROTEIN-CALORIE MALNUTRITION

Parathyroid Function.—***Neck Vein Catheterization.***—In general, an increase of the parathyroid hormone (PTH) level from veins in only one side of the neck suggests parathyroid tumor, whereas an increase on both sides suggests secondary hyperparathyroidism or ectopic PTH. Even this procedure does not always disclose PTH elevation in parathyroid tumor or always differentiate primary hyperparathyroidism (PHPT) from secondary hyperparathyroidism with absolute accuracy. Results vary according to whether large or small vessels are catheterized and in what areas, and success thus depends on the skill and experience of the operator. Such procedures are therefore best carried out in an institution that has someone with an interest and extensive experience in this technique.

Chloride/Phosphate Ratio.—One group of investigators found that serum chloride value (in milliequivalents per liter) divided by serum phosphorus value (phosphate, in milligrams per 100 ml) was above 33 in nearly 95% of patients with PHPT and below 33 in about the same percentage of patients with hypercalcemia from other etiologies. The test is not useful if the serum calcium level is normal or if a significant degree of renal failure is present. Ectopic PTH syndrome would also give false results. Some reports indicate too much overlap between PHPT and other diseases to rely on the chloride/phosphate ratio. More evaluation is needed.

Urine Adenosine 3,5-Monophosphate Assay (Cyclic Adenosine Monophosphate).—One of the effects of PTH is production of cyclic adenosine monophosphate (cyclic AMP) in the renal tubules, which mediates conversion of calcidiol to calcitriol, which, in turn, affects renal tubule reabsorption of phosphate, calcium absorption from the GI tract, and calcium mobilization from bone. In PHPT, cyclic AMP excretion is increased in about 70% of cases (literature range, 48%–93%). The test is unreliable when the patient has poor renal function. There are few data on values found with metastatic tumor to bone. Cyclic AMP values are decreased or normal in most other patients with hypercalcemia from other causes. Cyclic AMP can be used to differentiate PHPT from pseudohypoparathyroidism (normal parathyroids but kidneys refractory to PTH). Injection of PTH will not increase cyclic AMP values in patients with pseudohypoparathyroidism. Cyclic AMP is reported by one investigator to follow a diurnal rhythm in most persons (peak either between 9 A.M. and 3 P.M. or between 3 and 9 P.M.), so that a 24-hour urine collection is preferred. However, another investigator did not find a diurnal rhythm.

Sensitivity and specificity of cyclic AMP assay were improved by introducing a modification called "nephrogenous cyclic AMP" (NCAMP). Urine cyclic AMP is the sum of cyclic AMP filtered through the glomeruli and cyclic AMP secreted by renal tubules. Measurement of plasma cyclic AMP, urine cyclic AMP, and the glomerular filtration rate (by creatinine clearance) permits estimate of the cyclic AMP fraction secreted by the kidneys, which is the portion of cyclic AMP affected by PTH. Preliminary results suggest NCAMP levels are elevated in 90%–95% of PHPT patients. However, reports have varied from 50%–100%. In hypercalcemia of malignancy, the few studies available have varied widely, with NCAMP levels being elevated in 0%–82%. The two investigators who specifically mention pseudohyperparathyroidism (ectopic PTH syndrome) found elevation in 65%–92% of cases. There seems to be a significant difference in NCAMP results, depending on how the data are reported (e.g., units per 100 ml of glomerular filtrate, units per gram of creatinine, percentage of total cyclic AMP). The NCAMP levels are said to be normal or low in diseases without elevated PTH values. The assay at present can be obtained only in large reference laboratories and certain medical centers. More data are needed to determine usefulness in the differential diagnosis of hypercalcemia.

Glucocorticosteroid Suppression.—A large dose of hydrocortisone or equivalent steroids (e.g., 40 mg of prednisone three times daily) for 10 days decreases the serum calcium level at least 1 mg/100 ml in most patients with sarcoidosis, hyperthyroidism, hypervitaminosis D, and myeloma. More than 95% of PHPT patients who do not have hand x-ray evidence of bone changes fail to suppress, as well as about two thirds of those with bone changes. In patients with metastatic carcinoma to bone, 30%–50% fail to suppress. In the United States, this test has been mostly superseded by PTH assay. It is sometimes useful in patients with possible sarcoidosis.

Calcium Infusion Tests.—Hypercalcemia from calcium infusion inhibits secretion of PTH; this, in turn, decreases renal tubule phosphate reabsorption, producing loss of phosphorus into the urine. Parathyroid tumors theoretically should not be influenced by serum calcium levels, and patients therefore would not display significant change in urinary excretion of phosphate, whereas calcium infusion should suppress the action of nonautonomous parathyroid glands and result in a decrease in urine phosphate. The original Ellsworth-Howard test has not proved to be sufficiently reliable, nor have rapid infusions and other test modifications. Newer suggestions are based on measuring urine phosphate values in the second 12-hour period after 4-hour calcium infusion or measuring serum PTH values instead of urine phosphorus values but have not yet been sufficiently evaluated.

Preoperative Hypokalemia.—In contrast to previous studies which indicated that hypokalemia during surgery is dangerous and potentially fatal, one recent study reported on patients with untreated preoperative hypokalemia, ranging from mild to moderate (9% with <3.0 mEq/L). There was no significant difference in intraoperatiave and postoperative course between these patients and normokalemic controls, and no mortality.

Serum Water.—Serum water can be estimated by a refractometer (total solids meter), which measures the effects of serum proteins on the refractive index. Serum proteins constitute the major determinant of serum colloid osmotic pressure, which regulates plasma and extracellular water equilibrium. Therefore, serum water estimates intravascular colloid osmotic pressure, in contrast to serum osmolality, which measures intravascular osmotic pressure, an entity responding to electrolyte changes but not influenced significantly by colloid (protein). Serum water is influenced by changes in either protein or water. Elevated serum water levels suggest excess water; decreased serum water levels indicate water deficit. Unfortunately, decreased serum protein levels also lead to increased water values, and since decreased albumin levels are common in seriously ill patients, this fact plus the rather high cost of the instrument has limited the use of the test. Nevertheless, even protein abnormality does not totally destroy the usefulness of serum water determination, because a relative dilution caused by hypoproteinemia may be treated by administration of albumin. Normal serum water values are 93–94 gm/100 ml.

BIBLIOGRAPHY

Hirsch IA, et al: The overstated risk of preoperative hypokalemia. *Anesth Analg* 1988; 67:131.

Levine MA: Laboratory investigation of disorders of the parathyroid glands. *Clin Endocrinol Metab* 1985; 14:257.

Rude RK, et al: Urinary and nephrogenous adenosine 3,5-monophosphate in the hypercalcemia of malignancy. *J Clin Endocrinol* 1981; 52:765.

Lafferty FW: Primary hyperparathyroidism. *Arch Intern Med* 1981; 141:1761.

Watson L, et al: Hydrocortisone suppression test and discriminant analysis in differential diagnosis of hypercalcemia. *Lancet* 1980; 1:1320.

Broadus AE: Nephrogenous cyclic AMP as a parathyroid function test. *Nephron* 1979; 23:136.

Aro A, et al: Hypercalcemia: Serum chloride and phosphate. *Ann Intern Med* 1977; 86:664.

Babka JC, et al: Nephrogenous cyclic AMP levels in primary hyperparathyroidism. *Arch Intern Med* 1976; 136:1140.

Eisenberg H, et al: Selective arteriography, venography, and venous hormone assay in diagnosis and localization of parathyroid lesions. *Am J Med* 1974; 56:810.

Mansberger AR, et al: Refractometry and osmometry in clinical surgery. *Ann Surg* 1969; 169:672.

CHAPTER 26. TESTS FOR DIABETES AND HYPOGLYCEMIA

Amended Insulin/Glucose Ratio for Diagnosis of Insulinoma.—Some investigators have proposed variants of the immunoreactive insulin/glucose (IRI/G) ratio to increase sensitivity or specificity for insulinoma. The most commonly used variant is the "amended ratio" of Turner, whose formula is:

$$\frac{\text{Serum insulin level} \times 100}{\text{Serum glucose} - 30 \text{ mg/100 ml}}$$

when serum insulin is reported in μU/ml and serum glucose in mg/100 ml. A ratio over 50 suggests insulinoma, while a ratio less than 50 is evidence against insulinoma. The serum levels of glucose and insulin are obtained after fasting, which may have to be long term (as described in chapter 27). The amended IRI/G ratio is reported to be a little more sensitive than the standard IRI/G, but at least one report indicates that it may be less specific (a few more false positive results).

BIBLIOGRAPHY

Bates HM: Insulinoma and pheochromocytoma. *Lab Mgmt* 1983; 21(5):11.

CHAPTER 28. THYROID FUNCTION TESTS

Thyroxine-Binding Globulin Quantitative Assay.—Methods are available for measuring actual thyroxine-binding globulin (TBG) levels by means of electrophoresis-isotope combination techniques. This was useful when thyroid test abnormalities due to TBG alterations were suspected. With use of the "corrected" thyroxine (T_4) by isotope or free T_4 index, TBG assay should rarely be needed.

Thyroid Tests Based on Measurement of Serum Iodine.—Under normal conditions, approximately 95% of serum iodine is located in serum T_4, of which more than 99% is bound to serum proteins. The protein-bound iodine (PBI) test precipitated these serum proteins, followed by destruction of the proteins and assay of the iodine that they contained. This provided a good indirect estimate of total serum T_4 values. The major difficulty with the PBI was contamination by iodine from medicines and x-ray contrast media. Alterations in T_4-binding proteins also affected results in a manner identical to other total T_4 assays. The butanol-extractable iodine (BEI) test employed butyl alcohol to eliminate most of the iodide from medicines (and also most circulating thyroxine precursors). Iodine from x-ray media was not extracted, however. The T_4 by column test used an ion exchange resin to eliminate most of the inorganic iodide and some (not all) of the x-ray media. Other than elimination of a certain amount of iodine contamination, results of the BEI and T_4 by column were similar to those of the PBI. In the United States the iodine measurement tests have been superseded by T_4 methods not affected by iodine contamination, such as radioassay or enzyme immunoassay.

Thyroid Tests Based on Tissue Utilization of Thyroid Hormone.—This group of tests included the Achilles tendon reflex (a physical measurement), basal metabolic rate, and serum cholesterol. These procedures are rarely used today as thyroid function tests.

Achilles Tendon Reflex.—Thyroid hormone status affects the speed of muscle reflex. Equipment is available to measure either contraction or relaxation time. Although a few investigators claim good results, the usual accuracy is 50%–75% in hypothyroidism and 20%–50% in hyperthyroidism. Diabetes mellitus, pernicious anemia, various neurologic disorders, and thiourea drugs prolong reflex time; estrogens and corticosteroids shorten it.

Basal Metabolic Rate.—The basal metabolic rate supposedly measures body reaction as a whole to circulating thyroid hormone. Most methods are indirect, utilizing rate of oxygen uptake by means of breathing a measured amount of oxygen in a closed-circuit tank apparatus. If increased amounts of oxygen are breathed, theoretically the patient has an abnormally high basal metabolic rate and vice versa for decreased metabolism. Unfortunately, too many variables are involved, and the test is not sufficiently reliable in mild thyroid disease or difficult diagnostic problems. A truly basal state is difficult to achieve and maintain. Anxiety, obesity, adrenal dysfunction, and equipment malfunction are some of the other major obstacles to accurate results. This test is rarely used today.

Serum Cholesterol.—The serum cholesterol level is an indirect measurement of metabolic rate; this reflects a not-well-understood effect of thyroid hormone on cholesterol synthesis. Cholesterol levels are often elevated in myxedema and much less frequently are decreased in hyperthyroidism (mostly in classic cases). Serum cholesterol measurement is, however, a poor test of thyroid function for several reasons:

1. Many diseases influence cholesterol metabolism in various ways.
2. Changes from reference range tend to occur only in far-advanced thyroid disease, more often in hypothyroidism than in hyperthyroidism.
3. Cholesterol reference range is so wide that many persons could be abnormal and still have values within the population reference range.

Thyroid-Stimulating Immunoglobulin (TSI) Assay.—A group of immunoglobulins (antibodies) of the IgG class that could prevent binding of thyroid-stimulating hormone (TSH) to TSH receptors on the thyroid cell membrane were discovered. The antibody also has the ability to stimulate adenylate cyclase to produce cyclic AMP production, which causes release of T_4 and triiodothyronine (T_3). The antibody can exert effect over a relatively prolonged period of time. The antibody was originally named "long-acting thyroid stimulator" (LATS) and was measured with a bioassay system (McKenzie) using mouse thyroid. The LATS was considered to be fairly specific for Graves' disease, although it was also found in a few patients with Hashimoto's disease and occasionally in low titer in some other conditions. It could be detected in only 40%–45% (range, 9%–55%) of patients with Graves' disease. It was present more frequently when the patients had pretibial edema or hyperthyroidism with eye signs (but it was found in only about 15% of patients with so-called isolated Graves' ophthalmopathy). The titer tended to decrease after 6–12 months of clinically active disease, after treatment was given, or when the disease became inactive. There was not a close relationship between titer and severity of illness.

It was subsequently found that LATS would bind to human thyroid tissue but could not stimulate it, so that the antibody was renamed "mouse thyroid stimulator." In addition, once serum containing LATS was incubated with human thyroid tissue, that serum no longer showed any LATS activity in the McKenzie mouse bioassay (i.e., the LATS activity was destroyed or neutralized).

More recently, other related IgG antibodies were found that prevented adsorption of LATS onto human thyroid tissue and (as a group) was therefore called "LATS protector." This abnormal IgG antibody (or antibodies) can be demonstrated by three different assay techniques. One technique used high-titer LATS antibody as the indicator system whose endpoint was to show that antibody in patient serum blocked uptake of the LATS antibody by human thyroid tissue; since the LATS antibody activity in the McKenzie bioassay would be neutralized by human thyroid tissue and the patient antibody prevented such neutralization, the patient antibody was called LATS protector antibody. A second technique measured the ability of patient antibody to inhibit or block the binding of radioactive TSH to human or animal thyroid acinar cell membranes. This has been called the "TSH-binding inhibiting immunoglobulin" (TBII) assay. The third technique measured the ability of the antibody to stimulate human or animal thyroid acinar cell membrane-bound adenylate cyclase, producing increased cyclic AMP activity. The original assay method used human thyroid tissue, so the antibody was originally called "human thyroid-stimulating immunoglobulin." Since animal thyroid tissue can be used, the assay now is simply called "thyroid-stimulating immunoglobulin" (TSI). For example, one modification of the TSI uses special TSH-dependent FRTL-5 rat tissue culture thyroid cells.

The LATS-protector assay is reported to detect about 75%–80% (range, 60%–90%) of patients with Graves' disease. The LATS-protector assay was very complicated; few laboratories performed the assay and few if any do now. The TBII technique is reported to detect about 70%–80% (range, 39%–100%) of Graves' disease, and the TBI detects about 75%–80% (range, 18%–100%). Neither the TBII nor the TBI are simple or easy. Most laboratories using either technique use "homemade" reagents, which accounts for much of the great variation in sensitivity reported in the literature. Since many nonresearch laboratories base their test performance claims on data from one or more research laboratories using the same technique but their own reagents, performance claims based on someone else's results may not be valid. Therefore, it is desirable to send specimens to laboratories that can verify better sensitivity based on adequate numbers of well-diagnosed patients with Graves' disease that they assayed themselves. Besides sensitivity, it is necessary to question specificity, since different laboratories may find different numbers of false positive results when patients with hyperfunctioning thyroid nodules, nonfunctioning nodules or goiter, thyroiditis, autoimmune disorders, and clinically normal status are tested.

At present, TSI assay is used mainly for patients with borderline or conflicting evidence of Graves' disease, patients who have some condition that affects the results of other tests, or patients who have "isolated Graves' ophthalmopathy" (a condition in which all standard thyroid tests are normal). However, a negative test result in most laboratories does not completely exclude the diagnosis, and there is a possibility of false positive results.

Perchlorate Discharge Test.—Perchlorate blocks thyroid uptake of iodide but also helps to discharge or "wash out" iodide within the thyroid that is not incorporated into thyroid hormone precursors or thyroglobulin. The patient is given a tracer dose of radioiodine. Radioactive iodine uptake (RAIU) is counted over the thyroid 1 hour after the dose is administered. Potassium perchlorate, 200 mg, is then given orally, and radioactivity is again counted over the thyroid 1 hour later (2 hours after the radioiodine is administered). Normally, RAIU continues to rise after the first hour. If there is a defect in iodide binding to tyrosine (organification), the nonbound radioiodine will leave the thyroid, and the 2-hour RAIU will be less than the 1-hour RAIU.

The major use of the test is in diagnosis of thyroid hormone synthesis defect involving binding of iodide to tyrosine due to congenital thyroid peroxidase enzyme deficiency. The test also gives abnormal results in many patients with chronic (Hashimoto's) thyroiditis, iodine-induced goiter, and treatment with the thionamide drugs. The perchlorate discharge test is rarely used today.

Menstrual Irregularity Associated With Occult Hypothyroidism.—One report indicates that some patients with persistent menstrual disturbance without known cause may have occult hypothyroidism. The disturbance could be hypermenorrhea or oligomenorrhea. Standard thyroid function tests (T_4, FTI, and TSH) were within reference range. The thyrotropin-releasing hormone (TRH) test disclosed an exaggerated response consistent with hypothyroidism, and the clinical symptoms disappeared with administration of thyroid hormone. Only the TRH test was sensitive enough to detect the abnormality.

BIBLIOGRAPHY

Morris JC, et al: Clinical utility of thyrotropin-receptor antibody assays. *Mayo Clin Proc* 1988; 63:707.

Zakarija M, McKenzie JM: The spectrum and significance of autoantibodies reacting with the thyrotropin receptor. *Endocrinol Metab Clin North Am* 1987; 16:343.

Massart C, et al: Assays for thyrotropin-receptor binding and thyroid-stimulating antibodies in sera from patients with Graves' disease. *Clin Chem* 1986; 32:1332.

Wall JR, Kuroki T: Immunologic factors in thyroid disease. *Med Clin North Am* 1985; 69:913.

Chopra IJ: Laboratory aids in the diagnosis of hyperthyroidism. *Thyroid Today* 1978; 1:1.

Stoffer SS: Menstrual disorders and mild thyroid insufficiency. *Postgrad Med* 1982; 72:75.

CHAPTER 29. ADRENAL FUNCTION TESTS

Tests in Primary Aldosteronism

The technical difficulty of aldosterone and renin determinations has led to various screening tests for Conn's syndrome and, in some instances, to procedures that might replace renin for diagnosis. Although RIA has improved renin and aldosterone assay, there are still problems with reliability, so that need for alternatives has decreased but not ended. Of the various screening procedures listed, most have not been sufficiently evaluated to confirm original good results. These procedures include furosemide (Lasix) test, saline infusion, 24-hour urine potassium, and plasma aldosterone with saline infusion.

Furosemide Test.—The patient remains upright for 4 hours following an oral dose of the diuretic furosemide. Plasma renin is then drawn. The original report states 80% agreement with low-salt diet renin response in hypertensive patients, with the 20% disagreement containing both false positives and false negatives.

Saline Infusion.—Large quantities of saline given intravenously over a 2-day period are said to suppress aldosterone to less than 50% of baseline values in conditions other than primary aldosteronism.

24-Hour Urine Potassium.—Patients with hypokalemia who have primary aldosteronism usually have normal potassium excretion (40 mEq/day), whereas most others have low excretion as the body attempts to conserve potassium.

Plasma Aldosterone With Saline Infusion.—Plasma aldosterone levels are reported to be suppressed to less than 50% of baseline (recumbent for 8 hours) values by infusion of 2 L of saline over a 2-hour period, whereas levels in primary aldosteronism remain greater than 50%. Saline infusion causes more marked suppression than does a high-salt diet.

17-Ketogenic Steroids

These are C21 compounds that can be oxidized to 17-ketosteroids (17-KS). The ketogenic steroids thus constitute the difference between 17-KS determinations done before and after oxidation. The 17-ketogenic compounds include the 17-hydroxycorticosteroid (17-OHCS) group and also pregnanetriol. Pregnanetriol is a metabolite of 17-hydroxyprogesterone (a precursor of cortisone). Since pregnanetriol elevation occurs only in a very few conditions (e.g., the adrenogenital syndrome) in which 17-OHCS are not also elevated, in most situations a urinary 17-ketogenic steroid determination could be used (if desired) instead of urinary 17-OHCS. Whereas the metabolite of 17-hydroxyprogesterone (pregnanetriol) is included in 17-ketogenic assays, the metabolite of progesterone (pregnanediol) is not a 17-KS.

A list of compounds that may interfere with 17-OHCS or 17-KS (and ketogenic) determinations is given in Table 36–2.

17-Ketosteroid Fractionation.—The 17-KS can be fractionated into alpha (androsterone and etiocholanolone) and beta (dehydroepiandrosterone). Increase of 17-KS in adrenal carcinoma is most often due to beta fraction increase. The normal ratio of beta to alpha is less than 0.2. Alternatively, the "Allen blue" test is a reasonable estimate of DHA. Not all carcinoma results are positive with either of these procedures, and neither is indicated if urine 17-KS levels are normal; therefore, the use of these tests is decreasing.

BIBLIOGRAPHY

Arteaga E, et al: Use of the saline infusion test to diagnose the cause of primary aldosteronism. *Am J Med* 1985; 79:722.

Drury PL: Disorders of mineralocorticoid activity. *Clin Endocrinol Metab* 1985; 14:175.

Wallach L, et al: Stimulated renin: Screening test for hypertension. *Ann Intern Med* 1975; 82:27.

Frawley TF: Cushing's syndrome, in *Clinician.* Chicago, GD Searle & Co, 1971, vol 1, p 37.

Kem DC, et al: Saline suppression of plasma aldosterone in hypertension. *Arch Intern Med* 1971; 128:380.
Biglieri EG, et al: A preliminary evaluation for primary aldosteronism. *Arch Intern Med* 1970; 126:1004.

CHAPTER 32. LABORATORY ASPECTS OF CANCER

Carcinoma Antigen 19-9.—Carcinoma 19-9 (CA 19-9) is a carbohydrate antigen segment of a glycoprotein that appears to be a sialylated derivative of the Lewis A blood group. It is detected by monoclonal antibody immunoassay and is reasonably (but not highly) specific for GI tract origin (Table 35–1).

Currently, although there is considerable research activity, CA 19-9 assay is not being widely used. Although it has reasonably good sensitivity in pancreatic carcinoma, it does not detect these tumors early enough to improve their current dismal prognosis, and it is not specific for pancreatic neoplasms. It might be useful in the workup of patients when pancreatic or gastric carcinoma is a possibility and more informative diagnostic procedures (e.g., ultrasound or CT) are not available or do not provide a definite answer. A definitely elevated CA 19-9 level result would favor carcinoma of GI or GI accessory organs. The specimen has to be sent to a reference laboratory in most cases, and the results would not be available for several days. The CA 19-9 assay could be used to follow pancreatic carcinomas after surgical resection to detect recurrence, but the question then arises as to what could be done if it does recur. Finally, CA 19-9 has been used in addition to carcinoembryonic antigen (CEA) in order to detect recurrence of colon cancer. In some cases, CA 19-9 values become elevated before CEA, and the combination of the two tests is said to be more reliable than either test alone. However, at present CA 19-9 is not widely used for this purpose. As noted in Table 35–1, CA 19–9 may be elevated in some persons who do not have cancer. Also, 5%–10% of the population is Lewis A (blood group) negative and will not react with CA 19–9, even if they have cancer.

TABLE 35–1.
CA 19–9 in Various Conditions

CA 19–9	% Detected (Range)
Pancreas adenocarcinoma	80–85 (69–93)
Gastric adenocarcinoma	40–50 (21–80)
Colorectal carcinoma	30–40 (11–70)
Hepatoma	50
Lung carcinoma	16–20
Breast carcinoma	14–27
Ovarian carcinoma	17
Non-GI carcinoma	3–16
Chronic pancreatitis	11 (3–27)
Acute pancreatitis	9–11
Pancreatic insufficiency	26
Inflammatory bowel disease	1.5
Colon polyps	2.5
Benign GI diseases	(3–11)
Extrahepatic jaundice (benign)	16
Normal control persons	(0.5–1.1)

Centocor CA 15–3 and Hybritech CA 549.—CA 15–3 detects membrane antigens against human milk globules. It is said to be elevated in 57% of preoperative breast cancer patients, 75% (68%–80%) of patients with breast cancer with metastases, 3%–9% of patients with benign breast tumors, 4.5%–10.5% of patients with various nonmalignant conditions, and 1% of clinically normal persons. It is said to correlate with the clinical course of about 75% of patients with metastatic breast cancer, more frequently correlating with tumor progression than tumor regression. CA 549 detects any antigen present both in milk fat globule membranes and also in tumor cytoplasm. CA 549 is reported to be abnormal in 53%–90% of patients with metastatic breast cancer and 1%–13% of patients with benign breast disease. Certain other metastatic tumors are also detected.

Flow Cytometry Test for Bladder Cancer.—One study reports standard urine cytology that detected 58% of high-grade bladder carcinomas and 33% of low-grade bladder carcinomas. Flow cytometry (see chapter 7) methods detected 76% of low-grade tumors and 100% of high-grade tumors. However, one study suggests that the technique is not reliable when intravesical chemotherapy is given (which is also the problem with standard urine cytology).

Urine Hydroxyproline.—Hydroxyproline is a collagen component whose urinary excretion is increased in various disorders with increased osteoblastic activity as well as in some diseases involving osteolysis and collagen metabolism. Significantly increased 24-hour excretion is reported in about one half of patients with tumors having bone metastases, and normal results are obtained in most patients with tumors who do not have bone involvement. Some of those with skeletal metastases and elevated urine hydroxyproline values have normal alkaline phosphatase levels. Some investigators use hydroxyproline/creatinine ratios. The test may be useful in some cancer patients by suggesting occult bone metastasis, although a bone scan is probably more sensitive.

Bone Marrow Acid Phosphatase.—Several studies have reported that acid phosphatase assay from bone marrow aspiration material detects bone metastasis from prostate carcinoma more often than serum acid phosphatase. However, other investigators have not confirmed greater sensitivity or have found that the procedure is not a substantial help in diagnosis over that obtained by serum assays.

BIBLIOGRAPHY

Parry WL, Hemstreet GP: Cancer detection by quantitative fluorescence image analysis. *J Urol* 1988; 139:270.

Chan DW, et al: A new serum marker for breast cancer—CA 549. *Clin Chem* 1988; 34:1293.

AMA Diagnostic and Therapeutic Assessment Panel (DATTA): Transrectal ultrasonography in prostatic carcinoma. *JAMA* 1988; 259:2757.

Steinberg WM, et al: Comparison of the sensitivity and specificity of the CA 19-9 and carcinoembryonic antigen assays in detecting cancer of the pancreas. *Gastroenterology* 1986; 90:343.

Del Favero G, et al: CA 19-9 and carcinoembryonic antigen in pancreatic cancer diagnosis. *Cancer* 1986; 57:1576.

Kelleher PC, Smith CJP: Collagen metabolites in the urine and serum of patients with cancer. *Clin Lab Med* 1982; 2:519.

Boehme W.M., et al.: Lack of usefulness of bone marrow enzymes and calcium in staging patients with prostatic cancer. *Cancer* 1978; 41:1433.

CHAPTER 33. CONGENITAL DISEASES

X-ray in Lactase Deficiency.—An upper GI tract series with small bowel follow-through may be helpful in suggesting lactase deficiency. Fifty grams of lactose is added to the barium suspension. Certain roentgenographic findings (e.g., barium-lactose dilution, intestinal dilatation, and intestinal "hurry") point toward need for additional studies. Gastrectomy procedures may produce false positive results.

Familial Dysautonomia (Riley-Day Syndrome).—Riley-Day syndrome is a familial disorder characterized by a variety of signs and symptoms, including defective lacrimation, relative indifference to pain, postural hypotension, excessive sweating, emotional lability, and absence of the fungiform papilli on the anterior portion of the tongue. Most of those affected are Jewish. Helpful laboratory tests include increased urine homovanillic acid value and decreased serum dopamine-beta-hydroxylase (DBH) value, an enzyme that helps convert dopamine to norepinephrine. Besides the Riley-Day syndrome, the DBH value may also be decreased in mongolism (Down's syndrome) and Parkinson's disease. It has been reported to be elevated in about 50% of patients with neuroblastoma, in stress, and in certain congenital disorders (results in the congenital disorders have not been adequately confirmed). There is disagreement as to values in patients with hypertension.

Cystic Fibrosis.—One investigator reports that the sweat sodium/chloride ratio is 1.1 or less in patients with cystic fibrosis and 1.1 or more in patients who do not have cystic fibrosis.

BIBLIOGRAPHY

Hammond KB: Sweat testing. *Clin Chem News* 1988; 14(7):27.

Henderson MF, et al: Interpretation of sweat sodium and chloride concentrations. *Ann Clin Biochem* 1986; 23:109.

Kopin IJ, et al: Dopamine-beta-hydroxylase. *Ann Intern Med* 1976; 85:211.

Rosenquist CJ, et al: Intestinal lactase deficiency: Diagnosis by routine upper gastrointestinal radiography. *Radiology* 1972; 102:275.

Laws JW, Neale G: Radiological diagnosis of disaccharidase deficiency. *Lancet* 1966; 2:139.

Preger L, Amberg JR: Sweet diarrhea: Roentgen diagnosis of disaccharidase deficiency. *AJR* 1967; 101:287.

Riley CM, Moore RH: Familial dysautonomia differentiated from related disorders: Case reports and discussion of current concepts. *Pediatrics* 1966; 37:435.

CHAPTER 34. ANALYSIS OF THERAPEUTIC AND TOXIC SUBSTANCES

Tests for Tobacco Use.—In some instances, such as in smoking-cessation clinics, life insurance company examinations, and tests to determine degree of passive exposure to tobacco smoke, it is desirable to detect and quantitate tobacco exposure. The modalities that have been investigated are carboxyhemoglobin (based on effect of carbon monoxide generated by tobacco combustion), thiocyanate (a metabolite of cyanide derived from tobacco tar), and cotinine (a metabolite of nicotine). Most current tests are based on thiocyanate or cotinine. Thiocyanate is absorbed in the lungs and has a biological half-life of about 14 days. Ingestion of certain vegetables can falsely elevate serum thiocyanate levels. Cotinine is specific for nicotine, is not affected by diet, has a serum within-day variation of about 15%–20%, and has a biological half-life of about 19 hours. Thus, cotinine tests become negative after tobacco abstinence of a week or less, whereas thiocyanate requires considerably longer before becoming nondetectable. Also, thiocyanate can be assayed chemically and less expensively than cotinine, which is done by immunoassay. Nevertheless, because cotinine is specific for nicotine and is affected only by active or passive exposure to tobacco, cotinine seems to be favored by investigators. Cotinine can be assayed in serum, saliva, or urine; the levels are higher in urine.

BIBLIOGRAPHY

Steinman GD: Thiocyanate vs cotinine as a marker to identify smokers. *Clin Chem* 1985; 31:1406.

Pojer R, et al: Carboxyhemoglobin, cotinine, and thiocyanate assay compared for distinguishing markers for nonsmokers. *Clin Chem* 1984; 30:1377.

DIAGNOSTIC PROCEDURES THAT COMPLEMENT AND SUPPLEMENT LABORATORY TESTS

The clinical pathologist frequently encounters situations in which laboratory tests alone are not sufficient to provide a diagnosis. If this happens, certain diagnostic procedures may be suggested to provide additional information. These procedures are noted together with the laboratory tests that they complement or supplement. Nevertheless, it seems useful to summarize some basic information about these techniques and some data that, for various reasons, are not included elsewhere.

Diagnostic Ultrasound

Ultrasound is based on the familiar principle of radar, differing primarily in the frequency of the sound waves. Very high-frequency (1–10 MHz) sound emissions are directed toward an object, are reflected (echo production) by the target, and return to the detector, with a time delay proportional to the distance traveled. Differences in tissue or substance density result in a series of echoes produced by the surfaces of the various tissues or substances that lie in the path of the sound beam.

In A-mode (amplitude) readout, the echo signals are seen as spikes (similar to an ECG tracing format) with the height of the spike corresponding to the intensity of the echo and the distance between spikes depending on the distance between the various interfaces (boundaries) of substances in the path of the sound beam. The A-mode technique is infrequently used today, but early in the development of ultrasound it was often used to examine the brain, since the skull prevented adequate B-mode (brightness-modulated, bistable) visualization.

In B-mode readout, the sonic generator (transducer) is moved in a line across an area while the echoes are depicted as tiny dots corresponding to the location (origin) of the echo. This produces a pattern of dots, which gives a visual image of the shape and degree of homogeneity of material in the path of the sound beam (the visual result is a tomographic slice or thin cross-section of the target, with a dot pattern form somewhat analogous to that of a nuclear medicine scan).

Gray-scale mode is a refinement of B-mode scan readout in which changes in amplitude (intensity) of the sonic beam produced by differential absorption through different substances in the path of the beam are converted to shades of gray in the dot pattern. This helps the observer recognize smaller changes in tissue density (somewhat analogous to an x-ray).

B-mode ultrasound (including gray-scale) is now the basic technique for most routine work. Limitations include problems with very dense materials that act as a barrier both to signal and to echo (e.g., bone or x-ray barium), and air, which is a poor transmitter of high-frequency sound (lungs, air in distended bowel or stomach, etc.).

In M-mode (motion) readout, the sonic generator and detector remain temporarily in one location, and each echo is depicted as a small dot relative to original echo location; this is similar to A mode, but it uses a single dot instead of a spike. However, a moving recorder shows changes in the echo pattern that occur if any structures in the sonic beam path move; changes in location of the echo dot are seen in the areas that move but not in the areas that are stationary. The result is a series of parallel lines, each line corresponding to the continuous record of one echo dot; stationary dots produce straight lines and moving dots become a wavy or ECG-like line. In fact, the technique and readout are somewhat analogous to those of the ECG, if each area of the heart were to produce its own ECG tracing and all were displayed together as a series of parallel tracings. The M-mode technique is used primarily in studies of the heart (echocardiography), particularly aortic and mitral valve function.

Real-time ultrasound is designed to provide a picture similar to B-mode ultrasound but that is obtained rapidly enough to capture motion changes. Theoretically, real-time means that the system is able to evaluate information as soon as it is received rather than storing or accumulating any data. This is analogous to a fluoroscope x-ray image compared to a conventional x-ray. M-mode ultrasound produces single-dimension outlines of a moving structure as it moves or changes shape, whereas real-time two-dimensional ultrasound produces an image very similar to that produced by a static B-mode scanner but much more rapidly (15–50 frames/second)—fast enough to provide the impression of motion when the various images obtained are viewed rapidly one after the other (either by direct viewing as they are obtained on a CRT screen or as they are recorded and played back from magnetic tape or similar recording device). At present the equipment available to accomplish this exists in two forms: a linear array of crystals, the crystals being activated in sequence with electronic steering of the sound beam; and so-called small contact area (sector) scanners, having either an electronically phased crystal array or several crystals that are rotated mechanically. A triangular wedge-shaped image is obtained with the sector scanner and a somewhat more rectangular image with the linear-array scanner, both of which basically resemble images produced by a static B-mode scanner. On sector scanning, the apex of the triangle represents the ultrasound transducer (the sound wave generator and receiving crystal). The field of view (size of the triangle) of a typical real-time sector scanner is smaller than that of a standard static B-mode scanner (although the size differential is being decreased by new technology). Real-time image quality originally was inferior to that of static equipment, but this too has changed. Real-time equipment in general is less expensive, more compact, and more portable than static equipment; the ultrasound transducer is usually small and hand held and is generally designed to permit rapid changes in position to scan different areas rapidly using different planes of orientation. Many ultrasonographers now use real-time ultrasound as their primary ultrasound technique.

Uses of Diagnostic Ultrasound.—With continuing improvements in equipment, capabilities of ultrasound are changing rapidly. A major advantage is that ultrasound is completely noninvasive; in addition, no radiation is administered, and no acute or chronic ill effects have yet been substantiated in either tissues or genetic apparatus. The following sections describe some of the major areas in which ultrasound may be helpful:

Differentiation of Solid From Cystic Structures.—This is helpful in the diagnosis of renal space-occupying lesions, nonfunctioning thyroid nodules, pancreatic pseudocyst, pelvic masses, and so on. When a structure is ultrasonically interpreted as a cyst, accuracy should be 90%–95%. Ultrasound is the best method for diagnosis of pancreatic pseudocyst.

Abscess Detection.—In the abdomen, reported accuracy (in a few small series) varies between 60% and 90%, with 80% probably a reasonable present-day expectation. Abscess within organs such as the liver may be seen and differentiated from a cyst or solid tumor. Obvious factors affecting accuracy are size and location of the abscess, as well as interference from air or barium in overlying bowel loops.

Differentiation of Intrahepatic From Extrahepatic Biliary Obstruction.—This is based on attempted visualization of common bile duct dilatation in extrahepatic obstruction. Present-day accuracy is probably about 80%–90%.

Ultrasound may be useful in demonstrating a dilated gallbladder when cholecystography is not possible or suggests nonfunction. It may also be helpful in diagnosis of cholecystitis. Reports indicate about 90%–95% accuracy in detection of gallbladder calculi or other significant abnormalities. Some medical centers advocate a protocol in which single-dose oral cholecystography is done first; if the gallbladder fails to visualize, ultrasonography is performed. Detection of stones would make double-dose oral cholecystography unnecessary. Some are now using ultrasound as the primary method of gallbladder examination.

Diagnosis of Pancreatic Carcinoma.—Although islet cell tumors are too small to be seen, acinar carcinoma can be detected in approximately 75%–80% of instances. Pancreatic carcinoma cannot always be differentiated from pancreatitis. In the majority of institutions where CT is available, CT is preferred to ultrasound. Computerized tomography generally provides better results in obese patients, and ultrasound usually provides better results in very thin patients.

Guidance of Biopsy Needles.—Ultrasound is helpful in biopsies of organs such as the kidney.

Placental Localization.—Ultrasound is the procedure of choice for visualization of the fetus (fetal position, determination of fetal age by fetal measurements, detection of fetal anomalies, detection of fetal growth retardation), visualization of intrauterine or ectopic pregnancy, and diagnosis of hydatidiform mole. Ultrasound is the preferred method for direct visualization in obstetrics to avoid irradiation of mother or fetus.

Detection and Delineation of Abdominal Aortic Aneurysms.—Ultrasound is the current method of choice for these aneurysms. Clot in the lumen, which causes problems for aortography, does not interfere with ultrasound. For dissecting abdominal aneurysms, however, ultrasound is much less reliable than aortography. Thoracic aneurysms are difficult to visualize by ultrasound with present techniques.

Detection of Periaortic and Retroperitoneal Masses of Enlarged Lymph Nodes.—Ultrasound current accuracy is reported to be 80%–90%. However, computerized tomography has equal or better accuracy, and is preferred in many institutions because it visualizes the entire abdomen.

Ocular Examinations.—Although special equipment is needed, ultrasound has proved useful for detection of intraocular foreign bodies and tumors, as well as certain other conditions. This technique is especially helpful when opacity prevents adequate visual examination.

Cardiac Diagnosis.—Ultrasound using M-mode technique is the most sensitive and accurate method for detection of pericardial effusion, capable of detecting as little as 50 ml of fluid. A minor drawback is difficulty in finding loculated effusions. Mitral stenosis can be diagnosed accurately, and useful information can be obtained about other types of mitral dysfunction. Ultrasound can also provide information about aortic and tricuspid function, although not to the same degree as mitral valve studies. Entities such as hypertrophic subaortic stenosis and left atrial myxoma can frequently be identified. The thickness of the left ventricle can be estimated. Finally, vegetations of endocarditis may be detected on mitral, aortic, or tricuspid valves in more than one half of patients. Two-dimensional echocardiography is real-time ultrasound. It can perform most of the same functions as M-mode ultrasound, but in addition it provides more complete visualization of congenital heart defects and is able to demonstrate left ventricle heart wall motion or structural abnormalities in about 70%–80% of patients.

Doppler ultrasound is a special variant that can image blood flow. The Doppler effect is the change in ultrasound sound wave frequency produced when ultrasonic pulses are scattered by red blood cells moving within a blood vessel. By moving the transducer along the path of a blood vessel, data can be obtained about the velocity of flow in areas over which the transducer moves. Most present-day Doppler equipment combines Doppler signals with B-mode ultrasonic imaging ("duplex scanning"). The B-mode component provides a picture of the vessel, whereas the Doppler component obtains flow data in that segment of the vessel. This combination is used to demonstrate areas of narrowing, obstruction, or blood flow turbulence in the vessel.

BIBLIOGRAPHY

Ferris EB III: Noninvasive testing for carotid artery atherosclerosis. *Postgrad Med* 1986; 80:105.

Merritt CRB: Doppler blood flow imaging: integrating flow with tissue data. *Diagn Imag* 1986; 8(11):146.

McMeekin JM, et al: Cardiac nuclear imaging in coronary disease. *Appl Radiol* 1985; 14(6):71.

Gould KL, Mullani N: Dynamic cardiac imaging. *J Nucl Med* 1984; 25:1380.

Reeder GS, et al: The role of two-dimensional echocardiography in coronary artery disease. *Mayo Clin Proc* 1982; 57:247.

Hadlock FP, et al: Real-time ultrasound in the evaluation of the obstetrical patient. *Perinatol Neonatol* 1981; 5:29.

Merritt CRB, et al: Abdominal ultrasound: Clinical application of real time. *Appl Radiol Ultrasound* 1981; 10:83.

Burney BT: The role of ultrasound in the examination of the GI tract. *Appl Radiol Ultrasound* 1980; 9:99.

Cooperberg PL, Burhenne HJ: Real-time ultrasonography: Diagnostic technique of choice in calculous gallbladder disease. *N Engl J Med* 1980; 302:1277.

Duncan JG: Radial scans of the extrahepatic biliary system in obstructive jaundice. *Appl Radiol Ultrasound* 1980; 9:88.

Heidorn A: Ultrasound in management of patients with abdominal aneurysms. *Appl Radiol Ultrasound* 1980; 9:153.

Shaff MI, Walker WJ: Ultrasound in pancreatic disease. *Appl Radiol Ultrasound* 1980; 9:88.

Pertcheck L, et al: Ultrasound evaluation of the liver. *Appl Radiol Ultrasound* 1978; 7:139.

Gorham J: Relationship between ultrasound and computed tomography in whole-body scans. *Appl Radiol Ultrasound* 1978; 7:127.

Smith GV: Ultrasound of the gallbladder. *Appl Radiol Ultrasound* 1978; 7:193.

Weissberg DL, Gosink G: Grey-scale evaluation of the gallbladder. *Appl Radiol Ultrasound* 1978; 7:127.

Wolson AH, Goldberg BB: Grey-scale ultrasonic cholecystography: A primary screening procedure. *JAMA* 1978; 240:2073.

Sanders AD, Sanders RC: The complementary use of B-scan ultrasound and radionuclide imaging techniques. *J Nucl Med* 1977; 18:205.

Williamson B, et al: Ultrasonic examination of the urinary tract. *Appl Radiol* 1976; 5:85.

Computerized Tomography

Originally known as computerized axial tomography (CAT), CT combines radiologic x-ray emission with nuclear medicine–type radiation detectors (rather than direct x-ray exposure of photographic film in the manner of ordinary radiology). Tissue density of the various components of the object or body part being scanned determines how much of the electron beam reaches the detector assembly, similar to conventional radiology. The original machines used a pencil-like x-ray beam that had to go back and forth over the scanning area, with each track being next to the previous one. Current equipment is of two basic types. Some manufacturers use a fan-shaped (triangular) beam with multiple gas-filled tube detectors on the opposite side of the object to be scanned (corresponding to the base of the x-ray beam triangle). The beam source and the multiple detector segment move at the same time and speed in a complete 360-degree circle around the object to be scanned. Other manufacturers use a single x-ray source emitting a fan-shaped beam that travels in a circle around the object to be scanned while outside of the x-ray source path is a complete circle of nonmoving detectors. In all cases a computer secures tissue density measurements from the detector as this is going on and eventually constructs a composite tissue density image similar in many aspects to those seen in ordinary x-rays. The image corresponds to a thin cross-section slice through the object (3–15 mm thick), in other words, a tissue cross-section slice viewed at a right angle (90 degrees) to the direction of the x-ray beam.

Computerized tomography scan times necessary for each tissue slice vary with different manufacturers and with different models from the same manufacturer. The original CT units took more than 30 seconds per slice, second-generation CT units took about 20 seconds per slice, whereas current models can operate at less than 5 seconds per slice.

Computerized tomography is currently the procedure of choice in detection of space-occupying lesions of the CNS. It is also very important (the procedure of choice for some) in detecting and delineating mass lesions of the abdomen (tumor, abscess, hemorrhage, etc.), mass lesions of organs such as the adrenals or pancreas, and retroperitoneal adenopathy. It has also been advocated for differentiation of extrahepatic vs. intrahepatic jaundice (using the criterion of a dilated common bile duct), but ultrasound is still more commonly used for this purpose due to lower cost, ease of performance, and scheduling considerations.

BIBLIOGRAPHY

Davidson AJ, Hartman DS: Imaging strategies for tumors of the kidney, adrenal gland, and retroperitoneum. *CA* 1987; 37:151.

Goodenough DJ, Weaver KE: A decade of progress in computed tomography. *Diag Imag* 1985; 7(11):211.

Freeny PC, et al: Impact of high-resolution computed tomography of the pancreas on utilization of endoscopic retrograde cholangiopancreatography and angiography. *Radiology* 1982; 142:35.

Silberstein EB: New perspectives on the relationship of radionuclide and CT brain imaging. *Appl Radiol* 1981; 10:35.

van Sonnenberg E, Mueller PR: Ultrasound, CT, and fluoroscopic guidance for percutaneous abdominal biopsy. *Appl Radiol* 1981; 10:121.

Kamin PD, et al: Comparison of ultrasound and computed tomography in the detection of pancreatic malignancy. *Cancer* 1980; 46:2410.

Sones PJ: Computed tomography of the retroperitoneum. *Appl Radiol* 1980; 9:40.

Koehler PR, Moss AA: Diagnosis of intra-abdominal and pelvic abscesses by computerized tomography. *JAMA* 1980; 244:49.

Heitzman ER, et al: The role of computerized tomography in the diagnosis of diseases of the thorax. *JAMA* 1979; 241:933.

Epstein AJ, et al: Computerized tomography of the adrenal gland. *JAMA* 1979; 242:2791.

Korobkin M, Palubinskas AJ: CT of the urinary tract. *Appl Radiol* 1978; 7:47.

Scherer U, et al: Computerized tomography and nuclear imaging of the liver. *Eur J Nucl Med* 1978; 3:71.

Brahme FJ: CT scans in cerebrovascular disease. *Appl Radiol* 1978; 7:46.

Goldberg HI, et al: Capability of CT body scanning and ultrasonography to demonstrate the status of the biliary ductal system in patients with jaundice. *Radiology* 1978; 129:731.

Jones SE, et al: Computed tomographic scanning in patients with lymphoma. *Cancer* 1978; 41:480.

Nuclear Medicine Scanning

Nuclear medicine organ scans involve certain compounds that selectively localize in the organs of interest when administered to the patient. The compound is first made radioactive by tagging with a radioactive element. An exception is iodine used in thyroid diagnosis, which is already an element; in this case a radioactive isotope of iodine can be used. An isotope is a different form of the same element with the same chemical properties as the stable element form but physically unstable due to differences in the number of neutrons in the nucleus, this difference producing nuclear instability and leading to emission of radioactivity. After the radioactive compound is administered and sufficient uptake by the organ of interest is achieved, the organ is "scanned" with a radiation detector. This is usually a sodium iodide crystal. Radioactivity is transmuted into tiny flashes of light within the crystal. The location of the light flashes corresponds to the locations within the organ from which radioactivity is being emitted; the intensity of a light flash is proportional to the quantity of radiation detected. The detection device surveys (scans) the organ and produces an overall pattern of radioactivity (both the concentration and the distribution of activity), which it translates into a visual picture of light and dark areas.

Rectilinear scanners focus on one small area; the detector traverses the organ in a series of parallel lines to produce a complete (composite) picture. A "camera" device has a large-diameter crystal and remains stationary, with the field of view size dependent on the size of the crystal. The various organ scans are discussed in chapters that include biochemical function tests referable to the same organ.

The camera detectors are able to perform rapid-sequence imaging not possible on a rectilinear apparatus, and this can be used for "dynamic flow" studies. A bolus of radioactive material can be injected into the bloodstream and followed through major vessels and organs by data storage equipment or rapid (1- to 3-second) serial photographs. Although the image does not have a degree of resolution comparable to that of contrast medium angiography, major abnormalities in major blood vessels can be identified, and the uptake and early distribution of blood supply in specific tissues or organs can be visualized.

Data on radionuclide procedures are included in areas of laboratory test discussion when this seems appropriate.

BIBLIOGRAPHY

Blahd WH (ed): *Nuclear Medicine*, ed 2. New York, McGraw-Hill Book Co, 1971.

Magnetic Resonance Imaging

Magnetic resonance (MR; originally called nuclear magnetic resonance) is the newest imaging process. This is based on the fact that nuclei of many chemical elements (notably those with an uneven number of protons or neutrons such as ^{1}H or ^{31}P) spin ("precess") around a central axis. If a magnetic field is brought close by (using an electromagnet) the nuclei, still spinning, line up in the direction of the magnetic field. A new rate of spin (resonant frequency) will be proportional to the characteristics of the nucleus, the chemical environment, and the strength of the magnetic field. If the nuclei are then bombarded with an energy beam having the frequency of radio waves at a 90-degree angle to the electromagnetic field, the nuclei are pushed momentarily a little out of line. When the exciting radiofrequency energy is terminated, the nuclei return to their position in the magnetic field, giving up some energy. The energy may be transmitted to their immediate environment (called the "lattice," the time required to give up the energy and return to position being called the "spin-lattice relaxation time," or T_1), or may be transmitted to adjacent nuclei of the same element, thus providing a realignment response of many nuclei (called "spin-spin relaxation time," or T_2). The absorption of radiofrequency energy can be detected by a spectrometer of special design. Besides differences in relaxation time, differences in proton density can also be detected and measured. Magnetic resonance proton density or relaxation time differs for different tissues and is affected by different disease processes and possibly by exogenous chemical manipulation. The instrumentation can produce computer-generated two-dimensional cross-section images of the nuclear changes that look like CT scans of tissue. Thus, MR can detect anatomical structural abnormality and changes in normal tissue and potentially can detect cellular dysfunction at the molecular level. Several manufacturers are producing MR instruments, which differ in the type and magnetic field strength of electromagnets used, the method of inducing disruptive energy into the magnetic field, and the method of detection and processing of results. Unlike CT, no radiation is given to the patient.

BIBLIOGRAPHY

NIH Consensus Conference: Magnetic resonance imaging. *JAMA* 1988; 259:2132.

Kent DL, Larson EB: Magnetic imaging of the brain and spine. *Ann Intern Med* 1988; 108:402.

Baker HL, et al: Magnetic resonance imaging in a routine clinical setting. *Mayo Clin Proc* 1985; 60:75.

Kulkarni MV, et al: Clinical magnetic resonance imaging with nuclear medicine correlation. *J Nucl Med* 1985; 26:611.

Koutcher JA, Burt CT: Principles of nuclear magnetic resonance. *J Nucl Med* 1984; 25:101.

Drew PG: The NMR phenomenon: Putting spinning nuclei to work. *Diagn Imag* 1983; 5(8):41.

36 Appendix: A Compendium of Useful Data and Information

TABLE 36–1.
Effects of Age on Laboratory Tests

Apparent age-related increase in abnormal results has been reported in a wide variety of tests in patients over age 50 yr

1. Antinuclear antibodies, rheumatoid factor; VDRL; serum globulin (*Br J Ven Dis* 1966; 42:40. *Ann Rheum Dis* 1969; 28:431.)
2. Cholesterol, triglyceride
3. BUN (*J Lab Clin Med* 1969; 73:825.)
4. Oral GTT values
5. ESR
6. Creatinine clearance
7. D-Xylose test
8. Serum calcium (*N Engl J Med* 1969; 281: 367. However, most investigators do not find any significant difference)
9. Gastric acidity
10. T_3-RIA

Reference ranges for premature infants often are different from those of full-term infants, which, in turn, are frequently different from those of adults. In some cases the values change rapidly within the first week of life; in others, there is a slow change to adult levels at some time during childhood or adolescence. In some cases, notably alkaline phosphatase, high values relative to adult norms persist throughout childhood and adolescence. (Selected references: *Am J Med Technol* 1982; 48:7. Meites S (ed): *Pediatric Clinical Chemistry*, ed 2. Washington, DC, American Association of Clinical Chemists, 1981.)

SUBSTANCES THAT INTERFERE WITH CERTAIN LABORATORY TESTS

(Compiled from various sources; see especially *Clin Chem* 1975; 21:1D, and *Am J Med Technol* 1981; 47:183.)

The following does not pretend to be an all-inclusive list. It should also be noted that a substance that is reported to interfere with a particular test may or may not interfere with every method for that test and may not interfere with all modifications of the same method. In some cases the degree of interference is dose related (a large amount of interfering substance may be necessary to produce a clinically significant degree of change). In most cases the laboratory does not have any data from its own testing or experience as to which substances or conditions interfere with the particular test methods that it uses. Most of this information is derived from the literature.

TABLE 36–2.

Substances That Interfere With Certain Laboratory Tests

- I. Pheochromocytoma tests
  - A. Catecholamines (elevated)
    - Poor preservation during collection
    - Large doses of B complex vitamins
    - Certain broad-spectrum antibiotics (ampicillin, Declomycin, Erythromycin, tetracyclines) which produce fluorescence
    - Formaldehyde-forming drugs (Mandelamine, Uritone) in urine
    - Ascorbic acid (vitamin C)
    - Bananas
    - Coffee or tea
    - Chlorpromazine (Thorazine)
    - Hydralazine (Apresoline)
    - Methyldopa (Aldomet)
    - Isuprel or epinephrine-like drugs (inhalation)
    - Quinine or quinidine
    - Reserpine
    - Theophylline (Aminophylline)
    - Chloral hydrate
    - Levodopa
    - Propranolol (Inderal)
    - Salicylates
    - Uremia (fluorescent substances)
  - B. Vanillylmandelic acid (VMA)
    1. Screening tests (Gitlow method, etc.)
       - Tea
       - Coffee
       - Citrus fruits
       - Vanilla
       - Bananas
       - Chocolate
       - Aspirin
       - 5-Hydroxyindoleacetic acid (5-HIAA)
    2. Fluorescent techniques
       - Same medications as catecholamines
       - Glyceryl guaiacolate (cough medicines)
  - C. Metanephrines
    1. Increase
       - Levodopa
       - Nalidixic acid
       - Bananas
       - Tetracyclines
       - MAO inhibitors
       - Chlorpromazine
       - Hydralazine (Apresoline)
       - Imipramine (Tofranil)
       - Phenacetin
    2. Decrease
       - Reserpine
       - Clonidine (Catapres)
       - Guanethidine
       - IVP contrast media that contain methylglucamide (Renografin, etc.)
- II. 5-Hydroxyindoleacetic acid (5-HIAA)
  - A. Substances that contain large amounts of serotonin (increases any method)
    - Tomatoes
    - Red plums
    - Avocado

(Continued.)

TABLE 36–2 (cont.).

- Eggplant
- Bananas

B. Method of Udenfriend

1. Increase
   - Methocarbamol (Robaxin)
   - Diazepam (Valium)
   - Glyceryl guaiacolate (many proprietary cough medicines)
   - Methenasin carbamate (several proprietary muscle relaxants)
   - Phenacetin
2. Decrease
   - Aspirin
   - Levodopa
   - Phenothiazines

III. 17-Hydroxycorticosteroids (17-OHCS)

A. Increase
- Acetone (in urine)
- Ascorbic acid (vitamin C)
- Atarax
- Chloral hydrate
- Colchicine
- Doriden
- Estrogens or contraceptive drugs
- Fructose (in urine)
- Glucose (in urine)
- Librium
- Mandelamine
- Meprobamate
- Monase
- Oleandomycin
- Paraldehyde
- Quinine or quinidine
- Reserpine
- Spironolactone
- Thorazine and similar phenothiazines
- Valmid
- Vistaril

B. Decrease
- Apresoline
- Phenergan
- Reserpine
- Salicylate

IV. 17-Ketosteroids (17-KS)
- Acetone (in urine)
- Amphetamine
- Atarax (Vistaril)
- Cephalothin
- Diamox
- Digitoxin
- Diuril
- Doriden
- Librium
- Meprobamate
- Metabolites of progesterone (in urine)
- Nalidixic acid (NegGram)
- Oleandomycin
- Penicillin
- Pyridium
- Quinine
- Reserpine
- Seconal
- Spironolactone
- Thorazine
- Valmid

V. Anticoagulants

A. Drugs that potentiate sodium warfarin (Coumadin) (increase PT)
- Acetaminophen (Tempra, Tylenol)
- Allopurinol (Zyloprim)
- *p*-Aminosalicylic acid
- Aspirin (>1 gm/day)
- Cephalosporin antibiotics (cefamandole, cefotetan, cefoperazone, moxalactam)
- Chloral hydrate
- Chlorpropamide (Diabinese)
- Cimetidine (Tagamet)
- Clofibrate (Atromid-S)
- Isoniazid
- Kanamycin
- MAO inhibitors
- Mefenamic acid (Ponstel)
- Methyldopa (Aldomet)
- Methylphenidate (Ritalin)
- Metronidazole (Flagyl)
- Nalidixic acid (NegGram)
- Nandrolone phenpropionate (Durabolin)
- Phenylbutazone (Butazolidin)

(Continued.)

TABLE 36–2 (cont.).

Dextran	Phenyramidol (Analexin)
Dextrothyroxine (Choloxin) and cholestyramine	Phenytoin (Dilantin)
	Probenecid (Benemid)
Diazoxide (Hyperstat)	Quinidine and quinine
Disulfiram (Antabuse)	Reserpine
Estrogens	Sulfas
Ethacrynic acid (Edecrin)	Thiouracil drugs
Glucagon	Thyroid hormone
Hepatotoxic agents	Tolbutamide (Orinase)
Ibuprofen	Trimethoprim-sulfamethoxazole
Indomethacin (Indocin)	Vitamin B complex
B. Drugs that decrease response to sodium warfarin (decrease PT)	
Antacids	Glutethimide (Doriden)
Barbiturates	Griseofulvin
Corticosteroids	Haloperidol (Haldol)
Digitalis	Meprobamate
Diuretics (except ethacrynic acid)	Paraldehyde
Estrogens	Rifampin
Ethchlorvynol (Placidyl)	
C. Drugs that antagonize action of heparin	
Antihistamine (large doses)	Phenothiazines (Thorazine, etc.)
Digitalis	Polymyxin B (Coly-Mycin)
Penicillin	Tetracycline
D. Drugs affecting platelets	
1. Drugs producing thrombocytopenia	
Acetazolamide	Gold compounds
Antihistamines	Heparin
Aspirin	Hydroxychloroquin
Amiodarone (10%–15% cases)	Isoniazid (INH)
Amrinone	Penicillin
Cephalothin	Phenothiazines
Chlorothiazide	Phensuximide
Cimetidine	Phenylbutazone
Carbamazepine (2% of cases)	Phenytoin
Barbiturates	Quinine
Desipramine	Quinidine
Diazepam	Rifampin
Digitoxin	Sulfas
Ethanol	Trimethoprim
2. Drugs interfering with platelet function	
Acetaminophen	Heparin
Ampicillin	Ibufenac
Azlocillin	Ibuprofen
Aspirin	Meclofenamic acid
Antihistamines	Mefenamic Acid
Atropine	Moxalactam
Atromide	Nafcillin
Beta-blocking agents	Naproxen
Carbenicillin	Nitrofurantoin
Cocaine	Phenergan
Clofibrate	Phenothiazines
Dextran	Phenylbutasine
Diphenhydramine	Piperacillin
Dipyridamole	Theophylline
Ethacrynic acid	Ticarcillin
Ethanol	Tricyclic antidepressants
Furosemide	Vincristine
Gentamicin	
Glycerol guaiacolate	

(Continued.)

TABLE 36–2 (cont.).

VI. Drugs that interfere with absorption
Phenytoin (Dilantin): blocks folic acid; decreases B12 and D-xylose
Cholestyramine: decreases digoxin
Colchicine: decreases B12, carotene, D-xylose
Kaolin (Kaopectate): decreases digoxin
Neomycin: blocks folic acid; decreases B12 and D-xylose

VII. Effects of estrogens (birth control pills)
Decrease albumin, glucose tolerance, T_3 uptake test, haptoglobin, plasma cholinesterase, vitamin B6, vitamin C; may decrease folic acid
Increase transferrin, TBG (thus alters various T_4- and T_3-RIA tests), triglycerides, total lipids, serum iron, iron-binding capacity, plasma cortisol, urine aldosterone, serum alpha-2 globulins, growth hormone, alpha-1 antitrypsin, neutrophil alkaline phosphatase, ceruloplasmin, RBC cholinesterase, serum vitamin A and carotene, GGT, HDL cholesterol, prolactin, plasma renin activity, triglycerides
Potentiates sodium warfarin (Coumadin) (increases PT); invalidates metyrapone test

VIII. Technicon Autoanalyzer drug effects
AST increased by diabetic acidosis, p-aminosalicylic acid, hydroxyzine pamoate (Vistaril), barbiturates
Glucose oxidase-peroxidase interference by vitamin C, hydralazine, iproniazid (Marsilid), isoniazid (INH), tolazamide (Tolinase), acetaminophen
Neocuproine glucose increased by reducing substances (15 mg/100 ml creatinine plus 10 mg/100 ml uric acid raises glucose 20 mg/100 ml)
Lipemia decreases cholesterol, bilirubin, albumin, LDH, alkaline phosphatase

IX. Miscellaneous
Alkaline phosphatase: increased by many brands of human serum albumin (derived from placental tissue)
Uric acid: increase in (phosphotungstate) reduction methods from aspirin, hemolysis, protein, and from theophylline, caffeine, theobromine (coffee, tea, colas)
Urinary estrogens: **increased** by drugs that stimulate hepatic microsomal pathway; diuretics, licorice, glucosuria, urinary tract infection, ampicillin, neomycin; **decreased** by adrenocorticosteroids, thyroxine, oral contraceptives (progestins), cholestasis, mandelamine, meprobamate
AST: erythromycin increases colorimetric methods, but not UV methods
Heparin: antagonized by ascorbic acid; may cause thrombocytopenia; increases T_4 up to 60 min after injection; increases free thyroxine; increases plasma insulin and decreases gentamicin when used as specimen anticoagulant
Plasma cortisol: spironolactone produces increase by fluorometric method
Lithium therapy: frequent slight elevation of TSH and decrease in T_4; occasional clinical hypothyroidism; increased neutrophils
Creatinine: increased by vitamin C (large doses): some cephalosporin antibiotics (Table 36–2, XX); bilirubin (kinetic Jaffe reaction); severe lipemia (increase or decrease is method dependent); severe hemolysis; methyldopa; ketones; indirectly affected by nephrotoxic drugs
Porphobilinogen: false positive from phenothiazines
Methyldopa: may increase bilirubin, reducing-substance methods for creatinine, uric acid and glucose, SMA 12/60 AST method, catecholamines or VMA; may produce lupus erythematosus (LE) syndrome
Levodopa: may produce elevated BUN, AST, ALT, LDH, bilirubin, uric acid (phosphotungstic acid method), alkaline phosphatase, and positive Coombs' test
Betadine skin antiseptic: may cause increase in serum potassium, phosphate, uric acid
Cimetidine (Tagamet): decreases metabolism (increases blood levels) of quinidine, procainamide, diazepam (Valium), chlordiazepoxide, sodium warfarin (Coumadin), theophylline, propranolol, phenytoin, prazepam (Centrax), clorazepate (Traxene); may decrease sperm count as much as 50%
Aspirin: increases bleeding time, increases VMA screening tests, 5-HIAA, PT time (large doses); decreases T_4, uric acid, amylase (about 20% each); interferes with urine HVA test
Lipemia effect (severe lipemia): The literature reports increased hemoglobin, MCH, and MCHC by the Coulter Counter methods, increased AST, ALT, albumin, total protein, bilirubin, calcium, creatinine, fibrinogen, glucose, iron, and BUN by spectrophotometric methods; glycosylated hemoglobin by column methods; and various RIA tests using dextran-coated charcoal or PEG separation methods. The literature reports decreased serum and urine amylase and serum lipase; and sodium by flame photometry. EMIT therapeutic drug assay may also be affected.

Effects of lipemia differ to some extent according to the composition of the lipid (triglyceride per

(Continued.)

TABLE 36–2 (cont.).

se or chylomicrons) and the test methodology. For example, total bilirubin is mildly decreased by lipemia when assayed on the Technicon SMAC, but is markedly increased when assayed on the Abbott VP. Each laboratory should determine the effects of lipemia on their own test systems, but few do so. Many do not even report that the serum is lipemic.

A current (but not yet completed) study in my laboratory has disclosed the following results (Abbott VP system):

Increased test results: total bilirubin (200%–800%), serum cholesterol (20%–200%), serum calcium (10%–60%), and serum LDH (5%–35%).

Decreased test results: serum creatinine (10%–60%).

Inconsistent changes: serum albumin, AST, uric acid, alkaline phosphatase.

Clinically insignificant changes: serum glucose, BUN; sodium and potassium using ionselective electrode methodology.

Clinically significant changes began to appear when the triglyceride value rose above 1,000 mg/100 ml and were invariably present when the triglyceride value was more than 1,500 mg/100 ml. There was a general trend (with some individual variation) toward increasing abnormality with increasing triglyceride level. Uncommonly, abnormality appeared at levels below 1,000 (lowest was 550).

Hemolysis effect (severe intravascular, or artifactual): increases LDH and potassium: may increase uric acid, AST, ALT, and serum iron to varying degree; decreases T_4; can interfere with EMIT methods

X. Digitalis
- A. Conditions that increase risk of digitalis toxicity
  - Renal function decrease (especially when serum creatinine is increased)
  - Hypokalemia (diuretic or steroid therapy, cirrhosis, diabetic acidosis)
  - Hemodialysis
  - Hypothyroidism
  - Liver disease (hypokalemia and thiamine deficiency)
- B. Drugs that potentiate digitalis effects
  - Adrenergic drugs (ephedrine, isoproterenol [Isuprel], etc.)
  - Amiodarone
  - Calcium intravenous therapy
  - Diuretics (except spironolactone)
  - Gallopamil
  - Guanethidine (Ismelin)
  - Indomethacin
  - Insulin
  - Intravenous glucose in water
  - Nifedipine
  - Propranolol
  - Quinidine
  - Reserpine (Serpasil)
  - Thyroid hormone
  - Verapamil (Calan)
- C. Drugs that may decrease digitalis effect
  - Cholestyramine
  - Diphenylhydantoin (Dilantin)
  - Kaopectate
  - Oral aminoglycoside antibiotics
  - Phenobarbital
  - Phenylbutazone

XI. Drugs that affect kidney function
- Amphotericin B
- Aminoglycoside antibiotics (gentamicin, kanamycin, neomycin, tobramycin, amikacin)
- Diuretics
- Guanethidine (Ismelin)
- Indomethacin (Indocin)
- Lithium (concentration ability)
- Methicillin
- Methyldopa (Aldomet)
- Polymyxin antibiotics (colistin, Coly-Mycin, polymyxin B)
- Tetracyclines (intravenous)

XII. Serum cholinesterase (decrease)
- Atropine
- Barbiturates
- Chloroquine
- Epinephrine

(Continued.)

TABLE 36–2 (cont.).

Opiates
Phenothiazines
Prostigmin
Quinidine

XIII. Effects of ascorbic acid (vitamin C) in large doses

A. Increased

Tests that depend on reducing-substance reactions: creatinine, blood glucose (neocuproine, Folin-Wu, ferricyanide methods), uric acid, urine glucose by Benedict's or Clinitest methods

B. Decreased

Antagonist to heparin
Serum or urine glucose using glucose oxidase dipsticks
Serum vitamin B12
Urine dipstick tests for nitrite, bilirubin, leukocyte esterase
Occult blood using orthotolidine (Hematest or Hemastix)

C. Interferes with blood volume determination using RBC tagging

XIV. Drugs that may affect liver function

A. Exclusively cholestatic (androgenic/anabolic steroids, estrogens)

Fluoxymesterone (Halotestin)
Methandrostenolone (Dianabol)
Norethandrolone (Nilevar)
Norethindrone (Norlutin)
Norethynodrel (Enovid)

B. Cholestatic plus hepatocellular toxic component

Chlordiazepoxide (Librium)
Erythromycin
Iproniazid (Marsilid)
Meprobamate
Methimazole (Tapazole)
Nicotinic acid
Norethandrolone (Nilevar)
Phenothiazines (Thorazine)
Phenylbutazone (Butazolidin)
Phenytoin (Dilantin)
Tetracycline (intravenous)

C. Cytotoxic

β-Aminosalicylic acid
Azathioprine (Imuran)
Chlorpropamide (Diabinese)
Docusate potassium (Dialose) (laxative)
Gold salts
Halothane
Indocin
Isoniazid (INH)
Methotrexate
Methyldopa
MAO inhibitor (Marsilid, Nardil)
Nitrogen mustards
Novobiocin
Oxacillin
Oxyphenisatin acetate (stool softener ingredient)
Phenacetylurea (Phenurone)
Probenecid
Zoxazolamine (Flexon)

D. Reported but not in detail

Allopurinol
Carbenicillin
Clofibrate
Florantyrone
Lincomycin
Metaxalone
Papaverine
Procainamide
Rifampin
Thiothixene
Tolazamide
Troleandomycin

XV. Drugs that increase renin activity

Hydralazine (Apresoline)
Diazoxide (Hyperstat)
Minoxidil
Sodium nitroprusside
Spironolactone (Aldactone)
Thiazide diuretics

XVI. Drugs other than hydralazine and procainamide reported to produce the LE syndrome (mostly case reports)

(Continued.)

TABLE 36–2 (cont.).

Various anticonvulsants (Dilantin, Mesantoin, Mysoline, Tridione, Zarontin), sulfonamides, estrogens, *p*-aminosalicylic acid, tetracyclines, streptomycin, griseofulvin, propylthiouracil, phenothiazines, Sansert, reserpine, phenylbutazone, quinidine, clofibrate, gold salts

XVII. Drugs that stimualte the hepatic microsome hydroxylation system (microsomal enzyme-inducing drugs)

Psychiatric	Phenobarbital (barbiturates)
	Glutethiamide (Doriden)
	Methaqualone
	Meprobamate
Anticonvulsant	Phenobarbital
	Phenytoin (Dilantin)
	Primadone
Antibiotic	Rifampin
Antifungal	Griseofulvin
Anticoagulant	Warfarin sodium (Coumadin)
Oral contraceptives	Progesterone agents
Anti-inflammatory	Phenylbutasone (Butazolidine)
	Aminopyrine
Others	Alcohol
	Marijuana
	Nikethamide
	Cigarette smoking

Drugs or substances that are not microsomal enzyme inducers but that can be affected by drugs which are inducers

Decreased: Propranolol
Serum bilirubin
Serum calcium (to some extent)

Increased: γ-Glutamyltransferase (GGT)

XVIII. Some medications that increase serum prolactin

Estrogens (including oral contraceptives)
Phenothiazines
Tricyclic antidepressants
Haloperidol (Haldol)
Cimetidine (Tagamet)
Opiates
Certain antihypertensives—methyldopa, reserpine
Serotonin
Norepinephrine

XIX. Medications reported to affect phenytoin (Dilantin) blood levels

A. Frequently produce increase
Disulfiram (Antabuse)

B. Sometimes or occasionally produce increase
Benzodiazepine tranquilizers (Librium, Valium)
Estrogens
Ethanol (acute intake)
Ethosuxamide (Zarontin)
Methylphenidate (Ritalin)
Isoniazid (INH)
Phenobarbital (large dose)
Phenothiazine tranquilizers (Thorazine, Compazine)
Phenylbutazone (Butazolidin)
Propoxyphene (Darvon)
Sodium warfarin (Coumadin)
Sulfamethizole (Thiosulfil)

C. Sometimes produce decrease
Carbamazepine (Tegretol)

(Continued.)

TABLE 36–2 *(cont.).*

Ethanol (chronic intake)
Phenobarbital (small dose)
Loxapine (Loxitane)
Salicylates
Sulfonylureas
Valproic acid (Depakene)

XX. Cephalosporin antibiotics that affect creatinine (Jaffe reaction)
A. Cephalosporins that falsely elevate creatinine
Cefoxitin
Cephalothin
Cephaloridine
Cefamandole
Cefazolin
B. Cephalosporins that do not affect creatinine assay
Cefotaxime
Cefalexin
Cephapirin
Moxalactam

XXI. Substances that may cause acute attacks in hepatic porphyrias
A. Antibiotics
Griseofulvin
Sulfonamides
B. Anticonvulsants
Phenytoin (Dilantin)
Primadone
Carbamazepine
Valproic acid
C. Hormones
Estrogens
Progesterone
D. Sedatives/hypnotics
Barbiturates
Glutethimide (Doriden)
Meprobamate
E. Other drugs
Methyldopa
Theophylline
Phenylbutazone
Methyprylon (Noludar)
Chlordiazepoxide (Librium)
Amphetamines
Sulfonylureas
Ergot medications
Ethanol
Arsenic
Amidopyrine

XXII. Substances that affect theophylline blood levels
A. Increases blood levels
Allopurinol (large doses)
Cimetidine
Ciprofloxacin
Erythromycin (>6 days of therapy)
Propranolol
Thiabendazole
B. Decreases blood levels
Cigarettes
Isoproterenol
Marijuana
Phenobarbital
Phenytoin

BIBLIOGRAPHY

Siest G, Galteau M-M: *Drug Effects on Laboratory Test Results.* Littleton, Mass, PSG Publishing Co., 1988.

Affrime MB, Lowenthal DT: Anticonvulsants and drug interactions. *Res Staff Phys,* March 1982, p 94.

Martin EW, et al: *Hazards of Medication,* ed 2. Philadelphia, JB Lippincott Co, 1978.

Weindling H, Henry JB: Drug interaction and clinical laboratory data. *Lab Med* 1975; 6:24.

Young DS, et al: Effects of drugs on clinical laboratory tests. *Clin Chem* 1975; 21:1D.

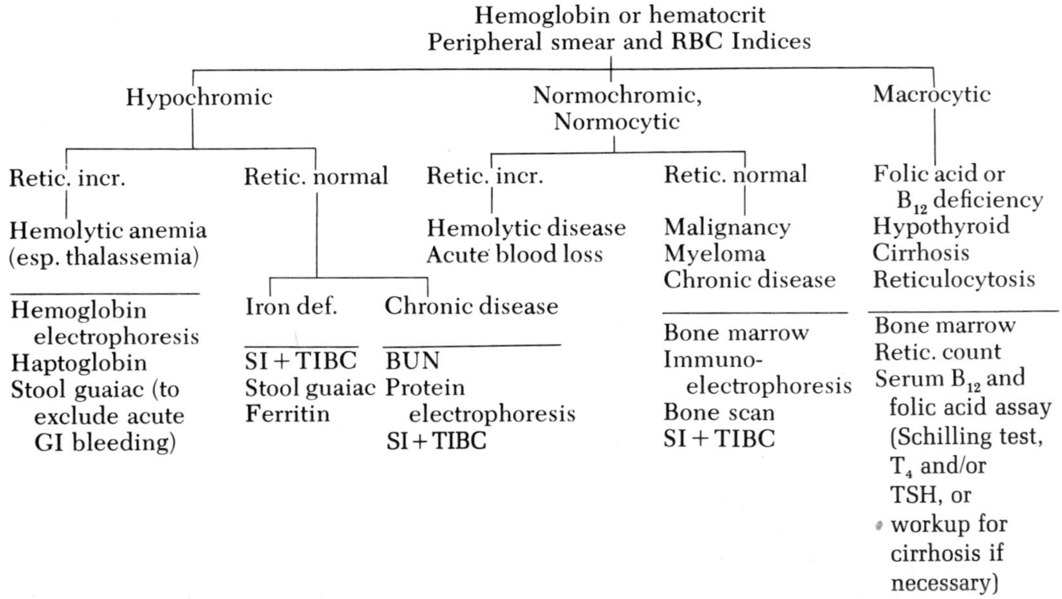

FIG 36–1.
Simplified guide to anemia diagnosis using a minimum of tests aimed at most important disease categories.

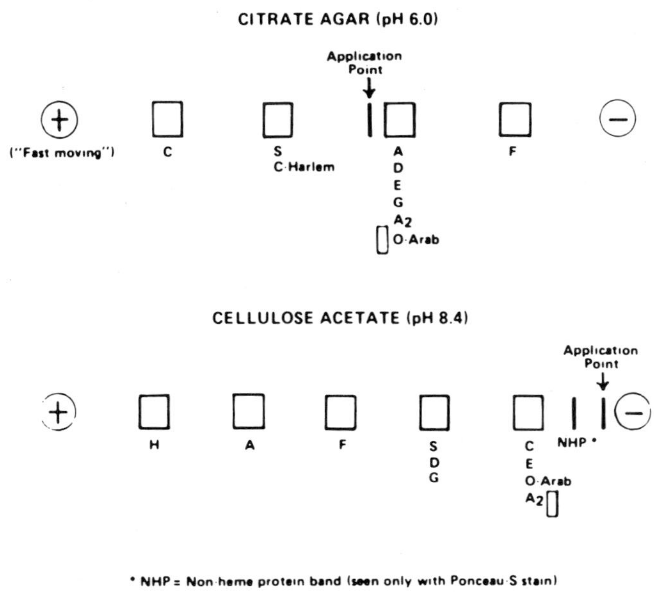

FIG 36–2.
Electrophoretic mobility of the most important hemoglobins on citrate agar and cellulose acetate. The hemoglobins are identified by letter, their position is shown by the square above the letter.

TABLE 36–3.
Normal Hematologic Blood Values at Various Ages*

	Cord	Day 1	Day 2	Day 3	Day 7	Day 14	Day 30
Hb (gm/100 ml, venous blood)	17.0 (13.5–22)	19.0† (14.5–23)	18.5 (15–23)	18 (14–23)	17.5 (13.5–22)	16.5 (13–21.5)	13.5 (10–17.5)
MCV (Fl)	110 (99–120)	109 (98–119)	115 (101–129)	116 (106–126)	114 (88–140)	106 (86–126)	102 (84–121)
Retics (%)	3–7	1.5–6.5	1.5–6.5	1–5	0–1	0–1	0–1
Nucleated RBCs (% of 100 WBCs)	2–5	1–3	0–1	0	0	0	
Platelets (1,000s)	100–290	140–300	150–400		200–470		150–450
WBCs (1,000s)	18.1 (9.0–30.0)	18.9 (9.4–34.0)			12.2 (5.0–21.0)	11.4 (5.0–20.0)	10.8 (5.0–19.5)
Neutrophils (% 100 WBCs)	55	60‡			50	40	35
Lymphocytes (% 100 WBCs)	30	30			35	50	55

(Continued.)

TABLE 36–3 (cont.).

	Month 2	Month 3	Month 6	Month 12	Year 5	Year 10	Adult
Hb (gm/100 ml, venous blood)	12.0 (10–13.5)	11.3 (9.7–13)	12.0 (10.1–14)	12.0 (10.5–13.5)	12.5 (10.7–14.7)	13.0 (10.8–15.5)	M: 14–18 F: 12–16
MCV (Fl)	96 (80–118)		88 (73–100)	79 (71–86)	80 (73–86)	81 (75–87)	90 (80–100)
Retics (%)	0–1						0–1.5
Nucleated RBCs (% of 100 WBCs)	0						0
Platelets (1,000s)							150–400
WBCs (1,000s)			11.9 (6.0–17.5)	11.4 (6.0–17.5)	8.5 (5.0–14.5)	8.1 (4.5–13.5)	7.5 (4.5–10.5)
Neutrophils (% 100 WBCs)			30	30	50	55	60
Lymphocytes (% 100 WBCs)			60	60	40	40	40

*Compiled from various sources. Numbers represent average values; numbers in parentheses indicate reference range.
†Capillary hemoglobin (Hb) is about 2 gm higher than venous; the gap then narrows and disappears by day 7. Neonatal Hb is influenced by amount of blood received from the umbilical cord at delivery.
‡Normal neutrophil count is about 25% higher in capillary than venous blood on day 1 and about 10% higher on day 2.

TABLE 36–4.

Classic Changes in Serum Iron (SI), Total Iron-Binding Capacity (TIBC), and Percent Transferrin Saturation (% TS) in Various Diseases*

	SI	TIBC	% TS
Chronic iron deficiency	Decr	Incr	Decr
Chronic infection	Decr	Decr	Decr
Malignancy (extensive)	Decr	Decr	Decr
Rheumatoid-collagen diseases (tissue inflammation)	Decr	Decr	Decr
Uremia	Decr	Decr	Decr
Starvation (protein malnutrition)	Decr	Decr	N/Incr
Nephrotic syndrome	Decr	Decr	N/Incr
Third trimester of pregnancy	Decr	Incr	Decr
Cirrhosis	Decr	Decr	N/Incr
Hemochromatosis	Incr	Decr	Incr
Iron overload	Incr	Decr	Incr
Oral contraceptives	Incr	Incr	N
Acute viral hepatitis	Incr	Incr	N/Incr
Thalassemia minor	Incr	Decr	Incr/N
Hemolytic anemias	Incr	Decr	Incr
Aplastic/sideroblastic/pyridoxine-deficient anemias	Incr	Decr/N	Incr/N
Megaloblastic anemia	Incr	Decr/N	Incr/N

*Incr, increase; decr, decrease; N, normal. It must be emphasized that some patients in each disease category will have normal values for one or more of SI, TIBC, or % TS, even though decrease or increase is more typical.

TABLE 36–5.

Laboratory Differences in Prothrombin Time (PT) Due to Reagents From Different Manufacturers*

Thromboplastin	Suggested Therapeutic Range (Seconds)†
1. Thrombotime (Pfizer)	24–30
2. Manchester (Poller)	30–53
3. Dried (Hyland)	22–36
4. Fibroplastin (BioQuest)	22–30
5. Simplastin (Warner-Lambert)	22–36
6. Brain (Ortho)	15–30
7. Dried (Dade)	17–26
8. Activated (Dade)	15–21
9. Simplastin-A (Warner-Lambert)	21–30

*From Miale JB: *Laboratory Medicine: Hematology*, ed 6. St Louis, CV Mosby Co, 1982, p 839. Reproduced by permission.

†Each therapeutic range listed represents a reduction of the factor VII level to 10% and to 20% of normal, as obtained by assay of reference plasmas in which factor VII is artificially depleted. The type of readout device (mechanical vs. photooptical clot detection and manual vs. automated methods) may influence results.

TABLE 36–6.
Primary Glomerular Disease (Simplified)*

	Light Microscope	Electron Microscope	Clinical
I. Lipoid nephrosis			
A. Minimal change (Nil disease)	Normal	Endothelial footplate fusion	NS
B. Focal sclerosis	Focal mesangial sclerosis	Footplate fusion + subepithelial deposits	NS
II. Membranous GN	Wire-loop BM thickening; spike and dome pattern in silver stains	1. Extramembranous: diffuse BM subepithelial deposits; EM spikes into deposits	Microscopic hematuria
		2. Membranous: diffuse BM thickening without subepithelial deposits or spikes	NS
III. Proliferative GN			
A. Postinfectious GN (acute poststreptococcal; mesangial GN)	Mesangial cell proliferation	Subepithelial humps	Hematuria; C3 low initially
B. Latent GN	Mild focal and segmental mesangial cell proliferation	Mesangial deposits	Mild hematuria
C. Rapidly progressive GN (subacute; crescentic)	Poststreptococcal lesions + epithelial crescents	1. Subepithelial humps	Hematuria and proteinuria, or NS; C3 low initially
		2. Fibrin deposition	Hematuria and proteinuria, or NS; C3 normal
D. Membranoproliferative GN (mesangiocapillary; hypocomplementary)	Mesangial proliferation + capillary wall thickening	1. Mesangial proliferation + either subepithelial deposits or BM double-contour appearance 2. Lobular GN; same as (1), but with mesangial thickening 3. Dense deposits within BM (dense deposit disease)	Many have persistently low C3; most have hematuria; majority have NS
E. Focal proliferative GN (IgA disease)	Focal cellular proliferation at edge of glomerulus	Focal mesangial hypercellularity	Hematuria
IV. Chronic GN	Widespread glomerular sclerosis; varying degrees of change in remaining glomeruli	Mesangial sclerosis and proliferation	Slowly progressive to renal failure; may have episodes of hematuria or NS

*GN = glomerulonephritis; NS = nephrotic syndrome; BM = basement membrane.

TABLE 36–7.
The Tribe Proteus and its Subdivisions*

Proteus Tribe	Indole +
Genus: *Proteus*	
P. vulgaris	Yes
P. Mirabilis	No
Providencia	
P. rettgeri	Yes
P. alcalifaciens	Yes
P. stuarti	Yes
Morganella	
M. morganii	Yes

*Resistance to ampicillin and cephalothin is characteristic of *Enterobacter, Serratia,* and indole-positive *Proteus* tribe organisms.

TABLE 36–8.
Nephritogenic Strains of Lancefield Group A Streptococci

4	25
12 (Most frequent)	Red Lake
18	

TABLE 36–9.
Enteropathogenic Strains of *E. coli*
(Serotypes Reported to Cause Infant Diarrhea)

O26:B6*	O119:B17
O55:B5	O125:B15
O86:B7	O126:B16
O111:B4	O127:B8
O119:B11	O127:B12

*O refers to somatic antigen, B to one of the "capsule antigens.

TABLE 36–10.
Classification of Legionella Organisms

Species	Strain*
L. pneumophilia	Philadelphia
	Pontiac
L. bozemanii	WIGA
L. dumoffii	Tex-KL
L. micdadei	TATLOCK
	HEBA
	Pittsburgh agent
L. gormanii	LS-13

*Not all strains are included.

TABLE 36–11.
Normal Body Flora

- **Mouth**
  - More common
    - Anaerobic streptococci
    - Aerobic streptococci (not group A)
    - Anaerobic *Spirochetes*
    - *Staph, epidermidis*
    - *Lactobacillus*
    - *Pneumococcus*
    - *Bramhamella catarrhalis*
    - *Bacteroides* sp., *Veillonella* sp.
    - Nonpathogenic *Neisseria*
    - *Candida* fungi
  - Less common
    - *Strep. pyogenes* (occasionally)
    - *Neisseria meningitidis*
    - *Staph. aureus*
    - *Haemophilus influenzae*
    - Enterobacteriaceae
    - *Actinomycetes*
- **Throat** (nasopharynx and oropharynx)
  - More common
    - Alpha- and nonhemolytic streptococci
    - Nonpathogenic *Neisseria*
    - *Staph. aureus*
    - *Diphtheroids (Corynebacteria* sp.)
    - *Haemophilus influenzae* (40%–80% population)
    - *Pneumococcus* (20%–40% population)
  - Less common
    - *Strep. pyogenes* (group A) (5%–20% of population*)
    - *Neisseria meningitidis* (5%–20% population)
    - Enterobacteriaceae
    - *Bacteroides*
    - *Candida* fungi
- **Nose**
  - More common
    - Diptheroids
    - *Staph. epidermidis*
    - Non–group A streptococci
    - *Staph. aureus* (20%–80% adult population)
    - *Haemophilus* sp.
  - Less common
    - *Pneumococcus* (5%–15% population)
    - *Haemophilus influenzae* (5%–10% population)
    - Neisseria meningitidis (5% [0%–15%] of population)
    - *Streptococcus pyogenes* (occasionally)*
- **Vagina**
  - More common
    - Gram-neg. anaerobes *(Bacteroides, Veillonella)*
    - Anaerobic streptococci (peptococcus)
    - Aerobic streptococci groups B and D
    - Lactobacilli (Doderlein's bacillus)
    - *Staph. epidermidis*
    - *Staph. aureus*
    - Diphtheroids *(Corynebacteria* sp.)
    - *Corynebacterium vaginalis (Gardnerella)*
    - *Candida* fungi
  - Less common
    - *Listeria monocytogenes*
    - *Mycoplasma (Ureaplasma* sp.)
    - *Neisseria* sp.
    - *Clostridium perfringens* (5% of population)
    - *Actinomyces*
- **Skin**
  - More common
    - *Staph. epidermidis*
    - *Staph. aureus*
    - Diphtheroids *(Corynebacterium* sp.)
    - *Pityrosporum* fungus
  - Less common
    - *Streptococcus* sp. (incl. group A)
    - *Bacillus* sp. (soil bacteria)
    - Anaerobic peptococcus
    - Nontuberculous mycobacteria
    - *Candida* fungi
    - *(Pseudomonas* and Enterobacteriaceae occ.)
- **Eye**
  - More common
    - *Staph. epidermidis*
    - *Haemophilus* sp.
    - Diphtheroids
  - Uncommon
    - *Strep. pyogenes*
    - *Sarcina*
  - *Moraxella* sp.
    - *Neisseria* sp.
    - Pneumococcus
    - Enterobacteriaceae
- **Sterile areas** (selected)
  - Larynx, trachea, bronchi
  - Cerebrospinal fluid
  - Joint fluid
  - Blood
  - Esophagus, stomach; small intestine down to midileum has few bacteria (excepting some non-TB mycobacteria in the stomach) but may be temporarily contaminated by food
- **Sputum**
  - Often contaminated from upper respiratory tract—including most commonly *Staph. aureus, H. influenzae,* diphtheroids, pneumococcus,

(Continued.)

TABLE 36–11 *(cont.)*.

Enterobacteriaceae, *Candida;* predominance of an organism is more important than its presence

Jejunum
- Lactobacilli
- Enterococci

Terminal Ileum
- Colon bacterial population

Colon (95% are anaerobes)
- More common
  - Gram-pos. anaerobic cocci (peptococcus and peptostreptococcus)
  - Gram-pos. anaerobic rods (*Clostridia,* all species)
  - Gram-neg. anaerobes (*Bacteroides* and fusobacterium)
  - Enterobacteriaceae (all species)
  - *Lactobacillus*
  - *Streptococcus* sp. (esp. *S. faecalis)*
- Less common
  - *Pseudomonas*
  - *Staph. aureus* and *epidermidis*
  - *Actinomyces*
  - Non-TB mycobacteria
  - *Treponema* sp.
  - Yeast (esp. *Candida)*
  - *Clostridium difficile*
  - *Bacillus subtilis*

*For clinical purposes not considered normal flora.

BIBLIOGRAPHY

Mackowiak PA: The normal microbial flora. *N Engl J Med* 1982; 307:83.

Larsen B, Galask RP: Vaginal microbial flora: Practical and theoretic relevance. *Obstet Gynecol* 1980; 55(suppl.):100S.

Traymont EC: General or nonspecific host defense mechanisms, in Mandell GL, et al (eds): *Principles and Practice of Infectious Diseases.* New York, John Wiley & Sons, 1979, pp 14–15.

Mikat DM, Mikat KW: *A Clinician's Dictionary Guide to Bacteria and Fungi,* ed 3. Indianapolis, Dista Products Co (Eli Lilly Co), 1978.

TABLE 36–12.

Classification of the Enterobacteriaceae

Tribe	Genera
Escherichieae	*Escherichia* (including Alkalescens-Dispar)
	Shigella
Edwardsielleae	**Edwardsiella*
Salmonelleae	*Salmonella*
	*Arizona
	**Citrobacter* (previous names of several organisms in this group were *E. freundii,* Bethesda-Ballerup, and *E. intermedium)*
Klebsielleae	*Klebsiella*
	Enterobacter (previous name was *Aerobacter)*
	**Hafnia* (sometimes included in *Enterobacter* genus)
	Serratia
Proteae	*Proteus* (including *P. vulgaris* and *P. mirabilis)*
	**Providencia* (includes several species previously included in the genus *Proteus)*
	Morganella (formerly included in the genus *Proteus)*
Yersinieae	*Yersinia* (previously named *Pasteurella)*
Erwinieae	*Erwinia*
	Pectobacterium

*These organisms were originally included in a group called Paracolons (Paracolon = resembles *E. coli* but are slow lactose or non-lactose fermenters).

TABLE 36–13.

Widal's Test—Serologic Groups (O Antigens) of the Pathogenic Salmonellae

Group	Organism
A	*paratyphi A*
B	*paratyphi B*
	typhimurium
C	*paratyphi C*
	choleraesuis
	Newport
D	*typhi (typhosa)*
	enteritidis
	sendai
E	*anatum*

TABLE 36–14.

Comparison of Tests for Hepatitis B Surface Antigen (HBsAg) (Approximate Sensitivity: CEP = 1)

Test	Sensitivity
Counterimmunoelectrophoresis (CEP)	1
Complement fixation (CF)	10–20
Reversed passive latex agglutination (Antigex)	20
Reversed passive hemagglutination (Auscell)	150
Radioimmunoassay (Ausria I)	200
Radioimmunoassay (Ausria II)	1,500

TABLE 36–15.

Causes of Myoglobinemia and Myoglobinuria

- Trauma and ischemic disease
  - Acute myocardial infarct
  - Muscle arterial ischemia
  - Surgical procedures
  - Muscle crush (trauma; pressure while immobile)
  - Burns; electric shock
- Metabolic disorders
  - Alcoholic myopathy
  - Potassium depletion
  - Hypothermia
  - Myxedema
- Muscle exertion
  - Convulsions
  - Delerium tremens
  - Severe exercise
  - Heat cramps
- Muscle disease/inflammation
  - Systemic lupus
  - Muscular dystrophies
  - Dermatomyositis/myositis
- Infections/fever
  - Viral influenza and various viral and bacterial infections
  - Tetanus
  - Gas gangrene
- Toxicity
  - Carbon monoxide
  - Certain drugs
- Miscellaneous
  - Myoglobinemia in renal failure (due to poor excretion)

TABLE 36–16.

Factors That Alter Results of the Overnight Dexamethasone Test for Melancholia

False Positive	False Negative
Conditions	Conditions
Severe physical illness	Addison's disease
Febrile illness	Hypopituitarism
Pregnancy or estrogen intake	
Cushing's syndrome	
Poorly controlled diabetes	
Malnutrition or anorexia nervosa	
Heavy alcohol intake	
Alcohol withdrawal (within 10 days)	
Electroshock (within 48 hours)	
Medications	Medications
Phenytoin	High-dose benzodiazepines
Barbiturates	Cyproheptadine
Meprobamate	
Methaqualone	
Glutethimide	
Methyprylon	
Carbamazepine	
Glucocorticosteroids	

Reference: Ritchie JC, Carroll BJ: A new test to identify depression. *Lab World* 1981; 32:25.

TABLE 36–17.
Rheumatoid Factor Tests

	Rose-Waaler Sensitized Sheep Cell	Poltz-Singer Latex	Hyland RA Test	Eosin Slide
Adult RA	64* (58–78)†	76 (53–94)	82 (78–98)	90 (88–92)
Normal	5.6 (0.3–13)	1.0 (0.2–3)	8 (0.7–15)	5 (0.2–8.6)
Collagen disease	15–39	17–20	14–67	10–50
Procedure	Tube	Tube	Slide	Slide

*Average % positive and reports from various publications.
†Numbers in parentheses refer to the range of values found in different reports.

TABLE 36–18.
Tests for Systemic Lupus Erythematosus (SLE) (Approximate % Positive)

	SLE	Scleroderma	Other Collagen Diseases	Rheumatoid Arthritis	Other
LE cell	60–80	0–20	<5	5–25	Lupoid hepatitis; drugs (hydralazine, procainamide)
Antinuclear antibody	95–100	75–80	10	10–500	Chronic liver disease Thyroid disease Acquired hemolytic anemia Old age
Serum complement (C′)	Low in 60% with active disease	Normal (rarely low)	Normal or high	Normal or high	Normal

TABLE 36–19.
Ideal Urinary Creatinine Excretion

Height		mg Creatinine/24 hr	
ft/in.	cm.	Men	Women
4′10″	147.3		830
4′11″	149.9		851
5′0″	152.4		875
5′1″	154.9		900
5′2″	157.5	1,288	925
5′3″	160	1,325	949
5′4″	162.6	1,359	977
5′5″	165.1	1,386	1,006
5′6″	167.6	1,426	1,044
5′7″	170.2	1,467	1,076
5′8″	172.7	1,513	1,109
5′9″	175.3	1,555	1,141
5′10″	177.8	1,596	1,174
5′11″	180.3	1,642	1,206
6′0	182.9	1,691	1,240
6′1″	185.4	1,739	
6′2″	188	1,785	
6′3″	190.5	1,831	

(Continued.)

TABLE 36–19 (cont.).

Height		mg Creatinine/24 hr	
ft/in.	cm.	Men	Women
6′6″	193	1,891	

Reference: Blackburn GL, Thornton PA: Nutritional assessment of the hospitalized patient. *Med Clin North Am* 1979; 63:1103.

TABLE 36–20.

Useful Fluid and Electrolyte Information*

Normal daily output
- Insensible loss (skin and lungs) 600–1,000 ml/day
- Urine 500–1,500 ml/day

Average composition of certain body fluids (±20%)

	Na	K	Cl (mEq/L)
Gastric	50	10	100
Bile	150	5	100
Small intestine	100	5	100
Perspiration (visible sweating)	30	0	30

Normal production of certain body fluids

Saliva	500–1,500 ml/day
Gastric	1,000–3,000 ml/day
Bile	300–1,000 ml/day
Pancreas	1,000–1,500 ml/day
Small intestine	1,000–2,000 ml/day
Visible sweating (at bed rest and/or high fever)	1,000–2,000 ml/day

Note: Normally, most GI secretions (fluid and electrolytes) are reabsorbed before they reach the rectum.

Daily nutritional requirements

A. Caloric requirements
   1st 10 kg body weight: 100 calories/kg
   10–20 kg body weight: 100 calories plus 50 calories for every kg over 10
   Over 200 kg body weight: 1,500 calories plus 20 calories for every kg over 20

B. Fluid requirements
   1 ml fluid for every calorie needed

C. Electrolyte requirements
   Na: 3 mEq/100 cal
   K: 2 mEq/100 cal
   Cl: 2 mEq/100 cal

*Compiled from various sources.

TABLE 36–21.

Data for Diabetes Tolerance Tests*

I. Intravenous glucose tolerance test
   Most investigators use a standard dose of glucose (in a 50% solution) amounting to 0.33 gm/kg of ideal body weight. Some use a standard dose of 25 gm, regardless of weight. For children, the recommended dose is 0.5 gm/kg.

II. Tolbutamide tolerance test
   Inject 20 ml of sterile Orinase Diagnostic (1 gm of water-soluble sodium tolbutamide) intravenously over 2–3 minutes' time. Blood samples are taken fasting and at 20 and 30 minutes after tolbutamide. At 20 minutes, normal values are less than 75% of FBS. Between 75% and 85% (of FBS) are considered borderline, between 85% and 89% highly suspicious (90% of patients in this group have diabetes), and over 89% are thought to show definite diabetes. At 30 minutes, over 76% of FBS are said to be virtually (99%) diagnostic. Either the 20- or 30-minute value is diagnostic when within the diabetic zone, even if the other is not.

*Note: These are not the normal values to be used when investigating hypoglycemia.

TABLE 36–22.
Blood Glucose Methods

I. Folin-Wu
   Technical: Copper reduction method. Manual only. Historically famous but little used today. Measures reducing substances such as creatinine, uric acid, glutathionine and ergothionine in addition to most sugars.
   Clinical: Performed on whole blood. Results 20–30 mg/100 ml higher than true glucose, but can fluctuate widely, as much as 10–70 mg/100 ml. False increases by metabolic reducing substances as noted and by vitamin C (large doses).
II. Neocuproine
   Technical: Reducing-substance method. Automated only, using serum, on Technicon SMA 12/60.
   Clinical: Results are 15% above manufacturer's stated 110 mg/100 ml fasting upper limit of normal for serum. Same basic interferences as Folin-Wu.
III. Somogyi-Nelson
   Technical: Needs protein-free filtrate. Manual method only. Time-consuming. Whole blood or serum.
   Clinical: Although not entirely specific for glucose, results are fairly close to true glucose values.
IV. Ferricyanide
   Technical: Widely used in Autoanalyzer equipment. Serum only.
   Clinical: Although a reducing method, results are within 5% of true glucose. A considerable increase in uric acid or vitamin C falsely increases values.
V. Orthotoluidine
   Technical: Need boiling apparatus. Manual or automated. Serum only.
   Clinical: Measures glucose and other aldoses; results close to true glucose. Dextran produces false increase.
VI. Glucose oxidase
   Technical: Manual or automated. Serum only. Enzymatic method.
   Clinical: True glucose method. However, in the oxidase-peroxidase modification, false decrease with vitamin C and false increase with hydralazine, iproniazid (Marsilid), INH, acetaminophen, tolazamide (Tolinase), oxazepam (Serax).
VII. Hexokinase
   Technical: Manual or automated. Serum only. Enzymatic method.
   Clinical: True glucose. To date, few interferences reported.

TABLE 36–23.
Criteria for Abnormal Oral Glucose Tolerance Tests Prior to 1979*

	U.S. Public Health Service			Fajans and Conn		University Group Diabetes Program	
	Blood	Serum	Points†	Blood	Serum	Blood‡	Serum‡
Fasting	110	130	1	—	—		
1 hour	170	195	$^1/_2$	160	185		
$1^1/_2$ hour	—	—	—	140	160		
2 hours	120	140	$^1/_2$	120	140	500 or more	600 or more
3 hours	110	130	1	—	—		

*Glucose values in mg/100 ml. *Note:* These criteria are being replaced by the NDDG criteria.
†Definite diabetes = 2 points; possible diabetes = 1 point
‡Sum of fasting, 1-, 2- and 3-hour values in mg/100 ml

BIBLIOGRAPHY

Fajans SS: What is diabetes? Definition, diagnosis, and course. *Med. Clin. North Am.* 1971; 55:793.

Standardization of the oral glucose tolerance test: Report of Committee on Statistics of the American Diabetes Association. *Diabetes* 1968; 18:299.

TABLE 36–24.
Compounds That Interfere With Results of Thyroid Tests*

	PBI or T_4		RAI Uptake		T_3 Uptake
	Effect	Duration	Effect	Duration	Effect
Inorganic iodides	*PBI (Not T_4)*				
Lugol's, KI, SSKI, etc. Ornade	Incr	1–4 wk	Decr	1–3 wk	None
Organic iodine	*PBI (Not T_4)*				
1. X-ray contrast media					
Teridax (gallbladder)	Incr	30 yr	None		None
Cholografin (gallbladder)	Incr	3–4 mo	Decr	3 mo	None
Telepaque (gallbladder)	Incr	6–12 mo	Decr	2 mo	None
Oragrafin (gallbladder)	Incr		Decr		None
Diodrast	Incr	2 wk	Decr	1–3 mo	None
Dionosil (bronchogram)	Incr	1–5 mo	Decr	2–5 mo	None
Lipiodol (bronchogram)	Incr	1–2 yr	Decr	1–3 yr	None
Pantopaque (myelogram)	Incr	3–12 mo	Decr	3–12 mo	None
Hypaque (IVP)	Incr	4–7 days	Decr	1–2 wk	None
Renografin (IVP)	Incr	1–4 wk (?)	Decr	1–2 wk	None
Salpix (uterosalpingogram)	Incr	2 wk	Decr	1 mo	None
2. Iodinated vaginal suppositories Floraquin, Vioform, etc. Betadine	Incr	4 wk	Decr	4 wk	None
3. Other					
Metrecal	Incr		?		?
Medications that affect T_4 (also affect PBI)					
Oragrafin (gallbladder)	Incr	?	Decr	?	None
Telepaque (gallbladder)	Incr	6 wk	Decr	8 wk	None
Amiodarone	Incr	4 mo	Decr		?
Thyroxine	Incr	2–4 wk	Decr	1–2 wk	Incr
Thyroid extract	Incr	4–6 wk	Decr	1–2 wk	Incr
Iodothiouracil	Incr	Several wk	Decr	2–8 days	Decr
Estrogens	Incr	2–4 wk	Occasional incr		Decr
Triiodothyronine (T_3)	Decr	2–4 wk	Decr		Decr/NL
Propylthiouracil (PTU) or methimazole (Tapazole)	Decr	5–7 days	Decr	2–8 days	Decr
Halothane	Incr		?		?
Barbiturates	NL/decr		None		NL/incr
Thiocyanate	Decr	2–3 wk	Decr	2–8 days	Decr
Dilantin	Decr	7–10 days	None		Incr[†]
Furosemide[‡]	Decr		?		Incr
Androgens	Decr	3 wk	None		Incr
Adrenal corticoids or ACTH	NL/decr	1–2 wk	Decr	1 wk	Incr
Salicylates (large doses)	Decr		Decr		Incr (?)
Phenylbutazone	Decr	2 wk	Decr		Incr
Perphenazine (Trilafon) after 6–10 wk of treatment	Occasional incr		?		Occ decr
Chlorpromazine (Thorazine)	NL/decr		Decr/NL		NL/decr
Heroin/methadone	NL/Incr		None		NL/decr
Heparin	NL/Incr[§]		None		None
Antihistamine (without iodine)	None		Decr	2–7 days	None

(Continued.)

TABLE 36–24 (cont.).

	PBI or T_4		RAI Uptake		T_3 Uptake
	Effect	Duration	Effect	Duration	Effect
Orinase	None		Decr	2–7 days	None
Dicumarol	None		None		Incr
Sulfonamides	Decr (?)		Decr	1 wk	?
p-Aminosalicylic acid or isoniazid (prolonged Rx)	Occasional decr		Decr	1–2 wk	?
Pentothal	?		Decr	1 wk	?
Penicillin (large doses only)	None		None		Incr
Gold salts	Decr	Several wk	None		None
Propranolol	NL/incr[‖]		?		None
Lithium carbonate	NL/decr		Incr		NL/decr

*Incr = increased; Decr = decreased; NL = normal.
†At least one report indicates no effect on T_3U.
‡High doses or low TBG or albumin levels.
§Increased only 15–60 min after administration.
‖Disagreement whether T_4 is unchanged or may be slightly elevated.

TABLE 36–25.
Interpretation of TRH Test*

	Baseline Serum TSH (μU/ml)	Increase in Serum TSH at 30 min (μU/ml)
Euthyroid	≤10 (97% of patients) [usually ≤6; 20% <1.5]	≥2 (95%) [usually 6–30]
Hyperthyroid	≤10 [usually ≤4]	<2
Primary hypothyroid	>10 (93%)	≥2 [usually ≥20]
Secondary hypothyroid (pituitary)	≤10 [usually ≤6]	<2 (60%) 2–50 (40%)
Tertiary hypothyroid (hypothalamus)	≤10 [often <2]	≥2 (95%) <2 (5%)

*500 μg of TRH intravenously.

TABLE 36–26.
Summary of Congenital Adrenal Hyperplasia Variants

Pathways Affected	17-OH-Progesterone to 11-Desoxycortisol		Progesterone to DOC 17-OH-Progesterone to 11-Desoxycortisol		DOC to Corticosterone 11-Desoxycortisol to Cortisol	
Enzyme defect	21-alpha-hydroxylase (partial)		21-alpha-hydroxylase (complete)		11-beta-hydroxylase	
Type	I		II		III	
Genetic sex	Male	Female	Male	Female	Male	Female
Genitalia appearance	Male	Ambiguous	Male	Ambiguous	Male	Ambiguous
Later virilization	Yes	Yes	Yes	Yes	Yes	Yes
Salt-losing crises	No	No	Yes	Yes	No	No
Hypertension	No	No	Yes	No	Yes	Yes
Pathway blocked	Cortisol		Mineralocorticoid Cortisol		Mineralocorticoid after DOC Cortisol	

(Continued.)

TABLE 36–26 (cont.).

Pathways Affected	Pregnenolone to Progesterone 17-OH Pregnenolone to 17-OH-Progesterone DHA to Androstenedione		Pregnenolone to 17-OH-Pregnenolone Progesterone to 17-OH-Progesterone		Cholesterol to Pregnenolone	
Enzyme defect	3-beta-OH dehydrogenase		17-alpha-hydroxylase		Cholesterol 20-alpha-hydroxylase	
Type	IV		V		VI	
Genetic sex	Male	Female	Male	Female	Male	Female
Genitalia appearance	Ambiguous	Female (clitoromegaly)	Female or ambiguous	Female	Female	Female
Later virilization	Yes	±	No (sexual infantilism at puberty)		No (sexual infantilism at puberty)	
Salt-losing crises	Yes	Yes	No	No	Yes	Yes
Hypertension	No	No	Yes	Yes	No	No
Pathway blocked	Mineralocorticoid Cortisol Androgens after DHA		Cortisol Androgens		Mineralocorticoid Cortisol Androgens	

Notes: 1. Refer to Figure 29–2 for the metabolic pathway involved.
2. The pathway 17-OH pregnenolone to 17-OH progesterone is not shown in Figure 29–2.
3. When one metabolic pathway is blocked, production tends to be increased in the other pathways.
4. When a metabolic pathway is blocked, the precursor compound tends to pile up.

BIBLIOGRAPHY

Wenzel KW: Pharmacological interference with in vitro tests of thyroid function. *Metabolism* 1981; 30:717.

PLASMA RENIN

Plasma renin determination may be very helpful in the diagnosis (or exclusion) of primary aldosteronism. However, to interpret results, one must keep in mind certain technical aspects of current methods. Renin is an enzyme. Most enzymes cannot be measured directly but are estimated indirectly by observing their effect on a known quantity of substrate. In the case of renin, the situation is even more complex, since the substrate (which results in production of angiotensin) cannot be directly measured and must be estimated indirectly by observing its effect on an indicator system and comparing the results with a known amount of angiotensin. In addition, renin is a very unstable enzyme and must be kept at freezing temperature as much as possible to preserve its activity. Collection methods are very important; if the specimen is not collected and processed correctly, a false low value may result.

An outline of one possible collection protocol follows. It incorporates a provocative test—low-sodium diet plus upright posture—to help differentiate primary from secondary aldosteronism. Urinary aldosterone determinations should not be collected during a low-salt diet because sodium deficiency stimulates aldosterone secretion. In fact, urine sodium should be obtained on all aldosterone specimens as a check on possible sodium deficiency. The protocol, therefore, incorporates a section with a high-salt diet to ensure proper collection of aldosterone. If desired, a plasma renin specimen may be obtained during this time to help rule out unilateral renal disease. If unilateral renal disease is not a possibility, step 2 may be omitted. If aldosterone collection is not desired, steps 1–3 may be omitted.

It is surprising how little well-documented information of this type is available in recent years. Most, but not all, of the data are derived from autopsy material and therefore presumably represent the maximum chance for organ involvement. However, the data are not uniform in terms of patient clinical course (treatment or no treatment). In the case of bone, the statistics almost certainly underestimate true incidence, because autopsy usually includes only the spine. The purpose of this review is to provide some framework for preoperative

TABLE 36–27.

Protocol for Plasma Renin and Urine Aldosterone Determinations

1. Patient off medications, placed on 9-gm (180-mEq) high-sodium (normal potassium) diet for 4 days. (Note: can use normal diet plus 6 gm salt tablets extra per day.)
2. Fasting plasma renin specimen drawn the morning of the 4th day before patient stands or sits up (specimen 1). (Note: this can be omitted if unilateral renal disease screening is not desired.)
3. Twenty-four-hour urine for aldosterone and sodium collected during the 4th day. (Note: can also get metanephrine determination on the same specimen to rule out pheochromocytoma.)
4. Patient then placed on a 0.5-gm (10-mEq) low-sodium (normal potassium) diet for 3 days.
5. After awakening the morning of the 4th day, the fasting patient is placed upright (standing or leaning; not allowed to sit or lie down) for 2 hours. Lab notified when the 2-hour period will end; patient kept upright until lab draws blood specimen.
6. Plasma renin specimen drawn while patient is still upright (specimen 2); test ends.

Note: Heparinized collection tube is placed in ice water before the specimen is obtained and kept in ice bath as long as possible before the blood is actually drawn. The tourniquet should be released for a few seconds before blood is drawn, since it has been reported that venous stasis may decrease blood renin. The tube is returned to the ice bath immediately after the specimen is drawn and kept in ice water. It is centrifuged still packed in ice and the plasma is withdrawn, frozen immediately and sent to the reference laboratory packed in dry ice (do not send specimen on weekend).

A high-sodium diet decreases aldosterone secretion in normal persons. In patients with hypertension due to primary aldosteronism or unilateral renal disease, aldosterone is elevated. Plasma renin levels should be decreased in normal persons and those with primary aldosteronism, and increased in hypertension due to unilateral renal disease. A low-sodium diet should confirm results. Renin levels should be high in normal persons, whereas the previous elevated renin level seen in unilateral renal disease remains elevated and the decreased level seen in primary aldosteronism remains decreased. (Although some rise in plasma renin may occur, even in primary aldosteronism, values do not reach normal range.)

TABLE 36–28.

Semen Analysis Reference Ranges

Color	Grayish white
pH	7.3–7.8 (literature range, 7.0–7.8)
Volume	2.0–5.0 ml (literature range, 1.5–6.0 ml)
Sperm count	20–250 million/ml (literature range for upper limit varies from 100–250 million/ml)
Motility	>60% motile <3 hours after specimen is obtained (literature range, >40% to >70%)
% Normal sperm	>60% (literature range, >60% to >70%)
Viscosity	Can be poured from a pipet in droplets rather than a thick strand

TABLE 36–29.

Survey of Pregnancy Tests

Pregnancy Test	Sensitivity IU/L (or mIU/ml)	Sensitivity IU/ml	Test Time	Positive (Weeks From Conception)	Positive (Days from LMP)
Ascheim-Zondek (mouse)	600–700	.6–.7	96 hr	2.5–3.0	30–40
Friedman (rabbit)	1,000–5,000	1.0–5.0	48 hr	3.0–4.0	35–41
Male frog	1,000–5,000	1.0–5.0	2 hr	3.0–4.0	35–41
hCG Slide	1,500–3,000	1.5–3.0	2 min	3.0–4.0	35–41
hCG Tube	500–2,000	.5–2.0	2 hr	2.5–4.0	30–40
Modified hCG tube (Neocept, Sensi-Tex)	200–250	.2–.25	1.5–2 hr	2.0–3.0	28–35
Beta-hCG Slide (1st generation)	500–2,000	.5–2.0	2 min	2.5–4.0	30–40

(Continued.)

TABLE 36–29 *(cont.).*

Pregnancy Test	Sensitivity IU/L (or mIU/ml)	Sensitivity IU/ml	Test Time	Positive (Weeks From Conception)	Positive (Days from LMP)
Beta-hCG Tube (1st generation) (UCG Beta-Stat, Beta-Neocept)	150–200	.15–.2	1 hr	2.0–3.0	28–35
Radioreceptor—serum (Biocept-G)	200	.200	1 hr	1.5–2.5	26–35
Beta-hCG (current)—serum/urine	3–50	.003–.050	1–2 hr	1.0–2.0	21–30

TABLE 36–30.

Some Acid Phosphatase Assay Systems With Relative Specificity for Prostatic Acid Phosphatase (No System Is Completely Specific)

Method	Substrate
Less Specific	
King-Armstrong	Phenyl phosphate
Bessey-Lowry	Paranitrophenyl phosphate
Babson-Read	Alpha-naphthyl phosphate
More Specific	
Bodansky	Beta-glycerophosphate
Roy	Thymolphthalein monophosphate

TABLE 36–31.

Frequency of Metastases to Certain Organs (%)*

Primary Site	Lymph Nodes	Liver	Lungs	Bone	Brain
Urinary bladder	30–40 (12–85)	15–30 (9–43)	20–30 (15–40)	15–40 (2–55)	Rare
Prostate	65–85 (65–100)	20 (20–24)	40 (13–66)	70 (33–92)	Uncommon
Lung	70–80 (64–93)	30–40 (30–58)	—	20–40 (15–45)	15–20 (11–41)
Breast	70–75 (65–80)	40–60 (33–65)	55–60 (54–61)	45–65 (44–78)	10–15 (6–29)
Colon	50 (12–58)	30–60 (24–83)	10–20 (5–38)	6 (3–11)	2 (1–4)
Uterus (corpus)	14	1–28	3–30	3	Rare
Uterus (cervix)	65 (46–77)	20–40 (9–42)	15–40 (4–52)	5–15 (1–20)	Uncommon
Melanoma	Frequent	39–68	7	2	5–39
Stomach	60–80 (50–89)	35–45 (33–68)	10–25	5–7 (3–10)	1–12
Kidney	40 (16–89)	35–45 (12–49)	50–60 (34–71)	30–40 (23–81)	7–10 (3–15)

*Parentheses enclose range found in the literature. Lack of parentheses indicates average expected frequency.

workup in patients with cancer. If an organ has low metastatic potential as reflected in autopsy findings, presumably at an early stage the metastatic potential would be still lower, and scan of that organ would probably have a low cost/benefit ratio.

ECTOPIC TUMOR HORMONE PRODUCTION

Tumors may develop in certain organs that produce hormones and as a result are frequently associated with clinical syndromes.

TABLE 36–32.
Ectopic Tumor Hormone Production

Syndrome	Usual Etiology	Hormone Secreted	Ectopic Tumor
Hyperthyroidism	Graves' or Plummer's disease	T_3/T_4	Ovarian teratoma (T_4) Choriocarcinoma (TSH)
Elevated calcitonin	Thyroid medullary carcinoma	Calcitonin	Lung carcinoma
Cushing's syndrome	Adrenal or pituitary tumor	Cortisol or ACTH	Lung small cell carcinoma (ACTH) Thymoma Various other tumors
Hypoglycemia	Pancreatic beta islet cell tumor (insulinoma)	Insulin	Massive fibrosarcomas Hepatoma
Hypercalcemia	Parathyroid adenoma	Parathyroid hormone	Lung small cell carcinoma PTH) Hypernephroma Myeloma Metastatic carcinoma to bone
Inappropriate ADH syndrome	Hypothalamic disorder	ADH	Lung carcinoma
Polycythemia	Polycythemia vera	Erythropoietin	Hepatoma Hypernephroma Cerebellar hemangioblastoma
Elevated gonadotropin	Choriocarcinoma	hCG	Testicular tumors Lung carcinoma
Elevated catecholamines	Adrenal pheochromocytoma	Catecholamines	Neuroblastoma
Carcinoid syndrome	GI tract carcinoid	Serotonin	Lung small cell carcinoma Lung carcinoid
Virilization	Adrenal carcinoma	Androgens	Testis Leydig cell tumor Ovarian arrhenoblastoma

TABLE 36–33.
Glycogen Storage Diseases (Glycogenoses)

Type I:	Glucose-6-phosphatase deficiency (hepatorenal; von Gierke's)
Type II:	Acid maltase deficiency (Pompe's)
Type III:	Debranching enzyme deficiency (limit dextranosis; Cori)
Type IV:	Branching enzyme deficiency (amylopectinosis; Anderson)
Type V:	Myophosphorylase deficiency (McArdle)
Type VI:	Liver phosphorylase deficiency (Hers)
Type VII:	Phosphofructokinase deficiency
Type VIII:	Hepatic phosphorylase kinase deficiency

Diagnosis: Liver in types I, III, IV, VI and VIII; muscle in types II, III, V and VII (glycogen content and enzyme analysis).

TABLE 36–34.
Muscular Dystrophies

Duchenne's
Limb-girdle
Fascioscapulohumeral
Myotonic dystrophy/atrophy
Myotonia congenita
Ocular myopathies
Congenital muscular dystrophy

TABLE 36–35.
Congenital Myopathies

Central core disease
Nemaline (rod) myopathy
Myotubular (centronuclear) myopathy

TABLE 36–36.
Sphingolipid Storage Diseases

Disease	Lipid	Diagnosis by WBC	Diagnosis by Fibroblast Culture	Diagnosis by Serum Enzyme Assay
A. Glycolipid storage diseases				
1. Ganglioside storage				
Tay-Sachs	GM_2	Yes	Yes	Yes
Sandhoff (hexosamidase A + B deficiency)	Globoside and GM_2	Yes	Yes	Yes
Metachromatic leukodystrophy	Sulfatide	Yes	Yes	Yes
Generalized gangliosidosis	GM_1	Yes	Yes	No
2. Ceramide storage				
Gaucher's	Glucosyl	Yes	Yes	No
Krabbe's (globoid leukodystrophy)	Galactosyl	Yes	Yes	No
Fabry's*	Trihexoside	Yes	Yes	Yes
Lactosyl ceramidosis	Lactosyl	No	Yes	No
Niemann-Pick	Sphingomyelin	Yes	No	No
Farber's	Ceramide	?	Yes	?
Fucosidosis	H-isoantigen	Yes	Yes	Yes
B. Other lipid storage diseases				
Wolman's†	Triglyceride (neutral lipid) and cholesterol esters	No	?	Yes
Refsum's‡	Phytanic acid	No	Yes	Yes

*Fabry's disease is transmitted as a sex-linked (X-linked) trait; all of the remainder are transmitted as an autosomal recessive trait.
†Calcification in adrenals on x-ray is typical.
‡Plasma fatty acids can be analyzed for phytanic acid.

TABLE 36–37.
Disorders of Connective Tissue (Mucopolysaccharidoses)

Name	Physical Anomalies	Mental Deficiency	Urinary Mucopolysaccharides	Diagnosis by Fibroblast Culture	Diagnosis by WBC	Diagnosis by Serum Enzyme Assay
Hurler	Marked	Moderate	Dermatan sulfate (chondroitin sulfate B) Heparan (heparitin) sulfate (approx. 2:1)	Yes	No	No
Hunter	Moderate	Variable or none	Dermatan sulfate and heparan sulfate (approx. 1:1)	Yes	No	No
Sanfillipo A and B	Mild	Marked	Heparan sulfate	Yes	No	No (Type A) Yes (Type B)
Morquio	Marked	None	Karatan sulfate	Yes	No	No
Scheie	Mild	None	Dermatan sulfate and Heparan sulfate (approx. 2:1)	No	No	No
Maroteaux-Lamy	Moderate	None	Dermatan sulfate	Yes	No	Yes

Note: All are transmitted as autosomal recessive except for Hunter, which is sex-linked.

TABLE 36–38.
Selected Skin Tests

Disease	Test	Antigen	Time	Positive
Brucellosis*	Brucellin	Brucellergen (killed bacteria)	24–48 hr	>5 mm reaction
Tularemia	Foshay	Killed bacteria	48 hr	>5 mm reaction
Lymphogranuloma venereum	Frei	Killed virus	48 hr	
Echinococcosis	Casoni	Fluid from hydatid cyst	15–30 min	"Immediate" reaction
Scarlet fever	Schultz-Charlton	Antitoxin	24 hr	Blanched area
Diphtheria susceptibility	Schick	Diphtheria toxin	3–6 days	Reaction >10 mm
Scarlet fever susceptibility	Dick	Erythrogenic toxin	24 hr	Reaction >10 mm
Sarcoidosis	Kveim	Sarcoid tissue	6 wk	
Tuberculosis	Mantoux	PPD or OT	24–48 hr	
Systemic fungal infection	Histoplasmin, etc.	Killed fungi	48 hr	
Trichinosis*	*Trichinella*	Killed larvae	15 min	

*Deleted by Center for Disease Control (CDC) from list of recommended tests (1976).

Tumors from other locations may also produce these hormones. It might be useful to list some of these syndromes, the associated tumor, the principal hormones secreted, and the most commonly reported ectopic hormone-secreting neoplasms.

SPECIMEN COLLECTION

To a pathologist, nothing is quite as upsetting as listening to an outraged complaint about laboratory results and tracing the difficulty to improper specimen collection. Sometimes the wrong type of specimen is obtained. Another possibility is the right specimen that was not collected at the proper time or in the proper way. Even when these criteria are met, the specimen may appear in the laboratory with inadequate identification or instructions or may be delayed in transit enough to cause damage. Finally, at times the test or specimen ordered is not what would be best in the particular situation. It is surprising, although understandable, how one can order the most complicated series of diagnostic manipulations and not realize that the specimens on which all results depend are being collected by personnel who may not have the slightest idea how to perform their task. Urine collection has additional problems, since even when written or verbal directions for collection are optimal, the patient may be confused, be incontinent, or may otherwise fail to provide the specimen in its entirety without close supervision. This is especially important for 24-hour samples. In some cases, such as clearance tests, exact timing to the minute is essential to calculate results.

For 24-hour urine specimens patient should void and discard the urine (this represents urine already in the bladder). Immediately afterward, the collection period begins. At the end of the time period, the patient voids again, but this specimen is added to the others collected during the time period. Most 24-hour urine specimens should be refrigerated or kept in an ice water bath during the collection to control bacterial growth. In some cases, a preservative may be added instead. The specimen container may be placed in a plastic bag while in the refrigerator.

It is usually advisable to have a creatinine excretion determination done to provide an additional check on completeness of collection. A 24-hour creatinine value below normal range suggests incomplete collection. Although there is moderate fluctuation in daily excretion, 24-hour creatinine values should vary less than 10%–15% from day to day.

Fresh specimens are needed in some cases, such as culture, cytology, or enzyme tests.

A partial list of special collection situations in the book is located in Table 36–40.

TABLE 36–39.
Therapeutic Drug Monitoring Data*

	% Protein Bound	Half-life		Time to Peak Plasma Level†	Liver Metabolism	Time to Steady State		Therapeutic Range		Toxic Levels
		Adults	Children			Adults	Children	Adults	Children	
Lithium carbonate	0	8–35 hr	—	1–3 hr	No	2–7 days	—	0.8–1.4 mEq/L	—	2.0 mEq/L
Amitriptyline	82–96	17–40 hr	—	4–8 hr	Yes	4–8 days	—	120–250 ng/ml	—	500 ng/ml
Desipramine	73–92	12–54 hr	—	2–8 hr	Yes	2.5–11 days	—	150–250 ng/ml	—	500 ng/ml
Imipramine	80–95	9–24 hr	—	1–2 hr	Yes	2–5 days	—	150–250 ng/ml	—	500 ng/ml
Nortriptyline	93–95	18–93 hr	—	4–8 hr	Yes	4–19 days	—	50–150 ng/ml	—	500 ng/ml
Acetysalicylic acid	50–90	2–4.5 hr	2–3 hr	1–2 hr	Yes	10–22.5 hr	10–15 hr	Depends on use	Same	300 μg/ml
Acetaminophen	20–30	2–4 hr	2–4 hr	0.5–1.0 hr	Yes	10–20 hr	10–20 hr	Depends on use	Same	250 μg/ml
Theophylline	55–65	3–8 hr	[illegible]–8 hr	1–3 hr	Yes	15–20 hr	5–40 hr	10–20 μg/ml	Same	20 μg/ml
Methotrexate	50–70	1.5–15 hr	[illegible].5–15 hr	1–2 hr	No	Varies	Varies	>0.01 μmol	—	10 μmol/24 hr
Carbamazepine‡	65–85	10–30 hr	8–19 hr	6–18 hr	Yes	2–6 days	2–4 days	8–12 μg/ml	Same	15 μg/ml
Ethosuximide	0	40–60 hr	30–50 hr	1–2 hr	Yes	8–12 days	6–10 days	40–100 μg/ml	Same	150 μg/ml
Phenobarbital	45–50	50–120 hr	40–70 hr	6–18 hr	Yes	11–25 days	8–15 days	15–40 μg/ml	Same	50 μg/ml
Phenytoin	87–93	18–30 hr	12–22 hr	4–8 hr	Yes	4–6 days	2–5 days	10–20 μg/ml	Same	20 μg/ml
Primidone	0–20	4–12 hr	4–6 hr	2–4 hr	Yes	16–60 hr	20–30 hr	5–12 μg/ml	Same	15 μg/ml
Valproic acid	90–95	8–15 hr	6–15 hr	0.5–1.5 hr	Yes	40–75 hr	30–75 hr	50–100 μg/ml	Same	200 μg/ml
Digoxin	10–40	32–51 hr	11–50 hr	1.5–5 hr	20%	7–11 days	2–10 days	0.1–2.0 ng/ml	Same	2.4 ng/ml
Disopyramide	10–80	5–6 hr	—	1–3 hr	Yes	25–30 hr	—	2–5 μg/ml	—	7 μg/ml
Lidocaine	60–70	1–2 hr		15–30 min (IM)	Yes	5–10 hr	—	1.5–5.0 μg/ml	—	7 μg/ml
Procainamide (PA)	15	2.2–4 hr	—	1–2 hr	Yes	11–20 hr	—	4–10 μg/ml	—	16 μg/ml
NAPA	10	4–8 hr	—	—	No	22–40 hr	—	9–20 μg/ml	—	—
PA + NAPA	—	—	—	—	—	—	—	10–30 μg/ml	—	30 μg/ml
Propranolol	90–96	2–6 hr	—	1–2 hr	Yes	10–30 hr	—	50–100 ng/ml	—	Variable
Quinidine sulfate	80–90	4–7 hr	—	1.5–2 hr	Yes	20–35 hr	—	2–5 μg/ml§	—	10 μg/ml
Amikacin	0–11	2–3 hr	—	1 hr (IM)	No	10–15 hr	—	15–25 μg/ml	—	35 μg/ml peak 5 μg/ml residual
Gentamicin	0–10	2–3 hr	2–3 hr	1 hr (IM)	No	10–15 hr	10–15 hr	5–10 μg/ml	—	12 μg/ml peak 2 μg/ml residual
Tobramycin	0–10	2–3 hr	—	1 hr (IM)	No	10–15 hr	—	5–10 μg/ml	—	Same as gentamicin

*Compiled from various sources. IM = intramuscular.
†Oral dose unless otherwise specified.
‡See text (chapter 34).
§More specific methods (HPLC or EMIT)

TABLE 36–40.
Specimen Collection Problem Areas

ALA, chapter 34.
Aldosterone (urine), chapter 29; Table 36–27.
Bacterial culture, anaerobic, chapter 14.
Bacterial culture, routine, chapter 14.
Bacterial meningitis, chapter 18.
Blood culture, chapter 14.
Blood glucose, chapter 27.
Cryptococcus, chapter 15, 18.
Cytomegalic inclusion disease, chapter 16.
Entamoeba histolytica, chapter 17.
Fungus, chapter 15.
Gastric contents for cytology, chapter 32.
Growth hormone, chapter 30.
Hemolysis effects on blood specimens, Table 36–2.
Lactic acid, chapter 35.
Lipoproteins, chapter 21.
Renin, chapter 29; Table 36–27.
Sputum for cytology, chapter 32.
Trichomonas, chapter 17.
Tuberculosis culture, chapter 14.
Urine culture, chapter 14.
Urine urobilinogen, chapter 19.
Uterus carcinoma cytology, chapter 32.
Venous blood pH specimens, chapter 23.
Virus culture, chapter 16.

REPRESENTATIVE "NORMAL VALUES" (TABLE 36–41)

There actually is little justification to provide a table of reference values for clinical chemistry procedures. There are usually several methods for assaying any substance; and with exceptions such as electrolytes, BUN and a few others, each method has different normal values. For example, enzyme procedures yield different results depending on temperature, pH and other conditions of assay. In addition, modifications of every basic technique inevitably appear (sometimes modifications of modifications), each with its own normal range. In addition, there may be local population factors that alter normal range data provided by kit manufacturers. Therefore, each laboratory must provide its own reference range for the particular techniques that it uses and the population it serves. Attempts to apply the same reference range blindly to a test that is performed in different laboratories will frequently be misleading. In spite of these comments, however, sufficient demand for a reference-value table has been generated so that one has been provided here. The figures listed represent "classic" procedures. The values are in some cases rounded off to be representative rather than exact transcription of a single method. In some cases the reader is referred to passages in the text. These values are derived from clinically healthy young adults, and may not be valid for certain tests in neonatal, childhood, or aged populations.

A new system of units of chemical and physical measurement (Système International d'Unités, or SI) has been proposed. It is based on the metric system, and it is designed to create uniformity in the type of reporting system used in clinical chemistry assays. To date, relatively few laboratories in the United States have adopted the SI system, because most chemistry instruments are programmed at the factory to read out in traditional units. The SI system, although useful to chemists, does little, if anything, to assist the physician, who still must contend with a multiplicity of reference ranges from different assays and from different methods for the same assay. In fact, while the transition from currently employed units to SI units is taking place, there will be yet another set of values to contend with. What is needed is a system such as the Centrinormal, in which ranges of most clinical chemistry assays (especially those whose critical values involve elevation from normal) are reported with the upper normal range set at 100. This eliminates memorization of normal ranges, bypasses the confusion that results when a different method with different reference range is substituted for a current test or a new test is introduced, and allows physicians who have patients with laboratory results from different hospitals to obtain comparable data. In addition, one can readily note the degree of abnormality in terms of multiples of the upper limit of normal.

TABLE 36–41.

Representative "Normal Values"

A. Blood	
1. Chemistry	
A/G ratio	1.5–2.5
Albumin	4.0–5.5 gm/100 ml (Biuret) (40–55 g/L) 3.5–5.0 gm/100 ml (electrophoresis)
Ammonia	30–70 μg/100 ml (17.6–41 μmol/L)
Bilirubin: total	0.2–1.5 mg/100 ml (3.42–25.7 μmol/L)
direct	0.1–0.5 mg/100 ml (1.71–8.56 μmol/L)
BSP (45 min)	0%–5%
BUN	10–20 mg/100 ml (3.57–7.14 mmol/L)
Calcium	8.5–10.5 mg/100 ml (2.12–2.62 mmol/L)
Chloride	98–109 mEq/L (mmol/L)
Cholesterol: total	150–200 mg/100 ml (chapter 21) (3.87–5.17 mmol/L)
esters	65%–75%
CO_2 (comb. power)	20–30 mEq/L (mmol/L)
Cortisol, plasma	5–20 μg/100 ml (138–552 nmol/L)
Creatinine, serum	0.8–2.0 mg/100 ml (70.1–176.8 μmol/L)
Folic acid (serum)	3–15 ng/ml (6.80–3.40 nmol/L)
Gamma glutamyl transferase:	
males	0–30 mU/ml at 25 C (0–0.5 μkat/L)
females	0–20 mU/ml at 25 C (0–0.33 μkat/L)
Globulin	1.2–3.0 gm/100 ml
Glucose (fasting)	70–110 mg/100 ml (chapter 27) (3.89–6.11 mmol/L)
Iron, serum	60–150 mg/100 ml (10.7–26.9 μmol/L)
Iron-binding capacity	250–350 mg/100 ml (44.8–62.7 μmol/L)
Lipids: total	400–1,000 mg/100 ml (4.0–10.0 g/L)
phospholipids	200–300 mg/100 ml
triglycerides	30–190 mg/100 ml (chapter 21)
Magnesium	1.5–2.5 mEq/L (0.62–1.03 mmol/L)
Osmolality, serum	278–295 (lit. range, 275–305) mOsm/L (mmol/kg)
Phosphorus (inorg.)	2.5–4.5 mg/100 ml (0.81–1.45 mmol/L)
Potassium	3.6–5.5 mEq/L (mmol/L)
Sodium (serum)	135–145 mEq/L (mmol/L)
Total protein	6–8 gm/100 ml (60–80 g/L)
Triglyceride	<200 mg/100 ml (<2.26 mmol/L)
Uric acid	M 3.0–8.5 mg/100 ml (178–506 μmol/L); F 2.5–7.0 mg/100 ml (149–416 μmol/L)
Vitamin B_{12}	200–1,000 pg/ml (147–738 pmol/L)
2. Thyroid tests	
BEI or T_4 by column	3–7 μg/100 ml
PBI	4–8 μg/100 ml
RAI uptake	10%–35% (chapter 28)
T_3 uptake	Below 0.87, hyper; above 1.13, hypo (Res-O-Mat) 25%–35% (Triosorb) 39%–64% (Trilute) 90%–110% (Thyopac)
T_3-RIA	100–200 ng/100 ml
T_4 by immunoassay	4–100 μg/100 ml (Murphy-Pattee) 5.5–14.5 μg/100 ml (Tetrasorb) (70.8–186.6 nmol/L) 5.3–12.2 μg/100 ml (Tetralute and Res-O-Mat)
TSH	1.5–9.0 μU/ml (mU/L)
3. Serologies	
Antistreptolysin-O	0–200 units

(Continued.)

TABLE 36–41 (cont.).

Febrile agglutinins (Weil-Felix)	0–1:40
Cold agglutinins	0–1:32
4. Enzymes	
Amylase	60–180 units/100 ml (Somogyi)
Acid phosphatase	0.5–2 units/100 ml (Bodansky)
	0.1–5 units/100 ml (King-Armstrong)
	0.1–0.8 units/100 ml (Bessey-Lowry)
	0.1–2 IU/L (Babson) (1.67–13.3 μkat/L)
	0.1–2 units/100 ml (Gutman)
Alkaline phosphatase	1–4 units/100 ml (Bodansky)
	4–13 units/100 ml (King-Armstrong)
	0.8–2.5 units/100 ml (Bessey-Lowry)
	30–110 mU/ml (SMA 12/60) (0.5–1.8 μkat/L)
CPK	1–12 IU/L (Okinaka-activated)
males	5–50 mU/ml (Oliver-Rosalki) (0.08–0.83 μkat/L)
females	5–30 mU/ml (Oliver-Rosalki)
	0–12 units (Sigma)
	0–1.5 IU/L (Tanzer-Gilvarg–nonactivated)
	1–12 IU/L (Tanzer-Gilvarg–activated)
males	5–70 IU/L (Hughes-activated)
females	5–45 IU/L (Hughes-activated)
	25–145 mU/ml SMA 12/60
HBD: males	150–300 units/100 ml (Rosalki-Wilkerson)
females	95–210 mU/ml (Rosalki-Wilkerson)
	55–125 units (Sigma)
LAP: males	75–230 units (Goldberg-Rutenberg)
females	80–210 units (Goldberg-Rutenberg)
	70–200 units (Sigma)
LDH, total	200–500 units/ml (Wroblewski-LaDue)
	200–600 OD units (Teller)
	25–80 IU/L Babson)
	5–50 IU/L (Wacker UV)
	30–100 mU/ml (Wacker UV)
	100–225 mU/ml (SMA 12/60) (1.67–3.75 μkat/L)
LDH, heat stable	20%–40% of total
Lipase	0–1.0 Sigma units
SGOT (AST)	8–40 units/100 ml (Reitman-Frankel)
	1–12 IU/L (Reitman-Frankel)
	15–36 units/ml (Henry)
	9–36 IU/L (Babson)
	5–40 units/100 ml (Karmen UV)
	5–20 mU/ml (Karmen UV)
	10–40 mU/ml (SMA 12/60) (0.17–0.67 μkat/L)
SGPT (ALT)	5–35 units/ml (Reitman-Frankel)
	1–12 IU/L (Reitman-Frankel)
	12–55 units/ml (Henry)
	5–25 mU/ml (Wroblewski) (0.08–0.42 μkat/L)
5. Blood gases (arterial)	
pH	7.38–7.42
P_{CO_2}	35–45 mm Hg

(Continued.)

TABLE 36–41 (cont.).

Po_2	80–90 mm Hg (<65 yr) 75–85 mm Hg (>65 yr)
O_2 sat.	96%–97% (room air)
BE	0 ± 2
6. Clearances	
Urea: standard	40–65 ml/min
maximum	60–100 ml/min
Creatinine	90–120 ml/min (1.5–2.0 mL/s)
Phosphate reabsorption (TRP, PRI)	Over 80%
7. Hematology and coagulation	
Hgb: males	14–18 gm/100 ml (140–180 g/L)
females	12–16 gm/100 ml (120–160 g/L)
Hematocrit: males	40%–54%
females	37%–47%
RBC: males	4.5–6.0 million (4.5–6.0 × 10^{12}/L)
females	4.0–5.5 million (4.0–5.5 × 10^{12}/L)
MCH	26–34
MCHC	31%–37%
MCV	80–100 cu μ (fL)
Platelets	150,000–400,000 (150–400 × 10^9/L)
WBC	4,500–11,000/cu mm (4.5–11.0 × 10^9/L)
Dif: lymphs	20%–40%
seg	50%–70%
bands	0–7
eos	0%–5%
monos	0%–7%
Sed rate: males	0–15 mm/hr (>60 yr, 0–25)
females	0–20 mm/hr (>60 yr, 0–30)
Fibrinogen (quant)	200–400 mg/100 ml (2.0–4.0 g/L)
Coagulation time (Lee-White)	5–15 min
PT	Control ± 2 sec
PTT	40–100 sec (nonactivated)
APTT (activated PTT)	30–45 sec
Bleeding time	2.5–10 min (Simplate method)
PRT	90–130 sec
8. Protein electrophoresis (cellulose acetate)	
Albumin	3.5–5.0 gm (50%–65%)
$Alpha_1$	0.2–0.4 gm (2.5%–5.5%)
$Alpha_2$	0.6–1.0 gm (7%–12%)
Beta	0.6–1.0 gm (7%–15%)
Gamma	0.7–1.3 gm (11%–21%)
B. Spinal fluid (CSF)	
Glucose	40–70 mg/100 ml (2.22–3.89 mmol/L)
Protein	20–45 mg/100 ml (0.20–0.45 g/L)
WBC	0–5 mononuclears
RBC	0
Colloidal gold	No number more than 1
Chloride	20 mEq/L higher than serum
C. Urine	
1. Adrenal chemistry	
Aldosterone	2–26 μg/24 hr (Kliman and Peterson)
Catecholamines	5–150 μg/24 hr 5–100 μg/25 hr (Lund)

(Continued.)

TABLE 36–41 (cont.).

Metanephrines	0.3–0.9 mg/24 hr (Pisano)
VMA	0.5–12 mg/24 hr
	0.5–7 mg/24 hr (Pisano)
17-KS male	10–25 mg/24 hr (34.7–86.7 μmol/d)
female <50 yr	5–15 mg/24 hr
female >50 yr	4–8 mg/24 hr
17-OHCS: male	3–12 mg/24 hr (8.3–33.1 μmol/d)
female	3–10 mg/24 hr
17-KG: male	8–25 mg/24 hr (27.7–86.7 μmol/d)
female	5–18 mg/24 hr
2. Miscellaneous urine chemistry	
Amylase	Up to 300 units/hr
Amylase clearance/creatinine clearance ratio	1%–4% (chapter 26)
Calcium	Less than 250 mg/24 hr (reg. diet) (6.23 mmol/d)
	Less than 150 mg/24 hr (low-calcium diet)
Creatinine	1.0–1.8 gm/24 hr (8.84–7.07 mmol/d)
Glucose	0–0.3 gm/24 hr
Phosphate (phosphorus)	400–1,300 mg/d (varies greatly with diet) (12.9–42.0 mmol/d)
Potassium	25–120 mEq/24 hr (mmol/d)
Protein	0–0.1 gm/24 hr (0.0–0.01 g/d)
Sodium	30–90 mEq/L
	40–220 mEq/24 hr (mmol/d)
Urea nitrogen	6–17 gm/day (normal BUN) (214–607 mmol/d)
Uric acid	250–800 mg/24 hr (normal diet) (1.49–4.76 mmol/d)
	Less than 600 mg/24 hr (low-purine diet) (<3.57 mmol/d)
5-HIAA	1–7 mg/24 hr (Goldenberg)
3. Urinalysis	
Protein	0–30 mg/100 (random)
	0–0.1 gm/24 hr
WBC	0–5/HPF
RBC	0–1/HPF
Urobilinogen	0–1 Ehrlich unit
	0–1:20
Sugar	Neg
Acetone	Neg

TABLE 36–42.

Conversion of Traditional Units to SI Units*

	Current Unit	SI Unit	Conversion Factor
Albumin	g/100 ml	g/L	10
Aspartate aminotransferase	U/L (mU/ml)	μkat/L	0.0167
Ammonia	μg/100 ml	μmol/L	0.587
Bicarbonate (HCO_3)	mEq/L	mmol/L	1.0
Bilirubin	mg/100 ml	μmol/L	17.1

(Continued.)

TABLE 36–42. (cont.)

	Current Unit	SI Unit	Conversion Factor
BUN	mg/100 ml	mmol/L	0.357
Calcium	mg/100 ml	mmol/L	0.25
Chloride	mEq/L	mmol/L	1.0
Cholesterol	mg/100 ml	mmol/L	0.026
Cortisol	μg/100 ml	μmol/L	0.0276
Creatinine	mg/100 ml	μmol/L	88.4
Creatinine clearance	ml/min	mL/s	0.0167
Folic acid	ng/ml	nmol/L	2.27
Glucose	mg/100 ml	mmol/L	0.0555
Iron	mg/100 ml	μmol/L	0.179
Lithium	mEq/L	μmol/L	1.0
Magnesium	mEq/L	mmol/L	0.5
Osmolality	mOsm/kg	mmol/kg	1.0
Phosphorus	mg/100 ml	mmol/L	0.323
Potassium	mEq/L	mmol/L	1.0
Sodium	mEq/L	mmol/L	1.0
Thyroxine (T_4)	μg/100 ml	nmol/L	12.9
Total protein	g/100 ml	g/L	10
Triglyceride	mg/100 ml	mmol/L	0.0113
Uric acid	mg/100 ml	mmol/L	0.0595
Vitamin B12	ng/ml	pmol/L	0.0738
PCO_2	mm/Hg	kPa	0.133
PO_2	mm/Hg	kPa	0.133
Hemoglobin	g/100 ml	g/L	10
Hematocrit	vol %	none	0.01
MCV	μ^3	fL	1.0
WBC count	cu mm	10^9/L	0.001
Platelet count	cu mm	10^9/L	0.001

*Current unit X conversion factor = SI unit; SI unit ÷ conversion factor = current unit.

BIBLIOGRAPHY

Young DS: Implementation of SI units for clinical laboratory data. *Ann Intern Med* 1987; 106:114.

Lehmann HP: Recommended SI units for the clinical laboratory. *Lab Med* 1980; 11:473.

Doumas BT: IFCC documents and interpretation of SI units—a solution looking for a problem. *Clin Chem* 1979; 25:655.

Index

A

Abdominal aortic aneurysms, detection/delineation of, 669
Abetalipoproteinemia, 55
ABO blood group system, 121
ABO incompatibility, hemolytic disease of newborn due to, 144–145
Abscess(es)
  brain, cerebrospinal fluid findings in, 293–294
  detection of, ultrasound in, 669
  intra-abdominal, 231
  intracerebral, radioisotope studies of, 653
Abuse
  drugs of, 627–631
  ethanol, chronic, laboratory screening for, 638
Acanthocytes in peripheral smear, 15
Accelerated arteriolar nephrosclerosis, kidney in, 168–169
Accuracy of laboratory test data, 2–3
Acetaminophen, toxicology of, 634–635
Acetone acid in urinalysis, 156–159
Acetylcholine receptor antibodies, assays of, myasthenia gravis diagnosis, 339
Acetylcholinesterase (ACE), amniotic fluid, in open neural tube defect detection, 558
Acetylsalicylic acid, toxicology of, 635
Achilles tendon reflex for thyroid function testing, 661–662
Acid phosphatase
  assay systems for, 696
  bone marrow, in cancer diagnosis, 666
  immunoassay of, in prostate carcinoma detection, 571
  in prostate carcinoma detection, 570–571
Acid phosphatase stain in hairy cell leukemia diagnosis, 77
Acid-base compensation, 398
Acid-base problems
  comments on, 399
  laboratory tests for, 394–395
  summary of, 397–398
Acid-base studies, data from, interpretation, 398–399
Acid-base tests, specimens for, 395
Acid-gaining acidosis, 395
Acid-losing alkalosis, 396
Acidosis
  acid-gaining, 395
  base-losing, 395–396
  diabetic, electrolyte problems in, 406–407
  metabolic, 395–396
    anion gap in, 400–401
  renal, 396
  respiratory, 396
Acquired immunodeficiency syndrome (AIDS), 267–271
  clinical findings in, 267–268
  diagnosis of, 269–271
  laboratory findings in, 269
  risk factors for, 268
  transmitted by blood transfusions, 149
Acromegaly, 535–536
  glucose tolerance and, 469
Actinomyces israelii, 220
Activated partial thromboplastin time (APTT)
  in hemorrhagic disorders, 94–95
  whole blood, in heparin therapy monitoring, 644
Activated whole blood clotting time in hemorrhagic disorders, 95
Acute tubular necrosis (ATN), 170
  and prerenal azotemia, differentiation of, 647
Acute viral hepatitis, laboratory findings in, 312
Addis count, 184
Addison's disease, 522–524
  hyperkalemia in, 415
Adenitis, mesenteric, 201–202
Adenocarcinoma
  exocrine, laboratory aspects of, 579–580
  renal cell, laboratory aspects of, 569
Adenomas, pituitary, prolactin-secreting, 534–535

Adenosine 3,5-monophosphate, urine, assay of, in parathyroid function evaluation, 659–660
Adrenal cortex, dysfunction of, effects of, 408
Adrenal cortex hormones, 509–512
Adrenal cortical steroids neutrophilic leukocytosis due to, 65
Adrenal function tests, 664
  for Addison's disease, 522–524
  for adrenal medulla dysfunction, 525–528
  for congenital adrenal hyperplasia, 512–513
  for Cushing's syndrome, 513–519 (*see also* Cushing's syndrome)
  furosemide, 664
  for hyporeninemic hypoaldosteronism, 525
  17-ketogenic steroids in, 664
  17-ketosteroid fractionation in, 664
  plasma aldosterone with saline infusion in, 664
  for primary aldosteronism, 519–522 (*see also* Aldosteronism, primary)
  saline infusion, 664
  for secondary adrenal insufficiency, 524–525
  24-hour urine potassium, 664
  for virilization syndrome, 513
Adrenal glands
  hyperplasia of, congenital, 512–513
    female hirsutism and, 547
    variants of, 693–694
  hypertension related to, 528
  localization of, in primary aldosteronism diagnosis, 522
Adrenal insufficiency, secondary, 524–525
Adrenal medulla, dysfunction of, 525–528
Adrenal precocious puberty, 541
Adrenocorticotropic hormone (ACTH)
  deficient production of, secondary adrenal insufficiency from, 524–525
  plasma, assay of, for Addison's disease, 524
  serum, in Cushing's syndrome confirmation, 517–518
Adrenocorticotropic hormone stimulation tests
  for Addison's disease, 523–525
  in Cushing's syndrome confirmation, 517
Adrenogenital syndrome, 512–513
Agammaglobulinemia in pediatric patient, tests for, 332
Age
  advanced, glucose tolerance test and, 464
  drug blood levels and, 614
  hematologic blood values by, 682
Agglutinin(s)
  definition of, 118
  febrile, in infectious disease diagnosis, 225–226
Agglutinogen, definition of, 118
Agnogenic myeloid metaplasia (AMM), 79
  differential diagnosis of, 80–81
Alanine aminotransferase, serum levels of, in liver/biliary tract evaluation, 305
Albumin
  serum
    electrophoretic visualization of, 344–345
    in liver/biliary tract evaluation, 308
    in protein-calorie nutritional status assessment, 432
  therapeutic administration of, alkaline phosphatase evaluation in, 303
  for transfusion, 134
Albumin-bound bilirubin in hemolytic disease of newborn, 145–146
Alcohol, ethyl, toxicology of, 636–638 (*see also* Ethanol)
Alcoholism
  folic acid deficiency and, 33
  iron deficiency anemia and, 24
  laboratory screening for, 638
Aldosterone
  overproduction of, 519–522 (*see also* Aldosteronism)
  plasma
    with saline infusion in adrenal function testing, 664
    or urine, in primary aldosteronism diagnosis, 520–521
Aldosteronism
  primary, 519–522
    adrenal localization procedures in, 522
    diagnosis tests, 520–522
    glucose tolerance and, 468
    laboratory findings in, 520
    tests in, 664
  secondary, 519
Alkaline phosphatase (ALP)
  of bone origin, 303
  in liver/biliary tract evaluation, 301–303, 315
  of liver origin, 302–303
  in metastases to liver, 314
  in metastatic bone cancer, 585
  serum
    in differential diagnosis of hypercalcemia, 420
    in prostate carcinoma detection, 572
Alkaline phosphatase isoenzymes in liver disease testing, 654
Alkalosis
  acid-losing, 396
  hypokalemic, 396–397, 414
  metabolic, 396–397
  respiratory, 397
Alkaptonuria, 600
Allergic bronchopulmonary aspergillosis, 242
Allergic purpura, 114
Allergic reactions from blood transfusions, 148
Allergic vasculitis, 381
Allergy
  acute, eosinophilia and, 66
  tests for, 336–337
Alloantibodies, definition of, 118
Alpha-fetoprotein (AFP)
  amniotic fluid, in open neural tube defect detection, 558
  maternal serum, in open neural tube defect detection, 557–558

serum levels of, in liver/biliary tract evaluation, 309–310
Alpha-1 antitrypsin deficiency, 609–610
Alpha-1 globulins, electrophoretic visualization of, 345
Alpha-2 globulins, electrophoretic visualization of, 345
Aluminum, 430–431
Amebiasis
extraintestinal, 279–280
intestinal, 279
Amebic encephalitis, 280
Amenorrhea
primary, 542–544
secondary, 544–545
Amino acid metabolism, defects in, 598–600
Aminoacidopathies, 598–600
primary, 598–600
secondary, 600
γ-Aminolevulinic acid, urine, assay of, in lead toxicity, 632
γ-Aminolevulinic acid dehydrase (ALA-D) in lead toxicity, 632
Aminophylline, analysis of, 625–626
Amiodarone, effects of, on thyroid function tests, 494
Ammonia, blood levels of, in liver/biliary tract evaluation, 308–309
Amniocentesis
in hemolytic disease of newborn, 146
laboratory problems with, 557
Amniotic fluid
acetylcholinesterase, in open neural tube defect detection, 558
alpha-fetoprotein in, in open neural tube defect detection, 558
Amphetamines, 630–631
Amylase
serum
in acute pancreatitis diagnosis, 454–455
in chronic pancreatitis diagnosis, 458
urine, in acute pancreatitis, 455
Amylase/creatinine clearance ratio, in acute pancreatitis diagnosis, 455–456
Amylase isoenzyme fractionation in acute pancreatitis diagnosis, 456–457
Amyloid, nephrotic syndrome and, 168
Amyloidosis, 352
urinalysis in, 172
Anaerobic bacteria, 207–210
Anaerobic infections, laboratory diagnosis of, 210
Anaerobic streptococci, 210
Anaphylactoid purpura, 114
Androgens, serum, in gonadal function testing, 537
Androstenedione in female hirsutism investigation, 546
Anemia(s), 19–21
aplastic, 36–38
associated with systemic disease, 38–40
causes of, by red blood cell morphology, 20
in chronic liver disease, 39–40
in chronic renal disease, 38
classification of, 19–20
Cooley's, 49–50
depletion, 42–59 (*see also* Hemolytic anemias)
diagnosis of, guide to, 681
factor deficiency, 23–24
false, conditions producing or contributing to, 19
hemolytic, 42–59 (*see also* Hemolytic anemias)
hypochromic, 26
in hypothyroidism, 40
of infection, 39
investigation of patient with, 20–21
jogger, 24
macrocytic, in liver disease, 39
megaloblastic
serum iron in, 26
thrombocytopenia in, 112
of neoplasia, 38–39
nonspherocytic, congenital, 52–53
pernicious
diagnosis of, 32
gastric analysis in, 445–446
Schilling test for, 31–32, 440–442
production-defect, 36–40
in rheumatoid arthritis, 369
in rheumatoid-collagen disease, 39
runner, 24
sickle cell, 46–47
urinalysis in, 172
sideroblastic, 34
Aneurysms, aortic, abdominal, detection/delineation of, ultrasound in, 669
Angioedema, hereditary, complement and, 356
Angiography
in central nervous system evaluation, 652–653
coronary, CPK-MB fraction in, 326
Angioplasty, coronary, CPK-MB fraction in, 326
Angiotensin-converting enzyme (ACE), assay of, in sarcoidosis diagnosis, 330
Anion gap, 400–401
Anisoylated plasminogen-streptokinase activator complex to dissolve thrombi, 109
Ankylosing spondylitis, 372
Anovulation, secondary amenorrhea and, 545
Anthropometric nutritional status assessment, 432
Antiarrhythmic drugs
analysis of, 621–625
digitoxin as, 625
digoxin as, 623–625
flecainide as, 623
lidocaine as, 621–622
procainamide as, 621
quinidine as, 622–623
tocainide as, 622
Antibiotic sensitivity testing, 231–234
disk diffusion method of, 231–232
serial dilution method of, 232–233
Antibiotics
analysis of, 626
bacterial resistance to, 233–234
removal of, for bacterial, 234
for septicemia, 227
serologic tests for syphilis and, 563

Antibody(ies)
- against other streptococcal enzymes in acute rheumatic fever diagnosis, 383
- antimitochrondrial, in biliary cirrhosis diagnosis, 309
- anti-smooth muscle, in chronic active hepatitis diagnosis, 309
- antistreptococcal, in acute glomerulonephritis, 166–167
- bivalent, definition of, 118
- complete, definition of, 118
- definition of, 118
- detection of
  - in human immunodeficiency virus I infection diagnosis, 269–270
  - and identification of, 120
  - methods for, 119–120
  - in viral disease infections, 246–247
- factor VIII, 108
- incomplete, definition of, 118–119
- to intrinsic factor, assay for, 642
- serologic tests for, in herpes simplex virus infection diagnosis, 266–267
- univalent, definition of, 118–119

Antibody-coated bacteria test for bacterial disease diagnosis, 649
Antibody elution in antibody detection and identification, 120
Antibody screen on serum, 124
Anticoagulant(s)
- citrate, in massive blood transfusions, 150
- coumarin, 101–102
- plasmin/fibrinolysin, 104–106

Anticoagulant systems, 101–115
- bone marrow deficiency and, 111–112
- coumarin, 101–102
- disseminated intravascular coagulation and, 106–107
- heparin/antithrombin III, 102–104
- hypersplenism and, 111
- immunologic-type coagulation factor inhibitors as, 107–108
- miscellaneous, 108–109
- plasmin/fibrinolysin, 104–106
- platelet defects and, 110
- platelet function and, 112–114
- protein C/protein S, 104
- thrombocytopenia and, 110–111
- vascular defects and, 114–115

Anticonvulsants, analysis of, 617–619
Antidepressants, tricyclic, analysis of, 620
Antidiuretic hormone, secretion of, inappropriate, 409–410
- disorders simulating, 410

Anti-DNA assay for systemic lupus erythematosus, 377–378
Anti-ENA antibody in systemic lupus erythematosus, 378
Antigen(s)
- bacterial, latex agglutination tests for, 290
- carcinoembryonic (*see* Carcinoembryonic antigen)
- cytomegalovirus, detection of, 260
- definition of, 118
- detection of
  - in human immunodeficiency virus I infection diagnosis, 269
  - in viral disease diagnosis, 246
- HSV, detection of, in herpes simplex virus infection diagnosis, 266
- platelet, transfusion and, 131–132
- prostate-specific, in prostate carcinoma detection, 571–572
- white blood cell, 126–127

Antigen reactions, immunoglobulin A, from blood transfusions, 148
Antimitochondrial antibodies in biliary diagnosis, 309
Antinuclear antibody test for systemic lupus erythematosus, 374–375
- patterns of, 375

Anti-nuclear glycoprotein (Sm) antibody in systemic lupus erythematosus, 378
Anti-RNP antibody in systemic lupus erythematosus, 378
Anti-smooth muscle antibodies in chronic active hepatitis diagnosis, 309
Anti-sNP antibody in systemic lupus erythematosus, 377–378
Antisperm antibody, serum, studies on, in male infertility investigation, 540–541
Anti-SS-A antibody in systemic lupus erythematosus, 378
Anti-SS-B antibody in systemic lupus erythematosus, 378
Antistreptococcal antibodies in glomerulonephritis, 166
Antithrombin III (AT-III), 102–103
- deficiency of, transfusions for, 133–134

Apheresis in transfusion therapy, 134–135
Aplastic anemia, 36–38
Aplastic crisis, transient, 650–651
Apnea, succinylcholine, 609
Apoprotein assay in coronary heart disease risk assessment, 362
Arteriosclerosis, benign, urinalysis in, 172
Arteritis
- giant cell, 381–382
- temporal, 381–382

Artery, renal, occlusion of, 170
Arthritis
- associated with inflammatory bowel disease, 372
- conditions associated with, 386–387
- from crystal deposition, 384–386
- psoriatic, 372
- rheumatoid, 369–371
- septic, 386

Arthropathy, crystalline, 384–386
Artifactual thrombocytopenia, 112
Aseptic meningitis, cerebrospinal fluid findings in, 292–293
Asparate aminotransferase (AST)

in acute myocardial infarction, 320–321
serum levels of, in liver/biliary tract evaluation, 303–305, 314–315
Aspergilloma, 242
Aspergillus, 242–243
Aspiration, bone marrow, 18
Aspirin
anticoagulant properties of, 108
toxicology of, 635
Atrias syndrome, 656
Auer rods in monocytic leukemia, 69–70
Autoagglutinins, hemolytic anemias due to, 55–56
Autoantibodies, 120–121
definition of, 118
hemolytic anemias due to, 55–56
thyroid, 505
Autoimmune hemolytic anemia, 55
secondary acquired, 56
Automated cell counters
differential counts with, 64–65
Autotransfusion, 130
Azotemia
chronic renal disease with, glucose tolerance and, 469
classification of, 177–178
differential diagnosis of, 183–184
prerenal
and acute tubular necrosis, differentiation of, 647
etiologies of, 178
renal failure and, 183–184
Azulfidine, folic acid deficiency and, 33

B

Babesiosis, 278
Bacilli, enteric, 199
Bacillus cereus, diarrhea due to, 229
Bacteremia, 226–227
Salmonella, 200
Bacteria
anaerobic, 207–210
antibiotic sensitivity procedures for, 231–234
associated with contamination of specimens, 221
on blood agar, hemolytic reactions of, 648
culture of, 221–225 (*see also* Culture of bacteria)
detection of, direct methods of, 188–189
hemolytic anemia due to, 59
infectious diarrhea due to, 299–230
infectious diseases caused by, 188–234
laboratory classification of, 189–215
resistance of, to antibotics, 233–234
Bacterial antigens, latex agglutination tests for, 290
Bacterial infections
eosinophilia and, 66
general concepts of, 226
Bacteriocidal concentration in serum, 234
Bacteriostatic concentration in serum, 234
Bacteriuria
in pregnancy, 171–172
screening tests for, 223
Bacteroides, 209–210
Band granulocyte in white blood cell maturation, 61, 62
Barbiturates, toxicology of, 634
Barr Body test for chromosome abnormalities, 601
Basal metabolic rate (BMR) in thyroid function testing, 662
Base excess, 398
Base-losing acidosis, 395–396
Basophilia, 66
Basophilic strippling
in lead poisoning, 58
in red blood cells, 16
of reticulocytes, 17
Basen-Kornsweig syndrome, 55
Bentiromide test in chronic pancreatitis diagnosis, 458–459
Beta globulins, electrophoretic visualization of, 345–346
Beta-lactamase test for bacterial resistance, 233–234
Beta subunit antibody tests for pregnancy, 550
Beta-2 microglobulin
assay of, for renal function, 647
in human immunodeficiency virus I infection diagnosis, 271
Bicarbonate, serum, 394
Bicarbonate-carbonic acid system, 392–394
Bile in urinalysis, 160
Bile acids, serum levels of, in liver/biliary tract evaluation, 307–308
Bile duct
obstruction of, 317
stones in, 316–317
Biliary cirrhosis
diagnosis of, antimitochondrial antibodies in, 309
primary, laboratory findings in, 313
Biliary tract
disease of
immunoglobulin levels in, 654
tests for
5-nucleotidase in, 654
leucine amino peptidase in, 654
extrahepatic, 316–318
obstruction of
intrahepatic vs. extrahepatic, differentiating, ultrasound in, 669
jaundice from, 300
laboratory findings in, 312–313
Bilirubin
albumin-bound, in hemolytic disease of newborn, 145–146
conjugated, in urinalysis, 160
levels of, in hemolytic disease of newborn, 145
metabolism of, inherited defects in, 655–656
serum levels of, tests for, 299–301
unconjugated
effects of renal function of, 300
serum levels of, in hemolytic anemia diagnosis, 44
urine, in liver/biliary tract evaluation, 301
Biochemical methods of blood glucose assay, 463
Biochemical tests

Biochemical tests *(cont.)*
  for congenital anomalies, 557–558
  for pregnancy, 549
Biopsy
  lymph node, in sarcoidosis diagnosis, 329–330
  needle, guidance for, ultrasound in, 669
  renal, 184
  skin, with immunofluorescence staining
    in Rocky Mountain spotted fever diagnosis, 651
    for systemic lupus erythematosus, 378
  small intestine, in malabsorption assessment, 444
  testicular, in male infertility investigation, 540
Biotinidase deficiency, 610
Bite cells in peripheral smear, 15
Bivalent antibody(ies), definition of, 118
Bladder cancer, flow cytometry test for, 665
Blast in white blood cell maturation, 61, 62
Blastomycosis, 238
Bleeding
  disorders of, investigation of, 115–116
  problems with, in surgery, 115
Bleeding time in hemorrhagic disorders, 92–93
Blood
  ammonia levels in, in liver/biliary tract evaluation, 308–309
  donation of, 130
  gastric, tests for, 450–451
  glucose in
    assay of, methods of, 462–463
    regulation of, 462
  loss of, iron deficiency from, 23, 24
  pH of, 392–394
  in urinalysis, 159–160
  volume of, measurement of, in transfusion therapy, 135–137
  whole
    activated partial thromboplastin time for, in heparin therapy monitoring, 644
    recalcification time for, in heparin therapy monitoring, 644
    for transfusion, 129–130
Blood bank screening for hepatitis B virus, 258
Blood coagulation, 90–116
  fibrinolysin tests and, 643–644
  Fletcher factor screening test and, 644
  heparin therapy monitoring test and, 644
  hexadimethrine bromide neutralization test and, 645
  mean platelet volume and, 645
  sodium warfarin therapy, monitoring and, 645
  theory of, 90–91
  thrombocytosis and, 645
  thromboplastin geneation time and, 643
Blood cultures
  for infective endocarditis, 225–229
  for septicemia, 227
Blood gas values, interpretation of, effects of physiologic patient variation on, 401–402
Blood group system
  ABO, 121
  Rh, 122–123
Blood group antigen systems, 123–124
Blood oxygen (PO_2), noninvasive measurement of, 402
Blood oxygen studies, 401
Blood smear, peripheral
  in Epstein-Barr infection diagnosis, 261–262
  examination of, limitations of, 16
  in sickle hemoglobin detection, 45
  Wright-stained, examination of, 14–16
Blood transfusions, 129–137
  of albumin, 134
  apheresis and, 134–135
  autologous, 130
  blood volume measurement and, 135–137
  of coagulation factor materials, 133–134
  of cryoprecipitate, 133
  of fibrinogen, 134
  filters for, 135
  of granulocytes, 132
  infections transmitted by, 148–149
  massive, 150–151
  neonatal cytomegalovirus infection acquired by, 651
  of packed red blood cells, 130–131
  of plasma, 132–133
  of platelets, 131–132
  procedures relevant to, 134–137
  of purified plasma protein fraction, 134
  reactions for, 139–140
    febrile, 147–148
    graft vs. host disease as, 146–147
    hemolytic, 139–146
    infectious, 148–149
    platelet, 147
    problems of, 149–151
  of red blood cell substitutes, 134
  tests before, considerations on, 126
  of whole blood, 129–130
Blood urea nitrogen (BUN)
  elevated (*see* Azotemia)
  for glomerular and tubular damage, 177–178
Blood volume measurements in polycythemia diagnosis, 82
Bone(s)
  alkaline phosphatase originating in, 303
  disorders of, 369–390, 598
  metastatic carcinoma to, laboratory aspects of, 585–586
  radionuclide scan of, 388–390
    in breast cancer diagnosis, 574–575
    in metastatic bone cancer, 585–586
  x-ray studies of
    for growth disorders, 533–534
    in metastatic bone cancer, 585
Bone marrow

acid phosphatase in, in cancer diagnosis, 666
aspiration of, 18
for aplastic anemia diagnosis, 37–38
in multiple myeloma diagnosis, 350–351
in polycythemia diagnosis, 82
deficiency of, thrombocytopenia in, 111
examination of
in differentiation of chronic myelogenous leukemia, agnogenic myeloid metaplasia, and leukemoid reaction, 80
leukemoid reaction, CML, AMM, 80–81
in metastatic bone cancer, 586
in vitamin B12 deficiency diagnosis, 31
hypoplastic, 36–38
replacement of
by fibrosis, 36
by neoplasm, 36
Bone marrow iron stain in chronic iron deficiency diagnosis, 29
Bordatella pertussis, 204
Botryomycosis, 220
Botulism, 209
Bowel disease, inflammatory, arthritis associated with, 372
Brain
abscess of, cerebrospinal fluid findings in, 293–294
diseases of, cerebrospinal fluid findings in, 291–297
radionuclide scanning of, in brain disease detection, 291
tumor of
cerebrospinal fluid findings in, 294
detection of
computerized tomography in, 290–291
magnetic resonance imaging in, 291
radionuclide brain scanning in, 291
laboratory aspects of, 581–582
radioisotope studies in, 652
Breast cancer, laboratory aspects of, 574–576
Brill-Symmer's disease, 83
Broad casts in urinary sediment, 163
Bromsulphalein (BSP) in liver disease testing, 655
Bronchopulmonary aspergillosis, allergic, 242
Bronchoscopy in lung cancer detection, 578–579
Brucella, 205–206
Brucellosis, 205–206
Buccal smear, indications for, 603
Buffer base, 398
Burkitt's lymphoma, 84–85
Burns
extensive, hyponatremia in, 406
glucose tolerance test and, 464

C

C-reactive protein (CRP), 331
Calcidiol, assays of, in hypocalcemia, 427
Calcitonin, assay of, in parathyroid hormone evaluation, 425
Calcitriol, assays of, in hypocalcemia, 427
Calcium
disorders of
hypercalcemia as, 414–425 (*see also* Hypercalcemia)
hypocalcemia as, 425–427
tests in, 417–427
excretion of, urinary, in differential diagnosis of hypercalcemia, 420–421
ionized, in differential diagnosis of hypercalcemia, 419–420
serum levels of, regulation of, 417
in urine, test for, 165
Calcium ions, 97–98
Calculi, urinary tract, laboratory evaluation in, 645–646
Calymmatobacterium granulomatis, 203
Campylobacter, 204–205
Cancer
anemia and, 38–39
of breast, laboratory aspects of, 574–576
of central nervous system, laboratory aspects of, 581–582
of cervix, laboratory aspects of, 576
colon
predisposition to, 450
sensitivity of tests for, 450
of endometrium, laboratory aspects of, 576–577
gastric, diagnosis of, gastric analysis in, 446
gastrointestinal tract, 447–450 (*see also* Gastrointestinal tract, cancer of)
jaundice from, 300
of kidney, laboratory aspects of, 569–570
laboratory aspects of, 665–666
bone marrow acid phosphatase in, 666
carcinoma antigen 19-9 in, 665
centocor CA 15-3 in, 665
hybritech CA 549 in, 665
urine hydroxyproline in, 665–666
of liver, laboratory aspects of, 581
of lung, laboratory aspects of, 578–579
metastatic
to bone, laboratory aspects of, 585
to liver, laboratory findings in, 314
of ovary, laboratory aspects of, 577
of pancreas
diagnosis of, ultrasound in, 669
laboratory aspects of, 579–581
of prostate, laboratory aspects of, 570–572
of sympathetic nervous system, laboratory aspects of, 582
of testis, laboratory aspects of, 580
tests for
carcinoembryonic antigen in, 588–590
effusions and, 586–588
serum lactic dehydrogenase in, 588

Cancer (cont.)
of thryroid, laboratory aspects of, 582–584
of uterus, laboratory aspects of, 576–577
Cancer antigen 125 (CA 125) in ovarian cancer diagnosis, 577
Candida infections, 241–242
of central nervous system, cerebrospinal fluid findings in, 292
Cannabis, 628–629
Carbamazepine, analysis of, 619
Carbohydrate metabolism, diseases of, genetic, 594–597
Carbon dioxide
noninvasive measurement of, 402
partial pressure of (PCO_2), 394
as measure of respiratory function, 398
Carbon dioxide combining power, 394
Carbon dioxide content of blood, 394
Carbon monoxide
poisoning from, glucose tolerance and, 469
toxicology of, 635–636
Carcinoembryonic antigen (CEA)
in colon cancer, 589
in gastrointestinal tract cancer detection, 449–450
in pleural effusion, 588
in recurrent tumor detection, 589–590
in tests for cancer, 588–590
Carcinoid syndrome, laboratory aspects of, 572–573
Carcinoids, laboratory aspects of, 572–574
Carcinoma antigen 19-9 (CA 19-9) in cancer diagnosis, 665
Cardiolipin tests for syphilis, 562–563
Carotene, plasma, in malabsorption assessment, 440
Casts in urinary sediment, 162–164
Cat-scratch disease, 206–207
Catacholamine/vanillymandelic acid/metanephrine assay for pheochromocytoma, 526–527
Catecholamines, plasma, assay of, for pheochromocytoma, 527
Catheterization, neck vein, in parathyroid function evaluation, 659
Cell component autoantibodies in liver-biliary tract evaluation, 309
Cell count in cerebrospinal fluid, 287–288
Cell counting instrument artifacts, 14
Cellular casts in urinary sediment, 162–163
Centocor CA 15-3 in cancer diagnosis, 665
Central nervous system (CNS)
cancer of laboratory aspects of, 581–582
Candida infection CA, cerebrospinal fluid findings in, 292
syphilis, 567–568
Central venous pressure measurement (CVP) in transfusion therapy, 137
Centromere pattern in antinuclear antibody test, 376–377
Cerebral infarction, radioisotope studies in, 652–653
Cerebral lesions, glucose tolerance and, 469
Cerebral thrombosis, cerebrospinal fluid findings in, 295
Cerebral vascular accident, radioisotope studies of, 653
Cerebrospinal fluid (CSF)
appearance of, 285
artifacts in, 297
cell count in, 287
examination of
colloidal gold reaction in, 651–652
oligoclonal vs. serum bands in, 652
radioisotope studies in, 652–653
findings in
in septic meningitis, 292–293
in brain abscess, 293–294
in brain diseases, 291–297
in brain tumor, 294
in *Candida* CNS infection, 292
in cerebral thrombosis, 295
in cryptococcal meningitis, 292
in human immunodeficiency virus meningitis, 293
in intracerebral hemorrhage, 295
in lead encephalopathy, 296–297
in multiple sclerosis, 295–296
in mycobacterial meningitis, 291–292
in subarachnoid hemorrhage, 295
in subdural hematoma, 294–295
in viral meningitis, 292–293
glucose in, 285–286
lactate in, in bacterial meningitis diagnosis, 290
pressure of, 285
protein in, 286–287
reference ranges in neonate compared to childhood and adult values, 288
tests of, 285–288
for syphilis, 288–289
Ceruloplasmin, plasma, assay of, in Wilson's disease diagnosis, 605–606
Cervix, cancer of, laboratory aspects of, 576
Chemical(s)
hemolytic anemia due to, 58–59
neutrophilic leukocytosis due to, 65
Chemstrip-L for white blood cells in urine, 160
Chest x-ray films
in lung cancer detection, 578
in tuberculosis, 212
Childhood, hypoglycemia in, 470–480
Children
oral glucose tolerance for, criteria for, 466
younger, white blood cell counts in, problems with, 65
Chlamydiae, 216–219
conjunctivitis from, 218–219
Chlamydia psittaci, 216–217

Chlamydia trachomatis, 217, 219
endocervicitis from, 217–218
infections from, diagnosis of, 218
urethritis from, 197, 217–218
Chloride, serum, 416
in parathyroid hormone evaluation, 424–425
Chloride/phosphate ratio in parathyroid function evaluation, 659
Chlorothiazide diuretics, glucose tolerance and, 468
Cholangiography, transhepatic, percutaneous, 311
Cholangiopancreatography, endoscopic retrograde
in acute pancreatitis, 457–458
in chronic pancreatitis diagnosis, 459
Cholecystitis
acute, 316
radiologic diagnosis of, 317–318
Cholecystography in cholecystitis diagnosis, 317
Choledochopancreatography, endoscopic retrograde, 311
Cholesterol
esters of, in liver disease testing, 654–655
high-density lipoprotein, in coronary heart disease risk assessment, 361–362
in liver disease testing, 654–655
low-density lipoprotein, in coronary heart disease risk assessment, 361
serum, in thyroid function testing, 662
total, serum, in coronary heart disease risk assessment, 358–361
Cholesterol/high density lipoprotein cholesterol ratio in coronary heart disease risk assessment, 362
Cholinesterase deficiency, congenital, 609
Cholinesterase inhibitors, toxicology of, 634
Choriocarcinoma, diagnosis of, 552
Chromosomes
abnormalities of, 600–603
analysis of, 600–601
in leukemia, 643
fragile X, 602–603
karyotyping of, indications for, 603
Philadelphia, in chronic myelogenous leukemia, 78
Chronic mononucleosis syndrome, 264–265
Chylomicrons, metabolism of, 358
Circulating immune complexes (CICs), 382–383
Cirrhosis
biliary
diagnosis of, antimitochrondrial antibodies in, 309
laboratory findings in, 313
electrolyte abnormalities in, 408
far-advanced, pattern of, in serum protein electrophoresis, 347–348
laboratory findings in, 313–314
Citrate anticoagulant in massive blood transfusions, 150
Clearance tests for glomerular function, 175
Clomiphene in testicular function stimulation, 540
Clinistix for urinary glucose, 157
Clinitest for urinary glucose, 157–158
Clonidine suppression test for pheochromocytoma, 526
Clostridia, 207–209
Clostridium botulinum, diarrhea due to, 229
Clostridium botulinus, 209
Clostridium difficile, 208–209
diarrhea due to, 229
Clostridum perfringens, 207–208
diarrhea due to, 229
Clostridium tetani, 208
Clot lysis test, 643–644
Clot retraction in hemorrhagic disorders, 92
Coagulation, blood, 90–116 (*see also* Blood coagulation)
Coagulation factors, 96–101
I (Fibrinogen), 96–97
II (Prothrombin), 97
III (Tissue Thromboplastin), 97
IV (Calcium Ions), 97–98
V (Labile Factor), 98
VII (Stable Factor), 98
VIII/von Willebrand factor complex, 98–99
IX (Plasma Thromboplastin Component), 100
X (Stuart Factor), 100–101
XI (Plasma Thromboplastin Antecedent), 101
XII (Hageman Factor), 101
XIII, 101
deficiency of, in massive blood transfusions, 150–151
high molecular weight kininogen as (HMWK; Fitzgerald Factor), 101
inhibitors of, immunologic-type, 107–108
prekallikrein as, 101
for transfusion, 133–134
Cocaine, 629–630
Cocci, Gram-positive, 190–196
Coccidioidomycosis, 238
Codeine, 631
Cold agglutinins in *Mycoplasma pneumoniae* infection, 219
Cold autoantibodies, 121
Colitis
Clostridium difficile, 208
hemorrhagic, 201
Collagen-vascular diseases, 372–380
mixed connective tissue disease as, 379–380
progressive systemic sclerosis as, 379
Sjögren's syndrome as, 380
systemic lupus erythematosus as, 373–379 (*see also* Systemic lupus erythematosus)
Colloidal gold reaction in cerebrospinal fluid examination, 651–652
Colon, cancer of
predisposition to, 450
sensitivity of tests for, 450
Colonoscopy, fiberoptic, in cancer detection, 449
Coma
diabetic, diagnosis of, 474
hyperosmolar nonketotic, 474

Coma (cont.)
prehepatic, 308–309
Complement, serum, 356–357
in systemic lupus erythematosus, 379
Complement fixation test for syphilis, 562
Compliance, patient, drug blood levels and, 615
Computerized tomography (CT), 670–671
for acute pancreatitis, 458
for brain disease detection, 290–291
in cholecystitis diagnosis, 318
in Cushing's syndrome confirmation, 518
in liver/biliary tract evaluation, 310–311
in lung cancer detection, 579
Confirmatory antibody detection methods in human immunodeficiency virus I infection diagnosis, 270
Congenital adrenal hyperplasia (CAH), 512–513
female hirsutism and, 547
variants of, 693–694
Congenital anomalies, biochemical tests for, 557–558
Congenital cholinesterase deficiency, 609
Congenital diseases of skeletal muscle, 603–605
Congenital hyperbilirubinemias, 655–656
Congenital nonspherocytic anemias, 52
Congenital rubella syndrome, 248, 249–250
Congenital syphilis, 566–567
Congestive heart failure, electrolyte abnormalities in, 408
Conjugated bilirubin in urinalysis, 160
Conjunctivitis, chlamydial, 218–219
Connecting peptide measurement serum for fasting hypoglycemia, 477
Connective tissue disorders, 598, 698
Conn's syndrome, 519–522 (*see also* Aldosteronism, primary)
Cooley's anemia, 49–50
Coomb's test
direct
for antibody detection, 119–120
in hemolytic anemia diagnosis, 44
indirect, in antibody detection and identification, 120
Copper, serum and urine levels of, in Wilson's disease diagnosis, 606
Coproporphyrins, in urine, tests for, 15
Coronary angiography, CPK-MB fraction in, 326
Coronary angioplasty, CPK-MB fraction in, 326
Coronary heart disease, risk assessment for
apoprotein assay in, 362
high-density lipoprotein cholesterol in, 316–362
laboratory tests for, 358–363
low-density lipoprotein cholesterol in, 361
serum cholesterol in, 358–361
serum cholesterol/high-density lipoprotein, 361–362
triglyceride measurement in, 362–363
Corticotropin-releasing hormone test in Cushing's syndrome conformation, 517
Cortisol
plasma, 511–512
diurnal variation in Cushing's syndrome screening, 515
urine free
in Cushing's syndrome screening, 515
in female hirsutism investigation, 547
Corynebacteria, 218–221
Corynebacterium diphtheriae, 216
Corynebacterium vaginalis, 198–199
Coumarin anticoagulants, 101–102
Counterimmunoelectrophoresis (CIE) technique for bacterial disease diagnosis, 648–649
Creatine clearance, tests of, 176–177
Creatine phosphokinase (CPK)
in acute myocardial infarction, 323–327
BB fraction of, 326
isoenzymes of, measurement of, 324
in malignant hyperpyrexia diagnosis, 605
MB fractions of (CPK-MB)
in acute myocardial infarction, 324–326, 657
in myocardial infarct size estimation, 657
technical problems with pseudo-MB substances and, 326–327
MM fractions of, in acute myocardial infarction, 324
total, elevation of, vs. CPK-MB fraction values, 326
Creatinine
serum, for glomerular and, 178–179
urinary excretion of, ideal, 689–690
Creatinine height index (CHI) in protein-calorie nutritional status assessment, 433
Crigler-Najjar syndrome, 656
Crithidia method of anti-DNA assay for systemic lupus erythematosus, 377
Crossmatch
major, of blood, 124–126
problems with, 126
Cryoglobulins in myeloma, 355–356
Cryoprecipitate for transfusion, 133
Cryptococcal meningitis, cerebrospinal fluid findings in, 292
Cryptococcosis, 238–239
Cryptosporidium, 821
Crystal deposition, arthritis due to, 384–385
Crystalline arthropathies, 384–386
Crystals in urinary sediment, 164
Culture(s)
in acute rheumatic fever diagnosis, 383
of bacteria
blood, for septicemia, 227

problems with, 225
specimens for, obtaining, 222
sputum, 224–225
urine, 222–224
for bacterial detection, 188–189
blood, for infective endocarditis, 228–229
of cerebrospinal fluid in bacterial meningitis diagnosis, 289
for cytomegalovirus infection, 260
of effusions, 587
fungal, 243
in herpes simplex virus infection diagnosis, 266
in human immunodeficiency virus I infection diagnosis, 269
of *Mycoplasma pneumoniae*, 219
in tuberculosis, 213–214
in viral disease diagnosis, 246
specimens for, 247–248
Cushing's syndrome, 513–519
computerized tomography for, 518
confirmatory tests for, 516–518
glucose tolerance and, 468
screening tests for, 514–516
standard test abnormalities in, 514
Cyanocobalamin (*see* Vitamin 12)
Cyclic adenosine monophosphate assay in parathyroid function evaluation, 659–660
Cyclosporine, analysis of, 626–627
Cystic fibrosis, 459, 607–609
sweat sodium/chloride ratio in, 666
Cysticercus cellulosa, 282
Cystitis-urethritis, urinalysis in, 172
Cytochemical stains in acute leukemia differentiation, 71–72
Cytology
of effusions, 587–588
sputum, in lung cancer detection, 578
Cytomegalic inclusion virus (CMV) disease, 258–260
laboratory abnormalities in, 259
laboratory diagnosis of, 259–260
Cytomegalic inclusion virus transmitted by blood transfusion, 149
Cytomegalovirus antigen, detection of, 260
Cytomegalovirus inclusion (CMV) body cytology, 260
Cytomegalovirus infection, neonatal, transfusion-acquired, 651
Cytometry, flow, for bladder cancer diagnosis, 665

D

D-Dimer test for fibrin degradation products, 106
D-Xylose test in malabsorption assessment, 442–444
Darkfield examination for syphilis, 561
Davidsohn differential test in Epstein-Barr infection diagnosis, 262–263
Dawn phenomenon, glucose tolerance, 470
de Quervain's disease, 504
Decision levels in applying reference ranges to medical action, 640
Defibrillation, CPK-MB fraction in, 326
Degmacytes in peripheral smear, 15
Dehydroepiandrosterone-sulfate (DHEA-S) in female hirsutism investigation, 546
Delta hepatitis, 253
Depletion anemia, 42–59 (*see also* Hemolytic anemias)
Depression, laboratory tests for, 338–339
Dermatophytes, 243
Dexamethasone suppression test
48-hour, in Cushing's syndrome confirmation, 516–517
single-dose, in Cushing's syndrome screening, 515–516
Dexamethasone test, overnight
low-dose, for melancholia, 338
for melancholia, factors altering results of, 688
Di Guglielmo's syndrome, 74
Diabetes insipidus, antidiuretic hormone secretion in, 409
Diabetes mellitus, 461–474
blood glucose assay methods of, 462–463
blood glucose regulation and, 462
categories of, 461
gestational, 466–467
glucose tolerance test of, 462–463
kidneys in, 171
laboratory tests for, 461–462
postprandial hypoglycemia in, 478
screening tests for, 467–468
tolerance tests for, data for, 690
Diabetic acidosis, electrolyte problems in, 406–407
Diabetic coma, diagnosis of, 474
Diabetic ketoacidosis
hyperkalemia in, 415
hypokalemia from, 414
Diabetic nephropathy, red blood cell casts in, 645
Diacetic acid in urinalysis, 156–159
Diagnostic ultrasound, 667–670 (*see also* Ultrasound, diagnostic)
Diamond-Blackfan congenital hypoplastic anemia, 38
Diarrhea
differential tests for, 447
infectious, due to bacterial agents, 229–230
nonbacterial causes of, 230
severe, hyponatremia in, 406
Diet, iron-deficient, iron deficiency anemia from, 24
Differential absorption test in Epstein-Barr infection diagnosis, 262–263
Differential hemoglobin solubility tests in sickle hemoglobin detection, 45–46
Digitoxin, analysis of, 625
Digoxin, analysis of, 623–625
Dihydrotestosterone (DHT) in female hirsutism investigation, 546–547

Dilantin
- analysis of, 617–618
- glucose tolerance and, 470
- therapy with, alkaline phosphatase elevation in, 303

Dilutional syndromes, electrolyte abnormalities in, 408
Diphtheroids, 216
Diplococci, Gram-negative, 196–199
Diplococcus pneumoniae, 193
Dipstick method
- for urinary glucose, 157
- for urinary protein, 156

Direct Coombs test for antibody detection, 119–120
Direct smear methods in herpes simplex virus infection diagnosis, 266
Direct visualization techniques in gastrointestinal tract cancer detection, 449
Disaccharide malabsorption, 595–596
Disk diffusion method of antibiotic sensitivity testing, 231–232
Disseminated intravascular coagulation (DIC), 106–107
- laboratory diagnosis of, 107
- protamine sulfate test for, 105–106

Diuretics, chlorothiazide, glucose tolerance and, 468
Diurnal variations
- glucose tolerance test and, 464
- in serum iron levels, 26
- in white blood cell counts, 63

DNA linkage analysis in cystic fibrosis diagnosis, 608
DNA probe for bacterial detection, 189
Donovania granulomatis, 203
Doriden, toxicology of, 634
Down's syndrome, 602
Drug(s)
- of abuse, 627–631
- coagulation and, 108
- effects of, on laboratory test data, 7
- hemolytic anemia, induced by, 56–57
- hyperkalemia induced by, 415–416
- hypokalemia induced by, 414–415
- jaundice from, 300
- neutrophilic leukocytosis due, to, 65
- other, drug blood levels and, 614
- systemic lupus erythematosus induced by, 379
- therapeutic, monitoring of, 612–617 (*see also* Therapeutic drugs)
- thrombocytopenia induced by, 110

Dubin-Johnson syndrome, 656
Duchenne's muscular dystrophy, 603
Duffy blood group antigens, 124
Duodenum, ulcer of, and gastric ulcer, differentiation of, gastric analysis, in 446
Dysautonomia, familial, laboratory tests for, 666
Dysproteinemia, coagulation and, 108

E

E-B early antigen (EA) complex, antibody against, 264
E-B nuclear antigen (EBNA), antibody against, 264
Echinococcus, 282
Echinocytes in peripheral smear, 15
Eclampsia, urinary findings in, 171
Ectopic parathyroid hormone syndrome, 424
Ectopic pregnancy, diagnosis of, 551–552
Ectopic tumors, hormone production by, 696–697
Effusions, tests for cancer and, 586–588
Electrocardiogram (ECG) in acute myocardial infarction, 320
Electrolyte(s)
- excretion of, urinary, in tubular function evaluation, 182
- imbalance of, clinical symptoms of, 416
- physiology of, kidney in, 407–408
- serum, panels on, 416

Electrophoresis, serum protein, 343–349
- for acute reaction proteins, 343–344
- for alpha-1 globulins, 345
- for alpha-2 globulins, 345
- for beta globulin, 345–346
- for gamma globulins, 346
- patterns of, typical, 346–349
- for serum albumin, 344–345

Electrophoretic mobility of hemoglobins, 707
Elliptocytes in peripheral smear, 15
Elliptocytosis
- hereditary, 55
- stomatocytic, 55

Elution, antibody, in antibody detection and identification, 120
Embolic glomerulonephritis, 171
Embolic purpura, 114–115
Embolism
- fat, urinalysis in, 173
- pulmonary, 328–329
- renal artery, 170

Embolization, fat, 331–332
Emotional hyperglycemia, glucose tolerance and, 469
Encephalitis, 245
- amebic, 280
- measles, 250
- test specimens for, 247

Encephalopathy, hepatic, 308–309
Endocarditis, infective, 227–229
Endocervicitis, chlamydial, 217–218
Endocrine metaplasias, multiple, 590
Endocrinologic syndromes, hyperkalemia in, 415
Endocrinopathies, hypokalemia from, 414
Endometrium, cancer of, laboratory aspects of, 576–577
Endoscopic retrograde choledochopancreatography (ERCR), 311
- in acute pancreatitis diagnosis, 457–458
- in chronic pancreatitis diagnosis, 459

Entamoeba histolytica, 279
Enteric bacilli, 198–202
Enteric fever, 200
Enterobacter, 200–201

Enterobacteriaceae, 199–202
  classification of, 687
  "opportunistic," 202
Enterobius vermicularis, 281–282
Enzyme(s)
  Hex-A, deficiency of, in Tay-Sachs disease, 597–598
  in myocardial infarct size estimation, 657
Enzyme deficiency diseases, 609–610
Eosinophilia, 66
  in allergy, 337
Eosinophilic granuloma, 87–88
Epithelial cells in urinary sediment, 164
Epstein-Barr (E-B) virus, 260–265 (*see also* Infectious mononucleosis)
Epstein-Barr virus
  infection with, laboratory diagnosis of, 261-265
  serologic tests for, 264–265
Erythema infectiosum, 650–651
Erythrocyte epimerase, deficiency of, galactosemia from, 595
Erythrocyte sedimentation rate (ESR), 330–331
  in acute myocardial infarction, 320
  limitations of, 330–331
  procedure for, 330
Erythroleukemia, 74
Erythropoiesis, inadequate, anemias due to, 36–40
Erythropoietin hormone assay in polycythemia diagnosis, 82
Escherichia coli, 201
  enteropathogenic strains of, 685
Estriol
  unconjugated, in placental function evaluation, 554–555
  urine, in placental function evaluation, 553–554
Estrogen receptor assay (ERA) in breast cancer diagnosis, 575
Estrogens
  serum, in gonadal function testing, 538
  total, in placental function evaluation, 553–554
Ethanol
  abuse of, chronic, laboratory screening for, 638
  blood
    assay of, legal use of, 637
    previous levels of, estimating, 637
  clinical and laboratory effects on, 637–638
  measurement of, 636–637
  toxicology of, 636–638
Ethanol gelation in test for fibrinolysin, 644
Ethyl alcohol, toxicology of, 636–638 (*see also* Ethanol)
Euthyroidism, false laboratory hyperthyroidism with, 498
  in hypothyroid patient, 501–502
Excretion, drug, blood levels and, 614
Exocine pancreatic adenocarcinoma, laboratory aspects of, 579–580
Extracorpuscular agents, hemolytic anemias due to, 55–59
Extrahepatic biliary tract, 316–318
  obstruction of, jaundice from, 300
Extraintestinal amebiasis, 279–280
Extrinsic system pathway of coagulation, 90, 91
Eye, examination of, ultrasound in, 669

F

Factor deficiency anemia, 23–24
  formiminoglutamic acid determination for, 641
  methylmalonic acid determination for, 641
  therapeutic trials for, 641–642
Factor I (Fibrinogen), 96–97
Factor II (prothrombin), 97
Factor III (tissue thromboplastin), 97
Factor IV (calcium ions), 97–98
Factor V (labile factor), 98
Factor VII (stable factor), 90, 98
Factor VIII
  antibodies against, 108
  concentrate of, for transfusion, 133
Factor VIII/von Willebrand factor complex, 98–100
Factor IX (plasma thromboplastin component), 100
  concentrate of, for transfusion, 133
Factor X (Stuart factor), 90, 100–101
Factor XI (plasma thromboplastin antecedent), 101
  deficiency, transfusions for, 133
Factor XII (Hageman factor), 90, 101
Factor XIII (fibrin stabilizing factor), 101
Familial dysautonomia, laboratory tests for, 666
Fanconi's anemia, pancytopenia in, 38
Fasting hypoglycemia, 475–478
Fat embolism, urinalysis in, 173
Fat embolization, 331–332
Fatty casts in urinary sediment, 163
Fatty liver, laboratory findings in, 313
Febrile agglutinins in infectious disease diagnosis, 225–226
Febrile transfusion reactions, 147–148
Fecal fat
  qualitative, in malabsorption assessment, 439
  quantitative, in malabsorption assessment, 439
Female delayed puberty, 542–544
Female hirsutism, 545–548 (*see also* Hirsutism, female)
Ferric chloride test for phenylpyruvic acid in urine, 165
Ferritin, serum levels of
  in chronic iron deficiency diagnosis, 27–28
  results of, interpretation of, 28
Fetal function, tests of, 553–555
Fetal maturity, tests of, 555–557
Fetoprotein test in liver/biliary tract evaluation, 309–310
Fever

Fever (cont.)
enteric, 200
glucose tolerance test and, 464
paratyphoid, 200
urinalysis in, 172
Fiberoptic colonoscopy in cancer detection, 449
Fibrin degradation product assay, immunologic, 106
Fibrin stabilizing factor, 101
Fibrinogen, 96–97
plasma, in hemorrhagic disorders, 96
for transfusion, 134
Fibrinogen/fibrin split products, 105–106
Fibrinolysin(s)
to dissolve thrombi, 109
primary vs. secondary, distinguishing between, 107
tests for, 105, 643–644
Fibrocystic disease of pancreas, 607–609
Fibronectin for transfusion, 134
Fibrosis, marrow replacement by, 36
"Fifth disease," 650–651
Filters, blood transfusion, 135
Fine-needle aspiration
in breast-cancer diagnosis, 575
cytology from, in thyroid cancer diagnosis, 584
Fisher-Race Rh system theory, 122–123
Fitzgerald factor, 101
Flecainide, analysis of, 623
Fletcher factor, 101
screening test for, 644
Flocculation reaction in test for syphilis, 562
Flora, body, normal, 686–687
Flow cytometry test for bladder cancer, 665
Fluids and electrolytes, information of, useful, 690
Fluorescent treponemal antibody-absorbed test for syphilis, 564–565
Foam stability index (FSI) in fetal maturity testing, 556–557
Foam test for urinary white blood cells, 160
Folate
deficiency of, 33–34
serum levels of, assay of, 33–34
Folic acid
deficiency of, 33–34
anemia from, therapeutic trial for, 641–642
formiminoglutamic acid determination for, 641
methylmalonic acid determination for, 641
serum levels of, assay of, 33–34
therapeutic trial with, for folic acid deficiency anemia, 641–642
Follicle-stimulating hormone (FSH)
in gonadal function testing, 536
testicular function and, 538–539
Follicular lymphoma, giant, 83
Formiminoglutamic acid determination in factor deficiency anemia, 641
Fouchet's reagent for urinary white blood cells, 160
Fraction of excreted sodium (FE_{Na}) in tubular function evaluation, 182–183
Fractures, radionuclide bone scanning for, 389
Fragile X chromosome, 602–603
Francisella, 206
Franklin's disease, 352
Free erythrocyte protoporphyrin in chronic diagnosis, 28–29
Free T_4 assay in thyroid function assessment, 488
Free thyroxine index (FTI) in thyroid function assessment, 487–488
Free water clearance test in tubular function evaluation, 182
French-American-British classification
of acute leukemias, 70–71
of myelodysplastic syndromes, 16
Fresh frozen plasma for transfusion, 133
Frozen red blood cells for transfusion, 131
Fructosamine assay serum in diabetes, 473
Fungal infections, 237–243 (*see also* Mycotic infections)
Fungi
cultures of, 243
opportunistic, 241–243
Furosemide test of adrenal function, 664

G

Galactokinase, deficiency of, galactosemia from, 595
Galactosemia, 594–595
in childhood, 480
Gallbladder stones, 316–317
Gallium 67 citrate in tumor scanning, 590–591
Gamma globulins, electrophoretic visualization of, 346
Gammopathies, monoclonal, 352–356
Gardnerella vaginalis, 198–199
Gas gangrene, 208
Gastric acidity, analysis of, 445
Gastric analysis, 445–447
in Zollinger-Ellison syndrome diagnosis, 580
Gastric blood, tests for, 450–451
Gastrin, serum, in Zollinger-Ellison syndrome diagnosis, 580–581
Gastrin stimulation tests in Zollinger-Ellison syndrome diagnosis, 581
Gastroenteritis
Salmonella, 200
viral, 245
test specimens, 247–248
Gastrointestinal tract
bleeding from, deficiency anemia from, 24
cancer of, 447–450
detection of, 447–450
carcinoembryonic antigen in, 449–450
direct visualization techniques in, 449
guaiac stool tests in, 448–449
interfering substances in, 448
nonguaiac stool tests in, 449
stool occult blood in, 448
x-rays in, 449
laboratory aspects of, 572–574

diarrhea in, 447
function of, 437–451
gastric analysis in, 445–447
malabsorption from, 437–445 (*see also* Malabsorption)
parasites of, 278–283
postprandial hypoglycemia originating in, 478
potassium loss from, hypokalemia from, 413–414
Gastroscopy in cancer detection, 449
Gaucher's disease, 598
Gender, hemoglobin levels and, 9
Genetic disorders, 593–610
of amino acid metabolism, 598–600
of carbohydrate metabolism, 594–597
chromosomal, 600–603
diagnostic methods for, 593
of enzyme deficiency, 609–610
of glandular secretion, 607–609
hematologic, 593
lysosomal storage, 597–598
of mineral metabolism, 605–607
of skeletal muscle, 603–605
Genitourinary tract obstruction, urinalysis in, 172
Gentamicin, analysis of, 626
German measles, 248–250
in pregnancy, 245–246, 248
Gestational diabetes, 466–467
Giant cell arteritis, 381–382
Giant follicular lymphoma, 83
Giardia lamblia, 280
Gilbert's syndrome, 655–656
Glandular secretion, abnormalities of, 607–609
Globulin(s)
alpha-1, electrophoretic visualization of, 345
alpha-2, electrophoretic visualization of, 345
beta, electrophoretic visualization of, 345–346
gamma, electrophoretic visualization of, 346
Rh immune, for Rh incompatibility prophylaxis, 143–144
Glomerular damage, severe, tests for, 177–179
Glomerular disease, primary, 684
Glomerular function tests, 175–177
summary of, 179
Glomerulonephritis, 166–167
chronic, nephrotic syndrome and, 168
embolic, 171
membranoproliferative, 168
membraneous, 168
Glucocorticoids, assay of, single-specimen, in Cushing's syndrome screening, 514–515
Glucose
blood
assay methods for, 462–463
methods for, 691
regulation of, 462
cerebrospinal fluid, 285–286
in effusions, 587
synovial fluid, 386–387
in urinalysis, 156–158
Glucose tolerance test (GTT)
in diabetes diagnosis, 463–466
factors affecting, 464–465
standardization of, 464
intravenous, 470–471
oral
abnormal criteria for, 691
clinical relevance of, 470
in other diseases, 468–470
Glucose-6-phosphate dehydrogenase (G-6-PD) defect, 52–53
screening test for, 53
Glucosuria, 156–157
in diabetes, 473–474
in pregnancy, 171
γ-Glutamyl transferase, serum levels of, in liver/biliary tract evaluation, 306
Glutethimide, toxicology of, 634
Glycogen storage disease, 596–597, 697
Glycosylated hemoglobin assay in diabetes, 471–473
Goiter, iodine deficiency, effects of, on thyroid function tests, 493
Gonadal function tests, 536–549
Gonadal precocious puberty, 541
Gonadotropin-releasing hormone (GTRH) in testicular function stimulation, 540
Gonococci, 196–197
Gout, 384–385
Graft vs. host disease, blood transfusion and, 146–147
Gram-negative diplococci, 196–199
Gram-positive cocci, 190–196
Gram-positive rods, 207
Gram stain
in bacteria diagnosis, 225
of cerebrospinal fluid in bacterial meningitis diagnosis, 289–290
Granulocytes
for transfusion, 132
in white blood cell maturation, 61, 62
Granulocytic leukemia, chronic, 78–79
Granulocytopenia, 67
Granuloma, eosinophilic, 87–88
Granuloma inguinale, 203
Granulomatous disease of childhood, chronic, 332
Granulomatous thyroiditis, 504
Granulomatous vasculitis, 381
Graves' ophthalmopathy, isolated, 498–499
Growth hormone
assay of, 532
deficiency of, 531–534
Growth hormone stimulation tests, 533
Guaiac stool tests in gastrointestinal tract cancer detection, 448–449
Gynecomastia, 548–549

H

Haemophilus (see also Hemophilus), 203
Hageman factor, 101
Hairy cell leukemia, 76–77
Hand-Schuller-Christian disease, 88
Haptoglobin, serum levels of
in hemolytic anemia diagnosis, 43
in tests for hemolytic transfusion reaction, 141
Heart
disorders of, diagnosis of, ultrasound in, 669–670
failure of, congestive, electrolyte abnormalities in, 408

Heart (cont.)
valves of, infection of, 227–229
Heavy chain disease, 352
Heavy metals, toxicology of, 634
Hemastix for urinary hemoglobin, 159
Hematest for urinary hemoglobin, 159
Hematocrit, 10
Hematologic blood values, normal, by age, 682
Hematologic disease, genetic, 593
Hematologic findings in metastatic bone cancer, 585
Hematologic tests
basic, 9–21
comments on, 18–20
Hematoma, subdural
cerebrospinal fluid findings in, 294–295
radioisotope studies of, 653
Hematuria
biochemical methods versus microscopic examination for, 159–160
problem of, 186
in renal cell adenocarcinoma, 569
Hemochromatosis, 606–607
urinalysis in, 173
Hemodimethrine bromide neutralization test in coagulation assessment, 645
Hemoglobin(s), 9–10
electrophoretic mobility of, 707
free, in plasma or urine in hemolytic anemia diagnosis, 43–44
glycosylated, assay in diabetes, 471–473
mean corpuscular, 12
plasma free, in tests for hemolytic transfusion reactions, 140
sickle, 45–48 (*see also* Sickle hemoglobin)
solubility of, differential, in sickle hemoglobin detection, 45–46
structure of, abnormalities of, in hemolytic anemia, 44–49
synthesis of, abnormalities of, 49–52
unstable, 48–49
in urinalysis, 159–160
Hemoglobin C disease, 48
Hemoglobin C trait, 48
Hemoglobin casts in urinary sediment, 163
Hemoglobin-Köln, 48
Hemoglobin SC disease, 47–48
Hemoglobin SS disease, 46–47
Hemoglobin-Zurich, 48
Hemoglobinopathies
detection of, comments on, 48
in hemolytic anemia, 44–48
Hemoglobinuria, paroxysmal
cold, 56
nocturnal, 57–58
Hemolysin, definition of, 118
Hemolysis, jaundice from, 299–300
Hemolytic anemia(s), 42–59
from autoagglutinins, 55–56
from autoantibodies, 55–56
autoimmune, 55–56
secondary acquired, 56
drug-induced, 56–57
from extracorpuscular agents, 55–59
from extracorpuscular defects, 42
hemoglobin structure abnormalities in, 44–49
hemoglobin synthesis abnormalities in, 49–52
in hypersplenism, 59
from intracorpuscular defects, 42
laboratory tests in, 42–44
microangiopathic, 57
from parasites, 59
red blood cell enzyme deficiencies in, 52–53
red blood cell membrane abnormalities in, 53–55
from toxins, 58–59
traumatic, 5
Hemolytic disease of newborn, 142–146
ABO-induced, 144–145
albumin-bound bilirubin in, 145–146
amniocentesis in, 146
bilirubin levels in, 145
laboratory criteria for, 145
laboratory tests in, 144
from Rh incompatibilities, 142–143
Hemolytic reactions of bacteria on blood agar, 648
Hemolytic transfusion reactions, 139–146
possible, nursing station action in, 141–142
tests for, 140–141
sensitivity of, 141
Hemophilia A
clinical aspects of, 99
laboratory tests in, 100
and von Willebrand's disease, differentiation of, 99–100
Hemophilus vaginalis, 198–199
Hemorrhage
intracerebral, cerebrospinal fluid findings in, 295
subarachnoid, cerebrospinal fluid findings in, 195
Hemorrhagic colitis, 201
Hemorrhagic disorders
basic tests in, 91–96
urinalysis in, 173
Henderson-Hasselbalch equation, 393
Henoch-Schonlein syndrome, urinalysis, 173
Henoch's purpura, 114
Heparin, 103–104
to dissolve thrombi, 109
therapy with, monitoring of, 644
Heparin/antithrombin III anticoagulant system, 102–104
Hepatic amebiasis, 279–280
Hepatic encephalopathy, 308–309
Hepatitis
chronic active, diagnosis of, anti-smooth muscle antibodies in, 309
delta, 253
non-A, non-B, tests for, 651
viral, acute, laboratory findings in, 312
Hepatitis B surface antigen, tests for, comparison of, 688
Hepatitis virus
A, 252
infection from, diagnosis of, 253–254
B, 252–253
blood bank screening for, 258
infection with
chronic, 257–258
diagnosis of, 254–257

D, 253
infection from, transmitted by blood transfusion, 148–149
non-A, non-B, 253
Hereditary angioedema, complement and, 356
Hereditary elliptocytosis, 55
Heroin, 631
Herpes simplex virus (HSV) infection, 265–267
diagnosis of, 266–267
Heterophil agglutination tube test in Epstein-Barr infection diagnosis, 262–263
Heterophil-negative infectious mononucleosis, 263
Hex-A enzyme, deficiency of, in Tay-Sachs disease, 597–598
High-density lipoprotein cholesterol in coronary heart disease risk assessment, 361–362
High molecular weight kininogen (HMWK), 101
Hirsutism, female, 545–548
conditions producing, 545
laboratory tests for, 545–547
polycystic ovary disease and, 547–548
Histiocytosis
Langerhans' cell, 87–88
X, 87–88
Histologic classification on non-Hodgkin's lymphomas, 83
Histoplasmosis, 239–240
Hodgkin's disease, 85–86
Homogeneous pattern in antinuclear antibody test, 376
Hookworm, 282
Hormone(s)
adrenal cortex, 509–512
production of, by tumors, 591
ectopic, 696–697
thyroid, (*see also under* Thyroid)
production of, 482, 483
thyroid-releasing, test of, interpretation of, 693
Hospital working procedures, effects of, on laboratory test data, 7–8
Howell-Jolly bodies in red blood cells, 16
Human chorionic gonadotropin (hCG)
neoplasms producing, diagnosis of, 552–553
in pregnancy testing, 549–550
technical problems with, 550–551
in testicular function stimulation, 540
Human immunodeficiency viruses (HIVs)
infection with, 267–271
clinical findings in, 267–268
diagnosis of, 269–271
laboratory findings in, 269
risk factors for, 268
meningitis from, cerebrospinal fluid findings in, 293
Human immunodeficiency virus transmitted by blood transfusion, 149
Human leukocyte-A (HLA) system in blood grouping, 126–127
Hurler's syndrome, 598
Hyaline casts in urinary sediment, 162–163
Hybritech CA 549 in cancer diagnosis, 665
Hydatid cyst infection, 282
Hydatidiform mole, diagnosis of, 552
Hydrocephalus, radioisotope studies of, 653
Hydrogen breath test in malabsorption assessment, 444
Hydroxybutryic acid dehydrogenase (HBO) in acute myocardial infarction, 323
17-Hydroxycorticosteroids, 509
5-Hydroxyindoleacetic acid (5-HIAA), urine, assay of, in carcinoid syndrome diagnosis, 573–574
Hydroxyproline, urine, in cancer diagnosis, 665–666
Hyperbilirubinemias, congenital, 655–656
Hypercalcemia, 414–415
differential diagnosis of, tests in, 419–425
etiologies of, 417
in malignancy, 418–419, 425
nonneoplastic causes of, 419
primary hyperparathyroidism and, 417–418
serum calcium levels regulation and, 417
Hyperglycemia
emotional, glucose tolerance and, 469
posthypoglycemic, glucose tolerance and, 470
Hyperkalemia, 415–416
drug-induced, 415–416
Hypernatremia, 413
Hypernephroma, laboratory aspects of, 569
Hyperosmolar nonketotic coma, 474
Hyperparathyroidism
primary, hypercalcemia in, 417–418
tertiary, hypercalcemia in, 419
Hyperphosphatemia, 430
Hyperplasia, adrenal, congenital, 512–513
Hyperprolactinemia, secondary amenorrhea in, 545
Hyperpyrexia, malignant, 604–605
Hypersegmentation, neutrophil, in megaloblastic anemia detection, 642
Hypersegmented granulocyte in white blood cell maturation, 62
Hypersensitivities, urinalysis in, 173
Hypersplenism
hemolytic anemia in, 59
thrombocytopenia in, 111
Hypertension
adrenal and nonadrenal causes of, 528
malignant, kidneys in, 168–169
of pregnancy, thrombocytopenia in, 112
Hyperthyroidism, 483
alkaline phosphatase elevation in, 303
confirmatory tests for, 499
with false laboratory euthyroidism, 498
glucose tolerance and, 468
laboratory test patterns in, 494–500
pseudo-T_3, 496–497
pseudo-T_4, 497

Hyperthyroidism (cont.)
pseudo-thyroxine/triiodothyronine, 495–496
thyrotropin-releasing hormone results in, 492
urinalysis in, 173
Hyperuricemia, disorders of, 384
Hypoaldosteronism, hyporeninemic, 525
Hypocalcemia, 425–427
Hypochromia, 14
Hypochromic anemias, 26
Hypogammaglobulinemia pattern in serum protein electrophoresis, 347, 348
Hypoglycemia, 474–480
fasting, 475–478
idiopathic, of infancy, 479–480
neonatal and childhood, 479–480
postprandial, 478–479
Hypogonadism, investigation of, 538–541
Hypokalemia, 413–415
medication-induced, 414–415
preoperative, studies on, 660
urine potassium assay in, 415
Hypokalemic alkalosis, 396–397, 414
Hyponatremia, 405–413
iatrogenic sources of, 405–406
laboratory findings in, 412–413
laboratory investigation of, 410–412
Hyponatremic depletional syndromes, 406–407
Hypophosphatemia, 429
Hypoplastic marrow, 36–38
Hyporeninemic hypoaldosteronism, 525
Hypothalamic precocious puberty, 541
Hypothyroid patients, false laboratory euthyroidism in, 501–502
Hypothyroidism, 483–484
anemia of, 40
laboratory test patterns in, 499–500
neonatal, screening for, 505–506
occult, menstrual irregularity with, 663
thyroid tests in, 500–502
thyrotropin-releasing hormone results in, 492

I

I-(IH) blood group antigens, 124
Ictotest tablets for urinary white blood cells, 160
Idiopathic monoclonal gammopathy, 353
Idiopathic thrombocytopenic purpura, 110
IgM monoclonal proteins, 659
Immune complexes, circulating, 382–383
Immune status tests in protein-calorie malnutrition, 434
Immunoassay in sickle hemoglobin detection, 46
Immunocytochemical estrogen receptor methods in breast cancer diagnosis, 576
Immunofluorescence staining, skin biopsy with
in Rocky Mountain spotted fever diagnosis, 651
in systemic lupus erythematosus diagnosis, 378
Immunoglobulin(s), 349
levels of
in biliary tract disease testing, 654
neonatal, 332
thyroid-stimulating, assay of, 662–663
Immunoglobulin A antigen reactions from blood transfusions, 148
Immunoglobulin D myeloma, 351–352
Immunoglobulin E levels in allergy testing, 336–337
Immunoglobulin M monoclonal proteins, 659
Immunologic classification of acute lymphocytic leukemia, 73
Immunologic fibrin degradation product assay, 106
Immunologic methods for bacterial detection, 189
Immunologic status tests in human immunodeficiency virus I infection diagnosis, 270–271
Immunologic tests
for pregnancy, 549–550
for syphilis, 562
Immunologic thrombocytopenia, 110–111
Immunologic-type coagulation factor inhibitors, 107–108
Immunophenotyping, lymphocyte, 72
Immunoreactive trypsin, serum
in acute pancreatitis diagnosis, 457
in chronic pancreatitis diagnosis, 458
Inactivity, glucose tolerance test and, 464
Inappropriate ADH (IADH) syndrome, 409–410
Indirect Coombs' test in antibody detection and identification, 120
Infancy, hypoglycemia of, ideopathic, 479–480
Infant, iron deficiency in, 23–24
Infection(s)
acute leukemia differentiated from, 75
anemia of, 39
deviation from white blood cell pattern in, 64
mycotic, 237–243 (see also Fungi; Mycotic infections)
neutrophilic leukocytosis due to, 64–65
pregnancy, bacteriuria in, 171–172
renal, 169
rubella, diagnosis of, 649–650
thrombocytopenia in, 112
transmitted by blood transfusions, 148–149
Infectious lymphocytosis, acute leukemia differentiated from, 75
Infectious mononucleosis, 260–265
acute leukemia differentiated from, 74–75
diagnosis of, 263–264
heterophil-negative, 263
laboratory diagnosis of, 261–265
laboratory findings in, 261
urinalysis in, 173
Infective endocarditis, 227–229

Infertility, male, investigation of, 538–541
Inflammation, neutrophilic leukocytosis due to, 64–65
Inflammatory bowel disease, arthritis associated with, 372
Inflammatory pattern, chronic, in serum protein electrophoresis, 347, 348
Instruments, cell counting, artifacts from, 14
Insulin, plasma, assay of, in diabetes, 471
Insulin/glucose ratio
  amended, for insulinoma diagnosis, 661
  in fasting hypoglycemia evaluation, 475–476
Insulinoma
  diagnosis of, amended insulin/glucose ratio for, 661
  localization of, 477–478
Intestine, small, biopsy of, in malabsorption assessment, 444
Intra-abdominal abscess, 231
Intracerebral abscess, radioisotope studies of, 653
Intracerebral hemorrhage, cerebrospinal fluid findings in, 295
Intrahepatic biliary tract obstruction, jaundice from, 300
Intravenous glucose tolerance test (IVGTT), 470–471
Intravenous pyelogram (IVP) in tubular function evaluation, 181–182
Intrinsic factor, assay for, 642
Intrinsic system pathway of coagulation, 90–91
Iodine
  deficiency of, effects of, on thyroid function tests, 493
  effects of, on thyroid tests, 493–494
  excess of, effects of, on thyroid function tests, 493–494
  serum, measurement of, thyroid tests based on, 661
Iodine function tests, 493–494
Ion-selective electrodes (ISEs) in sodium measurement, 404
Ionized calcium, in differential diagnosis of hypercalcemia, 419–420
Iontophoresis for sweat test for cystic fibrosis, 608
Iron
  deficiency of, 23–24
    chronic
      diagnosis of, 29
      laboratory tests for, 24–29
      Thalassemia minor vs., 51
    diagnosis of, 29
    zinc protoporphyrin, 28
  laboratory studies of, in hemochromatosis diagnosis, 607
  metabolism of, 23
  serum levels of
    changes in, by disease, 683
    in chronic iron deficiency diagnosis, 25–26
    conditions affecting, 26
    decrease in, 26
    increase in, 26
    in megaloblastic anemia, 26
  therapeutic trial with, for iron deficiency anemia, 641
Iron-binding capacity, total, changes in, by disease, 683
Iron stain, bone marrow, in chronic iron deficiency diagnosis, 29
Irradiated red blood cells for transfusion, 131
Isoagglutinins, hemolytic anemias due to, 55
Isoantibodies
  definition of, 118
  hemolytic anemias due to, 55–56
Isocitric dehydrogenase in liver disease testing, 654

J

Jaundice, causes of, 299–301
Jogger anemia, 24
Joint(s)
  disorders of, 369–390
  radionuclide scanning of, 387–388
Joint fluid aspiration in diagnosis of gout, 385
Juvenile rheumatoid arthritis, 371

K

Karyotyping, chromosome, indications for, 603
Kell blood group antigens, 123–124
Ketoacidosis, diabetic
  hyperkalemia in, 415
  hypokalemia from, 414
17-Ketogenic steroids in adrenal function testing, 664
Ketone bodies in urinalysis, 156–159
Ketonuria, 158–159
Ketosis in childhood, 480
17-Ketosteroids (17-KS), 509, 511
  fractionation of, in adrenal function testing, 664
  urine
    assay of, in Cushing's syndrome screening, 514
    in female hirsutism investigation, 546
Kidd blood group antigens, 124
Kidney(s)
  biopsy of, 184
  cancer of, laboratory aspects of, 569–570
  chronic passive congestion (CPC) in, urinalysis in, 172
  developmental anomalies of, 170
  in disease, 166–172
    anemia and, 38
    chronic, with azotemia, glucose tolerance and, 469
    congenital, 170
  in electrolyte physiology, 407–408
  failure of
    azotemia and, 183–184
    hyperkalemia in, 415
  function of
    effect of, on serum unconjugated bilirubin, 300
    tests of, 175–186 (*see also* Renal function tests)
  in glomerulonephritis, 166–167
  infections of, 169
  neoplasia of, 170

Kidney(s) *(cont.)*
  in nephrotic syndrome, 167–168
  polycystic, 170
  potassium loss through, hypokalemia from, 414
Kimmelstiel-Wilson syndrome, nephrotic syndrome and, 168
Kingsbury-Clark procedure for urinary protein, 155–156
Kininogen, high molecular weight, 101
Kirby-Bauer method of antibiotic sensitivity testing, 231–232
Klebsiella, 200–201
  pneumonia due to, 231
Klinefelter's syndrome, 539, 601
Kvein skin test in sarcoidosis diagnosis, 329

L

Labile factor, 98
Laboratory test data
  accuracy of, 2–3
  hospital working procedures affecting, 7–8
  interpretation of, 1–8
  medical literature and, 8
  medications affecting, 7
  normal ranges in, 3–6
  physiologic variables affecting, 7
  predictive value of, 1–2
  problems with laboratory specimens in, 6–7
  reproducivility of, 2
  sensitivity of, 1
  specificity of, 1
Laboratory tests, substances interfering with, 674–681
Lactase deficiency, 595–596
  x-ray in, 666
Lactase intolerance, 595–596
Lactate, cerebrospinal fluid, in bacterial meningitis diagnosis, 290
Lactic acidosis syndrome, 474
Lactic dehydrogenase (LDH)
  in acute myocardial infarction, 321–323
  in effusions, 587
  in hemolytic anemia diagnosis, 43
  serum
    in liver/biliary tract evaluation, 305
    in tests for cancer, 588
    in vitamin B12 deficiency diagnosis, 31
Lactogen, placental, in placental function evaluation, 555
Lactosuria, 596
Lancefield group A streptococci, 191
Lancefield group B streptococci, 191–192
Lancefield group C streptococci, 192
Lancefield group D streptococci, 192
Lancefield group F streptococci, 192
Lancefield group G streptococci, 192
Langerhans' cell histiocytosis, 87–88
Latex agglutination (LA) tests for bacterial antigens, 290
Lavage, peritoneal, for traumatic injury, 588
Lead
  blood, assay of, in lead toxicity, 632
  encephalopathy from, cerebrospinal fluid findings in, 296–297
  exposure to, detecting, 632–633
  toxicology of, 631–634
Lead poisoning
  diagnosis of, 633–634
  hemolytic anemia in, 58–59
Lecithin/sphingomyelin (L/S) ratio in fetal maturity testing, 555–556
Legionella, 205
  pneumonia due to, 231
Legionella organisms, classification of, 685
Leptospirosis, 210–211
Letterer-Siwe disease, 87
Leucine amino peptidase in biliary tract disease testing, 654
Leucine sensitivity in childhood, 480
Leukemia(s)
  acute, 67, 70–75
    blastic, 69
    differential diagnosis of, 74–75
    differentiation of, cytochemical stains in, 71–72
    French-American-British classification of, 70–71
    lymphocytic, 72–73
      immunologic classification of, 73
    nonlymphocytic, 72
  aleukemic, 67
  chromosome analysis in, 643
  chronic, 67
    lymphocytic, 77–78
    myelogenous, 78–79
      differential diagnosis of, 80–81
  definition of, 69
  granulocytic, 78–79
  hairy cell, 76–77
  monocytic, 67, 73–74
  myelomonocytic, 74
  stem cell, 67
  subleukemic, 67
Leukemic reticuloendotheliosis, 76
Leukemoid reaction, 66, 79–80
  differential diagnosis of, 80–81
Leukoagglutinin reaction from blood transfusions, 147–148
Leukocyte alkaline phosphatase (LAP)
  in differentiation of chronic myelogenous leukemia, agnogenic myeloid metaplasia, and leukemoid reaction, 80
  in polycythemia diagnosis, 82
Leukocyte esterase in urinalysis, 160
Leukocyte-poor packed cells for transfusion, 130
Leukocytes, 61–67 (*see also* White blood cells)
Leukocytosis
  in acute myocardial infarction, 320
  neonatal, 63–64
  neutrophilic, from infection and inflammation, 64–65
  in rheumatoid arthritis, 369
Leukoerythroblastosis, 67
Leukopenia in aplastic anemia, drugs causing, 37
Levothroid, therapy with, monitoring of, 503–504
Lewis blood group antigens, 124

Lidocaine, analysis of, 621–622
Lipase, serum, in acute pancreatitis diagnosis, 457
Lipid metabolism, disordered, 597–598
Lipoid nephrosis, 168
Liproprotein(s), 357–367
  disorders of, laboratory tests in, 363–367
  metabolism of, 358
  phenotyping of, 363
  subgroups of, 357
Lipoproteinemia(s)
  classification of, 364–365
  type IV, glucose tolerance and, 469
Listeria monocytogenes, 207
Literature, medical, laboratory tests and, 8
Lithium carbonate
  analysis of, 619–620
  neutrophilic leukocytosis due to, 65
Lithium therapy, hypercalcemia in, 419
Liver
  alkaline phosphatase originating in, 302–303
  amebiasis of, 279–280
  biopsy of, 311–312
  cancer of, laboratory aspects of, 581
  disease of
    chronic, anemia of, 39–40
    glucose tolerance and, 469
    laboratory findings in, 312–315
    laboratory test patterns in, 314–315
    tests for, 653–656
      alkaline phosphatase isoenzymes in, 654
      bromsulphalein in, 655
      cholesterol and cholesterol esters in, 654–655
      isocitric dehydrogenase in, 654
      ornithinine carbamyl transferase in, 653–654
  fatty, laboratory findings in, 313
  function of, tests of, selection of, 315–316
  metastatic carcinoma to, laboratory findings in, 314
  scan of, radionuclide, 310
  toxic effects of acetaminophen on, 634–635
  viral infections of, jaundice from, 301
Low-density lipoprotein cholesterol in coronary heart disease risk assessment, 361–362
Lukes-Collins classification of malignant lymphomas, 84
Lung(s)
  cancer of, laboratory aspects of, 578–579
  function of, tests of, radioisotope, 658
Lupus erythematosus
  kidneys in, 170–171
  systemic (*see* Systemic lupus erythematosus)
Luteinizing hormone (LH)
  in female hirsutism investigation, 547
  in gonadal function testing, 536–537
  testicular function and, 539
Lutheran blood group antigens, 124
Lyme disease, 211
Lymph nodes
  biopsy of, in sarcoidosis diagnosis, 329–330
  enlarged, periaortic and retroperitoneal masses of, detection of, ultrasound in, 669
Lymphocyte(s)
  B and T, identification of, 72
  subgroups of, monoclonal antibody identification of, 72–73
Lymphocyte count, total, for immune status in protein-calorie malnutrition, 434
Lymphocyte immunophenotyping, 72
Lymphocytic leukemia
  acute, 72–73
    immunologic classification of, 73
  chronic, 77–78
Lymphocytosis, 66–67
  infectious, acute leukemia differentiated from, 75
Lymphoma(s)
  Burkitt's, 84–85
  giant follicular, 83
  malignant, 82–87 (*see also* Malignant lymphomas)
  non-Hodgkin's, classification of, 642–643
Lysosomal storage diseases, 597–598

M

Macrocytes in peripheral smear, 14
Macrocytic anemia in liver disease, 39
Macrocytosis, causes of, 10–11
Macroglobulinemia, Waldenström's, 352–353
Magnesium
  deficiency of, 428
  excess, 428
  serum, abnormalities of, 427–428
Magnetic resonance imaging (MRI), 672
  for brain disease detection, 290–291
Major crossmatch of blood, 124–126
Malabsorption, 437–445
  classification of, 438–439
  clinical findings in, 437
  laboratory findings in, 437, 439
  laboratory tests for, 439–444
    D-xylose, 442–444
    fecal fat, 439
    hydrogen breath, 444
    of plasma carotene, 440
    radioisotope, 440
    Schilling, 440–442
    small intestine biopsy as, 444
    x-ray 440
  workup for, 444–445
Malaria, 278
Male infertility, investigation of, 538–541
Malignancy
  glucose tolerance and, 469
  hypercalcemia and, 418–419, 425
Malignant hyperpyrexia, 604–605
Malignant hypertension, kidneys in, 168–169
Malignant lymphomas, 82–87
  Burkitt's, 84–85
  clinical findings in, 86–87
  diagnosis of, 87
  differential diagnosis of, 87

Malignant lymphomas (cont.)
Hodgkin's disease as, 85–86
immunologic characterization of, 83–84
laboratory findings in, 87
Lukes-Collins classification of, 84
National Cancer Institute Lymphoma Panel Working Formulation on, 84
non-Hodgkin's histologic classification of, 83–84
Rappaport's classification of, 83
Malnutrition
categories of, differentiating, 435
protein-calorie
classification of, 431
current status of, 434–435
degree of deficiency in, assessment of, 434
immune status and, 434
metabolic indices and, 433
nutritional therapy for, 435
patient screening for, 434
patients with, tests in, 431–435
tests for, 431–435
visceral protein status, 432–433
Mammography in breast cancer diagnosis, 574
Mantoux test in tuberculosis, 213–214
Marginal ulcer, diagnosis of, gastric analysis in, 441
Marijuana, 628–629
Mattingly fluorescent procedure of serum cortisol measurement, 512
Mean corpuscular hemoglobin (MCH), 12
Mean corpuscular hemoglobin concentration (MCHC), 12
in chronic iron deficiency, 25
Mean corpuscular volume (MCV), 10–12
in chronic iron deficiency, 25
in megaloblastic anemia, 31
Mean platelet volume (MPV) in coagulation assessment, 645
Measles, 250–251
German, 248–250
in pregnancy, 245–246, 248
Medical literature, laboratory tests and, 8
Medication (see Drugs)
Megaloblastic anemia
diagnosis of
bone marrow examination in, 31
mean corpuscular volume in, 31
serum lactic dehydrogenase in, 31
serum iron in, 26
thrombocytopenia in, 112
Megaloblastic changes in vitamin B12 deficiency, 30–31
Melanocholia
laboratory tests for, 338
overnight dexamethasone test for, factors altering results of, 688
Membranoproliferative glomerulonephritis, 168
Membranous glomerulonephritis, 168
Meningitis
aspetic, cerebrospinal fluid findings in, 292–293
bacterial, diagnosis of
cerebrospinal fluid cultures in, 289
cerebrospinal fluid lactate in, 290
Gram staining of CSF in, 289–290
cryptococcal, cerebrospinal fluid findings in, 292
human immunodeficiency virus, cerebrospinal fluid findings in, 293
mycobacterial, cerebrospinal fluid findings in, 291–292
viral, 244–245
cerebrospinal fluid findings in, 292–293
test specimens for, 247
Meningococci, 196
Menstrual bleeding, iron deficiency anemia from, 24
Menstrual irregularity with occult hypothyroidism, 663
Mesenteric adenitis, 201–202
Metabolic acidosis, 395–396
anion gap in, 400–401
Metabolic alkalosis, 396–397
Metabolic indices in protein-calorie nutritional status assessment, 433
Metabolic toxic states, neutrophilic leukocytosis due to, 65
Metabolism
amino acid, defects in, 598–600
bilirubin, inherited defects in, 655–656
carbohydrate, diseases of, genetic, 594–597
drug, blood levels and, 613–614
iron, 23
mineral, diseases of, 605–606
Metals, heavy, toxicology of, 634
Metamyelocyte in white blood cell maturation, 61, 62
Metaplasia, agnogenic myeloid, 79
differential diagnosis of, 80
Metastatic carcinoma
to bone, laboratory findings in, 585–586
to liver, laboratory findings in, 314
to organs, frequency of, 696
Methacillin-resistant *S. Aureus* (MRSA), 231
3-Methoxy-4-hydroxyphenylglycol (MHPG) in depression evaluation, 338–339
Methylmalonic acid determination in factor deficiency anemia, 641
Metyrapone test in Cushing's syndrome confirmation, 517
Microalbuminuria, 156
Microangiopathic hemolytic anemia, 57
Microcytes in peripheral smear, 14
Microcytosis, causes of, 11
Microhemagglutination test for syphilis, 565
Mikulicz's syndrome, 380
Miliary tuberculosis, 214–215
Mineral metabolism, diseases of, 605–607
Minimal inhibitory concentration (MIC) in antibiotic sensitivity testing, 232–233

Mixed connective tissue (MCT) disease, 379–380
MN blood group antigens, 124
Mongolism, 602
Monitoring, therapeutic drug, 612–617 (*see also* Therapeutic drugs)
Monoclonal antibody identification of lymphocyte subgroups, 72–73
Monoclonal gammopathy(ies), 352–356
  benign and malignant, differentiation of, 354–355
  diagnostic techniques for, 353–354
  idiopathic, 353
  secondary, 353–356
Monoclonal gammopathy spike in serum protein electropheresis, 347, 348
Monocyte in white blood cell maturation, 63
Monocytic leukemia, 73–74
Monocytosis, 66
Mononucleosis, infectious, 260–265 (*see also* Infectious mononucleosis)
Morphine, 631
Moschcowitz's disease, 111–112
Mucin clot in synovial fluid analysis, 386
Mucopolysaccharidoses, 598, 698
Mucormycosis, 243
Mucoviscidosis, 607–609
Multiple endocrine neoplasia syndromes, 590
Multiple myeloma, 349–352
  anemia in, 36
  bone marrow diagnosis of, 350–351
  immunoglobulins in, 351
  laboratory test findings in, 350
  protein abnormalities in, 351
  x-ray findings of, 350
Multiple sclerosis, cerebrospinal fluid findings in, 295–296
Mumps, 251
Muscles, skeletal
  congenital diseases of, 603–605
  CPK-MB fraction, 325–326
Muscular dystrophies, 603–604, 697
Myasthenia gravis (MG), 339
Mycobacteria
  atypical, classification of, 215
  nontuberculosis, 215–216
Mycobacterial disease, 211–215 (*see also* Tuberculosis)
Mycobacterial meningitis, cerebrospinal fluid findings in, 291– 292
Mycobacterium tuberculosis, 211–215 (*see also* Tuberculosis)
Mycoplasma pneumoniae, 219–220
  pneumonia due to, 230–231
Mycoplasmas, 219–220
Mycotic infections, 237–243 (*see also* Fungi)
  of central nervous system, cerebrospinal fluid findings in, 292
  cultures for, 243
  diagnosis of, 237–238
  opportunistic, 241–243
  systemic, 237–241
Myelocyte in white blood cell maturation, 61, 62
Myelodysplastic syndrome, 75–76
Myelofibrosis, 36
Myelogenous leukemia, chronic, 78–79
  differential diagnosis of, 80–81
Myeloid metaplasia, 36
Myeloid spot in nucleus in white blood cell maturation, 61
Myeloma
  cryoglobulins in, 355–356
  diagnosis of, 353–354
  immunoglobulin D, 351–352
  multiple, 349–352 (*see also* Multiple myeloma)
Myelomonocytic leukemia, 74
Myelophthisic anemia, 36
Myocardial infarct, size of, enzymatic estimation of, 657
Myocardial infarction (MI)
  acute, 320–328
    creatine phosphokinase-MB isoforms in, 657
    glucose tolerance test and, 464, 469
    radionuclide heart scan in, 327–328
    reperfusion after thrombolytic agents for, detection of, 658
    tests in, 320–327
  diagnosis of, myoglobin in, 656–657
Myoglobin in myocardial infarction diagnosis, 656–657
Myoglobinemia, causes of, 688
Myoglobinuria, causes of, 688
Myopathies, congenital, 697
Mysoline, analysis of, 618
Myxedema
  glucose tolerance and, 468
  in thyroid deficiency, 483–484
  urinalysis in, 173

N

National Cancer Institute Lymphoma Panel Working Formulation, 84
Neck vein catheterization in parathyroid function evaluation, 659
Necrotizing papillitis, 169
Neisseria gonorrhoeae, 196–197
Neonatal hypocalcemia, 426–427
Neonatal hypoglycemia, 479–480
Neonatal hypothyroid screening, 505–506
Neonatal immunoglobulin levels, 332
Neonatal thrombocytopenia, 111
Neonate (*see* Newborn)
Neoplasia
  anemia of, 38–39
  renal, 170
Neoplasm(s)
  marrow replacement by, 36
  producing human chorionic gonadotropin diagnosis of, 552–553
Nephropathy, diabetic, red blood cell casts in, 645
Nephrosclerosis, accelerated arteriolar, kidneys in, 168–169
Nephrosis, primary, 168
Nephrotic syndrome, 167–168
Nephrotic syndrome pattern in serum protein electrophoresis, 347, 348

Nesidioblastosis in childhood, 480
Neural tube defects, open, biochemical tests for, 557–558
Neurology, laboratory test in, 339
Neutropenia, 67
Neutrophil cytoplasmic inclusions, 65
Neutrophil hypersegmentation in megaloblastic anemia detection, 642
Neutrophilic leukocytosis
  from drugs and chemicals, 65
  from infection and inflammation, 64–65
  from metabolic toxic states, 65
  from tissue destruction, 65
Neutrophils for transfusion, 132
Newborn
  hemoglobin levels in, 9–10
  hemolytic disease of, 142–146 (*see also* Hemolytic disease of newborn)
  leukocytosis in, 63–64
  white blood cell counts in, problems with, 65
Niemann-Pick disease, 598
Nitrite in urinalysis, 160
Nitroblue tetrazolium test for pediatric patient, 332–333
Nitrogen balance estimates in protein-calorie nutritional status assessment, 433
Nocardia, 220–221
Nongonococcal urethritis, 197–198
Nonguaiac stool tests in gastrointestinal tract cancer detection, 449
Non-Hodgkin's lymphomas, histologic classification of, 83
Nonlymphocytic leukemia, acute, 72
Nonspherocytic anemias, congenital, 52–53
Nontuberculous mycobacteria, 215–216
Normal values, representative, 701–705
Nosocomial infections, 231
Nuclear medicine scanning, 671–672
Nucleic acid probe (DNA) probe
  for bacterial detection, 189
  in hepatitis B virus detection, 257
  in tuberculosis, 213
Nucleolar pattern in antinuclear antibody test, 376
5-Nucleotidase in biliary tract disease testing, 654
Nutritional therapy for malnutrition, 435

O

Obesity, glucose tolerance test and, 464
Obstetrics, tests in, 549–557
  for ectopic pregnancy, 551–552
  for fetal maturity, 555–557
  for fetal or placental function, 553–555
  for neoplasms producing human chorionic gonadotropin, 552–553
  for pregnancy, 549–551
Occultest for urinary hemoglobin, 159
Ochronosis, 600
Ocular examination, ultrasound in, 669
Oligoclonal bands vs. serum bands in cerebrospinal fluid examination, 652
Oliguria in azotemia, 183
Ophthalmopathy, Graves', isolated, 498–499
"Opportunistic" enterobacteriaceae, 202
Opportunistic fungi, 241–243
Oral glucose tolerance test (OGTT)
  abnormal, criteria for, 691
  clinical relevance of, 470
  in diabetes diagnosis, 465–466
Organic phosphates, toxicology of, 634
Ornithinine carbamyl transferase in liver disease testing, 653–654
Osmolality
  serum, in hyponatremia investigation, 411–412
  urine
    in hyponatremia investigation, 411, 412
    in tubular function evaluation, 181
Osteomyelitis
  radionuclide bone scanning for, 389
  Salmonella, 200
Ova, stool examination for, 278
Oval fat bodies in fatty casts, 163
Ovalocytes in peripheral smear, 15
Ovalocytosis, 55
Ovarian agenesis, 601–602
Ovary(ies)
  cancer of, laboratory aspects of, 577
  polycystic, female hirsutism and, 547–548
Oxygen saturation, noninvasive measurement of, 402
Oxyuris vermicularis, 281–282

P

P blood group antigens, 124
Packed red blood cells for transfusion, 130–131
Pancreas
  cancer of
    diagnosis of, ultrasound in, 669
    laboratory aspects of, 579–581
  cystic fibrosis of, 459
  fibrocystic disease of, 607–609
  function of, 453–459
Pancreatic stimulation tests in chronic pancreatitis diagnosis, 459
Pancreatitis
  acute, 453–458
    amylase isoenzyme fractionation in, 456–457
    amylase/creatinine clearance ratio in, 455–456
    computerized tomography in, 458
    endoscopic retrograde cholangiopancreatography in, 457–458
    glucose tolerance and, 469
    laboratory tests for, 453–458
    serum amylase measurement in, 454–455
    serum immunoreactive trypsin assay in, 457
    serum lipase measurement in, 457

ultrasound in, 458
urine amylase measurement in, 455
chronic, 458–459
Pancytopenia
acute leukemia differentiated from, 75
in aplastic anemia, drugs causing, 37
in hairy cell leukemia, 76
Papanicolaou (PAP) smear in cervical cancer diagnosis, 576
Paper strip methods of blood glucose assay, 463
Pappenheimer bodies in red blood cells, 16
Paracetamol, toxicology of, 634–635
Parasites
eosinophilia and, 66
gastrointestinal, 278–283
hemolytic anemia due to, 59
stool examination for, 278
Parasitology, medical, 276–283
Parathyroid gland function
chloride/phosphate ratio for, 659
neck vein catheterization for, 659
urine adenosine 3,5-monophosphate assay in, 659–660
Parathyroid hormone
assay of
interpretation of, 424
problems in, current solutions to, 422–423
measurement of, in differential diagnosis of hypercalcemia, 421–425
Paratyphoid fever, 200
Parinaud's oculoglandular syndrome, 206
Paroxysmal cold hemoglobinuria, 56
Paroxysmal nocturnal hemoglobinuria (PNH), 57–58
Parvovirus B19 infection, 650–651
Pasteurella, 203–204
Paul-Bunnell test in Epstein-Barr infection diagnosis, 262–263
Pediatrics, tests of interest in, 332–333
Pelger-Huët anomaly of WBC, 63
Percentile system of applying reference ranges to medical action, 640
Perchlorate discharge test for thyroid function, 663
Percutaneous transhepatic cholangiography, 311
Peripheral blood smear
abnormalities of, 14–16
in chronic iron deficiency diagnosis, 25
in Epstein-Barr infection diagnosis, 261–262
examination of, limitations of, 16
in sickle hemoglobin detection, 45
Wright-stained, examination of, 14-16
Peripheral pattern in antinuclear antibody test, 375–376
Peritoneal lavage for traumatic injury, 588
Pernicious anemia
diagnosis of, 32
gastric analysis in, 445–446
Schilling test for, 31–32, 440–442
Pertussis, 204
pH
clinical disturbances of, 395–397
of effusions, 587
laboratory determination of, 394–395
measurement of, 394–395
in urinalysis, 153
Phencyclidine (PCP), 630
Phenistix for phenylpyruvic acid in urine, 165
Phenobarbital, analysis of, 618–619
Phenolsulfonphthalein (PSP) excretion test
for renal function, 646–647
in tubular function evaluation, 180
Phenothiazine tranquilizers, toxicology of, 634
Phenylketonuria (PKU), 598–600
Phenylpyruvic acid in urine, tests for, 165
Phenytoin
analysis of, 617–618
folic acid deficiency and, 33
glucose tolerance and, 470
therapy with
alkaline phosphatase elevation in, 303
thyroid tests in, 494
Pheochromocytomas
adrenal medulla dysfunction from, 525–528
glucose tolerance and, 468
localization methods for, 527–528
tests for, 526–528
Philadelphia chromosome in chronic myelogenous leukemia, 78
Phosphate(s)
abnormalities of, 429–430
excretion of, urinary, in differential diagnosis of hypercalcemia, 421
organic, toxicology of, 634
serum, in differential diagnosis of hypercalcemia, 420
tubular reabsorption of, in parathyroid hormone measurement, 423–424
Phosphate reabsorption index in parathyroid hormone measurement, 423–424
Phosphatidylglycerol in fetal maturity testing, 556
Phosphorus, abnormalities of, 429–430
Physiologic variable, effects of, on laboratory test data, 7
Pinworms, 281–282
Pituitary function
stimulation tests of, 531
suppression tests of, 531
tests of, 530–536
Pituitary hormones, asssay of, 530
Pituitary insufficiency, 530–531
Pituitary precocious puberty, 541
Placenta, localization of, ultrasound in, 669
Placental function, tests of, 553–555
Placental lactogen in placental function evaluation, 555
Plague, 201
Plasma
recalcification time of, in heparin therapy monitoring, 644
for transfusion, 132–133
Plasma fibrinogen in hemorrhagic disorders, 96

Plasma free hemoglobin in tests for hemolytic transfusion reaction, 140
Plasma insulin assay in diabetes, 471
Plasma protein fraction (PPPE), purified, for transfusion, 134
Plasma thromboplastin antecedant, 101
Plasma thromboplastin component, 100
Plasmacytoma, solitary, 352
Plasmin to dissolve thrombi, 109
Plasmin/fibrinolysin anticoagulant, 104–106
Platelet(s)
  defects in, 110
  function of, defects in, 112–113
  in massive blood transfusions, 150–151
  reactions to, in blood transfusions, 147
  for transfusion, 131–132
  in whole blood, 129
Platelet count, 18
  in hemorrhagic disorders, 91–92
Platelet factor 3 (PF-3), 90–91
Platelet volume, mean, in coagulation assessment, 645
Pleural effusion, carinoembryonic antigen in, 588
Pneumocystis carinii, 280–281
Pneumonia, 230–231
  measles and, 250–251
  viral, 244
Polyarteritis nodosa, 380–381
  kidneys in, 170–171
Polychromatophilia, 17
Polychromatophilic red blood cells, 14–15
Polyclonal gamma-globulin elevation pattern in serum protein electrophoresis, 347, 348
Polycystic kidney, 170
Polycystic ovary (PCO) disease, female hirsutism and, 547–548
Polycythemia, 81–82
Polycythemia vera, vitamin B12 and unsaturated vitamin B12 binding capacity in, 642
Polymorphonuclear neutrophil in white blood cell maturation, 61
Polymyalgia rheumatica, 382
Porphobilinogen, urine
  in acute intermittent porphyria, 336
  test for, 165
Porphyria(s), 333–336
  acute intermittent, 334–336
  classification of, 334
  porphyrin excretion in, 335
Porter-Silber colorimetric technique of serum cortisol measurement, 512
Posthypoglycemic hyperglycemia, glucose intolerance and, 470
Postpartum transient toxicosis, 504
Postprandial hypoglycemia, 478–479
Postrenal obstruction, azotemia from, etiologies of, 178
Posttransfusion purpura, 110–111
Potassium
  abnormalities of, 413–416
    hyperkalemia as, 415–416
    hypokalemia as, 413–415
  intake of
    exogenous, hyperkalemia and, 415
    inadequate, hypokalemia from, 413
  serum loading of, in primary aldosteronism diagnosis, 520
  sources of, endogenous, hyperkalemia and, 415
  24-hour urine, in adrenal function testing, 664
P&P test in sodium warfarin therapy monitoring, 645
Prealbumin, serum, in protein-calorie nutritional status assessment, 433
Precocious puberty, 541–542
Predictive value of laboratory test data, 1–2
Preeclampsia, urinary findings in, 171
Pregnancy
  alkaline phosphatase elevation in, 303
  cytomegalovirus infection in, 258
  ectopic, diagnosis of, 551–552
  folic acid deficiency in, 33
  glucose tolerance and, 469
  hypertension of, thrombocytopenia in, 112
  iron deficiency anemia in, 24
  rubella in, 245–246, 248
  tests for, 549–551
    survey of, 695
  urinary findings in, 171–172
  viral infections in, 245–246
Pregnanediol, urine, in gonadal function testing, 537
Prehepatic coma, 308–309
Prekallikrein, 90, 101
Prematurity, iron deficiency and, 23–24
Prerenal azotemia
  and acute tubular necrosis, differentiation of, 647
  etiologies of, 178
Pressure, cerebrospinal fluid, 285
Primidone, analysis of, 618
Procainamide, analysis of, 621
Proctoscopy in cancer detection, 449
Production-defect anemia, 36–40
17-OH-Progesterone (17-OH-P) in female hirsutism investigation, 547
Progesterone receptor assay (PRA) in breast cancer diagnosis, 575–576
Progranulocyte in white blood cell maturation, 61, 62
Progressive systemic sclerosis, 379
Proinsulin for fasting hypoglycemia, 476–477
Prolactin
  pituitary tumors secreting, 534–535
  secretion of, abnormalities of, 534–535
  stimulation tests for, 535
  suppression tests for, 535
Promyelocyte in white blood cell maturation, 61, 62
Prostate, cancer of, laboratory aspects of, 570–572
Prostate-specific antigen (PSF) in prostate carcinoma detection, 571–572
Protamine sulfate test for secondary fibrinolysin, 105–106

Protein(s)
C-reactive, 331
in cerebrospinal fluid, 286–287
in effusions, 586–587
monoclonal, IgM, 659
reaction, acute, electrophoretic visualization of, 343–344
retinol-binding, in protein-calorie nutritional status assessment, 433
serum, 342–367
assay methods for, 342–349
laboratory application of, 343–349
electrophoresis of, 343–349 (*see also* Electrophoresis, serum protein)
in liver/biliary tract evaluation, 308
tests for, in urinalysis, 155–156
in urinalysis, 154–156
visceral, status of, tests for, in protein-calorie nutritional status assessment, 432–433
Protein C/protein S anticoagulant system, 104
Protein-calorie malnutrition, 431–435 (*see also* Malnutrition, protein-calorie)
Protein-calorie nutritional status, evaluation of, 431–435
Protein S, 104
Proteinuria
etiology of, 154–155
in pregnancy, 171
problem of, 185–186
Proteus, 201
Proteus tribe, subdivisions of, 685
Prothrombin, 57
Prothrombin complex concentrate for transfusion, 133
Prothrombin time (PT)
in hemorrhagic disorders, 93–94
laboratory differences in, from reagents, 683
in liver/biliary tract evaluation, 306–307
Pro-urokinase (P-UK) to dissolve thrombi, 109
Pseudogout, 385–386
Pseudohyperkalemia, 415
Pseudohypothyroidism, 501
Pseudomonas, 202–203
Pseudo-T_3 hyperthyroidism, 496–497
Pseudo-T_4 hyperthyroidism, 497–498
Pseudo-thyroxine/triiodothyronine hyperthyroidism, 495–496
Psitticosis, 216–217
Psoriatic arthritis, 372
Psychiatric medications, analysis of, 619–620
Psychiatric patients, thyrotropin-releasing hormone results in, 492–493
Psychiatry, laboratory tests in, 337–339
Puberty
female, delayed, 542–544
precocious, 541–542
Pulmonary embolism, 328–329
Pulmonary function tests, radioisotope, 658
Pulse oximetry in oxygen saturation measurement, 402
Purpura
allergic, 114
anaphylactoid, 114
embolic, 114–115
Henoch's, 114
laboratory investigation of, 115
posttransfusion, 110–111
senile, 114
thrombocytopenic
idiopathic, 110
thrombotic, 111–112
urinalysis in, 173
Pyelogram, intravenous, in tubular function evaluation, 181–182
Pyelonephritis, kidneys in, 169
Pyridoxine, 34
Pyrogenic reactions from blood transfusion, 148
Pyuria, correction of, with urine culture, 161–162

Q

Quinidine, analysis of, 622–623

R

Rabies, 271–272
Race
hemoglobin levels and, 9
white blood cell counts and, 63
Radioactive iodine uptake (RAIU) in thyroid function assessment, 484–485
Radioallergosorbent test (RAST) in allergy testing, 337
Radioimmunoassay (RIA) of serum cortisol, 512
Radioisotope studies
in cerebrospinal fluid examination, 652–653
in malabsorption assessment, 440
in pulmonary function testing, 658
Radiology (*see also* X-ray studies)
in cholecystitis diagnosis, 317–318
Radionuclide scanning
of bones, 388–390
in breast cancer diagnosis, 574–575
in metastatic bone cancer, 585–586
of brain for brain disease detection, 291
in cholecystitis diagnosis, 318
of heart in acute myocardial infarction, 327–328
of joints, 387-388
of liver, 310
of lungs in lung cancer detection, 579
of thyroid in thyroid cancer diagnosis, 582–583
Radiopharmaceuticals, tumor-seeking, 590–591
Ranges
normal, of laboratory test data, 3–6
problems derived from, 4–6
reference
medical action based on, systems for, 640
nonparametric calculation of, 640
Rapid plasma reagin (RPR) test for syphilis, 562
Rappaport's classification of malignant lymphomas, 83
Red blood cell(s) (RBC)
basophilic stippling in, 16
count of, 10

Red blood cell(s) (RBC) *(cont.)*
- frozen, for transfusion, 131
- Howell-Jolly bodies in, 16
- inclusions in, 16
- indices for, 10–13
  - in chronic iron deficiency diagnosis, 25
  - factors affecting interpretation of, 13–14
  - in vitamin B12 deficiency diagnosis, 31
- irradiated, for transfusion, 131
- mean corpuscular hemoglobin and, 12
- mean corpuscular hemoglobin concentration and, 12
- mean corpuscular volume and, 10–12
- membrane of, abnormalities of, 53–55
- packed, for transfusion, 130–131
- Pappenheimer bodies in, 16
- substitutes for, for transfusion, 134
- survival studies on, in hemolytic anemia diagnosis, 44
- for transfusion, storage of, 149–150
- in urinary sediment, 161
- washed, for transfusion, 130–131

Red blood cell casts in diabetic nephropathy, 645
Red blood cell crenation in peripheral smear, 15
Red blood cell distribution width, 12–13
Red blood cell enzyme deficiencies, 52–53
Reed-Sternberg (R-S) cells in Hodgkin's disease, 85
Reference range
- medical action based on, systems for, 640
- nonparametric calculation of, 640

Refractory dilutional syndrome, 410
Regitine test for pheochromocytoma, 526
Reidel's struma, 504
Reiter protein complement fixation test for syphilis, 564
Reiter's syndrome, 372
- urethritis and, 198

Renal acidosis, 396
Renal artery, occlusion of, 170
Renal cell adenocarcinoma, laboratory aspects of, 569
Renal embolism, 170
Renal function tests, 175–186
- in acute glomerulonephritis, 166
- of glomerular function, 175–177
- of glomerular and/or tubular damage, 177–179
- phenolsulfonphthalein excretion in, 646–647
- in pregnancy, 171
- of tubular function, 179–183

Renal papillary necrosis, 164
Renal potassium loss, hypokalemia from, 414
Renal tuberculosis, 215
Renin, plasma
- determination of, 694–695
- in primary aldosteronism diagnosis, 521

Renin-aldosterone patterns in conditions, 522
Reproducibility of laboratory test data, 2
Reset osmostat syndrome, 410
Respiratory acidosis, 396
Respiratory alkalosis, 397
Respiratory function, partial pressure of carbon dioxide as measurement of, 398
Respiratory syncytial virus (RSV), 251
Respiratory tract
- upper, viral diseases of, test specimens for, 247
- viral diseases of, 244

Reticulocyte count, 16–18
- in hemolytic anemia diagnosis, 42–43

Reticulocyte response in vitamin B12 deficiency diagnosis, 32
Reticulocytes in chronic iron deficiency diagnosis, 25
Reticulocytosis, causes of, 17
Reticuloendotheliosis, leukemia, 76
Retinol-binding protein in protein-calorie nutritional status assessment, 433
Reye's syndrome, 272
Rh blood group system, 122
Rh immune globulin for Rh incompatibility prophylaxis, 143–144
Rh incompatibility, hemolytic disease of newborn due to, 142–143
Rheumatic fever, acute, 383–384
Rheumatoid arthritis (RA), 369–371
- juvenile, 371

Rheumatoid arthritis precipitin (RAP) in systemic lupus erythematosus, 378
Rheumatoid-collagen disease group, anemia of, 39
Rheumatoid-collagen diseases, thrombocytopenia in, 112
Rheumatoid diseases, 369–372
Rheumatoid factor
- in rheumatoid arthritis, 370
- tests for, 689

Rickettsial diseases, 272–273
Riley-Day syndrome, laboratory tests for, 666
Rim pattern in antinuclear antibody test, 375–376
Rocky Mountain spotted fever, 273
- diagnosis of, skin biopsy with immunofluorescence for, 651

Rods, Gram-positive, 207
Rotavirus, 251–252
Rotor syndrome, 656
Rouleaux in peripheral smear, 16
Roundworms, 282–283
- eosinophilia and, 66

Rubella, 248–250
- diagnosis of, 649–650
- in pregnancy, 245–246, 248

Rubeola, 250–251
Runner anemia, 24

S

Salicylate, overdose of, glucose tolerance and, 469–470
Saline infusion in adrenal function testing, 664
Salmonella, 199–200
- gastroenteritis from, 200
- pathogenic, serologic groups of, 688

Sarcoidosis, 329–330
- hypercalcemia in, 419

Shilling test

in malabsorption assessment, 440–442
in Vitamin B12 deficiency diagnosis, 31–32
Schistocyte(s)
in hemolytic anemias, 45
in peripheral smear, 15
Schistosoma mansoni, 281
Schlichter test for bacteria, 234
Sclerocystic ovary syndrome, female hirsutism and, 547
Scleroderma, 379
Sclerosis, progressive systemic, 379
Screening tests
for bacteriuria, 223
in sickle hemoglobin detection, 45–46
for thalassemia, 52
Secondary acquired autoimmune hemolytic anemia, 56
Segmented granulocyte in white blood cell maturation, 61, 62
Semen analysis
in male infertility investigation, 540
reference ranges for, 695
Senile purpura, 114
Sensitivity of laboratory test data, 1
Septic arthritis, 386
Septicemia, 227
jaundice from, 300–301
Serial dilution method of antibiotic sensitivity testing, 232–233
Serologic tests
for amebiasis, 279
for antibody in herpes simplex virus infection diagnosis, 266–267
for cytomegalovirus infection, 260
in Epstein-Barr infection diagnosis, 262–263
for Epstein-Barr virus, 264–265
for *Mycoplasma pneumoniae*, 219–220
in rheumatoid arthritis diagnosis, 370
for *Toxoplasma*, interpretation of, 277–278
Seronegative spondyloarthropathies, 371–372
Serum
antibody screen for, 124
osmolality of, in hyponatremia investigation, 411–412
Shigellae, 200
SI units, conversion of traditional units to, 705–706
Sickle cell anemia, 46–47
urinalysis in, 172
Sickle cell trait, 47
Sickle cells in peripheral smear, 15
Sickle hemoglobin
definitive diagnosis of, 46
in hemolytic anemia, 45–48
tests to detect, 45
Sickle hemoglobin-hemoglobin C disease, 47–48
Sickle thalassemia, 51–52
Sideroblastic anemias, 34
Sigmoidoscopy in cancer detection, 449
Sjögren's syndrome, 380
Skeletal muscle
congenital diseases of, 603–605
CPK-MB fraction and, 325–326
Skin
biopsy of, with immunofluorescence staining
in Rocky Mountain spotted fever diagnosis, 651
for systemic lupus erythematosus, 378
diseases of, chronic, eosinophilia and, 66
Skin test(s)
for immune status in protein-calorie malnutrition, 434
selected, 699
in tuberculosis, 213–214
Slide latex tests for systemic lupus erythematosus, 378–379
Small intestine, biopsy of, in malabsorption assessment, 444
Smoking
hemoglobin levels and, 9
neutrophilic leukocytosis due to, 65
tests for, 667
Sodium
excreted, fraction of, in tubular function evaluation, 182–183
filtered, fraction of, in tubular function evaluation, 182–183
serum
abnormalities of, 404–413
hypernatremia as, 413
hyponatremia as, 405–413 (*see also* Hyponatremia)
measurement of, problems with, 404–405
urine, in hyponatremia investigation, 410–411
Sodium/chloride ratio, sweat, in cystic fibrosis, 666
Sodium warfarin therapy monitoring, 645
Solid pattern in antinuclear antibody test, 376
Solitary plasmacytoma, 352
Somatomedin-C, assay of, 532–533
Somatomedins, growth hormone and, 531
Somogyi phenomenon, glucose tolerance and, 470
Sparganosis, 282
Specific gravity
of effusions, 586
in urinalysis, 153–154
of urine in tubular function evaluation, 180–181
Specificity of laboratory test data, 1
Specimens
collection of, 700
contamination of, bacteria associated with, 221
laboratory, problems with, 6–7
Speckled pattern in antinuclear antibody test, 376
Spermatozoa in urinary sediment, 164
Spherocytes in peripheral smear, 14
Spherocytosis
causes of, 14
congenital, 53–55
Sphingolipid storage diseases, 698
Sphingolipidoses, 597–598
Spirochetal diseases, 210–211
Spondyloarthropathies, seronegative, 371–372

Sporotrichosis, 240–241
Sputum, culture of, for bacteria, 224–225
Sputum cytology in lung cancer detection, 578
Sputum smear in tuberculosis, 212–213
Stable factor, 98
Stain(s)
  cytochemical, in acute leukemia differentiation, 71–72
  gram, 225
Staphylococci, 193–196
Staphylococcus, pneumonia due to, 230, 231
Staphylococcus aureus, 194
  diarrhea due to, 229
  methacillin-resistant, 234
Staphylococcus epidermidis, 195–196
Steatorrhea, 439
  diagnosis of, fecal fat assessment in, 439
Stein-Leventhal syndrome, female hirsutism and, 548
Stem cell leukemia, 69
Steroids
  adrenal cortical, neutrophilic leukocytosis due to, 65
  17-ketogenic, in adrenal function testing, 664
Stomach
  cancer of
    diagnosis of, gastric analysis in, 446
    laboratory aspects of, 572
  contents of, blood in, tests for, 450–451
  resection of, determining type and extent of, gastric analysis in, 446
  ulcer of, and duodenal ulcer, differentiation of, gastric analysis in, 446
Stomatocytes in peripheral smear, 15–16
Stomatocytic elliptocytosis, 55
Stomatocytosis, congenital, 55
Stool, examination of, for ova and parasites, 278
Stool occult blood in gastrointestinal tract cancer detection, 448–449
Stool tests, nonguaiac, in gastrointestinal tract cancer detection, 449
Streptococcal enzymes, antibodies against, in acute rheumatic fever diagnosis, 383
Streptococci, 190–193
  anaerobic, 210
  Group A, nephritogenic strains of, 685
  Lancefield classification of, 190–192
  nutritionally deficient, 229
Streptococcus agalactiae, 191–192
Streptococcus anginosus, 192
Streptococcus bovis, 192
Streptococcus faecalis, 192
Streptococcus MG in bacterial disease diagnosis, 649
Streptococcus milleri, 192
Streptococcus pneumoniae, 193
Streptococcus pyogenes, 191
Streptokinase to dissolve thrombi, 109
Streptolysin-O tests in acute rheumatic fever diagnosis, 383
Stress, glucose tolerance test and, 464
String sign in synovial fluid analysis, 386
Strongyloides stercoralis, 283
Stuart factor, 100–101
Subarachnoid hemorrhage, cerebrospinal fluid findings in, 295
Subdural hematoma
  cerebrospinal fluid findings in, 294–295
  radioisotope studies of, 653
Substances interfering with laboratory tests, 674–681
Succinylcholine apnea, 609
Sucrase enzyme, deficiency of, 596
Sulfasalazine, folic acid deficiency and, 33
Sulfur granules in actinomycosis, 220
Sweat, sodium/chloride ratio in, in cystic fibrosis, 666
Sweat test in cystic fibrosis, 607–608
Sweating, excessive, hyponatremia in, 406
Sympathetic nervous system, cancer of, laboratory aspects of, 582
Synovial fluid
  analysis of, in arthritis, 386–387
  findings in, 388
  glucose in, 386–387
  microbiologic studies of, 387
  specimens of, collection of, 387
  white blood cell count in, 387
Synthroid, therapy with, monitoring of, 503–504
Syphilis, 210
  central nervous system, 567–568
  congenital, 566–567
  darkfield examination for, 561
  tests for, 561–568
    cardiolipin, 562–563
    on cerebrospinal fluid, 288–289
    immunologic, 562
    selection of, 566
    sensitivity and specificity of, 565–568
Systemic disease, anemia associated with, 38–40
Systemic lupus erythematosus (SLE), 373–379
  antinuclear antibody tests for, 374–378
  autoantibodies and autoantibody tests in, 373
  drug-induced, 379
  laboratory findings in, 373
  lupus erythematosus cell preparation test for, 373–374
  nephrotic syndrome and, 168
  serum complement in, 379
  skin biopsy with immunofluorescence staining for, 378
  slide latex tests for, 378–379
  tests for, 689
Systemic mycoses, 237–241

T

t-PA to dissolve thrombi, 109
Tambocor, analysis of, 623
Tapeworm, 282
Target cells in peripheral smear, 15
Tay-Sachs disease, 597–598
Teardrop cells in peripheral smear, 15
Temporal arteritis, 381–382

Tes-Tape for urinary glucose, 157
Testicular biopsy in male infertility investigation, 540
Testicular function tests in male infertility investigation, 538–540
Testis, cancer of, laboratory aspects of, 582
Testosterone
  serum
    in female hirsutism investigation, 546
    in gonadal function testing, 537–538
  testicular function and, 539–540
Tetanus, 208
Thalassemia, 49
  screening for, 52
  sickle, 51–52
Thalassemia major, 49–50
Thalassemia minor, 500–501
  vs. chronic iron deficiency, 51
Theophylline, analysis of, 625–626
Therapeutic drugs
  absorption of, blood levels and, 613
  blood levels of
    factors influencing, 613–615
    rationale for obtaining, 612–613
  distribution of, extent of, blood levels and, 613
  excretion of, blood levels and, 614
  metabolism of, blood levels and, 613–614
  monitoring of, 612–617
    data in, 699–700
    for digoxin, data on, 623–625
    specimens for, obtaining, 615–616
  peak levels of, assay of, 614–615
  residual levels of, assay of, 614–615
  therapeutic and toxic ranges of, 615
  tissue utilization of, blood levels and, 615
  transport of, blood levels and, 613
  uptake of, by target tissues, blood levels and, 613
Thorn test for Addison's disease, 524
Thrombin time
  in hemorrhagic disorders, 96
  in heparin therapy monitoring, 644
Thrombocytopenia, 110–112
  in aplastic anemia, drugs causing, 37
  artifactual, 112
  drug-induced, 110
  immunologic, 110–111
  neonatal, 111
Thrombocytopenic purpura
  idiopathic, 110
  thrombotic, 111–112
Thrombocytosis
  in coagulation assessment, 645
  of platelet function defects, 114
Thrombolytic therapy
  for acute myocardial infarction, reperfusion after, detection of, 658
  coagulation and, 109
Thromboplastin generation time (TGT) for coagulation defect detection, 643
Thrombosis
  cerebral, cerebrospinal fluid findings in, 295
  conditions predisposing to, 109
  renal, 170
Thrombotest in sodium warfarin therapy monitoring, 645
Thrombotic thrombocytopenic purpura, 111
Thyroglobulin, serum, assay of, in thyroid cancer diagnosis, 583
Thyroid autoantibodies, 505
Thyroid disease
  replacement therapy for, monitoring of, 502–504
  signs and symptoms of, 482–484
Thyroid dysfunction, urinalysis in, 173
Thyroid function tests, 484–493, 661–663
  based on tissue utilization of thyroid hormone in, 661–662
  comments on, 502
  free T_4 assay in, 488
  free thyroxine index, 487–488
  in hypothyroidism, 500–502
  iodine, effects of, 493
  perchlorate discharge, 663
  in phenytoin therapy, 494
  radioactive iodine uptake as, 484–485
  serum iodine measurement in, 661
  serum thyrotropin assay as, 489–491
  thyroid hormone-binding ratio in, 485–486
  thyroid scan as, 493
  thyroid-stimulating immunoglobulin assay in, 662–663
  thyroid suppression, 491–492
  thyrotropin-releasing hormone, 492–493
  thyrotropin stimulation, 491
  thyroxine-binding globulin quantitative assay in, 661
  total serum thyroxine in, 486–487
  total serum triiodothyronine in, 488–489
  triiodothyronine withdrawal, 491
Thyroid gland
  cancer of, laboratory aspects of, 582-584
  medullary carcinoma of, 584
  scan of, in thyroid function assessment, 493
Thyroid hormone
  glucose tolerance and, 468
  production of, 482, 483
Thyroid hormone-binding ratio (THBR)
  in hypothyroidism assessment, 500
  in thyroid function assessment, 485–486
Thyroid-releasing hormone (TRH), test of, interpretation of, 693
Thyroid-stimulating immunoglobulin (TSI) assay, 662–663
Thyroid suppression test in thyroid function assessment, 491–492
Thyroid tests, results of, compounds interfering with, 692–693
Thyroiditis, 504–505

Thyrotoxicosis, 483
thrombocytopenia in, 112
in thyroiditis, 496
Thyrotropin assay (TSH), serum
in hypothyroidism assessment, 500–501
in thyroid function assessment, 489–491
Thyrotropin-releasing hormone (TRH) test
for depression, 338
in hypothyroidism assessment, 501
in thyroid function assessment, 492–493
Thyrotropin stimulation test in thyroid function assessment, 491
Thyroxine (T_4)
assay of, free, in thyroid function assessment, 488
serum, in hypothyroidism assessment, 500
total serum, in thyroid function assessment, 486–487
L-Thyroxine, therapy with, monitoring of, 503–504
Thyroxine-binding globulin quantitative assay, 661
Thyroxine index, free, in thyroid function assessment, 487–488
Tissue destruction, neutrophilic leukocytosis due to, 65
Tissue thromboplastin, 97
Tobacco use, tests for, 667
Tocainide, analysis of, 622
Tolbutamide tolerance test for fasting hypoglycemia, 476
Tomography, computerized, 670–671 (*see also* Computerized tomography)
Tonocard, analysis of, 622
Torulopsis glabrata, 242
Torulosis, 238–239
Total iron-binding capacity (TIBC), serum, in chronic iron deficiency diagnosis, 26–27
Tourniquet test in hemorrhagic disorders, 92
Toxemia of pregnancy, urinary findings in, 171
Toxic shock syndrome, *Staphylococcus aureus* and, 194–195
Toxicology, 631–638
Toxicosis, postpartum transient, 504
Toxins, hemolytic anemia due to, 58–59
Toxoplasmosis, 276–278
Trace elements, 430–431
Trachoma, 219
Tranquilizers, phenothiazine, toxicology of, 634
Transcutaneous electrode systems of PCO_2 and PO_2 measurement, 402
Transferase, deficiency of, galactosemia from, 594–595
Transferrin
levels of, serum iron levels and, 26
serum, in protein-calorie nutritional status assessment, 433
Transferrin saturation
changes in, by disease, 683
in chronic iron deficiency diagnosis, 26–27
Transfusions, blood, 129–137 (*see also* Blood transfusion)
Translocation in Down's syndrome, 602
Trauma, glucose tolerance test and, 464
Traumatic hemolytic anemia, 57
Treponema pallidum immobilization test for syphilis, 563–564
Trichinella infection, eosinophilia and, 66
Trichinella spiralis, 282–283
Trichomonas in urinary sediment, 164
Trichomonas vaginalis, 283
Tricyclic antidepressants, analysis of, 620
Triglycerides
measurement of, in coronary heart disease risk assessment, 362–363
metabolism of, 358
Triiodothyronine (T_3), total serum, in thyroid function assessment, 488–489
Triiodothyronine-radioimmunoassay (T_3-RIA) in hypothyroidism assessment, 500
Triiodothyronine (T_3) withdrawal test in thyroid function assessment, 491
Trypsin, serum, in cystic fibrosis diagnosis, 609
Tuberculosis, 211–215
military, 214–215
renal, 215
Tubular damage, severe, tests for, 177–179
Tubular function, tests of, 179–183
Tubular necrosis, acute, 170
chronic renal failure differentiated from, 184
and prerenal azotemia, differentiation of, 647
Tubular reabsorption of phosphate in parathyroid hormone measurement, 423–424
Tumor(s)
bile duct obstruction by, 317
brain
cerebrospinal fluid findings in, 294
radioisotope studies in, 652
ectopic, hormone production by, 696–697
hormone production by, 591
metastatic to bone, radionuclide bone scanning for, 389–390
pancreatic, localization of, 477–478
Tumor-seeking radiopharmaceuticals, 590–591
Turner's syndrome, 601–602
24-Hour measurement for urinary protein, 156
24-Hour urine potassium in adrenal function testing, 664
Type and screen, pretransfusion, 126

U

Ulcer(s)
gastric and duodenal, differentiation of, gastric analysis in, 446
marginal, diagnosis of, gastric analysis in, 446
Ultrasound, diagnostic, 667–670
A-mode readout in, 667

for abdominal aortic aneurysm detection/ delineation, 669
for abscess detection, 669
for acute pancreatitis, 458
B-mode readout in, 667–668
for biopsy needle guidance, 669
for cardiac diagnosis, 669–670
for cholecystitis, 317–318
for differentiation
of intrahepatic from extrahepatic biliary obstruction, 669
of solid from cystic structures, 669
M-mode readout in, 668
for ocular examination, 669
for pancreatic carcinoma diagnosis, 669
for periaortic and retroperitoneal mass of enlarged lymph node detection, 669
for placental localization, 669
real-time, 668
Unconjugated bilirubin, serum levels of, in hemolytic anemia diagnosis, 44
Univalent antibody, definition of, 118–119
Urea clearance, tests of, 175–176
Ureaplasma urealyticum, urethritis and, 197–198
Uremia, thrombocytopenia in, 112
Urethral syndrome, acute, 197–198
Urethritis
chlamydial, 218–219
nongonococcal, 197–198
Uric acid, serum levels of
in gout diagnosis, 384–385
in polycythemia diagnosis, 82
Urinalysis, 153–166
acetone in, 158–159
appearance in, 153
bile in, 160
diacetic acid, 158–159
glucose in, 156–158
hemoglobin in, 159–160
interpretation of, 165–166
ketone bodies in, 158–159
leukocyte esterase in, 160
microscopic examination of urinary sediment in, 161–165
in miscellaneous disease, 172–173
nitrite in, 160
pH in, 153
protein in, 154–156
red blood cell casts in diabetic nephropathy in, 645
specific gravity in, 153–154
in tests for hemolytic transfusion reaction, 141
in urinary tract calculi, 645–646
urine test in, 165
urobilinogen in, 160–161
Urinary calculi, urinalysis in, 172
Urinary sediment, microscopic examination of, 161–165
pitfalls in, 164–165
Urinary tract calculi, laboratory evaluation in, 645–646
Urine
bilirubin in, in liver/biliary tract evaluation, 301
calcium excretion in, in differential diagnosis of hypercalcemia, 420–421
collection of, for Schilling test, 441
culture of
for bacteria, 222–224
quantitative, drawbacks of, 224
pyuria correlated, 161–162
electrolyte excretion in, in tubular function evaluation, 182
17-ketosteroid in, assay of, in Cushing's syndrome screening, 514
osmolality of
in hyponatremia investigation, 411, 412
in tubular function evaluation, 181
phosphate excretion in, in differential diagnosis of hypercalcemia, 421
potassium assay in, in hypokalemia, 415
protein in, test methods for, 155–156
sodium in, in hyponatremia investigation, 410–411
specific gravity of, in tubular function evaluation, 180–181
Urine adenosine 3,5-monophosphate assay in parathyroid function evaluation, 659–660
Urine tests, 165
Urobilinogen
in liver/biliary tract evaluation, 301
in urinalysis, 160–161
Urokinase in dissolve thrombi, 109
Uroporphyrinogen-I-synthetase, decreased, in acute intermittent porphyria, 334–335
Uterus, cancer of, laboratory aspects of, 576–577

V

Vagotomy status evaluation, gastric analysis in, 446–447
Valproic acid, analysis of, 619
Valves, heart, infection of, 227–229
van denBergh reaction in serum bilirubin measurement, 229
Vancomycin, analysis of, 626
Vascular defects, 114–115
Vasculitis
allergic, 381
granulomatous, 381
syndromes due primarily to, 380–383
Vel blood group antigens, 124
Veneral Disease Research Laboratory (VDRL) test for syphilis, 562–563
Venous clotting time in hemorrhagic disorders, 95–96
Vibrio parahaemolyticus, diarrhea due to, 229
Vibrios, 207
Vincent's angina, 210
Viral capsid antigen (VCA), antibody against, 264
Viral diseases, 244–272
acute leukemia differentiated from, 75
diagnosis of, 246–247
specimens for, 247–248
in pregnancy, 245–246
of upper respiratory tract, 244
test specimens for, 247

Viral gastroenteritis, 245
test specimens for, 247–248
Viral infections of liver, jaundice from, 301
Viral meningitis, 244–245
cerebrospinal fluid findings in, 292–293
test specimens for, 247
Viral pneumonia, 244
Viridans streptococci, 192–193
Virilization syndrome, 513
Virus(es)
classification of, 245
culture of, for cytomegalovirus infection, 260
pneumonia due to, 230
Viscosity in synovial fluid analysis, 386
Vitamin B6, 34
Vitamin B12
assay of, 30
deficiency of, 29–32
anemia in, therapeutic, trial for, 641–642
diagnosis of, 32
formiminoglutamic acid determination for, 641
methylmalonic acid determination for, 641
serum levels of, in polycythemia vera, 642
therapeutic trial with, for vitamin B12 deficiency anemia, 641–642
Vitamin B12-binding capacity, unsaturated, in polycythemia vera, 642
Vitamin D compound assays in hypocalcemia, 427
Vitamin D disorders, laboratory findings in, 428
Vitamin K in prothrombin synthesis, 306–307
von Willebrand factor, 98–00
von Willebrand's disease
and hemophilia A, differentiation of, 99–100
platelet function defects in, 113–114

W

Waldenström's macroglobulinemia, 353–354
Warfarin sodium, therapy with, monitoring of, 645
Warm autoantibodies, 121
Washed red blood cells for transfusion, 130–131
Water, serum, estimation of, 660
Weight
deficiency of, in protein-calorie nutritional status assessment, 432
drug blood levels and, 614
Weil-Felix reaction in rickettsial disease diagnosis, 272–273
Weil's disease, 210
urinalysis in, 172–173
Weiner's Rh system theory, 122, 123
Whipple's triad for insulinoma screening, 475
White blood cells (WBC), 61–67
antigens of, 126–127
automated cell counter counts of, 64–65
basophilia of, 66
in cerebrospinal fluid, 287–288
counts of, 18
in acute myocardial infarction, 320
special problems in, in neonates and children, 65
in synovial fluid, 387
eosinophilia of, 66
leukemoid reaction of, 66
leukoerythroblastosis of, 67
lymphocytosis of, 66–67
maturation sequence for, 61–63
monocytosis of, 66
neonatal leukocytosis of, 63–64
neutropenia of, 67
pattern of, deviation from, in infection, 64
Pelger-Hüet anomaly of, 63
in urinalysis, 160
in urinary sediment, 161–162
Whole blood for transfusion, 129–130
Whole blood clotting time in hemorrhagic disorders, 95
Whooping cough, 204
Widal's test, 688
Wilson's disease, 605
Wintrobe indices, 10–13
interpretation of, factors affecting, 13–14
Wright blood group antigen-antibody system, 124
Wright-stained peripheral blood smear, examination of, 14–16

X

X-ray findings
in multiple myeloma, 350
in parathyroid hormone evaluation, 424
X-ray studies
of bone
for growth disorders, 533–534
in metastatic bone cancer, 585
of chest in lung cancer detection, 578
in gastrointestinal tract cancer detection, 449
in lactase deficiency, 666
in malabsorption assessment, 440
Xylocaine, analysis of, 621–622

Y

Yeast cells in urinary sediment, 164
Yersinia, 201–202
Yersinia enterocolitica, 202
Yersinia pestis, 201
Yersinia pseudotuberculosis, 201–202

Z

Zeta sedimentation rate (ZSR), 331
Zieve's syndrome, 40
Zinc, 430
Zinc protoporphyrin (ZPP)
assays of, problems with, 28–29
in chronic iron deficiency diagnosis, 28–29
in iron deficiency, 28
Zollinger-Ellison (Z-E) syndrome
diagnosis of, gastric analysis in, 446
laboratory aspects of, 580
Zygomycosis, 243